Second Edition

Rehabilitation of the Spine
A Practitioner's Manual

DVD Index

Note:
Throughout the DVD when a common dysfunction is contrasted with normal function—either during a test or exercise—the Pain icon will be shown as a visual cue signifying that the dysfunction represents a "weak link" which can cause biomechanical overload and eventual pain.

Pain Icon

Introduction

I. Physical Performance Evaluation
- Vele Forward Lean
- 1 Leg Standing Balance
- Squat
- One Leg Squat
- Vleeming Hip Flexion
- Janda Hip Extension
- Janda Hip Abduction
- Side Bridge Endurance
- Wall Angel
- Respiration
- Push-Up
- Arm Abduction
- Neck Flexion

II. Sparing Strategies
- Micro Breaks
  - McGill Overhead Arm
  - Brügger's Postural Re-Position
- Hip Hinge Advice
  - Sit to Stand
  - Standing
  - Putting on Socks
  - Putting on Shoes
- Psoas Stretch
- Mid-Thoracic Extension Mobilization
  - Foam Roll: Supine
  - Foam Roll: Upper Back
  - Foam Roll: Horizontal Stretch
- Health Club Tips
  - Hamstring Curl
  - Hip Extension Multi-Machine
  - Hip Abduction Multi-Machine
  - Rowing
  - Hanging Leg Raise
  - Incline Sit Ups
  - Seated Abdominal Crunch
  - Lat Pull Down & Lateral Raises
  - Sit Up
  - Pec Dec & Sit Up

III. Stabilizing Strategies
- Functional Bracing
- Quadruped
  - Cat Camel
  - Bracing
  - Quadruped Leg Raise
  - Quadruped Arm Leg Raise (Bird Dog)
- Side Bridge
  - On Knees
  - On Ankles
  - Roll Over

- Dead Bug
  - Floor
  - Half Foam
  - Full Foam
- McGill's Abdominal Curl Up
- Superman
- Wall Ball
- Hamstring Curls
- Balance Training
  - Rocker Board
- Push-Up with Plus
- Deep Neck Flexors
- Scapulo-Thoracic Facilitation

IV. Functional Integrated Training (FIT)
- Squats

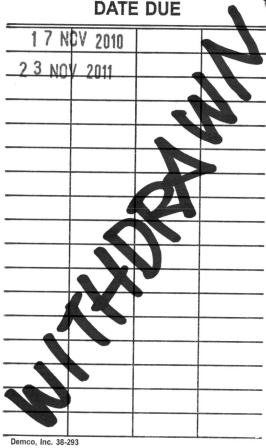

- with Stick
  - Core Twist

V. Czech School of Manual Medicine
- Jiri Cumpelik—Spinal Exercises
  - Ready—Supine Position
  - Supine Position with Legs Semi-Flexed
  - Supine Twist—Supine Position with Legs Flexed and Lifted
  - Side Lying
  - The Sphinx
  - The Cobra
- Pavel Kolar—Developmental Kinesiology
  - Postural Ontogenesis

- First Homolateral Pattern, e.g. the Development of Grasping Supine
  - Reflex Locomotion
    - Reflex Turning
  - The Deep Stabilizing System of the Spine
    - Palpation of Lateral Group of the Deep Abdominal Muscles
    - The Deep Stabilizing System of the Spine—Treatment
  - Examination and Mobilization of the Lumbar Spine
- Karel Lewit—Mobilization, Soft Tissue and Relaxation Techniques
  - Mobilization of the Fascia on the Back in a Cranial Direction
  - Mobilization of the Fascia on the Back in a Caudal Direction
  - Palpation of the Pelvic Floor
  - PIR: Pelvic Floor Plus M. Transversus Abdominis
  - Examination and Mobilization of the Thoracic Spine into Extension
  - Mid Thoracic Spine Self Mobilization
- Dagmar Pavlu—Brügger Concept
  - The Agistic-Eccentric Contraction to Influence the Fingers Flexors
  - Agistic-Eccentric Contraction Influence the Wrist Flexors
  - Thera-Band Exercises to Improve Function of the Thigh Adductors and Plantar Flexors and Supinators of the Foot
  - "Great" Combined Exercise with a Thera-Band
  - Activities of Daily Living
- Misa Veverkova—Sensory Motor Stimulation/Movement Pattern Assessment
  - Sensory Motor Stimulation Stability Test Standing on One Leg
    - Standing on One Leg with Eyes Closed
    - Standing on One Leg on a Firm Mattress
    - Standing on One Leg on a Firm Mattress with the Eyes Closed
  - The "Small Foot"
    - Passive Modeling of the "Small Foot"
    - Modeling the Small Foot with Patient's Cooperation
    - Active Small Foot Exercise
  - Balance Sandals
    - Sensory Motor Stimulation Walking with Balance Sandals
    - Walking Under Supervision
    - Walking by Oneself
  - Hip Extension Movement Pattern
    - Movement Pattern Assessment–Motor Stereotype of Hip Extension
    - Motor Stereotype of Hip Extension Walking
  - Arm Abduction Movement Pattern

Second Edition

Rehabilitation of the Spine
A Practitioner's Manual

Craig Liebenson, Editor

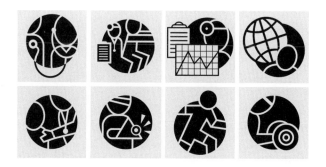

Lippincott Williams & Wilkins
a Wolters Kluwer business
Philadelphia • Baltimore • New York • London
Buenos Aires • Hong Kong • Sydney • Tokyo

Acquisitions Editor: Pete Darcy
Managing Editor: Laura Horowitz
Marketing Manager: Christen Murphy
Production Editor: Christina Remsberg
Designer: Risa Clow
Compositor: Circle Graphics
Printer: Quebecor—Dubuque

351 West Camden Street
Baltimore, MD 21201

530 Walnut Street
Philadelphia, PA 19106

Printed in the United States of America

First Edition, 1996

Library of Congress Cataloging-in-Publication Data

CIP data has been requested and is available from the Library of Congress.

The publishers have made every effort to trace the copyright holders for borrowed material. If they have inadvertently overlooked any, they will be pleased to make the necessary arrangements at the first opportunity.

To purchase additional copies of this book, call our customer service department at **(800) 638-3030** or fax orders to **(301) 824-7390.** International customers should call **(301) 714-2324.**

Visit Lippincott Williams & Wilkins on the Internet: http://www.LWW.com. Lippincott Williams & Wilkins customer service representatives are available from 8:30 am to 6:00 pm, EST.

08 09 10
5 6 7 8 9 10

Dedication

To my wife, Deannie, and children Justine and Zachary, who have given up so much so that this book could see the light of day.

Foreword

It is a pleasure and a privilege to welcome the second edition of *Rehabilitation of the Spine*. It is difficult to believe that nearly 10 years have passed since the first edition. So much that seemed revolutionary then is now accepted as the standard for good back care, and Liebenson's textbook has become a classic.

The goal remains to improve clinical management of spinal pain; more specifically, to integrate relief of symptoms with restoration of function. There is now broad agreement on the importance of rehabilitation and the need to improve functional and occupational outcomes. There is also growing recognition that rehabilitation is not a separate, second-stage intervention after "proper" treatment has no more to offer yet recovery remains incomplete. Rather, rehabilitation should be an integral part of good clinical management. *Every* health professional who cares for these patients should accept at least some responsibility for their functional and occupational outcomes. That does not

mean we should all become rehabilitation specialists: rather, it goes to the heart of what health care is all about.

The basic approach of this book remains the same. It updates the evidence base for an active approach, integrates it with clinical experience, and shows how it can be applied to routine practice. Every chapter is completely re-written and there are many distinguished new authors. The new format incorporates modern teaching aids and a DVD. Ten years on, the philosophy is more developed and more mature, but it remains true to the original. We are now more confident that we really can improve clinical management of spinal pain: the challenge remains to deliver that to every patient with spinal pain. I am confident this new edition will continue to deliver that message and help to make it a reality.

Gordon Waddell, MD, FRC
Western Infirmary
Glasgow, Scotland

Preface

In the 10 years that have passed since this book's first edition was published, rehabilitation for patients with activity-limiting pain of spinal origin has become the standard of care. The latest scientific evidence has identified patient reassurance and reactivation as the first steps in the self-management journey.

A team approach involving patients, health care providers, employers, and payors all working together is needed to alter the course of distressing or disabling back and neck pain. *Rehabilitation of the Spine, Second Edition,* sheds light on various iatrogenic risk factors of current practice approaches, in particular, the routine recommendation of bed rest, excessive diagnostic testing, overprescription of narcotic analgesics, and inappropriate selection criteria for spinal surgery. With new preemptive societal measures, via the Internet and mass media, providing the momentum, this book hopes to offer a practical manual for health care providers to shift towards a confident, empathetic, self-management approach to spinal disorders.

A New Paradigm

A new strategy utilizing the mass media to educate consumers directly about the positive benefits of physical activity and the dangers of deconditioning has been undertaken in both Australia and Scotland. This book supports this approach by giving health care providers a guide to the modern principles of evidence-based, outcome-based, patient-centered, functional, and active self-care for patients suffering disabling musculoskeletal spinal pain.

Many of the architects of this new paradigm—Steven Linton, Stuart McGill, and Nikolai Bogduk—have been added as contributors to this second edition to distill the new literature into a practical framework. Accordingly, each and every chapter has been entirely re-written. However, the book's basic premise of focusing on active care, outcomes, and psychosocial factors remains unchanged.

Organization

The book's organization is similar to the first edition, with the most significant addition being a new regional application section (Part VI).

Part I: Overview introduces readers to the new paradigm.

Part II: Basic Science covers the mechanisms of injury, restabilization, and pain.

Part III: Assessment covers diagnostic triage, functional assessment, psychosocial screening, and outcomes management.

Part IV: Acute Care Management outlines the modern approach for managing the acute phase of spine disorders.

Part V: Recovery Care Management focuses on the tools and techniques needed for recovery, including such topics as sensory-motor training, yoga, functional stability training, cognitive–behavioral training, and nutrition.

Part VI: Practical Application by Region contains a Visual Atlas of key assessment and training techniques designed to give the reader the full landscape and context of key rehab "tools of the trade."

Part VII: Implementing the Functional Paradigm sums up the book by covering implementation of the new paradigm in practice.

Pedagogical Features

Icons: An icon system has been designed for this second edition to guide readers to essential topics. You will find these icons highlighted on the chapter openers, and they will let you know what topics will be covered.

 Diagnosis

 Functional evaluation

 Classification

Psychosocial factors

Reassurance

Pain

Reactivation

Reconditioning

Learning Objectives: Each chapter starts with a list of Learning Objectives to emphasize the most relevant information in the chapter.

Audit Process: Each chapter ends with an Audit Process box—a self-check of the learning objectives.

Clinical Pearls: This special feature is found throughout the book and contains "pearls" of wisdom from experienced practitioners.

Practice-Based Problems: Found in many chapters, these boxes present common clinical dilemma encountered in practice, wherein clinical decision making is highlighted.

Illustrations: The second edition utilizes a highly illustrative presentation style, and many new line drawings and photographs have been added.

Design: The second edition has been completely redesigned. The hierarchy of the content is more clearly delineated, and the special features are easier to find and access.

The book is designed to have a visual emphasis. It is not designed to be read from beginning to end. The key to the book is **Part VI Practical Application by Region.** In this section are numerous *atlases* providing an overview of the rehabilitation landscape presented throughout the book. Chapter **32 An Integrated Approach to Regional Disorders** presents 2 *atlases* that show in one place a single representative picture of the major **tests** and **exercises** presented in the book.

Chapter 34 **Integrated Approach to the Lumbar Spine** and Chapter 35 **Integrated Approach to the Cervical Spine** delve into the practical, clinical management of lumbar, cervical, thoracic, and oro-facial problems. The first major *visual atlas* in these chapters shows the indication, procedure, scoring, and treatments to consider for each **Functional screen**. The second important *atlas* visually shows an integrated model of care from the view of important **Diagnostic cases** (e.g. herniated disc, spinal stenosis, headache, etc.) Each case is presented in a common format covering the kinetic chain approach and goals or continuum of care (e.g. palliative, sparing, stabilizing, functional).

The other key *visual atlas* is found in Chapter 26 on Functional Stability Training. Here the most important **exercises** are described in terms of indications, procedure, progression, evaluation/audit, and troubleshooting.

Accompanying DVD

To support the hundreds of illustrations of assessment and self-care techniques, a DVD is included to better demonstrate the correct application of the most important methods. A DVD icon in the book indicates methods that are shown on the DVD. Some of the methods included are:

- Vleeming's active straight leg raise test
- McGill's side bridge endurance test
- Hip hinge advice
- Brügger's micro-break
- Abdominal bracing
- Lewit's examination and mobilization of the thoracic spine
- Vojta's basic reflex locomotion positions
- Balance sandal training
- Star lunges
- Functional training with pulleys

Rehabilitation of the Spine is a practical guidebook for identification of rehabilitation candidates and solutions. Hopefully, restoring function in the locomotor system will become the standard of care for managing patients with complex neuromusculoskeletal disorders.

Craig Liebenson
Los Angeles, California

Acknowledgments

I have had the good fortune to have had my chiropractic education complemented by an introduction to a broader paradigm of care, Many conversations with one of the grandfathers of spinal surgery and pioneers of taking a functional view of spinal problems William Kirkaldy-Willis helped sharpen this author's view of the locomotor system.

In the mid 1980s I was fortunate to begin my studies with the great Czech neurologists and manual medicine practitioners, Karel Lewit and Vladimir Janda. This laid the groundwork for integrating rehabilitation with manipulative therapy. In particular, they have contributed to our approach, a comprehensive analysis of the locomotor system, which enables clinicians to see how various functional pathologies such as stiff joints, tight muscles, and weak muscles are all part of a chain of events amendable to a specific prescription of manipulation and rehabilitation.

In the late 1980s another great pioneer, from San Francisco, Dennis Morgan showed me how spine stabilization training had sprung forth from P.N.F.. Stabilization training has spread around the world, and I have been fortunate to have had the chance to spend a great deal of time over the last decade with Pr. Stuart McGill one the preeminant researchers of the spine stability system. In the past few years, I have begun visiting him at the University of Waterloo where many of the ideas of Pr. Janda and Dennis Morgan are being researched with "state of the art" biomechanical and neurophysiological techniques.

Institutions such as the Los Angeles College of Chiropractic, Anglo-European College of Chiropractic, and Charles University, and organizations such as Chiropractic Education of Australia have all contributed greatly to this work through their support of educational programs designed to expand the musculoskeletal paradigm to include a more functional, biopsychosocial approach to rehabilitation of the locomotor system.

Certainly, I could not have accomplished this task without the tremendous support of Dr.'s Sylvia Deily and Tanya Broaded in proofreading and commenting on hundreds upon hundreds of manuscript pages. My first and second edition editors, Linda Napora, Laura Horowitz, and Christina Remsberg under the stewardship of Pete Darcy have been a regular source of support and encouragement driving me on to the finish line. My photographer Howard Linton and artists Jirí Hlaváèek and Joseph DePinho have done exceptional work, along with my amazingly patient and persistant videographer and DVD editor Robert Fisher.

Craig Liebenson
Los Angeles, California

Contributors

Charles Aprill, MD
New Orleans, LA

Cindy Bailey, DPT, ATC
Associate Professor of Clinical Physical Therapy
University of Southern California
Los Angeles, CA

Nikolai Bogduk, PhD
Professor of Pain Medicine, University of Newcastle
Head, Department of Clinical Research,
Royal Newcastle Hospital, Newcastle,
New South Wales, Australia

Jennifer Bolton, PhD
Anglo-European College of Chiropractic
Bournemouth, England

Mark R. Bookhout, PT
Physical Therapy Orthopaedic Specialists
Minneapolis, MN

Alan Breen, DC, PhD
Institute for Musculoskeletal Research and
Clinical Implementation
Anglo-European College of Chiropractic
Bournemouth, UK

Wendy Burke, DPT
Assistant Professor of Clinical Research
University of Southern California
Department of Biokinesiology and Physical Therapy
Department of Orthopaedic Surgery
Los Angeles, CA

Micheal A. Clark, DPT
National Academy of Sports Medicine
Calabasas, CA

Jonathan Cook, DC
Anglo-European College of Chiropractic
Bournemouth, UK

Neil Craton, MD
Assistant Professor, University of Manitoba,
Faculty of Medicine
Director, Legacy Sport Medicine
Winnipeg, Manitoba Canada

Jirí Čumpelík, PT
Faculty of Physical Education and Sport
Faculty of Dance, Academy of Performing Arts
Charles University
Prague, Czech Republic

George DeFranca, DC
W. Boylston, MA

Sylvia Deily, DC
Los Angeles, CA

Scott Fonda, DC
Rehabilitation Institute of Chicago
Chicago, Illinois

Clare Frank, DPT
Back in Balance Physical Therapy
Kaiser Permanente Orthopedic Physical Therapy
Residency and Movement Science Fellowship
Los Angeles, CA

Michael C. Geraci, Jr., MD, PT
Buffalo Spine and Sports Institute
Buffalo, New York

Natalie Gluck-Bergman, DC
Los Angeles, CA

Steve Heffner, DC
Williamsport, PA

Alena Herbenová, PhD
Institute for Postgraduate Medical Education
Charles University
Prague, Czech Republic

Helena Hermach, PT
Gmünd, Austria

Paul W. Hodges, BPhty(Hons) PhD, MedDr
Professor and NHMRC Senior Research Fellow
Division of Physiotherapy
The University of Queensland
Brisbane, Australia

Gary Jacob, DC, LAc, MPH
Los Angeles, CA

Vladimír Janda, MD
Former Chief, Department of Rehabilitation
Medicine in Prague
Postgraduate Institute of Medicine
University Hospital
Prague, Czech Republic

Gwendolen A. Jull, PT, PhD
Head of Division of Physiotherapy
School of Health and Rehabilitation Sciences
The University of Queensland
Brisbane, Australia

William H. Kirkaldy-Willis, MD, BChir, FRCS (E and C),
FACS, LLD (Hon), FICC (Hon)
Emeritus Professor of Orthopaedic Surgery
Royal University Hospital
University of Saskatchewan
Saskatoon, Saskatoon Canada

Alena Kobesová, MD
2nd Medical Faculty
University Hospital Motol
Charles University, Prague, Czech Republic

Pavel Kolář, PaedDr
2nd Medical Faculty
University Hospital Motol
Charles University, Prague, Czech Republic

Martin Lambert, PT
Buffalo, NY

Ellen Lee, PhD
School of Physical Therapy
Texas Woman's University
Houston, Texas

Karel Lewit, MD, DSc
2nd Medical Faculty
University Hospital Motol
Charles University, Prague, Czech Republic

Craig Liebenson, DC
Los Angeles Sports and Spine
Los Angeles, CA

Steven J. Linton, PhD
Örebro University
Department of Behavioral, Social and Legal Sciences-Psychology
Örebro, Sweden

Leonard Matheson, PhD
Washington University School of Medicine
St. Louis, MO

Stuart M. McGill, PhD
Professor of Spine Biomechanics
Faculty of Applied Health Sciences
Department of Kinesiology
University of Waterloo, Canada

Robin McKenzie, PT
President McKenzie Institute International
Raumati Beach, New Zealand

Vert Mooney, MD
Clinical Professor Orthopaedics
University of California, San Diego
Medical Director of Spine & Sport Centers
San Diego, CA

Donald R. Murphy, DC
Rhode Island Spine Center
Providence, RI

Chris Norris, PT
Manchester, UK

Neil Osborne, DC, FRSH, FCC(Orth)
Anglo-European College of Chiropractic
Bournemouth, UK

Dagmar Pavlu, PaedDr, PhD
Faculty of Physical Education and Sport
Charles University
Prague, Czech Republic

Maria Perri, DC
Highland Mills, NY

Sibyle Petak-Krueger, PT
Switzerland

Charles Poliquin
Poliquin Performance Center
Tempe, AZ

Joel Press, MD
Medical Director, Spine and Sports Rehabilitation Center
Rehabilitation Institute of Chicago
Chicago, IL

David R. Seaman, DC
Palmer College of Chiropractic Florida
Port Orange, FL

Maureen J. Simmonds, PhD, PT
School of Physical and Occupational Therapy
McGill University
Montreal, Quebec, Canada

Clayton Skaggs, DC
Central Institute for Human Performance
St. Louis, MO

John J. Triano, DC, PhD, FCCS(c)
Texas Back Institute
Plano, TX

Pamela Tunnell, DC
Ridgefield, CT

Marie Vávrová, PT
Prague, Czech Republic

František Véle, MD, PhD
Faculty of Physical Education and Sport
Charles University, Prague, Czech Republic

Howard Vernon, DC, PhD
Director, Center for the Study of the Cervical Spine
Canadian Memorial Chiropractic College
Toronto, Ontario, Canada

Michaela Veverková, PT
Institute for Postgraduate Medical Education
Prague, Czech Republic

Robert Watkins, MD
Los Angeles Spine Surgery Institute
Professor of Clinical Orthopaedic Surgery
University of Southern California
Los Angeles, CA

Steven Yeomans, DC
Yeomans-Edinger Chiropractic Center
Ripon, WI

Contents

PART I

Overview

Editor's Note

A new patient-centered model is being applied to spine disorders. Rather than focusing merely on pathology and symptoms, the emphasis is on recovery, reactivation, and self-management. Passive care approaches utilizing medication, modalities, and manipulation are being replaced with an active self-care paradigm. This first section of the book lays out the added value to patients of a reactivation approach. The overwhelming evidence in support of this new direction is reviewed along with the reasons why a traditional biomedical way of thinking is far from ideal for a multifactorial problem such as spine pain. This section concludes with a discussion of why, when, and how to integrate the basic steps of this broad new biopsychosocial model into everyday clinical practice.

1

Active Care: Its Place in the Management of Spinal Disorders

Craig Liebenson

Learning Objectives

After reading this chapter you should be able to understand:

- The current state of knowledge for the diagnosis and classification of patients with low back disorders
- The relationship between functional disturbances and spinal disorders
- The relationship between psychosocial factors, such as fear–avoidance behavior, and deconditioning syndrome
- The distinction between impairments such as losses of strength or mobility and disability such as walking or sitting intolerances
- The evidence for the effectiveness of active care in the treatment of spinal disorders

"One of the most tragic events of our time is that we know more than ever before about the pains and sufferings of the world, and yet are less and less able to respond to them."

Henri Nouwen

Introduction

Activity has been shown to be effective for preventing or treating many of the most common chronic ailments in our society today (77). In particular, active care or patient reactivation plays a decisive role in the modern management of disorders of the cardiovascular and locomotor systems (75,94,95,161,183,189,195, 200,201). From simple, uncomplicated reactivation advice to comprehensive, multidisciplinary rehabilitation, the goal is to restore function. The functional goal is an essential hinge for guiding clinicians in the decision-making process. Biomechanical, neurophysiological, psychosocial, and biochemical rationales exist for the benefits of active care. However, the most important justification for making reactivation a primary focus of care is that patients in pain tend to accept the adage "let pain be your guide," with the result being they decondition as a result of their pain.

Persistent pain reinforces negative attitudes about the relationship of activity and pain as the patient takes on the "sick" role (147). Diagnostic tests that focus on pathoanatomy are frequently ordered to find the "cause" of the pain. Unfortunately, these tests have high false-positive rates for coincidental structural findings, such as degenerative joint disease or herniated discs, and thus reinforce the patients self-image as having a "bad" back or needing to "learn to live with it" (14,15,23,96,99,111,239,255,271). The result is further activity avoidance and deconditioning. Unfortunately, excessive immobilization interferes with the healing, coping, and recovery process. Thus, health care professionals are being urged by each successive international guideline on spinal disorders to first perform a diagnostic triage to rule out "red flags" of rare but serious disease, and then to reassure patients of the benign nature of their back pain and the safety and value of gradually resuming activities (2,25,38,94, 148,217).

The evidence in favor of reactivation for spine patients is strong. Reactivation advice to resume near-normal activities is both safe and effective for acute low back pain (LBP) patients (148). Similarly, early activation has been found to be effective for neck pain after a whiplash injury (18,166,213). Deconditioning normally accompanies acute LBP and its prevention has been shown to reduce recurrence rates (82,83, 234). Active therapies involving such diverse exercise methods as cognitive–behavioral, stabilization, and strengthening have demonstrated their effectiveness for subacute and chronic LBP (11,58–60,83,94,95,113, 128,150,190). Therefore, at each phase of the acute to chronic pain continuum, patient reactivation has been shown to play a fundamental role.

The Functional Paradigm in Diagnosis and Therapy

Practice-Based Problem

LBP is a subjective symptom that correlates poorly with objective findings. Less than 15% of LBP patients can be given a precise pathoanatomical diagnosis. These patients are labeled with general terms such as sprain/strain, "non-specific," or idiopathic LBP. Fortunately, most low back conditions have a favorable natural history. However, patients who don't recover rapidly with "tincture of time" can become frustrated. The physician shares in this frustration with the result being that tests are ordered that have low predictive value and thus are unlikely to make a difference in patient care. In fact, the reservoir of coincidental structural pathology (false-positive results) in patients is so high that performing advanced imaging injudiciously has the unwanted side effect of increasing anxiety and propagating an undesirable, interventionist cascade in pursuit of the cause of the pain (177,269,275).

The problem of back pain then is not what to do for the majority of patients who have a satisfactory outcome, but rather what to do for the disproportionately costly minority who do not. Because the goal of care is to restore function, are we able to identify the impairments and cognitive–behavioral factors that limit performance so that treatment decisions can be guided by a valid, logical reasoning process?

The Diagnostic Dilemma in Back Pain

The Problem

Optimal clinical management depends on accurate diagnosis. Unfortunately, only a minority of back pain patients can be given a clear diagnosis of their pain generator or relevant pathoanatomy (2). The conundrum of the LBP problem is that whereas most patients do well despite this diagnostic failure, the vast majority of the costs arise from the minority of those who become chronically disabled (80).

Current "state-of-the-art" guidelines suggest performing a diagnostic triage to classify patients with low back problems into three distinct groups. First, caused by "red flags" of serious disease, e.g., tumor, infection, fracture, or serious medical disease (<2%); second, caused by nerve root compression (<10%); or third, caused by "non-specific" mechanical factors (85%–90%) (2,38,217) (see Chapter 7). This "state of the art" will hopefully evolve because the most crucial of all "stake holders"—the patients—are dissatisfied with the diagnosis "non-specific" back pain (20,25).

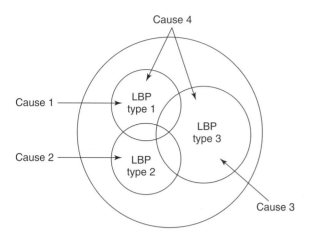

Figure 1.1 Non-specific LBP may consist of subtypes of LBP with different causes. From Laboeuf-Yde C, Lauritsen JM, Lauritzen T. Why has the search for causes of low back pain largely been nonconclusive? Spine 1997;22:878.

Although a precise pathoanatomic diagnosis of the pain generator remains elusive, emerging evidence shows a strong association between psychosocial factors and chronic LBP. These psychosocial illness traits (i.e., fear–avoidance behavior, anxiety) have been termed "yellow flags" to distinguish their relative importance from "red flags" of potentially serious disease processes (see Chapter 9). Individuals with a preponderance of "yellow flags" are at heightened risk for chronic symptoms and disability (26,53,110,165,202) and thus require a carefully mapped out management strategy. The strength of the association between "yellow flags" and spinal pain syndromes is reinforced by the prospective studies involving asymptomatic individuals which have shown that they predicted both future acute episodes (133) and who will have chronic problems (240). Importantly, there is preliminary evidence that psychosocial illness behavior can be improved merely by active rehabilitation alone without a structured cognitive–behavioral component (152).

A burning question in the low back field continues to be how to identify the patients who will respond best to individual interventions. Whereas general guidelines adhering to a biopsychosocial model have emerged that point out past errors and suggest a new path, there are still many unanswered questions (21). For instance, which patients respond best to manipulation, reactivation advice, exercise, medication, cognitive–behavioral approaches, or to various combinations of these? A report from the 2nd International Forum of Primary Care Researchers on LBP concluded that achieving a validated classification

system for "non-specific" LBP was their top research priority (19).

Subclassification of "Non-Specific" Low Back Pain

Contemporary research on the effectiveness of different treatments has assumed that "non-specific" back pain is a homogenous group (256). LaBouef has urged researchers to appreciate that patients lacking either "red flags" or nerve root signs or symptoms are most likely a heterogenous group (117,118) (Figs. 1.1 and 1.2). She points out that research that assumes this large patient population is homogenous and would fail to show statistical clinical effectiveness for specific interventions beneficial for a certain smaller subgroup. The result is that a promising treatment would be erroneously assumed to be ineffective. The Cochrane Back Review Group refers to identification of subgroups as "the Holy Grail" (22) (see Chapter 34).

Work at the University of Pittsburgh has convincingly shown that subclassification of the "non-specific" group is possible with an evaluation consisting of a thorough history, disability questionnaires, and examination using a battery of low-tech yet reliable tests (i.e., sacroiliac, McKenzie) (Table 1.1) (46,55,56). They have shown that treatment that is matched to the appropriate subclassification is superior to unmatched treatments (46). Furthermore, a recent randomized, clinical trial (RCT) shows that treatment driven by subclassification is superior to the "generic" treatment recommended by the Agency for Health Care Policy and Research (AHCPR) for the

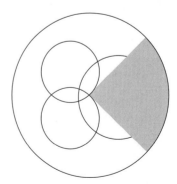

Figure 1.2 A positive association between a suspected risk factor and non-specific LBP will become apparent only if the study sample contains a sufficient number of people with the "right" subtype of LBP that matches the risk factor undergoing study. From Laboeuf-Yde C, Lauritsen JM, Lauritzen T. Why has the search for causes of low back pain largely been nonconclusive? Spine 1997;22:878.

Table 1.1 Treatment-Based Classification System (34, 41)

- Immobilization
- Mobilization
  - Sacroiliac mobilization
  - Lumbar mobilization
- Specific Exercise
  - Extension syndrome
  - Flexion syndrome
- Lateral shift
- Traction

broad "non-specific" category (57). Outcomes included reduced disability and accelerated return to work. Treatment classifications included manipulation/mobilization of lumbar or sacro-iliac joints, centralization (McKenzie) with flexion/extension, stabilization, and traction for nerve root syndromes not exhibiting a centralization phenomena.

The McKenzie method by itself has been shown to be a promising classification system (56,112,206,270) (see Chapter 15). Kilopikoski and colleagues demonstrated that classification of 39 chronic LBP patients, by two highly trained individuals, into the specific McKenzie syndromes (posture, dysfunction, and derangement) was possible with 95% agreement (κ=0.6; P=0.000) (112). The classic McKenzie approach of using repeated movements and end-range loading strategies to identify: (a) if the centralization phenomenon was present and (b) the patient's movement bias (i.e., directional preference) had agreement of 95% (κ=0.7; P=0.002) and 90% (κ=0.9; P<0.00), respectively. However, a limitation of the study was that most patients (35 out of 39) were classified into one syndrome—the derangement syndrome. Having such a homogenous sample can over-inflate the kappa value. Another study that used an abbreviated training program did not show acceptable inter-examiner reliability (210).

Long et al compared patients treated after the McKenzie classification system (directional preference) to a group treated with opposite directional exercise and another group after evidence-based care (EBC) (140). Ninety-five percent of the McKenzie group improved or resolved; 44% of EBC group improved or resolved. Only, 25% of opposite group improved or resolved. Previous work on the McKenzie system has also demonstrated the validity of the centralization phenomena (56,206).

Researchers at Washington University, applying the methods of Shirley Sahrman, P. T., have also begun validating a subclassification scheme based on

identifying the posture or movement that is consistently associated with increasing the patient's LBP (149,251–254). Similarly, in Toronto, a group associated with the Canadian Back Institute showed the reliability of a pain pattern system using key elements from the history and examination (273). They demonstrated 78.9% agreement among examiners using their approach. Furthermore, unlike the successful McKenzie study mentioned, only minimal training was required.

Table 1.2 highlights the steps required to evaluate diagnostic/classification procedures. The emerging evidence shows great promise for the ability to determine mutually exclusive categories of mechanical LBP that can guide the treatment decision-making process.

The Rationale for Active Care

Because the realization has dawned that there are no "quick fixes" for back pain, there has been an increasing realization that teaching patients what to do for themselves–self-management–is a growing priority. Is this merely an acceptance of our failure to cure LBP, or is it an acknowledgment of the physician's ancient role as teacher and helper?

Active care adheres to psychosocial principles by providing unambiguous cognitive and behavioral advice to enhance coping ability and motivate patients to gradually resume normal activities. Patients who worry about their functional status or fear their pain are more likely to have chronic problems (201, 207,240). They are particularly vulnerable to being "labeled" with an injured back (i.e., ruptured disc) or degenerative condition (16,40). Patients who expect an activity to be painful or disabling are less likely to perform at a normal level (5,119,120). Thus, one's per-

Table 1.2 Evaluation of Diagnostic Procedures

1. Establish interobserver reliability of individual tests
2. Establish reproducibility of combinations of reliable tests to identify homogenous LBP subgroups associated with specific syndromes
3. Determine sensitivity and specificity—predictive validity—of identification of LBP subgroups
4. Perform RCT of individualized care matched to the subgroup vs unmatched or generic treatment using clearly defined patient populations, well-accepted outcomes, and follow-up data

Modified from The International Federation for Manual/Musculoskeletal Medicine Scientific Committee Meeting The Hague, March 2000. J Orthop Med 2001;23:33–35.

formance is limited by psychological as well as physical factors. Stress, muscle tension, and pain are interrelated (147,171). It is the physician's role to inform the patient that fear and/or stress increase muscle tension, which in turn can exacerbate pain (94). Insight into this relationship helps to reassure patients that their pain is largely caused by factors that are potentially controllable.

Active care adheres to biomechanical principles by advising when and how to stabilize the back. LBP is just as likely to occur in individuals who move their back too little as in those who move too much. In fact, a trivial load encountered at a time of vulnerability such as in the early morning or after prolonged sitting is a typical mechanism of injury (71,162,225, 226).

Active care adheres to neurophysiological principles by training motor control patterns that are protective of the spine. Spinal instability has been shown to result from poor endurance and coordination of the trunk flexors and extensors (31,32, 61,66,193). In particular, low-intensity activation of key stabilization muscles has been shown to enhance joint stiffness and thus stability (31,209). Recent research shows that agonist–antagonist muscle coactivation is disturbed in LBP patients, thus compromising stability mechanisms involved in reacting to unexpected loads or perturbations (33,204,205,272).

Active care adheres to biochemical principles by advising patients to avoid the debilitation of bed rest and inactivity while encouraging them regarding the safety and value of resuming activities with simple biomechanical modifications. Pain and tissue healing are related to metabolic and nutritional issues. The disc is a relatively hypovascular tissue that contributes to its poor healing ability (87). In fact, some pain treatments such as epidural injections, although they clearly de-inflame the nerve root and initially reduce pain, have recently been shown to cause a rebound pain later, perhaps as a result of interfering with the body's natural resorption process for the herniated disc (106). Resorption or regression of herniated discs—even in large disc herniations—is a common finding and is consistent with the normal process of tissue repair and remodeling (28,29,107,116,172,203). Further evidence for this is the finding that macrophages are present in high concentration with disc herniations (72,78,93). Inactivity slows the recovery process because the disc is dependent on diffusion for its nutrition.

Rest, inactivity, or overly "guarded" movements are deleterious to the recovery of activity tolerance. Conversely, reassurance that the spine is not injured or damaged and that gradual reactivation will actually speed recovery is necessary to dispel the patient's disabling feelings and cognitions (i.e., worry, anxiety, and fear) (94,95,197,262).

The Deconditioning Syndrome—Functional and Cognitive-Behavioral Aspects

The Clinical Examination of Function and Performance

LBP is a subjective symptom that unfortunately correlates poorly with most pathoanatomical (MRI, x-ray) investigations including disc bulges, facet joint degeneration, endplate changes, and mild spondylolisthesis (97). Notable exceptions are disc extrusions, moderate or severe canal stenosis, and nerve root compression (97). In fact, most back problems are not caused by structural pathology (arthritis, herniated disc) or serious disease (tumor, infection, fracture) and benefit from prompt reassurance and early, reactivation advice. Therefore, one of the primary goals of care is to reassure patients about the benign nature of their pain and the safety and value of resuming normal activities. Prevention of deconditioning, both physical and psychological, is a fundamental goal of the modern management of spinal disorders.

What is deconditioning? Deconditioning is the diminished ability or perceived ability to perform tasks involved in a person's usual activities of daily living. In the Agency for Health Care Policy and Research (AHCPR) low back pain guidelines (2), it is stated that "the main goal for treatment of back pain has shifted from treatment of pain to treatment of activity intolerances related to pain." The plight of clinicians in this field is that because pathoanatomy only weakly correlates with symptoms, there is a dearth of objective findings to aid the clinician in navigating a safe and speedy course for the patient who is recovering slowly. This has led spine scientists to search for relevant, quantifiable features of LBP.

Measurable abnormalities whether structural or functional are considered impairments (275). Historically, impairment was viewed as objective and disability as primarily subjective. However, it is now recognized that impairments (isolated strength/mobility measures) are also related to psychological (cognitive–behavioral) issues such as self-efficacy, fear–avoidance, or pain expectancies, and that disability can at least in part be measured with "subjective" questionnaires (Oswestry, Neck Disability Index) or tests of actual activities (i.e., walking speed, reaching tests, sit-to-stand tests) (222).

The World Health Organization (WHO) has been classifying the consequences of disease, from a biomedical perspective, as impairments, disability, and handicap since 1980 (92). This work was updated recently as the International Classification of Functioning, Disability, and Health (ICF) document, from a biopsychosocial perspective, to take better account of the functional status of the individual (275). The ICF classifies functional status in three interrelated dimensions:

a. Functions—specific structural and functional impairments

b. Activities—actions that a person performs/ functional limitations

c. Participation—social or work involvement

Activity level pertains to functional limitations while impairments are isolated functional deficits (Table 1.3). Functional activities or limitations are further defined as what the patient can or can't do (or perceives he or she can't do!) in his or her daily life (Fig. 1.3). In contrast, specific functional deficits are found only with clinical examination and are often unrelated to the patient's symptoms or actual functional abilities (activity level and limitations) (Fig. 1.4).

Participation is dependent on the physical ability to perform an activity, but it also encompasses social and attitudinal factors. It can be measured with a subset of questions from the Chronic Pain Grading Scale (232,263,275).

1. To what extent did you perform any activities in or around your home during this episode of low back pain (not being work or household activities)?

2. To what extent did you participate in any work and/or household activities during this episode of low back pain?

3. To what extent did you participate in sport activities during this episode of low back pain?

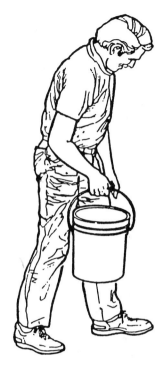

Figure 1.3 Spinal function sort—carrying a 30-lb bucket 30 feet. Reprinted with permission from Matheson L, Matheson M. Spinal Function Sort. Wildwood, MO: Employment Potential Improvement Corporation, 1989.

4. To what extent did you participate in any leisure time activities, besides sports, during this episode of low back pain?

5. To what extent did you participate in any social and/or family activities during this episode of low back pain?

Each question was answered on a 0–10 scale, with 0 indicating "no participation" and 10 indicating to "full normal participation."

What Is The Relationship Between Symptoms, Impairments, Disability, and Distress?

Impairments show a tenuous correlation to both pain and activity intolerances (e.g., disability) (115,180, 183,265). Far from being the so-called objective medical factors, they are related as much to an individual's motivation to perform as to their actual physical performance ability (34,37,119,120)! The American Medical Association's (AMA) (6) guide for assessing physical impairment allows only spinal range of motion (ROM), even though its reliability (185) and validity (180,196,279) are questionable and it doesn't discriminate chronic LBP patients from asymptomatic individuals (115,194). Fortunately, newer more promising methods have emerged (Table 1.4).

Table 1.3 Impairment vs Disability

Impairments—Specific functional deficits	Disability—Functional ability/limitations
ROM	
Strength	Walking tolerance
Endurance	Sitting tolerance
Cardiovascular fitness	Standing tolerance
Balance	Lifting ability
Muscle reaction time	Carrying ability
Fatigue-ability	
Measurable with physical performance testing	Measurable with activity intolerance questionnaires or simulated activity testing

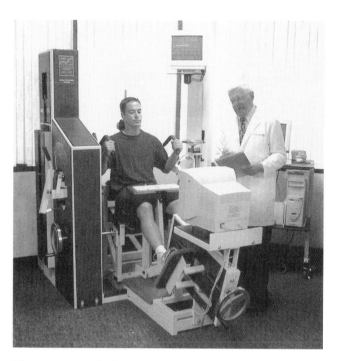

Figure 1.4 MedX lumbar extension machine.

Practice-Based Problem

The patient's goal is to resume activity with less pain. Can the clinician identify impairments that are related to the patient's symptoms or functional abilities (i.e., disability)? Impairments (i.e., specific dysfunctions) such as hypomobile joints, trigger points, and weak or tight muscles are frequent findings. How do we determine which impairments are clinically relevant?

For instance, can it be determined which impairments are responsible for biomechanical overload (pathomechanics) or are participating in clinically significant functional adaptations or compensations (pathophysiology)? Making this determination is at the heart of shifting care from one that is symptom-based (rest, medication, etc.) to one that is functionally oriented (reassurance, reactivation) (see Chapter 32).

The clinician must be careful not to make the goal of finding and correcting impairments an end in itself. This should be used as a means to achieving the end of symptom reduction and activity restoration.

The most popular measurement of disability (or ability) is a patient's self-report of activity limitations or perceived functional ability (i.e., Oswestry, Roland-Morris, Neck Disability Index). Whereas such questionnaires may be reliable and responsive, they do not correlate well with actual measurements of functional performance ability (49,222). Furthermore, they do not measure fundamental work behaviors important for vocational qualification (participation) or specific work behaviors relevant to the question of return to previous work ability (participation) (62,157). Thus, questionnaires, although valuable outcomes of care, may not be sufficient guides for determining appropriate treatment strategies or ability to return to work.

Recently, actual testing of **functional** abilities has been studied (186,222) (see Chapter 12). Simmonds and colleagues have shown how general functional ability can be measured with simple, reliable, inexpensive, time-efficient tests (186,187,222). Examples of such tests include sit-to-stand, rollover tasks, functional reach, loaded reach, distance walked, etc. These tests are proving to be valuable tools for both identifying functional limitations and establishing realistic goals in the management of LBP patients (60).

Matheson and colleagues have shown the continuum from observed signs and symptoms to structural diagnosis, impairments, and the inability to perform specific work behaviors (62,157). Figs. 1.5 and 1.6 show the features of this model along with specific measurements used.

The relationship between impairment (specific functional deficits), disability (general functional ability, perceived or actual), and pain is poorly understood. Every clinician can think of patients with severe pain and disability who have minimal impairment and others who are very impaired and yet avoid being disabled. Unfortunately, testing ability is more a test of one's performance than their true capacity, because effort is influenced by pain (actual or expectancy) and psychological factors (fear–avoidance, self-efficacy) (36,51). Human performance literature indicates that the goals one sets for task performance influence the performance itself (119).

Waddell was the first to quantify the relationship between these variables (Fig. 1.7) (265). More recently, Mannion showed that 51.4% of an individual's disability could be explained by performance,

---

Table 1.4 Performance Attributes Related to Chronic LBP

- Trunk extensor endurance
- Flexion–relaxation phenomena
- Spinal motion
- Back muscle fatigueability (EMG)
- Position sense
- Reaction times when exposed to unexpected perturbations
- Reaction times of trunk muscles with voluntary upper or lower limb movements
- Incoordination
- Balance ability

Work Disability Model

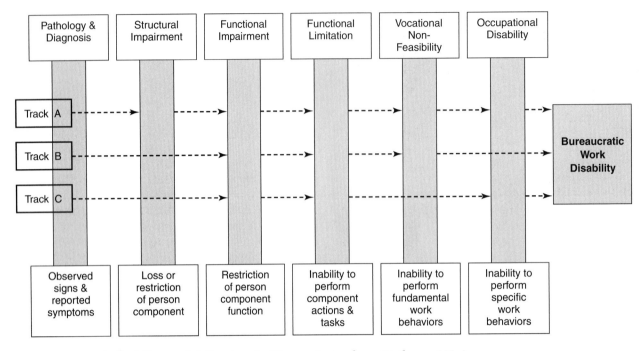

Figure 1.5 Work disability model. Reprinted with permission from Matheson LN. A new model for disability determination. Keynote Address, United Kingdom Society of Occupational Medicine Annual Scientific Meeting. Belfast Northern Ireland, June, 2001.

psychological, and pain factors (Fig. 1.8) (152). The performance factors alone accounted for 24.5% of the variance. Other studies have shown a similar relationship between functional performance deficits and disability (67,168,211,265). Turner et al recently showed that pain intensity scores measured with a visual analog scale (VAS) predicted disability as measured with the Roland-Morris questionnaire (246).

The authors concluded that back pain rated as 5 or higher is much more likely to be disabling. Swinkels also found that pain intensity along with specific pain-related fear significantly predict disability (232).

Mannion suggests that because one-half of self-reported disability before treatment and more than half of it afterwards is unaccounted for by structural, psychological, voluntary performance, or electromyo-

W.H.O.'s ICF Hierarchy

Unit of Analysis	Effect on Person	Case Example
Impairment	• Structural • Functional	• Disc herniation with nerve root compression • Strength/ROM deficits
Activity	Functional Limitations	Walking, standing, sitting
Participation	Vocational	Operating equipment

Figure 1.6 World Health Organization's ICF hierarchy. Modified from Matheson LN. A new model for disability determination. Keynote Address, Work Special Interset Section, American Occupational Therapy Association, Indianapolis, April, 1999.

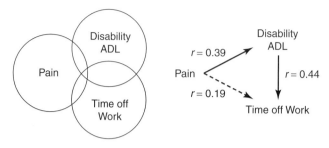

Figure 1.7 The quantitative relationship between the clinical presentation of pain, disability, and objective physical impairment and the correlation coefficients (r) between them when 0 is no correlation and 1 is complete correspondence. Reproduced with permission from Waddell G. The Back Pain Revolution. Edinburgh: Churchill Livingstone, 1989.

graphic (EMG) fatigue findings, then new aspects of physical function relating to motor control are worthy of future investigation (152). These include those aspects of function involved in non-voluntary, reflex control of movement such as position sense, delayed reaction times, and balance tests listed in Table 1.4 (153,163). The next section of this chapter discusses the evidence linking motor control and other functional deficits to spinal disorders.

Correlation Between Specific Performance Deficits and Low Back Pain

The relation between functional deficits or impairments and LBP has been studied extensively. Many features are identified by cross-sectional analysis to be present in greater incidence in pain patients than in asymptomatic patients. However, in such cases the associated impairment may be a result of pain rather than its cause. A better type of research uses prospective longitudinal analysis, thus providing evidence of the risk of future low back or neck pain when a certain dysfunction is present. Another valuable type of research is to determine if treatment of a specific dysfunction alters patient outcomes. Such research is ideally performed as a randomized controlled trial.

Isokinetic Strength A reduced ratio of trunk extensor to flexor strength/endurance discriminates between LBP patients and control subjects. The normal ratio is approximately 1.3:1, with the extensors being stronger (158). Mayer and colleagues demonstrated that patients chronically disabled with LBP frequently had a decreased trunk extensor/flexor strength ratio and that a comprehensive, multidisciplinary functional restoration program (including an emphasis on trunk extensor training)

successfully returned many of these individuals to work. (161)

Flexion–Relaxation Phenomena The flexion–relaxation phenomenon occurs when the erector spinae muscles relax involuntarily in terminal stage of a standing trunk flexion maneuver. It has been shown through EMG recordings to correlate with low back pain (153,220,245,267). However, despite significant reductions in pain ratings after active therapy, no improvement in flexion–relaxation was found by Mannion (153).

Spinal Motion ROM is an integral component in the evaluation of LBP patients (6). Although reliable, its validity is questionable. Various studies have failed to find a correlation between ROM deficits and pain or disability (67,194). The quality of motion seems more important than its quantity (164). In particular, velocity measurements have shown to be a more valid measure of LBP impairment (156) and to correctly predict which asymptomatic manual material handlers would have future LBP (231).

Back Muscle Fatigueability With EMG This is a unique functional measure because it is involuntary and theoretically not subject to psychophysical issues such as pain expectancy or motivation. Chronic LBP patients show a median frequency shift (increased rate of decline) during sustained contractions that control subjects do not (12,115,214,215). Reliability has been shown to be high when 80% of the maximum voluntary contraction (MVC) is performed (45). This same finding is reported to correctly predict which asymptomatic manual material handlers will report future LBP (231).

It has been shown in certain studies that these profiles can be improved with rehabilitation (103,104,

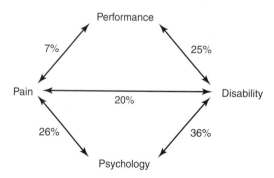

Figure 1.8 Interrelationship between performance, psychological, pain factors, and disability (explained proportion of variance using multiple regression analyses). From Mannion AF, Junge A, Taimela S, Muntener M, Lorenzo K, Dvorak J. Active therapy for chronic low back pain. Part 3. Factors influencing self-rated disability and its change following therapy. Spine 2001;26:920–929.

115,159,216,241). However, in other studies no improvement was found (153,174,198,274).

Position Sense Kinesthetic awareness of position sense (24,64,182,235) has been shown to be compromised in LBP individuals and in those with spinal stenosis (127). This is the ability to reproduce positions in space and is called repositioning ability or error. Similar results are also seen in the cervical spine (81,141,208,230,244).

Delayed Reaction Times

a) *When exposed to unexpected perturbations* Like the EMG studies mentioned, reactions to unexpected perturbations are largely involuntary. Altered reaction times of muscles have been correlated with LBP. Wilder showed that slow reaction time, decreased peak output, and increased peak output after discharges when irregular load is handled is typical of LBP subjects (272). After treatment, the reactions improved. Sitting was shown to disturb these variables and a brief walking break was shown to improve them again.

A recent study by Leinonen using similar methods as Wilder reported that there was a slower reaction time to anticipated, sudden loading in patients with sciatica than in healthy controls (126). This was theorized because of an impairment in the patient's central processing of information. It was concluded that chronic sciatica can impair lumbar feed-forward control.

Radebold and colleagues also found that a motor control signature discriminates LBP patients from asymptomatics—namely a slow reaction time, increased muscle activation, and slow relaxation of muscles after unexpected perturbations (33,204,205).

b) *With voluntary upper or lower limb movements* A delayed activation of the transverse abdominus muscle during arm or leg movements has been found to distinguish LBP patients from asymptomatic individuals (85,86). A rehabilitation program designed to improve this dysfunction has been shown to be effective for chronic LBP patients (190).

c) *To external visual stimuli* Reaction times to visual stimuli have been shown to be slower in chronic LBP patients than in asymptomatic individuals (143, 144,236).

Incoordination Incoordination is correlated with LBP. Paarnianpour showed that a loss of control of the center of rotation during resisted trunk movements in the sagittal plane occurred in LBP patients, but not in normal patients (193). Increases in rotation and side-bending and a decrease in sagittal motion occurred during the resisted movement. Similarly,

Grabiner reported that asymmetric muscle output during isokinetic-resisted trunk extension did not reduce torque production, but was abnormal (65).

Arendt-Nielson found over- and under-activity in muscles during different phases of gait in chronic LBP subjects, but not in asymptomatic patients (7). Overactivity of back muscles was found during the swing phase of gait and decreased agonist peak muscle activity during the double-stance phase was found in LBP patients (7). Simmonds has reported that stride length is decreased during the gait of LBP individuals compared to normal subjects (90,91). Lamoth and colleagues recently found that pelvis–thorax coordination in the LBP group differed significantly from that in the control group (121). Specifically, they reported that the gait of LBP patients was characterized by a more rigid, less flexible pelvis–thorax coordination and slower gait velocity than in asymptomatic subjects. In asymptomatic individuals at gait velocities more than 3.0 km/h, coupled transverse plane rotation of the pelvis and thoracic regions becomes uncoupled because of counter-rotation. However, in LBP subjects this uncoupling did not occur.

O'Sullivan found that an increased ratio of rectus abdominus to transverse abdominus/oblique abdominal activation is correlated with LBP (190). Control subjects were able to preferentially activate the internal oblique and transverse abdominus muscles without significant rectus abdominus activation, whereas LBP patients could not do this. Individuals who automatically perform a trunk curl fast instead of slow also showed a greater ratio of rectus abdominus to transverse abdominus/oblique abdominal activation (191).

An active straight leg raise test (ASLR) has been shown to be associated with postpartum sacroiliac (SI) pain. The test involves lifting one leg 20 cm up from a relaxed supine position. It is positive if significant heaviness of the leg is noted and if on repetition when a manual compressive force is applied through the ilia, or with a belt tightened around the pelvis, the ability to raise the leg improves (169,170). It has been shown that altered kinematics of the diaphragm and pelvic floor are present in those with a positive test (192). Additionally, manual compression through the ilia normalizes these altered motor control strategies (192).

Edgerton found that an altered muscle activation ratio of synergist spinal muscles during a variety of motor tasks was common in chronic neck pain patients after whiplash injury (44). Underactivity of agonists and overactivity of synergists was able to discriminate pain patients with 88% accuracy. He stated, "The nervous system apparently can detect a reduced capacity to generate force from a specific muscle or group of muscles and compensate by recruiting more motoneurons. This compensation can be made by recruiting motor units from an uninjured area of the muscle or from other muscles capable of performing the same tasks . . ." Nedherhand found that a decreased ability to relax the upper trapezius muscles during static tasks and after exercise distinguished between chronic whiplash-associate disorder (WAD) classification II patients and healthy control subjects (181).

Jull has shown that a cranio-cervical flexion test can differentiate both chronic headache and chronic neck pain patients after whiplash from asymptomatic individuals (100,101). During the test, patients showed over-activation of the superficial neck muscles (sternocleidomastoid), an inability to hold a constant pressure with the head against a pressure sensor at all test levels, and an inability to target higher pressure levels (26–30 mmHg) (230). Individuals with mild or moderate/severe pain and disability had significant overactivity of the superficial neck muscles during the flexion test at 1 month (230). This persisted at 3 months regardless of whether pain persisted (230). Treatment directed at improving cranio-cervical flexion has recently been shown to achieve lasting results in terms of improved function and reduced symptoms (102).

Endurance Endurance has been shown to correlate with LBP. Decreased endurance of the trunk extensors has not only been shown to correlate with pain (13,124,184) but also prospectively to predict recurrences (13), as well as first time onset of episodes in healthy individuals (88,142). Some studies have disputed that this test correlates with low back trouble (238). The test, if performed in the manner described by Biering-Sorensen, has been shown to be reliable in various populations—asymptomatic (124), symptomatic (175), and those with a past history of LBP (124). One study claimed the test was unreliable, but a small sample (12 subjects) and a different procedure using a Roman Chair was used (160).

Decreased endurance of the deep neck flexors has been correlated with chronic neck pain and headaches (10,221,243,268).

Balance Ability Balance deficits have been demonstrated to be related to LBP (30,145,238,176). Byl showed that excessive anterior to posterior body sway on an unstable surface or poor single-leg standing balance ability is correlated with LBP (30). Mok has shown that when compared with age- and gender-matched pain-free controls, study participants with LBP had poorer balance (176). Poor balance was also prospectively correlated with future LBP by Takala (238).

Structural Characteristics of Muscles Structural characteristics of the back such as fat content of the lower

erector spinae accounts for 30% of the variance in severely disabled men (3). Atrophy, demonstrated as a decreased cross-sectional analysis, of the multifidus in the low back has been shown to occur in patients with acute LBP (82), those recovered from acute LBP (84), and those having surgery for nerve root compression caused by a herniated disc (277,278). The acute patient's atrophy was ipsilateral to the pain and at the same segmental level as palpable joint dysfunction (82). Recovery from acute pain did not automatically result in restoration of the normal girth of the muscle (84). However, spinal stabilization exercises successfully restored the muscle's size in one study (84), whereas in another various exercise strategies did not (108). In the study that showed that the exercise did restore the muscle's girth, follow-up data demonstrated a decreased recurrence rate in those who performed the exercises versus those who did not (83).

Similarly atrophy has been shown in the suboccipital muscles of chronic neck pain patients (76,167).

Cognitive–Behavioral Components

Patients who equate hurt with harm have a disabling form of thinking. This is part of fear–avoidance behavior that promotes deconditioning (Fig. 1.9) (258,259). It is important to identify the patient who is fearful and avoid encouraging them to take on a "sick role" (147). Fear–avoidance beliefs (FAB) and distress have recently been shown to account for approximately 50% of the variation in self-rated disability (Oswestry Disability Index) in acute and chronic LBP patients (68). FABs were shown to be much higher in chronic than acute patients (68). In another study, psychological variables were demonstrated to account for 26% of self-reported pain and 36% of self-reported disability (Roland-Morris scale) (152) (Fig. 1.8). The most important psychological characteristics in this study were the use of negative coping strategies, self-efficacy beliefs, fear–avoidance behavior, and distress. Interestingly, in this study of three different active care approaches, none of which consisted of psychological or cognitive–behavioral approaches, all three improved the patient's psychological coping strategies, as well as their pain and disability (152).

FABs impact performance by limiting effort. Individuals who perceive that an activity will be painful have been shown to have reduced physical performance abilities (119,120). In fact, the cognitive association of activity with pain or anticipation of pain has been shown to be more predictive of physical performance than purely nociceptive factors (7). Council et al examined the association between pain expectancies and illness behavior by asking patients to anticipate how much pain they would experience when

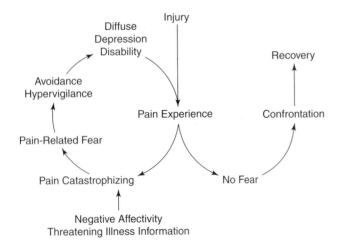

Figure 1.9 Fear–avoidance behavior. Reprinted with permission from Vlaeyen JWS, Linton S. Fear-avoidance and its consequences in chronic musculoskeletal pain. A state of the art. Pain 2000;85:317–332.

performing a number of simple motor tasks (36). They found substantial correlations between pain expectancies and self-rated physical disability (58).

It is well accepted that psychosocial variables such as depression are significantly correlated with illness behavior in patients with chronic pain (34,35,114, 146). However, of even greater importance are Ciccione's findings that show that pain expectancies accounted for 33% of the variance in acute subjects ($P < 0.001$) but for only 16% of the variance in the chronic patients ($P < 0.001$) (34). Fritz et al has also confirmed that initial fear–avoidance beliefs were significant predictors of subacute status at 4 weeks independent of pain intensity, physical impairment, disability, or therapy received (54). Thus, fear–avoidance beliefs such as pain expectancies are present even before acute pain becomes chronic!!

Psychosocial and physical deconditioning go hand-in-hand because many individuals have the belief that they will be unsuccessful gaining control over symptoms (locus of control) or regaining lost function (self-efficacy). Such beliefs have been shown to delay recovery (26,229,276). Asghari in a 9-month prospective trial in chronic pain patients demonstrated that self-efficacy beliefs—confidence in the ability to perform a variety of tasks despite pain—was predictive of pain behavior and avoidance behavior independent of pain, distress, or personality variables (8).

How a patient copes with acute pain has a lot to do with whether they will have a chronic problem (110). They may tend to catastrophize their illness and feel there is nothing that they can do themselves (26). Patients who fear pain or catastrophize it by fearing

an inevitable poor outcome are also less likely to perform exercise (258,259) and more likely to avoid activities (63). Thus, patients with fear–avoidance behavior can easily become deconditioned through activity avoidance, rest, symptomatic care, etc.

According to Vlaeyen (259), fear–avoidance behavior leads to deconditioning in the following manner:

a) Negative views about pain (i.e., viewing it as a threat rather than an annoyance) and its causes lead to catastrophization

b) Fear and anxiety in turn lead to the tendency to avoid the perceived threat.
  • Activities of daily living become restricted

c) Psychophysical reactivity (sympathetic activation, muscle tension) occurs when activities are encountered that are perceived as harmful.

d) Fearful patients become hypervigilant because they cognitively put increased attention on possible sources of pain.

e) Because avoidance behaviors are anticipatory, they are self-perpetuated since the individual rarely comes into contact with the actual (non-harmful) consequences of the feared situation.
  • "Guarded movements" such as an impaired flexion–relaxation phenomenon are correlated with fear–avoidance beliefs, NOT actual pain (267)
  • Anxious patients predict pain earlier during the performance of physical tasks such as ROM or straight leg raise tests (34,37,119,120)

f) Long-standing avoidance of physical activity leads to the "disuse syndrome" or deconditioning syndrome affecting both musculoskeletal and cardiovascular systems

The FAB model may be less applicable in repetitive strain injuries because of overuse (261). DeFier did not observe a similar relationship between pain-related fear and task performance in fibromyalgia patients as in chronic LBP (39). Whereas some people catastrophize pain and avoid activities, others may try to ignore pain and overexert (79). People use different "stop rules" with activities.

Teaching patients what they can do for themselves is an essential part of caring for the person with pain. A simple technique for getting a patient to become active in their own rehabilitation program is to shift them from being pain avoiders to pain managers (25,212). More comprehensive programs have traditionally involved cognitive–behavioral approaches focusing on "graded exposure" to generalized movements (50,128,129) (see Chapters 14 and 31). This has recently been modified by exposing the patient to the specific movements or activities avoided and addressing the fearful beliefs and emotions that accompany them (9,135,178,249,260,262). According to Vlaeyen (259), "graded exposures" have the following effects:

- Pain expectancies are corrected with repeated performance of the movements/exercises on subsequent days
- After multiple exposures, over-predictions of pain intensity tend to match actual pain experience

Another progressive strategy teaches patients to approach LBP in a problem-solving manner by: (a) taking an active role; (b) reducing modifiable risk factors; and (c) avoiding impulsively seeking mainly symptomatic relief (219,250).

The Negative Effects of Immobilization and Bed Rest

Immobilization

Why doesn't rest or inactivity allow tissues that are irritated to become less painful? Prolonged immobilization results in compromise of the musculotendinous, ligamentous–articular, osseous, cardiovascular, and central nervous systems (Figs. 1.10 and 1.11 and Table 1.5). Bed rest leads to a loss of muscle strength of 10% per week (179). The loss is reversible; however, reconditioning time is longer than deconditioning time (17).

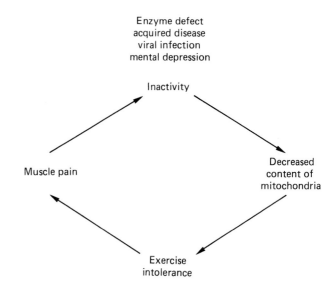

Figure 1.11 Effects of musculoskeletal immobilization. Reprinted with permission from Troup JDG, Videman T. Inactivity and the etiopathogenesis of musculoskeletal disorders. Clin Biomech 1989;4:175.

Prolonged immobilization after an injury can lead to scar tissue formation and lowered fatigue tolerance of injured tissues (Fig. 1.12). Soft tissue healing has three phases: inflammation, repair, and remodeling. Some form of local tissue immobilization is usually advisable during the inflammatory phase, which usually peaks at approximately the third day after injury. Toward the end of the inflammatory phase, fibroblasts are found in increasing numbers in the injured area. These fibroblasts contribute to scar formation. In a study of calf contusions in rats, Lehto and colleagues found that connective tissue scar formation will persist and become fibrotic rather than be absorbed if the acute inflammatory reaction is allowed to persist (125). These authors suggest early, aggressive management of injuries to limit enlargement of the injured area.

During the repair phase, passive and active motion of the tissues positively affects the injured tissues. Classic work on knee cartilage by Salter and co-workers showed that after 3 weeks of immobilization, intra-articular adhesions complicate the repair phase of soft tissue healing (218). Either intermittent active motion or continuous passive motion prevented such adhesion formation.

The remodeling phase involves lysis of adhesions and reorientation of collagen fibers along the lines of imposed stress. Again, prolonged immobilization is a negative factor in proper healing. In studies of rhesus monkeys, Noyes studied the effects of 8 weeks of immobilization on ligament stiffness and failure rate

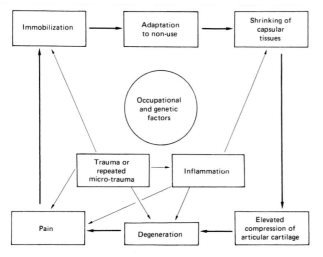

Figure 1.10 Biochemical changes associated with reduced physical activity. Reprinted with permission from Troup JDG, Videman T. Inactivity and the etiopathogenesis of musculoskeletal disorders. Clin Biomec 1989;4:175.

Table 1.5 Negative Effects of Immobilization

Joints
  Shrinks joint capsules
  Increases compressive loading
  Leads to joint contracture
  Increases synthesis rate of glycosaminoglycans
  Increase in periarticular fibrosis
  Irreversible changes after 8 weeks of
    immobilization
Ligament
  Lowers failure or yield point
  Decreased thickness of collagen fibers
Disk biochemistry
  Decreases oxygen
  Decreases glucose
  Decreases sulfate
  Increases lactate concentration
  Decreases proteoglycan content
Bone
  Decreases bone density
  Eburnation
Muscle
  Decreased thickening of collagen fibers
  Decreased oxidative potential
  Decreased muscle mass
  Decreased sarcomeres
  Decreased cross-sectional area
  Decreased mitochondrial content
  Increased connective tissue fibrosis
  Type 1 muscle atrophy
  Type 2 muscle atrophy
  20% loss of muscle strength per week
Cardiopulmonary
  Increased maximal heart rate
  Decreased VO$_2$ max
  Decreased plasma volume

From Liebenson C. Pathogenesis of chronic back pain.
J Manipulative Physiol Ther 1992;15:303.

(188). Ligament stability was only 31% of normal after 8 weeks. After 5 months of reconditioning, stability recovered to 93% of normal levels. Five months of reconditioning improved the tissue failure rate to 80% of normal, and after 12 months of reconditioning, the rate was completely normal.

Bed Rest

Of all the traditional treatment methods, none has fared worse than bed rest. Deyo performed a controlled clinical trial that compared 2 days of bed rest against 2 weeks and concluded that not only was 2 days of bed rest as effective as 2 weeks but the negative effects of prolonged immobilization were also limited (41). A Cochrane Collaboration review concluded that bed rest (74):

- has no positive effect for LBP
- may have slightly harmful effects
- yields no improvement with 7 days over 2 to 3 days in LBP or sciatica

This is similar to an earlier review that concluded there was no evidence in favor of bed rest (256). The Danish guidelines concluded that there is insufficient evidence of a positive effect in relation to the resources used for the bed rest (38). Vroomen found that there was no evidence of effectiveness of bed rest for sciatica (264).

The Paris Task Force on Back Pain recommended that "bed rest should neither be enforced nor prescribed, but may be authorized if pain indicates it (1). If authorized, it should be of as short a duration as possible and should be intermittent rather than continuous. After 3 days of bed rest, patients must be strongly encouraged to progressively resume their activities." The Danish guidelines concurred, suggesting that bed rest can be considered a pain-relieving measure for 1 to 2 days for severe pain (38).

When recommended for severe pain, it should be made clear that brief bed rest is recommended as a consequence of the pain, but not a treatment for the pain (217).

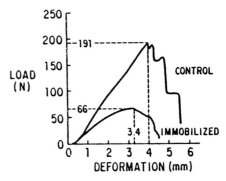

Figure 1.12 The strength of rested tissue deteriorates dramatically compared to normal tissue. In this medial collateral ligament of a rabbit knee that rested for 9 weeks, two-thirds of the strength has been lost. From Mooney V. The subacute patient: To operate or not to operate. In: Mayer TG, Mooney V, Gatchel RJ, eds. Contemporary Conservative Care for Painful Spinal Disorders. Baltimore: Lippincott, Williams & Wilkins, 1997.

A Patient-Centered Approach

The functional re-activation model is "patient-centered," because the patient's symptoms, dysfunction (impairment, abilities, and participation), and distress are all addressed (Table 1.6 and Fig. 1.13). If a patient's recovery is unsatisfactory, evaluation of each of these components is indicated.

Symptoms do not arise in a vacuum. Injury or pathology is certainly a factor, but one that is not nearly as important as has been assumed. The fact that advanced imaging modalities show that a large percent of asymptomatic individuals have herniated discs means that their presence in symptomatic individuals is often coincidental. Clearly, individuals can compensate for them. As Figure 1.13 shows, each of the major components can influence the other. Symptoms can be distressing (26,50,94,129) and lead to changes in how one performs activities such as walking (90,91) and specific functions (impairments) such as the body's ability to respond to a sudden load efficiently (272). In turn, psychological distress such as fear–avoidance behavior negatively influences impairments (119,120), activity tolerance (34), and pain reporting (249). Finally, specific dysfunctions such as poor trunk extensor endurance have been shown to be prospectively linked to the development of acute LBP in asymptomatic individuals (88,142,238) and recurrent LBP in acute LBP subjects (13). Thus, the relationship between function, psychological wellness, and symptoms is an important one to appreciate when caring for suffering individuals.

A typical LBP scenario involves a patient with persistent pain expecting that imaging be performed so they can learn what "the cause" of the pain is (47,98,111). Predictably, there is no dearth of structural pathology present that can easily be ascribed as being "the cause of the pain" (16,40). The patient is

Table 1.6 *The Patient-Centered Approach*

- Symptoms—Pain
- Dysfunction
  - ° Impairments—ROM
  - ° Functional abilities—walking tolerance
  - ° Participation—work activity
- Psychosocial—distress, fear, anxiety, disability

then given the label of having a herniated disc or degenerative arthritis and is informed that they have the option to learn to live with their pain with the help of medication, manipulation, or injections or to have surgery to correct the problem. Unfortunately, if a patient does not recover, after either symptomatic or surgical management, their distress in the form of frustration increases and they are now labeled as having psychogenic pain (43). In such cases, whose failure is this—the patient's or the health care system's? LaRocca (122) in his Presidential address to the Cervical Spine Research Society said, "An assumption is made that there is a pathological entity operating in the spine to produce pain which, if eliminated or controlled, should result in pain relief in every instance . . . The error here is the automatic leap to psychology. It assumes that all organic factors have been considered, when in reality the clinician's appreciation of the complexity of such factors is often severely limited."

In a patient-centered, self-management approach, non-responsive patients would receive an evaluation to rule out relevant pathoanatomy ("red flags") combined with an evaluation of psychosocial ("yellow flags") and functional/physiological factors.

Ironically, function—if evaluated at all—is usually limited to less valid measures such as ROM. A

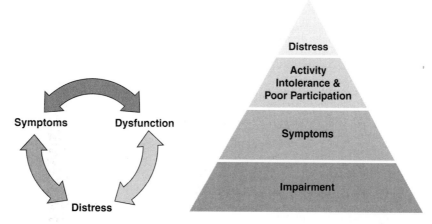

Figure 1.13 The patient-centered approach.

dichotomy exists in which function is either ignored completely or given too much credit for causing pain. Most parameters of dysfunction identified in LBP patients have not been shown to precede the pain, but rather only to accompany it. In other words, many dysfunctions are adaptive to the problem rather than part of its source. Important exceptions are trunk extensor endurance and balance function, which can predict future LBP in asymptomatic individuals (88,142,238). The challenge for clinicians is to strike a balance between ignoring function and blindly believing that every hypomobile joint, trigger point, or weak muscle requires treatment.

Evidence of Active Care's Effectiveness: Does It Exist?

Presented here is a summary of some evidence comparing active care to "tincture of time" or other modalities for the treatment of spine-related conditions. The most common criteria for recovery are symptom reduction and return to work. However, other criteria such as satisfaction, health care utilization, activity intolerances, participation, and distress have also been applied. Active care includes a variety of approaches, from basic advice to stay active to supervised machine-based exercise routines.

Prevention

A recent review of the preventive literature by Linton and van Tulder offered the following conclusions (130):

- Education including information oriented toward preventing fear–avoidance and promoting coping ability was more effective than no intervention (233).
- Advice to exercise and a free membership to a health club were at least as effective as an exercise program (131).
- Exercises were found by one study to be more effective than a back school (42).
- Exercises seem to be the only consistently proven effective preventive intervention, although most studies on which this is based are methodologically flawed, and the effects are only weak (42,70,109,237).
  - A high-quality study demonstrated with a randomized, controlled trial that an intervention group that received a 40-minute lesson on back problems and ergonomics and then performed passive prone extensions daily reported fewer back problems in the subsequent year than a

control group receiving no education or exercise advice (33% vs 51%) (123)
  - Adolescents who walk or bike more than 8 km per week were significantly less likely to have future LBP than those who were less active (223).
- There is strong and consistent evidence that back schools are not effective in preventing neck and back pain.
- There are no good-quality studies evaluating the effectiveness of ergonomics.

Acute Phase (First 4–6 Weeks)
Advice to Stay Active

Information and advice emphasizing the value of fitness and the safety of resuming activities achieved superior outcomes to advice that reinforced rest, activity restrictions, and the notion that the spine was injured or damaged (arthritis, herniated disc) (25). Reassuring workers and encouraging resumption of ordinary activities was superior to medication, bed rest, or mobilization exercises (148). Little et al recently demonstrated that educational advice that encourages early exercise (not just advice to stay active) or endorsement by a physician of a self-management booklet has been shown to increase patient satisfaction and function while reducing pain (137). Interestingly, combining advice to exercise with a take-home booklet was less effective than either intervention by itself. This is believed to be because of the fact that the written and verbal information presented was not consistent (27).

Exercise

The role of exercise in acute LBP is controversial. In a Cochrane Collaboration (257), systematic analysis it was concluded that "there is strong evidence that exercise therapy is not more effective than inactive treatments or other treatments for acute low back pain. Specific exercises are not recommended for acute low back pain patients . . ." One notable study that influenced these conclusions was by Faas et al, who reported that exercise was no better than usual care by a general practitioner in the treatment of uncomplicated, acute LBP (48). It has been argued that the Cochrane Collaboration researchers believe the null hypothesis has been fulfilled on the basis of results from only three studies, yet the null hypothesis requires much stronger evidence and thus appears spurious (151).

The studies considered to be of high methodological quality by the Cochrane Collaboration evaluated exercise that was prescribed on a "generic" basis rather than being customized to the needs of each patient. Such an approach to exercise prescription is not considered high-quality by most experts in the rehabilitation field (57,151,228). If a specific type of exercise is given to a large, heterogenous group and it fails to outperform other treatments, this may not suggest the exercise is ineffective for LBP (117). For instance, if extension exercise is given to a large heterogenous group of patients, some of whom respond well to extension and others who respond better to flexion, the exercise will not be shown to be effective (140).

Evidence that customizing exercises to the unique functional needs of the patient enhances outcomes was shown by researchers studying the McKenzie approach (228). The study had certain methodological flaws that weakened its conclusions, but the value of customization is not minimized. The Danish guidelines—based on technology assessment, ethical issues, and evidence-based review gave a favorable rating for McKenzie type exercises, generally recommending them for acute LBP (38).

Studies that compared individuals performing exercises matched to them versus unmatched concluded that the matched groups achieved significantly better results (46,140). A recent study found that the general reactivation recommendations of the AHCPR guidelines yielded inferior results to matched treatment (including exercise groups) based on a functional subclassification scheme (57).

Other recent studies not evaluated in the Cochrane review show that future meta-analysis will likely strengthen the place of exercise as a treatment for acute LBP. Little et al's study shows the value of exercise early on (137). An Australian study has shown that if acute LBP patients perform specific spinal stabilization exercises, multifidus muscle atrophy can be prevented (84). Although initial symptomatic and functional recovery (Oswestry) is not improved as a result of this intervention, the training has a secondary preventive effect by reducing future recurrences (83).

Studies evaluating behavioral strategies have also shown substantial improvements with early active care approaches. Early behavior modification through exercise reduced disability 1 year later than it did in the control group (50). An eight-fold reduction in the risk of becoming chronic was achieved from information designed to reduce fear and anxiety and provide self-care advice (129). A recent randomized, controlled trial verified the results of these early studies (134). What each of these cognitive-behavioral approaches has in common is that return to activity was quota-based, rather than being contingent on absence of symptoms. Quota-based exercise is exercise performed for a specific duration or frequency independent of symptoms.

It is striking that early active care methods have been put in such a negative light when such weak evidence of their ineffectiveness exists. On the contrary, when new evidence is considered and all of the literature is evaluated from a fresh perspective, the value of properly recommended exercises from the very beginning of care becomes overwhelmingly clear.

Passive Modalities

Many of the most popular treatments for acute LBP lack evidence of effectiveness. The recent Danish guidelines (38) (page 60) state, "One of the greatest errors in the treatment of LBP in this century has been the unquestioned usage of passive treatments, oftentimes initiated when spontaneous recovery has already begun." Passive modalities such as electrical muscle stimulation were recommended only as optional. Such passive modalities may engender higher levels of patient satisfaction, but they have not been demonstrated to improve outcomes related to recovery (89). Thus, similar to taking x-rays, patients may like it but because it doesn't improve outcomes, better patient education about appropriate management techniques for acute LBP are needed (47,98,111).

Subacute Phase Reactivation and Exercise (From 4–12 Weeks)

The subacute phase is the ideal time for both active and aggressive treatment (52,132,266). In cases of disability, the return to work curve declines steeply between 6 and 20 weeks (227,266). The longer patients with LBP are off work, the more difficult it is for them to return to work (227,266). For this reason, most guidelines recommend exercise therapy/fitness for LBP of more than 6 weeks (38). In patients with subacute LBP, light multidisciplinary treatment programs have been shown to be more effective than treatment as usual for return to work (73,94,95,128, 138). A Cochrane Collaboration review concluded that there is moderate evidence that multidisciplinary rehabilitation is effective for subacute LBP (105).

Two studies found that either lay-led or professional-led instruction in self-care and worry reduction were both successful in reducing back-related worry, fear–avoidance beliefs, pain severity, and activity intolerances (173,260). A long-term follow-up study led by Indahl focused on education designed to reduce fear (94,95). Patients were informed that light activity would not injure the disc, but instead speed recovery. The return to work rate was double that of the control group. Hagen reported at 1-year follow-up that light activity, education about the benign nature of pain, and encouragement to stay active achieved a significantly greater return to work rate than for those who received more traditional management (73). These studies used graded exposures, which means that patients exercise included movements that were perceived as threatening by the patient. Loisel's group demonstrated that a work site visit improved the success of the program (138,139).

A recent randomized, controlled trial of 160 LBP patients found that adding manual therapy to reactivation advice was shown to be superior to reactivation advice alone (69). Similarly, a pragmatic study of "best care" versus manipulation followed by exercise, exercise alone, or manipulation alone for 1334 subacute LBP patients in England was recently published (247). "Best care" involved giving advice to gradually resume near-normal activities along with a copy of *The Back Book.* Relative to "best care," the manipulation followed by exercise group had the best patient outcomes (disability, pain, adverse back pain beliefs, and general physical health) at both 3- and 12-month follow-up, whereas the manipulation alone group was the most cost-effective (247, 248).

Chronic Phase Reactivation and Exercise (After 12 Weeks)

A large number of well-controlled studies have shown that exercise is an effective treatment for chronic LBP. A Cochrane Collaboration review of exercise (257) concluded that, " . . . there is strong evidence (Level 1) that exercise therapy is more effective than usual care by a general practitioner for chronic low back pain." Two recent studies strongly suggest that exercise has a long-term beneficial effect in the management of chronic LBP (83,234). Both studies used exercise programs that focused on training coordinated movements and included evaluation of results during a prolonged follow-up period.

O'Sullivan et al showed that specific spine stabilization exercises achieved superior outcomes to isotonic exercises in chronic patients with spondylolisthesis (190). Manniche et al demonstrated that an isotonic regime emphasizing endurance training was successful in improving outcomes (150). In a large, randomized controlled clinical trial, Timm showed that exercise was superior to passive care in treating failed back surgery patients (242). In this study a further comparison of exercise types showed that low-technology exercise (McKenzie and stabilization) was superior to high-technology exercise (isotonics & Cybex).

The McKenzie method was shown to be as effective as an isotonic strengthening program in a recent randomized, controlled trial of subacute and chronic patients (pain duration of at least 8 weeks) (199). The course of treatment was 8 weeks of supervised training. McKenzie was superior at a 2-month follow-up, but no differences were noted at 8-month follow-up.

Mannion reported that low-cost exercise programs are more effective than one-on-one physical therapy for chronic LBP at 12-month follow-up (154). The key is "challenging the patient's misconception that exercise is contraindicated in LBP" (155). Aerobic exercise was one-sixth the cost. Dependence on the physical therapist was believed to be the cause of regression to the mean at 12 months (154).

General exercise programs using a cognitive–behavioral approach have been shown to be effective in both hospital and primary care settings (58–60,113, 134–136). Each of these programs encouraged reactivation and addressed fear–avoidance beliefs and behaviors by progressing exercises by quota independent of pain as well as used "graded exposures" to feared stimuli. Another publication regarding a light multidisciplinary program with a similar emphasis not only reduced chronic LBP but also showed it enhanced return to work in males (224). This was demonstrated to be superior to a more traditional and expensive multidisciplinary pain management–rehabilitation approach. Multidisciplinary functional restoration programs have demonstrated that they can enhance return to work in chronically disabled individuals with LBP, but their costs are generally higher (4,11,161).

The common denominators of care for chronic LBP that have been demonstrated to optimize outcomes are summarized in Table 1.7.

Active Care and the Neck

The Quebec Whiplash-Associated Disorders (WAD) guidelines recommended early, active intervention (including manipulation) (227) (Table 1.8).

Treatment following these guidelines has recently been shown to be much more effective than traditional passive-based care (213). Clinically important

---

Table 1.7 Common Denominators of Successful Care for Chronic Patients (132)

- Thorough physical and functional examination performed
- Report of findings given
- Emphasis on self-care
- Reduce any unfounded fear or anxiety about pain
- Crystal-clear recommendations about activities/exercise
- Avoidance of excessive "high-tech" testing or bed rest prescription

Table 1.8 WAD Guidelines (see also Table 35.5)

- Clinical diagnosis
- Reassurance
- Immobilization (<4 days for WAD classifications II & III)
- Activation
- Manipulation, mobilization/traction, exercise, postural advice, passive modalities (first 3 weeks only)
- Multidisciplinary team management (between 6 and 12 weeks)

Audit Process
Self-Check of the Chapter's Learning Objectives

- What lines of evidence suggest that the "non-specific" LBP classification can be more clearly defined?
- What specific functional disturbances are prospectively related to spinal disorders?
- How is fear–avoidance behavior related to deconditioning?
- What is quota-based exercise or graded-exposures and is it shown to be effective?
- Describe the controversy over the effectiveness of active care for acute LBP patients?

symptoms at 6 months after accident were present in only 10% of properly managed patients (early active intervention with submaximal movements identified by McKenzie evaluation) as compared with greater than 50% of those given standard care (soft collar, initial rest, gradual mobilization).

Similar positive results for early activation were found in two other studies. Encouragement to continue with activities of daily living had a superior outcome than prescription of sick leave and immobilization (18). Physical therapy or exact instruction in self-mobilization was better than 2 weeks of rest with a soft collar at 1-month, 2-month, and 2-year follow-ups (166).

Jull has recently demonstrated that a combination of manual therapy and exercise training that improves deep neck flexor function correlates with improved recovery in chronic neck pain patients after a whiplash injury (102).

■ CONCLUSION

The patient-centered reactivation approach is focused on the patient's dysfunction and distress rather than various signs of often coincidental structural pathology or the patient's subjective symptoms. A paradigm shift from a traditional biomedical model to a biopsychosocial one has taken firm hold in the spine field. The biopsychosocial approach teaches us that the old adage "let pain be your guide" can actually reinforce illness behavior such as fear–avoidance behavior. The more modern report of findings reassures patients that they do not have a disease (tumor, infection, and fracture) and that staying active will actually speed recovery. Learning that pain does not always warn of impending harm or damage can empower patients to remain active, avoid disability, and prevent the transition from acute to chronic pain.

■ REFERENCES

1. Abenheim L, Rossignol M, Valat JP, et al. The role of activity in the therapeutic management of back pain: Report of the International Paris Task Force on Back Pain. Spine 2000;25(4):1S–33S.
2. Agency for Health Care Policy and Research (AHCPR). Acute low-back problems in adults. Clinical Practice Guideline Number 14. Washington DC, U.S. Government Printing, 1994.
3. Alaranta H, Tallroth K, Soukka A, Heliaara M. Fat content of lumbar extensor muscles in low back disability: a radiographic and clinical comparison. J Spin Dis 1993;6:137–140.
4. Alaranta H, Rytokoski U, Rissanen A, et al. Intensive physical and psychosocial training program for patients with chronic low back pain: a controlled clinical trial. Spine 1994;19:1339–1349.
5. Al-Obaidi SM, Nelson RM, Al-Awadhi S, Al-Shuwaie N. The role of anticipation and fear of pain in the persistence of avoidance behavior in patients with chronic low back pain. Spine 2000;25(9):1126–1131.
6. American Medical Association. Guides to the evaluation of permanent impairment. 4th ed. Chicago: American Medical Association, 1994.
7. Arendt-Nielson L, Graven-Nielson T, Svarrer H, Svensson P. The influence of low back pain on muscle activity and coordination during gait. Pain 1995;64:231–240.
8. Asghari A, Nicholas MK. Pain self-efficacy beliefs and pain behavior. A prospective study. Pain 2001;94:85–100.
9. Balderson BHK, Von Korff M. The stepped care approach to chronic back pain. In: Linton SL, ed. New avenues for the prevention of chronic musculoskeletal pain and disability. Amsterdam: Elsevier, 2002.
10. Barton PM, Hayes KC. Neck flexor muscle strength, and relaxation times in normal subjects and subjects with unilateral neck pain and headache. Arch Phys Med Rehabil 1996;77:680–687.
11. Bendix AF, Bendix T, Labriola M, et al. Functional restoration for chronic low back pain: two-year

follow-up of two randomized clinical trials. Spine 1998;23:717–725.

12. Biedermann HJ, Shanks GL, Forrest WJ, et al. Power spectrum analyses of electromyographic activity discriminators in the differential assessment of patients with chronic low back pain. Spine 1991;16(10):1179–1184.

13. Biering-Sorensen F. Physical measurements as risk indicators for low-back trouble over a one-year period. Spine 1984;9:106–119.

14. Boden SD, Davis DO, Dina TS, et al. Abnormal magnetic-resonance scans of the lumbar spine in asymptomatic subjects. J Bone Joint Surg [Am] 1990;72:403.

15. Boden SD, McCowin PR, Davis DO, Dina TS, Mark AS, Wiesel S. Abnormal magnetic-resonance scans of the cervical spine in asymptomatic subjects. J Bone Joint Surg 1990a;72A:1178–1184.

16. Bogduk N. What's in a name? The labeling of back pain. Med J Australia 2000;173:400–401.

17. Booth FW. Physiologic and biochemical effects of immobilization on muscle. Clin Orthop 1987;219:15–20.

18. Borchgrevink GE, Kaasa A, McDonoagh D, et al. Acute treatment of whiplash neck sprain injuries. Spine 1998;23:25–31.

19. Borkan JM, Koes BW, Reis R, Cherkin DC. A report from the second international forum for primary care research on low back pain: Reexamining priorities. Spine 1998;23:1992–1996.

20. Borkan J, Reis S, Hermoni D, et al. Talking about the pain: a patient-centered study of low back pain in primary care. Soc Sci Med 1995;40:977–988.

21. Borkan J, Van Tulder M, Reis S, Schoene ML, Croft P, Hermoni D. Advances in the field of low back pain in primary care: A Report from the Fourth International Forum. Spine 2002;27:E128–E132.

22. Bouter LM, Pennick V, Bombarider C, Editorial Board of the Back Review Group. Cochrane back review group. Spine 2003;28:1215–1218.

23. Brandt-Zawadzki MN, Jensen MC, Obuchowski N, et al. Interobserver and intraobserver variability in interpretation of lumbar disc abnormalities: a comparison of two nomenclatures. Spine 1995;20:1257–1263.

24. Brumagne S, Cordo P, Lysens R, Verschueren S, Swinnen S. The role of paraspinal muscle spindles in lumbosacral position sense in individuals with and without low back pain. Spine 2000;25:989–994.

25. Burton K, Waddell G. Information and advice to patients with back pain can have a positive effect. Spine 1999;24:2484–2491.

26. Burton AK, Tillotson K, Main C, Hollis M. Psychosocial predictors of outcome in acute and subacute low back trouble. Spine 1995;20:722–728.

27. Burton AK, Waddell G. Educational and informational approaches. In: Linton SL, ed. New avenues for the prevention of chronic musculoskeletal pain and disability. Amsterdam: Elsevier, 2002.

28. Bush K, Cowan N, Katz DE, et al. The natural history of sciatica associated with disc pathology: A prospective study with clinical and independent radiologic follow-up. Spine 1992;17:1205.

29. Bush K, Chaudhuri R, Hillier S, Penny J. The pathomorphologic changes that accompany the resolu-

tion of cervical radiculopathy. Spine 1997;22(2):183–187.

30. Byl NN, Sinnot PL. Variations in balance and body sway. Spine 1991;16:325–330.

31. Cholewicki J, McGill SM. Mechanical stability of the in vivo lumbar spine: Implications for injury and chronic low back pain. Clin Biomech 1996;11(1):1–15.

32. Cholewicki J, Panjabi MM, Khachatryan A. Stabilizing function of the trunk flexor-extensor muscles around a neutral spine posture. Spine 1997;22:2207–2212.

33. Cholewicki J, Simons APD, Radebold A. Effects of external loads on lumbar spine stability. J Biomech 2000;33:1377–1385.

34. Ciccione DS, Just N. Pain expectancy and work disability in patients with acute and chronic pain: A test of the fear avoidance hypothesis. J Pain 2001;2:181–194.

35. Ciccone DS, Just N, Bandilla EB. Non-organic symptom reporting in patients with chronic non-malignant pain. Pain 1996;68:329–341.

36. Council JR, Ahern DK, Follick MJ, Kline CL. Expectancies and functional impairment in chronic low back pain. Pain 1988;33:323–331.

37. Crombez G, Vlaeyen JW, Heuts PH, et al. Pain-related fear is more disabling than pain itself: Evidence on the role of pain-related fear in chronic back pain disability. Pain 1999;80:329–339.

38. Danish Health Technology Assessment (DIHTA). Manniche C, et al. Low back pain: Frequency Management and Prevention from an HAD Perspective, 1999.

39. DeFier M, Peters ML, Vlaeyen JWS. Fear of pain, physical performance, and attentional processes in patients with fibromyalgia. Pain 2003;104:121–130.

40. Deyo RA. Back pain and disability conference, New York City as reported in The Back Letter 2001;16:13.

41. Deyo RA, Diehl AK, Rosenthal M. How many days of bed rest for acute low back pain? N Engl J Med 1986;315:1064.

42. Donchin M, Woolf O, Kaplan L, et al. Secondary prevention of low-back pain: A clinical trial. Spine 1990;15:1317–1320.

43. Dworkin S. Perspectives on psychogenic versus biogenic factors in orofacial and other pain states. Am Pain J 1992;1:172–180.

44. Edgerton VR, Wolf SL, Levendowski DJ, Roy RR. Theoretical basis for patterning EMG amplitudes to assess muscle dysfunction. Med Sci Sp Exer 1996;28:744–751.

45. Elfving B, Dedering A, Nemeth G. Lumbar muscle fatigue and recovery in patients with long-term low-back trouble—electromyography and health-related factors. Clin Biomech 2003;18:619–630.

46. Erhard RE, Delitto A. Relative effectiveness of an extension program and a combined program of manipulation and flexion and extension exercises in patients with acute low back syndrome. Phys Ther 1994;74:1093–1100.

47. Espeland A, Baerheim A, Albrektsen G, Korsbrekke K, Larsen JL. Patients views on importance and usefulness of plain radiography for low back pain. Spine 2001;26:1356–1363.

48. Faas A, Chavannes AW, van Eijk J Th M, Gubbels JW. A randomized, placebo-controlled trial of exercise therapy in patients with acute low back pain. Spine 1993;18:1388–1395.

49. Fordyce WE, Lansky D, Calshyn DA, Shelton JL, Stolov WC, Rock DL. Pain measurement and pain behavior. Pain 1984;18:53–69.

50. Fordyce WE, Brochway JA, Bergman JA, et al. Acute back pain: A control-group comparison of behavioral vs. traditional management methods. J Behav Med 1986;9:127.

51. Fordyce WE (ed). Back pain in the workplace: management of disability in non-specific conditions. Seattle: International Association for the Study of Pain (IASP) Press, 1995.

52. Frank J, Sinclair S, Hogg-Johnson S, et al. Preventing disability from work-related low-back pain. New evidence gives new hope—if we can just get all the players onside. Can Med Assoc J 1998;158:1625–1631.

53. Fransen M, Woodward M, Norton R, Coggan C, Dawe M, Sheridan N. Risk factors associated with the transition from acute to chronic occupational back pain. Spine 2002;27:92–98.

54. Fritz JM, George SZ, Delitto A. The role of fear-avoidance beliefs in acute low back pain: Relationships with current and future disability and work status. Pain 2001;94:7–15.

55. Fritz JM, George S. The use of a classification approach to identify subgroups of patients with acute low back pain. Spine 2000;1:106–114.

56. Fritz JM, Delitto A, Vignovic M, et al. Interrater reliability of judgments of the centralization phenomenon and status change during movement testing in patients with low back pain. Arch Phys Med Rehabil 2000;81:57–60.

57. Fritz JM, Delitto A, Erhard RE. Comparison of classification-based physical therapy with therapy based on clinical practice guidelines for patients with acute low back pain: A randomized clinical trial. Spine 2003;28:1363–1371.

58. Frost H, Lamb SE, Shackleton CH. A functional restoration program for chronic low back pain: A prospective outcome study. Physiotherapy 2000;86(6):285–293.

59. Frost H, Lamb S, Klaber Moffett JA, Faribank JCT, Moser JS. A fitness program for patients with chronic low back pain: Two-year follow-up of a randomized controlled trial. Pain 1998;75:273–279.

60. Frost H, Klaber Moffett JA, Moser JS, Faribank JCT. Randomized controlled trial for evaluation of fitness program for patients with chronic low back pain. Br Med J 1995;310:151–154.

61. Gardner-Morse MG, Stokes IAF. The effects of abdominal muscle coactivation on lumbar spine stability. Spine 1998;23:86–92.

62. Gaudino WA, Matheson LM, Mael F. Development of the functional assessment taxonomy. J Occup Rehabil 2001;11:155–175.

63. Geisser ME, Haig AJ, Theisen ME. Activity avoidance and function in persons with chronic back pain. J Occup Rehabil 2000;10:215–228.

64. Gill KP, Callaghan MJ. The measurement of lumbar proprioception in individuals with and without low back pain. Spine 1998;23(3):371–377.

65. Grabiner MD, Koh TJ, Ghazawi AE. Decoupling of bilateral paraspinal excitation in subjects with low back pain. Spine 1992;17:1219.

66. Granata KP, Marras WS. Cost-benefit of muscle cocontraction in protecting against spinal instability. Spine 2000;25:1398–1404.

67. Gronblad M, Hurri, Kouri JP. Relationships between spinal mobility, physical performance tests, pain intensity and disability assessments in chronic low back pain patients. Scan J Rehabil Med 1997;29:17–24.

68. Grotle M, Vollestad NK, Veierod MB, Ivar Brox J. Fear-avoidance beliefs and distress in relation to disability in acute and chronic low back pain. Pain 2004;112:343–352.

69. Grunnesjo MI, Bogefeldt JP, Svardsudd KF, Blomberg SIE. A randomized controlled clinical trial of stay-active versus manual therapy in addition to stay-active care: Functional variables and pain. JMPT 2004;27:431–441.

70. Gundewall B, Liljeqvist M, Hansson T. Primary prevention of back symptoms and absence from work: A prospective randomized study among hospital employees. Spine 1993;18:587–594.

71. Gunning J, Callaghan JP, McGill SM. The role of prior loading history and spinal posture on the compressive tolerance and type of failure in the spine using a porcine trauma model. Clin Biomech 2001;16:471–480.

72. Habtemariam A, Gronblad M, Virri J, et al. A comparative immunohistochemical study of inflammatory cells in acute-stage and chronic-stage disc herniations. Spine 1998;23:2159–2165.

73. Hagen EM, Eriksen HR, Ursin H. Does early intervention with a light mobilization program reduce long-term sick leave for low back pain? Spine 2000;25:1973–1976.

74. Hagen KB, Hilde G, Jamtvedt G, Winnem MF. The Cochrane review of bed rest for acute low back pain and sciatica. Spine 2000;25:2932–2939.

75. Hakim AA, Curb D, Petrovitch H, et al. Effects of walking on coronary heart disease in elderly men: The Honolulu Heart Program. Circulation 1999;100:9–13.

76. Hallgren R, Greenman P, Rechtien J. Atrophy of suboccipital muscles in patients with chronic pain: A pilot study. J Am Osteopath Assoc 1994;94:1032–1038.

77. Hamilton MT, Booth FW. Skeletal muscle adaptation to exercise: a century of progress. J Appl Physiol 2000;88:327–331.

78. Haro H, Komori H, Okawa A, et al. Sequential dynamics of monocyte chemotactic protein-1 expression in herniated nucleus pulposus resorption. J Orthop Res 1997;15:734–741.

79. Hasenbring M. Attentional control of pain and the process of chronification. In: Sandkuhler J, Bromm B, Gebhart GF, eds. Progress in brain research, vol 129. Amsterdam: Elsevier, 2000:525–534.

80. Hashemi L, Webster BS, Clancy EA, Volinn E. Length of disability and cost of workers' compensation low back pain claims. J Occup Environ Med 1998;40:261–269.

81. Heikkila H, Astrom PG. Cervicocephalic kinesthetic sensibility in patients with whiplash injury. Scand J Rehab Med 1996;28:133–138.

82. Hides JA, Stokes MJ, Saide M, Jull Ga, Cooper DH. Evidence of lumbar multifidus muscle wasting ipsilateral to symptoms in patients with acute/subacute low back pain. Spine 1994;19(2):165–172.

83. Hides JA, Jull GA, Richardson CA. Long-term effects of specific stabilizing exercises for first-episode low back pain. Spine 2001;26:e243–e248.

84. Hides JA, Richardson CA, Jull GA. Multifidus muscle recovery is not automatic after resolution of acute, first-episode of low back pain. Spine 1996;21(23):2763–2769.

85. Hodges PW, Richardson CA. Altered trunk muscle recruitment in people with low back pain with upper limb movement at different speeds. Arch Phys Med Rehabil 1999;80(9):1005–1012.

86. Hodges PW, Richardson CA. Delayed postural contraction of transversus abdominis in low back pain associated with movement of the lower limb. J Spinal Disord 1998;11(1):46–56.

87. Holm S, Nachemson A. Nutritional changes in the canine intervertebral disc after spinal fusion. Clin Orthop 1982;169:243–258.

88. Holm SM, Dickenson AL. A comparison of two isometric back endurance tests and their predictability of first-time back pain: A pilot study. J Neuromusculo Sys 2001;9(2):46–53.

89. Hurwitz EL, Morgenstern H, Harber PL, et al. The effectiveness of physical modalities among patients with low back pain randomized to chiropractic care: Findings from the UCLA low back pain study. J Manip Physiol Ther 2002;25:10–20.

90. Hussein TM, Simmonds MJ, Etnyre B, et al. Kinematics of gait in subjects with low back pain with and without leg pain. Scientific Meeting & Exposition of the American Physical Therapy Association. Washington, D.C., 1999.

91. Hussein TM, Simmonds MJ, Olson SL, et al. Kinematics of gait in normal and low back pain subjects. American Congress of Sports Medicine 45th Annual Meeting. Boston, MA, 1998.

92. ICDH-2. International Classification of Functioning and Disability. Beta-2 Draft. Full Version, World Health Organization, Geneva. 1999.

93. Ikeda T, Nakamura T, Kikuchi T, et al. Pathomechanism of spontaneous regression of the herniated lumbar disc: Histologic and immunohistochemical study. J Spinal Disord 1996;9:136–140.

94. Indahl A, Velund L, Eikeraas O. Good prognosis for low back pain when left untampered: A randomized clinical trial. Spine 1995;20:473–477.

95. Indahl A, Haldorsen EH, Holm S, Reikeras O, Hursin H. Five-year follow-up study of a controlled clinical trial using light mobilization and an informative approach to low back pain. Spine 1998;23:2625–2630.

96. Jarvik JG, Deyo RA. Imaging of lumbar intervertebral disc degeneration and aging, excluding disc herniations. Radiology Clinics of North America 2000;38:1255–1266.

97. Jarvik JG, Hollingworth W, Heagerty P, Haynor DR, Deyo RA. The longitudinal assessment of imaging and disability of the back (LAIDBack) study. Spine 2001;26:1158–1166.

98. Jarvik JG. Editorial. Don't duck the evidence. Spine 2001;26:1306–1307.

99. Jensel MC, Brant-Zawadzki MN, Obuchowki N, et al. Magnetic resonance imaging of the lumbar spine in people without back pain. N Engl J Med 1994;2:69.

100. Jull GA. Deep cervical flexor muscle dysfunction in whiplash. J of Musculoskel Pain 2000;8:143–154.

101. Jull G, Barret C, Magee R, Ho P. Further clinical clarification of the muscle dysfunction in cervical headache. Cephalgia 1999;19:179–185.

102. Jull G, Trott P, Potter H, et al. A randomized control trial of physiotherapy management of cervicogenic headache. Spine 2002;27:1835–1843.

103. Kankaanpää M, Taimela S, Airaksinen O, Hanninen O. The efficacy of active rehabilitation in chronic low back pain: Effect on pain intensity, self-experienced disability, and lumbar fatigability. Spine 1999;24:1034–1042.

104. Kankaanpää M, Taimela S, Laaksonen D, et al. Back and hip extensor fatigability in chronic low back pain patients and controls. Arch Phys Med Rehabil 1998;79:412–417.

105. Karjalainen K, Malmivaara A, van Tulder M, et al. Multidisciplinary biopsychosocial rehabilitation for subacute low back pain in working age adults. A systematic review within the framework of the Cochrane Back Review Group. Spine 2001;26:262–269.

106. Karppinen J, Malmivaara A, Kurunlahti M, et al. Periradicular infiltration for sciatica. A randomized controlled trial. Spine 2001;26:1059–1067.

107. Kawaguchi S, Yamashita T, Yokogushi K, Murakami T, Ohwada O, Sato N. Immunophenotypic analysis of the inflammatory infiltrates in herniated discs. Spine 2001;26:1209–1214.

108. Käser L, Mannion AF, Rhyner A, Weber E, Dvorak J, Müntener M. Active therapy for chronic low back pain. Part 2. Effects on Paraspinal Muscle Cross-Sectional Area, Fiber Type Size, and Distribution. Spine 2001;26:909–919.

109. Kellett KM, Kellett DA, Nordholm LA. Effects of an exercise program on sick leave due to back pain. Phys Ther 1991;71:283–293.

110. Kendall NAS, Linton SJ, Main CJ. Guide to assessing psychosocial yellow flags in acute low back pain: Risk factors for long-term disability and work loss. Accident Rehabilitation & Compensation Insurance Corporation of New Zealand and the National Health Committee. Wellington, NZ (http://www.nhc.govt.nz), 1997.

111. Kendrick D, Fielding K, Bentler E, Kerslake R, Miller P, Pringle M. Radiography of the lumbar spine in primary care patients with low back pain: randomized controlled trial. BMJ 2001;322:400–405.

112. Kilpikoski S, Airaksinen O, Kankaanpaa M, Leminen P, Videman T, Alen M. Interexaminer reliability of low back pain assessment using the McKenzie method. Spine 2002;27:E207–E214.

113. Klaber Moffet J, Torgerson D, Bell-Syer S, et al. A randomized trial of exercise for primary care back pain patients: Clinical outcomes, costs and preferences. BMJ 1999;319:279–283.

114. Klapow JC, Slater MA, Patterson TL, et al. Psychosocial factors discriminate multidimensional clinical groups of chronic low back pain patients. Pain 1995;62:349–355.

115. Klein AB, Snyder-Mackler L, Roy SH, et al. Comparison of spinal mobility and isometric trunk extensor forces with electromyographic spectral analysis in identifying low back pain. Phys Ther 1991;71(6):445–454.

116. Komori H, Shimoyama K, Nakai O, et al. The natural history of herniated nucleus pulposus with radiculopathy. Spine 1996;21:225–229.

117. Laboeuf-Yde C, Manniche C. Low back pain: time to get off the treadmill. JMPT 2001;24:63–65.

118. Laboeuf-Yde C, Lauritsen JM, Lauritzen T. Why has the search for causes of low back pain largely been nonconclusive? Spine 1997;22:877–881.

119. Lackner JM, Carosella AM, Feuerstein M. Pain expectancies, pain, and functional self-efficacy expectancies as determinants of disability in patients with chronic low back disorders. J Consulting and Clin Psych 1996;64:212–220.

120. Lackner JM, Carosella AM. The relative influence of perceived pain control, anxiety, and functional self-efficacy on spinal function among patients with chronic low back pain. Spine 1999;24:2254–2261.

121. Lamoth CJC, Meijer OG, Wuisman PIJM, van Dieën JH, Levin MF, Beek PJ. Pelvis-thorax coordination in the transverse plane during walking in persons with nonspecific low back pain. Spine 2002;27:E92–E99.

122. LaRocca H. A taxonomy of chronic pain syndromes. 1991 Presidential Address. Cervical Spine Research Society Annual Meeting. December 5, 1991. Spine 1992;10:S344.

123. Larsen K, Weidick F, Leboeuf-Yde C. Can passive prone extensions of the back prevent back problems?: A randomized, controlled trial of 314 military conscripts. Spine 2002;27:2747–2752.

124. Latimer J, Maher CG, Refshauge K, Colaco I. The reliability and validity of the Biering-Sorensen test in asymptomatic subjection and subjects reporting current or previous non-specific low back pain. Spine 1999;24:2085–2090.

125. Lehto M, Jarvinen M, Nelimarkka O. Scar formation after skeletal muscle injury. Arch Orthop Trauma Surg 1986;104:366–370.

126. Leinonen V, Kankaanpää M, Luukkonen M, Hänninen O, Airaksinen O, Taimela S. Disc herniation-related back pain impairs feed-forward control of paraspinal muscles. Spine 2001;26:E367–E372.

127. Leinonen V, Määttä S, Taimela S, et al. Impaired lumbar movement perception in association with postural stability and motor- and somatosensory-evoked potentials in lumbar pinnal stenosis Spine 2002;27(9):975–983.

128. Lindstrom A, Ohlund C, Eek C, et al. Activation of subacute low back patients. Physical Therapy 1992;4:279–293.

129. Linton SL, Hellsing AL, Andersson D. A controlled study of the effects of an early active intervention on acute musculoskeletal pain problems. Pain 1993;54:353–359.

130. Linton SJ, van Tulder MW. Preventive interventions for back and neck pain problems. What is the evidence? Spine 2001;26:778–787.

131. Linton SJ, Hellsing AL, Bergström G. Exercise for workers with musculoskeletal pain: Does enhancing compliance decrease pain? J Occup Rehabil 1996;6:177–190.

132. Linton SJ. The socioeconomic impact of chronic back pain: is anyone benefiting? Editorial. Pain 1998;75:163–168.

133. Linton SJ, Buer N, Vlaeyen J, Hellsing AL. Are fear-avoidance beliefs related to a new episode of back pain? A prospective study. Psychology and Health, 2000;14:1051–1059.

134. Linton SJ, Andersson T. Can chronic disability be prevented? A randomized trial of a cognitive-behavioral intervention for spinal pain patients. Spine 2000;25:2825–2831.

135. Linton SJ. Cognitive-behavioral therapy in the prevention of musculoskeletal pain: description of a program. In: Linton SL, ed. New avenues for the prevention of chronic musculoskeletal pain and disability. Amsterdam: Elsevier, 2002.

136. Linton SJ, Ryberg M. A cognitive-behavioral group intervention as prevention for persistent neck and back pain in a non-patient population: a randomized controlled trial. Pain 2001;90:83–90.

137. Little P, Roberts L, Blowers H, et al. Should we give detailed advice and information booklets to patients with back pain? A randomized controlled factorial trial of a self-management booklet and doctor advice to take exercise for back pain. Spine 2001;26:2065–2072.

138. Loisel P, Abenhaim L, Durand P, et al. A population-based, randomized clinical trial on back pain management. Spine 1997;22:2911–2918.

139. Loisel P, Gosselin L, Durand P, Lemaire J, Poitras S, Abenhaim L. Implementation of a participatory ergonomics program in the rehabilitation of workers suffering from subacute back pain. Appl Ergon. 2001;32(1):53–60.

140. Long A, Donelson R, Fung T. Does it matter which exercise? Spine 2004;29:2593–2602.

141. Loudon JK, Ruhl M, Field E. Ability to reproduce head position after whiplash injury. Spine 1997;22:865–868.

142. Luoto S, Heliovaara M, Hurri H, Alaranta H. Static back endurance and the risk of low-back pain. Clin Biomech 1995;10:323–324.

143. Luoto S, Taimela S, Hurri H, et al. Mechanisms explaining the association between low back trouble and deficits in information processing. A controlled study with follow-up. Spine 1999;24(3):255–261.

144. Luoto S, Taimela S, Hurri H, et al. Psychomotor speed and postural control in chronic low-back pain patients: A controlled follow-up study. Spine 1996;21:2621–2627.

145. Luoto S, Aalto H, Taimela S, et al. One-footed and externally disturbed two-footed postural control in chronic low-back pain patients and healthy controls: A controlled study with follow-up. Spine 1998;23:2081–2090.

146. Macfarlane GJ, Thomas E, Croft PR, Papageorgiou AC, Jayson MIV, Silman AJ. Predictors of early improvement in low back pain amongst consulters to general practice: The influence of pre-morbid and episode-related factors. Pain 1999;80:113–119.

147. Main CJ, Watson PJ. Psychological aspects of pain. Manual Therapy 1999;4:203–215.

148. Malmivaara A, Hakkinen U, Aro T, et al. The treatment of acute low back pain—bed rest, exercises, or ordinary activity? N Engl J Med 1995;332:351–355.

149. Maluf KS, Sahrmann SA, Van Dillen LR. Use of a classification system to guide non-surgical treatment of a patient with chronic low back pain. Phys Ther 2000;80:1097–1111.

150. Manniche C, Lundberg E, Christensen I, et al. Intensive dynamic back exercises for chronic low back pain. Pain 1991;47:53–63.

151. Manniche C, Jordan A. Letter to the editor. Spine 2001;26:840–844.

152. Mannion AF, Junge A, Taimela S, Muntener M, Lorenzo K, Dvorak J. Active therapy for chronic low back pain. Part 3. Factors influencing self-rated disability and its change following therapy. Spine 2001;26:920–929.

153. Mannion AF, Taimela S, Muntener M, Dvorak J. Active therapy for chronic low back pain. Part 1. Effects on back muscle activation, fatigability, and strength. Spine 2001;26:897–908.

154. Mannion AF, Muntener M, Taimela S, et al. A randomized clinical trial of three active therapies for chronic low back pain [In Process Citation]. Spine 1999;24:2435–2448.

155. Mannion AF, et al. Changes in pain and disability one year after active therapy for chronic low back pain. Inter Soc Study of Lumbar Spine, Adelaide, Australia, 2000.

156. Marras WS, Ferguson SA, Gupta P, et al. The quantification of low back disorder using motion measures. Methodology and validation. Spine 1999;24(20):2091–2100.

157. Matheson LM, Gaudino WA, Mael F, Hesse BW. Improving the validity of the impairment evaluation process: A proposed theoretical framework. J Occupa Rehabil 2000;10:311–320.

158. Mayer TG, Smith S, Keeley J, Mooney V. Quantification of lumbar function part 2: Sagittal plane trunk strength in chronic low back patients. Spine 1985;10:765–772.

159. Mayer TG, Kondraske G, Mooney V, et al. Lumbar myoelectric spectral analysis for endurance assessment. A comparison of normals with deconditioned patients. Spine 1989;14(9):986–991.

160. Mayer TG, Gatchel R, Betancur J, Bovasso E. Trunk muscle endurance measurement: Isometric contrasted to isokinetic testing in normal subjects. Spine 1995;20:920–927.

161. Mayer TG, Gatchel RJ, Mayer H, et al. A prospective two-year study of functional restoration in industrial low back injury. JAMA 1987;258:1763–1767.

162. McGill SM. ISB Keynote Lecture—The biomechanics of low back injury: Implications on current practice in industry and the clinic. J Biomech 1997;30:465–475.

163. McGill SM. Study in progress

164. McGregor AH, McCarthy ID, Dore CJ, et al. Quantitative assessment of the motion of the lumbar spine in the low back pain population and the effect of different spinal pathologies of this motion. Eur Spine J 1997;6(5):308–315.

165. McIntosh G, Frank J, Hogg-Johnson S, Bombardier C, Hall H. Prognostic factors for time receiving workers' compensation benefits in a cohort of patients with low back pain. Spine 2000;25:147–157.

166. McKinney LA. Early mobilization and outcome in acute sprains of the neck. BMJ 1989;299:1006–1008.

167. McPartland JM, Brodeur RR, Hallgren RC. Chronic neck pain, standing balance, and suboccipital muscle atrophy: A pilot study. J Manipulative Physiol Ther 1997;20:24–29.

168. Mellin G. Chronic low back pain in men 54–63 years of age. Correlations of physical measurements with the degree of trouble and progress after treatment. Spine 1986;11(5):421–426.

169. Mens JM, Vleeming A, Snijders CJ, et al. The active straight-leg-raising test and mobility of the pelvic joints. Eur Spine J 1999;8:468–474.

170. Mens JMA, Vleeming A, Snijders CJ, et al. Active straight-leg-raise test: A clinical approach to the load transfer function of the pelvic girdle. In: Vleeming A, Mooney V, Dorman T, et al, eds. Movement, Stability, and Low Back Pain: The Essential Role of the Pelvis. Edinburgh: Churchill Livingstone, 1997:425–431.

171. Mense S, Simons DG. Muscle Pain Understanding Its Nature, Diagnosis, and Treatment. Pain associated with increased muscle tension. Baltimore: Lippincott, Williams & Wilkins, 2001: 99–130.

172. Mochida K, Komori H, Okawa A, et al. Regression of cervical disc herniation observed on magnetic resonance images. Spine 1998;23:990–997.

173. Moore JE, Von Korff M, Cherkin D, et al. A randomized trial of a cognitive-behavioral program for enhancing back pain self-care in a primary care setting. Pain 2000;88:145–153.

174. Moffroid MT, Haugh LD, Haig AJ, Pope M. Endurance training of trunk extensor muscles. Phys Ther 1993;73:10–17.

175. Moffroid MT, Reid S, Henry S, Haugh LD, Ricamato A. Some endurance measures in persons with chronic low back pain. J Ortho Sports Phys Ther 1994;20:81–87.

176. Mok NW, Brauer S, Hodges PW. Hip strategy for balance control in quiet standing is reduced in people with low back pain. Spine 2004;29:E107–E112.

177. Mold JW, Stein HF. The cascade effect in the clinical care of patients. N Engl J Med 1986;314:512–514.

178. Moore JE, Von Korff M, Cherkin D, Saunders K, Lorig K. A randomized trial of a cognitive-behavioral program for enhancing back pain self-care in a primary care setting. Pain 2000;88:145–153.

179. Muller EA. Influence of training and of inactivity on muscle strength. Arch Phys Med Rehabil 1970;51:449–462.

180. Nattrass CL, Nitschke JE, Disler PB, et al. Lumbar spine range of motion as a measure of physical and functional impairment: An investigation of validity. Clin Rehabil 1999;13(3):211–218.

181. Nederhand MJ, Ijzerman MJ, Hermens HK, Baten CTM, Zilvold G. Cervical muscle dysfunction in the chronic whiplash associated disorder Grade II(WAD-II). Spine 2000;15;1938–1943.

182. Newcomer KL, Laskowski ER, Yu B, Johnson JC, An KN. Differences in repositioning error among patients with low back pain compared with control subjects. Spine 2000;25:2488–2493.

183. Newton M, Thow M, Somerville D, et al. Trunk strength testing with iso-machines: Part 2: Experi-

mental evaluation of the Cybex II Back Testing System in normal subjects and patients with chronic low back pain. Spine 1993;18(7):812–824.

184. Nicolaisen T, Joregnesen K. Trunk strength, back muscle endurance and low back trouble. Scand J Rehabil Med 1985;17:121–127.

185. Nitschke JE, Nattrass CL, Disler PB, et al. Reliability of the American Medical Association Guide's model for measuring spinal range of motion. Spine 1999;24(3):262–268.

186. Novy DM, Simmonds MJ, Olson SL, Lee E, Jones SC. Physical performance: Differences in men and women with and without low back pain. Arch Phys Med Rehabil 1999;80:195–198.

187. Novy DM, Simmonds MJ, Lee E. Physical performance tasks: What are the underlying constructs? Arch Phys Med Rehabil 2002;83:44–47.

188. Noyes F: Functional properties of knee ligaments and alterations induced by immobilization. Clin Orthop 1977;123:210–242.

189. O'Reilly SC, Muir KR, Doherty M. Effectiveness of home exercise on pain and disability from osteoarthritis of the knee: a randomized controlled trial. Ann Rheum Dis 1999;58:15–19.

190. O'Sullivan P, Twomey L, Allison G. Evaluation of specific stabilizing exercise in the treatment of chronic low back pain with radiologic diagnosis of spondylolysis or spondylolisthesis. Spine 1997;24:2959–2967.

191. O'Sullivan P, Twomey L, Allison G, et al. Altered patterns of abdominal muscle activation in patients with chronic low back pain. Aust J Physio 1997;43:91–98.

192. O'Sullivan PB, Beales DJ, Beetham JA, et al. Altered motor control strategies in subjects with sacroiliac joint pain during the active straight-leg-raise test. Spine 2002;27:E1–E8.

193. Paarnianpour M, Nordin M, Kahanovitz N, Frank V. The triaxial coupling of torque generation of trunk muscles during isometric exertions and the effect of fatiguing isoinertial movements on the motor output and movement patterns. Spine 1998;13:982–992.

194. Parks KA, Crichton KS, Goldford RF, McGill SM. A comparison of lumbar range of motion and functional ability scores in patients with low back pain. Spine 2003;28:380–384.

195. Pate R, Pratt M, Blair SN, et al. Physical activity and public health. A recommendation from the Centers for Disease Control and Prevention and the American College of Sports Medicine. JAMA 1995;273:402–407.

196. Pengel LHM, Refshauge KM, Maher CG. Responsiveness of pain, disability, and physical impairment outcomes in patients with low back pain. Spine 2004;29:879–883.

197. Pfingstein M, Kroner-Herwig B, Harter W, et al. Fear-avoidance behavior and anticipation of pain in patients with chronic low back pain—a randomized controlled study. Pain Med 2001;2:259–266.

198. Peach JP, McGill SM. Classification of low back pain with the use of spectral electromyogram parameters. Spine 1998;23:1117–1123.

199. Petersen T, Kryger P, Ekdahl C, Olsen S, Jacobsen S. The effect of McKenzie Therapy as Compared with that of intensive strengthening training for the treatment of patients with subacute or chronic low back pain: A randomized clinical trial. Spine 2002;27:1702–1709.

200. Physical Activity and Health: A Report of the Surgeon General. Atlanta, GA: U.S. Department of Health and Human Services, Centers for Disease Control and Prevention, National Center for Chronic Disease Prevention and Health Promotion, 1996.

201. Physical activity and cardiovascular health. NIH Consensus Development Panel on Physical Activity and Cardiovascular Health. JAMA 1996;276:241–246.

202. Pincus T, Burton AK, Vogel S, Field AP. A systematic review of psychological factors as predictors of chronicity/disability in prospective cohorts of low back pain. Spine 2000;27:E109–E120.

203. Postacchini F. Management of herniation of the lumbar disc. J Bone Joint Surg [Br] 1999;81:567–576.

204. Radebold A, Cholewicki J, Panjabi MM, Patel TC. Muscle response pattern to sudden trunk loading in healthy individuals and in patients with chronic low back pain. Spine 2000;25:947–954.

205. Radebold A, Cholewicki J, Polzhofer BA, Greene HS. Impaired postural control of the lumbar spine is associated with delayed muscle response times in patients with chronic idiopathic low back pain. Spine 2001;26:724–730.

206. Razmjou H, Kramer JF, Yamada R. Intertester reliability of the McKenzie evaluation in assessing patients with mechanical low back pain. J Orthop Sports Phys Ther 2000;30:368–383.

207. Reis S, Hermoni D, Borkan J, et al. The RAMBAM–Israeli Sentinel Practice Network The LBP PATIENT PERCEPTION SCALE. A new predictor of chronicity and other episode outcomes among primary care patients. (In Preparation).

208. Revel M, Minguet M, Gergoy P, Vaillant J, Manuel JL. Changes in cervicocephalic kinesthesia after a proprioceptive rehabilitation program in neck pain: A randomized controlled study. Arch Phys Med Rehabil 1994;75:895–899.

209. Richardson CA, Snijders CJ, Hides JA, Damen L, Pas MS, Storm J. The relation between the transversus abdominis muscles, sacroiliac joint mechanics, and low back pain. Spine 2002;27:399–405.

210. Riddle DL, Rothstein JM. Intertester reliability of McKenzie's classifications of the syndrome types present in patients with low back pain. Spine 1993;18:1333–1344.

211. Rissanaen A, Alaranta H, Sainio P, et al. Isokinetic and non-dynamometric tests in low back pain patients related to pain and disability index. Spine 1994;19(17):1963–1967.

212. Roland M, Waddell G, Moffett JK, Burton K, Main C, Cantrell T. The Back Book. London: The Stationary Office, 1996.

213. Rosenfeld M, Gunnarsson R, Borenstein P. Early intervention in whiplash-associated disorders: A comparison of two treatment protocols. Spine 2000;25(14):1782–1787.

214. Roy SH, De Luca CJ, Casavant DA. Lumbar muscle fatigue and chronic lower back pain. Spine 1989;14:992–1001.

215. Roy SH, DeLuca CJ, Emley M, et al. Spectral electromyographic assessment of back muscles in patients with low back pain undergoing rehabilitation. Spine 1995;20:38–48.

216. Roy SH, DeLuca CJ, Snyder-Mackler L, et al. Fatigue, recovery and low back pain in varsity rowers. Med Sci Sports Exer 1990;22:463–469.

217. Royal College of General Practitioners (RCGP). Clinical Guidelines for the Management of Acute Low Back Pain. London, Royal College of General Practitioners (www.rcgp.org.uk), 1999.

218. Salter R, Simmonds DR, Malcolm BW, et al. The biological effect of continuous passive motion on the healing of full-thickness defects in articular cartilage. 1980;62A:1232–1251.

219. Shaw WS, Feuerstein M, Haufler AJ, Berkowitz SM, Lopez MS. Working with low back pain: problem-solving orientation and function. Pain 2001;93:129–137.

220. Shirado O, Ito T, Kaneda K, et al. Flexion-relaxation phenomenon in the back muscles: A comparative study between healthy subjects and patients with chronic low back pain. Am J Phys Med Rehabil 1995;74:139–144.

221. Silverman JL, Rodriguez AA, Agre JC. Quantitative cervical flexor strength in healthy subjects and in subjects with mechanical neck pain. Arch Phys Med Rehabil 1991;72:679–681.

222. Simmonds MJ, Olson SL, Jones S, et al. Psychometric characteristics and clinical usefulness of physical performance tests in patients with low back pain. Spine 1998;23(22):2412–2421.

223. Sjolie AN. Active or passive journeys and low back pain in adolescents. Eur Spine J 2003;12:581–588.

224. Skouen JS, Grasdal AL, Haldorsen EMH, Ursin H. Relative cost-effectiveness of extensive and light multidisciplinary treatment programs versus treatment as usual for patients with chronic low back pain on long-term sick leave: randomized controlled study. Spine 2002;27(9):901–909.

225. Snook SH, Webster BS, McGorry RW, Fogleman MT, McCann KB. The reduction of chronic non-specific low back pain through the control of early morning lumbar flexion, Spine 1998;23:2601–2607.

226. Snook SH, Webster BS, McGorry RW. The reduction of chronic, nonspecific low back pain through the control of early morning lumbar flexion: 3-year follow-up. J Occupa Rehabil 2002;12:13–20.

227. Spitzer WO, Skovron ML, Salmi LIR, et al. Scientific monograph of the Quebec Task Force on Whiplash-Associated Disorders: Redefining "Whiplash" and its management. Spine 1995;20(Supp):S1–S73.

228. Stankovic R, Johnell O. Conservative treatment of acute low-back pain. A prospective randomized trial. McKenzie method of treatment versus patient education in "mini back school." Spine 1990;15:120–123.

229. Stenstrom CH, Sandberg A. Home exercise and compliance in inflammatory rheumatic diseases—a prospective clinical trial. J Rheumatol 1997;24(2):470–476.

230. Sterling M, Jull G, Vicenzino B, Kenardy J, Darnell R. Development of motor system dysfunction following whiplash injury. Pain 2003;103:65–73.

231. Stevenson JM, Weber CL, Smith JT, Dumas GA, Albert WJ. A longitudinal study of the development of low back pain in an industrial population. Spine 2001;26:1370–1377.

232. Swinkels-Meewisse IEJ, Roelofs J, Verbeek ALM, Oostendorp RAB, Vlaeyen JWS. Fear of movement/(re)injury, disability and participation in acute low back pain. Pain 2003;105:371–379.

233. Symonds TL, Burton AK, Tillotson KM, et al. Absence resulting from low back trouble can be reduced by psychosocial intervention at the work place. Spine 1995;20:2738–2745.

234. Taimela S, Diederich C, Hubsch M, Heinricy M. The role of physical exercise and inactivity in pain recurrence and absenteeism from work after active outpatient rehabilitation for recurrent or chronic low back pain. A follow up study. Spine 2000;25:1809–1816.

235. Taimela S, Kankaanpää M, Luoto S. The effect of lumbar fatigue on the ability to sense a change in lumbar position. A controlled study. Spine 1999;24 (13):1322–1327.

236. Taimela S, Österman K, Alaranta H, et al. Long psychomotor reaction time in patients with chronic low-back pain—preliminary report. Arch Phys Med Rehab 1993;74:1161–1164.

237. Takala EP, Viikari-Juntura E, Tynkkynen EM. Does group gymnastics at the workplace help in neck pain? A controlled study. Scand J Rehabil Med 1994;26:17–20.

238. Takala EP, Vikari-Juntura E. Do functional tests predict low back pain. Spine 2000;25(16):2126–2132.

239. Teresi LM, Lufkin RB, Reicher MA, et al. Asymptomatic degenerative disk disease and spondylosis of the cervical spine: MR Imaging. Radiology 1987;164:83–88.

240. Thomas E, Silman AJ, Croft PR, Papageorgiou AC, Jayson MIV, Macfarlane GJ. Predicting who develops chronic low back pain in primary care: A prospective study. BMJ 1999;318:1662–1667.

241. Thompson DA, Biedermann H-J, Stevenson JM, et al. Changes in paraspinal electromyographic spectral analysis with exercise: two studies. J EMG Kinesiol 1992;2(3):179–186.

242. Timm KE. A randomized-control study of active and passive treatments for chronic low back pain following L5 laminectomy. JOSPT 1994;20:276–286.

243. Treleavan J, Jull G, Atkinson L. Cervical musculoskeletal dysfunction in post-concussion headache. Cephalalgia 1994;14:273–279.

244. Treleaven J, Jull G, Sterling M. Dizziness and unsteadiness following whiplash injury: Characteristic features and relationship with cervical joint position error. J Rehabil Med 2003;35:36–43.

245. Triano JJ, Schultz AB. Correlation of objective measure of trunk motion and muscle function with low-back disability ratings. Spine 1987;12:561–565.

246. Turner JA, Franklin G, Haegerty PJ, et al. The association between pain and disability. Pain 2004; 112:307–314.

247. UK BEAM Trial Team. United Kingdom back pain exercise and manipulation (UK BEAM) randomized trial: Effectiveness of physical treatments for back pain in primary care. BMJ 2004;doi:10.1136/bmj. 38282.669225.AE.

248. UK BEAM Trial Team. United Kingdom back pain exercise and manipulation (UK BEAM) randomized trial: Cost effectiveness of physical treatments for back pain in primary care. BMJ 2004;doi:10.1136/bmj.38282.607859.AE.

249. van den Hout JHC, Vlaeyen JWS, Houben RMA, Soeters APM, Peters ML. The effects of failure feedback and pain-related fear on pain report, pain tolerance, and pain avoidance in chronic low back pain patients. Pain 2001;92:247–257.

250. Van den Hout JHC. Vlaeyen JWS. Problem-solving therapy and behavioral graded activity in the prevention of chronic pain disability. In: Linton SL, ed. New avenues for the prevention of chronic musculoskeletal pain and disability. Amsterdam: Elsevier, 2002.

251. Van Dillen LR, Sahrmann SA, Norton BJ, et al. The effect of active limb movements on symptoms in patients with low back pain. J Orthop and Sports Phys Ther 2001;31:402–413.

252. Van Dillen LR, McDonnell MK, Fleming DA, Sahrmann SA. The effect of hip and knee position on hip extension range of motion measures in individuals with and without low back pain. J Orthop and Sports Phys Ther 2000;30:307–316.

253. Van Dillen LR, Sahrmann SA, Norton BJ, et al. Reliability of physical examination items used for classification of patients with low back pain. Phys Ther 1998;78:979–988.

254. Van Dillen LR, Sahrmann SA, Norton BJ, Caldwell CA, McDonnell MK, Bloom NJ. Movement system impairment-based categories for low back pain: Stage 1 validation. J Orthop Sports Phys Ther 2003;33:126–142.

255. van Tulder MW, Assendelft JJ, Koes BW, Bouter LM. Spinal radiographic findings and nonspecific low back pain: A systematic review of observational studies. Spine 1997;22:427–434.

256. Van Tulder MW, Koes BW, Bouter LM. Conservative treatment of acute and chronic nonspecific low back pain: A systematic review of randomized controlled trials of the most common interventions. Spine 1997;22(18):2128–2156.

257. Van Tulder MW. Malmivaara A, Esmail R, Koes B. Exercise therapy for low back pain. A systematic review within the framework of the Cochrane Collaboration Back Review Group. Spine 2000;25(21):2784–2796.

258. Vlaeyen JWS, Crombez G. Fear of movement/(re)injury, avoidance and pain disability in chronic low back pain patients. Manual Therapy 1999;4:187–195.

259. Vlaeyen JWS, Linton S. Fear-avoidance and its consequences in chronic musculoskeletal pain. A state of the art. Pain 2000;85:317–332.

260. Vlaeyen JWS, De Jong J, Geilen M, Heuts PHTG, Van Breukelen G. Graded exposure in the treatment of pain-related fear: a replicated single case experimental design in four patients with chronic low back pain. Behav Res Ther 2001;39:151–166.

261. Vlaeyen JWS, Morley S. Active despite pain: the putative role of stop-rules and current mood. Pain 2004;110:512–516.

262. Von Korff M, Moore JE, Lorig K, et al. A randomized trial of a lay-led self-management group intervention for back pain patients in primary care. Spine 1998;23:2608–2615.

263. Von Korff J, Ormel FJ, Keefe SF, Dworkin. Grading the severity of chronic pain. Pain 1992;50:133–149.

264. Vroomen PCAJ, de Krom MCTFM, Wilmink JT, Kester ADM, Knottnerus JA. Lack of effectiveness of bed rest for sciatica. N Engl J Med 1999;340:418–423.

265. Waddell G, Somerville D, Henderson I, et al. Objective clinical evaluation of physical impairment in chronic low back pain. Spine 1992;17:617–628.

266. Waddell G. The Back Pain Revolution. Edinburgh: Churchill Livingstone, 1998.

267. Watson P, Booker CK, Main CJ, et al. Surface electromyography in the identification of chronic low back pain patients: The development of the flexion relaxation ratio. Clin Biomech 1997;12:165–171.

268. Watson DH, Trott PH. Cervical headache: An investigation of natural head posture and cervical flexor muscle performance. Cephalgia 1993:13;272–284.

269. Wennberg DE, Kellet MA, Dickens JD, Malenka DJ, Keilson LM, Keller RB. The association between local diagnostic testing intensity and invasive cardiac procedures. JAMA 1996;275:1161–1164.

270. Werneke M, Hart DL. Discriminant validity and relative precision for classifying patients with nonspecific neck and back pain by anatomic pain patterns. Spine 2003;28:161–166.

271. Wiesel SE, Tsourmans N, Feffer HL, et al. A study of computer-assisted tomography. I. The incidence of positive CAT scans in an asymptomatic group of patients. Spine 1984;9:549.

272. Wilder DG, Aleksiev AR, Magnusson ML, Pope MH, Spratt KF, Goel VK. Muscular response to sudden load. A tool to evaluate fatigue and rehabilitation. Spine 1996;21:2628–2639.

273. Wilson L, Hall H, McIntosh G, Melles T. Intertester reliability of a low back pain classification system. Spine 1999;24:248–254.

274. Wood KA, Standell CJ, Adams MA, et al. Exercise training to improve spinal mobility and back muscle fatigability: A possible prophylaxis for low back pain? Physical Medicine Research Foundation Symposium: Clinical Approaches to Spinal Disorders. Prague, 1997.

275. World Health Organization. International Classification of Human Functioning, Disability and Health: ICF. Geneva: WHO, 2001.

276. Yordi GA, Lent RW. Predicting aerobic exercise participation: social, cognitive, reasoned action, and planned behavioral models. J Sports Exer Psychol 1993;15:363–374.

277. Yoshihara K, Shirai Y, Nakayama Y, Uesaka S. Histochemical changes in the multifidus muscle in patients with lumbar intervertebral disc herniation Spine 2001;26:622–626.

278. Zhao WP, Kawaguchi Y, Matsui H, Kanamori M, Kimura T. Histochemistry and morphology of the multifidus muscle in lumbar disc herniation. Comparative study between diseased and normal sides. Spine 2000;25:2191–2199.

279. Zuberbier OA, Hunt DG, Kozlowski AJ, et al. Commentary on the American Medical Association Guides' lumbar impairment validity checks. Spine 2001;26:2735–2737.

2

The Role of Muscles, Joints, and the Nervous System in Painful Conditions of the Spine

Craig Liebenson

Introduction

The Biomechanics of the Spine Stability System

Spine Instability and Injury

The Role of Agonist-Antagonist Muscle Co-activation in Maintaining Spine Stability

Injury Prevention

Neurophysiological Aspects of Stability and Pain

Agonist-Antagonist Muscle Imbalance

The Neurodevelopmental Basis for Muscle Imbalance

Neuropathic Pain and Central Sensitization

Learning Objectives

After reading this chapter you should be able to understand:

- The clinical relevance of the concepts of spine stability and instability
- What the "neutral zone" concept means scientifically and clinically
- How agonist and antagonist muscle co-activation stabilizes the spine
- How central sensitization can explain how an individual can perceive pain in the absence of tissue damage or injury
- How pain leads to predictable adaptations in the muscular system involving muscle imbalance

"Yet all experience is an arch where through gleams that untraveled world whose margin fades, Forever and forever when I move."

Lord Alfred Tennyson

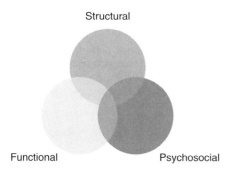

Structural

Functional   Psychosocial

Figure 2.1 The major sources of a patient's failure to recover.

Introduction

Musculoskeletal disorders are related to structural, psychosocial, biomechanical, and neurophysiological factors. Most patients recover with a minimalist approach that de-emphasizes the importance of structural pathology and prevents psychosocial illness behavior from emerging. This occurs mostly as a result of the fairly straightforward act of unambiguously reassuring patients and re-activating them. Unfortunately, structural pathology has been the focus of the biomedical model for generations. Clinicians and patients alike are mesmerized by modern imaging technology's ability to visualize the anatomic substrate of the patient's pain. However, just as a picture of a phone does not tell you if it is ringing, the ability of imaging modalities to inform us about the spine's function is limited. In fact, it is an individual's functional abilities or tolerances that are at the heart of the "patient-centered" approach.

The modern goal of care is to restore function. The means to that end involves overcoming any barriers to patient re-activation that may be present. This includes avoiding the type of overly aggressive management, from both a diagnostic and therapeutic standpoint, that erects new barriers! Recently, psychosocial factors have been recognized as significant impediments on the road to recovery. This has revolutionized spine care as the emerging biopsychosocial model (5,29,128).

Although structural factors explain far less of spine pain than had been hoped for, this does not mean that most pain is by default psychogenic. As chapter 1 demonstrated, inadequate function of the locomotor system, in particular poor motor control, is intimately associated with pain of spinal origin. Simple reactivation or self-care advice should be grounded in an understanding of what constitutes "safe back" activities and exercises. Additionally, patients not recovering from an acute episode within a few weeks should be evaluated not only for structural and psychosocial problems but also for functional pathology of the motor system (Fig. 2.1).

Functional pathology is not just altered biomechanics, it also involves motor control errors that are part of the central nervous system's response to pain and dysfunction.

The Biomechanics of the Spine Stability System

Management of patients with spinal disorders is built on an understanding of how the spine is injured, how it responds to pain or injury, and how it can be stabilized (see Chapter 5). When the emphasis is only on what the spine looks like anatomically, rather than how it functions then patient and doctor alike tend to become frustrated leading to psychosocial illness behavior.

Spine Instability and Injury

Practice-Based Problem
How can we explain to the patient what caused the pain if there is not a history of antecedent trauma or relevant imaging findings?

Spinal and whole-body stability are two distinct, but related, phenomena. Whole-body stability is the body's ability to maintain equilibrium, especially after being subjected to external forces that temporarily destabilize it (114). Equilibrium is the ability to maintain the body's center of mass over a stable base of support. The spine is likened to an inverted pendulum, and thus a highly unstable system (Fig. 2.2). In

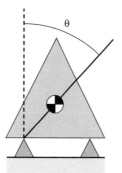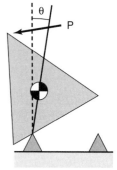

Figure 2.2 From a stability perspective, the body and each vertebrae is an inverted pendulum. Stability is increased by widening the base of support. A larger value of θ, which is modulated by the base width, increases the ability to survive a perturbation (P) and therefore is more stable. From McGill SM. Biomechanical basis for stability: An explanation to enhance clinical utility. J Orth Sports Physical Therapy 2001;31:97.

fact, it has been suggested that each vertebrae is an inverted pendulum (10,17,77,114)! According to Winter (131), "Because two-thirds of our body mass is two-thirds of body height above the ground we are an inherently unstable system, unless a control system is operating." Both muscle forces and ligamentous tension operating within a control system are necessary to maintain equilibrium.

Spine stability is defined more narrowly as the ability of the spinal column or its components to resist buckling when undergoing load. Various forces such as stretch, compression, shear, or torsion can be involved. According to Panjabi, three subsystems work together to maintain spine stability (94). They are the central nervous subsystem (control), an osteoligamentous subsystem (passive), and a muscle subsystem (active) (Fig. 2.3). He says "The neural subsystem receives information from the transducers, determines specific requirements for spinal stability, and causes the active subsystem to achieve the stability goal."

Panjabi has shown that minor trauma can stretch tissues beyond their elastic limit without causing rupture or tearing (95,96). Because there is no tissue failure, this "injury" is undetected by imaging procedures looking for hypermobility caused by ligamentous insufficiency (95,96). However, as a result of stretching of the passive–elastic components, an expansion of the joint's "neutral zone" occurs (Fig. 2.4) (94–96). The "neutral zone" is defined as the inner region of a joint's range of motion (ROM) where minimal resistance to motion is encountered (94). This inner region's mobility is restricted by passive ligamentous factors alone, and not by active muscular forces.

When the "neutral zone" is expanded, joint instability is said to exist. This is because with an expanded zone of non-resisted motion greater demands are placed on muscles that must stabilize a joint. Thus, the most observable and measurable sign of instability is not joint hypermobility, but rather excessive agonist–antagonist muscular co-activation (18).

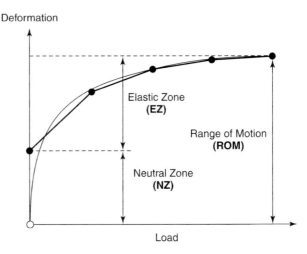

Figure 2.4 The neutral zone (NZ). This is a region of high flexibility. The elastic zone (EZ) is a region of high stiffness. The two zones together constitute the physiological range of motion (ROM) of a joint. The NZ is where spinal motion encounters minimal resistance. A joint with increased laxity will have an increased NZ. From Panjabi MM. The stabilizing system of the spine. Part 2. Neutral zone and instability hypothesis. J Spinal Disorders 1992;5:391.

Clinical Pearl

Minimal ligamentous tension is produced when movement occurs in a "neutral range." Gradually increasing tension occurs when movement enters an "elastic range." Ligamentous tension is greatest and so is injury when movement occurs at the anatomical limit of motion. Good motor control and appropriate activities maintain movements in the neutral or early elastic range. Poor motor control or inappropriate activities allow movement to repetitively reach the terminal elastic range.

McGill has defined the "neutral posture" as "one where the joints and surrounding passive tissues are in elastic equilibrium and thus at an angle of minimal joint load."

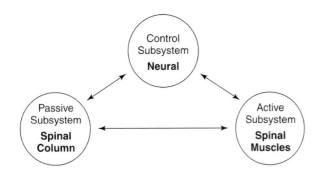

Figure 2.3 The spine stability system. From Panjabi MM. The stabilizing system of the spine. Part 1. Function, dysfunction, adaptation, and enhancement. J Spinal Disorders 1992;5:384.

Injury occurs when load exceeds tissue tolerance. The spinal column devoid of its musculature has been found to buckle at a load of only 90 Newtons (approximately 20 pounds) at L5 (26,27). However, during routine activities, loads 20-times this are encountered on a routine basis. Panjabi (94) says, "This large load-carrying capacity is achieved by the participation of well-coordinated muscles surrounding the spinal column." Surprisingly, the motor control system functions well when undergoing load. Muscles stabilize joints by stiffening, like rigging on a ship. But when load is at a minimum, such as when the body is relaxed or a task is trivial, the motor control system is often "caught off guard" and injuries are precipitated.

The Role of Agonist–Antagonist Muscle Co-activation in Maintaining Spine Stability

How does the body resist injury? According to Cholewicki and McGill, spine stability is greatly enhanced by co-contraction of antagonistic trunk muscles (17). Early work on the elbow (110) and knee (9) showed that antagonist muscle co-activation is necessary for aiding ligaments in maintaining joint stability during loaded tasks. Even though energetically costly, such co-contractions have been shown to occur during most daily activities (74). Co-contractions do increase spinal compressive load, as much as 12% to 18% or 440 N, but they increase spinal stability even more by 36% to 64% or 2925 N (44). Therefore, if injury risk is viewed as the ratio of tissue tolerance to external load, then a substantial increase in stability occurs as a result of co-activation. This mechanism is present to such an extent that without co-contraction the spinal column is unstable in upright postures (39)!

In particular, these co-contractions are most obvious during reactions to unexpected or sudden loading (66,75). Cholewicki showed an increased electromyographic (EMG) activation of the rectus abdominus in upright postures versus flexed postures as a mechanism to maintain stability in neutral postures (18). Stokes has described how there are basically two mechanisms by which this co-activation occurs (114). One is a pre-contraction to stiffen and thus dampen the spinal column when faced with unexpected perturbations. The second is a sufficiently fast speed of contraction of the muscles to react quick enough to prevent excessive motion that would lead to buckling after either expected or unexpected perturbations (16,24,66,75,114,122,129). Wilder et al (129) concluded in a study of body's reaction to sudden, unexpected loads that "the muscles will respond rapidly to stabilize the body, i.e., they will try to maintain balance and posture." This has also been verified by Radebold and Cholewicki in a series of studies (19,20,100,101).

Cholewicki et al demonstrated that antagonistic trunk muscle co-activation is necessary to provide mechanical stability to the lumbar spine around a neutral posture (18). The authors found that antagonistic muscle co-activation increased in response to increased axial load on the spine. EMG measurements were gathered from three flexors—external oblique, internal oblique, and rectus abdominus; and three extensors—multifidus, lumbar erector spinae, and thoracic erector spinae. The subjects were asked to perform slow trunk flexion and extension movements in a semi-seated position with hip motion restricted, but trunk motion free. Weights were then added to the torso. One conclusion was that "increased levels of

muscle co-activation may constitute an objective indicator of the dysfunction in the passive stabilizing system of the lumbar spine."

Trunk Muscle Recruitment Patterns in LBP Patients Differ From Those in Asymptomatic Subjects

- Increased antagonist muscle activation is a sign of muscle co-contraction consistent with elevated spine stability requirements

- A variety of dynamic and static trunk tasks were performed

- The ratio of lumbar erector spinae (intersegmental—antagonist) to thoracic erector spinae (multisegmental) muscle activation was greater in LBP individuals than in healthy subjects

- Stability index modeling showed that the observed patient recruitment patterns enhanced spinal stability

- The authors cautioned that increased antagonist muscle co-activation patterns in patients may not be the cause of LBP, but could be a compensatory adaptation.

van Dieen JH, Cholewicki J, Radebold A. Trunk muscle recruitment patterns in patients with low back pain enhance the stability of the lumbar spine. Spine 2003;28:834–841.

Various studies have pointed out how important the motor control system is for preventing spinal injury. Inappropriate muscle activation sequences during seemingly trivial tasks (only 60 Newtons of force), such as bending over to pick up a pencil, can compromise spine stability and potentiate buckling of the passive ligamentous restraints (2). This motor control skill has also been shown to be compromised under challenging aerobic circumstances (78). When a spinal stabilization and respiratory challenge is simultaneously encountered, the nervous system will naturally select maintenance of respiration over spine stability. An example of this occurs when during repetitive bending or lifting activities the back becomes vulnerable because of poor aerobic fitness even if the motor control system is well-trained. Studies have shown during a mildly aerobic challenge such as repetitive limb movements that tonic activity of the diaphragm and transverse abdominus muscles can be maintained (53,54).

Good abdominal strength without proper coordination between the abdominals and diaphragm can lead to spine instability during challenging aerobic activities (92,55). Normally during exhalation, the abdominals increase their activity while the diaphragm decreases its activity. It has been demonstrated that this reciprocal relationship can become dysfunctional if respiratory disease is present or aerobic demand is too great (55).

Injury Prevention

To avoid injury, conditioning or adaptation must keep pace as exposure to external load increases (Fig. 2.5). Exposure to load must also be temporarily removed so that the normal healing/adaptation process can fullfill its objective of increasing the failure tolerance of the tissues. Too little or infrequent exposure to external load and conditioning never raises the tissue failure tolerance. Too much, frequent, or prolonged exposure and adaptation can't keep pace. McGill has shown this relationship between tissue loading and risk of injury as "u"-shaped (1,82) (Fig. 2.6).

Most low back injuries are not the result of a single exposure to a high-magnitude load, but instead a cumulative trauma from subfailure magnitude loads (Fig. 2.7). For instance, repeated small loads (e.g., bending) or a sustained load (e.g., sitting). According to McGill, low back injury is usually a result of "a history of excessive loading which gradually, but progressively, reduces the tissue failure tolerance" (79).

The lumbar spine has been shown to be particularly vulnerable to repetitive motion at end range. Disc

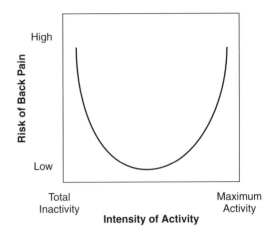

Figure 2.6 Relationship between activity history and injury. From Abenheim L, Rossignol M, Valat JP, et al. The role of activity in the therapeutic management of back pain: Report of the International Paris Task Force on Back Pain. Spine 2000;25:1S–33S.

herniation is related to repeated flexion motion (15), especially if coupled with lateral bending and twisting (4,42). Injuries to the posterior elements including the facet joints and pars have been shown to be related to cyclic full flexion and extension (14,50), as well as excessive shear forces (25,132).

Practice-Based Problem

Should exercise be performed in a "neutral" or end-range? According to McGill "evidence from tissue-specific injury generally supports the notion of a neutral spine (neutral lordosis) when performing loading tasks to minimize the risk of low back injury.... Avoiding spine end range of motion, during activity, can reduce the risk of several types of injury" (79).

A current controversy involves whether to prescribe exercises in a "neutral" or full ROM. Some approaches such as the McKenzie model advocate biased end-range movements, whereas other "stabilization" systems suggest training patients to control the "inner range." In reality, these approaches are not as much at odds as it appears. The evidence points to an integrated approach based on evaluation of the patient's sensitivity to different types of motion (McKenzie approach) as well as an understanding of the load profile of different movements and activities (stabilization approach).

For those in acute pain or "at risk," limiting ROM is preferred. For instance, a bias involving avoiding end-range flexion motions in younger disc patients and avoiding end-range extension motions in elder stenosis patients would be consistent with both McKenzie and
(continued)

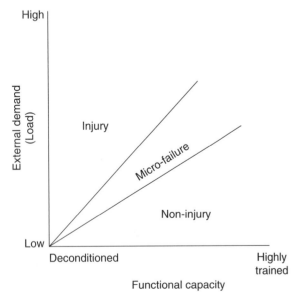

Figure 2.5 Relationship between external demand and functional capacity.

stabilization approaches. As recovery progresses and return to normal activities occurs, training must expand to a full ROM. However, as this occurs, peripheral mobility gains should be achieved in concert with "core" or proximal stability so that repetitive strain to key spinal joints can be avoided. Such "grooved motor programs" that promote "load sharing" during functional tasks (bending, kneeling, squatting, reaching, pushing, pulling, lifting, carrying, etc) are the ultimate goal of training designed to speed recovery, prevent re-injury, and enhance performance.

Increased end-range flexion loading of the spine has been shown to occur as a result of a fatiguing repetitive task such as lifting (112). Increases in spinal flexion and decreases in knee and hip motion were shown to occur as a stoop-lifting strategy replaced squat lifting. Sixteen subjects performed with a submaximal load at maximum lifting rate to study the effects of fatigue. Fatigue was associated with a decrease in knee and hip motion and an increa (see Chapter 14) se in peak lumbar flexion, indicating a change from a squat lift to a stoop lift strategy. Decreased postural stability documented by a greater anterior to posterior excursion of the trunk center of mass was also noted.

Etnyre et al showed that LBP patients alter their sit-to-stand motions by reducing their hip motion during this movement stereotype (34). In a trunk movement involving isoinertial resisted trunk movements in the sagittal plane (flexion/extension), Paarnianpour showed that loss of control of the center of rotation occurred in LBP patients, but not in normal subjects (93). This loss of control was observed as an increased rotation and side bending motions during resisted flexion/extension in the pain group versus non-pain group.

Patient Advice

Knowledge of when injury is most likely to occur can also influence the type of advice clinicians give (see Chapter 16). The early morning or after prolonged sitting are particularly vulnerable times. Reilly et al (102) showed that 54% of the loss of disc height (water content) occurs in the first 30 minutes after arising. Disc bending stresses are increased by 300% and ligaments by 80% in the morning (2,3). It has been shown that after just 20 minutes of full flexion of the spine, ligamentous creep or laxity occurs, which persists even after 30 minutes of rest (110)! In

a porcine model, just 2 minutes of full flexion has been shown to lead to a substantial loss of the normal spinal ligamentous stiffness (46).

According to Bogduk and Twomney, "After prolonged strain ligaments, capsules, and IV discs of the lumbar spine may creep, and they may be liable to injury if sudden forces are unexpectedly applied during the vulnerable recovery phase" (12). Therefore, avoidance of high-risk activities early in the morning or after sitting or stooping in full flexion is crucial to injury or re-injury prevention. Not surprisingly, Snook demonstrated that avoidance of early morning flexion facilitated recovery from acute LBP (108,109).

Suggestions to teach workers to lift with their knees and not their backs are overly simplistic. Most workers have learned various techniques to avoid injury that are inconsistent with this advice. Better advice is consistent with the following principles: avoid early morning lifting; avoid lifting after prolonged sitting or flexion activities; rotate jobs to vary loads; allow frequent rest breaks; maintain lumbar lordosis; and keep loads close to the spine (81).

Neurophysiological Aspects of Stability and Pain

Agonist–Antagonist Muscle Imbalance

The relationship between specific functions (i.e., impairments), pain, and activity intolerances is unknown. If clues can be obtained about how the body typically responds to pathology, injury, or repetitive strain, this would aid clinicians in determining if a patient's impairments are a cause of pain or its consequence. The evidence presented in "The Role of Agonist–Antagonist Muscle Co-activation in Maintaining Spine Stability" shows that the signature

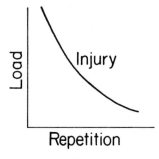

Figure 2.7 A fatigue curve illustrates the importance of repetition and load to fatigue failure. Reproduced with permission from Andersson GBJ. Occupational Biomechanics. In: Weinstein JN, Wiesel SW, eds. The Lumbar Spine. Philadelphia: WB Saunders, 1990.

response of the motor control system to biomechanically challenging situations is agonist–antagonist muscle co-activation. Therefore, a clinical "shortcut" in determining whether an impairment is clinically significant would be determining if it contributes to agonist–antagonist muscle imbalance.

Profiles of how individual muscles react to injury or inflammation are beginning to emerge. Certain muscles have a predictable tendency to become inhibited, whereas others become tense. Specific muscles in the knee (vastus medialis oblique) (30, 113,115), lumbar spine (multifidus) (52,133,134), or cervical spine (deep neck flexors, suboccipitals) (49,61,62,83) respond to inflammation or injury by becoming inhibited and atrophying. Other muscles such as the upper trapezius (7,8,47,71,90), sternocleidomastoid (SCM) (61,62), infraspinatus (65), or lumbar erector spinae (loss of flexion–relaxation phenomena) (37,73,107,124) respond to injury or overload by tensing or becoming overactive.

Lund proposed the pain adaptation theory to explain these muscle imbalances (68). He hypothesized that when pain is present, there is a decreased activation of muscles during movements in which they act as agonists and increased activation during movements in which they are antagonists (68,91). This model is in stark contrast to the pain–spasm–pain model, which suggests that muscle tension is necessarily increased when painful stimuli are present. Rather, it appears that muscle imbalance is the rule, with certain muscles tending toward hyperactivity and others toward inhibition. Arendt-Nielson found that overactivity of antagonist back muscles during the ipsilateral swing phase of gait and decreased agonist peak muscle activity during the double-stance phase distinguished those with chronic LBP from controls (6). Graven-Nielson showed that if the lower leg muscles are subjected to saline injection, gait coordination is altered by a decrease in EMG activity in agonist muscles and increase in EMG activity of antagonists (45). Similar dysfunctions in coordinated movement have been shown when experimental muscle pain was produced by saline injection in the masseter muscles (87,119–121).

Vogt et al found that reduced hip extension range of motion and early and prolonged activation of the gluteus maximus and lumbar erector spinae muscles can distinguish between back pain subjects and asymptomatic individuals (126). Because of the difficulty with clinical assessment of gait, the authors proposed that Janda's prone test of hip (hyper)extension should be evaluated to determine if it can be used as a valid assessment of pathological muscle coordination in the lumbo-pelvic region.

Perhaps as a result of agonist–antagonist muscle imbalance, another common finding is synergist substitution. Edgerton reported that strength is not always decreased in pain patients because synergists substitute for inhibited agonists (33). He found that synergist substitution, not muscle weakness, distinguished chronic neck pain patients from asymptomatics after whiplash injury (33). Sparto demonstrated that spinal loading forces were increased during a fatiguing isometric trunk extension effort without a loss of torque output (111). Torque output remained constant because as the erector spinae fatigued substitution by secondary extensors such as the internal oblique and latissimus dorsi muscles occurred.

> ## Muscle Response to Pain May Depend on Psychophysical Factors
>
> Nederhand et al reported in a recent study that acute patients who later had the greatest amount of neck disability tended to minimize the use of painful upper trapezius muscles (91). In fact, there was an inverse relationship between EMG activity during an isometric and a dynamic task and future (6 months later) disability (measured with the Neck Disability Index) (91)! In contrast, in a group with higher levels of disability and chronicity (10–53 months), elevated levels of muscle reactivity were recorded (90). This was concluded by the authors to be caused by a psychophysical response to prolonged exposure to chronic pain.

Synergist substitution may be a "sign" of compensatory strategies. Prospective studies are necessary to establish a causal relationship. Synergist substitution may be the bodies attempt to compensate for an inhibited muscle or agonist–antagonist pair that is not adequately stabilizing a key joint. A myofascial trigger point demonstrates the problem of assuming an area of tension or sensitivity is the "cause" of a problem. Treatment of a trigger point in the upper trapezius muscle is unlikely to give lasting pain relief if perpetuating factors responsible for maintaining the trigger point and possibly its existence in the first place, such as inputting on a keyboard that is too high or inhibited lower scapular stabilizers, are not addressed. Similarly, would repeated chiropractic adjustments or anesthetic injections to a primary pain generator without identification and correction of the underlying source of biomechanical overload (i.e., muscle imbalance, faulty ergonomics) or fear–avoidance behavior likely have a lasting effect?

Is the common clinical finding of tension in the lumbar paraspinals the cause or effect of pain? Musculoskeletal health care specialists commonly find and treat erector spinae tension. Yet soft tissue work and physical therapy modalities applied directly to this muscle may not be the "key" treatment. To determine if erector spinae tension is a cause of pain prospective, longitudinal studies are required. When prospective studies on this muscle have been performed, what has been discovered is that that poor trunk extensor endurance is correlated with future or recurrent LBP (11,57,69). The tension that is commonly palpated or observed is likely compensatory to the muscle being fatigued. Thus, a treatment that would address the primary dysfunction is endurance training to improve the muscle's fatigue resistance.

The Neurodevelopmental Basis for Muscle Imbalance

The fact that muscles respond predictably to pain and/or injury offers clinicians a valuable way to sort out which functional pathologies are clinically significant. That some muscles tend to become tight and others weak has long been observed in both neurological (i.e., cerebral palsy, stroke) and orthopedic (i.e., nerve root compression) problems. Rood was one of the first to propose classifying muscles on the basis of their functional characteristics as stabilizers or mobilizers (41). Janda (59,60) and Sahrmann (104) have championed this way of thinking that finally came under scientific scrutiny with Bergmark (10), who proposed that muscles could be broadly classified as deep, local stabilization muscles or superficial, global mobilization muscles.

Janda has suggested that there is a group of "postural" muscles (i.e., gastrocnemius, upper trapezius, SCM, erector spinae) that are involved in static tasks such as standing or sitting (60). These muscles have a tendency to become overactive. He describes another group as "phasic" because they are involved in stabilizing or producing dynamic movements such as head flexion, arm elevation, or trunk curling (i.e., deep neck flexors, inferior scapular fixators, abdominals). These muscles have a tendency to become inhibited. This notion emerged from his observation among individuals with neurologic disease that spasticity (e.g., cerebral palsy) usually favored certain muscles (i.e., extremity flexors, adductors, and internal rotators) and paralysis (e.g., stroke) favored other muscles (i.e., extremity extensors, abductors, and external rotators). Janda described how the postural

muscle system was needed for preservation of basic functions and its muscles were usually spared, whereas those required for more dynamic activities were more fragile and easily compromised. He also noted that these same tendencies were seen in individuals without neurological disease, who either remained in constrained, sitting postures for prolonged periods of time or were training their muscles inappropriately.

This theory has a neurodevelopmental basis (see Chapter 23). In the infant younger than 1 month old, the fetal position is maintained by "tonic" contraction of trunk and extremity flexors along with extremity adductors and internal rotators. Reciprocal inhibition (Sherrington's law) that is present in early infancy inhibits the antagonists of the "tonic" muscle chains. As the infant develops reciprocal inhibition becomes dampened, thus allowing the "phasic" muscle system to activate (fails in cerebral palsy). As the "reflex-bound" infant begins to develop its postural control system, "tonic" activity of muscles that maintains the fetal posture is superceded by agonist–antagonist co-activation of muscles necessary for movement control and production of the upright posture. Thus, extensors, abductors, and external rotators co-activate with their fetal partners to stabilize joints and allow neurodevelopment of posture.

For instance, orientation movements of the head and neck begin between 4 and 6 weeks as the deep cervical flexors activate to coordinate movement with the cervical extensors (127). Similarly, the inferior scapular fixators begin to activate in the following months to balance the activity of the upper trapezius and levator scapulae and allow for scapulothoracic stabilization during arm movements (grasping, prehension, pushing, pulling, etc.). A typical example of a failure of this agonist–antagonist co-activation occurs in Sprengel's deformity in which the scapula fails to descend.

Vojta, who developed a rehabilitation system for treatment of neurological diseases such as cerebral palsy, stroke, and spinal cord injury, formulated the idea that the fetal muscles were more primitive and thus better insulated, whereas the muscles needed for development of the upright posture were younger phylogenetically and thus biologically more fragile (Table 2.1) (127). Preliminary investigations suggest that imbalances between these systems of muscles may be present in 30% of young children without neurological disease (127)!

It is easy to see how the modern posture of slumping at a desk will influence muscles and joints. Brügger has described how the spinal column is part of a mechanical linkage system. He showed how the slumped sitting posture brings about changes in lumbo-pelvic, thoracic, and head and neck posture

Table 2.1 Neurodevelopmental Kinesiology

Global—"Tonic"	Local—"Phasic"
Phylogenetically older Dominant • Intrauterine & early infancy • Sedentarism • Deconditioning • Injury • Aging	Phylogenetically younger Not active intrauterine & early infancy Requires higher CNS control Fragile, easily inhibited

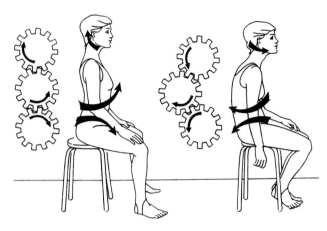

Figure 2.8 Cog wheel model of joint centration in upright posture. Reproduced with permission from: Brügger A. Lehrbuch der funktionellen Störungen des Bewegungssystems. Zollikon/Benglen: Brügger-Verlag, 2000:150.

and function. In particular, the muscles associated with the fetal position will be maintained in shortened lengths, whereas their antagonists will be lengthened (Fig. 2.8).

Bergmark divided muscles into two broad categories based on their function one functioning to produce movement and the other to control it (10). Superficial muscles are responsible for producing voluntary movement or torque production, whereas deep muscles are responsible for maintaining joint stability. The deep ("intrinsic") muscles are responsible for joint stability on an involuntary or subcortical basis, whereas movement production is largely a voluntary act.

The following charts show the different divisions of muscles according to their dysfunctional tendencies (Table 2.2).

During neurodevelopment, the infant learns to support his or herself using different points of support that facilitates a wide variety of postures and movements. The ensuing muscle co-activation centrates joints in a position of maximum congruence of joint surfaces. This allows for maximum load-bearing potential and thus facilitates further functional development of the infant. The first sign of this is in the head and neck by the end of the first month of life and progresses in the sagittal plane until the infant has

Table 2.2 Muscle System Classifications (after Bergmark, 1989)

Global—Superficial Muscles:	Local—Deep Muscles:
Typically become overactive or shortened	*Typically become inhibited or lengthened*
Gastro-soleus	Quadratus plantae
Adductors	Peronei
Hamstrings	Vastus medialis
Tensor fascia lata	Gluteals
Hip flexors	Transverse abdominus
Piriformis	Internal oblique
Quadratus lumborum (lateral)	Multifidus
Rectus abdominus	Quadratus lumborum (medial)
External obliques	Medial & lower erector spinae
Lateral & thoraco-lumbar erector spinae	Lower & middle trapezius
Upper trapezius	Serratus anterior
Levator scapulae	Deep neck flexors
Pectorals	Digastricus
Subscapularis	
Suboccipitals	
SCM	
Lateral pterygoids	
Masseter	

assumed a full squat position, although not weight-bearing, by the end of the fourth month of life (Fig. 2.9). Between the fourth and sixth months of life, oblique muscles begin to work together, which cross the midline and allow for creeping, crawling, and turning-over motions. Table 2.3 summarizes this neurodevelopment.

As a rule, muscle and joint dysfunction are inter-related. Various theories to explain this have been proposed. For instance, that there is decreased muscle stretch sensitivity when type III or IV high-threshold, non-adapting pain fibers are stimulated by either painful irritation of muscles or joints (Fig. 2.10). Also, that joint inflammation or pathology initiates a complex neuromuscular response in the dorsal horn of the spinal cord, resulting in flexor facilitation and extensor inhibition (Figs. 2.11 and 2.12).

Muscle imbalance typically alters the performance of movement patterns, including activities of daily living, with the ultimate result being increased instabil-

Table 2.3 Postural Ontogenesis and Higher CNS Function (see Chapter 23)

- Muscle co-activation → functional joint centration → maximum load-bearing
- Starts at head and neck (C0–1): 4 weeks
- By the fourth month the sagittal plane motor program is in place: full squat position (supine)
- Months 5–7 trunk rotation: oblique muscle chains develop
- 4 years: balanced upright posture is achieved

ity. Because of substitution patterns, the quality of movement at individual joints may be affected without any loss of strength (6,33,43,93,111). Muscle imbalance brings about typical postures such as the slumped posture described by Brügger (Fig. 2.8). Other examples of commonly observed patterns of

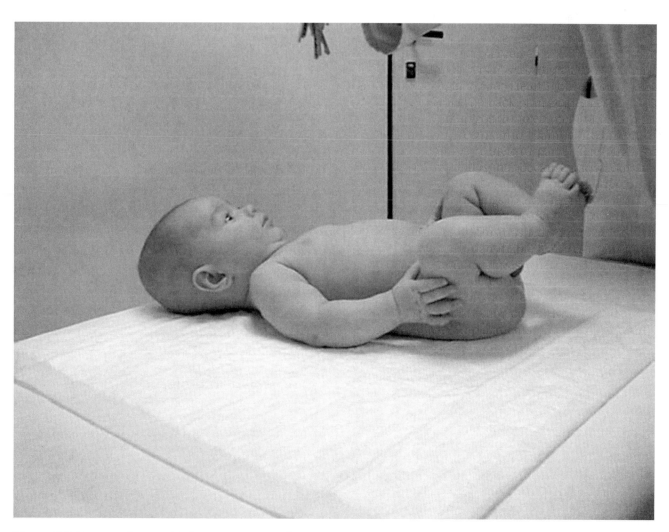

Figure 2.9 Posture of normal infant at 3 to 4 months.

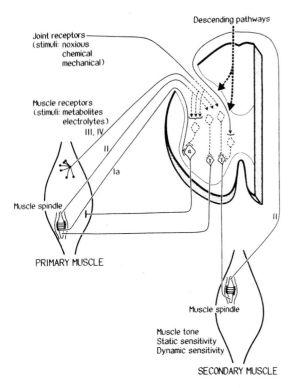

Joint receptors
(stimuli: noxious
chemical
mechanical)

Descending pathways

Muscle receptors
(stimuli: metabolites
electrolytes)
III, IV

Muscle spindle

PRIMARY MUSCLE

Muscle spindle

Muscle tone
Static sensitivity
Dynamic sensitivity

SECONDARY MUSCLE

Figure 2.10 Pathophysiologic model for mechanisms possibly involved in the genesis and spread of muscular tension in occupational muscle pain and chronic musculoskeletal pain syndromes. Reproduced with permission from Johansson H, Sokja P. Pathophysiological mechanisms involved in genesis and spread of muscular tension in occupational muscle pain and in chronic musculoskeletal pain syndromes. A hypothesis. Med Hypothesis 1991;35:196.

poor posture and muscle imbalance have been described by Janda. These include the lower crossed syndrome, upper crossed syndrome, and layer or stratification syndrome (Figs. 2.13, 2.14, and 2.15).

Neuropathic Pain and Central Sensitization

Pain casts a long shadow in the nervous system. Pain can be "learned" in the nervous system so that it is maintained independent of injury, pathology, expectations, or dysfunction. Such pain is called neuropathic and is an important under-recognized dimension of the chronic problem. Failure to appreciate when pain has become conditioned will lead to an overemphasis on coincidental structural pathology, functional deficits, and psychosocial factors.

Neuropathic pain is centrally maintained and therefore does not require peripheral sources of pain-

ful irritation or injury. Typically, it arises as a result of a prolonged, intensive afferent bombardment from peripheral nociceptive pathways (Fig. 2.16). However, because of central sensitization, altered processing of input from secondary neurons (after exiting the dorsal horn) occurs so that pain can be experienced in the absence of peripheral injury, inflammation, or irritation. The most obvious example of this is phantom limb pain where the painful source is not present, but the central pathways that carry nociceptive information are not inhibited, so that even non-noxious stimuli are interpreted as painful!

Two important aspects of neuropathic pain are hyperalgesia, an exaggerated pain response, and allodynia, pain to non-noxious stimuli. Neuropathic pain is an important construct that can explain the common clinical presentation of persistent pain, hypersensitivity, and poor motor control in the absence of or disproportionate to pathoanatomical or neurological disorders.

Hall and Quintner showed that in chronic pain patients, light pressure elicits a widespread increase in EMG activity (47). Sunderland was the first to propose that increased muscle tone would act to protect the nervous system from tensile forces (118). Hall has shown that the flexor withdrawal response is easier to activate in chronic pain patients (48). Increased upper trapezius tension has been demonstrated when stretch is applied to the brachial plexus (7). Upper trapezius and levator scapulae have been reported to have increased EMG activity in subjects with neck pain (8). Such elevations in muscular tension are consistent with the central sensitization syndrome.

Because of the poor correlation between presenting symptoms and objective physical signs chronic pain patients are commonly mislabeled as psychogenic. According to Merskey (85,86), "There is increasing evidence that signs and symptoms that were taken to be proof of hysteria—or of behavioral disorder—

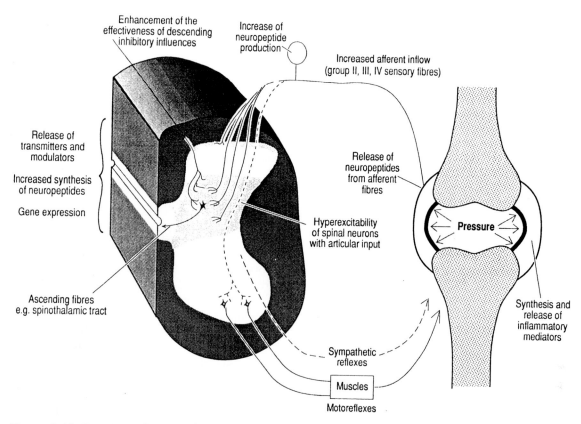

Figure 2.11 Overview of neuronal events in the course of inflammation in the joint. Reproduced with permission from Schaible HG, Grubb BD. Afferent and spinal mechanisms of joint pain. Pain 1993;55:5.

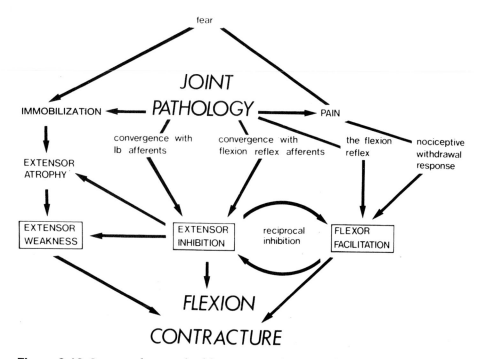

Figure 2.12 Suggested network of factors contributing to fixed flexion of a damaged joint. Reproduced with permission from Young A, Stokes M, Iles JF. Effects of joint pathology on muscles. Clin Orthop 1987;219:21.

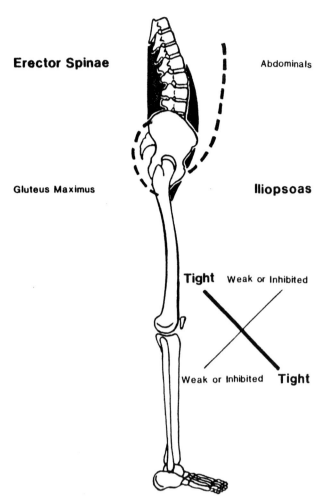

Erector Spinae

Abdominals

Gluteus Maximus

Iliopsoas

Tight Weak or Inhibited

Weak or Inhibited **Tight**

Figure 2.13 The lower crossed syndrome. Reproduced with permission from Jull G, Janda V. Muscles and motor control in low back pain. In: Twomney LT, Taylor JR, eds. Physical Therapy for the Low Back, Clinics in Physical Therapy. New York: Churchill Livingstone, 1987.

(98) and Kenshalo (63) made the initial experiments that showed that noxious sensory stimuli produced heightened sensitivity of dorsal horn neurons to future stimuli.

Osteopaths termed this neuro-mechanical phenomenon the "facilitated segment." Patterson (97) says of the facilitated segment that ". . . because of abnormal afferent sensory inputs to a particular area of the spinal cord, that area is kept in a state of constant increased excitation. This facilitation allows normally ineffectual or subliminal stimuli to become effective in producing efferent output from the facilitated segment . . ." (Fig. 2.17). The myofascial trigger point, osteopathic lesion, and chiropractic subluxation hypotheses long attacked on the basis that they were not scientific are now better-appreciated in this context (85). This includes pain often considered psychogenic because it does not correlate with pathoanatomy, the healing time for an injury, or does not match dermatomal referred pain pathways.

Neuropathic pain is well-accepted in causalgia, reflex sympathetic dystrophy, post-herpetic neuralgia, stroke, syringomyelia, syringobulbia, multiple sclerosis, "phantom limb" pain, and spinal cord injury. Neuropathic pain has also been proposed to result from a repetitive strain initiating strong afferent nociceptive barrage to dorsal horn neurones, eventually leading

such as a failure of complaints to observe anatomical boundaries, may have a physical basis . . . Regional pain syndromes and regional loss of sensitivity can have a pathophysiological origin related to expansion of receptor fields through the responses to peripheral injury of spinal cord neurones." According to Nachemson (89), "various pools of nerve cells in the dorsal columns can be hypersensitized and thus can signal a painful condition even though there is very little peripheral input."

As long ago as 1883, Sturge suggested that an injury could trigger a change in the central nervous system such that normal inputs would evoke an exaggerated response (116). MacKenzie in 1893 proposed that referred pain could result after sensory impulses from injured tissue have created an "irritable focus" in specific spinal cord segments (70). Perl

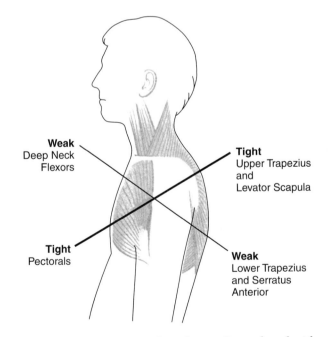

Weak Deep Neck Flexors

Tight Upper Trapezius and Levator Scapula

Tight Pectorals

Weak Lower Trapezius and Serratus Anterior

Figure 2.14 Upper crossed syndrome. Reproduced with permission from Liebenson C. Manual Resistance Techniques in Rehabilitation in Muscle Energy Techniques, 2nd ed. Chaitow L. Edinburgh: Churchill Livingstone, 2001.

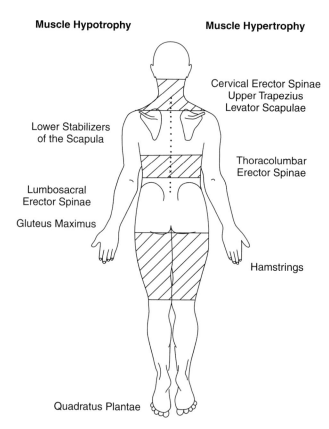

Muscle Hypotrophy

Muscle Hypertrophy

Cervical Erector Spinae
Upper Trapezius
Levator Scapulae

Lower Stabilizers
of the Scapula

Thoracolumbar
Erector Spinae

Lumbosacral
Erector Spinae

Gluteus Maximus

Hamstrings

Quadratus Plantae

Figure 2.15 The layer or stratification syndrome. Reproduced with permission from Jull G, Janda V. Muscles and motor control in low back pain. In: Twomney LT, Taylor JR, eds. Physical Therapy for the Low Back, Clinics in Physical Therapy. New York: Churchill Livingstone, 1987.

to sensitization of those neurones caused by central nervous system plasticity (23). As a result of sensitization of secondary dorsal horn neurones or a decreased threshold for primary peripheral afferents—including normally pain-insensitive groups I and II afferents—normal mechanoreceptor afferent input can be interpreted as nociceptive (23). This results in allodynia, deep hyperalgesia, and an expansion of the receptor field (RF). The RF is dermatomal representation zone where nociceptive irritation of a spinal nerve is felt.

Neuropathic pain is not simply a sensory phenomenon. With increased tissue sensitivity and increased muscle tension, motor control will also be affected. Movement patterns may change to reduce strain on the sensitive tissues. This process occurs on an involuntary basis but can have a large impact on body's ability to recover.

Neuropathic symptoms have been shown in part to be caused by convergent input in the dorsal horn from skin and/or deep somatic (visceral and non-visceral)

structures. Stimulation of viscera does not always produce pain, but visceral afferents projecting into the dorsal horn do typically converge with skin and/or deep somatic structures (38,40). Convergence and central neural plasticity provide the neuroanatomical basis for pain referral. It has been reported that many afferent units when noxiously stimulated elicit pain in two distinct RFs (84). Branching of the afferent fiber near its termination point is the likely anatomical explanation. According to Mense (84) this would, "reduce the spatial resolution of the nociceptive system and thus could contribute to the diffuse nature of deep pain." Dorsal horn neurons have been found to be able to change the size, number, and sensitivity of their RFs under the influence of noxious stimuli (56,58).

Under noxious stimuli, referred pain into new RFs has been shown experimentally to typically take a few minutes to occur (35). Neuroplasticity seems to be operating as new central nervous connections are formed after peripheral injury. It has been shown that visceral pain such as from a coronary infarct can be referred to a muscle like the pectoralis major (123). The muscular target for referred pain may also show signs of hyperalgesia (125).

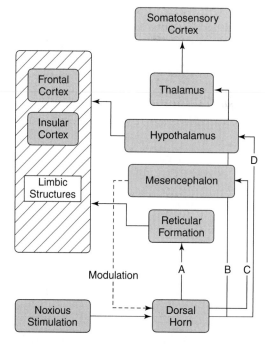

Figure 2.16 Multiple pathways of corticopetal nociceptive transmission (A, spinoreticular; B, spinothalamic; C, spinomesencephalic; D, spinohypothalamic tracts). From Chapman CR. The psychophysiology of pain in Bonica's Management of Pain, Third ed. In: Loeser JD, ed. Philadelphia: Lippincott Williams & Wilkins, 2001.

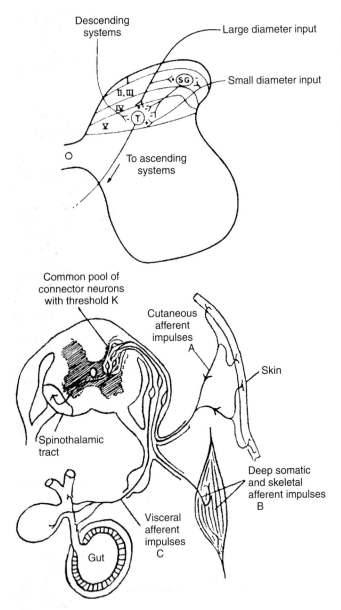

Figure 2.17 Physiologic mechanism of the "irritable focus" in the grey matter of the spinal cord. Reproduced with permission from Grieve GP. Simulated visceral disease. In: Grieve GP, ed. Modern Manual Therapy of the Vertebral Column. Edinburgh: Churchill Livingstone, 1986.

The presence of non-dermatomal referred pain and hyperalgesia implies that central changes independent of convergence are operative (22). An example is the situation in which referred pain spreads to the site of an old injury. An angina attack has been shown to refer pain directly to an old vertebral fracture (51). It has also been demonstrated that 1 week after dental surgery, pin prick of the nasal mucosa can produce referred pain to the treated teeth (103). Distant referral of pain to a non-dermatomal area can

also occur as in cardiac pain referring to the ear (13). A decrease in the flexion withdrawal reflex threshold has been demonstrated in women after gynecological surgery (28).

> ## Central Sensitization Demonstrated in Fibromyalgia Patients
>
> - Fibromyalgia patients had lower cold threshold tolerance along with an increased nociceptive flexion reflex compared to control subjects.
> - Cold threshold—immersion of the hand in an ice water bath. Minimum amount of stimulation that caused pain
> - Cold tolerance—the time a continuous painful immersion ion ice water bath could be endured
> - Nociceptive flexion reflex—surface electrode stimulated sural nerve near lateral malleolus. EMG used to measure biceps femoris muscle contraction
>
> Desmeules JA, Cedraschi C, Rapiti E, et al. Neurorphysiologic evidence for a central sensitization in patients with fibromyalgia. Arthritis Rhem 2003;48:1420–1429.

What is Sensitization?

Sensitization is a change in the stimulus–response profile of dorsal horn neurones so that they respond to normal mechanoreceptive afferents as if they were nociceptors (65,76,130). Willis explains that a nociceptive barrage leads to central sensitization of dorsal horn neurones (130), "If these nociceptive neurons have convergent input from mechanoreceptors, their responses to both innocuous and noxious mechanical stimuli will then be increased. . . . Sensitization then causes formerly subthreshold responses to reach threshold and trigger discharges." According to Mayer (76), "Overwhelming evidence supports the conclusion that a change in the central processing of input from low-threshold mechanoreceptors is responsible for secondary hyperalgesia to light touch." Silent nociceptors that are mechano-insensitive can become mechano-sensitive once sensitized (105). Table 2.4 lists the neural changes associated with sensitization.

How Do Mechanoreceptor Afferents Cause Pain? The Neurochemistry of Neuropathic Pain The pathophysiology of neuropathic pain involves peripheral and central neural events (Fig. 2.18). Sustained activity in type III and IV (small diameter) primary afferents leads to a release of excitatory amino acids (glutamate) and neuropeptides (substance P) in the

Table 2.4   The pathophysiology of sensitization

- Increased spontaneous activity of types III and IV primary afferents
- Prolonged after discharges of afferents to repeated stimulation
- Decreased threshold to afferent input
- Expanded receptive fields of dorsal horn neurons

dorsal horn. Increased concentration of these neurochemical mediators will lower the firing threshold for primary sensory afferents (65,130). In the presence of certain neurotransmitters, secondary dorsal horn neurons may become hyper-responsive because of excitatory amino acids acting at N-methyl-D-aspartate (NMDA) receptor sites and activating dorsal horn nociceptive neurons (65,131). Secondary neuron hyper-responsiveness after repeated stimulation is called "wind-up" and is often short-term. Inhibitory amino acids like GABA are present to dampen this but, over time, segmental inhibition is

deactivated by the flood of excitatory amino acids (31,99). Long-lasting changes appear to be the result of oncogene activation by strong nociceptive input (130). Oncogenes such as c-fos enter the nucleus of the neuron and regulate other gene activity. According to Willis (130), "The implications of this chain of events are still unclear, but a potential result could be long-term changes in the responsiveness of nociceptive neurons."

Pathoanatomical Changes in Neuropathic Pain Peripheral nerves can sprout after peripheral nerve injury so that low threshold mechanoreceptors can extend to terminate within the superficial dorsal horn and make direct connection with nociceptors (31,99). Peripheral nerve damage according to Dubner leads to an expansion of the low threshold portion of wide dynamic range (WDR) neurons caused by a loss of surrounding inhibition (31). Increased excitability leads to excitotoxicity (32,76,117). The most sensitive neurons are small local circuit inhibitory neurons (31). Morphological changes have been demonstrated in the rat dorsal horn after partial nerve injury (31, 117).

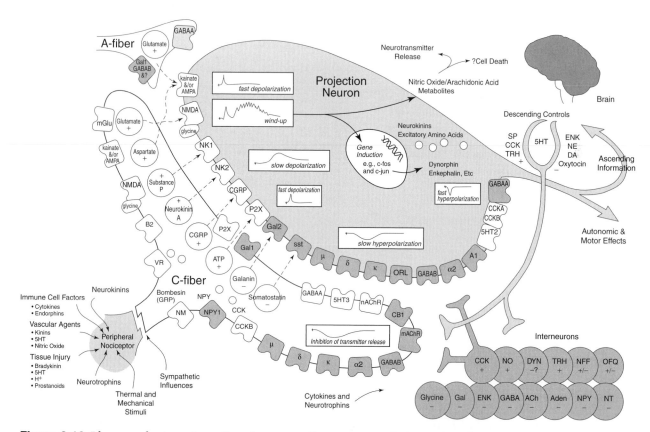

Figure 2.18 Pharmacologic systems thought to contribute to transmission and modulation of nociception in the dorsal horn of the spinal cord. From Terman GW, Bonica JJ. Spinal mechanisms and their modulation. Bonica's Management of Pain, Third ed. In: Loeser JD, ed. Philadelphia: Lippincott Williams & Wilkins, 2001.

Magnetoencephalographic and evoked potential studies in chronic low back pain patients have demonstrated central nervous system (CNS) hyper-responsiveness in the primary somatosensory cortex (Fig. 2.16) (35,36). Magnetoencephalography has also shown somatotopic cortical map reorganization in patients who underwent reconstructive surgery (88). That the spinal cord and CNS are involved in painful musculoskeletal disorders is no longer a question.

Neurophysiologic (Neuromagnetic) Abnormalities Documented in Chronic Upper Limb Pain

Clinical Findings

- allodynia

- decreased strength

- decreased mobility

Neurophysiologic Findings

From whole head magnetoencephalography

- Increased primary somatosensory (SI) responses to tactile stimulation of the affected side

- 25%–55% greater than on non-affected side

- Shortened distance between thumb and little finger SI representation zones corresponding to the affected hand

- Shortened duration of the tactile evoked 20-Hz rebound in the motor cortex (reflective of functional state of the motor cortex)

Conclusion

- Chronic pain patients typically have altered central tactile processing

- Somatosensory changes are likely to be related to motor findings as well

Juottonen K, Gockel M, Silén T, Hurri H, Hari R, Forss N. Altered central sensorimotor processing in patients with complex regional pain syndrome. Pain 2002;98:315–323.

Can Central Sensitization and Expanded Receptor Fields be Modulated? The interaction of descending neuromodulatory and segmental activity on spinal cord neurons indicates there is a high degree of modifiability of the sensory integration phenomena

termed neuropathic pain. Alongside the long-lasting spinal cord excitability produced by sustained, intense nociciceptive activity, depression of spinal cord excitability has been shown to be possible via descending serotonergic pathways (21,106). In particular, 5-hydroxytryptamine (5-HT) exerts a descending control on nociception via presynaptic inhibition of primary afferents (64). Shay and Hochman have also demonstrated that serotonin (5-HT) depresses multi-segmental sensory convergent input or receptive field size in laminae IV-VII spinal neurons (106).

The descending modulation of neuropathic pain by serotonergic strategies is a promising new approach for managing neuropathic pain. Other strategies designed to disinhibit the spinal cord excitability include cognitive–behavioral training and affective methods (i.e., meditation, relaxation training), which influence the hypothalamic–pituitary axis and limbic centers. Additionally, stabilization approaches designed to improve function of agonist–antagonist muscles during daily tasks may reduce nociceptive input to the dorsal horn, and over time help to re-establish more normal stimulus-response profiles in the pain system.

■ CONCLUSION

Co-activation of agonist and antagonist muscles is an essential motor control trait that develops over time in the infant and allows for a balanced, upright posture to be achieved by 4 years of life (127). In adults, this muscular co-activation is an essential feature of joint stability (17,18). Poor motor control—as demonstrated by synergist substitution (6,33,43,111), slow reaction time of muscles (19,100,101,129), or inadequate agonist–antagonist co-activation (17,18)—goes hand-in-hand with decreased joint stability. Mannion suggests that this faulty motor control is the most likely source of the approximately 50% of LBP syndromes that are still unexplained (72). Lewit said that this functional pathology of the motor system is the most common clinical finding in pain patients presenting to orthopedists, rheumatologists, and neurologists, yet it is routinely overlooked (67).

A study of the biomechanics and neurophysiology of spine stability demonstrates that rehabilitation approaches should focus on developing coordination between agonist and antagonist muscles, a fast speed of contraction of stabilizers, aerobic conditioning, and muscle endurance. The final common pathway of rehabilitation of the motor system is to train improved motor control in a patient's activities of daily living.

Audit Process
Self-Check of the Chapter's Learning Objectives

- Describe how agonist–antagonist muscle co-activation stabilizes the spine.

- What is the difference between whole body and spinal stability?

- How can chronic pain patients feel pain from non-noxious stimuli?

- Which muscles have a tendency to become inhibited and which overactive?

- How does neurodevelopmental kinesiology shed light on the problem of agonist–antagonist co-activation in adults?

■ REFERENCES

1. Abenheim L, Rossignol M, Valat JP, et al. The role of activity in the therapeutic management of back pain: Report of the International Paris Task Force on Back Pain. Spine 2000;25:1S–33S.
2. Adams MA, Dolan P. Recent advances in lumbar spine mechanics and their clinical significance. Clin Biomech 1995;10:3–19.
3. Adams MA, Dolan P, Hutton WC. Diurnal variations in the stresses on the lumbar spine. Spine 1987;12:130.
4. Adams MA, Hutton WC. Gradual disc prolapse. Spine 1985;10:524–531.
5. Agency for Health Care Policy and Research (AHCPR). Acute low-back problems in adults. Clinical Practice Guideline Number 14. Washington D.C.: US Government Printing, 1994.
6. Arendt-Nielson L, Graven-Nielson T, Svarrer H, Svensson P. The influence of low back pain on muscle activity and coordination during gait. Pain 1995;64:231–240.
7. Balster SM, Jull GA. Upper trapezius muscle activity during the brachial plexus tension test in asymptomatic subjects. Man Ther 1997;2:144–149.
8. Bansevicius D, Sjaastad O. Cervicogenic headache: The influence of mental load on pain level and EMG of shoulder-neck and facial muscles. Headache 1996;36:372–378.
9. Baratta R, Solomonow M, Zhou BH, Letson D, Chuinard R, D'Ambrosia R. Muscular coactivation. The role of antagonist musculature in maintaining knee stability. Am J Sports Med 1988;16:113–122.
10. Bergmark A. Stability of the lumbar spine. A study in mechanical engineering. Acta Orthop Scand 1989;230:20–24.
11. Biering-Sorensen F. Physical measurements as risk indicators for low-back trouble over a 1-year period. Spine 1984;9:106–119.
12. Bogduk N, Twomney L. Clinical Anatomy of the Lumbar Spine and Sacrum, 3rd ed. Edinburgh: Churchill Livingston, 1997.
13. Brylin M, Hindfelt B. Ear pain due to myocardial ischemia. Am Heart J 1984;107:186–187.
14. Burnett AF, Elliot BC, Foster DH, Marshall RN, Hardcastle P. Thoracolumbar disc degeneration in young fast bowlers in cricket: A follow-up study. Clin Biomech 1996;11:305–310.
15. Callaghan J, McGill SM. Intervertebral disc herniation: Studies on a porcine spine exposed to highly repetitive flexion/extension motion with compressive force. Clin Biomech 2001;16:28–37.
16. Carlson H, Nilsson J, Thorstensson A, Zomlefer MR. Motor responses in the human trunk due to load perturbations. Acta Physiol Scand 1981;111:221–223.
17. Cholewicki J, McGill SM. Mechanical stability of the in vivo lumbar spine: Implications for injury and chronic low back pain. Clin Biomech 1996;11(1):1–15.
18. Cholewicki J, Panjabi MM, Khachatryan A. Stabilizing function of the trunk flexor-extensor muscles around a neutral spine posture. Spine 1997;22:2207–2212.
19. Cholewicki J, Simons APD, Radebold A. Effects of external loads on lumbar spine stability. J Biomech 2000;33:1377–1385.
20. Cholewicki J, Greene HS, Polzhofer GK, Galloway MT, Shah RA, Radebold A. Neuromuscular function in athletes following recovery from a recent acute low back injury. J Orthop Sports Phys Ther 2002;32:568–575.
21. Cui M, Fen Y, McAdoo DJ, Willis WD. Periaqueductal gray stimulation-induced inhibition of nociceptive dorsal horn neurons in rats is associated with the release of norepinephrine, serotonin, and amino acids. J Pharmacol Exp Ther 1999;289:868–876.
22. Coderre TJ, Katz J, Vaccarino AL, Melzak R. Contribution of central neuroplasticity to pathological pain: Review of clinical and experimental evidence. Pain 1993;52:259–285.
23. Cohen ML, Champion GD, Sheaterh-Reid R. Comments on Gracely et al. Painful neuropathy: Altered central processing maintained dynamically by peripheral input. (Pain 1992;51:175–194) Pain 1993;54:365–366.
24. Cresswell AG, Oddsson L, Thorstensson A. The influence of sudden perturbations on trunk muscle activity and intraabdominal pressure while standing. Exp Brain Res 1994;98:336–341.
25. Cripton P, Berleman U, Visarino H, et al. Response of the lumbar spine due to shear loading. Injury Prevention Through Biomechanics. Symposium proceedings, May 4–5. Wayne State University, Detroit, MI, 1995.
26. Crisco JJ, Panjabi MM. Euler stability of the human ligamentous lumbar spine. Part 1: Theory. Clin Biomech 1992;7:19–26.
27. Crisco JJ, Panjabi MM, Yamamoto I, Oxland TR. Euler stability of the human ligamentous lumbar spine. Part 2: Experimental. Clin Biomech 1992;7:27–32.
28. Dahl JB, Erichsen CJ, Fuglsang-Frederiksen A, Kehlet H. Pain sensation and nociceptive reflex excitability in surgical patients and human volunteers. Br J Anesth 1992;69:117–121.
29. Manniche C, et al. Danish Health Technology Assessment (DIHTA). Low back pain: Frequency

Management and Prevention from an HAD Perspective, 1999.

30. DeAndrade JR, Grant C, Dixon A. Joint distension and reflex muscle inhibition in the knee. J Bone Joint Surg 1965;47:313–322.

31. Dubner R. Neuropathic pain. Am Pain Soc J 1993;1:8–11.

32. Dubner R, Sharav Y, Gracely RH, Price DD. Idiopathic trigeminal neuralgia: Sensory features and pain mechanisms. Pain 1987;31:23–33.

33. Edgerton VR, Wolf SL, Levendowski DJ, Roy RR. Theoretical basis for patterning EMG amplitudes to assess muscle dysfunction. Med Sci Sp Exer 1996;28:744–751.

34. Etnyre BR, Simmonds MJ, Radwan H, et al. Hip and knee displacements during sit-to-stand movements between low back pain patients and a control group. 13th International Congress of World Confederation for Physical Therapy. Yokohama, Japan, 1999.

35. Flor H, Birbaumer N, Furst M, et al. Evidence of enhanced peripheral and central responses to painful stimulation in states of chronic pain. Psychophysiology 1993;30:S9.

36. Flor H, Birbaumer N, Braun C, et al. Chronic pain enhances the magnitude of the magnetic field evoked by painful stimulation. In: Deecke L, Baumgartner C, Stroink G, Williamson SJ, eds. Recent advances in biomagnetism. 9th International Conference on Biomagnetism, Vienna, 1993:72–73.

37. Floyd WF, Silver PHS. Function of the erector spinae muscles in certain movements and postures in man. J Physiol 1955;129:184–203.

38. Foreman RD, Balir RW, Weber RN. Viscerosomatic convergence onto T2-T4 spinoreticular, spinoreticular-spinothalamic, and spinothalamic tract neurons in the cat. Exp Neurol 1984;85:597–619.

39. Gardner-Morse MG, Stokes IAF. The effects of abdominal muscle coactivation on lumbar spine stability. Spine 1998;23:86–92.

40. Gebhardt GF, Ness TJ. Central mechanisms of visceral pain. Can J Physiol Pharmacol 1991;69:627–634.

41. Goff B. The application of recent advances in neurophysiology to Miss M. Rood's concept of neuromuscular facilitation. Physiotherapy 1972;58:409–415.

42. Gordon SJ, Yang KH, Mayer PJ, et al. Mechanism of disc rupture-a preliminary report. Spine 1991;16:450–456.

43. Grabiner MD, Koh TJ, Ghazawi AE. Decoupling of bilateral paraspinal excitation in subjects with low back pain. Spine 1992;17:1219–1223.

44. Granata KP, Marras WS. Cost-benefit of muscle cocontraction in protecting against spinal instability. Spine 2000;25:1398–1404.

45. Graven-Nielsen T, Svensson P, Arendt-Nielsen L. Effects of experimental muscle pain on muscle activity and co-ordination during static and dynamic motor function. Electroencephalogr Clin Neurophysiol 1997;105:156–164.

46. Gunning J, Callaghan JP, McGill SM. The role of prior loading history and spinal posture on the compressive tolerance and type of failure in the spine using a porcine trauma model. Clin Biomech 2001;16:471–480.

47. Hall T, Quintner J. Responses to mechanical stimulation of the upper limb in painful cervical radiculopathy. Aust J Physiother 1996;42:277–285.

48. Hall T, Zusman M, Elvey R. Manually detected impediments during the straight leg raise test. In: Jull G, ed. Manipulative Physiotherapists Association of Australia 9th Biennial Conference. Gold Coast: MPAA, 1995:48–53.

49. Hallgren R, Greenman P, Rechtien J. Atrophy of suboccipital muscles in patients with chronic pain: A pilot study. J Am Osteopath Assoc 1994;94:1032–1038.

50. Hardcastle P, Annear P, Foster DH, et al. Spinal abnormalities in young fast bowlers. J Bone Joint Surg (B) 1992;74:421–425.

51. Henry JA, Montushi E. Cardiac pain referred to site of previously experienced somatic pain. BMJ 1978;9:1605–1606.

52. Hides JA, Stokes MJ, Saide M, Jull Ga, Cooper DH. Evidence of lumbar multifidus muscle wasting ipsilateral to symptoms in patients with acute/subacute low back pain. Spine 1994;19:165–172.

53. Hodges P, Gandevia S. Activation of the human diaphragm during a repetitive postural task. J Physiol (Lond) 2000;522:165–175.

54. Hodges P, Gandevia S. Changes in intra-abdominal pressure during postural and respiratory activation of the human diaphragm. J Appl Physiol 2000;89:967–976.

55. Hodges PW, McKenzie DK, Heijnen I, Gandevia SC. Reduced contribution of the diaphragm to postural control in patients with severe chronic airflow limitation. In Proceedings of the Thoracic Society of Australia and New Zealand. Melbourne, Australia, 2000.

56. Hoheisel U, Mense S. Long-term changes in discharge behavior of cat dorsal horn neurones following noxious stimulation of deep tissues. Pain 1989;36:239–247.

57. Holm SM, Dickenson AL. A comparison of two isometric back endurance tests and their predictability of first-time back pain: A pilot study. J Neuroxmusculoskel Syst 2001;9(2):46–53.

58. Hu JW, Sessle BJ, Raboisson P, Dallel R, Woda A. Stimulation of craniofacial muscle afferents induces prolonged facilitatory effects in trigeminal nociceptive brain-stem neurones, Pain 1992;48:53–60.

59. Janda V. On the concept of postural muscles and posture in man. Aus J Physioth 1983;29:83–84.

60. Janda V. Muscles, central nervous motor regulation, and back problems. In: Korr IM, ed. The neurobiologic mechanisms in manipulative therapy. New York: Plenium Press, 1978:27–41.

61. Jull GA. Deep cervical flexor muscle dysfunction in whiplash. J Musculoskel Pain 2000;8:143–154.

62. Jull G, Barret C, Magee R, Ho P. Further clinical clarification of the muscle dysfunction in cervical headache. Cephalgia 1999;19:179–185.

63. Kenshalo DR Jr, Leonard RB, Chung JM, Willis WD. Facilitation of the responses of primate spinothalamic cells to cold and mechanical stimuli by noxious heating of the skin. Pain 1982;12:141–152.

64. Khasabov SG, Lopez-Garcia JA, King AE. Serotonin induced population primary afferent depolarization

in vitro: The effects of neonatal capsaicin treatment. Brain Res 1998;789:339–342.

65. LaMotte RH. Subpopulations of "nocifensor neurons" contributing to pain and allodynia, itch and allokinesis. APS J 1992;2:115–126.

66. Lavender SA, Mirka GA, Schoenmarklin RW, Sommerich CM, Sudhakar LR, Marras WS. The effects of preview and task symmetry on trunk muscle response to sudden loading. Human Factors 1989;31:101–115.

67. Lewit K. Manipulative therapy in rehabilitation of the motor system, 3rd ed. London: Butterworths, 1999.

68. Lund JP, Donga R, Widmer CG, et al. The pain-adaptation model: A discussion of the relationship between chronic musculoskeletal pain and motor activity. Can J Physiol Pharmacol 1991;69:683–694.

69. Luoto S, Heliovaara M, Hurri H, Alaranta H. Static back endurance and the risk of low-back pain. Clin Biomech 1995;10:323–324.

70. MacKenzie J. Some points bearing on the association of sensory disorders and visceral diseases. Brain 1893;16:321–354.

71. Madeleine P, Lundager B, Voight M, Arendt-Nielsen L. Shoulder muscle co-ordination during chronic and acute experimental neck-shoulder pain: An occupational pain study. Eur J Appl Physiol 1999;79:127–140.

72. Mannion AF, Junge A, Taimela S, Muntener M, Lorenzo K, Dvorak J. Active therapy for chronic low back pain. Part 3. Factors influencing self-rated disability and its change following therapy. Spine 2001;26:920–929.

73. Mannion AF, Taimela S, Muntener M, Dvorak J. Active therapy for chronic low back pain. Part 1. Effects on back muscle activation, fatigability, and strength. Spine 2001;26:897–908.

74. Marras WS, Mirka GA. Muscle activities during asymmetric trunk angular accelerations. J Orthop Res 1990;8:824–832.

75. Marras WS, Rangarajulu SL, Lavender SA. Trunk loading and expectation. Ergonomics 1987;30:551–562.

76. Mayer RA, Treed RD, Srinivas NR, Campbell JN. Peripheral versus central mechanisms for secondary hyperalgesia. APS J 1992:2;127–131.

77. McGill SM. Biomechanical basis for stability: An explanation to enhance clinical utility. J Orth Sports Phys Ther 2001;31:97.

78. McGill SM, Sharratt MT, Seguin JP. Loads on the spinal tissues during simultaneous lifting and ventilatory challenge. Ergonomics 1995;38:1772–1792.

79. McGill SM. Low back exercises: prescription for the healthy back and when recovering from injury. Resources Manual for Guidelines for Exercise Testing and Prescription, 3rd ed. Indianapolis, In: American College of Sports Medicine/Baltimore: Lippincott, Williams and Wilkins, 1998.

80. McGill SM, Brown S. Creep response of the lumbar spine to prolonged full flexion. Clin Biomech 1992; 7:43–46.

81. McGill SM, Norman RW. Low Back Biomechanics in Industry: The Prevention of Injury Through Safer Lifting. In: Grabiner M, ed. Current Issues in Biomechanics. Champaign, IL: Human Kinetics, 1993.

82. McGill SM. Low back disorders: The scientific foundation for prevention and rehabilitation. Champaign, IL: Human Kinetics, 2002.

83. McPartland JM, Brodeur RR, Hallgren RC. Chronic neck pain, standing balance and suboccipital muscle atrophy: A pilot study. J Manipulative Physiol Ther 1997;20:24–29.

84. Mense S. Sensitization of group IV muscle receptors to bradykinin by 5-hydroxytryptamine and prostaglandin E2. Brain Res 1981;225:95–105.

85. Merskey H. Limitations of Pain Behavior. APS J 1992;2:101–104.

86. Merseky H. Regional pain is rarely hysterical. Arch Neur 1988;45:915–918.

87. Michelotti A, Farella M, Martina R. Sensory and motor changes of the human jaw muscles during induced orthodontic pain. Eur J Orthop 1999;21:397–404.

88. Mogliner A, Grossman JA, Ribary U, et al. Somatosensory cortical plasticity in adult humans revealed by magnetoencephalography. Proc Natl Acad Sci USA 1993;90;3593–3597.

89. Nachemson AL. Newest knowledge of low back pain. Clin Orth Rel Res 1992;279:8–20.

90. Nederhand MJ, Ijzerman MJ, Hermens HK, Baten CTM, Zilvold G. Cervical muscle dysfunction in the chronic whiplash associated disorder Grade II (WAD-II). Spine 2000;15;1938–1943.

91. Nederhand MJ, Hermens HK, Ijzerman MJ, Turk DC, Zilvold G. Chronic neck pain disability due to an acute whiplash injury. Pain 2003;102:63–71.

92. O'Sullivan PB, Beales DJ, Beetham JA, et al. Altered motor control strategies in subjects with sacroiliac joint pain during the active straight-leg-raise test. Spine 2002;27:E1–E8.

93. Paarnianpour M, Nordin M, Kahanovitz N, Frank V. The triaxial coupling of torque generation of trunk muscles during isometric exertions and the effect of fatiguing isoinertial movements on the motor output and movement patterns. Spine 1998;13:982–992.

94. Panjabi MM. The stabilizing system of the spine. Part 1. Function, dysfunction, adaptation, and enhancement. J Spinal Dis 1992;5:383–389.

95. Panjabi MM, Nibu K, Cholewicki J. Whiplash injuries and the potential for mechanical instability. Eur Spine J 1998;7:484–492.

96. Panjabi MM, Moy P, Oxland TR, Cholewicki J. Subfailure injury affects the relaxation behavior of rabbit ACL. Clin Biomech 1999;14:24–31.

97. Patterson M. Model mechanism for spinal segmental facilitation. Colorado Springs, CO: Academy of Applied Osteopathy Yearbook, 1976.

98. Perl ER, Dumuzawa T, Lynn B, Kenins P. Sensitization of high threshold receptors with unmyelinated (C) afferent fibers. In: Iggo A, Liynsky I, eds. Somatosensory and Visceral Receptor Mechanisms, Progress in Brain Research 1974;43:263–278.

99. Perl ER. Multireceptive neurons and mechanical allodynia. APS J 1992;1;37–41.

100. Radebold A, Cholewicki J, Panjabi MM, Patel TC. Muscle response pattern to sudden trunk loading in healthy individuals and in patients with chronic low back pain. Spine 2000;25:947–954.

101. Radebold A, Cholewicki J, Polzhofer BA, Greene HS. Impaired postural control of the lumbar spine is associated with delayed muscle response times in patients with chronic idiopathic low back pain. Spine 2001;26:724–730.

102. Reilly T, Tynell A, Troup JDG. Circadian variation in the human stature. Chronobiol It 1984;1:121.

103. Reynolds OE, Hutchins HC. Reduction of central hyper-irritability following block anesthesia of peripheral nerve. Am J Physiol 1948;152:658–662.

104. Sahrmann S. Diagnosis and Treatment of Movement Impairment Syndromes. St. Louis, MO: Mosby, Inc, 2001.

105. Schiable HG, Grubb BD. Afferent and spinal mechanisms of joint pain. Pain 1993;55:5–54.

106. Shay BL, Hochman S. Serotonin alters multisegmental convergence patterns in spinal cord deep dorsal horn and intermediate laminae neurons in an in vitro young rat preparation. Pain 2002;95:7–14.

107. Shirado O, Ito T, Kaneda K, et al. Flexion-relaxation phenomenon in the back muscles: A comparative study between healthy subjects and patients with chronic low back pain. Am J Phys Med Rehabil 1995;74:139–144.

108. Snook SH, Webster BS, McGorry RW, Fogleman MT, McCann KB. The reduction of chronic nonspecific low back pain through the control of early morning lumbar flexion. Spine 1998;23:2601–2607.

109. Snook SH, Webster BS, McGorry RW. The reduction of chronic, nonspecific low back pain through the control of early morning lumbar flexion: 3-year follow-up. J Occup Rehab 2002;12:13–20.

110. Solomonow M, Guzzi G, Baratta, et al. EMG-force model of the elbows antagonistic muscle pair. The effect of joint position, gravity and recruitment. Am J Phys Med 1986;65:223–244.

111. Sparto PJ, Paarnianpour M, Massa WS, Granata KP, Reinsel TE, Simon S. Neuromuscular trunk performance and spinal loading during a fatiguing isometric trunk extension with varying torque requirements. Spine 1997;10:145–156.

112. Sparto PJ, Paarnianpour M, Reinsel TE, Simon S. The effect of fatigue on multijoint kinematics and load sharing during a repetitive lifting test. Spine 1997;22:2647–2654.

113. Spencer JD, Hayes KC, Alexander IJ. Knee joint effusion and quadriceps reflex inhibition in man, Arch Phys Med Rehab, 1984;65:171–177.

114. Stokes IAF, Gardner-Morse M, Henry SM, Badger GJ. Decrease in Trunk Muscular Response to Perturbation With Preactivation of Lumbar Spinal Musculature. Spine 2000;25:1957–1964.

115. Stokes M, Young A. Investigations of quadriceps inhibition: Implications for clinical practice. Physiotherapy 1984;70:425–428.

116. Sturge WA. The phenomena of angina pectoris and their bearing upon the theory of counter irritation. Brain 1883;5:492–510.

117. Sugimoto T, Bennett GJ, Kajander KC. Transsynaptic degeneration in the superficial dorsal horn after sciatic nerve injury: Effects of a chronic constriction injury, transection, and strychnine. Pain 1990;42:205–213.

118. Sunderland S. Features of nerves that protect them during normal daily activities. Proceedings of the Manipulative Physiotherapists Association of Australia. Adelaide, 1989:197–201.

119. Svensson P, Arendt-Nielsen L, Houe L. Sensory-motor interactions of human experimental unilateral jaw muscle pain: A quantitative analysis. Pain 1995;64:241–249.

120. Svensson P, Arendt-Nielsen L, Houe L. Muscle pain modulates mastication: An experimental study in humans. J Orofac Pain 1998;12:7–16.

121. Svensson P, Houe L, Arendt-Nielsen L. Bilateral experimental muscle pain changes electromyographic activity of human jaw-closing muscles during mastication. Exp Brain Res 1997;116:182–185.

122. Thelen DG, Schultz AB, Ashton-Miller JA. Quantitative interpretation of lumbar muscle myoelectric signals during rapid cyclic attempted trunk flexions and extensions. J Biomech 1994;27:157–167.

123. Travell J, Rinzler SH. The myofascial genesis of pain. Postgrad Med 1952;11:425–434.

124. Triano JJ, Schultz AB. Correlation of objective measure of trunk motion and muscle function with low-back disability ratings. Spine 1987;12:561–565.

125. Vecciet L, Giamberardino MA, Dragani L, Galletti R, Albe-Fessard D. Referred muscular hyperalgesia from viscera: clinical approach. In: Lipton S, et al, eds. Advances in Pain Research and Therapy, vol. 13. New York: Raven Press, 1990:175–182.

126. Vogt L, Pfeifer K, Banzer W. Neuromuscular control of walking with chronic low-back pain. Manual Ther 2003;8:21–28.

127. Vojta V, Peters A. Das Vojta princip. Heidelberg: Springer-Verlag, 1992.

128. Waddell G. The Back Pain Revolution. Edinburgh: Churchill Livingstone, 1998.

129. Wilder DG, Aleksiev AR, Magnusson ML, Pope MH, Spratt KF, Goel VK. Muscular response to sudden load. A tool to evaluate fatigue and rehabilitation. Spine 1996;21:2628–2639.

130. Willis WD. Mechanical allodynia A role for sensitized nociceptive tract cells with convergent input from mechanoreceptors and nociceptors? APS J 1993;1:23–33.

131. Winter DA. Human balance and posture control during standing and walking. Clin Biomech 1995;3:193–214.

132. Yingling VR, McGill SM. Mechanical properties and failure mechanics of the spine under posterior shear load: Observations from a porcine model. J Spinal Dis 1999;12:501–508.

133. Yoshihara K, Shirai Y, Nakayama Y, Uesaka S. Histochemical changes in the multifidus muscle in patients with lumbar intervertebral disc herniation. Spine 2001;26:622–626.

134. Zhao WP, Kawaguchi Y, Matsui H, Kanamori M, Kimura T. Histochemistry and morphology of the multifidus muscle in lumbar disc herniation. Comparative study between diseased and normal sides. Spine 2000;25:2191–2199.

3

Quality Assurance: The Scope of the Spine Problem and Modern Attempts to Manage It

Craig Liebenson

Learning Objectives
After reading this chapter you should be able to:

- Understand the course of spinal disorders
- Understand the risk factors for both acute and chronic low back pain
- Understand the benefits and limitations of management guidelines for low back pain and whiplash-associated disorders

"I am merely picking up pebbles from the seashore of knowledge"

Sir Isaac Newton

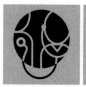

Introduction

Specialists in the management of spinal disorders have seen tremendous changes in the past decade. Whereas the low back pain (LBP) problem is acknowledged as an epidemic, a consensus has gradually emerged as to why this happened and what can be done about it (2,31,39,76,129,130,142). An overemphasis on the simplistic biomedical approach of identifying and treating the structural cause of pain has led to excesses in diagnostic testing, bed rest, narcotic analgesics, and surgery (29,52,65,167). Meanwhile, an underemphasis on illness behavior has led to an underuse of functional (reactivation advice, manipulation, and exercise) and cognitive–behavorial approaches (173). A wide variation in practice habits—not justified by evidence of effectiveness—has been the major motivation of the guidelines development players (2,29).

Patients with acute spinal problems tend to improve quickly, although recurrence is the norm and dissatisfaction is high (30,165). Those who have chronic, persistent pain or become disabled are failed by a health care system that characteristically falls into the trap of overemphasizing the structural cause of pain rather than early on providing reassurance that there is no serious disease and that the road to recovery is through gradually resuming normal activities and restoring function (19,74,104). Unfortunately, implementation of guidelines summarizing this modern self management approach has been poor (18,62). One possible explanation is that guidelines take an overly aggressive tone (1). Another proposed reason is that back pain lacks a defined specialty group such as cardiology that can be educated and partnered with to change practice behaviors (124). Finally, a third possibility is that it may be easier to educate patients who then will influence physician behavior rather than vice versa (18,21,134).

Acute LBP is one of the leading symptoms that leads an individual to seek health care services. From diagnostic triage to rehabilitation, the modern goal of care is to maintain or resume normal functional activities (2,23,167). Certain benchmark "tools of the trade" include diagnostic triage (without imaging unless "red flags" of serious disease are present), appropriate referral if there are "red flags," or reassurance that nothing serious is wrong, simple reactivation advice, and pain relief options such as medication (usually over the counter) and spinal manipulation.

The subacute patient has reached a different decision point. Beginning at the 4-week mark, a patient who has not significantly improved is "de-facto" at high risk for chronicity and thus requires a different "tool set." Structural (i.e., imaging), functional (physical performance ability), and psychosocial re-evaluation is necessitated. At this stage, exercise guided by a rehabilitation specialist is appropriate (167). This may include cognitive–behavorial education or exercise (i.e., McKenzie, stabilization, or isotonic), with no particular approach having been clearly shown to be superior to any other at present. New research has reinforced that it may not be so important exactly what is offered so long as it is matched to the patients activities and offered with worksite involvement if related to occupation (52, 99,100). Certainly, so long as appropriate indications—progressive neurologic deficit or significant non-responsive leg symptoms and confirmatory imaging findings—are present spinal surgery is an option at this stage (85).

A key question remains as to whom should receive which components of this "benchmark" and when. Because of the high prevalence and limited effectiveness of primary prevention, universal preventive care is not appropriate (136). Generally, too much care is withheld until patients have well-established chronic pain syndromes when costs are extremely high and effectiveness is low (97,106,136,167). However, can we afford early, aggressive strategies for everyone, or is it possible to stratify individuals into groups of who is either more or less likely to recover so that aggressive care can be targeted to those who need it most (25,26,52,53,57,76,89,90,93,94,95,97,104,109, 136,155)? The identification of psychosocial "yellow flags" indicative of a decreased likelihood of recovery have been proposed as a technique for early identification and thus matched appropriate management of those with a poorer prognosis (76,92,93,129,130,151).

Scope of the Problem

Epidemiology and Natural History

> **Practice-Based Problem**
>
> A common myth is that pain and activity intolerances are usually eliminated within 4 to 6 weeks of the onset of a typical low back pain episode. Although it is true that significant improvement is usually achieved quickly, pain and activity restrictions tend to persist and recur indefinitely. This being the case, what type of expectations should patients be given regarding their recovery in terms of pain, return to work, activity intolerances, and the likelihood of recurrence?

Incidence

Acute low back pain (LBP) affects most of the population at some time or another. By the age of 30, nearly one-half of the population will have experienced a significant episode of LBP (118).

The likelihood of someone having pain at any given time—the point prevalence—is between 15% and 30% (107,111). The Nuprin Pain Report found that LBP was second only to headache as the most common pain symptom affecting American adults over the previous year (149). This report showed that the 1-year prevalence rate (chances of having LBP in the past year) was 56% and the lifetime prevalence rate (chances of having LBP in one's lifetime) was 70% (64,149). Similarly, European studies have demonstrated 1-year prevalence rates of 35% to 40% (7, 71,79,107,119,169) and lifetime prevalence rates of between 60% and 80% (107,119,111,141,169).

Most patients with acute LBP have had it before (165). It typically runs a self-limiting course only to recur again in the future. Carey et al reported that only 5% of acute low back pain episodes become chronic (23). The General Survey on Living Conditions in Sweden and the General Household Survey in Britain came to similar conclusions (132,157). Unfortunately, even though the chronic problem affects a small percentage of individuals, it consumes the majority of the costs associated with this problem (68,142).

Course of Low Back Pain

It has been traditionally taught that for the majority of individuals (75%–90%), acute LBP episodes resolve within 4 to 6 weeks (65,142) (Fig. 3.1). This is based on insurance surveillance data that mostly tracked disability. Such an excellent natural history has led to the mistaken belief that acute LBP can be managed symptomatically (bed rest and medication) and left alone. However, there are two problems with this perspective. First, the view that most acute episodes resolve quickly and completely is disputed by a number of studies of primary care patients (36,165). Second, there is a growing body of evidence that it is more

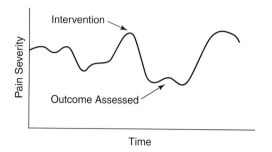

Figure 3.2 Actual course of LBP here. Reproduced from Deyo RA. Practice variations, treatment fads, rising disability. Do we need a new clinical research paradigm? Spine 1993;18:2153–2162.

cost-effective to attempt to prevent chronicity in those at risk for it rather than waiting to treat only those in whom it becomes fully apparent (97,106,122,136, 151,167).

One of the first studies that cast doubt on the often suggested rosey natural history for LBP was by Lloyd and Troup who presented evidence that showed that 70% of people continued to have have residual symptoms even after they returned to work (98). Berquist-Ullman and Larsson found that 62% of acute back pain patients had at least one recurrence during a 1-year follow-up (6). Similarly, Butler et al demonstrated that even though most disabled workers with LBP return to work within 1 month, 50% of them relapse within 1 year (20). Von Korff et al demonstrated in a non-occupational setting that after 1 month only 30% of neck and low back pain patients had achieved pain-free status and after 1 year one-half still reported recurrent or persistent pain (165)! Although this study is often criticized for not exclusively limiting itself to patients having their first-ever episode of acute LBP, it nonetheless served as a wake up call that the presumed natural history of LBP episodes was not what "experts" claimed. In fact, it could be said that because most of our acute patients have had symptoms before Von Korff's study is a more realistic look at the natural history clinicians in the trenches actually see!

In the past few years, a number of high-quality, prospective studies (23,30,36,160) have looked at the course of first-time acute LBP in non-occupational settings. These studies show that most acute episodes tend to improve rapidly, although not completely, and then run an intermittent, chronic course with less severe "flare-ups" (Fig. 3.2). The original episode frequently lasts for as long as 3 months, not 4 to 6 weeks, before it can be said to have remitted (30,36). The predictable "flare-ups" are mild to moderately activity-limiting and painful and lead to general dissatisfaction with the symptoms (30,36,165).

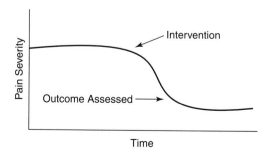

Figure 3.1 Presumed natural history of LBP. Reproduced from Deyo RA. Practice variations, treatment fads, rising disability. Do we need a new clinical research paradigm? Spine 1993;18:2153–2162.

When looking at the literature regarding the natural history of LBP, two important sources of error should be avoided. First, are the inception cohorts (study population) of each study similar enough to compare? Second, what criteria are being used to conclude that recovery has occurred?

Evaluating if inception cohorts are similar is performed to see if are we are comparing apples to apples. Some studies of recovery include in their inception cohort a mixed group of new-onset cases with pre-existing cases. Von Korff's study mixed the two (like in a real practice!), so naturally he shows a poorer natural history because he was already including in his cohort individuals with previous histories (165). Other studies like Carey's use very strict criteria to limit the cohort to only first-time sufferers, which is quite different than the make-up of most practices (23).

Another crucial difference in many studies is that they often use different outcomes to define "recovery." Symptoms, care-seeking, activity limitations, satisfaction, or disability have all been used and each constitutes something quite different.

Cherkin performed a prospective study with an inception cohort of 219 patients presenting to a primary care health maintenance organization (HMO) clinic in the state of Washington for care for the first time for a new episode of LBP (30). The criteria used for recovery included a novel measurement of how satisfied with care a patient would be if the current level of symptoms persisted. At 1 week, one-third were satisfied; at 3 weeks one-half were satisfied; at 7 weeks two-thirds were satisfied; and at 1 year 85% were satisfied. This certainly did not equate with traditional wisdom that 90% of LBP patients were recovered in 4 to 6 weeks. In fact, at 7 weeks, only 46% were symptom-free, 38% were free of dysfunction, and only 31% were both symptom-free and without dysfunction. Even at 1 year, only 39% were both symptom-free and without dysfunction, and fully 29% were considered to have poor outcomes.

In a related study, Croft et al performed a prospective study with an inception cohort of 463 adults presenting to general practitioner (GP) in England (36). These were patients having their first consultation for LBP in the past year. They could have had LBP, but not any consultations, within 1 year. The criteria for recovery were reduced pain and disability. At 3 months, although 91% stopped consulting, only 21% had completely recovered. At 1 year only 25% had completely recovered.

Jacob conducted a longitudinal, community-based study of 3350 individuals from a single town in Israel (75). Of these, 555 met the inclusion criteria of self-reported pain in the past month; 78.7% sought some health care at baseline. The outcomes of recovery studied were persistence of pain after 2 or 12 months. More than three-fourths of the pain group continued to report pain after 2 and 12 months.

The traditional view that most LBP patients are recovered in 4 to 6 weeks is not supported by the current literature (Table 3.1). Croft summarizes current thinking as, "The findings of our study are in sharp contrast to the frequently repeated assumption that 90% of episodes of low back pain seen in primary care will have resolved within a month" (36).

The Cherkin, Croft, and Jacob studies suggest that the 1-year data indicate a significant unrecognized problem (30,36,75). Croft et al says, "We should stop characterizing LBP as acute problems which recover, but rather as a chronic problem with frequent recurrences." Most striking is Croft's conclusion that more aggressive early treatment may be needed to address this rather non-benign natural history, "Since most consulters continue to have long term low back pain and disability, effective early treatment could reduce the burden of these symptoms and their social, economic, and medical impact."

Deyo and Weinstein agree saying, ". . . the emerging picture is that of a chronic problem with intermittent exacerbations, analogous to asthma, rather than an acute disease that can be cured" (44). Dutch findings confirm this by finding that at 12 months after initial consultation, even though only 10% of patients still had the same episode (chronic patients), 75% had reported at least one recurrence (160).

Table 3.1   Summary of the Natural History for LBP

The good news:

- For the majority, improvement begins rapidly
- Chronic, unremitting LBP affects a minority of patients
- Disability persists in a relatively small percentage of individuals, even in those with chronic LBP
- Most individuals don't seek care and when they do it does not last long
- Satisfaction with chiropractic care is very good
- The economic costs for managing most LBP is not that great

The bad news:

- Complete resolution of symptoms and activity intolerances does not occur rapidly
- The recurrence rate is high
- Satisfaction with medical care is not very good
- The economic costs related to the small minority of individuals with persistent, disabling occupational LBP are an enormous problem for society

Carey's study sheds significant light on the important question of what type of care is indicated by these data (23). Because persistent, chronic LBP occurs in less than 8% of new episodes of acute LBP and is usually not disabling, he suggests that the focus of care should be on disability prevention and functional recovery rather than symptom management, "The challenge for clinicians is to maintain patient functioning in the face of persistent symptoms that are not easily resolved with treatment." Thus, ". . . preservation of physical functioning, rather than symptom eradication, should be the paramount goal of health care for patients with chronic LBP."

Table 3.2 Table Percentage of Costs by Type of Treatment and Compensation

Back Pain Costs	Percent	Percent
Medical costs		33
Physician's fees	11	
Hospital costs	11	
Diagnostic tests	4	
Physical therapy	3	
Drugs	2	
Appliances	2	
Disability		67
Temporary	22	
Permanent	45	
Total costs		100

Adapted with permission from Pope MH, Frymoyer JW, Andersson G, eds. Occupational Low Back Pain. New York: Praeger, 1984:107.

Systematic Critical Review Evaluates Epidemiologic Data on Natural History and Course of Back Pain

- Finds no evidence for the popular claim that 90% of back pain episodes resolve spontaneously in 1 month

- Return to work does not equate with recovery because chronic patients may "move" in and out of employment or return to less demanding jobs

- Patients may stop consulting with their medical physician, but this does not mean they are recovered

- This study questions the value of short-term recovery as a valid outcome measure for a recurrent disorder such as back pain

- The authors propose long-term prevention of recurrences as a more relevant measure of the success of a therapeutic intervention

Hestbaek L, Leboeuf-Yde C, Manniche C. Low back pain: what is the long-term course? A review of studies of general patient populations. Eur Spine J 2003;12:149–165.

Costs

LBP is the second leading reason for visiting a physician after upper respiratory problems (40). Its cost represents a major under-appreciated health care failure. In the United States, the costs are estimated at $25 billion annually. This is approximately three-times the cost of all types of cancer!

Most of the costs related to back problems are associated with occupational back pain and are caused by disability (Table 3.2). Williams has shown that physical therapy, surgery, and diagnostic testing are the biggest health care contributors, with mental health

and chiropractic representing surprisingly small overall costs (0.5% and 3.4%, respectively) (173). The most expensive patients are the 1% who undergo surgery (173). Freidlieb concluded that 44% of CAT scans (CT) or magnetic resonance imaging (MRI) studies were unnecessary (55). New information also suggests medication abuse is a bigger cost problem than previously thought (158). Ursiny showed that narcotic use is the most significant cost factor from a treatment perspective (158).

In a study looking at 98 randomly selected disabled workers, Mahmud et al (102) concluded, "Disability was significantly associated with increased utilization of specialty referrals and provider visits, use of MRI, and use of opioids for more than seven days." The study found that 27% of uncomplicated acute LBP patients had an MRI scan in the first month and 33% had a CT scan; 38% received a prescription for narcotic opioids.

Even though only a small percentage (7%) of individuals with acute LBP develop chronic, unremitting pain and disability, this group demands our attention (68). They account disproportionately for the costs associated with the LBP problem with 7.4% of patients estimated to account for 75% of all the costs and 85% of the disability days (68,142) (Fig. 3.3). It is for this reason that identifying potential risk factors for acute pain becoming chronic has become an area of intense LBP research (see Chapter 9).

Care-seeking for LBP varies from country to country. In the United States, only 39% of acute patients sought care (23). In England 48% (174) sought care, in Belgium 63% (146) sought care, and in Israel 78% (75) sought care.

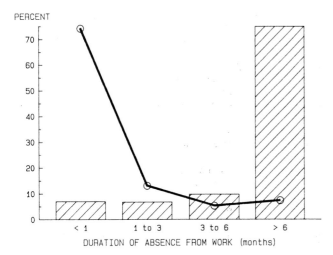
PERCENT

DURATION OF ABSENCE FROM WORK (months)

Figure 3.3 Compensation costs for back injury in groups with different durations of absence from work. Quebec, 1981. From Spitzer WO, Le Blanc FE, Dupuis M, et al. Scientific approach to the assessment and management of activity-related spinal disorders: A monograph for clinicians. Report of the Quebec Task Force on Spinal Disorders. Spine 1987;12(suppl 7):S1–S59.

Natural History for Spinal Disorders Other Than Low Back Pain

Sciatica is a common condition that typically lasts longer than LBP (44,156). The presence of leg pain has been shown prospectively to at least double the risk of a back problem becoming persistant (odds ratio, 2.55; 95% confidence interval, 1.3 to 5.1) (151). The lifetime prevalence for it is estimated to be between 14% and 40% (111,145,156). Surgery for sciatica is estimated to be necessary in between 1.3% and 3.1% of the population (41,86,156). In contrast, spinal stenosis does not have such a favorable prognosis (44). Approximately 15% of patients improve, 15% worsen, whereas the remainder remain fairly stable.

Neck and shoulder problems occur in nearly as many individuals as LBP, with a lifetime prevalence between 50% and 71% of the population (34,111). The 1-year prevalence rate is nearly 14.6 % in Saskatchewan (34) and 17.9% in England (38); 48% of neck pain episodes persist at 1 year (70). According to Makela (105), the chronic problem is frequent, affecting 9.5% of males and 13.5% of females. Like LBP, neck pain is generally persistant, with only one-third experiencing a complete resolution of symptoms (35). Headache has a high point prevalence of 16% to 22% and a lifetime prevalence of more than 90% (111). Whiplash injuries are common, but their duration is controversial (103). Many authors (59,102,117) estimate it to last approximately 2 to 3 months, whereas others have concluded that 20% to 70% of the time pain persists at least 6 months later (13,14).

Risk Factors: Etiology and Prognosis

Two quite distinct sets of risk factors can be identified in those with LBP. First are those that predict who will have acute LBP. Some of these may actually be predisposing or etiologic factors. Second are those factors that predict which acute LBP patients will have chronic pain. These can be thought of as perpetuating or prognostic factors. Prevention efforts are dependent on accurate risk factor identification. Because the cost of such preventive approaches is usually a consideration, groups at high risk are those who would be the likely targets. Prevention of acute LBP is considered primary prevention, whereas prevention of chronic LBP in those already having acute LBP is termed secondary prevention. Primary prevention efforts have been notably unsuccessful, whereas secondary prevention has become the focus of most recent guidelines statements (2,39,76,129,130).

The best studies of risk factors are those that are prospective, because they can infer more accurately causation. In contrast, cross-sectional or retrospective studies only reveal associations and often consequences rather than causes. There is a rapidly growing body of literature on risk factors for LBP, but very few for sciatica or neck pain.

Risk Factors Associated with the Onset of Acute LBP

> **Practice-Based Problem**
>
> Can factors related to the development of spinal pain and disability be identified so that better primary preventive efforts can be designed, investigated, and promoted?

Risk factors for the development of acute LBP have been divided into two general groups—individual and external. If risk factors for acute LBP can be identified, perhaps workers can be better-matched to occupations so as to reduce the incidence of costly, disabling episodes. Additionally, primary prevention measures depend on accurate identification of risk factors to be efficacious.

Individual The primary individual risk factors for onset of back pain are related to age, socio-economic class, education level, long-term activity levels, and self-rated health. Gender, genetics, congenital anomalies, degenerative conditions, muscle strength, and cardiovascular fitness have all been found to be unrelated to LBP onset. Smoking has been shown to be related, but the causal link is tenuous. Evidence that fitness and higher levels of physical activity over the long-term are correlated with reduced incidences of back pain exists, but so does short-term evidence to the contrary. Strength has not been shown to be related to LBP, but endurance has, although it is weak and controversial. Flexibility's relationship to LBP is controversial. Height and weight are often referred to as related to LBP episodes, but there is evidence to support and to reject the hypothesis. Table 3.3 summarizes the main categories of individual risk factors for acute onset LBP.

Psychosocial Fear–avoidance beliefs have been found to be prospectively related to the development of pain and dysfunction (96). The relative risk (RR) is 2.0 to 2.5 (96). The RR is the ratio of incidence rates for a condition in two distinct populations. Thus, individuals with substantial fear–avoidance beliefs are two-times to 2.5-times more likely to have LBP than those without such beliefs. High levels of distress have been shown to strongly predict that future episodes of LBP would be more likely to become chronic (151). In an asymptomatic group of 23-year-olds evaluated and then re-evaluated again 10 years later, psychological distress increased risk more than 2-fold for future LBP (odds ratio, 2.52; 95% confidence interval) (123). Depression was found to be an independent predictor of onset of an episode of neck or low back trouble (24).

Self-rated health is a potent predictor of new episodes of LBP (37,78). The relative risk in men is 1.5, whereas in women it is 2.2 (37). Below-average self-rated health has also been shown to predict that future episodes of LBP would be more likely to become chronic (151).

Table 3.3 Major Categories of Individual Risk Factors for Acute Onset LBP

- Psychosocial (self-rated health)
- Physical—functional (activity level—short-term and long-term, flexibility/motion characteristics, strength, endurance, balance, cardiovascular fitness, lifting capacity)
- Physical—structural (congenital anomalies, degenerative conditions)
- Work-related (some are also psychosocial or physical)—job satisfaction, low social support in the workplace
- Socio-demographic (age, socio-economic class, education level, gender, genetics, smoking, anthropometric—height, weight)

Physical–Functional

Activity level The relationship between overall fitness and LBP episodes is one of the more interesting potential risk factor. Cady showed in a large prospective study of 1652 fire fighters that higher levels of physical fitness were preventive of LBP episodes (22). Leino found that men with lower baseline levels of physical activity were at greater risk for LBP 10 years later (87). No such elevated risk was found in women. Harreby found that inactive teenagers were more likely to have LBP 25 years later than physically active ones (67). Similarly, Videman found that compared to elite athletes, matched controls had more LBP (163). In contrast, Croft (37) found that activity levels were not correlated with subsequent LBP in the short-term, over a 1-year period, except for the following:

- Regular sports activity in women is related to LBP: RR, 1.3
- Do-it-yourself activities in men are related to LBP: RR, 1.8.

In a related study, low levels of physical activity level were found to be strongly correlated with future development of chronic LBP in asymptomatic individuals (151).

Cardiovascular fitness Cardiovascular fitness has not been shown to be related to future onset of LBP (3,125,154).

Muscle strength and endurance There is some evidence that poor isometric endurance of the back muscles is predictive of LBP episodes (8,101). However, this has been disputed by Takala (148). Stevenson et al reported that the electromyographic median frequency shift (increased rate of decline) during sustained contractions of the erector spinae and quadriceps strength and endurance each predicted future LBP in workers involved in manual material handling (144).

Lifting capacity Isometric lifting capacity was not shown to be correlated by Battie (Battie 1989) but was correlated by Chaffin, Liles, and Takala. (27,91, 148).

Balance Poor balance was correlated with future LBP by Takala (148).

Flexibility Reduced flexibility was shown to be related by Battie (4). However, increased range of motion (ROM) has been identified as a risk factor in women and decreased ROM in men, according to Biering-Sorensen and Takala (8,148). A novel dimension of ROM is the patient's natural speed or acceleration during testing. Decreased thoracic acceleration during ROM testing was shown to be positively associated with future LBP (144).

Physical–structural (congenital anomalies, degenerative conditions) Spinal x-rays have been used for many years to screen workers in high-risk occupations for potential risk of disabling back conditions without finding any predictive value (146). The Occupational Health Guidelines (OHG) (12,15,168) from England summarize current scientific opinion on this subject quite succinctly, "It is important to address a very commonly held misconception about the relationship between various structural findings and spinal disorders. Historically, the public and clinicians have assumed that congenital abnormalities such as tropism or spina bifida, degenerative changes in discs or facets, spondylolisthesis, and herniated discs were all structural changes which if present would predispose a person to future LBP, sciatica, or neck pain episodes. To date the correlation is very weak. The likelihood of an asymptomatic individual with any of these structural pathologies developing clinical problems in the future is hardly greater than for someone without them."

Work-Related: Job Satisfaction, Low Social Support in the Workplace

Job satisfaction There is strong evidence for low job satisfaction as a risk factor for LBP. The magnitude of risk estimate (relative risk) is 1.7 to 3.0 (9,10,72, 120,122,127). This risk also extends to future acute episode being more likely to become chronic (151)!

Social support in the workplace There is also significant evidence that low social support in the workplace correlates with future onset of disabling LBP (72). The magnitude of risk is estimated to be 1.3 to 1.9 (10,126).

Sociodemographic (Age, Socio-Economic Class, Education Level, Gender, Genetics, Smoking, Anthropometric—Height, Weight)

Age It can be said that LBP is more common in those between late adolescence and the early 40s. After the age of 60, incidence rates begin to decline. New evidence suggests LBP may be more common than thought in even younger individuals (112,167).

Socio-economic class Lower socio-economic class is related, for a variety of reasons, such as external factors including heavier manual labor (167). In fact, the relationship is stronger for the duration of disability than it is for actual incidence of episodes.

Education level Low education level like socio-economic class is more related to duration of disability than actual incidence rates for LBP (167).

Smoking Smoking has clear effects on the anatomic structures of the low back. Decreased blood flow and nutrition to the disc, lowered pH of the disc, demineralization of the vertebral bodies, altered fibrinolytic activity, and increased degenerative changes have all been described. However, epidemiologic studies show there is only a very weak correlation between smoking and LBP and no correlation with sciatica (80,112). An exception is Croft's recent study, which showed that current smokers have more LBP than non-smokers or former smokers (37).

Height and Weight Anthropometric measures such as height and weight have been looked at in numerous studies reviewed by Nachemson (112). An early study of US military recruits found that those hospitalized for LBP were significantly taller and heavier than control subjects (73). Croft found that women in the shortest quintile had reduced risk (37). Kopec el al found height was correlated with LBP in men, but not women, whereas weight was not a factor for either sex (78). Deyo and Bass found that there was an increased likelihood of the heaviest individuals having LBP when compared with the lightest individuals (42). Shekelle found no relationship between body mass index (BMI) and back pain in 3000 adults (137). Croft found that both weight and body mass index were related to subsequent LBP in the next 12 months with borderline significance (37). They also found increased weight in women increased the risk. Women in the heaviest quintile had a relative risk of 1.8 compared to those in lowest quintile. No similar association was found for men. In this study, the risk associated with BMI was the same as for weight.

External Work activities have been studied extensively for their possible association with future onset of LBP. Whole-body vibration such as in truck and automobile drivers, as well as frequent bending (flexion) and twisting, have been shown to be related to both LBP and sciatica (164). Both repetitive work tasks (arm or neck movements) and manual handling (carrying, lifting, pushing, and pulling) have been shown to be related to future onset of LBP.

According to the Occupational Health Guidelines (OHG) (168) from England summary, "There is strong evidence that physical demands of work (manual materials handling, lifting, bending, twisting, and whole body vibration) are a risk factor for the incidence (onset) of LBP, but overall it appears that the size of the effect is less than that of other individual, non-occupational and unidentified factors."

Risk Factors for Neck Conditions Static load has been shown to be related to neck pain (i.e., heavy exposure to visual display unit work is correlated with neck pain) (164). Also, somewhat weaker evidence suggests that work tasks involving forceful arm movements are correlated with neck pain (164). Fatigue, sleep problems, less sports activity, and high psychosomatic score in those 15 to 18 years old predicted future neck and shoulder pain (7 years later) (140). Female sex, having given birth to more children, psychological distress, previous LBP, and previous neck injury are other risk factors for future neck pain (70). Depression has been prospectively linked to future neck pain (24). There is a trend toward a greater incidence of neck pain in women, and it peaks between the ages of 30 and 45 (34); 50% of all soft tissue neck injuries are related to automobile accidents, with a female preponderance (162). Other causes are accidental falls (25%), sports injuries (24%), and bicycle injuries, with a male preponderance (162).

Perpetuating Factors for Poor Recovery of LBP: Prognostic Factors

Practice-Based Problem

Because many acute LBP patients recover with minimal intervention, aggressive treatment of all acute LBP patients in the hope of reducing the expensive chronic problem is cost-inefficient. However, can primary care providers identify a subgroup of acute patients at high risk for chronicity so that an efficient allocation of resources can be used to prevent chronic pain before it is established?

Although long-term disability affects a small percentage of patients, they consume a disproportionate portion of the overall costs. Once chronic pain and disability is established, it is very resistant to treatment. Therefore, if it can be predicted who will be resistant to recovery, then more aggressive treatments given early on to those individuals may reduce the chronic problem.

Frymoyer was one of the first to focus on identification of high risk patients, "if a patient is identified early in the course of the low back pain episode to have a high risk for disability, early, aggressive rehabilitative efforts may be more successful and cost effective than permitting the patient to have a longer period of disability with its resultant economic, social and medical consequences" (45). Others have followed in Frymoyer's footsteps (11,53,54,89,90,92, 93,151).

To scientifically determine whom should receive more versus less aggressive care, Frank has presented the concept of the "number needed to treat" to determine the cutoff for when it would be more efficient and cost-effective to substitute more aggressive treatment for a less aggressive approach (52). Basically, because most individuals who are disabled by acute LBP have a low risk for chronic disability, it would be necessary to treat a very high percentage of all disabled individuals to even make a small difference in the return to work outcomes. Frank explains "the number needed to treat" to make a significant difference in outcomes declines quickly after the first month. This is because of the facts that: (a) the pool of individuals suffering is much smaller; and (b) these individuals' likelihood of spontaneous recovery is much smaller.

According to Frank, there are three distinct stages in terms of risk of an acute episode becoming chronic (52) (Fig. 3.4):

Acute—First 4 weeks: risk of chronicity is low

Subacute—Weeks 4 to 12: risk is high "ipso facto" and the survival curve suggests aggressive treatment will be cost-effective here

Chronic—After 12 weeks: recovery halts

Frank warns that a risk factor for acute pain becoming chronic is overly aggressive acute management (therapeutic or diagnostic) (52,102). Therefore, he states, "there is ample evidence that the prognosis for most patients with LBP (who have only ordinary low back strain) is so good, even without any medically prescribed treatment, that only minimal investigation and treatment, together with substantial reassurance, is warranted" (53). Staging patients uncovers the patients at greatest risk for chronicity by the mere presence of continued disability after 4 weeks.

Individual risk factors for acute pain becoming chronic are called "yellow flags" (Table 3.4). They are divided into those related to symptoms, examination, psychosocial, functional, and work-related factors. Most are subjective and they are predominately psychosocial. In contrast to "red flags," which require urgent attention, further testing, and possibly specialist referral, "yellow flags" only require a shift in the focus of care. These risk factors have been shown to predict future chronic pain or disability in acute LBP patients (19,30,54,69,76,92,93). Some have shown that they can predict future chronic LBP in individuals before they have an episode of acute LBP (151). It has been demonstrated that formal use of a questionnaire has higher sensitivity and predictive value for identifying distressed patients than simple history taking alone (63).

In the context of disabling back pain, the individual risk factors exist alongside health care provider, workplace, and compensation risk factors (116). Williams et al showed that whereas psychosocial factors are

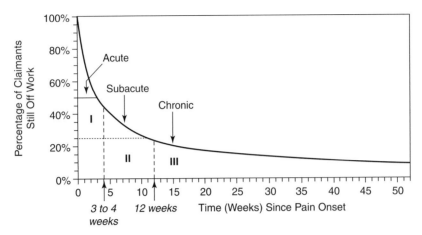

Figure 3.4 Three-phase model of low back pain natural history. From Frank JW, Kerr MS, Brooker AS, et al. Disability resulting from occupational low back pain. Part 2: What do we know about secondary prevention? Spine 1996;21:2918–2929.

Table 3.4 "Yellow Flags" Risk Factors of Chronicity

Symptoms (19,30,45,48,52,53,60,83,109,135,151,159):

- Duration of symptoms
- Sciatica
- Severe pain intensity
- Widespread pain

Physical Examination (19,33,66,77,84,148,149,170):

- Positive straight leg raise test
- Positive neurological examination (motor, sensory, reflex)
- Restriction in two or more spinal movements

Psychosocial Factors (30,43,45,66,77,92,93,109,151):

- Three or more Waddell signs of illness behavior
- Self-rated health as poor
- Fear–avoidance beliefs
- Anxiety
- Catastrophizing
- Self-efficacy
- Locus of control

Work-Related (25,26,30,33,66,69,72,92,93,109,151,173)

- Involved in compensation or litigation
- Physically demanding job (or perception of)
- Job dissatisfaction
- Disability in the previous 12 months

Functional (92,93,109)

- Light work or activity tolerance
- Sleep negatively affected by pain

significantly involved in those not returning to work, only 0.5% of workers disabled for 6 months had treatment that addressed these issues (173). Workplace dissatisfaction is a key element in those who are disabled, yet proactive policies at the workplace to facilitate return to work are not commonly seen (10,151,116). The compensation system itself is adversarial and this contributes to the problem (116).

Perpetuating Factors for Persistant Neck Conditions
Persistent neck pain is predicted by co-morbid LBP, cycling as a regular activity, older age, and being out of work (70). Whiplash Associated Disorders classification II patients with neuropsychologic problems have a worse prognosis over a 3-year follow-up period (150).

Evolution of Evidence-Based Healthcare

Practice-Based Problem

Clinicians and consumers are faced with the frustrating challenge of judging the veracity of often contradictory claims of effectiveness for a broad array of tests and treatments for spinal problems. How can one sift through the widely varying empirical claims and vast scientific literature to determine what is appropriate care?

What Is Evidence-Based Healthcare?

Introduction

Evidence-based health care (EBHC) is designed to evaluate the overwhelming volume of medical literature and disseminate the most valid and important findings to practitioners. EBHC helps clinicians to determine which management approaches (diagnostic and therapeutic) are proven effective, proven ineffective, or lacking in sufficient evidence to draw a conclusion. Those with evidence of effectiveness are typically ranked from weakest to strongest based on the quality of the studies, with RCTs given the greatest weight. Those neither proven nor unproven are usually called experimental and viewed skeptically if they are either expensive or potentially dangerous. Those that are proven ineffective are debunked and their use discouraged!

With the advent of EBHC, clinical or practice guidelines about the efficacy of different management approaches for a wide variety of health care conditions (e.g., breast cancer surgery, hysterectomy, hypertension, mammography screening) have emerged. The US Institute of Medicine (IOM) (51) defines such guidelines as "Systematically developed statements to assist practitioner and patient decisions about appropriate health care for specific clinical circumstances." Low back pain guidelines have been released throughout the world including Canada, the United States, England, Sweden, New Zealand, the Netherlands, and Denmark.

According to Chapman-Smith "the primary goal of guidelines is to improve standards of care by bringing the most up-to-date knowledge to clinical practice in a form that is easy to use" (28). Wiesel recommends that we distinguish guidelines from standards of care by virtue of their being based on expert consensus opinion rather than scientifically strong evidence (172). A major goal of guidelines players is to produce diagnostic and therapeutic protocols or algorithms with scientifically sound decision points. Eddy estimates that if strong evidence is present for all decision points that diagnosis and treatment will be appropriately directed for more than 95% of the patients of the specific disease entity (47). According to Wiesel, when only consensus-based decision points are available for algorithms, this figure decreases to 60% (172). He states that to use a guideline to influence management decisions, ". . . the physician must be prepared to modify the recommended care as the specific clinical setting dictates." This echoes the sentiments of Sackett (131) the pioneer of EBHC who says, "clinical expertise should be informed but not replaced by evidence."

The Agency for Health Care Policy and Research's (AHCPR's) introduction states the following reasons for LBP guidelines (2):

- High prevalence of low back problems in society
- High cost of the low back problem to society

- Increasing evidence that much of the care for low back problems is either inappropriate or suboptimal
  ○ Widespread variation in practice habits
- Growing body of scientific literature demonstrating evidence of ineffectiveness for certain commonly used assessment and treatment approaches

Cherkin et al surveyed a large group of medical physicians (nearly 1200 respondents) regarding their beliefs about the efficacy of different treatments for LBP (29). The only treatment that a majority recommended was physical therapy. Less than half of the physicians believed that spinal manipulation was effective, yet substantial minorities believed bed rest and narcotic analgesics were effective. The study highlighted that physicians lack a consensus on what is appropriate care for LBP. Furthermore, the only treatment they generally agreed is effective is considered by most systematic reviews and guidelines to be merely supportive (physical therapy). Most alarming is that a substantial minority believed in treatments such as bed rest and narcotic analgesics, which have been demonstrated to lack effectiveness, whereas missing from nearly half of the respondent's list was spinal manipulation—one of the only treatments that actually has evidence of effectiveness for LBP!

Summary of Major New Conclusions From Successive Guidelines

Many international teams of research methodologists, clinical scientists, and health care providers have been brought together to review the available "best evidence" for the management of low back and neck pain. Their consensus opinions do NOT represent a new standard of care, but the guidelines that have emerged have proposed a revolutionary new paradigm for managing spinal disorders. What follows is a brief summary of the most important of these international guidelines.

1987: Quebec Task Force (142)

- Specific diagnosis of acute LBP is possible in only 20% of cases
- Management different for acute stage than for later stage: 7 weeks was the cutoff
- Utility of diagnostic imaging limited and not recommended routinely
- Iatrogenic effects of bed rest prescription discussed

- Early return of patient to normal activity recommended even if pain is present

1994: Agency for Health Care Policy and Research (AHCPR) (2)

- Perform diagnostic triage with special emphasis on finding "red flags" requiring urgent attention
- Recommended very strict criteria be applied to the decision to have surgery
- Recommended spinal manipulation as one of the few primary treatment options for acute LBP requiring additional symptomatic relief

1994: Clinical Standards Advisory Group (CSAG) (31)

- Recommended biopsychosocial assessment at 6 weeks
- Described appropriate versus inappropriate use of medication

1995, 1999: Royal College of General Practitioners (RCGP) (129,130)

- Recommended consideration of referral to specialists if primary care failed (4–6 weeks)
- Recommended early identification of psychosocial risk factors of chronicity
- Recommended exercises for those not returning to normal activities within 6 weeks

1997: New Zealand (76)

- Described the psychosocial aspects of pain and how to uncover them from history
- Provided a screening questionnaire for identifying psychosocial "yellow flags" risk factors of chronicity

1999: Denmark—Danish Institute for Health Technology Assessment (39)

- First guidelines to include a health technology assessment that considered ethical issues, health care organization, and economics
- Recommended advice that emphasizes overcoming fear–avoidance behavior and that hurt does not equal harm, rather than traditional "back school" with more "careful" advice

- Specific recommendations regarding manual therapy are given
  - For patients with acute pain of more than 2 to 3 days
  - For acute recurrences or flare-ups of chronic pain
  - As part of an overall approach to manage chronic LBP
  - As part of the approach for nerve root problems
- The GP and DC are recommended as the portals to the system
- The emergency room should not be a portal except for trauma patients because such physicians lack the necessary evaluation skills

1995: Quebec Whiplash Associated Disorders (WAD) Guidelines 1995 (143)

- Recommended classification system based on signs and symptoms (see Table 1.8)
- Recommended early, active intervention (including manipulation) (see Table 35.5)

2002: Dutch Royal Physical Therapy Association and the Dutch Society of General Practitioners (133)

- Guidelines for WAD grades 1 and 2
- Active interventions such as education, exercise therapy, training of functions, and activities are recommended according to the length of time since the accident and the rate of recovery.

2003: Dutch Physiotherapy Guidelines for Low Back Pain (5)

- Distinguished between impairments, disabilities, and participation based on the International Classification of Human Functioning, Disability, and Health (171).
- Behavioral therapy incorporating a time-contingent rather than pain-contingent approach is recommended

2005: European Guidelines for the Management of Acute Nonspecific Low Back Pain in Primary Care—Preliminary Draft (50)

For Prevention of LBP

- There is limited evidence for prevention of LBP

- The most exists for physical activity/exercise and biopsychosocial eduction
- The emphasis should be on prevention of the consequences of LBP—care-seeking, disability, recurrence, work loss

For Acute LBP

- Be aware of psychosocial factors, and review them in detail if there is no improvement
- Multidisciplinary treatment programs in occupational settings may be an option for workers with subacute low back pain and sick leave for more than 4 to 8 weeks

For Chronic LBP

- Prognostic factors including psychosocial distress, depressive mood, severity of pain and functional impact, prior history, and patient expectations should be assessed
- Cognitive–behavioral, exercise, educational, and multidisciplinary (bio-psycho-social) treatment can be recommended; also, back schools and short courses of manipulative therapy
- Physical therapy modalities cannot be recommended
- Acupuncture, injections, intradiscal electrothermal therapy, spinal cord stimulation, radiofrequency lesioning of the dorsal root ganglion cannot be recommended
- Surgery cannot be recommended unless after 2 years of all other conservative measures have failed or are unavailable

Implementation of New Evidence

Practice-Based Problem

Guidelines have been published throughout the world, which summarize the scientific evidence and multidisciplinary expert consensus opinion about recent changes in clinical management. Has publication of guidelines actually improved the quality of health care for spinal disorders and if not, why not?

Although guidelines have flourished, practitioner's implementation of the suggested changes in practice has not occurred. The Fourth International Forum on Low Back Pain Research in Primary Care, in Israel in March 2000, recognized this problem and was thus entitled, "Implementation and Dissemination: Getting Research into Practice" (16). The focus of this meeting was on how to change behavior of health care providers (HCPs). Rainville showed that physician recommendations for activity restrictions and disability with chronic LBP patients vary widely and are frequently more restrictive than is recommended in consensus guidelines (124). The Paris Task Force (1) identified the following obstacles to clinical utilization of the guidelines:

- The primary care physicians seeing back patients are a diverse group difficult to reach with educational outreach
- Guidelines do not differentiate types of activity or define activity yet they all recommend it
- No discussion of tools that evaluate functional capacity
- Guidelines take a very aggressive tone with physicians in that they recommend physicians to alter behavior and admit failure
- No description of the clinical profile of the necessary specialists is given

Revolutionary changes in cardiac care incorporating early activation were readily incorporated into practice because heart patients are seen by a single speciality of physicians. In contrast, less than one-third of all patients with LBP seek care and when they do, they go to a diverse array of HCPs. In fact, the largest group are GPs who have widely differing views about proper management of LBP (29) and in whom education measures will not be nearly so simple as in cardiology (124).

According to Rossignol education must be part of a new system of care that is easy for the doctor (128). Most valuable is better explanations to patients and their participation in decision-making. Guidelines by themselves are not likely to improve quality; however, it is not because they are unnecessary. Rather, they are necessary just not sufficient.

The Danish guidelines emphasize for the first time that it is not just provider behavior that must change, but the entire health care milleau must undergo a transformation (39). Specifically, they endorse better interdisciplinary cooperation between different HCPs. They recommend that management methods should not differ substantially from HCP to HCP. To encourage these paradigm shifts common postgraduate courses should be offered for different HCPs involved in managing LBP.

Goldberg has "benchmarked" a novel approach to using education to reduce surgery rates (61). By targeting areas with high surgery rates and using a noncoercive approach, a 9% reduction in surgery rates was achieved. Surgeon study groups were used to review the scientific evidence on surgical indications and the implications of different rates of surgery. Surgeons and their patients participated in outcomes research to assess indications and outcomes of surgery. A 6-month follow-up was included and the surgeons received a report showing how they compared with their peers. Conferences for primary care providers were offered that explained what evidence-based spine care entailed. Emphasis on minimal bed rest, early return to normal activity, avoidance of early imaging, and appropriate criteria for surgical referral were all discussed. A local general physician presented essential facets of this new approach in what is called "academic detailing." Videodiscs were used for patient education of surgical candidates. An overview of the results of surgery were presented along with interviews of both satisfied and dissatisfied patients after a variety of surgical and non-surgical procedures. Lastly, a hospital intervention led by a health care economist was directed at administrative personnel and emphasized cost-effectiveness issues.

A recent Australian study revealed that significant changes in physician behavior could be achieved by a mass media campaign (18). Physicians appeared motivated partially by their more informed patients. They were found to give more reactivation advice and less prescribed bed rest than their peers who were not in a province exposed to the mass media campaign. Similar education, in Scotland, aimed directly at the consumer has shown promise (134).

Frank and Loissel have shown that in a highly complex and costly occupational setting, it may not matter as much what different strategies are offered as it does that the worksite is involved. Explicit involvement of the workplace includes workplace visits by rehabilitation specialists to negotiate individualized job modifications (52,99,100).

Shared decision-making is another proposed solution to meeting the needs of the various players involved in back pain. In shared decision-making, the patient is involved with the clinician in choosing among different options. This empowers patients by giving them some control over the decision-making process. By involving the patient in this process, it has the potential to increase their satisfaction with the process regardless of outcome. Studies involving patients with heart disease have shown that through shared decision-making patients become both more knowledgeable and confident (88,110). Such an approach was recently used with prospective surgical candidates for lumbar disc surgery. It was shown that an interactive video program facilitated patient decision-making about their treatment (121).

Von Korff proposed that HCPs should negotiate with their patients their respective roles, responsibilities, and expectations (166). The HCP is the trainer and the patient is the active participant. A key to the success of such active participation is mutually agreed on goals. Back problems with their recurrent natural histories are more like asthma or diabetes. Like such chronic illnesses, treatment is not likely to be successful without a self-care component (166).

Is EBHC actually better than traditional care?

EBHC may be based on the "best evidence," but is it *itself* evidence-based? A recent Australian trial compared evidence based care to traditional care (108). Patients were assessed at baseline, 3 months, 6 months, and 12 months. X-ray utilization was 7% in the experimental group compared to 30% in traditional care group. Bed rest was recommended only 2% of the time in the evidence-based group versus 40% in the traditional group. The traditional care group recommended opiates 25% of the time. At 12 months, 71% of the evidence-based patients were fully recovered, compared to 56% of the traditional care group. Most impressively, quality was achieved at a reduced cost. The traditional care costed 71% more than the evidence-based care.

Limitations of Evidence-Based Healthcare

Although guidelines have been a boon to clinicians and consumers alike, they are far from perfect. What if any are the specific limitations of low back pain guidelines? While they recommend the goal of increasing activity tolerance, there is very little in the guidelines about how to improve patient's activity tolerance (1)! There is insufficient evidence that they improve the quality or reduce the cost of care. In fact, in physical medicine there is often a scarcity of high-quality evidence. In such an instance, there is a danger of giving too much weight to the evidence and underestimating how little is actually known (152).

The Quebec Task Force acknowledged that an accurate diagnosis of LBP is possible less than 20% of the time (142). However, merely because it is difficult to diagnose subtypes of LBP does not mean they don't exist. Laboeuf-Yde has described how non-specific LBP is most likely made up of several specific subtypes that are not yet identified (81,82). As discussed in chapter 1, new classification schemes are emerging that show that improved care results from identification of the subclassifications of "non-specific" LBP patients (46,49,56).

Improving the Quality of Evidence-Based Guidelines

For EBHC to be the "benchmark" for quality in health care, a rigorous ongoing process called total quality improvement is needed. Of course, quality must be achieved at a reasonable cost. Frymoyer defined value as the ratio of quality to cost (58). Success depends on flexibility, ongoing review, and participation of all the "players." From the patient's perspective, effective guidelines must be clear, specific, and unambiguous (161).

According to the Institute of Medicine (51) and U.K. National Health Service (114), good guidelines should adhere to certain criteria:

- Define their target disorder
- Adhere to scientifically rigorous standards
- Be user-friendly
- Lend themselves to audit processes
- Include distribution plans
- Include implementation plans
- Include regular, future reviews

Important outcomes to measure to determine the usefulness of guidelines include (161):

a) Patient-centered outcomes such as pain reduction, function, return to work, and satisfaction
b) Health care utilization costs
c) Cost of developing, implementing, and updating guidelines

To stay abreast of new knowledge groups, the Cochrane Collaboration provides updates of new evidence (32). Periodic updates of guidelines are necessary. No established criteria for guideline revision exists. Shekelle suggests guidelines should be revised when (138):

- Significant changes occur in the scientific literature
- New methods emerge
- New outcomes are deemed appropriate
- There is a change in the availability of health care resources

On reviewing 17 different guidelines published by AHCPR between 1990 and 1996, Shekelle et al estimated that half of the guidelines were outdated after 5.8 years (139). The authors suggest that guidelines should be evaluated for validity every 3 years.

The Institute for Musculoskeletal Research and Clinical Implementation (IMRCI) developed an audit for use in England to help HCPs provide the highest possible quality care in the first 6 weeks of a low back episode (17) (see Chapter 39). The audit offers evidence-based recommendations on specific aspects of care. The audit may guide care or can be used retrospectively to see where changes could be made to optimize future care. Action steps, supportive evidence, and chart review are all described in detail. Another British group has formed to help GPs learn how to identify appropriate decision points for referring to specialists (115).

Guidelines are considered by many HCPs as merely a current trend. Such thinking is prejudiced by those who hold to untested belief systems (113,153). It is the challenge of those who believe in an unproven approach to secure funding for the necessary research to demonstrate the validity of the methods. However, lack of evidence of effectiveness is NOT the same thing as evidence of ineffectiveness. In fact, certain erroneous conclusions can be reached if it is assumed that all patients are alike. Researchers may prefer homogenous populations of individuals, but clinicians know that each patient is unique.

■ CONCLUSION

LBP is an epidemic problem in which certain advances are known but not generally used. The natural history is not as brief as has been believed, with most patients suffering prolonged symptoms and activity intolerances after acute episodes. Although it is not clear why most individuals have acute LBP, we now know that acute pain becomes chronic primarily as a result of psychosocial factors.

The focus in care has traditionally taken two contrasting paths. One path is typified by limiting care for acute and subacute patients (medication and rest). The other path involves maximizing care for chronic patients (i.e., diagnostic imaging and surgery).

The evidence points us in a different direction. Namely, that secondary preventive efforts should target individuals at "high risk" for chronic pain while they are in the subacute phase. This management does not necessitate aggressive imaging or surgery on these patients, but rather orients care toward restoring function and addressing psychosocial problems such as fear–avoidance beliefs and distress/depression.

How to improve implementation of this new evidence is a major question. Unlike cardiovascular problems in which only one specialty dominates care, patients with spine problems are seen by myriad HCPs. To get all the "players on the same side of the ball"—patients, HCPs, insurers, government, and employers—is a major challenge for those interested in solving this epidemic problem.

Audit Process
Self-Check of the Chapter's Learning Objectives

- What is the likelihood of your patient having achieved a satisfactory recover at 3 weeks and 7 weeks?

- What are examples of specific "yellow flag" risk factors of chronicity?

- What new information have the various international low back pain management guidelines given you regarding patient care?

- Are you aware of commonly used assessment and treatment approaches that are not recommended by the various guidelines?

  —For instance, x-rays for acute LBP without "red flags"

- Are you aware of assessment and treatment approaches that you were not previously using or referring for that are recommended by the various guidelines?

  —For instance, manipulation for acute LBP without "red flags"

■ REFERENCES

1. Abenheim L, Rossignol M, Valat JP, et al. The role of activity in the therapeutic management of back pain: Report of the International Paris Task Force on Back Pain. Spine 2000;25(4):1S–33S.

2. Agency for Health Care Policy and Research (AHCPR). Acute low-back problems in adults. Clinical Practice Guideline Number 14. Washington D.C.: U.S. Government Printing Office, 1994.

3. Battie MC, Bigos SJ, Fisher LD, et al. A prospective study of the role of cardiovascular risk factors and fitness in industrial back pain complaints. Spine 1989;14(2):141–147.

4. Battie MC, Bigos SJ, Fisher LD, et al. The role of spinal flexibility in back pain complaints within industry: A prospective study. Spine 1990;15: 768–773.

5. Bekkering GE, Hendrriks HJM, Koes BW, et al. Dutch physiotherapy guidelines for low back pain. Physiotherapy 2003;89:82–96.

6. Berquist-Ullman M, Larsson U. Acute low back pain in industry. Acta Orthop Scand Suppl 1977;170:1.

7. Biering-Sorensen F. A prospective study of low back pain in a general population. I. Occurrence, recurrence, and etiology. Scand J Rehabil Med 1983;15:71.

8. Biering-Sorensen F. Physical measurements as risk indicators for low-back trouble over a 1-year period. Spine 1984;9:106–119.

9. Biering-Sorensen F, Thomsen CE, Hilden J. Risk indicators for low back trouble. Scan J Rehabil Med 1989;21:151–157.

10. Bigos SJ, Battie MC, Spengler DM, et al. A prospective study of work perceptions and psychological factors affecting the report of back injury. Spine 1991;15:1–6.

11. Bolton JE. Evaluation and treatment of back pain patients. Eur J Chir 1994:42;29–40.

12. Boos N, Semmer N, Elfering A, et al. Natural history of individuals with asymptomatic disc abnormalities in magnetic resonance imaging predictors of low back pain-related medical consultation and work incapacity Spine 2000;25:1484–1492.

13. Borchgrevink GE, Leriem I. Symptoms in patients with neck injury after a car crash: A retrospective study. Tidsskr Nor Laegeforen 1992;112:884–886.

14. Borchgrevink GE, Kaasa A, McDonoagh D, et al. Acute treatment of whiplash neck sprain injuries. Spine 1998;23:25–31.

15. Borenstein G, et al. A 7-year follow-up study of the value of lumbar spine MR to predict the development of low back pain in asymptomatic individuals. Presented to International Society for the Study of the Lumbar Spine, Brussels, June 9–13, 1998.

16. Borkan J, Van Tulder M, Reis S, Schoene ML, Croft P, Hermoni D. Advances in the field of low back pain in primary care: A Report from the Fourth International Forum. Spine 2002;27:E128–E132.

17. Breen AC, Langworthy J, Vogel S, et al. Primary Care Audit Toolkit: Acute Back Pain. Bournemouth: Institute for Musculoskeletal Research and Clinical Implementation, (www.imrci.ac.uk) 2000.

18. Buchbinder R, Jolley D, Wyatt M. 2001 Volvo Award Winner in Clinical Studies: Effects of a media campaign on back pain beliefs and its potential influence on management of low back pain in general practice. Spine 2001;26:2535–2542.

19. Burton AK, Tillotson K, Main C, Hollis M. Psychosocial predictors of outcome in acute and subacute low back trouble. Spine 1995;20:722–728.

20. Butler RJ, Johnson WG, Baldwin ML. Managing work disability: Why first return to work is not a measure of success. Industrial and Labor Relations Review. 1995;48(3):452–469.

21. Burton AK, Waddell G. Educational and informational approaches. In: Linton SL, ed. New avenues for the prevention of chronic musculoskeletal pain and disability. Amsterdam: Elsevier, 2002.

22. Cady LD, Bischoff LP, O'Connel ER, et al. Strength and fitness and subsequent back injuries in firefighters. J Occup Med 1979;21:269.

23. Carey TS, Mills Garret J, Jackman AM. Beyond the good prognosis. Spine 2000:25:115–120.

24. Carroll LJ, Cassidy JD, Cote P. Depression as a risk factor for onset of an episode of troublesome neck and low back pain. Pain 2004;107:134–139.

25. Cats-Baril WL, Frymoyer JW. Demographic factors associated with the prevalence of disability in the general population: Analysis of the NHANES I database. Spine 1991;16:671–674.

26. Cats-Baril WL, Frymoyer JW. Identifying patients at risk of becoming disabled because of low-back pain. The Vermont Rehabilitation Engineering Center predictive model. Spine 1991;16:605–607.

27. Chaffin DB, Herrin GD, Keyserling WM. Preemployment strength testing: An updated position. J Occup Med 1978;20(6):403–408.

28. Chapman-Smith D. Back pain guidelines from Denmark. The Chiropractic Report 2000;14(5):3.

29. Cherkin DC, Deyo RA, Wheeler K, Ciol MA. Physician views about treating low back pain: The results of a national survey. Spine 1995;20(1):1–10.

30. Cherkin DC, Deyo RA, Street JH, Barlow W. Predicting poor outcomes for back pain seen in primary care using patients' own criteria. Spine 1996;21:2900–2907.

31. Clinical Standards Advisory Group (CSAG). Back Pain. Report of a CSAG committee on back pain. London: HMSO, 1994.

32. Cochrane library http://www.cochranelibrary.net (Health Communication Network).

33. Coste J, Delecoeuillerie G, Cohen De Lara A, Le Parc JM, Paolaggi J. Clinical course and prognositc factors in acute low back pain: An inception cohort study in primary care practice. BMJ 1994;308:577–580.

34. Cote P, Cassidy JD, Carroll L. The factors associated with neck pain and its related disability in the Saskatchewan population. Spine 2000;25(9):1109–1117.

35. Cote P, Cassidy JD, Carroll L, Kirstman V. The annual incidence and course of neck pain in the general population: A population-based cohort study. Pain 2004;112:267–273.

36. Croft PR, Macfarlane GJ, Papageorgiou AC, Thomas E, Silman AJ. Outcome of low back pain in general practice: A prospective study. BMJ 1998;316:1356–1359.

37. Croft PR, Papageorgiou AC, Thomas E, Macfarlane GJ, Silman AJ. Short-term physical risk factors for new episodes of low back pain: Prospective evidence from the South Manchester Back Pain Study. Spine 1999;24(15):1556–1561.

38. Croft PR, Lewis M, Papageorgiou AC, et al. Risk factors for neck pain: A longitudinal study in the general population. Pain 2001;93:317–325.

39. Danish Health Technology Assessment (DIHTA). Manniche C, et al. Low back pain: Frequency Management and Prevention from an HAD Perspective, 1999.

40. Deyo RA. Low back pain—A primary care challenge. Spine 1996;21:2826–2832.

41. Deyo RA, Rainville J, Kent DL. What can history and physical examination tell us about low back pain? J Am Med Assoc 1992;268:760–765.

42. Deyo RA, Bass JE. Lifestyle and low back pain. The influence of smoking and obesity. Spine 1989;14:501–506.

43. Deyo RA, Battie M, Beurskens AJ, et al. Outcome measures for low back pain research. Spine 1998;23:2003–2013.

44. Deyo RA, Weinstein JN. Low back pain. N Engl J Med 2001;344:363–370.

45. Dionne CE, Koepsell TD, Von Korff M, et al. Predicting long-term functional limitations amount back pain patients in primary care settings. J Clin Epidemiol 1997;30:31–43.

46. Dreyfuss P, Michaelsen M, Pauza K, McLarty J, Bogduk N. The value of medical history and physical examination in diagnosing sacroiliac joint pain. Spine 1996;21:2594–2602.

47. Eddy DM. A Manual for Assessing Health Practices and Designing Practice Policies: The Explicit Approach. Philadelphia: American College of Physicians, 1991.

48. Epping-Jordan JE, Wahlgren DR, Williams RA, et al. Transition to chronic pain in men with low-back pain: Predictive relationships among pain intensity, disability, and depressive symptoms. Health Psychol 1998;17:421–427.

49. Erhard RE, Delitto A. Relative effectiveness of an extension program and a combined program of manipulation and flexion and extension exercises in patients with acute low back syndrome. Phys Ther 1994;74:1093–1100.

50. European Guidelines for the management of acute nonspecific low back pain in primary care—preliminary draft—http://www.backpaineurope.org.

51. Field MJ, Lohr KN, eds. Guidelines for Clinical Practice: From Development to Youth. Institute of Medicine. Washington, DC: National Academy Press, 1992.

52. Frank J, Sinclair S, Hogg-Johnson S, et al. Preventing disability from work-related low-back pain. New evidence gives new hope—if we can just get all the players onside. Can Med Assoc J 1998;158:1625–1631.

53. Frank JW, Kerr MS, Brooker AS, et al. Disability resulting from occupational low back pain. Part 2: What do we know about secondary prevention? Spine 1996;21:2918–2929.

54. Fransen M, Woodward M, Norton R, Coggan C, Dawe M, Sheridan N. Risk factors associated with the transition from acute to chronic occupational back pain. Spine 2002;27:92–98.

55. Friedlieb OP. The impact of managed care on the diagnosis and treatment of low back pain. Am J Medi Qual 1994;9(1):24–29.

56. Fritz JM, George S. The use of a classification approach to identify subgroups of patients with acute low back pain. Spine 2000;1:106–114.

57. Frymoyer JW. Predicting disability from low back pain. Clin Orth 1992;279:107.

58. Frymoyer JW. Quality: An international challenge to the diagnosis and treatment of disorders of the lumbar spine. Spine 1993;18:2147–2152.

59. Gargan MR, Bannister GC. Long-term prognosis of soft-tissue injuries of the neck. J Bone Joint Surg (Br) 1990;72:901–903.

60. Gatchel R, Polatin PB, Kinney RK. Predicting outcome of chronic back pain using clinical predictors of psychopathology: A prospective analysis. Health Psychol 1995;14:415–420.

61. Goldberg HI, et al. Can evidence change the rate of back surgery? A randomized controlled trial of community-based education. Effect Clin Pract 2001:95–104.

62. Gonzalez-Urzelai V, Palacio-Elua L, Jopez de Munain J. Routine primary care management of acute low back pain: adherence to clinical guidelines. Eur Spine J 2003;12:589–594.

63. Grevitt M, Pande K, O'dowd J, Webb J. Do first impressions count? A comparison of subjective and psychologic assessment of spinal patients. Eur Spine J 1998;7:218–223.

64. Gyntelberg F. One year incidence of low back pain among male residents of Copenhagen age 40–59. Danish Medical Bulletin 1974;21:30–36.

65. Hadler NM. Regional back pain. N Engl J Med 1986;315:1090–2.

66. Haldorsen EMH, Inhalhl A, Ursin H. Patients with low-back pain not returning to work. A 12-month follow-up study. Spine 1998;23:1202–1208.

67. Harreby M, Hesselsoe G, Kjer J, Neergaard K. Low back pain and physical exercise in leisure-time in 38 year old men and women: A 25 year prospective cohort study of 640 school children. Eur Spine J 1997;6:181–186.

68. Hashemi L, Webster BS, Clancy EA, Volinn E. Length of disability and cost of workers' compensation low back pain claims. J Occup Environ Med 1998;40:261–269.

69. Hazard RG, Haugh LD, Reid S, Preble JB, MacDonald L. Early prediction of chronic disability after occupational low back injury. Spine 1996;21:945–951.

70. Hill J, Lewis M, Papageorgiou AC, Dziedzic K, Croft P. Predicting persistent neck pain. A 1-year follow-up of a population cohort. Spine 2004;29:1648–1654.

71. Hillman M, Wright A, Raujaratnam G, et al. Prevalence of low back pain in the community: Implications for service provision in Bradford, UK. J Epidemiol Commun Health 1996;50:347–352.

72. Hoogendoorn WE, van Poppel MNM, Bongers PM, Koes BW, Bouter LM. Systematic review of psychosocial factors at work and private life as risk factors for back pain. Spine 2000;25(16):2114–2125.

73. Hrubec A, Nashbold BS Jr. Epidemiology of lumbar disc lesions in the military in World War II. Am J Epidemiol 1975;102:366–376.

74. Indahl A, Haldorsen EH, Holm S, Reikeras O, Hursin H. Five-year follow-up study of a controlled clinical trial using light mobilization and an informative approach to low back pain. Spine 1998;23:2625–2630.

75. Jacob T, Baras M, Zeev A, Epstein L. A longitudinal, community-based study of low back pain outcomes. Spine 2004;29:1810–1817.

76. Kendall NAS, Linton SJ, Main CJ. Guide to assessing psychological yellow flags in acute low back pain: Risk factors for long-term disability and work loss. Wellington, New Zealand: Accident Rehabilitation & Compensation Insurance Corporation of New Zealand and the National Health Committee, 1997.

77. Klenerman L, Slade P, Stanley I, et al. The prediction of chronicity in patients with an acute attack of low back pain in a general practice setting. Spine 1995;20:478–484.

78. Kopec JA, Sayre EC, Esdaile J. Predictors of back pain in the general population. Spine 2003;29:70–78.

79. Leboef-Yde C, Lauritsen JM. The prevalence of low back pain in the literature: A structured review of 26 Nordic studies from 1954 to 1993. Spine 1995;20:2112–2118.

80. Laboeuf-Yde C. Smoking and low back pain: A systematic literature review of 41 journal articles reporting 47 epidemiologic studies. Spine 1999;24:1463–1470.

81. Laboeuf-Yde C, Manniche C. Low back pain: Time to get off the treadmill. JMPT 2001;24:63–65.

82. Laboeuf-Yde C, Lauritsen JM, Lauritzen T. Why has the search for causes of low back pain largely been nonconclusive? Spine 1997;22:877–881.

83. Lancourt J, Ketteljut M. Predicting return to work for lower back pain patients receiving worker's compensation. Spine 1992;17:629–640.

84. Lanier DC, Stockton P. Clinical predictors of outcome of actue episodes of low-back pain. J Fam Pract 1988;27:483–489.

85. Larequi-Lauber T, Vader JP, Burnand B, et al. Appropriateness of indications for surgery of lumbar disc hernia and spinal stenosis. Spine 1997;22(2):203–209.

86. Lawrence JS. Rheumatism in populations. London: Heinemann, 1977.

87. Leino P. Does lesiure time physical activity prevent low back disorders? A prospective study of metal industry employees. Spine 1993;18:863–871.

88. Liao L, et al. Impact of an interactive video on decision making of patients with ischemic heart disease. J Gen Intern Med 1996;11:373–376.

89. Liebenson C, Yeomans S. Identification of the patient at risk for persistent or recurrent low back trouble. In: Yeomans S, ed. The clinical application of outcomes assessment. Stamford, CT: Appleton & Lange, 1999.

90. Liebenson CS, Yeomans SG. Yellow Flags: Early identification of risk factors of chronicity in acute patients. J Rehabil Outcomes Meas 2000;4(2):31–40.

91. Liles DH, Deivanayagam S, Ayoub MM, Mahajan P. A job severity index for the evaluation and control of lifting injury. Hum Factors 1984;26:683–693.

92. Linton SJ, Hallden K. Risk factors and the natural course of acute and recurrent musculoskeletal pain: Developing a screening instrument. In: Jensen TS, Turner JA, Wiesenfeld-Hallin Z, eds. Proceedings of the 8th World Congress on Pain, Progress in Pain Research and Management, vol 8. ed. Seattle: IASP Press, 1997.

93. Linton SJ, Hallden BH. Can we screen for problematic back pain? A screening questionnaire for predicting outcome in acute and subacute back pain. Clin J Pain 1998;14:1–7.

94. Linton SJ. Psychological risk factors for neck and back pain. In: Nachemson A, Jonsson E, eds. Swedish SBU report. Evidence-based treatment for back pain. Stockholm/Philadelphia, Swedish Council on Technology Assessment in Health Care (SBU)/Lippincott (English translation), 2000:75.

95. Linton SJ. A review of psychological risk factors in back and neck pain. Spine 2000;9:1148–1156.

96. Linton SJ, Buer N, Vlaeyen J, Hellsing AL. Are fear-avoidance beliefs related to a new episode of back pain? A prospective study. Psychol Health 2000;14;1051–1059.

97. Linton SJ. Cognitive-behavioral therapy in the prevention of musculoskeletal pain: Description of a program. In: Linton SL, ed. New avenues for the prevention of chronic musculoskeletal pain and disability. Amsterdam: Elsevier, 2002.

98. Lloyd DCEF, Troup JDG. Recurrent back pain and its prediction. J Soc Occup Med 1983;33:66–74.

99. Loisel P, Abenhaim L, Durand P, et al. A population-based, randomized clinical trial on back pain management. Spine 1997;22:2911–2918.

100. Loisel P, Gosselin L, Durand P, Lemaire J, Poitras S, Abenhaim L. Implementation of a participatory ergonomics program in the rehabilitation of workers suffering from subacute back pain. Appl Ergon 2001;32(1):53–60.

101. Luoto S, Heliovaara M, Hurri H, Alaranta H. Static back endurance and the risk of low-back pain. Clin Biomech 1995;10:323–324.

102. Mahmoud MA, et al. Clinical management and the duration of disability for work-related low back pain. J Occup Environ Med 2000;42:1178–1187.

103. Maimaris C, Barnes MR, Allen MJ. 'Whiplash injuries' of the neck: A retrospective study. Injury 1988;19:393–396.

104. Malmivaara A, Hakkinen U, Aro T, et al. The treatment of acute low back pain—bed rest, exercises, or ordinary activity? N Engl J Med 1995;332:351–355.

105. Makela M, Heliovaara M, Sievers K, Impivaara O, Knekt P, Aromaa A. Prevalence, determinants, and consequences of chronic neck pain in Finland. Am J Epidemiol 1991;134:1356–1367.

106. Marhold C, Linton SJ, Melin L. Cognitive-behavioral return-to-work program: Effects on pain patients with a history of long-term versus short-term sick leave. Pain 2001;91:155–163.

107. Mason V. The prevalence of back pain in Great Britain. Office of Population C Censuses and Surverys, Social Survey Division (now Office of National Statistics). London: Her Majesty's Stationery Office, 1994:1–2.

108. McGuirk B, King W, Govind J, Lowry J, Bogduk N. Safety, efficacy, and cost-effectiveness of evidence-based guidelines for the management of acute low back pain in primary care. Spine 2001;26:2615–2622.

109. McIntosh G, Frank J, Hogg-Johnson S, Bombardier C, Hall H. Prognostic factors for time receiving workers' compensation benefits in a cohort of patients with low back pain. Spine 2000;25:147–157.

110. Morgan MW, Deber HA, Llewellyn-Thomas H, et al. A randomized trial of the ischemic heart disease shared decision making program: An evaluation of a decision aid (abstract). J Gen Intern Med 1997;12(Suppl):62.

111. Nachemson A, Waddell G, Norlund AI. Epidemiology of neck and low back pain. In: Nachemson A, Jonsson E, eds. Swedish SBU report. Evidence-based treatment for back pain. Stockholm/Philadelphia, Swedish Council on Technology

Assessment in Health Care (SBU)/Lippincott (English translation), 2000b.

112. Nachemson A, Vingard E. Influences of individual factors and smoking on neck and low back pain. In: Nachemson A, Jonsson E, eds. Swedish SBU report. Evidence-based treatment for back pain. Stockholm/Philadelphia, Swedish Council on Technology Assessment in Health Care (SBU)/Lippincott (English translation), 2000c.

113. Nachemson A, Jonsson E, eds. Swedish SBU report. Evidence-based treatment for back pain. Stockholm/Philadelphia, Swedish Council on Technology Assessment in Health Care (SBU)/Lippincott (English translation), 2000.

114. National Health Service Executive. Effective Health Care: Implementing Clinical Guidelines, N Report No. 8: Can guidelines be used to improve clinical practice? 1994:1–12, Leeds.

115. National Institute for Clinical Excellence. Referral Advice: A guide to appropriate referral from general to specialist services London, December 2001. www.nice.nhs.uk.

116. Nicholas MK. Reducing disability in injured workers: The importance of collaborative management. In: Linton SL, ed. New avenues for the prevention of chronic musculoskeletal pain and disability. Amsterdam: Elsevier, 2002.

117. Olsson I, Bunketorp O, Carlsson G, et al. An in-depth study of neck injuries in rear end collisions. IRCOBI 1990:269–280.

118. Papegeorgiu AC, Croft PR, Ferry S, et al. Estimating the prevalence of low back pain in the general population: Evidence from the South Manchester back pain survey. Spine 1995;20:1889–1894.

119. Papegeorgiu AC, Croft PR, Thomas E, et al. Influence of previous pain experience on the episode incidence of low back pain: Results from the South Manchester back pain survey. Pain 1996;66:181–185.

120. Papegeorgiu AC, Macfarlane GJ, Thomas E, et al. Psychosocial factors in the workplace: Do they predict new episodes of low back pain? Evidence from the South Manchester back pain survey. Spine 1997;22:1137–1142.

121. Phelan EA, Deyo RA, Cherkin DC, et al. Helping patients decide about back surgery: A randomized trial of an interactive video program. Spine 2001;26(2):206–212.

122. Pincus T, Vlaeyen JWS, Kendall NAS, Von Korff MR, KAlauokalani DA, Reis S. Cognitive-behavioral therapy and psychosocial factors in low back pain. Spine 2002;27:E133–E138.

123. Power C, Frank J, Hertzman C, Shierhout G, Li L. Predictors of low back pain onset in a prospective British study. Am J Public Health 2001;91:1671–1678.

124. Rainville J, Carlson N, Polatin P, Gatchel R, Indahl A. Exploration of physician's recommendations for activities in chronic low back pain. Spine 2000;25(17):2210–2220.

125. Ready AE. Boreskie SL, Law SA, Russell R. Fitness and lifestyle parameters fail to predict back injuries in nurses. Can J Appl Physiol 1993;18(1):80–90.

126. Riihimaki H, Viikari-Juntura E, Moeta G, Kuha J, Videman T, Tola S. Incidence of sciatic pain among

men in machine operating, dynamic physical work, and sedentary work: A 3-year follow-up. Spine 1994;19(2):138–142.

127. Rossignol M, Lortie M, Ledoux E. Comparison of spinal health indicators in predicting spinal status in a 1-year longitudinal study. Spine 1993;18(1):54–60.

128. Rossignol M. Coordination of Primary Health Care for Back Pain. Spine 2000;25: 251–259.

129. Royal College of General Practitioners (RCGP). The development and implementation of clinical guidelines. Report of the Clinical Guidelines Working Group. London, Royal College of General Practitioners, 1995:1–30.

130. Royal College of General Practitioners (RCGP). Clinical Guidelines for the Management of Acute Low Back Pain. London, Royal College of General Practitioners (www.rcgp.org.uk), 1999.

131. Sackett DL, Rosenberg WMC, Muir Gray JA, Haynes BA, Richardson W. Evidence-based medicine: What it is and what it isn't. Br Med J 1996;312:71–72.

132. SCB. Undersokningar av levnadsforhalleanden, ULF [National household surveys]. Stockholm, 1996.

133. Scholten-Peeters GGM, Bekkering GE, Verhagen AP, et al. Clinical Practice Guideline for the Physiotherapy of Patients With Whiplash-Associated Disorders. Spine 2002;27:412–422.

134. Scotland's Work Backs Partnership. Working Backs Scotland 2000, www.workingbacksscotland.com.

135. Selim AJ, Xinhua SR, Graeme F, et al. The importance of radiating leg pain in assessing health outcomes among patients with low back pain. Spine 1998;23:470–474.

136. Shaw WS, Feuerstein M, Huang GD. Secondary prevention in the workplace. In: Linton SL, ed. New avenues for the prevention of chronic musculoskeletal pain and disability. Amsterdam: Elsevier, 2002.

137. Shekelle PG, Markovich M, Louie R. An epidemiologic study of episodes of back pain care. Spine 1995;20:1668–1673.

138. Shekelle PG, Eccles MP, Grimshaw HM, Woolf SH. When should guidelines be updated? Br Med J 2001;323:155–157.

139. Shekelle PG, et al. Validity of the Agency for Health Care Policy and Research clinical practice guidelines: How quickly do guidelines become outdated? JAMA 2001;286:1461–1471.

140. Siivola SM, Levoska S, Latvala K, Horkio E, Vanharanta H, Keinanen-Kiukaanniemi S. Predictive factors for neck and shoulder pain: A longitudinal study in young adults. Spine 2004;29:1662–1669.

141. Skovron ML, Szpalski M, Nordin M, et al. Sociocultural factors and back pain: A population-based study in Belgian adults. Spine 1994;19:129–137.

142. Spitzer WO, Le Blanc FE, Dupuis M, et al. Scientific approach to the assessment and management of activity-related spinal disorders: A monograph for clinicians. Report of the Quebec Task Force on Spinal Disorders. Spine 1987;12(suppl 7):S1–S59.

143. Spitzer WO, Skovron ML, Salmi LIR, et al. Scientific monograph of the Quebec Task Force on Whiplash-Associated Disorders: Redefining "Whiplash" and its management. Spine 1995;20(Supp):S1–S73.

144. Stevenson JM, Weber CL, Smith JT, Dumas GA, Albert WJ. A longitudinal study of the development of low back pain in an industrial population. Spine 2001;26:1370–1377.

145. Svenssson HO, Andersson GBJ. A retrospective study of low back pain in 38 to 64 year old women: Frequency and occurrence and impact on medical services. Spine;1988;13:548–552.

146. Symmons DPM, van Hemert AM, Vandenbrouke JP, Valkenburg HA. A longitudinal study of back pain and radiological changes in the lumbar spines of middle-aged women.II. Radiographic findings. Annals of the Rheumatic Diseases 1991;50:162–166.

147. Szpalski M, Nordin M, Skovron ML, et al. Health care utilization for low back pain in Belgium. Influence of sociocultural factors and health beliefs. Spine 1995;20:431–442.

148. Takala EP, Vikari-Juntura E. Do functional tests predict low back pain. Spine 2000;25(16):2126–2132.

149. Taylor H, Curran NM. The Nuprin Pain Report. New York: Louis Harris and Associates, 1985:1–233.

150. Tenenbaum A, Rivano-Fischer M, Tjell C, Edblom M, Sunnerhagen KS. The Quebec Classification and a new Swedish classification for whiplash-associated disorders in relation to life satisfaction in patients at high risk of chronic functional impairment and disability. J Rehabil Med 2002;34:114–118.

151. Thomas E, Silman AJ, Croft PR, Papageorgiou AC, Jayson MIV, Macfarlane GJ. Predicting who develops chronic low back pain in primary care: a prospective study. BMJ 1999;318:1662–1667.

152. Tonelli MR. In defense of expert opinion. Academic Medicine 1999:74;1187–1192.

153. Trial and error. Economist 1998;93.

154. Troup JDG, Foreman TK, Baxter CE, Brown D. The perception of back pain and the role of psychophysical tests of lifting capacity. Spine 1987;12:645–657.

155. Truchon M, Fillion L. Biopsychosocial determinants of chronic disability and low-back pain: A review. J Occup Rehab 2000;10:117–142.

156. Tuback F, Leclerc A. Natural history of sciatica, presented at the annual meeting of the American College of Rheumatology, Philadelphia, 2000.

157. UK General Household Surveys. London: Office of National Statistics.

158. Ursiny J, et al. Managing the costs of care for low back pain: Experience within a large health care delivery system, presented at the annual meeting of the American College of Rheumatology, Philadelphia, 2000.

159. van den Hoogen HJM, Koes BW, Deville W, van Eijk JTM, Bouter LM. The prognosis of low back pain in general practice. Spine 1997;22:1515–1521.

160. van den Hoogen HJM, Koes BW, van Eijk JTM, Bouter LM, Deville W. On the course of low back pain in general practice: A 1-year follow-up study. Ann Rheum Dis 1998;57:13–19.

161. Van Tulder WE, Croft PR, van Splunteren P, et al. Disseminating and implementing the results of back pain research in primary care. Spine 2002;27:E121–E127.

162. Versteegen GJ, Kingma J, Miejler WJ, ten Duis HJ. Neck sprain not arising from car accidents: A retrospective study covering 25 years. Eur Spine J 1998;7:201–205.

163. Videman T, Sarna S, Battie MC, et al. The long-term effects of physical loading and exercise lifestyles on back-related symptoms, disability and spinal pathology among men. Spine 1995;20:699–709.

164. Vingard E, Nachemson A. Work related influences on neck and low back pain. In: Nachemson A, Jonsson E, eds. Swedish SBU report. Evidence-based treatment for back pain. Stockholm/Philadelphia, Swedish Council on Technology Assessment in Health Care (SBU)/Lippincott (English translation), 2000.

165. Von Korff M, Deyo RA, Cherkin D, Barlow W. Back pain in primary care: Outcomes at 1 year. Spine 1993;18:855–862.

166. Von Korff M. Collaborative care. Ann Intern Med 1997;127:187–195.

167. Waddell G. The Back Pain Revolution, 2nd ed. Edinburgh: Churchill Livingstone, 2004.

168. Waddell G, Burton AK. Occupational health guidelines for the management of low back pain at work—evidence review. London: Faculty of Occupational Medicine, 2000.

169. Walsh K, Crudda M, Coggon D. Low back pain in eight areas of Britain. J Epidemiol Commun Health 1992;46:227–230.

170. Werneke M, Hart DL. Centralization phenomenon as a prognostic factor for chronic low back pain and disability. Spine 2001;26:758–765.

171. World Health Organization. International Classification of Human Functioning, Disability and Health: IC, WHO, Geneva 2001.

172. Wiesel SW. 1999 International society for the study of the lumbar spine presidential address: Let the froth settle education and quality care: Our other missions. Spine 2000;25(12): 1468–1470.

173. Williams DA, Feuerstein M, Durbin D, Pezzulo J. Healthcare and indemnity costs across the natural history of disability in occupational low back pain. Spine 1998;23(21):2329–2336.

174. Williams RA, Pruitt SD, Doctor JN, et al. The contribution of job satisfaction to the transition from acute to chronic low back pain. Arch Phys Med Rehabil 1998;79:366–373.

4

Putting the Biopsychosocial Model into Practice

Craig Liebenson

Introduction

The Biopsychosocial Model

Overemphasis on a Structural Diagnosis

Overemphasis on Bed Rest

Overuse of Surgery

Abnormal Illness Behavior

Diagnostic Triage to Rehabilitation—The Benchmark

Reassurance/Diagnostic Triage

Reactivation Advice

Relief of Pain

Re-Evaluation of Structural, Functional, and Psychosocial Contributors to Continued Pain or Disability

Reconditioning

Referral

Practitioner Audit

Learning Objectives

After reading this chapter you should be able to:

- Understand the limitations of a biomedical approach in managing spine pain patients
- Understand the importance of functional reactivation as a guiding principle in spine patient care
- Understand the importance of psychosocial factors such as fear–avoidance behavior in a patient when there is failure to achieve a satisfactory outcome
- Understand the "decision points" of care when implementing the biopsychosocial model into clinical practice

"Let fear, then be a kind of pain or disturbance resulting from imagination of impending danger, either destructive or painful."

Aristotle

      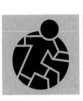

Introduction

Individuals with persistent activity limiting low back pain (LBP) generally assume that structural factors play a decisive role in their pain and disability. However, it is now acknowledged that most structural pathologies are present in asymptomatic individuals in nearly equal degree as they are in those who are symptomatic. This fact combined with the generally unsatisfactory results of traditional care for LBP has led to the critical evaluation of the biomedical model (49,66,97). According to the International Association for the Study of Pain (IASP), pain is not simply the result of structural injury or pathology but is "an unpleasant sensory and emotional experience associated with actual or potential tissue damage . . ." (63).

Pain has its origin in peripheral activation from physical sources; however, it is also modulated in the dorsal horn, and by descending influences largely of psychologic origin (57). Concurrent evaluation of both the sources of pain and the psycho-physical perceptions that lead one to fear and thus avoid activity should be addressed so that reactivation can occur (39,53,94).

Thus, musculoskeletal pain patients in general and LBP patients in particular require an approach that addresses the physical (biological) and psychosocial dimensions of their problem. This modern approach is called biopsychosocial (BPS) in that the total patient is our subject. Rather than focusing on structural causes and cures, this new paradigm emphasizes the goal of maintaining or restoring function. Such an approach is of value regardless of the pathoanatomic diagnosis. This BPS approach is the main subject of not only this chapter but also the entire book that follows.

The Biopsychosocial Model

> **Practice-Based Problem**
>
> Less than 20% of back pain is caused by structural factors. Does this mean that most pain is psychogenic?

Pain has been interpreted since the time of Descartes as signaling tissue damage (Fig. 4.1). The biomedical model of finding the structural cause and then treating it or "fixing" it to elicit a cure is based on this rather narrow view of pain. It is now acknowledged that a structural cause for pain does not usually exist and that a structural cure is not often successful. The Cartesian model leads one to assume if cure is not brought about, then the problem must be psychogenic. The dualism inherent in the early Renaissance notion of pain suggests that pain is either in the mind or body, but not both! According to the new IASP definition of

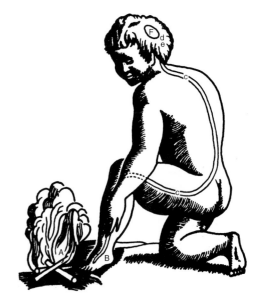

Figure 4.1 The Cartesian model of peripheral activation of pain pathways. From Descarte's L'Homme (Paris 1644).

pain, it is associated with both a disagreeable physical sensation and an emotional experience (58,59). Thus, it is sensorial (nociceptive) and affective (emotional) and should not be defined dichotomously as either physical or psychological.

The biopsychosocial model views pain as involving ascending nociceptive input from the periphery (Cartesian model), descending modulation that inhibits or facilitates nociception (Gate Control Theory of Melzack and Wall), and central processes with neurological, affective, and cognitive dimensions (Figs. 4.2–4.4) (57). Therefore, the perception of pain is heavily influenced both by nociception and by one's attitudes, beliefs, and social environment (Fig. 4.5).

Even though most patients begin improving from back pain episodes quickly, both the recurrence rate and dissatisfaction with medical care is high. Additionally, the minority in whom persistant chronic disabling pain develops account for by far the greatest percent of costs (85%). Therefore, the traditional biomedical model should be re-evaluated in light of its failure to successfully address the low back problem.

In patients who do not recover, the limitations of the biomedical approach are even more evident. In an attempt to find the structural cause of LBP, overly sensitive tests are ordered, with high false-positive rates. The patient either is told nothing is wrong and labelled psychogenic or is told about the pathology and to rest, take medicines, and learn to live with it. If they can't tolerate it anymore, then they are informed that they should have surgery.

The incidence rate, cost of chronicity and disability, general dissatisfaction, and high recurrence rate add up to a problem of epidemic proportions. Waddell

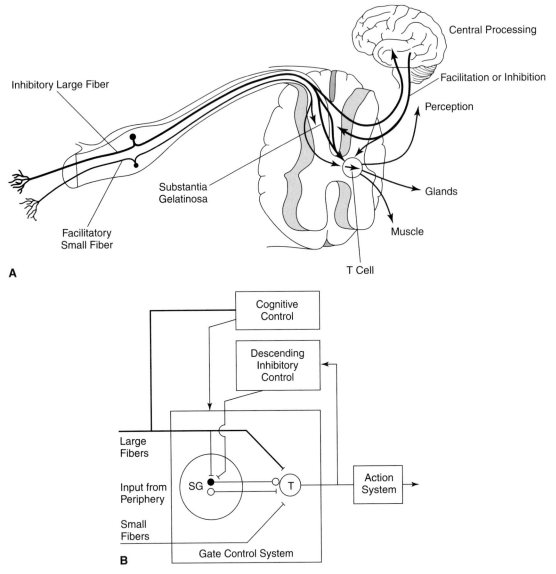

Figure 4.2 The gate control theory of pain. **(A)** Ascending pathways from small and large diameter fibers to the dorsal horn of the spinal cord and to higher centers. From Suchdev PK. Pathophysiology of pain. In: Warfield CA, Fausett JH, ed. Manual of Pain Management, 2nd ed. Philadelphia: Lippincott Williams & Wilkins, 2002. **(B)** The excitatory (white circle) and inhibitory (black circle) links from the substantia gelatinosa (SG) to the transmission (T) cells, as well as descending inhibitory control from brainstem systems. The round knob at the end of the inhibitory link implies that its actions may be presynaptic, postsynaptic, or both. All connections are excitatory, except the inhibitory link from SG to T cell. From Bonica JJ, Loeser JD. History of pain concepts and therapies. In: Loeser JD, ed. Bonica's Management of Pain, 3rd ed. Philadelphia: Lippincott Williams & Wilkins, 2001 (modified from Melzack R, Wall PD. The challenge of pain. New York: Basic Books, 1983.)

(97) in his Volvo award-winning paper stated, "Conventional medical treatment for low-back pain has failed, and the role of medicine in the present epidemic must be critically examined." The low back epidemic is caused by a number of factors. The reasons for this failure are presented in Table 4.1.

Overemphasis on a Structural Diagnosis

Many doctors overuse diagnostic imaging as part of the initial evaluation of a LBP patient. This is performed for two mistaken reasons. One is the belief that serious diseases (i.e., tumors, infections) can be missed

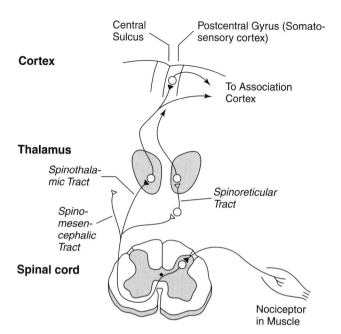

Figure 4.3 Ascending nociceptive pathways. From Mense S. Simons DG. Muscle Pain: Understanding Its Nature, Diagnosis, and Treatment. Baltimore: Lippincott Williams & Wilkins, 2001.

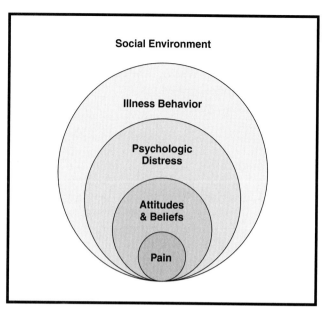

Figure 4.5 The biopsychosocial model. Reproduced with permission from Waddell G. The Back Pain Revolution. Edinburgh: Churchill Livingstone, 1998.

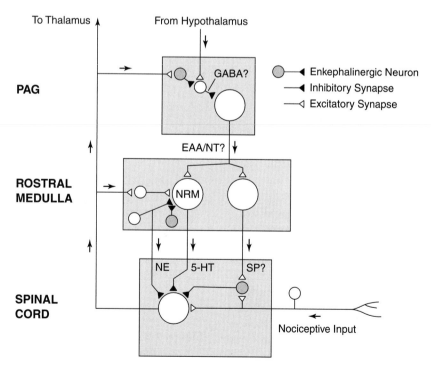

Figure 4.4 Descending antinociceptive modulation. From Mense S. Simons DG. Muscle Pain: Understanding Its Nature, Diagnosis, and Treatment. Baltimore: Lippincott, Williams & Wilkins, 2001 (redrawn from Basbarum AI, Fields HL. Endogenous pain control system: brainstem spinal pathways and endorphin circuitry. Ann Rev Neurosci 1984;7:309–338.).

Table 4.1 Medical Reasons for the Low Back Disability Epidemic

A) Overemphasis on a structural diagnosis
B) Overprescription of bed rest
C) Overuse of surgery

by a thorough history and physical examination. Second, the belief that structural pathologies (e.g., herniated discs, arthritis) that can only be identified with imaging are strongly correlated with symptoms.

History and examination are more than 99% sensitive for identifying "red flags" of serious disease (21,56,97,98).

No "Red Flags" of Tumor, Infection, or Fracture Were Missed as a Result of Not Routinely Imaging Acute Patients

- Long-term follow-up of 437 patients revealed no serious disorders were missed as a result of not performing routine imaging on acute patients

- A "red flag" checklist mostly from history alone was used

- 1.4% of patients did have serious conditions such as crush fracture, kidney carcinoma, and prostate carcinoma, but they were suspected on initial evaluation and referred for additional tests

McGuirk B, King W, Govind J, Lowry J, Bogduk N. Safety, efficacy and cost-effectiveness of evidence-based guidelines for the management of acute low back pain in primary care. Spine 2001;26:2615–2622

The false-positive rate for identifying clinically significant herniated discs or degenerative conditions with imaging (e.g., x-ray, MRI) is so high as to make the tests clinically inappropriate as screening procedures (Fig. 4.6). The problem is that many individuals who have pain unrelated to the structural findings will be mislabeled and potentially receive unnecessary treatments. They may think of themselves as "sick" when in fact most of these changes are related more to age than to symptoms.

After the discovery by Mixter and Barr that compression of a nerve root by a herniated disc could cause sciatica, the belief in the pathoanatomical basis for back and leg pain has been a fundamental dogma (1,64). Structural evidence of a lumbar disc hernia in a patient with appropriate symptoms is present more than 90% of the time (4,38,74,104).

Unfortunately, even when using advanced imaging techniques such as myelography, CAT scans, or magnetic resonance imaging, the same positive findings are also present in 28% to 50% of asymptomatic individuals (4,9,38,43,74,104). Similarly, in the neck, the false-positive rate for imaging has been reported to be as high as 75% in the asymptomatic population (5,81). Thus, imaging tests have high sensitivity (few false-negatives) but low specificity (high false-positive rate) for identifying symptomatic disc problems.

Furthermore, the presence of structural pathology in an asymptomatic individual does not predict a greater likelihood of future problems (6,16)! Borenstein et al performed MRI on 67 asymptomatic people; 31% has abnormality of disc or spinal canal (6). The MRI findings were not predictive of future LBP. Individuals with longest duration of LBP were not those with the greatest anatomical abnormalities. Carragee et al studied discograms and reported that a painful disc injection did not predict LBP on follow-up at 4 years (16). Though discograms have high sensitivity for identifying tears in asymptomatic patients, it was the psychometric profiles that were found to strongly predict future LBP and work loss.

Even when the diagnosis of disc herniation is relevant, such pathology has a tendency to resolve without surgical intervention. Bush et al (13) reported, "A high proportion of intervertebral disc herniations have the potential to resolve spontaneously. Even if patients have marked reduction of straight leg raising, positive neurologic signs, and a substantial intervertebral disc herniation (as opposed to a bulge), there is potential for making a natural recovery, not

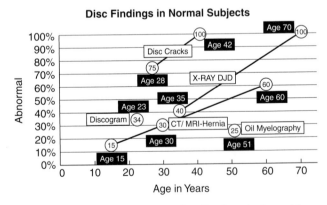

Figure 4.6 False-positive rates for disc herniation with various imaging modalities. Imaging findings of disc abnormalities increase in frequency with age in patients without symptoms. (CT, computed tomography; DJD, degenerative join disease; MRI, magnetic resonance imaging.) From Bigos S, Müller G. Primary care approach to acute and chronic back problems: Definitions and care. In: Loeser JD, ed. Bonica's Management of Pain, 3rd ed. Philadelphia: Lippincott Williams & Wilkins, 2001.

least due to resolution of the intervertebral disc herniation." This group found similar results in the cervical spine, concluding that most cervical disc herniations regress with time without resorting to surgery (14). Yukawa found that in sciatica patients treated conservatively and followed-up for 3 years that 57% had a reduction in the size of disc herniation and only 3% had an enlargement (107).

Other structural pathologies have also been overstated as causes of back pain. There is little relationship between radiological signs of degeneration and clinical symptoms (19,30,32,47,52,78,82,87). Nachemson (67) said, "Even when strict radiographic criteria are adhered to, 'disk degeneration' is demonstrated with equal incidence in subjects with or without pain." According to a recent review by Jarvik and Deyo, the prevalence of disc degeneration among asymptomatic individuals of at least middle age ranges from 46% to 93% (41). They conclude that findings such as bulges, dehydration, and loss of disc height should not automatically be viewed as abnormalities because they are strongly related to age. However, there are certain exceptions, such as disc extrusions, moderate or severe canal stenosis, and nerve root compression, which are significantly correlated with symptoms (42). Van Tulder in a systematic evaluation of the literature concluded that spondylosis, spondylolisthesis, spina bifida, transitional vertebrae, and Scheuermann disease are not associated with low back pain (87). Videman, in a study of cadaver specimens, found no correlation between structural pathology and a history of low back pain (91–93). Segmental instability and isolated disc resorption are other diagnosis that again cannot be validated (67).

Recently Kendrick reported that patients who received x-rays were more likely to report a longer duration and greater severity of pain, reduced functioning, and poorer health status than those who had not (44). They concluded that "radiography encourages or reinforces the patient's belief that they are unwell and may lead to greater reporting of pain and greater limitation of activities." Nearly two-thirds of the patients who underwent x-ray were found to have structural pathologies, yet no significant differences in outcome were noted between patients with normal versus abnormal x-rays. Because patient satisfaction was higher if x-rays were taken, the authors concluded that patient education regarding the inability of radiography to improve therapy, decision-making, or outcomes is important.

Most low back patients do not have structural pathology that can be clearly diagnosed as being the cause of their symptoms (3). For this reason, most of these patients are classified with the label non-specific back pain. According to Frymoyer (31), "most commonly, diagnosis is speculative and unconfirmed

by objective testing." An interesting exception to this involves patients with chronic pain in whom, according to Bogduk, the pain generator can be identified the majority of the time with the use of a double anesthetic block technique (see Chapter 6).

Overemphasis on Bed Rest

Because of the failure to pinpoint the specific pain generators in low back pain, bed rest and analgesics have become the typical treatment. The generally positive early course of most low back pain episodes has given justification to this practice of symptomatic treatment. As it turns out, this seemingly benign prescription of prolonged bed rest has now been shown to be one of the most costly errors in musculoskeletal care. Allan and Waddell (1) said, "Tragically, despite the best of intentions to relieve pain, our whole approach to backache has been associated with increasing low back disability. Despite a wide range of treatments, or perhaps because none of them provide a lasting cure, our whole strategy of management has been negative, based on rest. We have actually prescribed low back disability!"

Deyo performed a controlled clinical trial that compared 2 days of bed rest against 2 weeks and concluded that a shorter period of bed rest was as effective as a longer one (22). The negative effects associated with prolonged immobilization were not seen with brief bed rest. A more recent study confirmed Deyo's work by finding that 4 days of bed rest led to more sick leave than advice to continue normal activity (73).

The Danish guidelines concluded that bed rest should only be used for severe pain and then only for 1 to 2 days (20). They found there to be insufficient evidence of a positive effect. Van Tulder found that there was no evidence in favor of bed rest for acute LBP (88). Vroomen demonstrated that there was no evidence of effectiveness of bed rest for sciatica (96).

Cochrane Collaborations Review of Bed Rest Versus Advice to Stay Active

- "There is no evidence that advice to stay active is harmful for either acute LBP or sciatica"

- ". . . there are potential harmful effects of prolonged bed rest . . ."

- ". . . it is reasonable to advise people with LBP and sciatica to stay active."

Hagen KB, Hilde G, Jamtvedt G, Winnem MF. The Cochrane Review of advice as a single treatment for low back pain and sciatica. Spine 2002;27:1736–1741.

Overuse of Surgery

The overuse of surgery has been one of the most problematic interventions in back pain. Bigos and Battie (3) said, "Surgery seems helpful for at most 2% of patients with back problems, and its inappropriate use can have a great impact on increasing the chance of chronic back pain disability." Saal and Saal (75) supervised care for a group of patients referred by neurologists for surgery. They attempted rehabilitation for these patients and made the following observations, "Surgery should be reserved for those patients for whom function cannot be satisfactorily improved by a physical rehabilitation program . . . Failure of passive non-operative treatment is not sufficient for the decision to operate."

In 1970 Hakelius performed a study that revealed that the majority of sciatica patients responded to conservative care (37). Bush (13) in 1992 published that "86% of patients with clinical sciatica and radiologic evidence of nerve root entrapment were treated successfully by aggressive conservative management."

The Danish guidelines recommend spinal surgery for disc herniation, cauda equina syndrome, spinal stenosis, and stabilizing back surgery so long as appropriate indications are present (20). Table 4.2 summarizes the Danish guidelines indications for spinal surgery.

Table 4.2 Surgical Indications for Disc Herniation according to the Danish Guidelines (20)

- after 4–6 weeks of conservative care
- when there is a positive correlation between clinical findings and imaging reports
- and progressive weakness in the leg
- or severe leg symptoms in spite of medication

A Cochrane Collaboration systematic analysis found that there is considerable evidence on clinical effectiveness of discectomy for carefully selected patients with sciatica caused by lumbar disc prolapse that does not resolve with conservative management (33,34). They found that 65% to 90% of sciatica patients whose symptoms lasted 6 to 24 months had good to excellent outcomes. In contrast only, 36% of conservatively treated patients had good to excellent outcomes. Although this often is interpreted to defend the aggressive recommendation for surgery, this is not necessarily the case. A study of spinal stenosis patients found that there is no difference in surgical outcome in patients who delay surgery by opting for a trial of conservative care (2). In 1983, Weber reported that even in properly selected patients there is no difference in outcome between surgically and conservatively treated patients at 10 years (103). However, the study by Gogan and Fraser suggests the long-term results of surgery are superior to conservative care (35).

Gibson et al (33) concluded, "There is a serious lack of scientific evidence supporting surgical management for degenerative lumbar spondylosis." They found no acceptable evidence for the efficacy of any form of decompression for degenerative lumbar spondylosis or spinal stenosis. Also, that there is no acceptable evidence of the efficacy of any form of fusion for degenerative lumbar spondylosis, back pain, or "instability."

Failure rates with spine surgery are estimated to be between 10% and 30%. The only RCT is more than 25 years old (103), and this has recently come under methodological criticism (85). Improper selection of patients may be the most important factor. The most certain surgical criteria are:

- Cauda equina syndrome
- Paresis, rapidly progressive despite optimal treatment (trial of conservative care for 4 weeks to 3 months)

The RAND corporation convened a multidisciplinary expert panel to review the scientific literature and come to a consensus regarding the criteria for spine surgery as appropriate, equivocal, or inappropriate (Table 4.3) (86); 38% of surgeries performed in two university neurosurgery departments were prospectively evaluated using this criteria and were determined to be inappropriate (46). Agreement with these criteria was reached independently in Switzerland (85).

The notion that if there is a large disc extrusion that surgery is necessary is not supported in the literature. Bush et al (13) reported, "Indeed, the intervertebral disc pathomorphology that might seem best suited to surgical resection is in fact that which shows the most significant incidence of natural regression . . . These results confirm that if the pain can be controlled, nature can be allowed to run its course with the partial or complete resolution of the mechanical factor. . . . Lumbar herniated nucleus pulposus can be treated non-operatively with a high degree of success."

Carragee recently reiterated that preoperative MRI is not a highly reliable predictor of disc surgery outcome (15). But it was still possible to conclude

that the larger the disc herniation the greater the likelihood of a surgical success. In fact, 57% of patients with anterior–posterior (AP) disc herniation dimensions of less than 6 mm had poor clinical results, whereas only 2% with AP dimensions more than 9 mm were considered failures, although they did have the highest rehrniation rate.

Surgery clearly has its place for lumbar spine disorders, but this should be only when appropriate criteria are applied. Allan and Waddell (1) point out that unnecessary surgery has been a major problem for some time, "The rapid and enthusiastic expansion of disc surgery soon exposed its limitations and failures. It was accused of leaving more tragic human wreckage in its wake than any other operation in history." Schneider and Kahanovitz noted that even in patients who had an apparently successful operation for sciatica, if the problem is compensable (i.e., workman's compensation or personal injury), they are still at significant risk for recurrence and disability (76).

Abnormal Illness Behavior

According to Dworkin (24), "Pain report often occurs in the absence of pathophysiology or any discernible peripheral somatic changes. This finding implies the need to reexamine our limited understanding of pain, rather than leaping to the conclusion that such pains must be psychogenic." LaRocca in his Presidential Address to the Cervical Spine Research Society Annual Meeting in December of 1991 explained that if physicians assume pathology is the major cause of symptoms, then if a patient has not recovered with treatment, they incorrectly assume the problem must be psychogenic (48). Merskey (60) explained, "Slater & Glithero (77) showed that 60% of patients diagnosed by distinguished neurologists as having hysteria did suffer from, or develop, relevant physical disease that might account for their symptoms . . ." He goes on to conclude that most regional pain syndromes are not psychogenic in origin and are often mislabeled as such (40,61,62).

This is not to say that pain behavior does not accompany pain sensation. Dworkin (24) says "Finally, there is no inconsistency in accepting the likelihood that chronic pain patients experience distress in the form of depression, anxiety, and multiple nonspecific physical symptoms, without having recourse to the diagnosis or classification of their pain condition as psychogenic." Pain behavior is common and should be recognized and addressed. Whereas acute pain is directly related to painful stimuli, nociception, and tissue injury chronic pain is due only in part to physical events (40,51,71,99,108). Chronic illness behavior

---

Table 4.3 Surgical Indications for Disc Herniation or Spinal Stenosis according to the Rand Corporation (46)

Appropriate:
- Pain in lower limb, imaging positive for disc hernia or spinal stenosis, major or minor neurological findings, restricted activity for more than 6 weeks

Equivocal:
- Pain in lower limb, imaging positive for disc hernia or spinal stenosis, major neurological findings, restricted activity for less than 4 weeks
- Pain in lower limb, imaging equivocal for disc hernia or spinal stenosis, minor neurological findings, restricted activity for more than 6 weeks

Inappropriate:
- Pain in lower limb, imaging positive for disc hernia or spinal stenosis, minor neurological findings, restricted activity for less than 4 weeks

Minor neuro findings (2 or more items)
- Asymmetric ankle reflex
- Dermatomal sensory deficit
- Positive ipsilateral SLR (straight leg raise) test
- Sciatica

Major neurologic findings
- Progressive unilateral leg weakness, or
- Positive contralateral SLR test

and disability are only partially related to nociceptive influences (26,50,68,71). Psychosocial illness behavior, including depression, inactivity, and pain avoidance, is the rule with chronic pain sufferers (8,25,69, 80,100).

Because the majority of patients do not have a diagnosable structural cause of their symptoms, a functional disorder should be assumed. Pain in the locomotor system should be viewed as a sign of impaired function. Non-specific or idiopathic back pain most likely has to do with muscle or joint dysfunction combined with soft tissue irritation and pain generation. Treatments designed for injury states or disc lesions will inevitably fail, thus causing depression, despair, and illness behavior (27,28,79,102,105).

Abnormal illness behavior was defined by Pilowsky as a patient's inappropriate or maladaptive response to a physical symptom (Table 4.4) (72). This typically occurs in back pain when no organic cause for a patient's symptoms can be identified. Descartes' view of pain as a warning signal of impending harm has led to the advice to "let pain be your guide." This is helpful in acute situations when nociceptive factors predominate. However, in chronic cases behavior should be encouraged that focuses on functional reactivation, not pain avoidance. In fact, it is necessary for the chronic pain patient to focus on increasing their activities in spite of their pain.

Abnormal illness behavior contributes to a slower or inadequate recovery. For instance, fear–avoidance behavior leads to deconditioning (94). Patients who equate hurt with harm have a disabling form of thinking. They begin fear–avoidance behavior, which promotes deconditioning and thus leads to less stability in the low back patient (Fig. 4.7). It is important to identify the patient who is fearful and avoid encouraging that patient to take on a "sick role." According to Troup (83), "If fear of pain persists, unless it is specifically recognized and treated, it leads inexorably to pain-avoidance and thence to disuse."

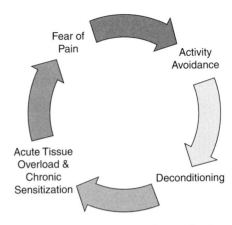

Figure 4.7 How fear–avoidance behavior leads to chronic sensitization.

Diagnostic Triage to Rehabilitation—The Benchmark

The overarching goals of modern care for neuromusculoskeletal problems has been succinctly described by the recent Clinical Framework document from the Victorian Workcover Authority in Australia (90). The aims and principles of care are summarized in the following goal statements:

1. Treatment must be based on the best evidence available
2. Treatment effectiveness must be demonstrated with outcome measurements
3. A biopsychosocial approach is essential
4. Treatment must focus on self-care or management skills
5. Treatment must be functional and focused on return-to-work or activities

Working Backs Scotland has focused on marketing a clear message to the public about how to manage back pain (106). The three key points are:

1. Stay active
2. Try simple pain relief
3. If you need it, get advice

An aggressive public media campaign (radio ads, free press); physician, employer, and union involvement; an informative web site; and distribution of brochures and posters led to a reversal in health care beliefs (rest vs. stay active) within 1 to 2 months (99). With the help of follow-up booster campaigns, this continued to improve for more than 2 years.

Table 4.4 Abnormal illness behavior

Affective (emotional)
- Anxiety
- Depression

Cognitive (coping)
- Fear–avoidance behavior
- Ignoring "stop rules"
- Catastrophizing the low back problem (labeling)
  - ruptured disc
  - degenerative arthritis

Does our failure to pinpoint the precise cause of LBP in 80% of cases mean that there is no decision-making process to guide care for these patients?

The first step in management is diagnostic triage. This establishes an algorithm or critical pathway for care (Fig. 4.8). Patients have two basic goals (84). First, to receive information about how to manage their LBP; and second, to receive advice on how to resume normal activities. The patient centered paradigm is goal-oriented, focusing on function, not just relief of symptoms. In the report of findings, it is important to mutually establish the following goals of care: reduce pain, restore function, and keep the patient independent. This requires a strategic program heeding "best practice" approaches incorporating reassurance, relief of pain, and reactivation (Table 4.5). Whereas this patient-centered approach

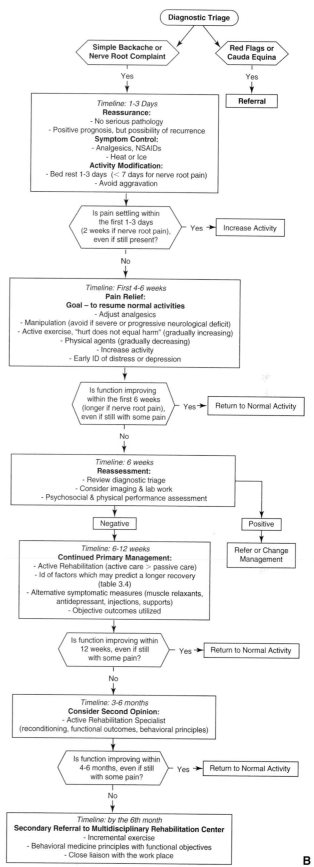

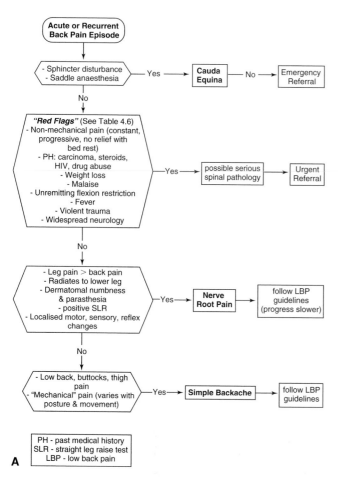

Figure 4.8 **(A)** Diagnostic triage algorithm. **(B)** Treatment guidelines algorithm

Modified from CSAG Clinical Standards Advisory Group report on Back pain. London: HMSO. 1994; 1-89.

Table 4.5 "Best Practice" Keys to Recovery—The 7 R's

1. **Rule out** "red flags" of serious disease
2. **Reassurance** that no serious disease is present and that improvement is likely to begin rapidly (within a few weeks)
3. **Reactivation** advice that normal activities can be resumed (walk, swim, bike, etc.) and education about simple activity modifications to reduce biomechanical strain (i.e., hip hinge, cats, abdominal bracing)
4. **Relieve** pain with medication or manipulation
5. **Re-evaluation** of those entering the subacute phase for structural, functional, or psychosocial pathology
6. **Rehabilitate/Recondition/Reeducate** muscles with McKenzie, stabilization, progressive strengthening, or cognitive-behavorial (indicated if high "yellow flags" score) approaches
7. **Refer** for specialist tests (i.e., "red flags") or treatments (i.e., "yellow flags") when indicated

is goal-oriented, traditional approaches are technique- or profession-driven (manipulation, injection, surgery). These traditional approaches have for the most part confused and frustrated the health care consumer.

The good natural history for acute problems necessitates a minimalist approach (29). Unless there are "red flags," reassure and reactivate the patient. If needed, provide pain relief treatments. Avoid unnecessary surgery, overmedication, and overexamination, especially with diagnostic imaging. In contrast, the subacute phase is a better time for more aggressive management than is the chronic phase, because it is easier to prevent than to treat chronic pain. The key time frame is between 4 and 12 weeks (29). Those

with "yellow flags" (i.e., fear–avoidance behavior) should be more aggressively managed, even as early as 3 weeks and certainly by 6 weeks. This still does not mean MRIs for every patient, but it does mean a rehabilitation specialist should be involved. The most important point is that when a full diagnostic workup is recommended, it should not be limited to MRIs or other structural evaluations. It should also include functional or physiological testing such as a functional capacity evaluation and a psychosocial workup.

Despite the fact that most patients begin improvement rapidly, 20% to 25% of patients are dissatisfied with their care for back and neck pain (21). Cherkin found that despite the much publicized rosy picture for back pain, one-third of patients are dissatisfied with recovery even after 7 weeks, and one-half of these continue to be so at 1 year (18). Carey reported that even in those who were returned to pre-injury functional levels, they were generally dissatisfied with their care (17). Thus, at least in terms of customer satisfaction, there is much room for improvement. Patients require an approach that demonstrates empathy with their situation. This is why prompt reassurance and pain relief options are important, along with education about the value of reactivation and possible reconditioning.

Reassurance/Diagnostic Triage

- **How**—diagnostic triage
- **What**— there is no serious disease and improvement is likely to begin rapidly (within a few weeks)
- **When**—on day 1
- **Why**—to dispel the myth that imaging is needed or the spine is damaged

Diagnostic triage validates that nothing bad or sinister is going on (Table 4.6). Klassen reported that a chief

Table 4.6 Red Flags of Serious Disease (tumor, infection, fracture, serious medical disease) (see Chapter 7)

- Age younger than 20 or older than 50 years
- Trauma
- History of cancer
- Night pain
- Fevers
- Weight loss
- Pain at rest
- Immune suppression (i.e., significant corticosteroid use)
- Recent infection
- Generalized systemic disease (diabetes)
- Failure of 4 weeks of conservative care
- Cauda equina
- Saddle anesthesia
- Sphincter disturbance
- Motor weakness lower limbs

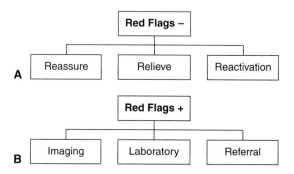

Figure 4.9 "Red Flags" action steps. A) Red flags negative. B) Red flags positive.

purpose for visiting a doctor for 43% of pain patients is the need for reassurance about the absence of serious disease (45). Those with "red flags" of serious disease require different action steps than those without them (Fig. 4.9). Explanation includes a discussion of pain relief options as well as what to avoid and what to do to speed recovery. It is important to help the patient to see that the goal is avoiding debilitating inactivity. This requires an interactive approach that alleviates fears and overcomes past misperceptions. The health care provider (HCP) should show concern as well as empathy for the patient's well-being and safety. Guidelines and patient booklets such as "The Back Book" can be used as aids (12).

The patient will hear the good news that we can confidently rule out sinister factors, even though we are not very accurate in identifying the exact cause of their pain. Their pain can be likened to a common cold or the pain from gardening for the first time after a long winter. Performing a novel activity such as gardening is expected to give rise to pain, because we realize we are not in shape. This pain is rarely a cause for concern, and LBP can be likened to it.

It may also be reassuring that the natural history is relatively good. Some improvement begins very rapidly such that there is approximately a 50% chance of returning to normal activities within 1 week and a 90% chance within 1 month. Even with sciatica there is a 50% chance of resuming normal activities within 1 month and a 90% chance within 3 months. However, this does not guarantee that your patient will be in those good outcome groups. We can't promise to have a magic wand, let alone a crystal ball!

Much of the early reassurance of acute patients is so that they don't feel they need an MRI or aggressive early treatment and vigilant self-protection of their back (29,55). Most recent systematic reviews of the literature suggest that the traditional back school emphasis on learning how to protect the back actu-

Australian Province of Victoria Demonstrates that the Message in "The Back Book" Can Change Social Behavior

- Multimedia campaign begun in 1997 in Victoria, Australia advised patients with back pain to stay active and exercise, and not to rest for prolonged periods or take time off from work.

- The campaign consisted of:
  - Television commercials during "prime time" during the first 3 months
  - International & national experts
  - Australian sporting and television stars with past history of LBP
  - Lower-key maintenance advertising including radio and print ads
  - "The Back Book" was widely available in 16 languages
  - All doctors in Victoria received evidence-based guidelines for managing LBP
  - Another intensive television campaign for 3 months starting in September 1999

- Study of 4730 individuals in the general population and 2556 general medical practitioners (GPs)

- The message of "The Back Book" was delivered in the province of Victoria, but not in New South Wales (NSW)

- Back pain beliefs changed in Victoria during the campaign, but not in NSW

- Among individuals who had back pain in the previous year, fear–avoidance beliefs about physical activity improved considerably in Victoria, but not in NSW

- GPs in Victoria improved their beliefs about back pain management as compared to their colleagues in NSW

- Previous studies have shown than only one-third of doctors are motivated to change behavior by continuing education

- Outside influences such as a mass media campaign and changed attitudes in their own patients appeared to motivate the doctors

Buchbinder R, Jolley D, Wyatt M. 2001 Volvo Award Winner in Clinical Studies: Effects of a media campaign on back pain beliefs and its potential influence on management of low back pain in general practice. Spine 2001;26:2535–2542.

ally promotes deconditioning through avoidance behavior (20,88,101). It seems back school may be too much of a good thing!

According to Deyo and Weinstein (23), the search for a precise anatomical diagnosis is often frustrating for physicians and patients. They state that it is more useful to address the following three questions:

1. Is systemic disease causing the pain?
2. Is there psychosocial distress present that will amplify or prolong the pain?
3. Is there a neurologic compromise present that may require surgical evaluation?

This requires a careful history and examination with imaging not typically being necessary.

One-half to two-thirds of acute patients have substantial worries about the safety of activity, whereas between one-quarter and one-half of subacute patients report having reduced their housework, sexual activity, and walking (65,95). Such unnecessary beliefs are often promoted by biomedical action (ordering imaging tests) or inaction (proposed bed rest or avoidance of activities that hurt). Thus, early reassurance is an integral part of the BPS approach. Table 4.7 illustrates the stark contrast between a traditional biomedical report of findings and a BPS one.

Reactivation Advice (see Chapter 14)

- **How**—an educational discussion about recovery goals and the means to reach those goals
- **What**—that normal activities can be resumed (walk, swim, bike, etc.) and education about simple activity modifications to reduce biomechanical strain (i.e., hip hinge, cats, abdominal bracing)
- **When**—day 1

- **Why**—dispel the myth that rest is required or that spine is vulnerable

Reactivation advice requires an educational discussion about recovery goals and the means to reach those goals. It starts with reassurance of the safety of gradually resuming normal activities such as walking, swimming, and biking. Normal activity is necessary to prevent the debilitating effects of inactivity. It is important to acknowledge that these activites may be uncomfortable, but the patient should be reassured that hurt does not necessarily equal harm. Most normal activities, while possibly uncomfortable, are actually less stressful than prolonged sitting. When someone has a flu their back hurts because they have been resting. Similarly, pain when returning to activity is not usually caused by harmful activity, rather it is a result of debilitation.

Along with advice to gradually resume normal activities education about simple activity modifications to reduce biomechanical strain (i.e., early-morning flexion, hip hinge, cats, abdominal bracing, etc.) is important. Basic activity modification advice for severe pain is to limit sitting to 20 minutes and limit unassisted lifting to 20 pounds. Although healthful biomechanics can hopefully facilitate recovery and prevent recurrences, it can also have an unanticipated negative effect of deconditioning the patient! Strict avoidance of bending, reaching, and lifting will certainly decondition. This is like wearing a brace or cast for too long.

If we modify activities to reduce harmful biomechanical stress and strain, then we must provide some prescribed therapeutic exercise to maintain conditioning of those important muscles. An example is if we advise patients to avoid lifting with their spine in full flexion, especially first thing in the morning or after prolonged sitting. In such a case it is important to also prescribe cat/camel exercises to maintain mobility throughout the entire functional range of motion and to teach patients NOT to over-

Table 4.7 Biomedical vs Biopsychosocial Approaches (adapted from (12))

Biomedical	Biopsychosocial
• Emphasize anatomy, injury & damage • "Let pain be your guide" • Emphasize further tests • Focus on pain rather than activity • Encourage passivity & dependency • Positive attitudes result in a speedier recovery	• Reassurance—no sign of serious disease • LBP is symptom that back is biomechanically unfit • Psychologic treatment can help, but long-term results depend on lifestyle • Recovery depends on restoring function—the sooner the better

protect their backs during otherwise routine safe activities.

According to the Occupational Health Guidelines (OHG) (101), the first treatment is generally acknowledged to be advice to remain active. "There is strong evidence that advice to continue ordinary activities of daily living as normally as possible despite the pain can give equivalent or faster symptomatic recovery from the acute symptoms, and leads to shorter periods of work loss, fewer recurrences and less work loss over the following year than 'traditional' medical treatment (advice to rest and 'let pain be your guide' for return to normal activity)."

Relief of Pain (see Chapters 21 and 38)

- **How**—the recommendation of over-the-counter or prescription medication, or delivery of skilled manipulation
- **When**—within a few days if discomfort is present
- **Why**—provide greater comfort until recovery begins

Although there are no magic bullets, pain relief options can take the edge off. If the pain can be softened, then it will be easier to encourage the patient to resume activities. The main goal is to avoid the debilitation of rest and build activity tolerance through safe conditioning. According to the Danish guidelines, the following are the recommended, optional, and recommended against acute pain relief treatments (20):

Recommended
- Acetaminophen, aspirin, ibuprofen
- Prescription NSAIDS
- Manipulation
- Surgery—for cauda equina syndrome

Optional
- Modalities
- Muscle relaxants
- McKenzie exercises
- Acupuncture
- Epidural—for sciatica

Recommended Against
- Sedatives, hypnotics, steroids
- Epidural—recommended against for LBP

- Surgery—recommended against for sciatica (in the acute phase)
- Surgery—recommended against for LBP

Nicholas has pointed out that if the focus is on pain relief before activation that this can actually reinforce avoidance behaviors (70). According to Main, the adage "let pain be your guide" is responsible for promoting unnecessary fear and functional limitations (54). Pain is likely to run a course and even come and go. The determining factors in recovery have to do with how a person copes with their pain. If all the focus on care is on pain relief, then avoidance behavior will be promoted with the result being that physical and psychological deconditioning will ensue. Patients should be informed that light activities, while uncomfortable, are not harmful. If patients are overly concerned about pain and fearful of activities, then a "stepped-up" approach including exercise and supervised exposure to feared activities is needed (65,95).

Re-Evaluation of Structural, Functional, and Psychosocial Contributors to Continued Pain or Disability

- **How**—comprehensive bio (structural and functional) and psychosocial (yellow flags) re-examination (see Chapters 9 and 11)
- **Who**—those entering the subacute phase
- **When**—in the subacute phase
- **Why**—to reassure the patient that there is no serious disease causing their pain or that something has not been missed that could help them. Also, to identify functional deficits that may be realistic targets for treatment or affective or cognitive behaviors that may impede recovery

Re-evaluation requires a comprehensive structural, functional, and psychosocial re-examination. For patients not satisfactorily recovering at the 4-week mark, it is important to once again reassure the patient that there is nothing seriously wrong. At this juncture rather than a minimalist approach being recommended, aggressive management strategies are needed to rule out structural pathologies, identify functional deficits, and evaluate for psychosocial "yellow flags." Frequently, only structural imaging is performed, thus boxing the doctor into a corner where he or she is forced to give greater credence to coincidental imaging findings. But if at the same time an MRI is performed on a non-responsive patient, a "yellow flags" questionnaire is administered and a functional capacity evaluation performed, then the doctor will be able to place imaging findings in context along with coping issues and functional deficits.

Reconditioning (see Chapters 26, 27, and 31)

- **How**—skilled assessment and training of patient
- **What**—McKenzie, stabilization, progressive strengthening, or cognitive-behavioral approaches
- **When**—in the subacute phase or earlier for those at risk of chronicity
- **Why**—dispel the myth that more aggressive treatment of symptoms is required; instead, focus on function/physiology not structure/pathology

Reconditioning exercise requires skilled assessment and training of patient. Exercises may involve McKenzie, stabilization, progressive strengthening, or cognitive–behavorial approaches. Patients should be educated that activity and conditioning will facilitate recovery. Conditioning is more important with increased age because we lose a significant percentage of our muscles protection between 20 and 50 years old.

The report of findings after re-evaluation should focus on the importance of building activity tolerance. That this requires training or conditioning should seem reasonable. Treatment with manipulation, medication, injection, or surgery will not condition the muscles needed to enhance performance or stability. A famous Groucho Marx story applies here:

Groucho Marx: "Doctor! After surgery will I be able to play violin?"
Doctor: "I would think so."
Groucho Marx: "Good! Cause I could never play it before."

Backs are like knees. Regardless of cause or treatment (even surgery), the road to recovery is through reactivation and reconditioning. This allows the patient to prevent debilitation and increase the body's compensatory ability for normal age related changes or deficits.

According to the OHG, a rehabilitation specialist will be working with a team that can offer the services described in Table 4.8 (101).

Referral (see Chapter 7)

Referral requires knowledge of assessment and treatment protocols

Table 4.8 OHG Recommendations for the Active Rehabilitation Program (101)

Education—directed at managing their pain and overcoming disability
Reassurance and advice—to stay active
Exercise—an active and progressive physical fitness program
Pain management—using behavioral principles
Work—in an occupational setting and directed strongly towards return to work
Rehabilitation—symptomatic relief measures should support and must not interfere with rehabilitation

- **When**—in the acute phase for laboratory or imaging tests or to specialists if "red flags" are present; in the subacute phase for rehabilitation especially if "yellow flags" are present
- **Purpose**—provide "best practice" care following protocols based on current care guidelines

Practitioner Audit (see Chapter 39)

The reflective practice-based model presented here can be facilitated by self-audit of your practice procedures (10). There is no more important player in the transformation of the paradigm for managing spinal conditions than the HCP. All the key players who need to work together are shown in Figure 4.10.

Chart review should reflect that diagnostic triage has been performed; "yellow flags" have been assessed

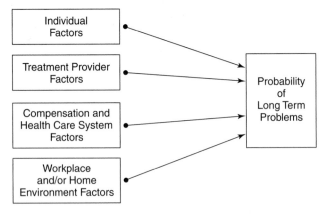

Figure 4.10 Key "players" driving chronic spinal problems. From Pincus T, Vlaeyen JWS, Kendall NAS, Von Korff MR, Kalauokalani DA, Reis S. Cognitive-behavioral therapy and psychosocial factors in low back pain: Directions for the future. Spine 2002;27:E133–E138.

(questionnaire); pain relief options (i.e., manipulation or medication) offered; the patient advised to stay active; self-treatment(s) recommended and instructed ("active care"); referral made if "red flags" of serious pathology, cauda equina, or unresolving neurological condition; and additional investigations or treatment arranged if back pain non-responsive within 6 weeks.

A number of decision points have emerged that are crucial to the modern management of the back pain patient. Guidelines allow us to formulate protocols and even algorithms of care incorporating decision points or care pathways. As further evidence accumulates these protocols will be "fine-tuned" and standards of care will gradually emerge. Presently the following 10 decision points can be identified for management of acute patients with LBP. These are the critical attributes of the new benchmark for managing LBP.

1. Diagnostic triage—patient should be triaged on day 1 into one of three main overarching categories. This involves history and examination without special tests. It is best performed by a primary care doctor such as a general practitioner or chiropractor.
   - Red flags of possible serious disease
   - Nerve root pain
   - Mechanical LBP

2. If there are no red flags, the patient should be reassured that the prognosis is good.

3. If there are red flags present, the patient should be referred for further tests or treatments.

4. Baseline outcome measurements of symptoms (e.g., visual analog scale), impairments (e.g., range of motion), and disability (e.g., activity intolerances) should be captured at the initial visit and monitored at regular intervals to monitor patent status and treatment effectiveness.

5. The patient should be advised to stay as active as possible and to gradually increase their physical activity. They can be encouraged that it is safe to do so, so long as pain is not peripheralizing. Explanation should include a discussion mentioning that hurt does not necessarily equal harm, but is just a sign that stiff areas are being mobilized.

6. Bed rest should not be prescribed unless the patient is in severe pain, and then it should not last more than 2 to 3 days.

7. If patient is failing to return to normal activities within 1 or 2 weeks or the patient needs additional help with pain relief then manipulation by a trained specialist (i.e., chiropractor) or medication (prescribed by a physician) is recommended.

8. Evaluation of "yellow flags"—does not need to wait until 4 or 6 weeks, but can be screened for on visit 1.

9. If there is an unresolving condition after 4 to 6 weeks of conservative care the patient should be referred for additional investigations. Structural tests such as imaging or laboratory work-up. Functional tests such as a physical performance or functional capacity evaluation and psychosocial evaluation, including a "yellow flags" screen and possibly a referral to a pain psychologist.

10. By week 6 if the patient is failing to resume normal activities, rehabilitation should be commenced by a rehabilitation specialist.

At a recent International Forum on Low Back Pain Research in Primary Care, the emphasis was on how to disseminate and implement the new guidelines (7,89). The difficulties of changing physician behavior and ideas on how to accomplish it were discussed. The recent Australian study shows that physician behavior can change, although it may take changes in patient behavior to stimulate it (11)! Goldberg found that physician education lowered spine surgery rates (36). A multipronged approach was used incorporating surgeon study groups, outcomes research, conferences for primary care physicians with a local physician presenting essential components of the model in what is called "academic detailing," and, lastly, a hospital intervention led by a health care economist aimed at discussing cost-effectiveness.

Audit Process
Self-Check of the Chapter's Learning Objectives

- Are you comfortable reassuring patients who have diagnosis such as degenerative arthritis or herniated discs that they can safely reactivate and that in fact this is the best way to recover?

- Are you able to identify when negative coping strategies such as fear–avoidance behavior are leading a patient to avoid activity and thus promote deconditioning?

- What shift in management is necessitated by the presence of "red flags"?

- What shift in management is necessitated by the presence of "yellow flags"?

- Is a structural and psychosocial reevaluation sufficient if a patient is not adequately recovered after 6 weeks?

■ REFERENCES

1. Allan DB, Waddell G. An historical perspective on low back pain and disability. Acta Orthop Scand Suppl 1989;60:1.

2. Amundsen T, Weber H, Nordal HJ, Magnaes B, Abdelnoor M, Lilleas F. Lumbar spinal stenosis: Conservative or surgical management? A prospective 10-year study. Spine 2000;25:1424–1436.

3. Bigos, S, Battie MC. Back disability prevention. Clin Orthop 1987;221:121.

4. Boden SD, Davis DO, Dina TS, et al. Abnormal magnetic-resonance scans of the lumbar spine in asymptomatic subjects. J Bone Joint Surg [Am] 1990a;72:403.

5. Boden SD. McCowin PR, Davis Do, Dina TS, Mark AS, Wiesel S. Abnormal magnetic-resonance scans of the cervical spine in asymptomatic subjects. J Bone Joint Surg 1990b;72A:1178–1184.

6. Borenstein DG, O'Mara JW, Boden SD, et al. The value of magnetic resonance imaging of the lumbar spine to predict low-back pain in asymptomatic subjects. J Bone and Joint Surg 2001;83-A:1306–1311.

7. Borkan J, Van Tulder M, Reis S, Schoene ML, Croft P, Hermoni D. Advances in the field of low back pain in primary care: A Report from the Fourth International Forum. Spine 2002;27:E128–E132.

8. Bortz WM. The disuse syndrome. West J Med 1984;141:691.

9. Brandt-Zawadzki MN, Jensen MC, Obuchowski N, et al. Interobserver and intraobserver variability in interpretation of lumbar disc abnormalities: A comparison of two nomenclatures. Spine 1995;20:1257–1263.

10. Breen AC, Langworthy J, Vogel S, et al. Primary Care Audit Toolkit: Acute Back Pain. Bournemouth: Institute for Musculoskeletal Research and Clinical Implementation. www.imrci.ac.uk, 2000.

11. Buchbinder R, Jolley D, Wyatt M. 2001 Volvo Award Winner in Clinical Studies: Effects of a media campaign on back pain beliefs and its potential influence on management of low back pain in general practice. Spine 2001;26:2535–2542.

12. Burton K, Waddell G. Information and advice to patients w/ back pain can have a positive effect. Spine 1999;24;2484–2491.

13. Bush K, Cowan N, Katz DE, et al. The natural history of sciatica associated with disc pathology: A prospective study with clinical and independent radiologic follow-up. Spine 1992;17:1205.

14. Bush K, Chaudhuri R, Hillier S, Penny J. The pathomorphologic changes that accompany the resolution of cervical radiculopathy. Spine 1997;22(2):183–187.

15. Caragee E, Alamin T, et al. Can MR scanning in patients with sciatica predict failure of open limited discectomy? Presented at the annual meeting of the International Society for the Study of the Lumbar Spine, Edinburgh, 2001.

16. Carragee EJ, Barcohana B, Alamin T, van den Haak E. Prospective controlled study of the development of lower back pain in previously asymptomatic subjects undergoing experimental discography. Spine 2004;29:1112–1117.

17. Carey TS, Mills Garret J, Jackman AM. Beyond the good prognosis. Spine 2000:25:115–120

18. Cherkin DC, Deyo RA, Street JH, Barlow W. Predicting poor outcomes for back pain seen in primary care using patients' own criteria. Spine 1996;21:2900–2907.

19. Dabbs VM, Dabbs LG. Correlation between disk height narrowing and low-back pain. Spine 1990;15:1366.

20. Manniche C, et al. Danish Health Technology Assessment (DIHTA). Low back pain: Frequency Management and Prevention from an HAD Perspective, 1999.

21. Deyo RA. Low back pain—A primary care challenge. Spine 1996;21:2826–2832.

22. Deyo RA, Diehl AK, Rosenthal M. How many days of bed rest for acute low back pain? N Engl J Med 1986;315:1064.

23. Deyo RA, Weinstein JN. Low back pain. N Engl J Med 2001;344:363–370.

24. Dworkin SF. Perspectives on psychogenic versus biogenic factors in orofacial and other pain states. APS J 1992;3:172.

25. Engel GL. Psychogenic pain and the pain prone patient. Am J Med 1959;26:899.

26. Fordyce WE, McMahon R, Rainwater G, et al. Pain complaint-exercise performance relationship in chronic pain. Pain 1981;10:311.

27. Fordyce WE, Fowler RS, Lehmann JF, et al. Operant conditioning in the treatment of chronic pain. Arch Phys Med Rehabil 1973;54:399.

28. Fordyce WE, Brochway JA, Bergman JA, et al. Acute back pain: A control-group comparison of behavioral vs. traditional management methods. J Behav Med 1986;9:127.

29. Frank J, Sinclair S, Hogg-Johnson S, et al. Preventing disability from work-related low-back pain. New evidence gives new hope—if we can just get all the players onside. Can Med Assoc J 1998;158:1625–1631.

30. Frymoyer JW, Newberg A, Pope MH, et al. Spine radiographs in patients with low-back pain: An epidemiological study in men. J Bone Joint Surg [Am] 1984;66:1048.

31. Frymoyer JW. Predicting disability from low back pain. Clin Orth 1992;279:103.

32. Fullenlove TM, Williams AJ: Comparative roentgen findings in symptomatic and asymptomatic backs. JAMA 1957;168:572.

33. Gibson JNA, Grant IC, Waddell G. The Cochrane Review of Surgery for Lumbar Disc Prolapse and Degenerative Lumbar Spondylosis. Spine 1999;24(17):1820–1832.

34. Gibson JNA, Grant IC, Waddell G. Surgery for Lumbar Disc Prolapse (Cochrane Review). The Cochrane Library 2004;3.

35. Gogan WH, Fraser RD. Chymopapain: A 10-year, double-blind study. Spine 1992;17:388–394.

36. Goldberg HI, et al. Can evidence change the rate of back surgery? A randomized controlled trial of community-based education. Effective Clinical Practice May/June, 2001:95–104.

37. Hakelius A. Prognosis in sciatica. Acta Orthop Scand Suppl 1970;129:1.

38. Hitselberger WE, Witten RM. Abnormal myelograms in asymptomatic patients. J Neurosurg 1968;28:204.

39. Indahl A, Haldorsen EH, Holm S, Reikeras O, Hursin H. Five-year follow-up study of a controlled clinical trial using light mobilization and an informative approach to low back pain. Spine 1998;23:2625–2630.

40. International Association for the Study of Pain. Pain terms: A list with definitions and notes on usage. Pain 1979;6:249.

41. Jarvik JG, Deyo RA. Imaging of lumbar intervertebral disc degeneration and aging, excluding disc herniations. Radiology Clinics of North America 2000;38:1255–1266.

42. Jarvik JG, Hollingworth W, Heagerty P, Haynor DR, Deyo RA. The longitudinal assessment of imaging and disability of the back (LAIDBack) study. Spine 2001;26:1158–1166.

43. Jensel MC, Brant-Zawadzki MN, Obuchowski N, et al. Magnetic resonance imaging of the lumbar spine in people without back pain. N Engl J Med 1994;2:69.

44. Kendrick D, Fielding K, Bentler E, Kerslake R, Miller P, Pringle M. Radiography of the lumbar spine in primary care patients with low back pain: Randomized controlled trial. BMJ 2001;322:400–405.

45. Klassen AC, Berman ME. Medical care for headaches. A consumer survey. Cephalgia 1991;11(suppl 11):85–86.

46. Larequi-Lauber T, Vader JP, Burnand B, et al. Appropriateness of indications for surgery of lumbar disc hernia and spinal stenosis. Spine 1997;22(2):203–209.

47. LaRocca H, Macnab IA. Value of pre-employment radiographic assessment of the lumbar spine. Can Med Assoc J 1969;101:383.

48. LaRocca H. A taxonomy of chronic pain syndromes. 1991 Presidential Address, Cervical Spine Research Society Annual Meeting, December 5, 1991. Spine 1992;10:S344.

49. Linton SJ. The socioeconomic impact of chronic back pain: Is anyone benefiting? Editorial. Pain 1998;75:163–168.

50. Linton SJ. The relationship between activity and chronic pain. Pain 1985;21:289.

51. Loeser JD, Fordyce WE. Chronic pain. In: Carr JE, Dendgerink HA, eds. Behavioral Science in the Practice of Medicine. New York: Elsevier, 1983.

52. Magora A, Schwartz A. Relation between the low back pain syndrome and x-ray findings. Scand J Rehabil Med 1976;8:115.

53. Main CJ, Watson PJ. Psychological aspects of pain. Man Ther 1999;4:203–215.

54. Main CJ. Concepts of treatment and prevention in musculoskeletal disorders. In: Linton SL, ed. New avenues for the prevention of chronic musculoskeletal pain and disability. Amsterdam: Elsevier 2002.

55. Malmivaara A, Hakkinen U, Aro T, et al. The treatment of acute low back pain—bed rest, exercises, or ordinary activity? N Engl J Med 1995;332:351–355.

56. McGuirk B, King W, Govind J, Lowry J, Bogduk N. Safety, efficacy and cost-effectiveness of evidence-based guidelines for the management of acute low back pain in primary care. Spine 2001;26:2615–2622.

57. Melzack R, Wall PD. Pain mechanisms: A new theory. Science 1965;150:978.

58. Melzack R. In: Gatchel RJ, Turk DC, ed. Psychological factors in pain. Critical perspectives. New York: The Guilford Press, 1999:3–17.

59. Merskey H. The definition of pain. Eur J Psychiatry 1991;6:153–159.

60. Merskey H. Limitations of pain behavior. APS Journal 1992;2:101.

61. Merskey H. The importance of hysteria. Br J Psychiatry 1986;149:23.

62. Merskey H. Regional pain is rarely hysterical. Arch Neurol 1988;45:915.

63. Merskey H, Bogduk N, eds. Classification of chronic pain: Description of chronic pain syndromes and definitions of pain terms, 2nd ed. Seattle, WA: IASP Press, 1994.

64. Mixter WJ, Barr JS. Rupture of the intervertebral disc with involvement of the spinal canal. N Engl J Med 1934;211:210.

65. Moore JE, Von Korff M, Cherkin D, Saunders K, Lorig K. A randomized trial of a cognitive-behavioral program for enhancing back pain self-care in a primary care setting. Pain 2000;88:145–153.

66. Nachemson A. Introduction. In: Nachemson A, Jonsson E, eds. Swedish SBU report. Evidence based treatment for back pain. Stockholm/Philadelphia: Swedish Council on Technology Assessment in Health Care (SBU)/Lippincott Williams & Wilkins (English translation), 2000.

67. Nachemson AL. Newest knowledge of low back pain. Clin Orthop 1992;279:8.

68. Nachemson A. Work for all, for those with low back pain as well. Clin Orthop 1983;179:77.

69. Naliboff BD, Cohen MJ, Swanson GA, et al. Comprehensive assessment of chronic low back pain patients and controls: Physical abilities, level of activities, psychological adjustment and pain perception. Pain 1985;23:121.

70. Nicholas MK. Reducing disability in injured workers: The importance of collaborative management. In: Linton SL, ed. New avenues for the prevention of chronic musculoskeletal pain and disability. Amsterdam: Elsevier, 2002.

71. Philips HC, Jahanshahi M. The components of pain behavior report. Behav Res Ther 1986;24:117.

72. Pilowsky I. A general classification of abnormal illness behavior. Br J Med Psychol 1979;51:131.

73. Rozenberg S, et al. French multicenter prospective, randomized, open study comparing advice to stay active and bed rest in acute low back pain, presented at the annual meeting of the International Society for the Study of the Lumbar Spine. Edinburgh, 2001.

74. Rothman RH, et al. A study of computer-assisted tomography. Spine 1984;9:548.

75. Saal JA, Saal JS. Nonoperative treatment of herniated lumbar intervertebral disc with radiculopathy. Spine 1989;14:431.

76. Schneider PL, Kahanovitz N. Clinical testing in chronic low back pain. Surg Rounds Orthop 1990;4:19.

77. Slater E, Glithero E. A follow-up of patients diagnosed as suffering from "hysteria." J Psychosom Res 1965;9:9.

78. Splithoff CA. Lumbosacral junction: Roentographic comparison of patients with and without back ache. JAMA 1953;152:1610.

79. Sternbach RA, Timmermans G. Personality changes associated with reduction of pain. Pain 1975;1:177.

80. Szasz TS. The painful person. Lancet 1968;88:18.

81. Teresi LM, Lufkin RB, Reicher MA, et al. Asymptomatic degenerative disk disease and spondylosis of the cervical spine: MR Imaging. Radiology 1987;164:83–88.

82. Torgeson WR, Dotler WE. Comparative roentgenographic study of the asymptomatic and symptomatic lumbar spine. J Bone Joint Surg [Am] 1976;58:850.

83. Troup JDG. The perception of pain and incapacity for work: Prevention and early treatment. Physiotherapy 1988;74:435.

84. Turner JA. Educational and behavorial interventions for back pain in primary care. Spine 1996;21:2851–2859.

85. Vader JP, Forchet F, Larequi-Lauber T, Dubois RW, Burnand B. Appropriateness of surgery for sciatica: Reliability of guidelines from expert panels. Spine 2000;25(14):1831–1836.

86. Value Health Science: Indications for Laminectomy–Physician Expert Panel. Santa Monica, California (Unpublished data), 1989.

87. van Tulder MW, Assendelft JJ, Koes BW, Bouter LM. Spinal radiographic findings and nonspecific low back pain: A systematic review of observational studies. Spine 1997;22:427–434.

88. van Tulder MW, Koes BW, Bouter LM. Conservative treatment of acute and chronic nonspecific low back pain: A systematic review of randomized controlled trials of the most common interventions. Spine 1997;22(18):2128–2156.

89. van Tulder WE, Croft PR, van Splunteren P, et al. Disseminating and implementing the results of back pain research in primary care. Spine 2002;27:E121–E127.

90. Victorian Workcover Authority. Clinical framework for the delivery of health services to injured workers. www.workcover.gov.au, 2004.

91. Videman T, Nurminen M, Troup JDG. Lumbar spinal pathology in cadaveric material in relation to history of back pain, occupation, and physical loading. Spine 1990;15:728.

92. Videman T, Sarna S, Battie MC, et al. The long-term effects of physical loading and exercise lifestyles on back-related symptoms, disability and spinal pathology among men. Spine 1995;20:699–709.

93. Videman T, Battié MC. The influence of occupation on lumbar degeneration. Spine 1999;24:1164–1168.

94. Vlaeyen JWS, Crombex G. Fear of movement/(re)injury, avoidance and pain disability in chronic low back pain patients. Manual Therapy 1999:4:187–195.

95. Von Korff M, Moore JE, Lorig K, et al. A randomized trial of layperson-led self-management group intervention for back pain patients in primary care. Spine 1998;23:2608–2615.

96. Vroomen PCAJ, de Krom MCTFM, Wilmink JT, Kester ADM, Knottnerus JA. Lack of effectiveness of bed rest for sciatica. N Engl J Med 1999;340:418–423.

97. Waddell G. A new clinical model for the treatment of low-back pain. Spine 1987;12:634.

98. Waddell G. A new clinical model for the treatment of low back pain. In: Weinstein JN, Wiesel SW, eds. The Lumbar Spine: The International Society for the Study of the Lumbar Spine. Philadelphia: WB Saunders, 1990:38–56.

99. Waddell G. The Back Pain Revolution, 2nd ed. Edinburgh: Churchill Livingstone, 2004.

100. Waddell G, Main CJ, Morris EW, et al. Chronic low back pain, psychological distress and illness behavior. Spine 1984;9:209.

101. Waddell G, Burton AK. Occupational health guidelines for the management of low back pain at work—evidence review. Faculty of Occupational Medicine. London, 2000.

102. Waddell G, Morris EW, DiPaoloa M, et al. A concept of illness tested as an improved basis for surgical decisions in low back disorders. Spine 1986;11:712.

103. Weber H. Lumbar disc herniation: A controlled, prospective study with 10 years of observation. Spine 1983;8:131–140.

104. Wiesel SE, Tsourmans N, Feffer HL, et al. A study of computer-assisted tomography. I. The incidence of positive CAT scans in an asymptomatic group of patients. Spine 1984;9:549.

105. Wiltse LL, Rocchio PF. Preoperative psychological tests as predictors of success of chemonucleolysis in the treatment of the low back syndrome. J Bone Joint Surg [Am] 1975;57:478.

106. Scotland's Working Backs Partnership 2000. Working Backs Scotland, www.workingbacksscotland.com

107. Yukawa U, Kato Fumihiko, Matsubara Y, Kajino G, Nakamura S, Nitta H. Serial magnetic resonance imaging follow-up study of lumbar disc herniation conservatively treated for average 30 months: Relation between reduction of herniation and degeneration of disc. J Spinal Disord 1996;9:251–256.

108. Zarkowska E, Philips HC. Recent onset vs. persistent pain: Evidence for a distinction. Pain 1987;25:365.

Basic Science

Editor's Note

The foundation of the reactivation self-care model is grounded in the sciences of biomechanics and neurophysiology. This section reviews the most common mechanisms of spine injury as well as the most likely sources of pain. How to improve stability patterns and the exercise science behind that are also key areas of discussion in this section.

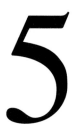

5

Lumbar Spine Stability: Mechanism of Injury and Restabilization

Stuart M. McGill

Learning Objectives

On completion of this chapter you should be able to:

- Explain stability and the foundation for clinical instability
- Understand injury mechanisms to ensure that injury exacerbating maneuvers are not unknowingly involved when prescribing therapeutic exercise
- Be able to prescribe basic stabilization exercises designed to coordinate muscular contraction to challenge both muscle and the motor system while simultaneously sparing the spine joints

      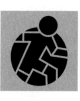

Introduction

Traditional emphasis on the enhancement of muscle strength and spine range of motion during rehabilitation protocols has not reduced back troubles; in fact, some evidence suggests a link to negative outcome in significant numbers of people. Scientific efforts to quantify the mechanisms of injury and of stability suggest that a spine must first be stable to minimize the risk of tissue overload and damage that result from either inappropriate muscle activation and/or spine joint position. The concept of stability, together with notions of design and application of stabilization exercise, is briefly synthesized. The objective is to challenge muscle systems to achieve sufficient functional stability, but to achieve this challenge in a way that spares the spine of excessive exacerbating load.

Lumbar stability, core stability, and low-back stabilizing exercises are popular topics related to optimal athletic/occupational performance and to the rehabilitation of painful backs. The objective of such exercise is to enhance the function of these critical torso muscles in a way that spares the spine from damage. The intention of this chapter is to develop a synthesis of the scientific foundation and formalization of the notion of stability as it pertains to the lumbar spine, and then to provide specific guidelines for enhancing stability to advance spine rehabilitation. Although a large book could be written to describe ideal exercise programs for the entire population including those with chronic low back pain, adolescents to geriatrics through to elite athletes, the focus of the exercises discussed here is more toward the beginner's program—developing the safest exercise for enhancing stability and for acquiring and maintaining low back health. For the interested reader, more extensive references together with tabulated data of specific muscle activation profiles, resultant spine loads, etc., can be found in the authors review chapters and original papers listed at www.ahs. uwaterloo.ca/kin/kinfac/mcgill.html or in my recent textbooks *Low Back Disorders: Evidence Based Prevention and Rehabilitation* (56) and *Ultimate Back Fitness and Performance* (58).

In most traditional approaches to designing low back exercise, an emphasis has been placed on the immediate restoration, or enhancement, of spine range of motion and muscle strength. Generally, this approach has not been sufficiently efficacious in reducing back troubles; in fact, a review of the evidence suggests only a weak link with improving back symptoms, whereas some studies suggest a link with negative outcome in significant numbers of people (51). It appears that the emphasis on early restoration of spine range of motion continues to be driven by legislative definitions of low back disability, namely loss of range of motion. Thus, therapeutic success is often judged on motion restored. Most recent work suggest little correlation between ROM and work versatility ratings (64). The underlying theme of this chapter, and in fact book, reflects the developing philosophy based on mechanisms of injury and stability that a spine must first be stable before moments and forces are produced to enhance performance but to do so in a way that spares the spine from potentially injurious load. Preliminary field evidence (although not yet definitive) suggests that the approach has promise.

The meaning of the words "spine stability" depends on the background of the individual; to the biomechanist, they pertain to a mechanical structure that can become unstable when a critical point is reached; a surgeon may view abnormal joint motion patterns as unstable but correctable by changing the anatomy; the manual medicine practitioner may interpret patterns of muscle coordination and posture and attempt to alter one, or a few, muscle activation profiles. Several groups have made contributions to the stability issue but only a very few have attempted to actually quantify stability and joint moment and force demands. This chapter is biased toward efforts to quantify stability and develop clinical notions based on direct biomechanical evidence of stability indexes, resultant joint and paraspinal tissue loads, and measurements of processed muscle activation and joint motion patterns. For this reason, the reader is familiarized with injury mechanisms first to minimize the risk of inadvertently prescribing routines that produce unnecessarily high loads on damaged tissues.

The Injury Process— Tissues Damage

There is a tendency among those reporting or describing the back injury to identify a single specific event as the cause of the damage, such as lifting a box and twisting. This description of low back injury is common, particularly among the occupational/medical community who are often required to identify a single event when filling out injury reporting forms. However, relatively few low back injuries occur from a single event. Rather, the culminating injury event was preceded by a history of excessive loading that gradually, but progressively, reduced the level of tolerance to tissue failure (49). Thus, other scenarios in which subfailure loads can result in injury are probably more important. For example, the ultimate failure of a tissue (i.e., injury) can result from accumulated trauma produced either by repeated application of load (and failure from fatigue) or of a sustained load that is applied for long durations or repetitively applied (and failure from deformation and strain). Thus, the injury process may not always be associated with loads of high magnitude. Finally, it goes without saying that loss of mechanical integrity in any load bearing tissue of the spine will result in stiffness losses and an increased risk of unstable behavior. Thus, documenting the injury process is a necessary foundation for understanding, formulating, and utilizing the concepts of spine instability and stability.

Whereas excellent progress has been made in the laboratory documenting specific instabilities in flexion–extension, lateral bend, and axial rotation modes in animal preparations (63), understanding the injury process in humans (the cause of back troubles in real life) has perhaps been hampered by the focus on exposure to a single variable, namely acute, or single maximum exposure to, lumbar compression. A few studies have suggested higher levels of compression exposure increased the risk of LBD (e.g., 31), although the correlation was low. Further, some studies show that higher rates of LBDs occur when levels of lumbar compression are reasonably low. Are there other mechanical variables that modulate the risk of LBDs?

There are many tissues in the lower back and many different modes of loading that occur when performing work and exercise. Apart from joint compression, joint shear has been shown to be very important as a metric for injury risk in the Norman et al. study (60), particularly cumulative shear over a work day. Shear is an interesting variable because whereas most studies report reaction shear (that is the action of gravity and load in the hands to shear forward the ribcage on the pelvis through the lumbar spine), this is not the form of shear load that is experienced by the lumbar joints. In a series of work, the Waterloo group (43,66,48) has shown that if the spine maintains a neutral curvature (the torso is flexed forward about the hips, neither flexing nor extending the spine itself), then the dominant low back extensors with their unique force vector direction (specifically longissimus thoracis and iliocostalis lumborum) support the shear reaction forces caused by the action of gravity on the flexed torso, resulting in a lowering of the shear load experienced by the joint. These forces would normally be borne by the disc and facet joints. However, if the individual elects to flex the spine itself when bending forward, sufficiently so to stretch the posterior ligaments with full spinal flexion, then the architecture of the interspinous ligaments cause anterior shear forces (32) to add to the shearing reaction from gravity. Furthermore, ligamentous involvement disables the lumbar muscles (specifically noted) from supporting the

reaction shear as they reorientate to a line of action more parallel to the compressive axis (54) (Fig. 5.1). With full spine flexion and a modest amount of gravitational reaction shear, it is not difficult to exceed shear failure loads of the spine, which have been found to be approximately 2,000 to 2,800 Newtons in adult cadavers (20). This paragraph suggests that personal work technique or, more specifically, spine motion can affect the risk of spine damage. Recent work by Yingling et al. (77) on pig spines has shown that load rate is not a major modulator of shear tolerance unless the load is very ballistic, such as what might occur during a slip and fall. Summarizing the lumbar sagittal motion and shear issue, evidence from tissue-specific injury studies generally supports the notion of avoiding full lumbar flexion when performing loading tasks to minimize the risk of low back injury. There is no evidence to support conscious effort to perform pelvic tilts (i.e., hyperlordosis or lumbar flexion) during lifting or exertion.

Although twisting has been named in several studies as a risk factor for low back injury, the literature appears confused by not making the distinction between the kinematic variable of twisting and the kinetic variable of generating twisting torque. Whereas many epidemiological surveillance studies link a higher risk of LBD with twisting, twisting with low twist moment results in relatively low muscle activity and correspondingly low spine load (45,46). Further, passive tissue loading is not substantial until the end of the twist range of motion (22). However, developing twisting moment places very large compressive loads on the spine because of the enormous co-activation of the spine musculature (46) and this can occur when the spine is not twisted, but in a neutral posture in which the ability to tolerate loads is higher. It would appear that either single variable (the kinematic act of twisting, or generating the kinetic variable of twist torque while not twisting) is less dangerous than may be suggested by epidemiological surveys. However, it would appear that elevated risk from very high tissue-loading occurs when the spine is fully twisted at the same time when there is a need to generate high twisting torque (46).

There are many personal factors that appear to affect spine tissue tolerance, for example age and gender. Jager et al. (35) compiled the available literature that passed their inclusion criteria on the tolerance of lumbar motion units to bear compressive load. Their results revealed that if males and females are matched for age, females were able to sustain only approximately two-thirds of the compressive loads of males. Furthermore, the data of Jager et al. showed that within a given gender, the 60-year-old spine was able to tolerate only approximately two-thirds of that tolerated by a 20-year-old. There are

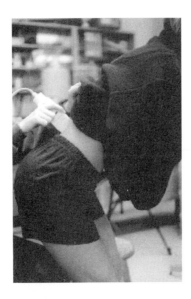
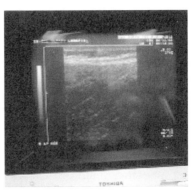
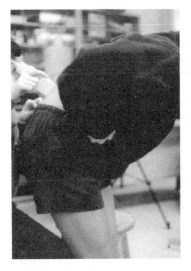
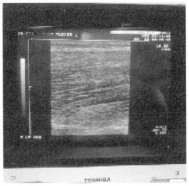

Figure 5.1 Subjects rotated about the hips while maintaining a neutral lordosis to activate the longissimus/iliocostalis complex. Note the oblique angle of the fibers in the ultrasound image with respect to the compressive axis suggesting these muscles produce large shear forces. This angle is lost, together with the protective shear forces, when the spine is flexed.

other personal factors such as motor control system fitness in which it appears a motor control error can lead to a back injury during very benign tasks such as picking up a pencil from the floor. (This is explained in a subsequent section.)

Many factors appear to modulate the risk of specific low back tissues damage other than load magnitude and loading mode. Although disc herniations have been produced under controlled conditions (e.g., 28), Callaghan and McGill (14) have been able to consistently produce disc herniations by mimicking spine motion and load patterns seen in workers

and in replicating the motion and loads of some lumber extension exercise machines. Specifically, it appears that only a very modest amount of spine compression force is required (only 800–1000 N) but the spine specimen must be repeatedly flexed—mimicking repeated torso–spine flexion from continual bending to a fully flexed posture. In these experiments, the progressive tracking of disc nucleus material traveling posteriorly through the annulus of the disc was documented with sequestration of the nucleus material approximately 18,000 to 25,000 cycles of flexion (fewer cycles were required for herniation with higher simultaneous compressive loads). This study included the utilization of a pig degenerative trauma model, which on one hand was an animal model but on the other, control over age, diet, and physical activity provided a unique opportunity. Spines and discs obtained from humans are typically older and have lost sufficient disc hydration to match the hydration levels, and potential for herniation, seen in the age groups of workers at risk for this specific type of event (typically 30–50-year-olds). But the important point here is that herniation appears to be more strongly linked to repeated flexion motion rather than load.

Another modulator for tissue damage appears to be the posture of the joint resulting from the curvature of the spine in vivo. For example, Adams et al. (3) showed that a fully flexed spine is weaker than one that is moderately flexed. In a most recent study, Gunning and McGill (29) have shown that a fully flexed spine (using a controlled porcine spine model) is 20% to 40% weaker than if it were in a neutral posture, and that hydration levels matched to the changes seen in peoples' discs throughout the work day also modulate the tolerance. For example, the spinal discs are more easily damaged first thing in the morning on rising from bed when they are fully hydrated. A fascinating study, reported by Snook and colleagues (70), demonstrated that of 85 patients randomly assigned to a group that controlled the amount of early morning lumbar flexion had significant reduction in pain intensity, compared to a control group. Then, when the control group received the experimental treatment they responded with similar reductions.

Collectively, the evidence suggests that the risk of spine tissue damage is a function of load magnitude, directional mode of the applied load, motion repetition, spine posture, hydration level and time of day, motor control and instantaneous stability, and individual age and gender. Injury history and tissue damage is an overlaying modulator. Collectively these data supports the notion of an envelope of motion and loading for optimal tissue health. In addition, it is well known that tissues adapt and remodel with load (e.g., bone, Carter (16); ligament, Woo et al. (76); disc, Porter (65); vertebrae, Brinckmann et al. (11)), which is at the core of any rehabilitation program. However, biological variability prevents the identification of specific levels of loading that either build tissue or initiate breakdown, together with the optimal rest periods and days off that promote healthy tissue adaption for a given individual. Thus, it would appear that the wisest philosophical approach for the optimal design of activity, either during the activities of daily living or during rehabilitation efforts, may be to adopt the notion that too much of any single activity is problematic. No rehabilitation program can be fully effective if patients undo the beneficial responses of therapy with inappropriate activities of daily living.

Summary of Specific Tissue Injury Mechanisms

A very brief description of tissue damage from excessive load is provided here. All injuries noted are known to be accelerated with repetitive loading.

Endplates Schmorls nodes are thought to be healed end plate fractures (75) that are linked to trauma (5). In fact, traumatic Schmorls node formation has been documented (via MRI) in a patient after forced lumbar flexion, which resulted in an injury (40). People apparently are not born with Schmorls nodes and their presence is associated with a more active lifestyle (30). Under excessive compressive loading of spinal units in the laboratory, the endplate appears to be the first structure to be injured (11,14), whereas Gunning and McGill (29) have shown discs hydrated to mimic conditions similar to just rising from bed fail at a much lower load (20%–40%), compared to the strength later in the day (they also observed that failure was reached at lower levels if the spines were fully flexed at the time of loading). Endplate avulsion has been observed under excessive anterior–posterior shear loading.

Vertebrae Vertebral cancellous bone is damaged under compressive loading (26) and often accompanies disc herniation and annular delamination (29).

Disc Annulus Several types of damage appears to occur. Classic disc herniation appears to be associated with repeated flexion motion with only moderate compressive loading required (14) and repeated full flexion with lateral bending and twisting (1,28). Avulsion of the lateral annulus, in particular, has been documented under anterior posterior shear loading (78). Annular damage during twisting has been noted in animal spines (e.g., 61) but the link remains a controversial issue in humans. Farfan et al. (23) concluded that axial twists were the most important factor in the initiation of damage to the annulus, whereas Adams and Hutton (2) suggested that healthy facet joints prevent such an occurrence.

Disc Nucleus Although Buckwalter (12) has stated "no other musculoskeletal soft tissue structure undergoes more dramatic alterations with age . . ." the relationship between loading, disc nutrition, decreasing concentration of viable cells, accumulation of degraded matrix molecules, and fatigue failure of the matrix remain obscure. However, recently Lotz et al. (41) has documented cell death (apoptosis) within the nucleus increases under excessive compressive load. It is interesting that these changes are not delectable or diagnosable in vivo.

Neural Arch (Posterior Bony Elements) Spondylitic fractures are thought to occur from repeated stress strain reversals associated with cyclic full flexion and extension (30,13). Excessive shear forces have been also documented to fracture parts of the arch (20,75).

Ligaments It appears that ligaments avulse at lower load rates but will tear in their midsubstance at higher rates of load (61). Landing on the buttocks from a fall has been hypothesized by McGill (49) to rupture the interspinous complex given the documented forces (52) and joint tolerance. Falling on the behind results in a higher risk for prolonged disability (73), which is consistent with the prolonged length of time for ligamentous tissue to regain structural integrity, if ever (76).

Summary of Injury Pathways

Avoidance of further tissue damage during rehabilitation exercise and activities of daily living is a critical objective. Evidence suggests that reduction in specific tissue damage could be accomplished by:

1. Reducing peak (and cumulative) spine compressive loads to reduce the risk of end-plate damage;
2. Reducing repeated spine motion to full flexion to reduce risk of disc herniation; reducing spine flexion in the morning reduces symptoms;
3. Reducing repeated full range flexion to full range extension to reduce the risk of pars (or neural arch) fracture;
4. Reducing peak and cumulative shear forces to reduce the risk of facet and neural arch damage;
5. Reducing slips and falls, or ballistic loading, to reduce risk of passive collagenous tissues such as ligaments;
6. Reducing length of time sitting, particularly exposure to seated vibration to reduce a risk of disc herniation or accelerated degeneration.

The Injury Process—Motor Changes

Those reporting debilitating low back pain conclusively have simultaneous changes in their motor control systems. Recognizing these changes is important because they effect the stabilizing system and, therefore, are a focal point for optimal rehabilitation. Richardson et al. (67) have produced quite a comprehensive review of this literature together with

making a case for targeting specific muscle groups during rehabilitation. Specifically, their objective is to re-educate faulty motor control patterns after injury. The challenge is to train the stabilizing system during steady-state activities together with stabilizing during rapid voluntary motions and to withstand sudden surprise loads.

A wide variety of motor changes have been documented with particular attention directed to the transverse abdominis and multifidus muscles. For example, during anticipatory movements like sudden shoulder flexion movements, the onset of transverse abdominis has been shown to be delayed in some individuals with back troubles (34,67,62), suggesting compromise of the ability to ensure spine stability. They have developed a rehabilitation protocol specifically intended to re-educate the motor control system for involvement of the transverse abdominis.

Changes to the multifidus complex in some individuals have also been well-documented by a number of laboratories. For example, Sihvonen et al. (69) documented diminished myoelectric activity around the unstable joints during concentric contractions. Jorgensen and Nicoliasen (37) and Nicoliasen and Jorgensen (59) have associated lower endurance in the spine extensors in general, whereas Roy et al. (68) established faster fatigue rates in the multifidus, in many individuals with low back troubles. Further, there is evidence that the structure of the muscle itself experiences change after injury or pain episodes, and several have documented selective atrophy in the type II fibers (24,25,38,42,79), whereas long-term outcome was associated with certain composition characteristics. Specifically, good outcome was associated with normal fiber appearance, whereas poor outcome was associated with atrophy in the type II fibers and a moth-eaten appearance observed in type I fibers. Further, even after symptoms have resolved, Hides et al. (33) have documented a smaller multifidus and suggested impaired reflexes as a mechanism. This theory appears tenable given documented evidence of this at other joints, particularly at the knee (36,71,72). It is this collection of evidence that supports stabilization exercises that promote patterns of muscular co-contraction observed with fit spines.

Instability as a Cause of Injury

Although biomechanists have been able to successfully explain how strenuous exertions cause specific low back tissue damage, explaining how injury occurs from tasks such as picking up a pencil from the floor has been more challenging. Recent evidence suggests that such injuries are real and result from the spine buckling or exhibiting unstable behavior. But this buckling mechanism can occur during far more challenging exertions as well.

A number of years ago we were investigating the mechanics of power-lifter spines while they lifted extremely heavy loads using video fluoroscopy to view their vertebrae in the sagittal plane. During their lifts, even though the lifters outwardly appeared to fully flex their spines, in fact their spines were 2 to 3 degrees per joint from full flexion, thus explaining how they could lift magnificent loads without sustaining injury—the risk of disc and ligamentous damage is greatly elevated when the spine is fully flexed (which the lifters skillfully avoided). We happened to capture one injury on the fluoroscopic motion film—the first such observation that we know of. During the injury incident, just as the semi-squatting lifter had lifted the load approximately 10 cm off the floor, only the L2/L3 joint briefly rotated to the full flexion calibrated angle and exceeded it by one-half a degree, whereas all other lumbar joints maintained their static positions (not fully flexed) (17). The spine buckled! Sophisticated modeling analysis revealed that buckling can occur from a motor control error in which a short and temporary reduction in activation to one, or more, of the intersegmental muscles would cause rotation of just a single joint so that passive or other tissues become irritated or possibly injured (18).

Adams and Dolan (4) have noted that passive tissues begin to damage with bending moments of 60 Nm—this occurs simply with the weight of the torso when bending over and a temporary loss of muscular support. This scenario is not an excessive task, but it is often reported to clinicians by patients as the event that caused their injury (i.e., picking up a pencil). However, reporting of such an event will not be found in the scientific literature. Medical personnel would not record this event because in many jurisdictions it would not be deemed a compensable injury—the medical report attributes the cause elsewhere.

Other evidence linking poor motor coordination with higher risks for the lumbar spine reaching critical points of instability exists and is revealing. Cholewicki and McGill (18) have identified through a modeling analysis, the nodal points, or specific spinal joint, where buckling could occur from specific motor control errors. Such inappropriate muscle sequencing has been observed in men who are challenged by holding a load in the hands while breathing 10% CO_2 to elevate breathing. On one hand, the muscles must co-contract to ensure sufficient spine stability, but on the other, challenged breathing is often characterized by rhythmic/contraction/relaxation of the abdominal wall (44). Thus, the motor system is

presented with a conflict—should the torso muscles remain active isometrically to maintain spine stability or will they rhythmically relax and contract to assist with active expiration (but sacrifice spine stability). Fit motor systems appear to meet the simultaneous breathing and spine support challenge—unfit ones may not. All of these deficient motor control mechanisms will heighten biomechanical susceptibility to injury or reinjury (18,19).

In vitro, a ligamentous lumbar spine buckles under compressive loading at approximately 90 Newtons (approximately 20 lb) highlighting the critical role of the musculature to stiffen the spine against buckling (with the critical work and analysis of he passive tissues being performed by Crisco and Panjabi (21)). Anatomical arrangement of muscle around the spine, coupled with critically important patterns of activation, enables the spine to bear a much higher compressive load as it stiffens and becomes more resistant to buckling but in so doing, the spine bears even more load because of the stiffening muscle activity. As noted, aberrant patterns of activation can result in instantaneous spine instability (18) and acute tissue overload. But over the longer-term, several groups including the Queensland group (66) have developed a tissue damage model which suggests chronically poor motor control (and motion patterns) initiates microtrauma in tissues, which accumulates leading to symptomatic injury. Injury leads to further deleterious change in motor patterns such that chronicity can only be broken with specific techniques to re-educate the local muscle–motor control system. Both acute and chronic instability tissue models have been proposed. But given the wide range of individuals and physical demands, questions remain as to what is the optimal balance in terms of stability, motion facilitation, and moment generation—if stability is achieved through muscular cocontraction, how much is necessary and how is it best achieved?

On Stability: The Foundation

This section shall formalize the notion of stability from a spine perspective. During the 1980s, Professor Anders Bergmark of Sweden, very elegantly formalized stability in a spine model with joint stiffness and 40 muscles (9). In this classic work he was able to formalize mathematically the concepts of energy wells, stiffness, stability, and instability. For the most part, this seminal work went unrecognized largely because the engineers who understood the mechanics did not have the biological–clinical perspective, and the clinicians were hindered in the interpretation and implications of the engineering mechanics. This pioneering effort, together with its continued evolution by several others, is be synthesized here—the current author has attempted to encapsulate the critical notions without mathematical complexity but directs the mathematically inclined reader to other sources (9,18).

The concept of stability begins with potential energy that, for the purposes here, is of two basic forms. In the first form, objects have potential energy by virtue of their height above a datum.

$$PE = mass * gravity * height$$

Critical to measuring stability are the notions of energy wells and minimum potential energy. If a ball is placed into a bowl it is stable, because if a force was applied to the ball (or a perturbation) the ball will rise up the side of the bowl but then come to rest again in the position of least potential energy at the bottom of the bowl, or the energy well. As noted by Bergmark, a stable equilibrium prevails when the potential energy of the system is at minimum. The system is made more stable by deepening the bowl and/or by increasing the steepness of the sides of the bowl (Fig. 5.2). Thus, the notion of stability requires the specification of the unperturbed energy state of a system followed by study of the system following perturbation—if the joules of work performed by the perturbation is less than the joules of potential energy inherent to the system, then the system will remain stable (i.e., the ball will not roll out of the bowl). The corollary is that the mechanical system will collapse if the applied load exceeds a critical value (determined by potential energy and stiffness).

The previous ball analogy is a two-dimensional example. This would be analogous to a hinged skeletal joint that only has the capacity for flexion/extension. Spinal joints can rotate in three planes and translate along three axes requiring a six-dimensional bowl for each joint—mathematics enables the examination of a 36-dimensional bowl (6 lumbar joints with 6 degrees of freedom) representing the whole lumbar spine. If the height of the bowl were decreased in any one of these 36 dimensions, the ball could roll

out. In clinical terms, a single muscle having an inappropriate force (and thus stiffness), or a damaged passive tissue, which has lost stiffness, can cause instability that is both predictable and quantifiable.

Whereas potential energy by virtue of height is useful for illustrating the concept, potential energy as a function of stiffness and storage of elastic energy is actually used for musculoskeletal application. Elastic potential energy is calculated from stiffness (k) and deformation (x) in the elastic element:

$$PE = 1/2 * k * x^2$$

In other words, the greater the stiffness (k), the greater the steepness of the sides of the bowl (from the previous analogy), and the more stable the structure. Thus, stiffness creates stability (Fig. 5.3). Active muscle produces a stiff member and in fact the greater the activation of the muscle, the greater this stiffness—it has long been known that joint stiffness increases rapidly and non-linearly with muscle activation such that only very modest levels of muscle activity create sufficiently stiff and stable joints. Furthermore, joints possess inherent joint stiffness as the passive capsules and ligaments contribute stiffness particularly at the end range of motion. The motor control system is able to control stability of the joints through coordinated muscle co-activation and to a lesser degree by placing joints in positions that modulate passive stiffness contribution. However, a faulty motor control system can lead to inappropriate magnitudes of muscle force and stiffness, allowing a valley for the ball to roll out or clinically and for a joint to buckle or undergo shear translation. But mechanical systems, and particularly musculoskeletal linkages, are limited to analysis of local stability since the energy wells are not infinitely deep and the many anatomical components contribute force and stiffness in synchrony to create surfaces of potential energy where there are many local wells. Thus, local minima are located from examination of the derivative of the energy surface (9,18). Spine

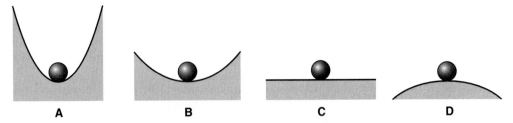

Figure 5.2 The continuum of stability. A is most stable whereas D is least stable. The ball in the bowl seeks the energy well or position of minimum potential energy (m*g*h). Deepening the bowl or increasing the steepness of the sides increases the ability to survive perturbation. This increases stability.

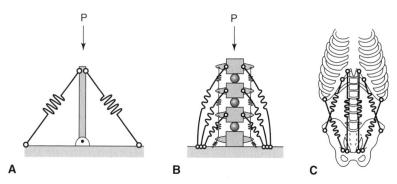

Figure 5.3 **(A)** Increasing the stiffness of the cables (muscles) increases the stability (or deepens the bowl) and increases the ability to support larger applied loads p without falling. **(B)** Spine stiffness (and stability) is achieved by a complex interaction of stiffening structures along the spine and **(C)** those forming the torso wall (right panel).

stability, then, is quantified by forming a matrix in which the total stiffness energy for each degree of freedom of joint motion is represented by a number (or Eigen value) and the magnitude of that number represents its contribution to forming the height of the bowl in that particular dimension. Eigen values less than zero indicate the potential for instability. The eigenvector (different from the Eigen value) can then identify the mode in which the instability occurred, whereas sensitivity analysis may reveal the possible contributors allowing unstable behavior. Gardner-Morse et al. (27) have initiated interesting investigations into eigenvectors by predicting patterns of spine deformation caused by impaired muscular intersegmental control or for clinical relevance—what muscular pattern would have prevented the instability?

Activating a group of muscle synergists and antagonists in the optimal way now becomes a critical issue. In clinical terms, the full complement of the stabilizing musculature must work harmoniously to ensure stability together with generation of the required moment and desired joint movement. But only one muscle with inappropriate activation amplitude may produce instability, or at least unstable behavior could result at lower applied loads.

How much stability is necessary? Obviously insufficient stiffness renders the joint unstable but too much stiffness and co-activation imposes massive load penalties on the joints and prevents motion. Sufficient stability is a concept that involves the determination of how much muscular stiffness is necessary for stability together with a modest amount of extra stability to form a margin of safety. Interestingly enough, given the rapid increase in joint stiffness with modest muscle force, large muscular forces are rarely required. In our recent papers, stabilization exercises were quantified and ranked for muscle acti-

vation magnitudes together with the resultant spine load (15,56). Quantification of individual tissue loads in the spine is a complex procedure and an issue outside the constraints of this article and is reported elsewhere (47) (see Table 26.1). Furthermore, Cholewicki's work (19) has demonstrated that sufficient stability of the lumbar spine is achieved, in an undeviated spine, in most people with modest levels of co-activation of the paraspinal and abdominal wall muscles. This means that people, from patients to athletes, must be able to maintain sufficient stability in all activities with low, but continuous, muscle activation. Thus, maintaining a stability margin of safety when performing tasks, particularly the tasks of daily living, is not compromised by insufficient strength but rather insufficient endurance. We are now beginning to understand the mechanistic pathway of those studies showing the efficacy of endurance training for the muscles that stabilize the spine. Having strong abdominals does not necessarily provide the prophylactic effect that had been hoped for, but several works suggest that endurable muscles reduce the risk of future back troubles (10).

A Philosophy of Low Back Exercise Prescription

Many traditional notions that exercise professionals consider to be principles for exercise prescription, particularly when dealing with the low back, may not be as well supported with data as generally thought. A review of the efficacy of traditional exercise versus stabilization programs both identified and motivated a re-examination of conventional thought (51). For example, there is a widely held view that sit-ups should be performed with bent knees, but it is becoming apparent that the resultant spinal loading (well more than 3000 N of compression to a fully flexed spine) suggests sit-ups are not suitable for most people at all. Other abdominal challenges are more effective and safer. Other examples include, contrary to the belief of many, adopting a posterior pelvic tilt when performing many types of low back exercise actually increases the risk of injury by flexing the lumbar joints and loading passive tissues.

Having stronger back and abdominal muscles appears to have no prophylactic value for reducing bad back episodes; however, muscle endurance has been shown to be protective (10). Greater lumbar mobility leads to more back troubles, not less (10)! And, in fact, ROM appears to have little correlation with work disability status (64). It is also troubling that replicating the motion and spine loads that occur during the use of many low back extensor machines used for training and therapy produces disc herniations when applied to spines in our laboratory! It is clear that some current clinical wisdom needs to be re-examined in the light of relatively recent scientific evidence (those interested in the literature evidence should consult my review in my textbooks) (56,58).

It appears that the safest and mechanically justifiable approach to enhancing lumbar stability through exercise entails a philosophical approach consistent with endurance, not strength; that ensures a neutral spine posture when under load, and that encourages abdominal cocontraction and bracing in a functional way. (A neutral posture is defined as one in which the joints and surrounding passive tissues are in elastic equilibrium and thus at an angle of minimal joint load). It is also acknowledged that optimal athletic performance, which demands reaction and prehension challenges, is not synonymous with health objectives and that additional risk is accepted for extreme ranges of motion and particular motor patterns. The most recent insights provided by Cholewicki suggest that whereas steady-state motor patterns are important for daily activity, the health of reflexive motor patterns is critical for maintaining stability during sudden events (19), achieving a fit and effective motor control system probably requires training in a variety of static and dynamic, expected and unexpected, and stable and labile conditions.

What are the Stabilizers of the Lumbar Torso?

Although many muscles have been regarded as primary spine stabilizers, confirmation of their role requires two levels of analysis. First, engineering stability analysis must be conducted on anatomically robust spine models to document the ability of each component to stiffen and stabilize. Second, electromyographic recordings of all muscles (even deep muscles requiring intramuscular electrodes) are necessary to confirm the extent that the motor control system involves each muscle to ensure sufficient stability. For some time, our limited intramuscular EMG and modelling studies, and those of others, suggested that virtually all torso muscles play a role in stabilization. (Our most recent quantification breakthroughs appear at the end of this section). However, whereas multifidus, the other extensors, and the abdominal wall, have been highlighted before, the architecture of quadratus lumborum (QL) suggests that it can be a stabilizer. This notion is further strengthened by some earlier observation that the motor control system involves this muscle together with the abdominal wall when stability is required in the absence of major moment demands. The fibers of QL cross-link the vertebrae. They have a large lateral moment arm via the transverse process attachments and traverse to the rib cage and iliac crests. Thus, the QL could buttress shear instability and could be effective in all loading modes, by design. Typically, the first mode of buckling is lateral—the QL can play a significant role in local lateral buttressing.

Further, activation profiles support the notion of the stabilizing role of quadratus. It is active during a variety of flexion-dominant, extensor-dominant, and lateral bending tasks. Specifically, Andersson et al. (7) found the QL did not relax with the extensors during the flexion–relaxation phenomenon. The flexion– relaxation phenomenon is an interesting task because there is no substantial lateral or twisting torques and the extensor torque appears to be supported passively, suggesting some stabilizing role for QL. Other very limited data suggest (our laboratory techniques to obtain QL activation were rather imprecise at the time) that in an experiment in which subjects stood upright, but held buckets in either hand in which load was incrementally added to each bucket, the QL appeared to increase its activation level (together with the obliques) as more stability was required. This task forms a special situation since only compressive loading is applied to the spine in the absence of any bending moments. The three layers of the abdominal wall are also important for stability together with muscles which attach directly to vertebra—the multisegmented longissimus and iliocostalis and the unisegmental multifidi. Cholewicki (18) has also presented an argument for the role of the small intertransversarii in producing small but critical stabilizing forces. However, psoas activation appears to have little relationship with low back demands—the motor control system activates it when hip flexor moment is required (6,39).

Most recently we have completed evolution of our model to quantify the role of individual muscles to contribute to stability. Once again the conclusion is that all muscles are important and that the most important muscle at any instant or task is a transient variable—they continually change their relative contribution. An example from one individual (Fig. 5.4) shows how the rank order of importance among muscles to stabilize changes with each task. In this case we have quantified the contribution to prevent buckling. It is interesting to observe how, in flexion tasks, the pars lumborum (in this example) plays a larger stabilizing role over the rectus abdominis. In contrast, during the extension tasks, the opposite holds true demonstrating the task dependent role reversal between moment generation and stability. In another example, we computed the stability index for a group of eight healthy men performing a variety of "stabilization" exercises, together with the resultant compression (Fig. 5.5). More stability is generally associated with more compression. So, which are the wisest ways to challenge and train these identified stabilizers?

Training Quadratus Lumborum

Given the architectural and electromyographic evidence for QL as a spine stabilizer, the optimal technique to maximize activation but minimize the spine load appears to be the **side bridge** (Fig. 5.6) —beginners bridge from the knees, whereas advanced bridges are from the feet. When supported with the feet and elbow the lumbar compression is a modest 2500 N, but the QL closest to the floor appear to be active up to 50% of MVC (the obliques experience similar challenge). Advanced technique to enhance the motor challenge is to roll from one elbow over to the other, with abdominally bracing (Fig. 5.7) rather than repeated hiking the hips off the floor

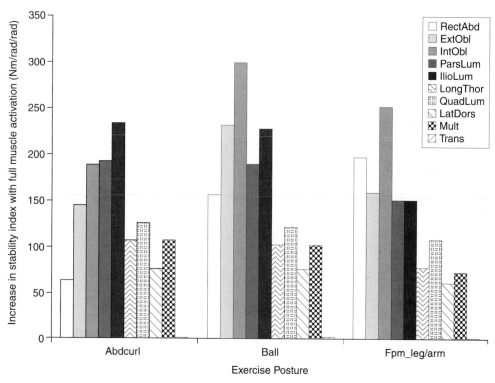

Figure 5.4 In an attempt to understand the contributions of each muscle pair on spine stability, the increase in the stability index is shown as a function of setting each muscle pair activation to 100% MVC; in this way their relative contribution could be assessed. This is an example from a single person; others will have different patterns. Note that the relative order of muscles that increase stability changes across exercises. Also, in flexion tasks, the pars lumborum (in this example) plays a larger stabilizing role over the rectus abdominis. In contrast, during the extension tasks the opposite holds true, suggesting a task dependent role reversal between moment generation and stability. The exercises were: abcurl, curl-up on the stable floor; ball, sitting on a gym ball; and fpn leg/arm, four-point kneeling while extending one leg and the opposite arm.

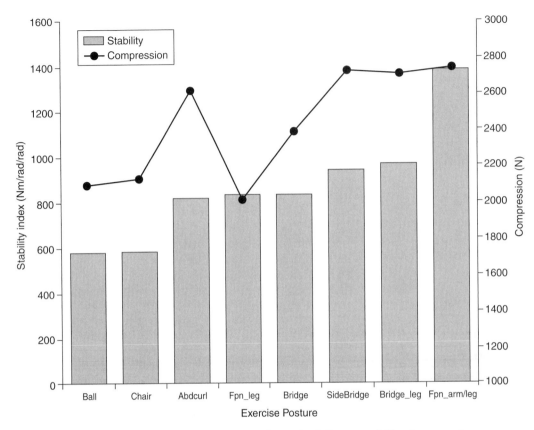

Figure 5.5 Stability versus L4-L5 compression for eight different stabilization exercises (averages from a group of eight healthy men). All exercises were performed with the abdominal wall active and were as follows: ball, sitting on a gym ball; chair, sitting on a chair; abcurl, curl-up on the floor; fpn leg, four-point kneeling while extending one leg at the hip; bridge, back bridge on the floor; side bridge, side bridge with the elbow and feet on the floor; bridge leg, back bridge but extending the knee and holding one leg against gravity; and fpn arm/leg, four-point kneeling while extending one leg and the opposite arm. Exercises are rank-ordered based on increasing lumbar spine stability.

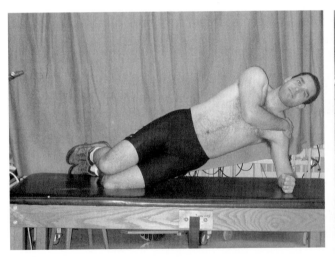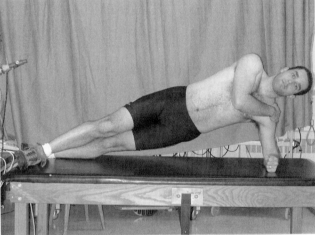

Figure 5.6 The horizontal isometric side bridge. Supporting the lower body with the knees on the floor reduces the demand further for those who are more concerned with safety while supporting the body with the feet increases the muscle challenge, but also the spine load.

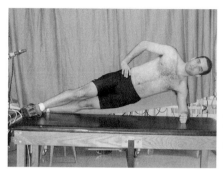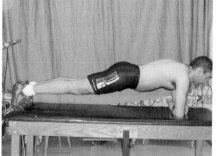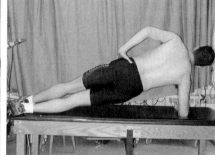

Figure 5.7 Advanced side bridge—following each side bridge hold, one rolls from one elbow to the other while abdominally bracing locking the pelvis and the rib cage.

into the bridge position. Higher levels of activation would be reached with the feet on a labile surface (71).

Training Rectus Abdominis, the Obliques, and Transverse Abdominis

Given the evidence for the obliques and transverse abdominis in ensuring sufficient stability, quantitative data have confirmed that there is no single abdominal exercise that challenges all of the abdominal musculature (8,39) requiring the prescription of more than one single exercise. Calibrated intramuscular and surface EMG evidence suggests that the various types of curl-ups challenge mainly rectus abdominis because psoas and abdominal wall (internal and external oblique, transverse abdominis) activity is relatively low. Sit-ups (both straight-leg and bent-knee) are characterized by higher psoas activation and higher low-back compressive loads that exceed NIOSH occupational guidelines, whereas leg raises cause even higher activation and also spine compression (8). It is also interesting that myoelectric evidence suggests that there is no functional distinction between an upper and lower rectus abdominis in most people but, in contrast, the obliques are regionally activated with upper and lower motor point areas together with medial and lateral components. Transverse abdominis is selectively activated by dynamically hollowing in the abdominal wall (67), whereas an isometric abdominal brace co-activates transverse abdominis together with the external and internal obliques to ensure stability in virtually all modes of possible instability (18).

Several relevant observations were made regarding abdominal exercises in our investigations. The challenge to psoas is lowest during curl-ups, followed by higher levels during the horizontal side bridge, whereas bent-knee sit-ups were characterized by

larger psoas activation than straight-leg sit-ups, through to the highest psoas activity observed during leg raises and hand-on-knee flexor isometric exertions. It is interesting to note that the often-recommended press-heel sit-up that has been hypothesized to activate hamstrings and neurally inhibit psoas was actually confirmed to increase psoas activation (39)! We note here that some clinicians and coaches who intentionally wish to train psoas and will find these data informative. Once again, the horizontal side support appears to have merit as it challenges the lateral obliques and transverse abdominis without high lumbar compressive loading.

Clearly, curl-ups excel at activating the rectus abdominis but produce relatively low oblique activity. Curl-ups with a twisting motion are expensive in terms of lumbar compression because of the additional oblique challenge. A wise choice for abdominal exercises, in the early stages of training or rehabilitation, for simple low back health objectives would consist of several variations of curl-ups for rectus abdominis and the side bridge for the obliques and quadratus, the variation of which is chosen commensurate with patient/athlete status and goals.

Training the Back Extensors (and Stabilizers)

Most traditional extensor exercises are characterized with very high spine loads that result from externally applied compressive and shear forces (either from free weights or resistance machines). From our search for methods to activate the extensors (including longissimus, iliocostalis, and multifidi) with minimal spine loading, it appears that the single leg extension hold minimizes the spine load (<2500 N) and activates one side of the lumbar extensors to approximately 18% of MVC. Simultaneous leg extension with contralateral arm raise (birddog) increases the unilateral extensor muscle challenge (approximately 27% MVC in one side of the lumbar extensors and 45% MVC in the other side of the thoracic extensors) but also increases lumbar compression to well more than 3000 N. This exercise can be enhanced with abdominal bracing and deliberate mental imaging of activation of each level of the local extensors. The often performed exercise of lying prone on the floor and raising the upper body and legs off the floor is contraindicated for anyone at risk for low back injury or re-injury. In this task the lumbar region pays a high compression penalty to a hyperextended spine (usually much higher than 4000 N), which transfers load to the facets and crushes the interspinous ligament.

Clinical Pearl
A Note on abdominal hollowing and bracing

In this author's opinion, there appears to be some confusion in the broad interpretation of the literature regarding the issue of abdominal hollowing and bracing. The Queensland group has evaluated hollowing—observing that the drawing in of the abdominal wall recruits transverse abdominis. Given that transverse abdominis has been noted to have impaired recruitment after injury (34,66), the Queensland group developed a therapy program designed to re-educate the motor system to activate transverse abdominis in a normal way in LBP patients. Hollowing was developed as a motor re-education exercise and not necessarily as a technique to be recommended to patients who require enhanced stability for performance of the ADL, which has perhaps been misinterpreted by some clinical practitioners. Rather, abdominal bracing that activates the three layers of the abdominal wall (external oblique, internal oblique, transverse abdominis) with no drawing-in is much more effective at enhancing spine stability (56). Specifically, the lumbar torso must prepare to withstand steady-state loading (which may be a complex combination of flexion–extension, lateral bend, and axial twisting moments), and withstand sudden unexpected complex loads together with loads that develop from anticipated and planned ballistic motion. The abdominal brace is required to ensure sufficient stability using the oblique cross bracing although high levels of cocontraction are rarely required—probably approximately 5% MVC cocontraction of the abdominal wall during performance of ADL and up to 10% MVC during rigorous activity.

The Beginner's Program for Stabilization

Some specific recommended low back exercises have been shown (50). We recommend that the program begin with the flexion–extension cycles—**cat– camel**—

(Fig. 5.8) to reduce spine viscosity and floss the nerve roots as they outlet at each lumbar level, followed by hip and knee mobility exercises. Note that the cat–camel is intended as a motion exercise, not a stretch, so the emphasis is on motion rather than pushing at the end ranges of flexion and extension. We have found that five to six cycles are often sufficient to reduce most viscous stresses. This is followed by anterior abdominal exercises, in this case the **curl-up** with the hands under the lumbar spine to preserve a neutral spine posture (Fig. 5.9), and one knee flexed but with the other leg straight to lock the pelvis–lumbar spine and minimize the loss of a neutral lumbar posture. Then, lateral musculature exercises are performed, namely the side bridge, for quadratus lumborum and muscles of the abdominal wall for optimal stability (Fig. 5.6). Advanced variations involve placing the upper leg–foot in front of the lower leg–foot to facilitate longitudinal rolling of the torso to challenge anterior and posterior portions of the wall. The extensor program consists of leg extensions and the **birddog** (Fig. 5.10) . In general, we recommend that these isometric holds be held no longer than 7 to 8 seconds given recent evidence from near-infrared spectroscopy indicating rapid loss of available oxygen in the torso muscles contracting at these levels; short relaxation of the muscle restores oxygen (55).

Motivated by the evidence for the superiority of extensor endurance over strength as a benchmark for good back health, we have recently documented normal ratios of endurance times for the torso flexors relative to the extensors (for example, it is normal to hold a flexor posture, approximately 0.77 of the maximum time holding a reference extensor posture) (53,58) and for the lateral musculature relative to the extensors (0.5) to assist clinicians to identify endurance deficits, both absolute values and for one muscle group relative to another. Our most recent evidence suggests that these endurance ratios (both right-to-left side and flexor to extensor) are significantly out of balance in those who have had a history of low back troubles with work loss (57). Finally, as patients progress with these isometric stabilization exercises, we recommend conscious simultaneous contraction of the abdominals (i.e., bracing—simply isometrically activating the abdominals for maximum stability).

Advanced Techniques

The beginner's program should be sufficient for daily spine health. Athletic performance demands higher challenges of low back training but is achieved with much higher risk of tissue damage from over-

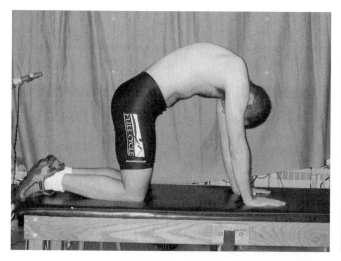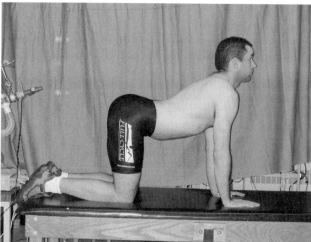

Figure 5.8 The flexion–extension (cat–camel) stretch is performed by slowly cycling through full spine flexion to full extension. Spine mobility is emphasized rather than pressing at the end range of motion. This exercise facilitates motion for the spine with very low loading of the intervertebral joints, reduces viscous stresses for subsequent exercise, and flosses the nerve roots through the foramina at each spine joint (hence coordination of full cervical, thoracic, and lumbar flexion–extension).

load. Furthermore, specific athletic objectives require specific training techniques (space restrictions do not permit their discussion here). The interested reader is directed to my textbook *Ultimate Back Fitness and Performance* for athletic progression of back exercise (58). But, for example, torsional moments are often required athletically but the question must address how to maximize stability and minimize injury during training for trunk tor-

sion. The fact that generating torque about the twist axis imposes approximately 4-times the compression on the spine than for an equal torque about the flexion extension axis cannot be dismissed. The technique we have found for producing low spine loads while challenging the torsional moment generators is to raise a hand-held weight while supporting the upper body with the other arm and abdominally bracing (Fig. 5.11) to resist the torsional torque with

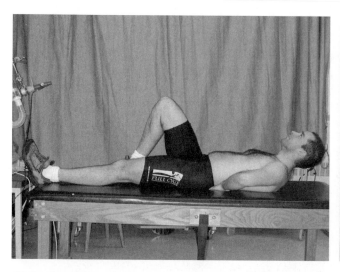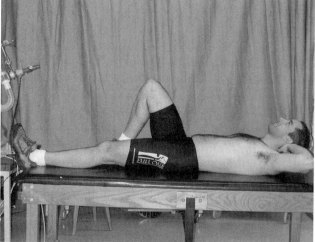

Figure 5.9 The curl-up, in which the head and shoulders are raised off the ground with the hands under the lumbar region to help stabilize the pelvis and support the neutral spine. Only one leg is bent to assist in pelvic stabilization and preservation of a neutral lumbar curve. Additional challenge can be created by raising the elbows from the floor and generating an abdominal brace or co-contraction.

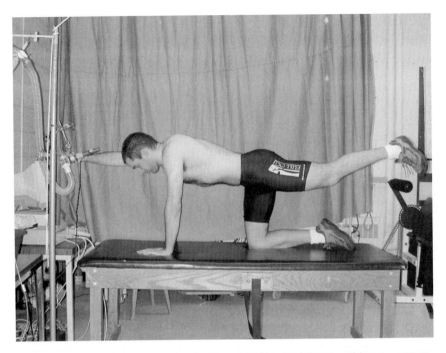

Figure 5.10 Single leg extension holds, while on the hands and knees, produces mild extensor activity and lower spine compression (<2500 N). Raising the contralateral arm (birddog) increases extensor muscle activity and also spine compression to levels more than 3000 N. Sufficient stability is ensured with mild abdominal bracing.

an isometrically contracted and neutral spine. Dynamic challenged twisting is reserved for the most robust of athlete backs.

Finally, it is recognized that challenges to the spine during daily activity include the maintenance of stability during stable, steady-state posture maintenance, and during unexpected loading events together with ballistic movement that is apprehensively planned. This has motivated some clinicians to utilize labile surfaces such as gym balls. Certainly, these labile surfaces challenge the motor system to meet the dynamic tasks of daily living. But is this

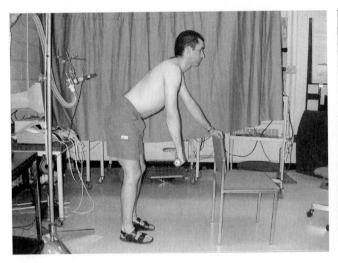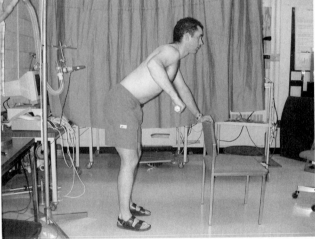

Figure 5.11 A challenge for the torsional components that produces low spine loads is to support the extensor moment of the flexed torso with one hand while the other raises a modest weight. The lumbar torso is braced (including all layers of the abdominal wall) in a neutral posture resisting the twisting moments generated by the weight.

type of training of concern for some patients? Our recent quantification of elevated spine loads and muscle co-activation when performing a curl-up on labile surfaces (74) suggests that the rehabilitation program should begin on stable surfaces. Labile surfaces should be introduced once the spine load bearing capacity has been sufficiently restored.

In summary, progression of a patient through rehab to function follows the three-step procedure:

1. Establish motion and motor patterns that avoid the injury mechanisms identified earlier in this chapter. Pain motion/motor patterns may have also been identified through provocative testing described in other chapters, which should be avoided at this step (see Chapters 15 and 26).
2. Enhance lumbar stability (see Chapter 26).
3. Progress to functional tasks while ensuring sufficient stability and ensuring commensurate tolerance to the elevated loads placed on the spine (see Chapters 26 and 29).

■ CONCLUSION

Rehabilitation endeavors are continuing to embrace techniques that consider notions of lower torso, or core stability. Whereas there is no question that first a system must be stable before presented with a physical challenge, the enhancement of low back health, and the avoidance of troubles have motivated scientific inquiry into the mechanics of stability. Many groups continue to work to understand the contributions to stability of various components of the anatomy at particular joints and the ideal ways to enhance their contribution; to understand what magnitudes of muscle activation are required to achieve sufficient stability; and to identify the best methods to re-educate faulty motor control systems to both achieve sufficient stability and reduce the risk of inappropriate motor patters occurring in the future. Motor patterns to achieve stability appear to be different depending on whether the activity is steady-state (with or without combined loads) or with dynamic motion, which may involve rapid voluntary motions or unexpected loading requiring reaction. Understanding stability in all of these unique conditions is the global goal. Finally, the efficacy studies to date, although promising, can only be considered to provide preliminary data. Rigorous efficacy trials are needed on populations of patients who have been sufficiently examined to be categorized into pathological groups and on athletes classified by performance goals. Much remains to be done.

■ ACKNOWLEDGMENTS

The author acknowledge the contributions of several colleagues who have contributed to the collection of works reported here: Daniel Juker, MD, Craig Axler, MSc, Sylvain Grenier, PhD, and Jack Callaghan, PhD and in particular Professor Jacek Cholewicki, who I consider to be the premier scientist in the world regarding the engineering analysis of spine stability. Also, the continual financial support from the Natural Science and Engineering Research Council, Canada has made this series of work possible.

Audit Process
Self-Check of the Chapter's Learning Objectives

- What is the role of the motor control system in injury prevention?
- What is the mechanism of injury for facet and disc tissues?
- Can exercises that do not place injured tissues at risk be prescribed to train the back?
- Give examples of basic stabilization exercises designed to coordinate muscular co-contraction to challenge both muscle and the motor system while simultaneously sparing the spine joints.

■ REFERENCES

1. Adams MA, Hutton WC. Gradual disc prolapse. Spine 1985;10:524–531.
2. Adams MA, Hutton WC. The relevance of torsion to the mechanical derangement of the lumbar spine. Spine 1981;6:241–248.
3. Adams MA, McNally DS, Chinn H, Dolan P. Posture and the compressive strength of the lumbar spine. Clin Biomech 1994;9:5–14.
4. Adams MA, Dolan P. Recent advances in lumbar spine mechanics and their clinical significance. Clin Biomech 1995;10:3–19.
5. Aggrawall ND, Karr R, Kumar S, Mathur DN. A study of changes in the spine in weight lifters and other athletes. Br J Sports Med 1979;13:58–61.
6. Andersson E, Oddsson L, Grundstrom H, Thorstensson A. The role of the psoas and iliacus muscles for stability and movement of the lumbar spine, pelvis and hip. Scand J Med Sci Sports 1995;5:10–16.
7. Andersson EA, Oddsson LIE, Grundström H, Nilsson J. EMG activities of the quadratus lumborum and erector spinae muscles during flexion-relaxation and other motor tasks. Clin Biomech 1996;11(7): 392–400.
8. Axler CT, McGill SM. Low back loads over a variety of abdominal exercises: Searching for the safest abdominal challenge. Med Sci Sports Exercise 1997;29:804–811.

9. Bergmark A. Mechanical stability of the human lumbar spine. Doctoral Dissertation, Department of Solid Mechanics. Sweden: Lund University, 1987.

10. Biering-Sorensen F. Physical measurements as risk indicators for low back trouble over a one year period. Spine 1984;9:106–119.

11. Brinckmann P, Biggemann M, Hilweg D. Prediction of the compressive strength of human lumbar vertebrae. Clin Biomech 1989;4(Suppl 2):s1–s27.

12. Buckwalter JA. Spine update: Aging and degeneration of the human intervertebral disc. Spine 1995;20: 1307–1314.

13. Burnett AF, Elliot BC, Foster DH, Marshall RN, Hardcastle P. Thoracolumabar disc degeneration in young fast bowlers in cricket: A follow-up study. Clin Biomech 1996;11:305–310.

14. Callaghan J, McGill SM. Intervertebral disc herniation: Studies on a porcine spine exposed to highly repetitive flexion/extension motion with compressive force. Clin Biomech 2001;16(1):28–37.

15. Callaghan JP, Gunning JL, McGill SM. Relationship between lumbar spine load and muscle activity during extensor exercises. Physical Ther 1998;78:8–18.

16. Carter DR. Biomechanics of bone. In: Nahum HM, Melvin J, eds. Biomechanics of trauma. Norwalk, CT: Appleton Century Crofts, 1985:135–165.

17. Cholewicki J, McGill SM. Lumbar posterior ligament involvement during extremely heavy lifts estimated from fluoroscopic measurements. J Biomech 1992; 25(1):17–28.

18. Cholewicki J, McGill SM. Mechanical stability of the in vivo lumbar spine: Implications for injury and chronic low back pain. Clin Biomech 1996;11(1): 1–15.

19. Cholewicki J, Simons APD, Radebold A. Effects of external trunk loads on lumbar spine stability. J Biomech 2000;33(11):1377–1385.

20. Cripton P, Berleman U, Visarino H, et al. Response of the lumbar spine due to shear loading. Injury Prevention Through Biomechanics. Symposium proceedings, May 4–5, Wayne State University, 1995.

21. Crisco JJ, Panjabi MM. Euler stability of the human ligamentous lumbar spine, Part I Theory and Part II Experiment. Clin Biomech 1992;7:19–26,27–32.

22. Duncan NA, Ahmed AM. The role of axial rotation in the etiology of unilateral disc prolapse: An experimental and finite-element analysis. Spine 1991;16: 1089–1098.

23. Farfan HF, Cossette JW, Robertson GH, Wells RV, Kracs H. The effects of torsion on the lumbar intervertebral joints: The role of torsion in production of disc degeneration. J Bone Joint Surg 1970;52A: 468–497.

24. Fidler MW, Jowett RL, Troup JDG. Myosin ATPase activity in multifidus muscle from cases of lumbar spinal derangement. J Bone Joint Surg 1975;57B: 220–227.

25. Ford D, Bagnall KM, McFadden HD, Greenhill B, Raso J. Analysis of vertebral muscle obtained during surgery for correction of a lumbar disc disorder. Acta Anatomica 1983;116:152–157.

26. Fyhrie DP, Schaffler MB. Failure mechanisms in human vertebral cancellous bone. Bone 1994;15: 105–109.

27. Gardner-Morse M, Stokes IAF, Laible JP. Role of the muscles in lumbar spine stability in maximum extension efforts. J Orthop Res 1995;13:802–808.

28. Gordon SJ, Yang KH, Mayer PJ, et al. Mechanism of disc rupture-a preliminary report. Spine 1991;16:450–456.

29. Gunning J, Callaghan JP, McGill SM. The role of prior loading history and spinal posture on the compressive tolerance and type of failure in the spine using a porcine trauma model. Clin Biomech 2001;16(6):471–480.

30. Hardcastle P, Annear P, Foster DH, et al. Spinal abnormalities in young fast bowlers. J Bone Joint Surg (B) 1992;74:421–425.

31. Herrin GA, Jaraiedi M, Anderson CK. Prediction of overexertion injuries using biomechanical and psychophysical models. Am Ind Hyg Assoc J 1986;47:322–330.

32. Heylings DJ. Supraspinous and interspinous ligaments of the human lumbar spine. J Anat 1978;123:127–131.

33. Hides JA, Richardson CA, Jull GA. Multifidus muscle recovery is not automatic following resolution of acute first episode low back pain. Spine 1996;21:2763–2769.

34. Hodges PW, Richardson CA. Inefficient muscular stabilization of the lumbar spine associated with low back pain: a motor control evaluation of transversus abdominis. Spine 1996;21:2640–2650.

35. Jäger M, Luttmann A. The load on the lumbar spine during asymmetrical bi-manual materials handling. Ergonomics 1992;35:783–805.

36. Jayson M, Dixon A. Intra-articular pressure in rheumatoid arthritis of the knee. III. Pressure changes during joint use. Ann Rheum Dis 1970;29:401–408.

37. Jorgensen K, Nicolaisen T. Trunk extensor endurance. Determination and relation to low back trouble. Ergonomics 1987;30:259–267.

38. Jowett R, Fidler MW, Troup JDG. Histochemical changes in the multifidus in mechanical derangement of the spine. Orthop Clin North Am 1975;6:145–161.

39. Juker D, McGill SM, Kropf P, Steffen T. Quantitative intramuscular myoelectric activity of lumbar portions of psoas and the abdominal wall during a wide variety of tasks. Med Sci Sports Ex 1998;30(2):301–310.

40. Kornberg M. MRI diagnosis of traumatic Schmorl's node. Spine 1988;13:934–935.

41. Lotz JC, Colliou OK, Chin JR, Duncan NA, Liebenberg E. Compression-induced degeneration of the intervertebral disc: An in vivo mouse model and finite-element study. Spine 1998;23(23):2493–2506.

42. Mattila M, Hurme M, Alaranta H, et al. The multifidus muscle in patients with lumbar disc herniation. A histochemical and morphometric analysis of intraoperative biopsies. Spine 1986;11:732–738.

43. McGill SM, Norman RW. Effects of an anatomically detailed erector spinae model on L4/L5 disc compression and shear. J Biomech 1987a;20:591–600.

44. McGill SM, Sharratt MT, Seguin JP. Loads on the spinal tissues during simultaneous lifting and ventilatory challenge. Ergonomics 1995;38(9):1772–1792.

45. McGill SM. Kinetic potential of the lumbar trunk musculature about three orthogonal orthopaedic axes in extreme postures. Spine 1991a;16:809–815.

46. McGill SM. Electromyographic activity of the abdominal and low back musculature during the generation of isometric and dynamic axial trunk torque: Implications for lumbar mechanics. J Orthop Res 1991b;0:91–103.

47. McGill SM. A myoelectrically based dynamic three-dimensional model to predict loads on lumbar spine tissues during lateral bending. J Biomech 1992;25:395–414.

48. McGill SM, Kippers V. Transfer of loads between lumbar tissues during the flexion-relaxation phenomenon. Spine 1994;19:2190–2196.

49. McGill SM. ISB Keynote Lecture—The biomechanics of low back injury: Implications on current practice in industry and the clinic. J Biomech 1997;30:465–475.

50. McGill SM. Low back exercises: Prescription for the healthy back and when recovering from injury. Resource manual for guidelines for exercise testing and prescription, American College of Sports Medicine, 3rd ed. Baltimore: Williams and Wilkins, 1998.

51. McGill SM. Low Back Exercises: Evidence for improving exercise regimens. Physical Ther 1998;78:754–765.

52. McGill SM, Callaghan JP. On the risk of injury from falling as a result of an unexpected removal of a chair while sitting. Accident Anal Prevent 1998;31:85–89.

53. McGill SM, Childs A, Liebenson C. Endurance times for stabilization exercises: Clinical targets for testing and training from a normal database. Arch Phys Med Rehab 1999;80:941–944.

54. McGill SM, Parks K, Hughson R. Changes in lumbar lordosis modify the role of the extensor muscles. Clin Biomech 2000;15(10):777–780.

55. McGill SM, Highson R, Parks K. Erector spinae oxygenation during prolonged contractions: Implications for prolonged work. Ergonomics 2000;43:486–493.

56. McGill SM. Low back disorders: Evidence based prevention and rehabilitation. Champaign, IL: Human Kinetics Publishers, 2002.

57. McGill SM, Grenier S, Bluhm M, Preuss R, Brown S, Russell C. Previous history of LBP with work loss is related to lingering effects in biomechanical, physiological, personal and psychosocial characteristics. Ergonomics 2003;46(7):731–746.

58. McGill SM. Ultimate Back Fitness and Performance. Wabuno Publishers, 2004. Available at: www.backfitpro.com

59. Nicolaisen T, Jorgensen K. Trunk strength, back muscle endurance and low back trouble. Scand J Rehabil Med 1985;17:121–127.

60. Norman RW, Wells R, Neumann P, Frank J, Shannon H, Kerr M. A comparison of peak vs. cumulative physical work exposure risk factors for the reporting of low back pain in the automotive industry. Clin Biomech 1998;13:561–573.

61. Noyes FR, De Lucas JL, Torvik PJ. Biomechanics of ligament failure: An analysis of strain-rate sensitivity and mechanisms of failure in primates. J Bone Joint Surg 1974;56A:236–253.

62. O'Sullivan P, Twomey LT, Allison GT. Altered pattern of abdominal muscle activation in chronic back pain patients. Aust J Physiother 1997;43:91–98.

63. Oxland TR, Panjabi MM, Southern EP, Duranceau JS. An anatomic basis for spinal instability: A porcine trauma model. J Orthop Res 1991;9:452–462.

64. Parks KA, Crichton KS, Goldford RJ, McGill SM. On the validity of ratings of impairment for low back disorders. Spine 2003;28(4):380–384.

65. Porter RW. Is hard work good for the back? The relationship between hard work and low back pain-related disorders. Int J Ind Ergonomics 1992;9:157–160.

66. Potvin J, McGill SM, Norman RW. Trunk muscle and lumbar ligament contributions to dynamic lifts with varying degrees of trunk flexion. Spine 1991;16(9):1099–1107.

67. Richardson C, Jull G, Hodges P, Hides J. Therapeutic exercise for spinal segmental stabilization in low back pain. Edinburgh: Churchill-Livingston, 1999.

68. Roy SH, DeLuca CJ, Casavant DA. Lumbar muscle fatigue and chronic low back pain. Spine 1989;14:992–1001.

69. Sihvonen T, Partanen J, Hanninen O, Soimakallio S. Electric behavior of low back muscles during lumbar pelvic rhythm in low back pain patients and healthy controls. Arch Physi Med Rehabil 1991;72:1080–1087.

70. Snook SH, Webster BS, McGorry RW, Fogleman MT, McCann KB. The reduction of chronic non-specific low back pain through the control of early morning lumbar flexion. Spine 1998;23:2601–2607.

71. Stokes M, Young A. The contribution of reflex inhibition to arthrogenous muscle weakness. Clin Sci 1984;67:7–14.

72. Stratford P. EMG of the quadriceps femoris muscles in subjects with normal knees and acutely effused knees. Physical Ther 1981;62:279–283.

73. Troup JDG, Martin JW, Lloyd DCEF. Back pain in industry—A prospective study. Spine 1981;6:65–69.

74. Vera Garcia FJ, Grenier SG, McGill SM. Abdominal response during curl-ups on both stable and labile surfaces. Phys Ther 2000;80(6):564–569.

75. Vernon-Roberts B, Pirie CJ. Healing trabecular microfractures in the bodies of lumbar vertebrae. Ann Rheum Dis 1973;32:406–412.

76. Woo SL-Y, Gomez MA, Akeson WH. Mechanical behaviors of soft tissues: Measurements, modifications, injuries, and treatment. In: Nahum HM, Melvin J, eds. Biomechanics of trauma. Norwalk, CT: Appleton Century Crofts, 1985:109–133.

77. Yingling VR, Callaghan JP, McGill SM. Dynamic loading affects the mechanical properties and failure site of porcine spines. Clin Biomech 1997;12:301–305.

78. Yingling VR, McGill SM. Mechanical properties and failure mechanics of the spine under posterior shear load: Observations from a porcine model. J Spinal Disord 1999;12(6):501–508.

79. Zhu XZ, Parnianpour M, Nordin M, Kahanovitz N. Histochemistry and morphology of erector spinae muscles in lumbar disc herniation. Spine 1989;14:391–397.

6

The Sources of Back Pain

Nikolai Bogduk and Charles Aprill

Learning Objectives
After reading this chapter you should be able to:

- Evaluate on what grounds you believe that certain conditions are the cause of back pain.
- Provided a list of philosophical criteria by which to judge if a condition can be credited as a cause of back pain.
- Offer a synopsis of conditions that fail to satisfy these criteria.
- Offer a summary of the evidence for conditions that do satisfy the criteria.
- Utilize a means by which to evaluate the extent to which past beliefs and future suggestions about the causes of back pain can be credited.

Introduction

How do you know what causes back pain? This is a philosophical question that few practitioners would have wrestled with. Few spine scientists have addressed this question in a systematic, and unbiased, manner. The convention has been for practitioners to be taught by senior practitioners and academics what the causes of back pain are. What has not been a tradition is to allow and to encourage students to ask, why do you say it is a cause of back pain; how do you know? This chapter addresses this issue and provides the answer to this question, as far as is currently known.

Tradition

In any textbook on back pain, one is likely to encounter lists of possible causes of back pain. These lists usually include, as common conditions, entities such as spondylosis, degenerative disease, and disc prolapse, and rare conditions such as metabolic disorders, ankylosing spondylitis, chondrocalcinosis, etc. Some lists might include conditions such as myofascial disorder, trigger points, postural abnormalities, or segmental dysfunction.

The basis for such lists is largely, if not exclusively, "I say so." The author creates the list from experience and education or copies it from other sources. Students learn the list and learn to reproduce it for their examinations.

Close scrutiny of such lists reveals that few of the entities satisfy contemporary standards of clinical science and critical reasoning. Those who espouse the lists, those who learn them, and those who set the lists as the correct answers to exam questions have not answered the question, how do you know?

Principles

Practice-Based Problem

Patients have a strong desire to know what the cause of their pain is. Are most diagnostic labels commonly given to patients based on actual knowledge of the pain's source or are they based on a number of less certain beliefs and assumptions? If the latter, what can clinicians do to improve the report findings given to patients?

There are various criteria that, logically, should be satisfied before an entity can be regarded as a cause of back pain. The more an entity satisfies the criteria, the more credible it is as a cause of back pain. Conversely, the less an entity satisfies the criteria, the less credible it is. If certain key criteria are not satisfied, or if the available evidence is contrary to the criteria, the entity cannot be held to be a cause of back pain.

Without resorting to jargon terms, such as plausibility, face validity, concept validity, and content validity, the criteria can be encapsulated by the questions:

1. Could it be a source of back pain?
2. Can it be a source of back pain?
3. Is it ever a cause of back pain?
4. Is it ever a source of back pain?

The first criterion is the easiest to satisfy. In essence, if a structure in the lumbar spine has a nociceptive nerve supply, it is potentially a source of back pain. The strength of this criterion lies not in what could be a source of pain, but in what cannot be a source. For example, it was long held, until approximately 1980, that intervertebral discs could not be a source of back pain because they lacked a nerve supply (2,39,70). Once that nerve supply was demonstrated, however, the discs were promoted to the list of possible sources of back pain. Anatomical studies have shown that the fascia (65), muscles (8), ligaments (8,34,35,56,71,72), vertebrae (3,17,25,32), synovial joints (8,17), and intervertebral discs (4,8,16,32,33,44,55,57,73) of the lumbar spine are all innervated. Any of these structures, therefore, could be a source of pain, in principle. Only the nucleus pulposus, in its natural state, lacks a nerve supply. So, it cannot be a source of pain. However, recent studies have shown that damaged discs obtain a neo-innervation (29). It may be that in damaged discs the nucleus becomes sensate.

This first criterion has paved the way for various suggestions, models, theories, and assertions that muscles, ligaments, joints, and fascia could be or are the source of back pain. However, the first criterion only satisfies that the structure could be a source of pain; it does not satisfy that the structure can be or ever is a source.

The second criterion is, to an extent, technical or ceremonial, for it may be superfluous when subsequent criteria are satisfied. However, it is included not only for the sake of completeness and to reinforce other criteria but also to dispel rhetorical cynicism. In other words, it is there as a vaccine to dispel arguments that can be raised by critics. The second criterion requires that it be shown that noxious stimulation of the structure in normal volunteers does, in fact, cause pain. It is the physiological correlate to the anatomical first criterion. Structures believed on the basis of traditional wisdom not to be sources of pain can be elevated into consideration if stimulation of them in normal volunteers produces pain of similar quality and distribution as that seen in patients. Showing that a structure can be a source of pain does not, of itself, prove that it does cause pain in patients, but it nevertheless enhances the plausibility of that structure being a possible source of pain. The strength of this criterion lies not in it being satisfied but more in when it is not satisfied. An assertion that particular structure can be a source of back pain is somewhat shallow if and when it has not been shown to be painful in normal volunteers. Doubts or reservations in this regard are dispelled once the formality of undertaking experiments in normal volunteers has been acquitted. Examples include the lumbar zygapophysial joints and the sacroiliac joint. Traditional wisdom long maintained that these structures could not be sources of back pain until experiments in normal volunteers showed that they could. Thereafter, subsequent investigations were undertaken to satisfy other, and more compelling, criteria.

The third criterion is the most traditional. It requires demonstration of a unique pathology on which the pain can be blamed. It is also the most abused criterion. A habit of the past has been to blame back pain on the most obvious, or any, pathology evident in a patient, usually on medical imaging. As a result, back pain has been blamed on degenerative joint disease, spondylosis, spondylolysis, spondylolisthesis, spina bifida, transitional vertebrae, etc. This is intellectually moribund and has caused a great disservice to patients, the health system, and the medicolegal system. For an evident pathology to be regarded, logically and responsibly, as a cause of back pain, an epidemiological requirement must be satisfied. If that requirement is not satisfied regarding the pathology to be the cause of pain is illogical because it defies the data.

The condition must be present in patients with pain but not present in patients without pain. This requires population surveys to collect data that complete a contingency table (Fig. 6.1). If the condition really is a cause of pain, the numbers A and D must be large. That means that when the condition is present so is pain, but pain is absent when the condition is absent. Reciprocally the numbers B and C must be small. That means that rarely does the condition occur in the absence of pain, and that pain is rarely present when the condition is absent. Statistically, the ratios of A to B and of D to C must be large and well in excess of values that might arise by chance alone.

When subjected to scrutiny in this manner, many popular and traditional entities fail the criterion. If a condition is equally present in patients with pain and in individuals without pain, it cannot logically be deemed to be a cause of pain. Abuses have arisen in this regard either when authorities have based their beliefs having seen only symptomatic patients and having never studied asymptomatic individuals (or read the literature), or when they have deliberately defied the evidence and have irresponsibly applied a false diagnosis just because it was convenient to do so.

The fourth criterion is the most novel. It is designed to accommodate circumstances when the causal pathology is not evident because it defies available means of detection. Back pain is not a lethal disorder and so patients rarely to come to postmortem, at which microscopic or molecular causes of pain might be identified. Contemporary techniques of medical imaging lack resolution for any but large abnormalities. Failure to detect pathology is not evidence of absence of pathology, especially if and when the wrong or inadequate techniques of investigation are used. Plain x-rays can show fractures or deformities, but they do not show intervertebral discs. Therefore, a normal x-ray does not exclude an abnormal (and painful) disc.

Pain cannot be seen. It is not a structure. It cannot be photographed. Pain is a sensory experience. Consequently, its detection requires a physiological test. The fourth criterion requires demonstration that investigations that selectively target the structure either aggravate or relieve the pain that it is presumed to cause. But stringent subsidiary criteria apply.

If a test is used to aggravate a patient's pain, it must be shown that the test stresses only the structure inferred to be the source of pain. If the test happens, inadvertently, to stress other structures it lacks specificity. Under these conditions, the test may be positive for reasons other than the professed or preferred reason. All too often tests have been promoted without validation. They may be said to be specific for a given source or cause of pain, but when subjected to scientific scrutiny they prove not to be. Yet many tests, particularly clinical examination tests, continue to be taught solely on the basis of assertion that they work when in fact they do not. Practition-

Pathology	Pain	
	Present	Absent
Present	A	B
Absent	C	D

Figure 6.1 A contingency table with data tests whether a pathology can be held to be a cause of pain. The strength of correlation is reflected by the magnitude of the A-to-B and D-to-C ratios.

ers prefer to believe the myths that they were taught or invented, rather than face the evidence and the reality that it reveals. It is beholding on anyone who invents, professes, or teaches a test to show objectively that it has specificity. Insistence and wishful thinking do not constitute evidence in this regard.

Similarly, relief of pain must be target-specific. A chestnut that arises in this regard is trial by treatment. Some people believe that if a theory maintains that a specific condition is the cause of pain, then a certain treatment is appropriate; and if that treatment works, it constitutes evidence that the theory is correct. This is wrong. The fallacy arises when the treatment works for reasons other than those expressed in the theory. Thus, if a theory maintains that the pain stems from a subluxated zygapophysial joint, and that manipulation is indicated, a successful manipulation is not necessarily evidence that the abnormal joint was the source of pain and was successfully treated. Relief might have arisen because of simultaneous manipulation of a painful disc, because of fortuitous stretch of the back muscles, or because of non-specific factors, such as attention and expectation of relief. Inferences drawn from trial of treatment require studies that control for these confounding effects and that show a consistent correlation between diagnosis and outcome of treatment. "It works sometimes" simply does not wash.

The most rigorously studied physiological tests that pertain to back pain are diagnostic blocks and discography. Diagnostic blocks involve anaesthetizing a target structure or its nerve supply. Discography involves provoking a target disc. All of these procedures involve the use of needles under fluoroscopic control. The advantages of needles are several.

- They are target-specific. Fluoroscopy shows that the needle is used to anaesthetize or stimulate selectively the target structure, and no other. Faith is not involved. Radiography shows where the needle is and where it is not.
- They can be controlled. Controls are critical for diagnostic procedures. They militate against false-positive (and false-negative) results. Thereby they secure correct inferences. The nature of the controls that should be used differs according to the test at hand (q.v.).
- They are less subject to observer bias than manual clinical tests. The drug injected does the work. Special perceptual skills that involve years of training and practice to master are not required. The only skills required are the ability to deliver the needle safely and accurately. Thereafter, the test is performed by the drug injected, and the patient announces the response, not the examiner.

Diagnostic Blocks

Diagnostic blocks are not a treatment. They are a means by which to test a diagnostic hypothesis. The investigator raises a suspicion about where the pain might be coming from. He or she then tests that suspicion by selectively anaesthetizing the suspected structure or its nerve supply. In this regard, the block does not test the patient or the veracity of the symptom. Blocks are a test of the investigator's acumen or how well they have guessed the source of pain. Investigators are allowed to be wrong; the test can be negative. But questions can be raised about the investigator's practice if all or most of their blocks are negative. Perhaps they are guessing wrongly too often and should change their perceptions about what are the likely sources of pain in their patients.

In the pursuit of low back pain, diagnostic blocks can be performed of the zygapophysial joints and the sacroiliac joint (10,15). Other structures might also be tested in the same manner, such as muscles or ligaments, but few studies of these latter structures have been undertaken to date.

Zygapophysial joints can be anaesthetized directly by intra-articular injections or indirectly by anesthetizing their nerve supply via the medial branches of the lumbar dorsal rami (10,15). The sacroiliac joint can be anaesthetized only by intra-articular injection (15).

"Face validity" means that anatomically the test does what it is alleged to do, that it affects the target structure and no other. The face validity of intra-articular injections is secured by performing an arthrogram of the target joint. The arthrogram should show that what is injected goes into the target joint not into any other structure and stays in the joint. This requires respect for the capacity of the joint, which, in the case of lumbar zygapophysial joints is approximately 1 ml and in the case of the sacroiliac joint is approximately 3 ml. If the injectant spills out of the joint, the target specificity of the test is corrupted and no legitimate inference can be drawn from a positive response.

The target specificity of lumbar medial branch blocks has been assiduously studied and established. When small volumes of injectant are accurately deposited onto the target nerve, they stay there and spread to no other structure that might confound the effect (22). Blocking medial branches in normal volunteers protects them from zygapophysial joint pain (36).

Controls are of paramount importance during the conduct of diagnostic blocks. Patients may report relief of their pain for reasons other than the action of the local anesthetic agent injected. Studies have shown that patients expecting to undergo diagnostic blocks of the zygapophysial joints can report complete relief of pain after just a subcutaneous injection (63). Such is the power of just simply "doing a procedure." Controls do not perfectly eliminate false-positive responses, but they guard against them and reduce the likelihood of a false-positive inferences being drawn about the source of pain.

For research purposes, the optimal control is placebo injections. Under double-blind conditions, the patient is injected with an agent that does not have the intended physiological effect. A positive response refutes the diagnostic hypothesis. The patient has obtained relief for reasons other than the intended effect of the block. Placebo controls, however, are not practical for conventional practice. They require informed consent and at least three procedures (i.e. "challenges") to provide an interpretable pattern of response (10,13).

More practicable are comparative blocks (6). On separate occasions, under double-blind conditions, the target joint is anaesthetized using local anesthetic agents with different durations of action. Double-blind conditions are essential to prevent the investigator cueing the patient as to what to expect, and thereby imposing the investigator's bias, usually for a positive response. A convincing positive response is one in which the patient reports long-lasting relief when a long-acting agent is used and short-lasting relief when a short-acting agent is used.

Comparative blocks are not perfect. They have a finite but small false-positive rate (14%) (41). For practical purposes this is more than acceptable. It is far more preferable than relying a single diagnostic blocks, which have a much higher false-positive rate that in context of lumbar zygapophysial joint pain means that for every three positive results two are wrong (58).

Provocation Discography

Provocation discography is a more vexatious procedure, for it relies on provoking pain rather than relieving it. Consequently, it cannot be controlled using injections of different agents or placebos. It involves introducing a needle into an intervertebral disc suspected of being the source pain and using the needle to distend the disc from the inside, with an injection of saline or of contrast medium (14). The test is positive if stressing the disc reproduces the patient's pain. But provocation discography is subject to false-positive responses.

Provocation may be positive if the patient has segmental hyperalgesia, i.e., something else, innervated by the same segmental nerves as supply the target disc is actually the source of pain and stressing the disc aggravates the pain from that other source rather than any pain from the disc. There are no expedient measures by which to guard against hyperalgesia. On assessing the patient, the investigator must be confident that there are no possible, or likely, confounding sources of pain. Diagnostic blocks of the zygapophysial joints or the sacroiliac joint may need to be performed before discography to exclude these other sources of pain. Or discography might be performed while these other structures are anesthetized. The latter combination has not yet been evaluated.

Provocation may also be positive for behavioral reasons. The patient may report a positive response to disc provocation because anything and everything hurts in the back. It is for this reason that the International Association for the Study of Pain (IASP) has required anatomical controls for provocation discography (48). For the diagnosis of discogenic pain, provocation of the target disc must reproduce the patient's pain, but stressing adjacent discs does not. Such a response refutes the competing hypothesis that anything and everything hurts in the patient's back.

Several studies have warned of possible false-positive responses to provocation discography (18,19). Patients with no back pain but with a painful iliac crest can have a positive response to discography (18). Some normal volunteers have a positive response to disc provocation (19). The incidence of false-positive responses is greater in patients with chronic pain and is even greater in patients with a somatization disorder diagnosed (19). However, if the IASP criteria for a positive response are rigorously applied, the putatively alarming published figures are deflated. In normal volunteers and in patients with chronic pain, the false-positive rate is only 10%. In patients with somatization disorder it is 25%. These data warn physicians to be careful with over-interpreting response to provocation discography, but they do not impugn the test. Read reciprocally, the data attest to a true positive rate of 90% in most patients and 75% in patients with somatization.

Confidence in a diagnosis of discogenic pain is enhanced if pathology can be demonstrated in a disc found to be painful. The cardinal pathology is that of internal disc disruption (IDD). This condition is characterized by radial fissures penetrating to the outer third of the anulus fibrosus but in a disc whose circumference is essentially intact, i.e., there is no herniation (9,11). Such fissures are demonstrated by performing CT of the disc soon after it has been injected with contrast medium. Large studies have shown that radial fissures correlate strongly with the affected disc being painful, but that they are not related to age changes or disc degeneration (49). Furthermore, it has been shown that IDD is associated with abnormal stress profiles in the nucleus pulposus and the anulus fibrosus of the affected disc (1), and that these abnormal profiles correlate strongly with the affected disc being painful (47).

Losers

Of the many sources and causes of back pain professed by conventional wisdom, few withstand philosophical scrutiny. They do not satisfy the criteria.

Back muscles have been made to hurt in normal volunteers (7,37), but no controlled studies using diagnostic blocks have shown if and how commonly the back muscles cause pain. Nor have any studies shown the pathology responsible. Muscle sprains might be inferred as a cause of acute low back pain, but no pathology of muscle is known to cause chronic low back pain.

Doubtless, patients exhibit tender areas in their back muscles, but the notion of trigger points is not sustainable. There is no evidence that trigger points are an explicit pathological entity. Clinically, the diagnosis of trigger points in the lumbar spine has been shown to lack reliability (52,53).

Ligament sprain is an entity easy to conceive of but difficult to prove. Stimulation of interspinous ligaments in normal volunteers does produce back pain and somatic referred pain (7,38), but no controlled studies have demonstrated relief of back pain on anesthetizing these ligaments. One uncontrolled study indicates that if interspinous ligaments are a source of back pain, its prevalence is less than 10% in primary care (68). No studies have provided evidence that other ligaments are a source of back pain, such as the iliolumbar ligament. That is not to say that these ligaments are never a source of pain; there is simply no evidence, yet, to credit the belief that they are.

Spondylosis or degenerative joint diseases are simply age changes. They occur increasingly with age and are not significantly more common in patients with back pain than in individuals with no pain (31,40,42,64,66,69). Egregious has been the habit of ascribing patients' pain to "pre-existing degenerative changes." Being contrary to the available epidemiological data, such behavior is heretical to the science of medicine.

Similar comments apply to spondylolysis and spondylolisthesis. The prevalence of spondylolysis is 7% in the asymptomatic population (51). Seeing a pars defect on a radiograph does not make it the source of pain. Such defects might be painful, but evidence other than radiographic presence is required. To test if a defect is painful it can be blocked in an attempt to relieve the patient's pain. Spondylolisthesis has a prevalence of 8% in men and 5% in women,

and may be totally asymptomatic (67). In men with spondylolisthesis, back pain is not significantly more common than in the general population, although women with spondylolisthesis are more likely to have back pain (67). Finding spondylolisthesis does not automatically render it the cause of pain. Radiographic investigation cannot and does not reveal the actual source of pain. It could lie in the disc or the posterior elements of the affected segments, or it might be anywhere else in the lumbar spine and be unrelated to the spondylolisthesis. Simply sighting the abnormality does not discriminate between these possibilities.

"Instability" is an abused term (12). It is invoked to convey the sense that something is wrong with the way the lumbar spine works, but no objective criterion for its diagnosis has been validated. The practitioner may believe that the patient's back is unstable, but he or she has no means by which to objectify that belief. Even spondylolisthesis is not unstable (54). High-precision studies have shown that the motion patterns of patients with spondylolisthesis are indistinguishable from those with degenerative disc disease (5).

Diagnosis such as segmental dysfunction and lumbar insufficiency are no more than metaphors. They say nothing about the source of pain or its cause. These words mean nothing more than "something must be wrong with the back, about here."

Winners

There are absolutely no data on the common causes of acute low back pain. Patients in primary care with acute low back pain have simply not been studied with techniques that might reliably identify a valid source of pain. For red flag conditions, such as tumors and infections, the evidence is that they are rare (<1%) (20,21). Moreover, red flag conditions usually provide cues that permit recognition, such as history of cancer, systemic disturbances, risk factors, or uncharacteristically severe pain. Back pain without such accompanying features is extremely unlikely to be caused by occult tumor or infection.

There are, however, data on the possible sources of chronic low back pain. These data come from studies using controlled diagnostic blocks or provocation discography. These procedures have not been applied to random or general populations. So, the prevalence figures may not be accurate in a true epidemiological sense. However, the figures stem from populations seen in specialist spine centers in Australia and in the US and reflect what is seen in such practices.

In normal volunteers, stimulation of the sacroiliac joint produces low back pain (28). In approximately

20% of patients with chronic low back pain the source of pain can be traced to the sacroiliac joints. Two studies have demonstrated this. The first used anatomical controls, in that all patients had negative responses to previous zygapophysial joint blocks (61). The second study used comparative local anesthetic blocks (43). Previously, belief in sacroiliac joint pain had been based purely on conjecture or wishful thinking. Now there are data that satisfy criteria 1, 2, and 4. The pathology of sacroiliac joint pain remains unknown.

In normal volunteers, stimulation of the lumbar zygapophysial joints produces low back pain and referred pain in the lower limb (30,46,50). Using controlled diagnostic blocks, in younger patients with chronic low back pain after some sort of injury, the prevalence of lumbar zygapophysial joint pain was found to be $15\% \pm 5\%$ (59). In older patients without a history of injury, the prevalence of lumbar zygapophysial joint pain may be as high as $40\% \pm 13\%$ (63). In a heterogeneous population it has been found to be 36% (45). The lumbar zygapophysial joints satisfy criteria 1, 2, and 4 as possible sources of back pain. The causative pathology is not known.

The single most common cause of chronic low back pain is IDD. A stringent study using IASP criteria found the prevalence of IDD to be $39\% \pm 10\%$ (59). This prevalence may be an underestimate because the diagnostic criteria were strictly applied. The patients had to have a positive response to provocation discography at one level and a negative response at least one adjacent level, and had to exhibit at radial fissure on CT discography. The criteria used did not admit IDD at multiple levels, which is one reason why the prevalence estimate might underestimate the true prevalence of IDD in all forms.

Conspicuously, these various prevalence figures add up to approximately 70%, which dispels the myth that the source of chronic low back pain cannot be diagnosed in more than 80% of cases. That myth obtains only if inappropriate diagnostic tests are used. X-rays do not show zygapophysial joint pain, sacroiliac joint pain, or IDD, nor do CT or MRI. Relying on such investigations serves a self-fulfilling prophesy: that no cause of back pain will be found. The opposite applies if diagnostic blocks and provocation discography are used.

Moreover, studies have shown little overlap between the cardinal sources of chronic low back pain. When investigated by zygapophysial joint blocks and/or sacroiliac joint blocks and/or provocation discography, few patients are positive to more than one test under controlled conditions (60,61). Despite prevailing wisdom to the contrary, zygapophysial joint pain, sacroiliac joint pain, and discogenic pain are separate entities and rarely co-exist at the same time in the one patient.

Readers who feel that their favorite condition has not been mentioned in this chapter are invited to assess for themselves to what extent there is evidence about that condition that satisfies the four criteria.

Future Players

There is room and opportunity for people to produce compelling evidence that muscles, ligaments, or other structures might be sources of acute or chronic low back pain. Individuals intent on promoting a particular belief need only satisfy the criteria outlined. That, however, has yet to be performed.

An intriguing proposition is that of torsion injury to the disc (9,11). In this condition, the nucleus pulposus is intact, and there are no internal radial fissures; it is not IDD. The condition is characterized by circumferential tears in the outer anulus fibrosus. Metaphorically, this condition may constitute the sprained ankle of the back. It has been produced experimental in cadavers (23,24). It has been described in case reports (26,27) but not in any substantive population studies. Its diagnosis requires the injection of contrast medium accurately into the anulus fibrosus to demonstrate the tear (which is not easy) and subsequently anesthetizing the tear with a very small volume of local anesthetic. The prevalence of this condition is currently being explored in some research centers. If validated, this condition would add to the prevalence of discogenic pain.

■ CONCLUSION

- In the past, proclamations about the causes and sources of back pain have been based on concept validity at best and hearsay at worst.
- The extent to which a particular entity might be credited as a cause of back pain depends on the extent to which it satisfies the criteria:

  1. Could it be a source of back pain?

  2. Can it be a source of back pain?

  3. Is it ever a cause of back pain?

  4. Is it ever a source of back pain?

- Conditions that fail to satisfy these criteria and that therefore are no more than conjectures include muscle sprain, myofascial pain, ligament pain, spondylosis, spondylolysis, and spondylolisthesis.
- Conditions that fulfill at least criteria 1, 2, and 4 are zygapophysial joint pain and sacroiliac joint pain (see p. 113). Internal disc disruption satisfies all four criteria.

- Collectively, these conditions account for more than 70% of chronic low back pain.
- What has prevented greater and earlier recognition of these conditions in the past is the preoccupation with imaging studies and the reluctance to use diagnostic blocks and provocation discography in the investigation of back pain.

Practice-Based Problem

Readers are invited to follow the approach outlined in this chapter on low back pain, and apply the principles to what they believe and know about neck pain and thoracic spinal pain.

They should find that although there is experimental evidence from normal volunteers that cervical and thoracic muscles, synovial joints, and intervertebral discs can hurt, there is a poverty of data on exactly how often any of these structures is the source of pain in patients.

Only the prevalence of cervical zygapophysial joint pain is known.

The available evidence refutes spondylosis as a cause of neck pain.

Conditions such as myofascial pain, cervical instability, and segmental dysfunction do not satisfy criteria 2, 3, or 4.

Audit Process
Self-Check of the Chapter's Learning Objectives

- What criteria have been presented to judge if a condition is the cause of back pain?
- What common diagnostic entities fail to meet these criteria?
- What diagnostic entities succeed in meeting these criteria?
- What conditions that you presently label your patients as having are based on "soft" criteria?

■ REFERENCES

1. Adams MA, McNally DS, Wagstaff J, Goodship AE. Abnormal stress concentrations in lumbar intervertebral discs following damage to the vertebral bodies: Cause of disc failure? Eur Spine J 1993;1:214–221.
2. Anderson J. Pathogenesis of back pain. In: Grahame R, Anderson JAD, eds. Low Back Pain. volume 2. Westmount: Eden Press, 1980:23–32.
3. Antonacci MD, Mody DR, Heggeness MH. Innervation of the human vertebral body: A histologic study. J Spinal Dis 1998;11:536–531.
4. Ashton IK, Roberts S, Jaffray DC, Polak JM, Eisentstein SM. Neuropeptides in the human intervertebral disc. J Orthop Res 1994;12:186–192.
5. Axelsson P, Johnsson R, Stromqvist B. Is there increased intervertebral mobility in isthmic adult spondylolisthesis? A matched comparative study using roentgen stereophotogrammetry. Spine 2000;25:1701–1703.
6. Barnsley L, Lord S, Bogduk N. Comparative local anaesthetic blocks in the diagnosis of cervical zygapophysial joints pain. Pain 1993;55:99–106.
7. Bogduk N. Lumbar dorsal ramus syndrome. Med J Aust 1980;2:537–541.
8. Bogduk N. The innervation of the lumbar spine. Spine 1983;8:286–293.
9. Bogduk N. The lumbar disc and low back pain. Neurosurg Clin North Am 1991;2:791–806.
10. Bogduk N. International Spinal Injection Society guidelines for the performance of spinal injection procedures. Part 1: Zygapophysial joint blocks. Clin J Pain 1997;13:285–302.
11. Bogduk N. Clinical Anatomy of the Lumbar Spine and Sacrum. 3rd ed. Edinburgh: Churchill Livingston, 1997:205–212.
12. Bogduk N. Clinical Anatomy of the Lumbar Spine and Sacrum. 3rd ed. Edinburgh: Churchill Livingston, 1997:215–225.
13. Bogduk N, Lord SM. Cervical zygapophysial joint pain. Neurosurg Q 1998;8:107–117.
14. Bogduk N, Aprill C, Derby R. Discography. In: White AH, ed. Spine Care, Volume One: Diagnosis and Conservative Treatment. St Louis: Mosby, 1995:219–238.
15. Bogduk N, Aprill C, Derby R. Diagnostic blocks of synovial joints. In: White AH, ed. Spine Care, Volume One: Diagnosis and Conservative Treatment. St Louis: Mosby, 1995:298–321.
16. Bogduk N, Tynan W, Wilson AS. The nerve supply to the human lumbar intervertebral discs. J Anat 1981;132:39–56.
17. Brown MF, Hukkanen MVJ, McCarthy ID, et al. Sensory and sympathetic innervation of the vertebral endplate in patients with degenerative disc disease. J Bone Joint Surg 1997;79B:147–153.
18. Carragee EJ, Tanner CM, Yang B, Brito JL, Truong T. False-positive findings on lumbar discography. Reliability of subjective concordance during provocative disc injection. Spine 1999;24:2542–2547.
19. Carragee EJ, Tanner CM, Khurana S, et al. The rates of false-positive lumbar discography in select patients without low back symptoms. Spine 2000;25:1373–1381.
20. Deyo RA, Diehl AK. Cancer as a cause of back pain: frequency, clinical presentation and diagnostic strategies. J Gen Intern Med 1988;3:230–238.
21. Deyo RA, Rainville J, Kent DL. What can the history and physical examination tell us about low back pain? JAMA 1992;268:760–765.
22. Dreyfuss P, Schwarzer AC, Lau P, Bogduk N. Specificity of lumbar medial branch and L5 dorsal ramus blocks: a computed tomographic study. Spine 1997;22:895–902.
23. Farfan HF, Cossette JW, Robertson GH, Wells RV, Kraus H. The effects of torsion on the lumbar

intervertebral joints: The role of torsion in the production of disc degeneration. J Bone Joint Surg 1970;52A:468–497.

24. Farfan HF, Huberdeau RM, Dubow HI. Lumbar intervertebral disc degeneration. The influence of geometrical features on the pattern of disc degeneration-a post mortem study. J Bone Joint Surg 1972; 54A:492–510.

25. Feinstein B, Langton JNK, Jameson RM, Schiller F. Experiments on pain referred from deep somatic tissues. J Bone Joint Surg 1954;35A:981–987.

26. Finch P M, Khangure MS. Analgesic discography and magnetic resonance imaging (MRI). Pain 1990; Suppl 5:S285.

27. Finch P. Analgesic discography in the diagnosis of spinal pain. Paper presented at "Spinal Pain": Precision diagnosis and treatment, Official Satellite Meeting of the VIth World Congress on Pain, Perth, 1990, April 8–10. Meeting Abstracts p 8.

28. Fortin JD, Dwyer AP, West S, Pier J. Sacroiliac joint: Pain referral maps upon applying a new injection/arthrography technique: Part I: Asymptomatic volunteers. Spine 1994;19:1475–1482.

29. Freemont AJ, Peacock TE, Goupille P, Hoyland JA, O'Brien J, Jayson MIV. Nerve ingrowth into diseased intervertebral disc in chronic back pain. Lancet 1997;350:178–181.

30. Fukui S, Ohseto K, Shiotani M, Ohno K, Karasawa H, Nagaauma Y. Distribution of referred pain from the lumbar zygapophyseal joints and dorsal rami. Clin J Pain 1997;13: 303–307.

31. Fullenlove TM, Williams AJ. Comparative roentgen findings in symptomatic and asymptomatic backs. Radiology 1957;68:572–574.

32. Groen G, Baljet B, Drukker J. The nerves and nerve plexuses of the human vertebral column. Am J Anat 1990;188:282–296.

33. Hirsch C, Ingelmark BE, Miller M. The anatomical basis for low back pain. Acta Orthop Scandinav 1963;33:1–17.

34. Jackson HC, Winkelmann RK, Bickel WH. Nerve endings in the human lumbar spinal column and related structures. J Bone Joint Surg 1966;48A: 1272–1281.

35. Jiang H, Russell G, Raso J, Moreau MJ, Hill DL, Bagnall KM. The nature and distribution of the innervation of human supraspinal and interspinal ligaments. Spine 1995;20:869–876.

36. Kaplan M, Dreyfuss P, Halbrook B, Bogduk N. The ability of lumbar medial branch blocks to anesthetize the zygapophysial joint. Spine 1998;23: 1847–1852.

37. Kellgren JH. Observations on referred pain arising form muscle. Clin Sci 1938;3:175–190.

38. Kellgren JH. On the distribution of pain arising from deep somatic structures with charts of segmental pain areas. Clin Sci 1939;4:35–46.

39. Lamb DW. The neurology of spinal pain. Phys Ther 1979;59:971–973.

40. Lawrence JS, Bremner JM, Bier F. Osteo-arthrosis. Prevalence in the population and relationship between symptoms and x-ray changes. Ann Rheum Dis 1966;25:1–24.

41. Lord SM, Barnsley L, Bogduk N. The utility of comparative local anaesthetic blocks versus placebo–controlled blocks for the diagnosis of cervical zygapophysial joint pain. Clin J Pain 1995;11:208–213.

42. Magora A, Schwartz A. Relation between the low back pain syndrome and x-ray findings. Scand J Rehabil Med 1976;8:115–126.

43. Maigne JY, Aivaliklis A, Pfefer F. Results of sacroiliac joint double block and value of sacroiliac pain provocation tests in 54 patients with low-back pain. Spine 1996;21:1889–1892.

44. Malinsky J. The ontogenetic development of nerve terminations in the intervertebral discs of man. Acta Anat 1959;38:96–113.

45. Manchikanti L, Pampati V, Fellows B, Bakhit CE. The diagnostic validity and therapeutic value of lumbar facet joint nerve blocks with or without adjuvant agents. Curr Rev Pain 2000;4:337–344.

46. McCall IW, Park WM, O'Brien JP. Induced pain referred from posterior lumbar elements in normal subjects. Spine 1979;4:441–446.

47. McNally DS, Shackleford IM, Goodship AE, Mulholland RC. In vivo Stress measurement can predict pain on discography. Spine 1996;21:2500–2587.

48. Merskey H, Bogduk N. Classification of Chronic Pain. Descriptions of Chronic Pain Syndromes and Definitions of Pain Terms, 2nd ed. Seattle: IASP Press, 1994.

49. Moneta GB, Videman T, Kaivanto K, et al. Reported pain during lumbar discography as a function of annular ruptures and disc degeneration. A re-analysis of 833 diskograms. Spine 1994;17:1968–1974.

50. Mooney V, Robertson J. The facet syndrome. Clin Orthop 1976;115:149–156.

51. Moreton RD. Spondylolysis. JAMA 1996;195:671–674.

52. Nice DA, Riddle DL, Lamb RL, Mayhew TP, Ruckler K. Intertester reliability of judgements of the presence of trigger points in patients with low back pain. Arch Phys Med Rehabil 1992;73:893–898.

53. Njoo KH, Van der Does E. The occurrence and interrater reliability of myofascial trigger points in the quadratus lumborum and gluteus medius: A prospective study in non-specific low back pain patients and controls in general practice. Pain 1994;58:317–323.

54. Pearcy M, Shepherd J. Is there instability in spondylolisthesis? Spine 1985;10:175–177.

55. Rabischong P, Louis R, Vignaud J, Massare C. The intervertebral disc. Anat Clin 1978;1:55–64.

56. Rhalmi S, Yahia L, Newman N, Isler M. Immunohistochemical study of nerves in lumbar spine ligaments. Spine 1993;18:264–267.

57. Roberts S, Eisenstein SM, Menage J, Evans EH, Ashton IK. Mechanoreceptors in intervertebral discs: morphology, distribution, and neuropeptides. Spine 1995;20:2645–2651.

58. Schwarzer AC, Aprill CN, Derby R, Fortin J, Kine G, Bogduk N. The false–positive rate of uncontrolled diagnostic blocks of the lumbar zygapophysial joints. Pain 1994;58:195–200.

59. Schwarzer AC, Aprill CN, Derby R, Fortin J, Kine G, Bogduk N. Clinical features of patients with pain stemming from the lumbar zygapophysial joints. Is

the lumbar facet syndrome a clinical entity? Spine 1994;19:1132–1137.

60. Schwarzer AC, Aprill CN, Derby R, Fortin J, Kine G, Bogduk N. The relative contributions of the disc and zygapophyseal joint in chronic low back pain. Spine 1994;19:801–806.

61. Schwarzer AC, Aprill CN, Bogduk N. The sacroiliac joint in chronic low back pain. Spine 1995;20:31–37.

62. Schwarzer AC, Aprill CN, Derby R, Fortin J, Kine G, Bogduk N. The prevalence and clinical features of internal disc disruption in patients with chronic low back pain. Spine 1995;20:1878–1883.

63. Schwarzer AC, Wang S, Bogduk N, McNaught PJ, Laurent R. Prevalence and clinical features of lumbar zygapophysial joint pain: A study in an Australian population with chronic low back pain. Ann Rheum Dis 1995;54:100–106.

64. Splithoff CA. Lumbosacral junction: Roentgenographic comparison of patients with and without backaches. JAMA 1953;152:1610–1613.

65. Stillwell DL. Regional variations in the innervation of deep fasciae and aponeuroses. Anat Rec 1957;127:635–653.

66. Torgerson WR, Dotter WE. Comparative roentgenographic study of the asymptomatic and symptomatic lumbar spine. J Bone Joint Surg 1976;58A:850–853.

67. Virta L, Ronnemaa T. The association of mild-moderate isthmic lumbar spondylolisthesis and low back pain in middle-aged patients is weak and it only occurs in women. Spine 1993;18:1496–1503.

68. Wilk V. Pain arising from the interspinous and supraspinous ligaments. Austral Musculoskel Med 1995;1:21–31.

69. Witt I, Vestergaard A, Rosenklint A. A comparative analysis of x-ray findings of the lumbar spine in patients with and without lumbar pain. Spine 1984;9:298–300.

70. Wyke B. The neurology of low back pain. In: Jayson MIV, ed. The lumbar spine and back pain, 2nd ed. Tunbridge Wells, Pitman, 1980:265–339.

71. Yahia LH, Newman N, Rivard CH. Neurohistology of lumbar spine ligaments. Acta Orthop Scandinav 1988;59:508–512.

72. Yahia LH, Newman NA. A light and electron microscopic study of spinal ligament innervation. Z mikroskop anat Forsch Leipzig 1989;103:664–674.

73. Yoshizawa H, O'Brien JP, Thomas-Smith W, Trumper M. The neuropathology of intervertebral discs removed for low-back pain. J Path 1980;132:95–104.

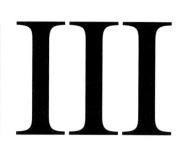

Assessment

Editor's Note

Pain is subjective, and unfortunately it is all we as clinicians have as a starting point in the evaluation of patients. Objectification of our patient's symptoms has proven remarkably elusive. This has even

Editor's Note (*Continued*)

led many to conclude that back problems are largely psychosomatic! However, this may point out more about the limitations of the biomedical model than about the source of our patient's pain.

The practice of using advanced diagnostic imaging, with its high false-positive rate for coincidental structural pathology, as a screening test on nearly all severe pain patients only confuses and frustrates the patient and doctor. The resulting "labeling" of the patient has too high a potential to foster illness behavior in patients with excessive fear–avoidance behavior.

The World Health Organization has described how symptoms, disability (activity level), and impairment are inter-related. Many people with substantial impairments are participating in high level activities (e.g., a person with an artificial limb competing in a marathon!). Disability in the sense of actual skills or activities we perform, dysfunction in the sense of impairments in mobility or strength identified, and distress that patients feel over slow or failed recoveries are all equally important to assess in the modern biopsychosocial paradigm.

Naturally, the first role of the clinician is to diagnose the patient. Unfortunately, this is only possible with certainty for a minority of spine patients. The next question is, can we at least classify patients into meaningful subgroups who will respond to or require specific interventions? Recent developments in diagnostic triage, outcomes management, assessment of "yellow flags" prognostic traits, and functional assessment enable clinicians to give patients a better explanation of what is causing their pain, what can we do for them, what can they do for themselves, and how long might it take.

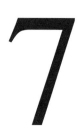

7

Diagnostic Triage in Patients with Spinal Pain

Neil Craton

Learning Objectives

After reading this chapter you should be able to:

- Define the "red flag" as it applies to the diagnostic triage of patients with spinal pain
- Define the "yellow flag" as it applies to the diagnostic triage of patients with spinal pain
- List five red flags for the presence of cancer in patients with spinal pain
- List two red flags for the presence of infection in patients with spinal pain
- Describe the role of plain radiography in the diagnostic triage algorithm for patients with spinal pain
- List the specific deep tendon reflex, myotome, dermatome, and dural stretch signs associated with radiculopathy from C5-T1 and L4-S1
- Describe the "patient in jeopardy" of chronic spinal pain associated with work loss and disability
- List 10 yellow flags for work loss and disability in patients with acute spinal pain.
- Describe the limitations associated with the clinical identification of a specific tissue label for patients with simple backache
- Describe the sensitivity and specificity of magnetic resonance imaging in the diagnosis of spinal pain

Diagnostic Triage in Patients with Spinal Pain

The diagnosis and treatment of spinal pain is a controversial and enigmatic subject. Many different paradigms have been developed to explain where back pain comes from and how to treat it. The treatment offered to patients is often based on tissue-specific, paradigm-specific diagnostic labels. Unfortunately, the same patient may receive distinctly different diagnoses from different practitioners to explain the same episode of spinal pain. Despite the use of differing diagnostic labels, clinicians from all paradigms are required to identify patients with serious underlying conditions responsible for the patient's back pain. This chapter discusses a process of diagnostic triage that can be used to characterize patients as falling into one of the following categories:

1. Possible serious pathology
2. Benign spinal problems with no neurologic deficit (simple backache)
3. Spinal causes with neurologic deficit
4. Non-spinal problems

The process of making a tissue-specific diagnosis for patients with chronic lumbar pain is also reviewed.

Most spinal clinicians pride themselves on the ability to conduct a comprehensive physical assessment of a patient with spinal pain. The identification of a pain generator, biomechanical anomalies, and other culprits forms a large part of the diagnostic process of most practitioners. However, the assessment of patients with acute spinal pain does not require the clinician to make a tissue-specific diagnosis. Even though a diagnosis might be made using elegant clinical assessments or invasive techniques, this is often only of academic interest, because many patients will recover regardless of diagnosis or management (4). This, combined with the fact that many common spinal conditions have no reliable or validated physical manifestations, limits the utility of a tissue-specific diagnosis in the triage of patients with spinal pain (6,12,21,23,27,36,39). Therefore, the diagnostic algorithm regarding patients with spinal pain focuses initially on the exclusion of serious pathology (Fig. 7.1). Patients with spinal pain that may be caused by malignant tumors, infections, fractures, or cauda equina syndrome require emergent triage to tertiary care institutions for definitive investigation and management. The diagnostic triage process then must exclude non-spinal pathology such as renal, abdominal, or gynecological disease. After ruling out serious or non-spinal pathology, the clinician can then conduct a musculoskeletal assessment to exclude spinal pathology and should distinguish a nerve root problem from simple backache (33).

The diagnostic triage process does not end with the simple determination of what is causing a patient's pain. The biopsychosocial model of spine care emphasizes that pain and suffering are different entities, and that emotional and social factors can strongly influence whether a person seeks care for a particular spinal problem and the outcome of that problem. The pandemic of spinal pain-related disability and work loss clearly points to the importance of preventing chronicity in people with spine pain, and psychosocial factors strongly influence the prognosis of organic spinal pathology.

The process of assessing patients with spinal pain has been the subject of substantial scholarship. Guidelines have been published throughout the world to assist the clinician in making evidenced-based cost-effective decisions to deal with the back and neck pain population (1,4,24,33,41,44). Multi-disciplinary diagnostic algorithms outlining the consensus opinion of researchers have been published with recommendations for the investigation and clinical treatment of patients with spinal pain (1,4,24,33,41,44).

The Red Flag

The red flag can be defined as a clinical symptom or sign that may indicate sinister pathology as a source of the patient's spinal pain (1,4). The identification of a red flag should trigger action steps that need to be individualized to each patient. The red flag may prompt advanced imaging, serological investigations, patient referral, or expectant observation (see Table 4.6).

The key tools used in determining which patients may have a serious underlying condition presenting as spinal pain are the patient history and physical examination. The identification of the "red flag" from a detailed history is the most important part of the diagnostic triage process. The majority of red flags are symptoms and can be elicited without a physical examination. Simple historical red flags serve as a sensitive diagnostic tool for the identification of tumor, infection, and fracture (11). The physical examination is typically less valuable in determining which patients have serious problems like cancer (1,4). The existing evidence show that no particular clinical constellation of physical signs elicited on physical examination allows a valid or reliable diagnosis to be made in anatomical or pathological terms (4).

The majority of patients with spinal pain will not have sinister pathology as the source of their spinal pain (1,4). Health care practitioners who see a high

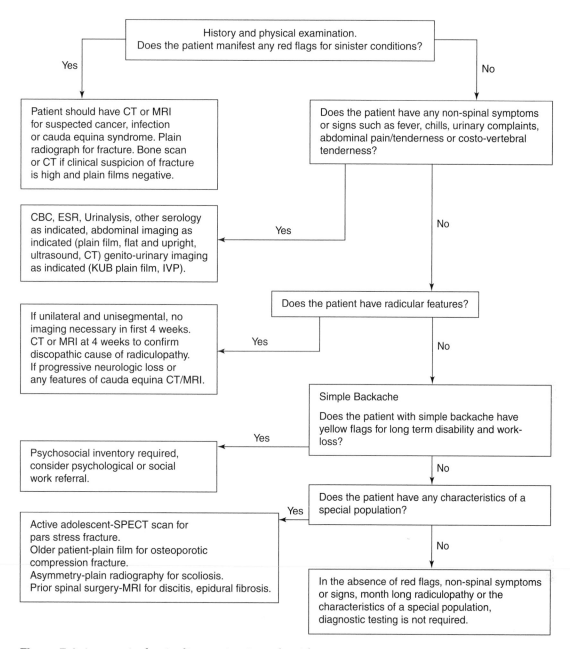

Figure 7.1 Acute spinal pain diagnostic triage algorithm.

volume of spinal pain patients will generally see benign mechanical low back pain, which can be referred to as simple backache (33). Still, the clinician needs to maintain a high level of vigilance to avoid missing sinister pathology among the many patients with benign spinal pain.

The Yellow Flag

The yellow flag is a symptom or sign that should raise the index of suspicion regarding the development of chronicity in a patient with spinal pain (24).

Although the red flag can be thought of as a physical problem worsening a patient's prognosis, the yellow flag can be thought of as a psychosocial factor that worsens prognosis. The yellow flag is not a harbinger of sinister pathology but should be considered a risk factor that the patient is in "jeopardy" of chronic spinal pain and disability. Yellow flags are often found in the patients' psychosocial, psychodynamic, or socioeconomic background (1,24) (see chapter 9). The process of diagnostic triage in patients with spinal pain should attempt to uncover such yellow flags. There is ample literature describing risk factors for the development of chronicity that can be elicited through a patient interview (1,24,43). The prevention of chronicity should be the foundation of the triage and management algorithm for all patients with spinal pain.

Sinister Conditions

The most serious conditions that may cause spinal pain include cancerous lesions, infections, unstable vertebral fractures, intra-abdominal vascular accidents, or a ruptured viscus. The triage process for these conditions should begin with the patient interview focusing on symptoms suggestive of sinister pathology (Table 7.1) (see also Chapter 35).

Malignancy

The probability of a patient presenting to a primary care practitioner with back pain having cancer is less than 1% (4,11). Most of these patients would be elderly. The most common presenting symptom of patients with spinal neoplasia is back pain (13). This is obviously of little use in the diagnostic triage process. The fact that patients with spinal neoplasia will often report an episode of trauma at the onset of their pain is also a challenge to the clinician. Symptoms that are suggestive of spinal malignancy are pain that is persistent, progressive, and worse at night. The lack of pain relief with recumbency is not typical of benign low back problems (7). Patients with low back pain and weakness of the lower extremities must also be considered to be at increased risk for harboring a spinal tumor. Up to 40% of people with primary neoplasms of the spine present with lower extremity weakness (49), whereas 30% of patients with metastatic lesions will present with a neural compression syndrome (28). Deyo and Diehl showed that age older than 50, cancer history, unexplained weight loss, pain lasting more than 1 month, and no improvement with initial therapy were symptoms significantly associated with back pain attributed to cancer (11). Other worrisome symptoms for malignancy include anorexia, fevers, chills, rigors, and night sweats. The presence of these red flags requires the clinician to undertake diagnostic tests to rule out a malignancy.

The majority of tumors that affect the lumbar spine are metastatic. Metastatic disease accounts for 40-times as many cases of spinal neoplasia as all other forms of bone cancer combined (13). Therefore, ascertaining other risk factors for malignancy can help guide the triage process. In females, the most common tumors to metastasize to the vertebrae are from the breast and lung (28). A personal history of breast cancer or a personal history of smoking would be considered important risk factors for these malignancies. In males, the most common tumors to metastasize to the vertebrae are from the prostate and lung. Advancing age and symptoms of prostatism such as urinary hesitancy, nocturia, and decreasing caliber of the urinary stream should prompt consideration of prostate disease. A rectal examination including assessment of the volume and consistency of the prostate will indicate which patients should be sent to the urologist for additional testing. Serological investigations including serum calcium, alkaline phosphatase, and acid phosphatase should be performed if metastatic prostate cancer is suspected. Prostatic serum antigen (PSA) blood levels can also be a useful screening test for prostatic malignancy.

Aside from imaging tests, simple laboratory tests including a complete blood count and erythrocyte sedimentation rate can aid the diagnostic process when there is a suspicion of infection or tumor being the causes for a patient's spinal pain (1). The higher the ESR and white blood cell count, the greater the probability of cancer, infection, or an inflammatory process being responsible for the patient's pain.

Infections of the Spine

The probability of a patient presenting to a primary health care practitioner with back pain having an infection as the cause is said to be less than 0.01% (4,10). However, in the past decade, the incidence of central nervous system infections has increased largely because of the epidemic of acquired immunodeficiency syndrome (AIDS). As a consequence, spinal infections have also increased (32). Therefore, the diagnostic triage process must include appropriate questions regarding the risk factors for HIV acquisition. Intravenous drug use, anal intercourse, multiple sexual partners, and hemophilia are important risk factors for HIV infection.

The most common symptoms of spinal infection include malaise and back pain (32). The most sensitive historical factors for the identification of spinal osteomyelitis in a patient with back pain are a history of intravenous drug use, a previous urinary tract infection, or a skin infection (48). Symptoms more specific for a spinal infection or an infection that is responsible for spinal pain may also include fevers, chills, rigors, and night sweats. Individuals with these symptoms need to be evaluated for osteomyelitis, discitis, or an epidural abscess (4). The compromised host, such as diabetic subjects, intravenous drug users, and the chronically ill are particularly susceptible to spinal infections. Previous spinal surgery should also raise the index of suspicion regarding an infectious process.

Table 7.1 Estimated accuracy of medical history in diagnosis of spine diseases causing low back problems:

References	Diseases to be detected	Medical history red flags	True-positive rate (sensitivity)	True-negative rate (specificity)
Deyo and Diehl	Cancer	Age >50	0.77	0.71
		Previous cancer history	0.31	0.98
		Unexplained weight loss	0.15	0.94
		Failure to improve with 1 month of therapy	0.31	0.90
		Bed rest no relief	>0.90	0.46
		Duration of pain >1 month	0.50	0.81
		Age >50, history of cancer or unexplained weight loss or failure of conservative Rx	1.00	0.60
Waldvogel and Vasey	Spinal osteomyelitis	Intravenous drug use, UTI, or skin infection	0.40	NA
	Compression fracture	Age >50	0.84	0.61
		Age >70	0.22	0.96
		Trauma	0.30	0.85
		Corticosteroid use	0.06	0.995
Deyo	Herniated disc	Sciatica	0.95	0.88
Turner, Ersek, Herron, et al.	Spinal stenosis	Pseudoclaudication	0.60	NA
		Age >50	0.90	0.70
Gran	Ankylosing spondylitis	Positive responses 4 out of 5	0.23	0.82
		Age at onset <40	1.00	0.07
		Pain not relieved in supine position	0.80	0.49
		Morning back stiffness	0.64	0.59
		Duration of pain >3 months		

From Bigos S, Bowyer O, Braen G. et al. Acute Low Back Problems in Adults. Clinical Practice Guidelines. No. 14. Rockville MD, Agency for Health Care Policy and Research, 1994, AHCPR publication 95-0642.

Patients who have had previous chemotherapy, radiotherapy, or used corticosteroids or other immune-suppressant drugs should be considered at increased risk for spinal infection when they present with back pain. Dysuria, urinary frequency, urinary urgency, and pain radiating to the groin increase the likelihood of a urinary tract infection.

There are few clinical signs that are sensitive and specific for the identification of a spinal infection. Fever, vertebral tenderness, and very limited spinal range of motion can suggest the possibility of a spinal infection but may also be present in other causes of spinal pain (1,32). The urinalysis is a simple non-invasive test that can be used to screen for hematuria or pyuria in the presence of urinary tract pathology. Subsequent mid-stream urine assessment for culture and sensitivity can confirm the presence of bacterial pathogens and guide subsequent anti-microbial treatment.

The evaluation of a patient suspected of having an infection as the source of their spinal pain should include a complete blood count (CBC) and an erythrocyte sedimentation rate (ESR). The ESR is a very sensitive tool for infection, although it is not specific and may be elevated in other systemic conditions like spondyloarthropathies and rheumatic conditions (4). Culture of the appropriate body fluids should precede any advanced imaging. The bone scan is the primary investigation for suspected spinal infection (4).

Spinal Fractures

Significant trauma is the most important historical factor that would lead the clinician to suspect a fracture in a patient with acute spinal pain. The age of the patient will influence the magnitude of trauma required to cause a spinal fracture and is the second most important factor in the assessment of these problems. In the general population, significant fractures presenting as back pain occur only in patients with a history of major trauma (4,35). A fall from a significant height or a high-velocity motor vehicle accident associated with acute low back pain should prompt the clinician to consider at least plain radiographic imaging to detect a fracture. In older individuals or in those with other constitutional difficulties, simple heavy lifting or a minor fall should raise the index of suspicion of a spinal fracture (1). Increasing age and osteoporosis are definite risk factors for spinal fractures with minimal identifiable trauma.

A patient with spinal pain after trauma needs to be considered to have an unstable spinal injury until proven otherwise. Any neurological symptoms or alteration in the patient's level of consciousness mandate that the patient be immobilized and emergently triaged for spinal imaging. Hard collar immobilization for cervical injuries and the use of a backboard with pelvic and cervical immobilization should be used for more caudal injuries. Practitioners who cover athletic events with a high risk of spinal trauma such as football and hockey need to rehearse the management of an athlete with a suspected spinal fracture. Any athlete who has bony tenderness, diminished range of motion, or even transient neurologic signs needs to be managed with great caution.

The triage of a patient with trauma and back pain should include plain radiography as the initial investigation. Screening for spinal injuries in which instability is a possibility is typically performed with lateral plain radiographs. The spine must be evaluated for evidence of soft tissue swelling and alignment. The lateral radiograph can be performed while the patient is in the appropriate immobilizing devices if a suspected unstable spine fracture is being evaluated (18). Focal kyphosis or other local alignment anomalies can be an important sign of injury. The lateral radiograph must include all of the spinal elements that may be at risk. Imaging of the lower cervical spine and the cervico-thoracic junction is a frequent problem because of the overlapping bony anatomy in that area.

The lateral radiograph alone is insufficient to rule out fracture and is the starting point in the triage of a patient with a potential spinal fracture. If the lateral film is normal, other views can be obtained.

If plain radiographs are normal and index of suspicion is high enough, either bone scan or CT should be performed. In a patient with persisting pain after trauma with an initial normal x-ray, the investigation should be repeated in 10 to 14 days.

When a fracture is identified on plain film, CT can be of particular value in demonstrating the relationship of the fracture fragments to the spinal canal (18). CT is also of particular value for imaging the posterior spinal elements.

Other Red Flags

Cauda Equina Syndrome Patients who manifest incontinence of stool or urine need to be considered as having cauda equina syndrome until proven otherwise. Associated symptoms include bilateral leg pain, urinary urgency, urinary retention, and sexual dysfunction. Physical signs that may accompany the historical red flags could include a perineal sensory disturbance often referred to as saddle anesthesia and decreased rectal tone. In these patients, it is believed that emergent surgical decompression of the cauda equina can prevent a neuropraxia from progressing to a more permanent neurologic deficit. Therefore, emergent advanced imaging with CT or MRI is necessary in this population.

Progressive Neurologic Loss The presence of progressive neurologic loss is another harbinger of sinister spinal pathology (13). Most spinal clinicians are quite comfortable after patients with unilateral and unisegmental lower motor neuron abnormalities. These findings are often associated with compressive discopathy or chemical radiculitis secondary to discopathy. Published guidelines state that such patients do not require advanced spinal imaging or referral if they improve with the initial clinical interventions and time (1,34). However, when patients have progressive loss of strength, sensation, or hyporeflexia, urgent imaging for an expanding space occupying lesion is indicated. Magnetic resonance imaging is the most sensitive tool for the investigation of this group of patients (34). Individuals with upper motor neuron findings of hyperreflexia, increasing muscle tone, up-going toes, and clonus also require urgent central nervous system imaging to rule out compressive myelopathy or other central nervous system anomalies. Patients manifesting these signs need to have a definitive diagnosis reached as soon as possible.

Non-Spinal Causes of Back Pain The most common systemic conditions that present with spinal pain are the spondyloarthropathies. Patients with spondyloarthropathies or other inflammatory conditions need to be identified as early as possible in the diagnostic process, because they often require specific investigations and pharmacologic therapy in addition to manual, modality, or exercise-based therapy. Psoriatic rashes are a clue to the presence of psoriatic spondyloarthropathy. Symptoms of diarrhea or inflammatory bowel disease also should prompt the clinician to consider Reiter disease and ankylosing spondylitis. Ankylosing spondylitis is characterized by morning stiffness, improvement with exercise, onset at younger than 40 years of age, and duration of more than 3 months. Recurring tendinoplasties or enthesitis should also increase the index of suspicion of this class of disorder. Initial blood work for the evaluation of a patient with a suspected rheumatic condition or spondyloarthropathy should include a complete blood count, an erythrocyte sedimentation rate, a rheumatoid factor, an anti-nuclear antibody screen, and a uric acid level. Concern regarding ankylosing spondylitis should prompt an HLA B27 histocompatability screen.

Diagnostic triage should distinguish patients with non-spinal causes of pain felt in the vertebral area. Pain emanating from intra-abdominal and retroperitoneal structures will frequently require non-primary care investigation and management.

Various intra-abdominal conditions can present with spinal pain. The most sinister would be a ruptured abdominal aortic aneurysm. These patients may have no specific features early in their presentation. A history of vascular disease or the presence of cardiovascular risk factors warrants assessment for this condition. Careful abdominal palpation should reveal a pulsatile mass, which may be tender. Any abdominal guarding, rebound tenderness, or vital sign anomaly would prompt emergent referral to a tertiary care institution via ambulance. En route to hospital, large-bore intravenous access will be established. At the hospital, definitive imaging will include CT, MRI, or ultrasound.

There are many other intra-abdominal conditions that can refer pain to the back. Peptic ulcer disease (with or without perforation), pancreatitis, biliary colic, endometriosis, pelvic inflammatory disease, ectopic pregnancy, and ovarian cysts can all cause back pain. Most of these conditions would be missed if the clinician fails to lay a hand on the patient's belly or considered gynecological problems in female patients.

Simple Backache Versus Nerve Root Problems

The term "simple backache" can be used to describe mechanical back pain that is musculoskeletal in origin. Pain receptors are present in bone, z-joints, muscle, connective tissue, periosteum, the outer third of the intervertebral disc, and in perivascular tissue. Pain receptors can be activated by mechanical strain or dysfunction, metabolites, or inflammation. Simple backache can be very painful and can refer pain to the leg, hip, or thigh, but generally not below the knee (33). The term simple backache implies that the nerve roots and spinal cord are not compromised, and that there is no evidence of sinister or non-spinal pathology. This group of patients can receive a wide array of different diagnostic labels depending on the training of the health care practitioner they visit. Patients with simple backache and no red flags do not require any diagnostic investigations in the first month of symptoms.

Simple backache can be considered from different perspectives in the process of diagnostic triage. Traditional medical diagnostic labels have involved structural changes purported to be pathoanatomic. Such changes have often been based on radiographic evidence. However, changes such as degenerative discs and osteophytes on plain radiography and other imaging are not sensitive or specific for patients with spinal pain. Clinicians from other disciplines use diagnostic labels based on a functional model, often involving manual palpation. Diagnostic labels such as subluxation, fixation, somatic dysfunction, myofascial trigger point, and others are often used to explain spinal pain episodes. Most of these labels have had difficulties with scientific validity, inter-rater reliability, and sensitivity and specificity for spinal pain. Other models for categorizing spinal pain patients involve movement patterns and impairments identified during physical examination associated with the patient's pain. The McKenzie protocol is one of the best known of these models. This method has been shown to be a useful way of classifying patients into groups that respond to a specific treatment (29). Although not having face validity for its purported pathoanatomic correlates, it is useful from a treatment perspective.

Modifications to the McKenzie method have been made and evaluated in a scientific fashion (14).

Table 7.2 Treatment-based classification system categories

- Immobilization
- Lumbar mobilization
- Sacro-iliac mobilization
- Extension syndrome
- Flexion syndrome
- Lateral shift
- Traction

From Fritz, JM, George S. The use of a classification approach to identify subgroups of patients with acute low back pain. Interrater reliability and short term outcomes. Spine 2000;25(1):106–114.

So-called treatment-based classification systems, which use information gathered from a physical examination, patient self-report of pain (pain diagram and pain scale), and Oswestry pain questionnaires, have been used to classify patients with acute spinal pain into groups for specific treatments. The classifications are not based primarily on a tissue-specific diagnosis or pathoanatomy, but rather the type of treatment indicated for the particular patient (Table 7.2). This type of classification system has been documented to have a moderate degree of inter-rater reliability but requires further investigation to establish its validity (14). Some of the premises in this classification system do not withstand close scientific scrutiny (see Chapter 6).

Nerve root pain commonly arises from a single nerve root, and is associated with unilateral pain radiating down the leg in a distribution that approximates a dermatome. The pain can refer to the foot. Leg pain is often more bothersome to the patient than the back pain. The pain is often associated with numbness or paresthesiae. There are often specific physical signs of nerve root irritation such as myotome weakness, diminished deep tendon reflexes, dermatomal sensory loss, and dural stretch signs (Tables 7.3 to 7.5). The finding of leg pain in the contralateral leg with straight leg raising is a very specific test for neurologic compromise with a herniated lumbar disc (1). This abbreviated neurologic examination of the lower extremities will allow detection of most clinically significant nerve root compromise, which makes up more than 90% of all radiculopathy of the lumbar spine. Such screening examination in the diagnostic triage may miss more cephalad discopathy and radiculopathy (25).

In the cervical spine, an accurate diagnosis regarding nerve root involvement can be obtained through the patient's history 75% of the time (47). Pain is often greater in the upper extremity than in the cervical region. The pain is often associated with paresthesiae and weakness. A lancinating quality to the pain is often reported. The distribution of the pain depends on the nerve root involved. C1 and C2 radiculopathies are

Table 7.3 Typical physical findings associated with the most common lumbar radiculopathies

Nerve root involved	Muscular weakness	Sensory loss	Reflex effected
L4	Quadriceps, tibialis anterior	Medial malleolus	Knee jerk
L5	Extensor hallucis longus	First web space of foot	Medial hamstring
S1	Gastrocnemius, soleus	Lateral malleolus	Ankle jerk

Table 7.4 Typical physical findings associated with the most common cervical radiculopathies

Nerve root involved	Muscular weakness	Sensory loss	Reflex effected
C5	Biceps, deltoid	Lateral arm	Biceps
C6	Biceps, wrist extensors	Lateral forearm	Brachioradialis
C7	Triceps, wrist extensors	Triceps	Middle finger
C8	Hand intrinsics	Medial forearm	
T1	Hand intrinsics	Medial arm	

Table 7.5 Estimated accuracy of physical examination for lumbar disc herniation among patients with sciatica

Physical Examination test	True-positive rate (sensitivity)	True-negative rate (specificity)	Comments
Ipsilateral SLR	0.80	0.40	Positive result: leg pain at <60 deg
Crossed SLR	0.25	0.90	Positive result: reproduction of contralateral pain
Ankle dorsiflexion weakness	0.35	0.70	HNP usually at L4-L5 (80%)
Great toe extensor weakness	0.50	0.70	HNP usually at L5-S1 (60%) or L4-L5 (30%)
Impaired ankle reflex	0.50	0.60	HNP usually at L5-S1: absent reflex increases specificity
Sensory loss	0.50	0.50	Area of loss poor predictor of HNP level
Patellar reflex	0.50	NA	For upper lumbar HNP only
Ankle plantar flexion reflex	0.06	0.95	—
Quadriceps weakness	<0.01	0.99	—

From Bigos S, Bowyer O, Braen G, et al. Acute Low Back Problems in Adults. Clinical Practice Guidelines. No. 14. Rockville MD, Agency for Health Care Policy and Research, 1994, AHCPR publication 95-0642. HNP, herniated nucleus pulposis; SLR, straight leg raise.

uncommon and can refer pain to the occipital and retro-orbital regions, respectively. The C3 root refers pain to the ear and jaw regions. C4 radiculopathies refer pain along the base of the neck. C5-T1 radiculopathies are listed in Table 7.4. Severe dermatomal loss of sensation is rare in cervical radiculopathies. Loss of manual dexterity, gait instability, generalized weakness, or urinary symptoms are red flags for cervical myelopathy and require emergent imaging with CT or MRI.

Aside from routine local musculoskeletal and neurological examination, some provocative physical examination tests are advocated for the evaluation of patients with suspected cervical radiculopathy. Spurling's neck compression test has a high sensitivity but low specificity. It involves axial compression with cervical extension and rotation provoking upper extremity or scapular pain. Relief of symptoms with cervical traction or glenohumeral abduction also implies the presence of nerve root pathology.

In the patient with suspected nerve root compromise, close clinical attention is required to ensure no progressive neurologic loss or cauda equina symptoms develop. In the absence of red flags, patients with unilateral, unisegmental nerve root findings do not require imaging or other diagnostic tests in the first month of symptoms, as long as they improve with clinical treatment and time. In patients with refractory nerve root compromise, diagnostic imaging is required to rule out non-disc-related nerve root compression, such as tumor or other space occupying lesion. To evaluate for such abnormalities, the clinician can utilize myelography, CT, CT myelography, or MRI. Most studies indicate no significant difference in the true positive and true negative rates for diagnosing lumbar disc herniation among CT, CT myelography, and MRI (1,22). Plain myelography was inferior to these three modalities. Because any myelographic procedure can expose the patient to complications of headache after spinal tap, reaction to contrast media, and meningeal infection, the noninvasive modalities of CT and MRI are likely a superior choice for diagnostic triage of the patient with suspected herniated nucleus pulposus with nerve root compression.

The Patient in Jeopardy

Disability associated with chronic spinal pain syndromes is a significant public health problem (40). Chronic low back pain causes more disability than all other health care problems combined for people younger than age 45 (40). Chronic cervical spine pain after whiplash is also a common cause of disability (44). There is evidence that the clinician can contribute to this disability in numerous ways (43). Primary care medical doctors often receive little training in the management of spinal pain, such that diagnosing and treating these problems is not their area of greatest clinical competency (8). The prescription of prolonged periods of rest, encouraging work absenteeism, the indiscriminate use of narcotics or sedatives, and facilitating dependence on passive care all can serve to increase the risk of the development of chronicity. Under-identifying at-risk patients may also result in inadvertently reinforcing factors that are disabling (24). For example, failure to understand that patients believe that movement will be harmful may result in them unnecessarily experiencing the negative consequences of withdrawal from social, vocational, and recreational activities. It is also important to note that cognitive and behavioral factors can produce important physiological consequences such as muscle wasting and joint stiffness, prompted by inactivity. Consistently missing yellow flags can be harmful and usually contributes to the development of chronicity (24).

To minimize the risk for chronicity, the triage process should include an effort to identify risk factors for the development of chronic spinal pain (see chapter 9) (24). Most risk factors are based on historical information and can be documented in a thorough patient interview. The identification of these yellow flags should lead to appropriate psychosocial interventions such as cognitive and behavioral management (24). Such management can in turn help with the patient's physical condition.

The New Zealand Ministry of Health commissioned a series of guidelines on the assessment of yellow flags for long-term disability and work loss (24). That group prepared a template on how to judge if a person is at risk for long-term disability or work loss because of psychosocial factors. They also compiled an extensive list of psychosocial factors that adversely affect the prognosis for patients with spinal pain. They emphasized that the most accurate identification of yellow flags required adequate time for evaluation. They also suggested that pain drawings and other pain-specific psychometric measures could assist in the triage process. The key question to be kept in mind while conducting the risk assessment in one's diagnostic triage is, "What can be done to help this person experience less distress and disability?" (24). These factors need to be considered in each patient presenting with spinal pain. There is greater risk to the patient in under-identifying these factors than over-identifying them. Patients may benefit from early cognitive and behavioral therapy as opposed to being

referred as a salvage procedure with so-called failed back syndrome (see chapter 15).

The person at the greatest risk for chronicity can be described as a "patient in jeopardy" (43). The patient in jeopardy of chronic pain cannot be identified by paradigm-based physical examination findings. Psychosocial factors are of greater prognostic value than traditional physical findings based on range of motion assessment, palpation, and alignment factors. However, in 1980, Gordon Waddell described non-organic physical signs that identified patients who required more detailed psychological assessment (46). Waddell described his non-organic physical signs as a simple and rapid screen to help identify patients who required more detailed assessment (Table 7.6).

The non-organic signs documented by Waddell were more common in patients without clear-cut pathology and were not present in normal patients. The nonorganic signs were equally common in medicolegal cases, compensation patients, and those who had no such third party involvement. Waddell suggested that the examination for the non-organic signs should form part of a routine preoperative screen. The signs did not indicate a patient was malingering or that they did not have a treatable lesion, but simply identified those patients who required formal psychological assessment prior to surgery. Given the ease of performing these signs on patients with chronic low back pain, they should be part of the diagnostic triage process of any patient with chronic spinal pain in whom surgery is contemplated (see Chapter 10).

Table 7.6 The Waddell nonorganic signs

- Superficial tenderness to light pinch
- Nonanatomic tenderness, which is not localized and often extends from lumbar spine to thorax or pelvis
- Axial loading pain, when low back pain is reported with vertical loading to the patients head
- Pain with whole body rotation, when shoulders and pelvis are rotated in the same plane
- Discrepancy between seated and lying straight leg raise
- Give-way or cogwheel weakness that cannot be explained on a localized neurologic basis
- Sensory disturbances in a stocking rather than a dermatomal distribution
- Disproportionate verbalization and facial expressions during examination

From Waddell G, McCulloch MD, Kummel E, Venner RM. Nonorganic physical signs in low back pain. Spine 1980;5(2):117–125.

Special Populations and Diagnostic Labels

The Elderly and Osteoporosis

Vertebral osteoporotic compression fractures are a common cause of spinal pain in the elderly. The progressive loss of spinal bone mass renders the vertebrae at risk for wedge fractures with activities of daily living. Clinical suspicion of a vertebral compression fracture should exist in all females older than age 65 and in the presence of risk factors in both men and women. Historical risk factors include smoking, corticosteroid use, premature or surgical menopause, small stature, and a positive family history of osteoporosis. Physical findings suggestive of vertebral compression fractures include an increased thoracic kyphosis (dowager hump), an increased lumbar lordosis, and a protuberant abdomen. In the triage of these patients, a plain radiograph is often all that is necessary to identify the osteoporotic compression fracture (35). Bone scintigraphy can determine whether the identified radiographic abnormality is recent (37).

The elderly typically have a lower incidence of acute herniated nucleus pulposus with nerve root compression. Therefore, any acute radiculopathy in the elderly should raise the clinical suspicion of a compressive lesion such as a tumor. The other condition that is more common in the elderly is spinal stenosis. The patient will typically report pain that increases with walking with relief with rest. These patients often have difficulty with standing and relief with sitting.

The Active Adolescent: Pars Interarticularis Stress Fractures

The majority of spinal pain in young athletes is not sinister. However, any evidence of neurological abnormality in a young patient should be considered a red flag for malignancy. Davids has shown that radiculopathy in the adolescent population is more commonly associated with malignancy than in adults (9).

The other condition that needs to be considered in the process of diagnostic triage in the active adolescent is a pars interarticularis stress fracture or acute spondylolysis. This condition is found in adolescents involved in activities characterized by repetitive spinal loading in flexion and extension. The pain is said to be exacerbated by spinal extension, particularly when performed on one leg (20). These patients can manifest an accentuated lumbar lordosis, shortened hamstrings, and a characteristic gait known as the pelvic waddle (20). These need to be differentiated from more generic mechanical spinal pain, because the management for this group requires the cessation of activities associated with pain. In addition, some

authors recommend spinal bracing with thoracolumbar spinal orthotics (TLSO) (16,45).

In the investigation of a patient with a suspected pars interarticularis stress fracture, plain radiography is of limited usefulness (2,35). Even with the use of oblique views, up to 50% of patients with an acute stress fracture will have normal films. The other complicating issue using plain radiographs alone is that an identified spondylolysis or spondylolisthesis may not be the patient's pain generator. It may be an old lesion and not currently metabolically active or experiencing bone stress. Therefore, bone scintigraphy with technetium 99M has been used as a more sensitive tool. Bone scintigraphy with computer enhancement or so-called single-photon emission computerized tomography (SPECT) scanning is even more sensitive for this condition than plain bone scintigraphy (31).

The Postoperative Lumbar Spine: Discitis, Arachnoiditis, and Epidural Fibrosis

The triage of patients who have had spinal surgery presents several unique challenges. This group of patients may have recurrent disc herniation, epidural fibrosis, spinal stenosis, arachnoiditis, or discitis. Other conditions such as osteomyelitis, nerve root injury, soft tissue infection, instrument failure, pseudarthrosis, and adjacent segment degeneration make this group of patients particularly difficult to evaluate clinically. The diagnostic process can be further clouded by the potential of psychosocial issues (see previous section) that may be involved in the genesis and perpetuation of the patients pain syndrome.

Plain radiography with weight-bearing views supplemented by flexion and extension are useful in the patient who has undergone a fusion procedure to evaluate integrity of the procedure (16). MRI is the imaging modality of choice for all postoperative patients except those with spinal instrumentation. MR provides the best evaluation of the soft tissue structures. MR is the most useful modality for the differentiation between recurring disc and fibrosis.

Most postoperative infections are related to the disc space and the adjacent vertebral bodies. These patients generally have unrelenting back pain after surgery. An elevated ESR is frequently found. In this population, MRI is the imaging modality of choice. MRI is more sensitive in this population than technetium bone scan or gallium scan (16).

Spinal fusion is a common operation in certain geographic areas. An increasing array of operative devices and techniques are being used for these procedures (16). The complications of fusion surgery include hardware malalignment, hardware failure, pseudarthrosis, adjacent segment disk degeneration, and infection. Plain radiographs can be the first diagnostic technique in this patient population. Lucency noted adjacent to pedicle screw hardware implies hardware loosening.

Spondylosis/Disc Degeneration/Spondyloarthrosis

This diagnostic label assumes that degenerative changes identified on imaging tests are pathoanatomic and related to a patient's pain. The purported pathologic changes include disc space narrowing, facet arthrosis, osteophytes, and subchondral sclerosis. However, whereas most patients improve with episodes of spinal pain, degenerative changes obviously do not. Many people have such changes but do not have spinal pain or dysfunction. These changes are simply age-related changes. They occur with increasing frequency with age and are not more prevalent in patients with spinal pain than in individuals with no pain.

The Old Spine: Spinal Stenosis

In most individuals, aging leads to a decrease in the spinal canal volume. The person's canal size and shape will determine which individuals are at greater risk for spinal canal compromise. Spinal canal compromise is referred to as spinal stenosis. Patients with spinal stenosis will often have had a long history of spinal pain. With increasing age, they will have leg pain, particularly with walking. Patients with central canal spinal stenosis typically manifest leg pain with walking variable distances, called neurogenic claudication. This differs from vascular claudication in that patients with vascular claudication tend to stop walking to alleviate the pain in the legs. Patients with neurogenic claudication tend to have to sit down or stoop forward to relieve the pain. Walking uphill is better for those with spinal stenosis, because it involves forward spinal flexion, whereas downhill walking with its relative spinal extension makes the problem worse.

Lateral canal spinal stenosis typically manifests itself as intense radicular pain rather than with neurogenic claudication. This pain may not be posture-related and may persist nocturnally during sleep. Physical examination may be unremarkable. Patients can be differentiated from radiculopathy associated with disc herniation because they will often have a lack of dural tension signs.

Diagnosis of spinal stenosis involves a careful history and physical examination and can be confirmed by CT, CT myelography, and MRI. Electromyography may be necessary to demonstrate denervation.

The Arching Spine: Scheuermann Kyphosis

Scheuermann kyphosis is a common condition affecting up to 8% of the population. The condition usually affects adolescents beginning at age 12 or 13. It generally affects the lower thoracic and upper lumbar vertebrae. It tends to present with pain and a thoracolumbar kyphosis. Other postural anomalies may be present, such as an increased lumbar lordosis and rounding of the shoulders. This condition is associated with an increased risk of pars interarticularis stress fractures and spondylolysis. The diagnosis is suggested by the appropriate history and physical findings combined with plain radiographic features. The x-ray findings include irregular vertebral endplates, anterior wedging of the involved vertebrae, and Schmorl nodes. Schmorl nodes are thought to represent vertebral endplate bulging into the vertebral body.

The Curving Spine: Scoliosis

Scoliosis refers to lateral deviation of the vertebral column in the coronal plane. The deviation in the coronal plane is often accompanied by rotation of the vertebral bodies. Often compensatory curves develop with the convexity in an opposite direction to the primary curve. The diagnosis of scoliosis is most important before the growth phase of adolescence, when the curves and subsequent deformity can increase in magnitude. The diagnosis of scoliosis can be made with a thorough history and physical examination. Careful attention for biomechanical factors that could be contributing to the scoliosis is necessary. Most scoliosis is idiopathic. Plain radiographs confirm the diagnosis.

Investigations in the Diagnostic Triage Process

The investigative process needs to be individualized for each patient with low back pain. Most patients can be managed without investigations as long as they do not manifest red flags and improve with treatment and time (1). The clinician's index of suspicion, the patient's demographics, and specific symptoms will influence the nature of the investigations performed. Although there are guidelines throughout the world to assist the clinician in the consideration of which tests are required in various situations, they cannot replace the intuition of the caregiver (1,41). Investigations generally include diagnostic imaging and serological tests. Neurophysiologic studies such as electromyography (EMG) and nerve conduction studies (NCS) are also of value in the triage of patients with spinal pain associated with potential neurological anomalies.

Plain Radiography

In patients presenting with acute spinal pain, radiographic, or other spinal imaging is generally unnecessary in the first several weeks (1,34,35,41). Plain radiographs have traditionally been ordered as the initial step in the diagnostic imaging of lumbar spinal pain. The purpose of plain x-rays is to identify bony and structural pathology that may be associated with back pain (Table 7.7). Unfortunately, spinal radiographs have limited usefulness in the triage process of patients with low back pain. Scavone showed that nearly 75% of plain x-rays provided no useful clinical information (35). They are of use to rule out spinal fracture after trauma but provide less soft tissue detail than computed tomography and magnetic resonance imaging. Conventional radiography may be valuable in the initial evaluation of suspected spine infection (32). However, bone scintigraphy is likely the best imaging modality in this patient population, because plain x-ray cannot rule out the presence of a spinal infection (1,32). Flexion–extension radiographs are a useful modality to rule out ligamentous instability after trauma (18). In the neck, translation of one segment on another more than 3 millimeters should be considered evidence of ligamentous disruption, and the patient should be managed as having an unstable cervical spine.

There are many plain radiographic findings that traditionally have been considered to be indicative of pathology and therefore associated with the presentation of acute back pain. An example of such a finding is an altered lumbar or cervical lordosis thought to be indicative of muscular hypertonicity associated with acute back pain. However, Hansson has shown that there is no difference in lumbar lordosis on x-ray among patients with acute low back pain, chronic low back pain, and asymptomatic subjects (17).

Degenerative changes of the spine have been considered to represent pathology by some clinicians. The presence of degenerative disc narrowing and osteophytes correlates poorly with the presence of low back pain. These findings are more likely related

---

Table 7.7   Indications for plain radiography

- To rule out a fracture in a well patient with significant trauma
- To rule out a fracture in a compromised patient with minor trauma
- To rule out spinal instability with flexion–extension views in the post-traumatic patient
- The evaluation of a patient for hardware failure in a post-fusion patient

---

Table 7.8   Indications for CT scanning

- To rule out tumor or other space occupying lesion in a patient with refractory radiculopathy (no improvement with 4–6 weeks of treatment)
- To rule out cauda equina syndrome in a patient with urinary anomalies, incontinence of stool or urine, bilateral leg symptoms, saddle anesthesia, or decreased rectal tone
- To confirm a match between disc herniation at a particular segment with nerve root compression at a particular segment in a case of radiculopathy when surgery is contemplated
- To evaluate for spinal fracture in cases where clinical suspicion of fracture remains high despite normal plain radiographs (head injury or altered level of consciousness)
- To evaluate spinal cord anatomy in a patient with neurologic symptoms or signs after trauma
- To evaluate a patient with suspected spinal stenosis
- To obtain the best image of bony lesions in patients with red flags or abnormal bone scans

---

to aging (1,33). Most patients with low back pain improve whether the plain radiograph reveals degenerative changes. Therefore, the finding of degenerative changes on plain films is not a decision point in the diagnostic triage algorithm.

The diagnostic significance of many other findings of plain radiographs remains unknown. Bigos et al showed that spondylolysis, transitional vertebrae, spina bifida occulta, lumbar lordosis, moderate scoliosis, and degenerative joint disease were not predictive factors for acute low back pain or chronicity (2).

Plain lumbar radiography is of limited usefulness in the diagnostic triage process. It can identify many structural anomalies that are not related to the cause of the patient's low back pain (2). It is also of insufficient sensitivity to rule out tumor or infection in the patient presenting with red flags (1). Most clinicians have seen patients who have become overly concerned with the presence of degenerative changes or other abnormalities on their x-rays. It is often difficult to convince the patient that these findings are of little import.

CT Scans

The objective of using a CT scan in a patient with spinal pain would be to identify anatomical pathology that is responsible for the patient's problem (Table 7.8). Unfortunately, the abnormalities most frequently documented in CT scans are common in asymptomatic individuals (50). Disc herniations, facet hypertrophy, and, to a lesser extent, spinal stenosis were all found in patients with no back or leg pain. As a result, CT scans are not part of the diagnostic triage process for patients with spinal pain alone, unless red flags are evident. CT scans can be used to confirm the presence of disc herniation in patients presenting with radiculopathy. This group of patients is relatively easy to separate from the patient with spinal pain alone. CT scans are not useful as a screening tool (4). CT scanning can be used to rule out tumor when red flags are present (1). The CT may be the optimal imaging modality for bone problems and in some geographical regions may be easier to access for some practitioners.

MRI

The purpose behind using MRI in the diagnostic triage of patients with spinal pain is to identify the anatomical or physiological pathology responsible for the patient's spinal pain syndrome (Table 7.9). As with other imaging tests, the MRI may reveal anatomical abnormalities in individuals who do not have spinal pain. Disc herniation, disc bulging, spinal stenosis, and disc degeneration are all commonly found in asymptomatic individuals (3) (Fig. 7.2). These findings occur with increasing frequency with age. Disc degeneration is virtually ubiquitous at age older than 60 on MRI (4). As a result, the MRI is not part of the diagnostic triage process for patients with spinal pain alone, unless red flags are evident. Some have stated that MRI is not justified for the investigation

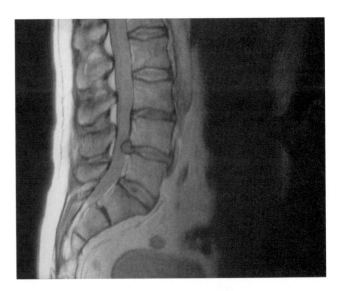

Figure 7.2 MRI abnormalities on an asymptomatic individual

of acute low back pain, even to screen for red flag conditions, because of cost and the relative paucity of red flag conditions rendered evident by this modality (4). MRI is the recommended imaging modality for patients who have had previous spinal surgery (1). MRI with contrast is the imaging test of choice to distinguish disc herniation from perineural fibrosis associated with previous surgery. MRI is the best modality for imaging neural tissues and bone marrow and for diagnosing tumor or infection.

Bone Scan

The purpose of using a bone scan in the evaluation of patients with spinal pain is to identify lesions manifesting hyperemia and increased metabolic activity (Table 7.10). The bone scan is an excellent tool to evaluate the metabolic activity in bone. Bone scintig-

---

Table 7.9 Indications for MRI

- To rule out tumor or other space occupying lesion in a patient with refractory radiculopathy (no improvement with 4–6 weeks of treatment)
- To rule out cauda equina syndrome in a patient with urinary anomalies, incontinence of stool or urine, bilateral leg symptoms, saddle anesthesia or decreased rectal tone
- To confirm a match between disc herniation at a particular segment with nerve root compression at a particular segment in a case of radiculopathy when surgery is contemplated
- To evaluate for post-operative complications such as discitis or perineural fibrosis
- To evaluate a patient for potential spinal infection
- To evaluate spinal cord compression in patients with equivocal findings on CT

Table 7.10 Indications for bone scan

- To evaluate for potential spinal infection
- To evaluate for spinal stress fractures, especially pars interarticularis stress fractures (consider SPECT scan with high index of suspicion because of greater sensitivity)
- To evaluate for spinal fracture in cases where clinical suspicion of fracture remains high despite normal plain radiographs
- To identify areas of skeletal metastases in patients with known cancer
- To identify sacroiliitis

raphy with 99M-radiolabeled technetium is an excellent screening test for potential spinal infection (48). Osteoblastic activity is increased in osteomyelitis, discitis, and other spinal infections. In the patient with a suspected spinal infection, bone scans rarely provide false-negative results. Bone scanning has also been recommended to evaluate patients with potential spinal tumor or occult fracture. The procedure is moderately sensitive in the detection of these conditions, but it cannot specify the diagnosis. The bone scan can help in the dating of an identified fracture on plain film, such as a compression fracture. Bone scanning is a useful screening tool in patients with known non-spinal malignancy who present with spinal pain (22). The use of bone scan is also recommended in the evaluation of patients with suspected pars interarticularis stress lesions or other stress fractures of the lumbar spine and pelvic region. The bone scan can also be used in the assessment of patients with potential inflammatory sacroiliitis. It is of note that the bone scan is often not a useful test in the presence of multiple myeloma, the most common primary tumor of spinal bone.

Electrophysiologic Testing

The electrodiagnostic medical consultation can play and important role in the diagnosis and management of patients with spinal pain and neurological problems. Electromyography (EMG) has the highest diagnostic yield in lumbosacral radiculopathy (Table 7.11)

Table 7.11 Indications for EMG

- To show the nature, location, distribution and severity of the nerve lesion; because not all extremity pain is based on nerve root injuries, this can be helpful in the diagnostic triage when nerve root signs are normal or equivocal
- To highlight pathologic processes such as peripheral neuropathy
- To localize a nerve lesion
- A properly timed EMG can differentiate a neuropraxic injury from active axonal degeneration; it can also determine the acuity of the problem
- To confirm whether identified pathoanatomy on imaging is causing any nerve root pathology; this can be valuable when surgical therapies are being considered
- To assist in the determination of whether a radiculopathy with myotome weakness will have a good prognosis for the return of muscle strength
- To determine whether the patient's problem is improving on a physiologic basis

---

(15). The EMG provides information regarding neurophysiologic abnormalities as opposed to the structural anomalies identified on most imaging studies. All nerve lesions are not caused by nerve root compression and can involve the root, the plexus, the peripheral nerve, or generalized neurologic function.

EMG can provide data that correlate more closely with patient symptoms than imaging studies do. However, the EMG provides data only regarding the motor root and in the cervical spine where there more spatial diversity between motor and sensory roots may not identify a purely sensory anomaly (15).

EMG is not recommended in the diagnostic triage of spinal pain alone or simple backache.

In summary, the use of electrodiagnostic studies is of value in the patient with radiculopathic findings where more specific information about the exact neurophysiology is required. Objective anomalies on EMG can also be useful in the patient with third party involvement.

Invasive Diagnostic Needling Techniques

The Tissue-Specific Diagnosis

The identification of the specific pain generator for patients with spinal problems was previously considered impossible in up to 85% of cases (30). More recent publications have stated that by using invasive diagnostic needling techniques, the clinician can determine the pain generator much more commonly (see Chapter 6). Because this is not practical, cost-effective, or even necessary, such procedures are not a key component of the diagnostic triage process in the acute spinal pain patient. They may play a greater role in the triage of chronic pain patients with disability.

Internal Disc Disruption and Discography

Discography is an invasive diagnostic procedure designed to determine whether a disc is intrinsically painful (5) (Fig. 7.3). Discography involves the injection of contrast material or saline into the nucleus pulposus of the inter-vertebral disc. Information can then be documented regarding the amount of contrast accepted, the pressure necessary to inject the material, the morphology the contrast assumes, and the reproduction of the patient's pain. Postdiscography computed tomography can be used to highlight the features of internal disc disruption, which is the most common known cause of discogenic pain in patients with chronic spinal problems (5).

The diagnostic goal of discography is to determine the structural anatomy of the disc, to characterize the pain response prompted by the injection of the disc,

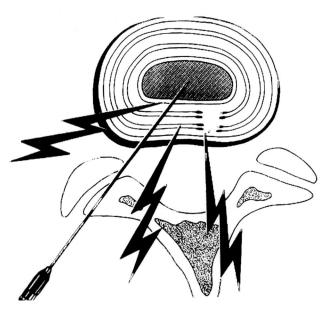

Figure 7.3 Pain provocation with discography

and to compare that to the patient's typical pain (1). To reduce the number of false-positive discograms, the diagnosis of discogenic pain requires that a patient must report reproduction of pain on stimulation of the target disc but no pain when an adjacent disc, and preferably two discs, are stimulated (5). Single-level discography is not clinically meaningful, because the lack of a control level prevents the investigator from concluding that a positive response is specific to disc disruption as opposed to other factors. In a similar fashion, triple-level positive disc stimulation should not be considered a true positive (5).

Holt has reported that discography is painful in normal volunteers (19). However, this position has been refuted in subsequent publications (5,42). It is believed that discogenic pain as manifest on discography correlates with substantial disruption in the annulus fibrosis (Fig. 7.4). Discogenic pain does not correlate with disc degeneration (5). The use of discography with this type of rigorous standard has shown that spinal pain caused by internal disc disruption is present in more than 39% of patients with chronic low back pain (38).

Given its invasive nature, potential complications, cost, and lack of availability in some regions, discography is not part of the diagnostic triage process for acute spinal pain. There is no red flag that would prompt discography. Discography is not recommended as a part of the diagnostic triage process for patients with suspected disc herniation (1). Discography can identify a particular disc as a pain generator and may allow better result in spinal surgery, which is planned on the basis of positive discography. This procedure can provide an anatomic diagnosis

for a patient with chronic spinal pain and establishes that a patient's pain is not imaginary (5). This can be of particular importance when third parties or litigation is involved, and when imaging studies such as CT or MR have been non-contributory.

The intervertebral disc can be a source of pain in the cervical spine also (36). Attempts to identify a characteristic marker of cervical discogenic pain with MRI have been largely unsuccessful. In cases of chronic cervical spine pain in which conservative treatment has not been effective and in which surgical procedures are being contemplated, the importance of cervical discography should be stressed (32a). Patients will often have their pain provoked by discography at morphologically inconspicuous discs, often after failed surgery on the morphologically more aberrant discs (36). Patients can have discogenic pain with normal CT and MR findings, and can also have annular tears that are asymptomatic.

The Sacroiliac Joint

It is generally accepted that the sacroiliac joint can be a source of spinal pain (12,26). Sacroiliac injections can prompt pain over the region of the joint which can radiate to the buttock and thigh. The sacroiliac joint can be involved in the spondyloarthropathies, fractures of the pelvis, childbirth, and pregnancy and in crystal-induced or pyogenic arthropathy (12). The

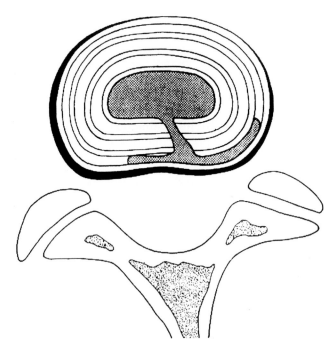

Figure 7.4 Depiction of discogram revealing substantial annular tear. This would appear normal on CT and on some MRI images.

paradigmatic constructs of sacroiliac joint dysfunction, fixation, or subluxation are more controversial. These terms are used to explain pain from a sacroiliac joint that is morphologically normal but that is presumed to have a biomechanical disorder that causes the pain (12). Some clinicians assert that they can identify the biomechanical anomalies on clinical examination alone (26). The validity of most of these physical examination techniques has not been established.

Intra-articular sacroiliac diagnostic injections can now be performed. The joint can be cannulated under fluoroscopic guidance, and contrast can be injected to perform arthrography. If a patient has pain emanating from the sacroiliac joint, traditional logic would indicate that this pain should be ablated with the injection of local anaesthetic (12). Using this as the criterion standard, 12 common physical findings have been evaluated for external validity (12). The diagnostic tests evaluated included joint play, sacral sulcus tenderness, thigh thrust, the Gillet test, Patrick test, Gaenslen test, a midline sacral thrust, and pain drawings over areas traditionally associated with sacroiliac pain referral. Traditional physical examination tests such as the Gillet test, the Patrick test, and Gaenslen test were demonstrated to be unreliable in the diagnostic triage of patients with potential sacroiliac pain (12). The Gillet test has also been demonstrated to have poor inter-rater reliability (6,12). With respect to medical history, no aggravating or alleviating factor is of value for diagnosing the presence of sacroiliac joint pain.

The Zygapophyseal Joint

Many clinicians believe that the zygapophyseal joint (z-joint) is an important source of spinal pain in both the cervical and lumbar regions (27,39). The primary pathology was thought to be that of osteoarthritis, chondromalacia, or occult fractures. Mechanical anomalies are also cited as potential factors involved in pain generation according to the fixation, subluxation, or somatic dysfunction models. In the process of diagnostic triage, the identification of z-joint pain is difficult on clinical grounds alone (21,39). There are no clinical features that are pathognomonic of z-joint pain (39). Fundamental to the diagnosis of lumbar z-joint pain is the use of diagnostic blocks. Radiologically controlled blocks of the joints performed under fluoroscopic guidance constitute the only gold standard for the diagnosis of z-joint pain (39). Multiple blocks with either extra-articular or variable-length local anesthetic controls are required to decrease the false-positive rate of z-joint blocks. When multiple blocks

are used in a chronic lumbar spinal pain population, 15% of patients appear to have the z-joint as the key pain generator. In this group, there are no clinical features that could distinguish the z-joint patient from those who did not respond to blocks (21,39).

The z-joint is an important pain generator in the cervical spine after whiplash (27). Patients with z-joint-mediated pain often have no significant findings on physical examination. These patients also have no consistent abnormalities on x-ray, CT, or MRI (23). Therefore, the diagnostic process requires the use of stringent methods involving fluoroscopically guided, placebo-controlled medial branch blocks if a diagnosis of z-joint pain is to be confirmed. Using such invasive techniques, it can be shown that the prevalence of z-joint pain after whiplash is up to 64% (Fig. 7.5) (27). The upper cervical z-joints often provoke head pain and the lower cervical z-joints often provoke shoulder girdle pain. Such testing has only been performed on patients with chronic neck pain after whiplash, and the relevance to the acute situation has yet to be determined. Therefore, given that the majority of patients with whiplash will return to usual activities within the first 2 months of injury, z-joint diagnostic blocks are

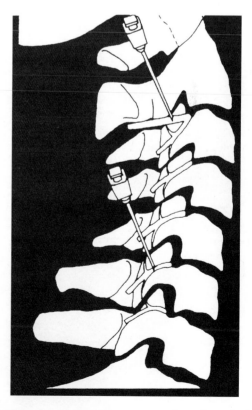

Figure 7.5 Diagrammatic representation of cervical medial branch block.

not part of the diagnostic triage process for acute whiplash injury (44). They are typically reserved for the evaluation and treatment of chronic pain and can be of particular uses in cases complicated by third party and litigation issues.

Clinical Vignettes

A 17-year-old elite athlete had been out all day mountain biking. He returned home and retired for the night. He awoke from sleep to urinate. He collapsed and struck his head and neck on the side of his bathtub and was rendered unconscious. He was taken by ambulance to a local emergency room. In emergency, he underwent routine cervical spine x-rays and was discharged, because the x-rays were interpreted as normal (Fig. 7.6). The next day, his mother called my office and described the situation. I saw him that afternoon, when he manifested no cervical spine motion in any plane and substantial paraspinal muscular hypertonicity. He was placed in a Philadelphia hard collar and sent for emergent CT scan. The CT revealed an unstable C 2–3 fracture (Fig. 7.7). He was treated by a neurosurgeon for 12 weeks in a cervicothoracic orthotic. He was left with a 3- to 4-mm slip at C2-3 but has no neurological findings and has returned to cycling. An MRI was performed by the neurosurgeon to evaluate for disc desiccation at C2-3

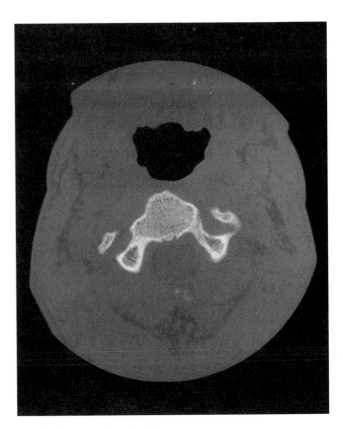

Figure 7.7 CT showing fracture

(Fig. 7.8). Significant disc desiccation would have increased the strength of the recommendation for spinal fusion.

Clinical Pearl

The trauma in this case was "significant" and should have merited more than plain radiographs in the diagnostic triage. Flexion–extension views, CT, or MRI should have been performed while the patient was in the emergency room. He had two red flags, significant trauma, and loss of consciousness. This case demonstrates that plain radiography alone is not sensitive enough for all cases of trauma, particularly when red flags are present. It demonstrates that CT is a sensitive modality for fracture identification. It shows that MR can have utility in planning follow-up care.

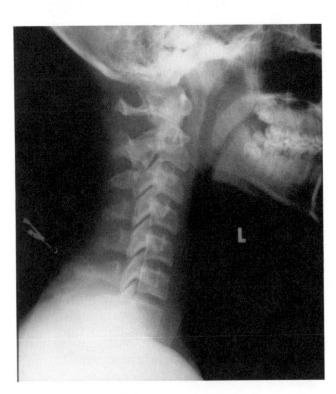

Figure 7.6 Original plain cervical radiographs.

An 18-year-old woman presented on referral from her family doctor. She had "scoliosis" that was worsening. She was getting pain with exercise. She had been receiving adjustive therapy from her chiropractor with no benefit. She had no other symptoms and no red or yellow flags. Her family doctor had won-

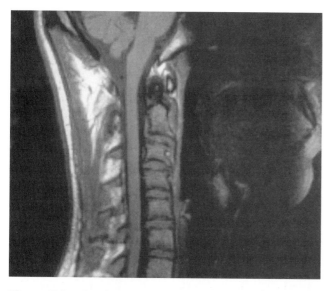

Figure 7.8 MRI showing small spondylolisthesis at C2-3.

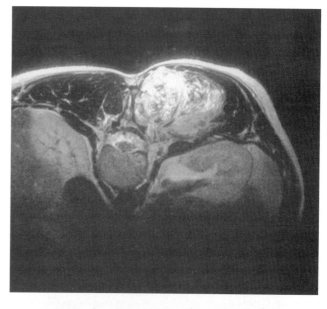

dered whether a trigger point injection might help her problem. Clinical examination revealed asymmetry in the musculature of her spine, but no true scoliosis. On palpation, the area presumed to be muscular hypertonicity in the paraspinal area was soft. An emergent MRI revealed an extensive arteriovenous malformation that had extended into her vertebrae and spinal canal, as well as the subcutaneous areas (Fig. 7.9). She was referred to several neurosurgeons, and at this time has had no definitive therapy. She is 24, and doing well, but she has a guarded prognosis.

Clinical Pearl

This patient "flew beneath the radar" based on her history alone. She had no true red flags. The only factor was her chronic pain. This emphasizes that whereas guidelines and algorithms can assist us in our management of patients with spinal pain, they are not a replacement for clinical evaluation and intuition.

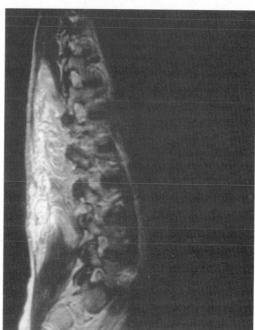

Figure 7.9 MRI showing extensive subcutaneous and intra-spinal arteriovenous malformation.

■ CONCLUSION

The clinical management of patients with spinal pain involves both the art and science of health care. There is much art and tradition surrounding many of the paradigms that diagnose and treat spinal disorders. As with art, these diagnostic and therapeutic techniques often bring the joy of relief from suffering to the patron. However, it is apparent that in the evidence-based, controlled care environment of the new millennium, art alone will not suffice. However, as we strive to allow science to enhance the validity and reliability of our art, we must remember our patrons with spinal pain. We must do everything in our power to survive the tension between therapeutic nihilism and overly invasive or poorly validated treatments. Through this tension, it is comforting to know that the most important information we can glean from our patients with spinal pain is that obtained through simple conversation.

Audit Process
Self-Check of the Chapter's Learning Objectives

- Are you inquiring about red flags for cancer and infection in your review of systems in patients who present with spinal pain?

- Are you facilitating disability and work loss through emphasizing passive care or ignoring yellow flags?

- Are you relying on plain radiographs to make a tissue-specific diagnosis such as degenerative disc disease or facet arthrosis in your patients?

- Do you use MRI as a primary diagnostic or screening tool in your patients with spinal pain?

- Do you routinely examine for deep tendon reflex abnormalities, weakness, sensory change, or dural irritability in patient with leg pain (leg begins at iliac crest)?

- Are you referring patients to mental health professionals when you think someone has a risk for chronicity because of psychosocial factors, or do you only do this as a last resort?

- Do you always make a tissue-specific diagnosis for your patients with low back pain based on your clinical assessment?

- Do you tell your patients that you know what is wrong with them after viewing their x-ray or MRI?

- Do you know which of your patients are at the greatest risk for chronic pain and disability after taking a history?

■ REFERENCES

1. Bigos S, Bowyer O, Braen G, et al. Acute Low Back Problems in Adults. Clinical Practice Guidelines. No. 14. Rockville MD, Agency for Health Care Policy and Research, 1994, AHCPR publication 95-0642.
2. Bigos SJ, Hansson T, Castillo RN, Beecher PJ, Wortley MD. The value of preemployment roentgenographs for predicting acute back injury claims and chronic back pain and disability. Clin Orthop Rel Res 1992;283:124–129.
3. Boden SD, Davis DO, Dina TS, Patronas NJ, Wiseel SW. Abnormal magnetic resonance scans of the lumbar spine in asymptomatic subjects. J Bone Joint Surg 1990;72A: 403–408.
4. Bogduk N. Evidence-based clinical guidelines for the management of acute low back pain. Draft. Submitted for endorsement by the NH&MRC, November 1999.
5. Bogduk N. The argument for discography. Neurosurg Q 1996;6(2):152–153.
6. Carmichael JP. Inter-and intra-tester reliability of palpation for sacro-iliac joint dysfunction. J Manipulative Physiol Ther 1987;10:164–171.
7. Cherkin DC, Deyo RA, Street JH, Barlow W. Predicting poor outcomes for back pain seen in primary care using patient's own criteria. Spine 1996;21:2900–2907.
8. Craton N, Matheson GO. Training and clinical competency in musculoskeletal medicine: Identifying the problem. Sports Med 1993;15(5):328–337.
9. Davids JR, Fulp T. Tumors and tumorlike conditions of the cervical spine and neck in children. Spine: State of the art reviews. 1996;10(1):144–166.
10. Deyo RA, Rainville J, Kent DL. What can the history and physical examination tell us about low back pain? JAMA 1992;268(6):760–765.
11. Deyo RA, Diehl AK. Cancer as a cause of back pain: Frequency, clinical presentation, and diagnostic strategies. J Gen Intern Med 1988;3(3):230–238.
12. Dreyfuss P, Michaelsen M, Pauza K, McLarty J, Bogduk N. The value of medical history and physical examination in diagnosing sacroiliac joint pain. Spine 1996;21(22):2594–2602.
13. Frank CJ, Brantigan JW, McGuire MH. Evaluation of patients with spinal column tumors. Spine: State of the art reviews. 1996;10(1):13–23.
14. Fritz, JM, George S. The use of a classification approach to identify subgroups of patients with acute low back pain. Interrater reliability and short-term outcomes. Spine 2000;25(1):106–114.
15. Grant PA. Electrodiagnostic medical consultation in lumbar spine problems. Occup Med: State of the art reviews 1998;13(1):97–120.
16. Gundry CR, Heithoff KB, Pollei SR. Imaging of the postoperative lumbar spine. Spine: State of the art reviews 1995;9(1):211–244.
17. Hansson T, Bigos S, Beecher P, Wortley M. The lumbar lordosis in acute and chronic low back pain. Spine 1985;10(2):154–155.
18. Hart BL, Orrison WW, Benzel EC. Imaging spinal trauma Spine: State of the art review 1995;9(1):93–118.
19. Holt EP. The question of lumbar diskography. J Bone Joint Surg 1968;50A:720–725.
20. Jackson DW, Wiltse LL, Dingeman RD. Stress reactions involving the pars interarticularis in young athletes. Am J Sports Med 1981;9:304–312.
21. Jackson RP. The facet syndrome myth or reality? Clin Orthop Rel Res 1992;279:110–120.
22. Jackson RP, Cain JE, Jacobs RR, Cooper BR, McManus GE. The neuroradiographic diagnosis of lumbar herniated nucleus pulposus: II. A comparison of computed tomography, (CT), myelography, CT-myelography, and magnetic resonance imaging. Spine 1989;14(12):1362–1367.
23. Kelroser DB. Whiplash, chronic neck pain and zygapophyseal joint disorders. A selective review. Minnesota Med 2000;83:51–54.
24. Kendall NAS, Linton SJ, Main CJ. Guide to assessing psychosocial yellow flags in acute low back pain: Risk factors for long-term disability and work loss. Accident Rehabilitation and Compensation Insurance Corporation of New Zealand and the National Health Committee. Wellington NZ.

25. Kortelainen P, Puranen, J, Koivisto E, Lahde S. Symptoms and signs of sciatica and their relation to the localization of the lumbar disc herniation. Spine 1985;10(1):88–92.

26. Laslett M, Williams M. The reliability of selected pain provocation tests for sacroiliac joint pathology. Spine 1994;19(11):1243–1249.

27. Lord SM, Barnsley L, Wallis BJ, Bogduk N. Chronic cervical zygapophyseal joint pain after whiplash. A placebo-controlled prevalence study. Spine 1996; 21(15):1737–1745.

28. Mardjetko SM., DeWald CJ. Management of metastatic spinal disease. Spine: State of the art reviews 1996;10(1):89–105.

29. McKenzie RA. The lumbar spine. Mechanical diagnosis and therapy. Waikanae, New Zealand: Spinal Publications Limited, 1989.

30. Nachemson AL. Low back pain. Its etiology and treatment. Clin Med 1971;78:18–22

31. Read MT. Single photon emission computed tomography (SPECT) scanning for adolescent back pain. A sine qua non? Br J Sports Med 1994;28(1):56–57.

32. Reddy S, Leite CC, Jinkins JR. Imaging of infectious disease of the spine. Spine: State of the art reviews 1995;9(1):119–140.

32a. Rogers C, Joshi J, Dreyfuss P. Cervical intrinsic disc pain and radiculopathy. Spine: State of the art reviews 1998;12(2):323–356.

33. Rosen M. Chair. Back Pain. Report of a Clinical Standards Advisory Group on Back Pain. May 1994.

34. Russo R, Cook P. Diagnosis of low back pain: Role of imaging studies. Occup Med: State of the art reviews 1998;13(1):P83–P96.

35. Scavone JC, Latshaw RF, Rohrar GV. Use of lumbar spine films: Statistical evaluation at a university teaching hospital. JAMA 1981;246:1105–1108.

36. Schellhas KP, Smith MD, Gundry CR, Pollei SR. Cervical discogenic pain. Prospective correlation of magnetic resonance imaging and discography in asymptomatic subjects and pain sufferers. Spine 1996;21(3):300–311.

37. Schutte HE, Park WM. The diagnostic value of bone scintigraphy in patients with low back pain. Skeletal Radiol 1983;10(1):1–4.

38. Schwarzer AC, Aprill CN, Derby R, Fortin J, Kine G, Bogduk N. The relative contributions of the disc and zygoapophyseal joint in chronic low back pain. Spine 1994;19:801–806.

39. Schwarzer AC, Aprill CN, Derby R, Fortin J, Kine G, Bogduk N. Clinical features of patients with pain stemming from the lumbar zygapophyseal joints: Is the lumbar facet syndrome a clinical entity. Spine 1994;19(10):1132–1137.

40. Shelerud R. Epidemiology of occupational low back pain. Occupational Medicine: State of the art reviews. 1998;13:1–22.

41. Simmons JW, Aprill CN, Dwyer AP, Brodsky AE. A reassessment of Holt's data on "the question of lumbar discography." Clin Orthop 1988;237:120–124.

42. Simmons ED Jr., Guyer RD, Graham-Smith A, Herzog R. X-ray assessment for patients with low back pain. Contemporary Concepts in Spine Care. Rosemont IL, North American Spine Society, 1993.

43. Sommer HM. The patient in jeopardy: how the low back pain patient becomes disabled. Occup Med: State of the art reviews. 1998;13:23–31.

44. Spitzer WO, Skovron ML, Salmi LR, et al. Scientific monograph of the Quebec Task Force on Whiplash-Associated Disorders: Redefining "whiplash" and its management. Spine 1995;20 (8 Suppl):1S–73S.

45. Steiner ME, Micheli LJ. Treatment of symptomatic spondylolysis and spondylolisthesis with the modified Boston Brace. Spine 1985;10:937–943.

46. Waddell G, McCulloch MD, Kummel E, Venner RM. Nonorganic physical signs in low back pain. Spine 1980;5(2):117–125.

47. Wainner RS, Gill H. Diagnosis and nonoperative management of cervical radiculopathy. J. Orthop Sports Phys Ther 2000;30(12):728–744.

48. Waldvogel FA, Vasesy H. Osteomyelitis: The pase decade. N Engl J Med 1980;303(7):360–370.

49. Weinstein JN, McLain RF. Primary tumors of the spine. Spine 1987;12:843–851.

50. Wiesel SW, Tsourmas N, Feffer HL, Citrin CM, Patronas N. A study of computer assisted tomography. I. The incidence of positive CAT scans in an asymptomatic group of patients. Spine 1984;9:549–551.

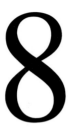

8

Outcome Assessment

Steven Yeomans, Craig Liebenson,
Jennifer Bolton, and Howard Vernon

Learning Objectives
After reading this chapter you should be able to understand:

- How to evaluate if outcome tools meet the minimum criteria for effective measurement instruments by possessing good validity, reliability, responsiveness, and practicality
- How to choose which outcomes to measure based on the needs of your practice
- How to administer and score simple questionnaires for many of the major domains of outcome assessment

Introduction

Outcomes assessment (OA) is essential in modern health care to assure quality and contain costs. It typically starts on the first visit with the establishment of baselines, and thus is an aid in goal setting. OA tools should be simple to administer and inexpensive, as well as being reliable, valid, and responsive. By utilizing them, health care providers (HCPs) can document patient status and progress over time, and thus enhance the quality of their decision-making by having the most accurate information regarding health status readily available.

OA is a component in promoting quality without sacrificing cost. Frymoyer defined value as the ratio of quality to cost (53). Cost containment has been a major focus of managed health care, but without quality assurance it may lead to dissatisfaction of health care consumers. In a patient-centered paradigm, the primary goals of care are pain reduction, functional restoration (i.e., prevention of disability), and avoidance of psychosocial distress.

How are these goals achieved? First, by keeping the focus of care on reducing disability or activity limitations/intolerances such as in walking, sitting, standing, etc. (79). Second, by addressing "yellow flags" barriers to recovery (26,44,72,123). And third, by utilizing quantifiable OA tools to establish baselines, document progress, assist in goal setting, and motivate patients. OA allows the value of the health care encounter to be audited. OA benefits all the players in the health care system—the patient, HCP, employer/government, and payer.

At the present time, it appears that health care has shifted to a customer-driven market (185). Health care "customers" now include patients, employers, unions, government, managed care organizations, and insurance companies (45,63). These customers want choice, value, and data to help them in their decisions (45, 104). Future competencies of HCPs likely will depend on their ability to work with these new information systems. Hansen explains, "The methods of outcomes assessment, even in their currently evolving form may help provide tools clinicians can use to learn to focus on important attributes of care that not only meet accountability demands, but enhances efficiency, quality and patient satisfaction" (64).

What Outcomes?

Traditional medical care has emphasized "objective" measures such as imaging and laboratory modalities. However, multifactorial conditions such as lower back pain are best explained by a biopsychosocial model of illness rather than a biomedical one of disease. This necessitates that "subjective" measures of pain, distress, and perception of functional abilities (i.e., disability) also be utilized (11,12,17,86).

In the spine care field in which patient dissatisfaction with care runs high, measuring outcomes that matter to the patients themselves is of paramount importance (11). Patient-centered outcomes include pain severity, distress, and ability to perform common activities of daily living (disability). Interestingly, the "objective" tests such as imaging, laboratory tests, and physical impairments (muscle strength and range of motion) correlate poorly with self-reported symptoms and functional status (i.e., disability) (1,106,171). Thus, patient-centered outcomes derived from self-administered questionnaires have achieved a surprisingly high level of significance (73,103,135,158).

Because of the multidimensionality of the biopsychosocial model, a broad spectrum of outcomes can be potentially measured. Deyo et al and Bombardier have listed the following domains as most relevant to a patient's clinical status—pain, disability, well-being, work status, and satisfaction (23,43). Psychosocial status, especially fear–avoidance beliefs, is another relevant area to document (92,101,102,123).

Criteria Regarding Outcomes Assessment

An effective outcome measure should be valid, reliable, responsive to clinical change, and practical (18–20,60,93). Ironically, the so-called subjective measures have been shown to be more psychometrically valid than the so-called objective measures. Many of the latter, such as muscle strength and mobility, are vulnerable to submaximal effort and impairment exaggeration (50,51,131) (see Chapters 11 and 12).

About Statistical Measures

<u>Pearson's</u> <u>Correlation</u> <u>Coefficient</u>: This is the degree to which two different tests are correlated. It is designated as a Pearson r value. The range is +1.0 (perfect positive or direct correlation) to –1.0 (perfect negative or inverse correlation). Values between 0.5 and –0.5 are considered of questionable reliability.

<u>Intra-Class</u> <u>Correlation</u> <u>Coefficient</u> <u>(ICC)</u>: The ICC is used to study the consistency and agreement between two or more examiners or ratings. It is calculated with repeated measures of analysis of variance (ANOVA). ICCs range from 0 to 1, with 1 representing the highest agreement. Scores more than 0.75 are considered good to excellent and those less than 0.50 are generally considered poor.

(continued)

About Statistical Measures (*Continued*)

<u>Cronbach's Alpha</u>: This measure is used to determine the degree of correlation between different items in a questionnaire. It is a measure of internal consistency. If all of the items of a particular questionnaire correlate very highly, then any one of them predicts the results of the others and, therefore, some of the items may be redundant. Researchers like to see the results of Cronbach alpha of at least 0.5. A value of 0.8 is considered good and a value of 0.9 is excellent. The higher the coefficient, the greater the likelihood that all the questions in the calculation are related to each other and therefore are measuring a similar underlying concept.

***p* value:** This is a standard measure of the probability that the results of a statistical test are caused by chance. Typical *p* values of 0.05 or 0.01 mean that the results of the statistical test have a 95% or 99% probability, respectively, of not having occurred by chance. Thus, the smaller the *p* value, the less likely the effect is a chance event, and the more likely it is an actual effect.

<u>Confidence intervals (CIs)</u>: Confidence intervals are normally given as either the 90% CIs or the 95% CIs. The 90% CIs of A to B means that there is a 90% probability that the actual mean value (for example) lies between the values of A and B. A 95% confidence interval means that the actual value of the test lies within that interval 19 times out of 20.

Validity

Validity refers to the ability of an outcome measurement (OM) to accurately quantify what it purports to measure.

Face validity: The extent to which a test appears to measure a purported construct.

Content validity: The extent to which the OM incorporates all relevant features of the domain in question.

Criterion validity: Generally refers to a comparison of a measure against some sort of "gold standard," or criterion measure. There are no gold standards for health status measures because health is a latent (or non-observable) trait, so one can never quantify it with certainty. In such a case, validity is established by testing a construct.

Construct validity: The extent to which the measurement corresponds to theoretical concepts (constructs) concerning how the phenomenon under study is expected to react (151).

Concurrent validity: The comparison of two measures completed at the same time. There are two subtypes: (i) convergent: the expectation that the scores between two related variables will be correlated. In other words, the scores of the two measures will increase (or decrease) together; and (ii) divergent or discriminative: this is tested when two or more variables that measure something totally unrelated are studied. Good discriminative validity is shown if two unrelated measures do not correlate with one another. For example, if anxiety is independent of intelligence, then we should not find a strong correlation between the two (151).

Predictive validity: The ability of a test to predict a future event/state (i.e., readmission rates to a hospital).

Reliability

Reliability is the amount of error associated with a measurement. It is defined as "the degree of stability exhibited when a measurement is repeated under identical conditions" (99). Thus, if a reliable measure is used, any change that occurs over time is caused by an actual change in patient status.

Test–retest reliability: demonstrated when repeated test scores on an individual whose health status is unchanged gives the same result. This is a measure of an instrument's standard error of measurement (SEM) (61).

Interobserver reliability: reflects the consistency of measurement application when different observers measure the same phenomenon.

Intraobserver reliability: a specific type of test–retest reliability in which the degree of consistency within the same examiner is evaluated.

Responsiveness

Responsiveness is defined as "the accurate detection of change when it has occurred" (37). If a tool is responsive to change, the score on a questionnaire should improve as a person's health status improves. This is clinically significant change that is not caused by a random occurrence. Responsiveness is essential when an OA tool is used by an HCP to show clinical improvement in health status as a result of care over time.

Minimal clinically important difference: The change score that maximizes the accurate classification of those patients who change (improved) an important amount from those who do not.

How Is the Minimal Clinically Important Change in an Outcome Determined?

A key dimension of responsiveness is the minimal clinically important change in an outcome in a specific patient population (48,81). This is the smallest change in the OA score that the patient perceives as beneficial. A patient's own global impression of change (PGIC) (improvement/deterioration) is the most commonly used external criterion to compare the outcome against (48,61) (see appendix form 1).

PGIC scores are calculated on the basis of the patients own perception of change with care. A PGIC may ask if the patient is very much improved, much improved, slightly improved, unchanged, or worse with care (48,61). The PGIC for improvement has been defined by subtracting the mean OA score of "unchanged" from "much improved" or "very much improved" (48,61). The PGIC for deterioration has been defined by the subtracting the mean OA score of "unchanged" from "worse" (61).

Another common way responsiveness is determined is by the effect size. This is the size of an effect from a treatment intervention (156). It is determined from a comparison of different instruments measuring the same thing. The larger the effect size, the greater the treatment effect (signal) as related to the variability (noise) in the sample. An effect size of 0.2 is small, 0.5 is moderate, and 0.8 or more is large.

Different methods are used to calculate effect size. They each use a ratio with the same numerator of the mean pretreatment score minus post-treatment score across the study population. The denominator is usually the range of scores or standard deviation of the entire group.

In individuals who classify themselves as having improved greatly, a responsive instrument should have a large effect size. Whereas in individuals who classify themselves as not improving, the effect size should be small. Thus, it would be expected that in chronic patients (who are less likely to show improvement) an instruments effect size would be much smaller than in acute patients (who are more likely to show improvement).

Another way of determining when meaningful change in an outcome instrument has occurred is from the minimal detectable change (MDC). This is the amount of error associated with a multiple measures on stable patients (expressed in the same units

as a measure). For a change to be significant, it must be equal to or greater than the MDC.

Ceiling and Floor Effects

A ceiling effect occurs when a respondent begins at a high level of function and therefore if they improve, the instrument cannot accurately detect this improvement. An example would be an athlete. A floor effect occurs when a respondent begins at a low level of function and further deterioration in function cannot be detected by the measure. An example is a frail or postoperative person. Ceiling or floor effects are caused by the inability of the instrument to discriminate at the higher or lower end of the dimension being measured. The impact of ceiling and floor effects is that clinically important change will not be measured or detected.

Practicality

An outcome tool should be simple to administer and understand, time-efficient, and easy to score and interpret. Disability questionnaires should have wording that is simple and unambiguous so that patients will easily be able to complete the entire form. Scoring should be possible with a simple computer program that shows a percent improvement over time. "Yes" and "no" responses are ideal for research questionnaires because they are easier to administer with telephonic follow-up. However, HCPs may prefer forms with 0-to-10 visual analog scales that give patients more options for their answers. A practical tool is time- and cost-efficient as well as valid, reliable, and responsive.

Domains

There are two broad categories into which OA tools can be assigned, subjective and objective (184). Subjective OA tools are patient-driven, whereas objective measures are driven by the HCP. This chapter discusses the subjective OA tools and the objective tools are discussed in chapters 11 to 13. There are several outcomes assessment tools included in the appendix to this chapter. When available, the MDC score is reported.

There have been several classifications of the various domains or groups of OA tools (184). Bombardier describes a core set of measures that should be considered when managing patients with spinal disorders—pain, generic health status, disability or functional status, work status, and patient satisfaction (Table 8.1) (23). Psychological distress is a sixth domain that should also be addressed.

Table 8.1 An Example of Recommended Outcomes Assessment Tools for Low Back Pain Patients

Domain	Instrument	Number of items	Score (best to worst)	Time to complete
Pain	NRS	1 item	0–10; clinically meaningful change = 30%	<1 minute
Generic health status (including well-being)	Single self-rated health question	1	0–10	<1 minute
Function/ disability	PSFS or Oswestry	3 10 (6 levels)	0–30 0–100	1 minute 3–5 minutes
Work status	Time off work	1	Number of days	<1 minute
Satisfaction	Satisfaction with care	10	1–5	2–3 minutes

Pain

In the assessment of pain, there are several measures to consider, including the pain severity, pain affect, pain location, and pain persistence (chronicity). The severity of pain is related to how much a person hurts, whereas pain affect measures the mental or emotional component of pain. When assessing pain severity for chronic and recurrent pain conditions, assessing the pain severity during a specified time period such as 1 week, 1 month, 6 months, etc., may be more important than reporting the pain status at a particular point of time (169). Von Korff describes key parameters of pain status based on a retrospective report to include: (a) the number of days pain is experienced during a specified time frame; (b) the average or usual pain intensity when in pain; (c) average interference with activities; and (d) the cumulative number of activity limitation days caused by pain (168).

Pain Severity/Intensity

Measuring pain intensity can be accomplished using verbal rating scales, visual analog scales (VAS), and/or numerical rating scales (NRS). Von Korff concludes that "... 0–10 NRSs have many advantages over the alternatives for clinical use and for research in clinical populations in which a simple and robust measurement method is needed" (169). Hence, a 0-to-10 NRS anchored by "no pain" at the "0" end and "extreme pain" at the "10" end (or vice versa) is a commonly used and practical approach.

A VAS of current pain has been shown to be less responsive than a rating of pain over the past 24 hours, week, or 2 weeks (20,54,85,139). Therefore, when asking a patient to rate pain, the usual or average

pain level may be the best choice when limiting the number of questions asked regarding pain intensity to one. The report of average pain intensity has been found to correlate with a 3-month daily pain diary in a number of studies (82,84,141). These validity studies support using measures of average or usual pain intensity for up to a 3-month recall period with acceptable discrimination. An example of a simple 0-to-10 NRS for pain intensity using the "usual," "typical," or "average" is depicted in Figure 8.1.

What is the Minimum Amount of Change in Pain Severity/Intensity that Is Clinically Significant?

Farra and colleagues demonstrated in patients with scores of at least 4 out of 10 that an improvement of 2 points or 30% was shown be a clinically meaningful improvement (48). This equates to the patient's own global impression of change (PGIC) of "much improved." A 50% improvement was shown to correspond to a PGIC of "very much improved." In those with scores less than 4 out of 10, an improvement of only 0.5 points indicated clinically meaningful improvement. Therefore, using percent improvement rather than numerical or "raw" scores is recommended. If the pain severity score at baseline has wide variability, such as including subjects with scores less than 4 out of 10, the raw change will not correlate with the PGIC, but the percent change will!

Clinically Meaningful Change in VAS or NRS

- 30% improvement = PGIC of "much improved"
- 50% improvement = PGIC of "very much improved"

What is your TYPICAL or AVERAGE pain?

0	1	2	3	4	5	6	7	8	9	10
no										Worst
pain										pain
										possible

Figure 8.1 The numerical rating scale (NRS) using the pain intensity at usual, typical, or average.

Hagg and colleagues found a change of 18 to 19 out of 100 in the VAS of chronic low back pain patients to be clinically significant (61). Turner studied the correlation of pain with disability (160). If the initial VAS was 5 or more, a change of at least 2 points was needed to influence disability scores significantly. If the initial VAS score was less than 5, then a VAS change of at least 1 point would have a clinically relevant effect on functioning.

Pain Affect

Pain intensity may be defined as the amount a person hurts, whereas pain affect can be defined as the emotional arousal and disruption created by the pain experience (49,56,117,127,169). The McGill Pain Questionnaire (MPQ) (113,114) includes 20 category scales of verbal pain descriptors categorized in order of severity and clustered into four subscales:

- Sensory discrimination
- Affective
- Evaluative
- Miscellaneous

A detailed description for scoring this instrument is described elsewhere (184).

Pain Diagrams

The pain diagram or drawing is perhaps the best way to obtain the patient's perception of the location of their symptom (94,128,184). Improvement or exacerbation can quickly be determined by comparing current to previously completed pain diagrams. Pain diagrams enhance the HCP's ability to differentiate between a mechanical low back, nerve root, and psychogenic problem (Fig. 8.2).

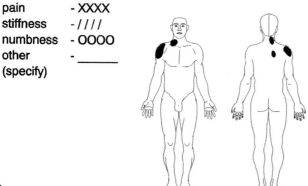

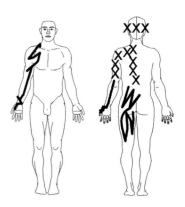

Figure 8.2 Pain diagram. **(A)** Example of a well-delineated, anatomically correct depiction. **(B)** Example of a poorly delineated, anatomically incorrect, exaggerated depiction.

Abnormal illness behavior or somatization is suggested if the pain diagram shows multiple types of pain qualities (achy, stabbing, burning, numbness, pins and needles, etc.) in all four extremities and the trunk, and/or if markings outside of the body such as lightening bolts are present. This can then be correlated with other subjective information such as psychometric "yellow flags" that include poor coping strategies, depression, and anxiety, as well as objective tools such as the Waddell Non-Organic Low Back Pain signs (see Chapter 9).

Though the pain drawing is usually used qualitatively, there are several validated methods for scoring pain drawings (119,120,155,161). The scoring procedure is usually accomplished by overlapping the patient's pain drawing with a transparency that includes the same drawing but with grid lines and adding up points based on the number of body regions/extremities marked and quantity of pain quality markings used.

Summary

The NRS and pain diagram have the greatest utility for the typical practitioner.

General Health

Patient-based general health outcome measures can be classified into two general categories: generic and disease or condition-specific measures (95,98). Generic measures include global ratings of health status and multidimensional measures of health-related quality of life, which include the Sickness Impact Profile (SIP) (9,10), SF-36 Health Survey (172), Nottingham Health Profile (NHP) (78), Dartmouth COOP Health Charts (118), and others. The strength of generic measures of general health is that these are not specific to any one condition or disease and, therefore, are applicable across populations regardless of their health status. However, this is also a weakness because they are not as responsive to change over time compared to condition-specific tools (184). An example of a highly responsive condition-specific version of the SIP general health questionnaire is the Roland-Morris questionnaire.

The SF-36 is a popular generic outcome tool that has been used in outcomes-based research has been translated into more than 40 languages as part of the International Quality of Life Assessment (IQOLA), and it is often utilized in clinical settings (25,176). The strength of the SF-36 lies in the fact that normative data exist for healthy and non-healthy populations (69,70). Both versions 1.0 and 2.0 are divided into eight scales representing different aspects of general health (172–174). Utilizing the eight individual scales, version 2.0 yields two composite scores, which include mental health and physical health. Table 8.2 lists the eight scale titles, the number of items or questions that are used to compute the

Table 8.2 The SF-36 Subscales

Scale (SF-36 scale titles in parentheses when different)	N of Items	Scale Items	Minimum N of Items Needed to Compute a Score
Health perception (general health)*	5	1, 33, 34, 35, 36	3
Physical functioning*	10	3, 4, 5, 6, 7, 8, 9, 10, 11, 12	5
Role limitations caused by physical health*	4	13, 14, 15, 16	2
Role limitations caused by emotional problems**	3	17, 18, 19	2
Social functioning**	2	20, 32	1
Mental health**	5	24, 25, 26, 28, 30	3
Bodily pain*	2	21, 22	1
Energy/fatigue (vitality)**	4	23, 27, 29, 31	2

*Four scales used to calculate the physical component.
**Four scales used to calculate the mental component.
Modified from Yeomans. The Clinical Application of Outcomes Assessment. McGraw-Hill, 2000.

score, the specific scale items, and the minimum number of items needed to compute a score.

The physical component summary (PCS) is made up of the following four scales: Physical Function, Role Physical, Bodily Pain, and General Health. The Mental Health component (MHC) is made up of Mental Health, Role Emotional, Social Function, and Vitality. The advantage of grouping all 36 questions into two rather than eight scales results in an improvement in the reliability. The mean score for a healthy adult population regarding both scales is 50 ± 10 points, which carries a reliability level of 0.92 and 0.88 for the PCS and the MHC, respectively.

The SF-36 has generally been shown to be a responsive instrument for measuring clinically meaningful change in low back pain and sciatica individuals in certain studies (121,156), whereas in others it has not (138). Even in the Taylor et al study in which it was found to be responsive, it was not as good as the Oswestry Disability Index (156). The scales with the greatest responsiveness were Physical Function, Bodily Pain, and Social Function (156). In fact, the Physical Function scale was more sensitive to change than the Oswestry Disability Index (156).

The SF-12 is an abbreviated version derived from the SF-36 that was designed to improve the practicality and utility of the longer 36-item version introduced (175). The SF-36 can also be utilized to form two distinct scales, the physical function and mental health scales. The advantage of the SF-12 over the SF-36 is the length of time needed to complete the form is only 2 to 5 minutes. Standard and acute versions of the SF-12 and 36 are available in multiple languages (176).

correlate very well with functional limitations (i.e., disability) or participation. Whereas clinical decisions are frequently guided by tests of specific dysfunction or impairments, it is important to realize that patient's goals are oriented toward general dysfunctions, functional limitations, or disability.

Low Back Pain

Oswestry Disability Index The Oswestry Disability Index (ODI) was developed from studying low back pain (LBP) patients attending hospital outpatient departments. Since Fairbank presented the original version in 1980, various revisions have been published, including the original author's updated version, version 2.0, as well as others (47,52,133).

One of these, the Revised ODI, published by Hudson-Cook et al. (77), was an attempt to enhance the sensitivity of the ODI for patients with less disabling LBP than those receiving hospital treatment (in other words, lower the floor of the instrument). A similar goal was sought by Fritz et al. in their revised ODI (52). Test–retest reliability, responsiveness, and construct validity were obtained and found superior when compared to the Quebec Back Pain Disability Scale.

The utility of the ODI is enhanced by the fact that it has been translated into a number of languages (47,133). It has been shown to be responsive to clinically meaningful change (11,88,105,110,133,156). The mean baseline scores for this instrument in different populations are shown in Table 8.3.

Summary

If the clinician is planning to assess other outcome domains, it may be more practical to use the SF-12 instead of the SF-36 for measuring general health status. If time is still deemed excessive, a single question about self-perceived health can be utilized as has been used in "yellow flags" questionnaires (157) (see Chapter 9).

Region-Specific Functional Disability Outcomes

Disability is defined as the ability of a person to perform common activities of daily living (ADL) (13). Thus, disability is an outcome of paramount importance in charting the progress of a patient undergoing treatment. The International Classification of Disabilities and Health has contrasted disability with impairment (79,182). Impairments such as range of motion or strength, although objective, do not always

---

What Is the Minimum Amount of Change in the Revised ODI that Is Clinically Significant?

- 8% (110)
- 10% (61)
- 12% (52)
- 16.3% (156)

How to Score the Revised ODI

It consists of 10 sections, each covering a different activity of daily living (for example, personal care, lifting, walking, and social life) and a 6-point rating scale for each section (from 0 to 5), which the patient uses to rate his or her ability to function (see appendix form 2). The disability score is obtained by adding the scores of each of the sections (maximum score 50), which is usually converted to a percentage. If one section is missed or not applicable, the score is calculated as a percentage from the remaining total possible score (e.g., 45) (see appendix form 2).

Table 8.3 How Does the Mean Baseline ODI Score Vary in Different Patient and Asymptomatic Groups (19,46,47,77)

- Asymptomatic individuals—10% (SD ± 2–12)
- Hospital outpatient patients—22%
- Chiropractic patients—27% (revised ODI 36%–47%)
- Mixed LBP—27% (SD ± 6–24)
- Chronic LBP—43% (SD ± 10–21)
- Sciatica—45% (SD ± 10–30)
- Orthopedic surgical patients—47%

Roland-Morris Disability Questionnaire The Roland-Morris Disability Questionnaire (RDQ) is a modification of the SIP with 24 items most relevant to LBP patients. Each of the 24 questions refers to the perceived effect of back pain on a particular daily activity and requires a simple yes or no answer. As with the ODI, the RDQ has been subjected to considerable psychometric testing over the years and shown to be reliable and valid (39,133). Shortened versions of the RDQ containing 18 and 11 items, respectively, have been shown to have good reliability and validity criteria (145,152). Responsiveness was compared to the SIP's physical subscales and were found to be similar (40,83) and others have also reported data on responsiveness (12,96,121,130,144,146,149,153).

What Is the Minimum Amount of Change in the RDQ that Is Clinically Significant?

- 2.5 to 5 points (12)

- 2 to 4 points (24,121,133)

- 1 to 2 points in those with little disability (114)

- 7 to 8 points in those with high levels of disability (146)

- 5 points in a mixed population (146)

- 4 to 5 points in acute and subacute LBP patients in an outpatient setting (144)

How to Score the RDQ

The score is a simple addition of the number of affirmative replies (maximum score 24). If a question is not answered, then only those responses answered are used to determine the percent (see appendix form 3).

Comparison of the Oswestry Disability Index and the Roland-Morris Disability Questionnaire The ODI has been directly compared with the RDQ in a number of studies (5,75,100,133,142). It has generally been found that the ODI tends to score higher than the RDQ. For this reason, the ODI may be better in detecting change in more severely disabled patients, whereas the RDQ is more sensitive in detecting change in less disabled patients. However, the Revised ODI was found to be more sensitive than the original ODI (75,77).

The questionnaires do address different aspects of daily functions, with the Revised ODI covering only approximately half of the functional categories of the RDQ. An interesting and unexpected finding from the study by Stratford et al. (142) was the frequency of blank and multiple response items associated with the ODI. This may be because of the fact that ODI uses a multiple choice format, whereas the RDQ has a more direct yes/no format. Other factors that may influence a decision to using one over the other include translation availability (either tool), telephonic administration necessary for long-term follow-up needed in research (favors the RDQ), ceiling effects (favors the ODI), whereas floor effects favor the RDQ. Fairbank and Roland suggest using the ODI in patients with persistent severe disability and the RDQ in those with relatively little disability (133). Studies regarding test–retest reliability and internal consistency show high correlation between the two (5,33,96).

The layout of the ODI more clearly depicts each activity of daily living in 10 clear-cut sections and therefore can be utilized as a goal-setting tool by the health care provider easier than the RDQ. When comparing patients who had reached their treatment goals versus those who did not, a corresponding significant change (improvement) versus lack of change in the ODI and RDQ score was noted, respectively, as noted in Table 8.4 (12,100,142).

Although the RDQ and ODI (or Revised ODI) are considered "gold standards" for functional measurement in LBP patients there are other validated tools available, as noted in Table 8.5.

Spinal Function Sort The Performance Assessment and Capacity Testing Spinal Function Sort (SFS), authored and developed by Leonard N. Matheson, PhD, and Mary L. Matheson, MS (1991), measures a patient's perception of his or her capacity to perform 50 different activities of daily living shown in picture form (108,116). These represent the positions or activities defined in the Dictionary of Occupational Titles (DOT). A total score referred to as the rating of perceived capacity (RPC) is calculated and reliability checks are made to determine internal consistency and effort. The score is compared to a chart listing the physical demand characteristics of work developed by the United Stated Department of Labor. Tasks that are utilized at work are identified and work-related lift/carry capacities are determined.

Table 8.4 The Mean Scores of the ODI and RDQ in Different Patient Populations

Study	RDQ	ODI
Patients recruited to trial, less than 3 out of 10 pain, no radiculopathy (100) (mean, range, and standard deviation)	10.9, 0–22, 4.7	33.0, 4–70, 14.7
EMG evidence of radiculopathy (100) (Canada) (mean, range, and standard deviation)	14.2, 0–24, 5.2	49.1, 6–86, 17.1
Patients referred to a physical therapist (142)	Pre-PT 11.8 ± 6.2 4 weeks: 7.1 ± 5.7	Pre-PT 40.5 ± 17.8 4 weeks: 24.4 ± 15.5
Patients with nonspecific LBP for >6 weeks (12)	Baseline: 12.1 5 weeks: 7.5 improved 12.1–4.3 unimproved: 11.8–10.6	Baseline: 27.6 5 weeks: 21.9 improved 26.2–14.3 unimproved: 29.1–29.5

Modified from Table 3 of Roland M and Fairbank J. Roland-Morris Disability Questionnaire and Oswestry Disability Questionnaire. Spine 2000;25:3115–3124.

Several important items are derived from this evaluation. These include:

- A score of RPC
- The RPC score categorizes the patient into one of the five physical demand characteristics (PDC) work levels (sedentary to heavy)
- A perceived maximum lift/carry
- Internal reliability is checked when the scores of similar tasks are compared
- The RPC score is compared to normative data collected on working and disabled/unemployed males and females
- The physical demand characteristics level that the RPC score places the patient is then compared to a Job Demands Questionnaire (which describes the demands of their

current job). This comparison allows the HCP to determine if the patient is capable of returning to their "normal" duty or current job versus to a more limiting PDC work level.

- Work-related duties are circled so that tolerance to specific work activities can be appreciated and separated from non-occupational duties. This can also be used to institute work-specific exercise protocols or work simulation in a rehabilitation setting.

The practicality and utility of the SFS is excellent because it takes only 5 to 7 minutes for the patient to complete and approximately 5 to 10 minutes to calculate the score, interpret the results of maximum lift/carry, and compare it to their current work demands (Job Demands Questionnaire) and to the normative data. Though the intention of the SFS is

Table 8.5 Other Validated Lumbar Spine Assessment Tools

Quebec Back Pain Disability Scale (QBPDS) (96,97)	Spinal Stenosis Questionnaire (SSQ) (153,154)
North American Spine Society Lumbar Spine Questionnaire (NASS-LSQ) (36)	Million Visual Analogue Scale (MVAS) (115)
Curtin Back Screening Questionnaire (CBSQ) (65)	Waddell Disability Index (WDI) (170)
Activities Discomfort Scale (ADS) (159)	Resumption of Activities of Daily Living Scale (RADL) (181)
Low-Back Outcome Score (LBOS) (58)	Clinical Back Pain Questionnaire (CBPQ) (138)

not to function as an OA tool, the RPC scores improve (increase) as the patient's disability decreases.

Neck Pain

Neck Disability Index The Neck Disability Index (NDI) (162) was designed using the ODI as a template. This instrument was initially studied using a sample of 17 consecutive whiplash-injured patients and showed good statistical significance (Pearson r = 0.89, $p \leq$ 0.05). The alpha coefficients were calculated from a pool of questionnaires completed by 52 patients resulting in all items having individual alpha scores more than 0.75 and a total index alpha of 0.80. Concurrent validity was reported with moderate correlations when assessed in two different ways (0.60 and 0.69–0.70). It has been studied in individuals with work-related neck pain as well (164).

More recently, Hains et al. (62) studied seven modified versions of the NDI against the original NDI and confirmed the validity of the original NDI items. The item presentation revealed a strong correlation with internal consistency reported at 0.92 (Cronbach alpha).

The NDI was utilized in monitoring the outcome of patients with whiplash-associated disorders (WAD) (165). The NDI favorably compared to other neck pain and disability self-report tools in a group of WAD patients (166,167). In this study, the NDI, Neck Pain Questionnaire, and the Copenhagen Neck Functional Disability Index were compared for assessing pain, impairment, and disability. The results of the study revealed numerous similarities in content and format and equally good basic psychometric efficacy. The NDI was found to be more extensively studied and, therefore, was the recommended tool for use in research settings.

Vernon et al. (163) compared WAD patients with three or more Waddell non-organic signs (NOS) versus those without and found that the mean scores of the NDI was over double for the high NOS group (17.6 ± 9.1 verses 36 ± 3.7). Additionally, it was found that strength was lower in the high NOS group.

Stratford et al. (147) evaluated the use of the NDI when evaluating individual patients. They reported on 49 initial and 48 follow-up patients using the standard error of measurement (SEM) and also applied this to 15 stable patients. Three primary questions were asked:

1) What is the variability for an obtained score value?

2) What is the minimal detectable change (MDC)?

3) What is a clinically important change?

After analysis, a 5-point change was reported as clinically important change with an internal consistency of 0.87 and test–retest reliability of 0.94. The SEM was estimated at 2.7 NDI points (95% confidence interval = 2.7 × 95% = ± 4.5points) (see appendix form 3). A typical range for patient scores on the NDI are reported to be between 35% and 39% (147,162).

> ### What Is the Minimum Amount of Change in the NDI that Is Clinically Significant?
>
> • 10% or 5 points out of 50 (115,129)
>
> #### How to Score the NDI
>
> Like the ODI it consists of 10 sections, each covering a different activity of daily living (for example, driving, and sitting), and a 6-point rating scale for each section (from 0 to 5), which the patient uses to rate his or her ability to functions. The disability score is obtained by adding the scores of each of the sections (maximum score 50), which is usually converted to a percentage (see appendix form 4).

Other Forms The Copenhagen Neck Functional Disability Scale has been found to have very good reliability, responsiveness, validity, and practicality (90). The Cronbach alpha coefficient for internal consistency was 0.9 for the entire scale, and the coefficients for individual items were all more than 0.88. Disability scale scores correlated strongly to pain scores as well as to doctor and patient global assessments, indicating good construct validity. Relative changes in disability scores demonstrated a moderately strong correlation to changes in pain scores after treatment. Another validated form is the Neck Pain and Disability Scale (179).

A Whiplash-Specific Disability Measure has recently been published (124). It was shown to have no significant floor or ceiling effects and high internal consistency (Cronbach alpha = 0.96). It covers items relevant to whiplash patients that are absent in the NDI such as emotional health, social activity, and fatigue (see appendix form 4).

Upper Extremity

The Shoulder

The Croft Index This questionnaire has good construct validity in that it is able to discriminate between those with shoulder pain of severity sufficient to make them seek health care versus those who did not (35). It has also been shown to discriminate between those with disabling shoulder pain and those with no disability (125). It has good concurrent validity because of its moderate correlation with the SPADI instrument (r = 0.79) (57). Its test–retest reliability is high (ICC 0.95) (57). A clinically significant change would require a change of 3 points to represent a change greater than the error associated with the instrument 95% of the time (57). It also has a high level of internal consistency (approximately 0.91) (57). However, the responsiveness of the tool is not yet assessed.

Shoulder Pain and Disability Index The Shoulder Pain and Disability Index (SPADI) covers the following domains: pain, mobility, and self-care. Test–retest reliability of the SPADI is very good in a surgical population (ICC = 0.91) and marginal in a primary care setting (ICC = 65, 95% confidence interval) (132,180). The internal consistency of the entire scale is very good (Cronbach alpha = 0.91), with the disability scale higher than pain scale (180). Its construct validity has been established in a variety of ways, including correlating it with the SIP (74) and SF-36 (7). The SPADI's responsiveness has also been established (74). The minimum amount of change that is clinically significant is 10% (57,74,180). Neither the SPADI nor Croft form correlates well with ROM (r = 0.24 to 0.56) (57).

Another popular questionnaire for use in this region is the Shoulder Evaluation Form (SEF). The SEF involves a 15-item activity of daily living questionnaire developed by the American Shoulder and Elbow Surgeons (6,136). The SEF was studied as a stand-alone instrument in the non-operative treatment of rotator cuff tears (68). It is not as well-studied as the other forms described.

The Wrist

The Carpal Tunnel Syndrome Questionnaire The Carpal Tunnel Syndrome Questionnaire (CTSQ) is a valid, reliable, self-administered outcome tool used with patients with carpal tunnel syndrome (4). The validity was tested against the SF36 and reliability (test–retest) was tested at 1 and 3 weeks. A strong internal consistency score of 0.8 to 0.95 (Cronbach alpha) was reported and the responsiveness ranged between 0.94 and 1.7.

Hand Function Sort The Hand Function Sort (HFS) is a patient self-report of their ability to perform 62 tasks involving a broad range of physical demands, including ADLs. The HFS has demonstrated construct validity by virtue of the HFS scores corresponding to impairment when the dominant hand was involved in the disability, but not if it was the non-dominant hand (107).

General Upper Quarter Function

Upper Extremity Function Scale The Upper Extremity Function Scale (UEFS) is an eight-item, self-

administered questionnaire used to measure the functional loss of upper extremity disorders (UEDs), including shoulder or elbow tendonitis or carpal tunnel syndrome (CTS) (126). This instrument was tested in two groups of patients in a prospective follow-up study using 108 patients with work-related UEDs and 165 patients with carpal tunnel syndrome (CTS). Good internal consistency (Cronbach alpha > 0.83), relative absence of floor effects, and excellent convergent and discriminant validity, compared with measures of symptom severity and clinical findings was reported. The UEFS was more responsive in the CTS group when compared to clinical measures such as grip and pinch strength.

What Is the Minimum Amount of Change in the UEFS that Is Clinically Significant?

- More than 15% (96)

How to Score the UEFS

Scoring of the questionnaire is simply the calculation of the sum of all responses. Not answering one response is allowed and is interpolated as the average of the other responses (see appendix form 5).

The Upper Extremity Functional Index (UEFI) The UEFI was designed as a single, all-purpose upper extremity functional outcome to cover patients with shoulder, elbow, wrist, or hand symptoms (150). It has good test–retest reliability (0.94). The standard error of measurement is 3.9. When compared to the UEFS, this form was found to have similar test–retest reliability and cross-sectional validity but better longitudinal validity. Longitudinal validity was determined by comparison with independent clinician impression of patient improvement.

What Is the Minimum Amount of Change in the UEFI that Is Clinically Significant?

- Nine scale points

How To Score The UEFI

Subjects check which answer best describes their abilities. There are 20 questions and scores range from 0 to 4 for each question, with the higher the score the less the dysfunction. The scoring range for the entire questionnaire is from 0 to 80, with 0 being the most dysfunction and 80 the least dysfunction (see appendix form 6).

The Lower Extremity

The Hip There are a number of hip outcome tools available for use (66,89,91,183,184). Some are designed with the objective of assessing pre- versus post-surgical hip arthroplasty function (184). A commonly used hip-related outcome tool in the United States is the Harris Hip Score (66). Many young active patients with activity-limiting hip pain require a modified outcome tool such as the Nonarthritic Hip Score (32). This form takes only approximately 5 minutes to complete. Its reproducibility, internal consistency, and validity have all been demonstrated (32). This is a modification of a general arthritis form called the Western Ontario and McMaster Universities Osteoarthritis Index (8).

The Knee

Functional Index Questionnaire (FIQ) A review of five methods of evaluating patellofemoral pain syndrome (PFPS) was conducted to investigate the psychometric properties of each tool (67). The five methods included the Functional Index Questionnaire (FIQ) (31); visual analogue scales for pain at worst, least, and usual; the Patellofemoral Function Scale (PFS) (129); a step test; and a subjective report of functional limitations. A sample of 56 patients with PFPS participated in a randomized clinical trial before treatment and 1 month after treatment. The Functional Index Questionnaire compared very favorably to the other measures and was concluded to be a practical easy-to-score tool with high utility for tracking the care of the knee-injured patient (67).

The FIQ was shown to have modest test–retest reliability and to have very good internal consistency of 0.85 before treatment and 0.88 after treatment (Cronbach alpha) (31). The FIQ was also found to be a good discriminator for measuring clinical change.

Other Questionnaires The Noyes and Lysholm Knee scoring questionnaires are commonly used in assessing the outcome of knee surgery in athletes (38). These questionnaires consist of activities of daily living consistent with knee function. The Lysholm Knee Rating Scale was also used along with the SF-36 in a study of 426 patients with knee impairment who were treated conservatively (87). The outcome after physical therapy revealed simultaneous improvements in the results obtained from both tools.

The International Knee Documentation Committee Subjective Knee Form is a relatively new but psychometrically robust outcome measure for health-related quality of life in knee patients (80). It has been shown to have very good test–retest reliability, internal consistency, convergent and discriminative validity, and responsiveness. However, it is a slightly longer form to complete than the FIQ.

Ankle A simple-to-administer 12-question form, The Ankle Joint Functional Assessment Tool (AJFAT), has been validated for assessing disability in ankle sprain patients (137). This is based on various validated knee outcome assessment tools (38,87). Ankle sprain patients' disability scores improve concurrently with impairment score improvements in balance ability (137).

General Lower Quarter Function

The Functional Assessment Scale (FAS) The FAS has been developed for assessing functional levels in the elderly with osteoarthritis of the knee(s) (177). It was devised from the mobility and physical activity components of the Arthritis Impact Measurement Scale (111), which has been shown to be reliable and valid (112).

The FAS has demonstrated internal consistency by being able to discriminate between an elderly group with osteoarthritis and one without it (Cronbach coefficient alpha = 0.83) (177). Arthritis sufferers' mean score was 13.0 (SD = 2.68), whereas a control groups mean score was 6.4 (SD = 1.35) out of maximum score of 25. The age range for the sample was 54 to 79 years. Age was not associated with functional score.

This form could also have utility for measuring functional status in any lower-quarter patient with marked functional limitations relating to standing, walking, stair-climbing, or those requiring aids such as a cane or crutches.

How to Score the FAS

Subjects circle the answer that best describes their abilities. There are five questions and scores range from 5 to 25 (for each scale, a = 1, b = 2, . . . f = 6). Higher scores indicate greater dysfunction (see appendix form 7).

The Lower Extremity Functional Scale (LEFS) The LEFS was designed as a single all-purpose lower extremity functional outcome to cover patients with joint replacement, patellofemoral disorders, arthritis, ankle sprain, joint instability, etc. (16). It has superior sensitivity to change in lower extremity patients than a general measure such as the SF-36 (16). The 90% confidence interval, or error, for a specific score is 6 scale points (16). Ninety percent of stable patients have an inherent variation of less than 9 scale points when tested on different occasions (16). Thus, the Minimal Detectable Change or Minimal Clinically Important Difference is 9 scale points (16). It is efficient to administer and score. An initial follow-up study validated this questionnaire on patients with lower functional levels—these were patients recovering from total hip or knee arthroplasties (149). A second follow-up study demonstrated the test–retest reliability, cross-sectional, and longitudinal validity of the LEFS on a more athletic population who had sustained an ankle sprain within the past 14 days (2). Because the LEFS was valid in highly disabled and high-performing individuals, this demonstrates both a strong "floor" and "ceiling" effect for this OA tool.

What Is the Minimum Amount of Change in the LEFS that Is Clinically Significant?

- 9 scale points (16)

How to Score the LEFS

Subjects check which answer best describes their abilities. There are 20 questions and scores range from 0 to 4 for each question, with the higher the score the less the dysfunction. The scoring range for the entire questionnaire is from 0 to 80, with 0 being the most dysfunction and 80 the least dysfunction (see appendix form 8).

Summary

A wide variety of region specific functional questionnaires are available that measure a patient's activity intolerances related to his or her chief symptom. Table 8.6 summarizes the author's recommendations for which forms to choose for which regions of the body.

Patient-Specific Functional Disability Outcome

Patient-Specific Functional Scale (PSFS)

The PSFS is an innovative OA tool that allows the patient to choose three activities they either are unable to perform or are having the most difficulty with as a result of their pain (27,143,148,178). The PSFS has been shown to be more responsive than other outcome tools or impairment tests (122).

Table 8.6 Recommended Outcome Forms

Any region—PSFS
Low back—Revised ODI, RDQ or Back BQ
Neck—NDI or Neck BQ
Upper Extremity—UEFI
Lower Extremity—LEFS

- PSFS effect size = 1.6
- Numerical pain scale effects size = 1.3
- RDQ effect size = 0.8
- Impairment evaluation (ROM) effect size = 0.1 to 0.6

What Is the Minimum Amount of Change in the PSFS that Is Clinically Significant?

- 3 scale points (178)

How to Score the PSFS

Subjects choose three activities that are giving them the most trouble. They then score them on a scale of 0 to 10, with 0 meaning "unable to perform activity" and 10 meaning "able to perform activity at pre-injury level" (see appendix form 9).

The PSFS was designed to be administered weekly. It is to measure progress (make ongoing clinical decisions) and outcome. It could be administered less often if slower change is expected.

The MDC of three is validated per item, rather than the average of all three items. Activities mentioned by patients are all of different levels of difficulty and averaging could mask potential improvement on one while others may change slower.

As an example, if a breast cancer patient has shoulder dysfunction, number one on her PSFS might be playing volleyball (not on most functional scales!), and combing her hair and washing floors are numbers two and three. Obviously, two and three will change faster and when number one increases to nine or 10 on the scale, it will likely mean that she is ready for discharge. The clinician should set short-term goals around the "easier" items with an "increased ability to play volleyball to more than eight out of 10" as a measurable long-term goal.

Summary

The PSFS is an excellent complement to the more well-known region specific functional disability scales.

Work Status

Many reasons exist for measuring work outcomes (71,109). Five that stand out include (3):

- To assess productivity loss in clinical trials
- To evaluate the effectiveness of health services

Table 8.7 Psychometrics of WL-26 Scales

Scales	Number of Items	Conbach Alpha	Scaling Success*
Work scheduling	6	0.88	100%
Physical demands	8	0.88	91%
Mental demands	4	0.92	94%
Social demands	3	0.08	92%
Output demands	5	0.90	95%

*Scaling success is the extent that an item correlates with the scale it is hypothesized to correlate with as opposed to another scale. A success rate greater than 90% is considered successful.
Reprinted with permission from Amick BC, et al. Spine 2000;25(24):3152–3160.

- To target injury and re-injury prevention programs
- To evaluate the effectiveness of work reorganization projects such as ergonomic changes
- To improve provider–worker and provider–safety engineer interaction

The Work Loss-26

The WL-26 is an example of a generic role-specific measure. Originally, it was designed for use in occupational illness and injury populations but has since been used in the clinical setting, especially those managing a variety of musculoskeletal disorders (Table 8.7).

The WL-26 scales can discriminate between workers with low or high hand–wrist symptom severity or upper extremity functioning. Also, construct validation is supported by emerging data on the relationship between work limitations and productivity. In general, when a worker's capacity to work is limited because of a condition, work performance is compromised. Amick et al. described a 20-point change in work limitations for Massachusetts workers with upper extremity musculoskeletal disorders as being associated with an additional 2.7 weeks of lost productivity (3).

Summary

The simplest measure by far of work status is the actual time off work. For most practitioners this may be the most practical outcome to obtain.

Patient Satisfaction Outcomes Assessment Tools

The fifth domain described by Deyo et al and Bombardier is patient satisfaction (23,43). This is an impor-

tant domain when assessing quality assurance issues (41). Table 8.8 represents a partial list of some of the patient satisfaction questionnaires available (15, 29,34).

By identifying the patient who is dissatisfied with care early on, realistic advice can be given to the patient, and frustration, disappointment, and even anger in patients who do not respond can be avoided (30). Deyo reported that most people treated for hypertension, cancer, and other serious medical diseases are satisfied with their care. However, 20% to 25% of patients presenting with back and neck pain for medical care are dissatisfied (42).

Symptom Satisfaction

Cherkin et al. (30) asked a novel question to a sample of 219 patients, "If you had to spend the rest of

Table 8.8 Examples of Various Patient Satisfaction Questionnaires

Test	Conditions Tested
1. Client Experience Survey	Patient satisfaction
2. Client Satisfaction Questionnaire	Patient satisfaction
3. Patient Experience Survey (PES)	Patient satisfaction
4. Chiropractic Satisfaction Questionnaire (34)	Patient satisfaction
5. Work APGAR (15)	Job satisfaction
6. Patient Satisfaction Subscales (29)	Patient satisfaction

your life with your <u>condition as it is right now,</u> how would you feel about it?". He found that at 1 week one-third were satisfied; at 3 weeks one-half were satisfied; at 7 weeks two-thirds were satisfied; and at 1 year 85% were satisfied.

In this sample, 82% of patients presented for their first visit of a recurrent low back pain episode in less than 3 weeks from the episode's onset.

Symptom Satisfaction Is a Novel and Highly Predictive Measure of Recovery

Cherkin showed that a patient's satisfaction with his or her current symptom status was as predictive of functional and symptomatic recovery as self-rated health, sciatica, and a history of frequent episodes of LBP (30). This can be determined with a single question—

"If you had to spend the rest of your life with your condition as it is right now, how would you feel about it?"

0   1   2   3   4   5   6   7   8   9   10

Delighted   Terrible

Job Satisfaction

Bigos and colleagues used the work APGAR in a longitudinal, prospective study of 3020 aircraft employees to identify risk factors for reporting acute back pain at work (15). At a 4-year follow-up point, 279 subjects reported back problems. Subjects who stated they "hardly ever" enjoyed their job tasks were 2.5-times more likely to report a back injury ($P = 0.0001$) compared to subjects who "almost always" enjoyed their job tasks. The authors conclude that ". . . a broader approach to the multifaceted problem of back complaints in industry helps explain why past prevention efforts focusing on purely physical factors have been unsuccessful."

The modified work APGAR is a seven-item tool derived initially from a family APGAR—a six-item family function questionnaire (55,140). Further modifications came based on findings from the retrospective analysis of the Boeing company work force (14), and two additional questions were added for this study (15), making the total number of questions to seven. A simple scoring method is based on the formula: Patient Score / Total Possible × 100 = % risk. Responses include "almost always," "some of the time," and "hardly ever" with points of 0, 1 and 2, respectively. A score of "0" represents no risk, whereas a maximum score of 14 ($7 \times 2 = 14$) divided by the highest possible score of 14 equals 1, multiplied by 100 equals 100%, which represents the highest risk possible.

The Patient Satisfaction Subscales (PSS)

The Patient Satisfaction Subscales (PSS) was designed for patients with lumbar spine problems (28,29,76). The PSS consists of 17 items, of which 10 are used that reflect three distinct dimensions of care: information (3 items), caring (4 items), and effectiveness (3 items). Table 8.9 includes the mean, standard deviation, and Cronbach alpha for each subscale. This tool was specifically recommended to be used in outpatient settings and because of its practicality of being short (10 items) and easy to score (76).

How to Score the Patient Satisfaction Subscales

Each of the three subscales are scored by calculating the mean of the items in each subscale. An overall total scale score is then obtained by adding the numerical value of the 10 subscale items (maximum score possible is 5 × 10 or, 50) (see appendix form 10).

Psychological Distress

Different questionnaires for evaluating psychosocial aspects of illness in back pain patients have been developed (92,101,102). Although there are numerous condition-specific questionnaires that measure pain and disability, most do not address affective or cognitive aspects of the pain experience (see also Chapter 9). It has been shown that utilizing a ques-

Table 8.9 Using a 305-Patient Sample, the Three Subscales of the PSS, and the Associated Mean, Standard Deviation and Chronbach Alpha Are Reported

PSS Subscales	Mean ± Standard Deviation	Cronbach alpha
Information	2.72 ± 0.92	0.75
Caring	2.09 ± 0.67	0.84
Effectiveness	2.59 ± 0.76	0.71
Overall score	NA	0.87

Reprinted with permission from Cherkin D, Deyo RA, Berg AO. Evaluation of a physician education intervention to improve primary care for low-back pain: II. Impact on patients. Spine 1991;16:1173–1178. NA, not available.

tionnaire for identifying psychosocial stress is more reliable than first impressions from a history (59).

The Back Bournemouth Questionnaire The Back Bournemouth Questionnaire (BQ) is a hybrid measuring instrument that consists of seven scales covering pain intensity, disability in activities of daily living and social life, anxiety, depression, fear–avoidance behavior, and locus of control (21). The back BQ has been shown to be valid, reliable, and responsive. The internal consistency (Cronbach alpha = 0.9) and test–retest reliability (ICC = 0.95) are very good (21). This is on the basis of two administrations in stable patients (n = 61), indicating strong agreement between total scores in these patients.

The back BQ has shown good construct validity because of its strong comparison to other outcome measures, especially the Revised ODI questionnaire (Pearson r = 0.78) (21). The back BQ is responsive to clinically significant change, as demonstrated by its high effect size. This was 1.29 for LBP, which was comparable to other established measures in the same study population such as the Revised ODI (1.07) (21). The effect size for the neck is 1.43 (22).

What Is the Minimum Amount of Change in the Back BQ that Is Clinically Significant?

Stable subjects were found to exhibit changes of between 2.6 and 4.5 points (or 3.7% to 6.4%) over time. Therefore, change scores more than 4.5 (6.4%) are indicative of real change beyond the variability in change scores in stable subjects who used this scale. The mean score before treatment in LBP subjects was 50.3 ± 18.8% (21).

How to Score the Back BQ

The individual items are summed to produce a total overall score. Because the seven dimensions each have a maximum score of 10, it is best to express the total score of the back BQ as a percentage (see appendix form 11).

The Neck Bournemouth Questionnaire The same seven core items used in the Back BQ are used in the Neck BQ. Some minor changes were made such as replacing activities like "walking," "climbing stairs," and "getting in/out of bed/chair" in the back BQ by activities "lifting," "reading," and "driving." The instrument demonstrated high internal consistency on 3 administrations (Cronbach alpha = 0.87, 0.91, 0.92) (22). The form demonstrated good reliability in test–retest administrations in stable subjects (ICC = 0.65) (22). The treatment effect size was found to be very good (1.43–1.67), contributing to its good

responsiveness (22). The effect size of the Neck BQ is considerably greater than for the NDI or Copenhagen scale (22).

Scoring of the Neck BQ is identical to the Back BQ (see appendix form 12).

■ CONCLUSION

Clinical Utility of OA Tools

OA tools can be used to establish mutually agreeable goals of care. If the NDI reveals that neck discomfort is greatest with driving, then improving this activity intolerance can be established as a primary goal of care. Utilizing OA tools helps to focus patients on functional goals such as reduction of activity intolerances so that symptom reduction is not the sole outcome of interest.

OA tools can be used on a weekly or monthly basis to review patient progress towards meaningful goals. If the ODI shows a prominent sitting or walking intolerance, then progress in these functional parameters can be monitored, discussed, and problem-solved on an ongoing basis. Such functional, outcome-based dialogues with the patient are an integral part of patient care. They allow clinician and patient to discuss if the patient has reached a key "decision point" in care such that a different treatment modality, diagnostic assessment, or referral is indicated. Such discussions are often necessary to avoid patient dissatisfaction with care that can arise when inappropriate expectations exist.

Outcome-based dialogues offer an opportunity to review mutually agreed on goals as well as the patient's prognosis and expected course of recovery. Functional outcomes allow for a discussion centered on expectations and achievements (61).

OA reports are invaluable for quantifiably demonstrating a patient's clinical status, improvement, or lack thereof. This is important for med-legal reporting, insurance review progress reports, or referral letters to other health care providers. The integrity of case management is preserved by utilizing reliable, valid, and responsive outcomes to measure a patient's progress over time.

All outcome, or evaluative, measures must be valid (measure what they purport to), reliable (reproducible in stable conditions), and responsive (able to detect clinically significant change in the status of the patient). Many outcome tools, although initially considered a burden by health care providers, are surprisingly simple to administer. They enhance doctor–patient communication and improve goal setting and decision-making.

Outcome measurements are essential to unmask ineffective treatments believed to be effective. If an outcome represents a mutually agreed on goal between provider and patient, then improvement in the outcome should demonstrate if treatment is successful. Regular re-evaluation with outcome measurements is thus important so that treatment that does not improve outcomes can be re-directed. Similarly, treatment that is effective but for which a provider is having difficulty justifying to a third party payer can now more easily be defended.

Audit Process
Self-Check of the Chapter's Learning Objectives

- What is the minimum amount of change that is clinically significant in the following OM tools— ODI, VAS or NRS, NDI, UEFS, LEFS, PSFS, and back/neck BQ?

- Do you know the mean scores in specific clinical populations for the OM questionnaires that you plan to use in your practice?

- How can measurement of activity intolerances such as with the ODI help establish realistic goals of care for a patient?

■ REFERENCES

1. Alaranta H, Hurri H, Heliovaara M, Soukka A, Harju R. Non-dynametric trunk performance tests: Reliability and normative data base. Scand J Rehab Med 1994;26:211–215.

2. Alcock GK, Stratford PW. Validation of the lower extremity functional scale on athletic subjects with ankle sprains. Physiotherapy Canada 2002;Fall: 233–240.

3. Amick III BC, Lerner D, Rogers WH, Rooney T, Katz JN. A review of health-related work outcome measures and their uses, and recommended measures. Spine 2000;25:3152–3160.

4. Atroshi I, Johnsson R, Sprinchorn A. Self-administered outcome instrument in carpal tunnel syndrome. Acta Orthop Scand 1998;69:82–88.

5. Baker D, Pynsent P, Fairbank J. The Oswestry Disability Index revisited. In: Roland M, Jenner J, eds. Back pain: New approaches to rehabilitation and education. Manchester, UK: Manchester University Press, 1989:174–186.

6. Barrett NWP, Franklin JL, Jackins SE, Wyss CR, Matsen FA. Total shoulder arthroplasty. J Bone Joint Surg 1987;69A:865–872.

7. Beaton DE, Richards RR. Measuring function of the shoulder. A cross-sectional comparison of five questionnaires. J Bone Joint Surg (Am) 1996;78(6): 882–890.

8. Bellamy N, Buchanoan WW, Goldsmith CH, Campbell J, Stitt LW. Validation study of WOMAC: A health status instrument for measuring clinically important patient relevant outcomes to antirheumatic drug therapy in patients with osteoarthritis of the hip or knee. J Rheumatol 1988;15:1833–1840.

9. Bergner M, Bobbitt RA, Kressel A, Pollard WE, Gilson BS, Morris JR. The Sickness Impact Profile: Conceptual formulation and methodology for the development of a health status measure. International J Health Services 1976;6:393–415.

10. Bergner M, Bobbitt RA, Carter WB, et al. The Sickness Impact Profile: Development and final revision of a health status measure. Med Care 1981;19: 787–805.

11. Beurskens AJ, de Vet HCW, Koke AJA, van der Heijden GJ, Knipschild PG. Measuring functional status of patients with low back pain: Assessment of the quality of four disease specific questionnaires. Spine 1995;20:1017–1028.

12. Beurskens AJ, de Vet HCW, Koke AJA. Responsiveness of functional status in low back pain: a comparison of different instruments. Pain 1996;65: 71–76.

13. Beurskens AJ, de Vet HC, Koke AJ, et al. A patient-specific approach for measuring functional status in low back pain. J Manipulative Physiol Ther 1999;22: 144–148.

14. Bigos SJ, Spengler DM, Martin NA, et al. Back injuries in industry: A retrospective study. II. Employee-related factors. Spine 1986;11:252–256.

15. Bigos S, Battie MC, Spengler DM, et al. A prospective study of work perceptions and psychosocial factors affecting the report of back injury. Spine 1991;16:1–6.

16. Binkley JM, Stratford POW, Lott SA, Riddle DL. The lower extremity functional scale (LEFS): Scale development, measurement properties, and clinical application. Phys Ther 1999;79:371–383.

17. Bolton JE. Future directions for outcomes research in back pain. Eur J Chiropractic 1997;45:57–64.

18. Bolton JE. On the responsiveness of evaluative measures. Eur J Chiropractic 1997;45:5–8.

19. Bolton JE, Fish RG. Responsiveness of the revised Oswestry Disability Questionnaire. Eur J Chiropractic 1997;45:9–14.

20. Bolton JE, Wilkinson RC. Responsiveness of pain scales: Comparison of three pain intensity measures in chiropractic patients. J Manipula Physiol Ther 1998;21:1–7.

21. Bolton JE, Breen AC. The Bournemouth Questionnaire: A short-form, comprehensive outcome measure. I Psychometric properties in back pain patients. J Manipula Physiol Ther 1999;22:503–510.

22. Bolton JE, Humphreys BK. The Bournemouth Questionnaire: A short-form comprehensive outcome measure. II. Psychometric properties in neck pain patients. J Manipula Physiol Ther 2002;25: 141–148.

23. Bombardier C. Outcome assessments in the evaluation of treatment of spinal disorders: Summary and general recommendations. Spine 2000;25:3100–3103.

24. Bombardier C, Hayden J, Beaton DE. Minimally clinically important difference. Low back pain: Outcome measures. J Rheumatol 2001;28:431–438.

25. Brazier JE, Harper R, Jones NM, et al. Validating the SF-36 health survey questionnaire: New outcome measure for primary care. BMJ 1992;305: 160–164.

26. Burton AK, Tillotson K, Main C, Hollis M. Psychosocial predictors of outcome in acute and sub-acute low back trouble. Spine 1995;20:722–728.

27. Chatman AB, Hyams SP, Neel JM, et al. The patient-specific functional scale: Measurement properties in patients with knee dysfunction. Phys Ther 1997;77: 820–829.

28. Cherkin D, MacCormack F. Patient evaluations of low-back pain are from family physicians and chiropractors. Western J Med 1989;150:351–355.

29. Cherkin D, Deyo RA, Berg AO. Evaluation of a physician education intervention to improve primary care for low-back pain: II. Impact on patients. Spine 1991;16:1173–1178.

30. Cherkin DC, Deyo RA, Street JH, Barlow W. Predicting poor outcomes for back pain seen in primary care using patients' own criteria. Spine 1996;21: 2900–2907.

31. Chesworth BM, Culham EG, Tata GE, Peat M. Validation of outcome measures in patients with patellofemoral syndrome. JOSPT 1989;11:302–308.

32. Christensen CP, Allthausen PL, Mittleman MA, Lee J, McCarthy JC. The nonarthritic hip score: Reliable and validated. Clinical orthopedics and related research. 2003;406:75–83.

33. Co Y, Eaton S, Maxwell M. The relationship between the St. Thomas and Oswestry disability scores and the severity of low back pain. J Manipula Physiol Ther 1993;16:14–18.

34. Coulter ID, Hays RD, Danielson CD. The chiropractic satisfaction questionnaire. Top Clin Chiro 1994;1(4):40–43.

35. Croft P, Pope D, Zonca M, O'Neill T, Silman A. Measurement of shoulder related disability: Results of a validation study. Ann Rheum Dis 1994;53:525–528.

36. Daltroy LH, Cats-Baril WL, Katz JN, et al. The North American Spine Society lumbar spine outcome assessment instrument: Reliability and validity tests. Spine 1996;21:741–749.

37. De Bruin AF, Diederiks JP, de Witte LP, et al. Assessing the responsiveness of a functional status measure: The Sickness Impact Profile versus the SIP68. J Clin Epidemiol 1997;50:529–540.

38. Demirdjian AM, Petrie SG, Guanche CA, Thomas KA. The outcomes of two knee scoring questionnaires in a normal population. Am J Sports Med 1998;26:46–51.

39. Deyo RA. Comparative validity of the Sickness Impact Profile. Spine 1986;11:951–954.

40. Deyo R, Centor R. Assessing the responsiveness of functional scales to clinical change: An analogy to diagnostic test performance. J Chronic Dis 1986;39: 897–906.

41. Deyo RA, Diehl AK. Patient satisfaction with medical care for low back pain. Spine 1986B;11:28–30.

42. Deyo RA. Low back pain—A primary care challenge. Spine 1996;21:2826–2832.

43. Deyo RA, Battie M, Beurskens AJ, et al. Outcome measures for low back pain research. A proposal for standardized use. Spine 1998;23:2003–2013.

44. Dionne CE, Koepsell TD, Von Korff M, et al. Predicting long-term functional limitations among back pain patients in primary care settings. J Clin Epidemiol 1997;30:31–43.

45. Enzmann, DR. Surviving in Health Care. St. Louis, MO: Mosby-Year Book, 1997.

46. Fairbank J, Davies J, Couper J, O'Brien. The Oswestry Low Back Pain Disability Questionnaire. Physiother 1980;66(18):271–273.

47. Fairbank JCT, Pynsent PB. The Oswestry Disability Index. Spine 2000;25:2940–2953.

48. Farra JT, Young JP, LaMoureauz L, Werth JL, Poole RM. Clinical importance of changes in chronic pain intensity measured on an 11-point numerical pain rating scale. Pain 2001;94:149–158.

49. Fernandez E, Turk DC. Demand characteristics underlying differential ratings of sensory versus affective components of pain. J Behav Med 1994;17: 375–390.

50. Fishbain DA, Khalil TM, Abdel-Moty A, et al. Physician limitation when assessing work capacity: A review. J Back Musculoskel Rehabil 1995;5:107–113.

51. Fishbain DA, Cutler R, Rosomoff HL, Rosomoff RS. Review: Chronic pain disability exaggeration/ malingering and sub maximal effort research. Clin J Pain 1999;15:244–274.

52. Fritz JM, Irrgang JJ. A comparison of a modified Oswestry Low Back Pain Disability Questionnaire and the Quebec Back Pain Disability Scale. Physical Therapy 2001;81:776–788.

53. Frymoyer JW. Quality: An international challenge to the diagnosis and treatment of disorders of the lumbar spine. Spine 1993;18:2147–2152.

54. Gaston-Johansson F. Measurement of pain: The psychometric properties of the Pain-O-Meter, a simple, inexpensive pain assessment tool that could change health care practices. J Pain Symptom Manage 1996;12:172–181.

55. Good MD, Smilkstein G, Good BJ, Shaffer T, Aarons T. The family APGAR index: A study of construct validity. J Fam Pract 1979;8:577–582.

56. Gracely RH, McGrath P, Dubner R. Ratio scales of sensory and affective verbal pain descriptors. Pain 1978;5:5–18.

57. Green S. Classification, treatment, and outcome assessment of shoulder disorders. Thesis. Monash University, Melbourne, 2000.

58. Greenough CG, Fraser RD. Assessment of outcome in patients with low back pain. Spine 1992;17:36–41.

59. Grevitt M, Pande K, O'Dowd J, Webb J. Do first impressions count? A comparison of subjective and psychologic assessment of spinal patients. Eur Spine J 1998;7:218–223.

60. Guyatt G, Walter S, Norman G. Measuring change over time: Assessing the usefulness of evaluative instruments. J Chron Dis 1987;40:171–178.

61. Hagg O, Fritzell P, Nordwall A. The clinical importance of changes in outcome scores after treatment for chronic low back pain. Eur Spine J 2003;12: 12–20.

62. Hains F, Waalen J, Mior S. Psychometric properties of the Neck Disability Index. J Manipulative Physiol Ther 1998;21:75–80.

63. Hansen DT, Vernon H. Applications of Quality Improvement to the Chiropractic Profession. In: Lawrence D, ed. Advances in Chiropractic, Vol 4. St. Louis, MO: Mosby-Year Book, 1997.

64. Hansen DT, Mior S, Mootz RD. Why Outcomes? Why Now? In: Yeomans S, ed. The Clinical Application of Outcomes Assessment. Stanford, CT: Appleton & Lange, 2000.

65. Harper AC, Harper DA, Lambert LJ, et al. Development and validation of the Curtin Back Screening Questionnaire (CBSQ). Pain 1995;6:73–81.

66. Harris WH. Traumatic arthritis of the hip after dislocation and acetabular fractures: Treatment by mold arthroplasty: An end-result study using a new method of result evaluation. J Bone Joint Surg 1969;51A:737–755.

67. Harrison E, Quinney AH, Magee D, Sheppard MS, McQuarrie A. Analysis of outcome measures used in the study of patellofemoral pain syndrome. Physiother Can 1995;47:264–272.

68. Hawkins RH, Dunlop R. Non-operative treatment of rotator cuff tears. Clin Ortho Rel Res 1995;321: 178–188.

69. Hays RD, Hayashi T, Carson S, et al. Users Guide for the Multitrait Analysis Program (MAP). A Rand Note: N-2786-RC. Santa Monica, CA: Rand, 1988.

70. Hays RD. Revised Multitrait Analysis Program Software (MAP-R). Memorandum. Boston, MA: Health Institute, New England Medical Center, 1991.

71. Hazard RG. Spine Update: Functional restoration. Spine 1995;21:2345–2348.

72. Hazard RG, Haugh LD, Reid S, Preble JB, MacDonald L. Early prediction of chronic disability after occupational low back injury. Spine 1996;21: 945–951.

73. Hazard RG, et al. Chronic spinal pain: The relationship between patient satisfaction, symptom and physical capacity outcomes, and achievement of personal goals following functional restoration. Presented at the annual meeting of the International Society for the Study of the Lumbar Spine, Edinburgh, 2001.

74. Heald SL, Riddle DL, Lamb RL. The shoulder pain and disability index: the construct validity and responsiveness of a region-specific disability measure. Phys Ther 1997;77:1079–1089.

75. Hsieh CJ, Phillips RB, Adams AH, Pope MH. Functional outcomes of low back pain: Comparison of four treatment groups in a randomized controlled trial. J Manipula Physiol Ther 1992;15:4–9.

76. Hudak PL. Wright JG. The characteristics of patient satisfaction measures. Spine 2000;25:3167–3177.

77. Hudson-Cook N, Tomes-Nicholson K, Breen AC. A revised Oswestry disability questionnaire. In: Roland M, Jenner J, eds. Back Pain: New Approaches to Rehabilitation and Education. Manchester, UK: University Press, 1989:187–204.

78. Hunt SM, McEwen J, McKenna SP. Measuring health status: A new tool for clinicians and epidemiologists. J R Coll Gen Pract 1985;35:185–188.

79. ICDH-2. International Classification of Functioning and Disability. Beta-2 Draft. Full Version. Geneva: World Health Organization, 1999.

80. Irrgang JJ, Anderson AF, Boland AL, et al. Development and validation of the International Knee Documentation Committee Subjective Knee Form. Am J Sports Med 2001;29:600–613.

81. Jaeschke R, Singer J, Guyatt GH. Measurement of health status. Ascertaining the minimally clinically important difference. Controlled Clinical Trials 1989;10:407–415.

82. Jensen MP, Karoly P, O'Riordan EF, et al. The subjective experience of acute pain: An assessment of the utility of 10 indices. Clin J Pain 1989:153–159.

83. Jensen MP, Strom SE, Turner JA, et al. Validity of the Sickness Impact Profile Roland Scale as a measure of dysfunction in chronic pain patients. Pain 1992;50:157.

84. Jensen MP, Turner JA, Romano JM. What is the maximum number of levels needed in pain intensity measurement? Pain 1994;58:387–392.

85. Jensen MP, Turner JA, Romano JM, Fisher L. Comparative reliability and validity of chronic pain intensity measures. Pain 1999;83:157–162.

86. Jette AM. Outcomes research: shifting the dominant research paradigm in physical therapy. Phys Ther 1995;75:965–970.

87. Jette DU, Jette AM. Physical therapy and health outcomes in patients with knee impairments. Phys Ther 1996;76:1178–1187.

88. Jette DU, Jette AM. Physical therapy and health outcomes in patients with spinal impairments. Phys Ther 1996;76:930–941.

89. Johanson NA, Charlson ME, Szatrowski TP, Ranawat CS. A self-administered hip-rating questionnaire for the assessment of outcome after total hip replacement. J Bone Joint Surg (Am) 1992;74: 587–597.

90. Jordan A, Manniche C, Mosdal C, Hindsberger C. The Copenhagen Neck Functional Disability Scale: A study of reliability and validity. J Manipula Physiol Ther 1998;21:520–527.

91. Katz JN, Phillips CB, Poss R, et al. The validity and reliability of a Total Hip Arthroplasty Outcome Evaluation Questionnaire. J Bone Joint Surg (Am) 1995;77:1528–1534.

92. Kendall NAS, Linton SJ, Main CJ. Guide to assessing psychosocial yellow flags in acute low back pain: Risk factors for long-term disability and work loss. Wellington, NZ: Accident Rehabilitation & Compensation Insurance Corporation of New Zealand and the National Health Committee, 1997. Available from http://www.nhc.govt.nz.

93. Kirshner B, Guyatt G. A methodological framework for assessing health indices. J Chron Dis 1985;38:27–36.

94. Kirkaldy-Willis WH. Managing low back pain. New York: Churchill Livingstone, 1983:635.

95. Kopec JA, Esdaile JM. Spine update: Functional disability scales for back pain. Spine 1995;20:1943–1949.

96. Kopec JA, Esdaile JM, Abrahamowicz M, et al. The Quebec Back Disability Scale. Spine 1995;20: 341–352.

97. Kopec JA, Esdaile JM, Abrahamowicz M, et al. The Quebec Back Pain Disability Scale: Conceptualization and development. J Clin Epidemiol 1996;49: 151–161.

98. Kopec JA. Measuring functional outcomes in persons with back pain: A review of back-specific questionnaires. Spine 2000;25:3110–3114.

99. Last JM. A dictionary of epidemiology, 3rd ed. New York: Oxford University Press, 1995.

100. Leclaire R, Blier F, Fortin L, Proulx R. A cross-sectional study comparing the Oswestry and Roland-Morris functional disability scales in two populations of patients with low back pain with different levels of severity. Spine 1997;22:68–71.

101. Linton SJ, Hallden K. Risk factors and the natural course of acute and recurrent musculoskeletal pain: Developing a screening instrument. In: Jensen TS, Turner JA, Wiesenfeld-Hallin Z, eds. Proceedings of the 8th World Congress on Pain, Progress in Pain Research and Management, Vol 8. Seattle: IASP Press, 1997.

102. Linton SJ, Hallden BH. Can we screen for problematic back pain? A screening questionnaire for predicting outcome in acute and subacute back pain. Clin J Pain 1998;14:1–7.

103. Long AF, Dixon P. Monitoring outcomes in routine practice: Defining appropriate measuring criteria. J Eval Clin Prac 1996;2:71–78.

104. Magnusson P, Hammonds K. Health care: The quest for quality. Business Week 1996;April 8:108.

105. Manniche, Asmussen K, Lauritsen B, et al. Low Back Pain Rating Scale: Validation of a tool for assessment of low back pain. Pain 1994;57:317–326.

106. Mannion AF, Junge A, Taimela S, Muntener M, Lorenzo K, Dvorak J. Active therapy for chronic low back pain. Part 3. Factors influencing self-rated disability and its change following therapy. Spine 2001;26:920–929.

107. Matheson LN, Kaskutas VK, Mada D. Development and construct validation of the hand function sort. J Occup Rehabil 2001;11:75–86.

108. Matheson LN. History, design characteristics, and uses of the pictorial activity and task sorts. J Occup Rehabil 2004;14:175–195.

109. Mayer TG, Polatin P, Smith B, et al. Contemporary concepts in spine care: Spine rehabilitation—secondary and tertiary non-operative care. Spine 1995;20:2060–2066.

110. Meade T, Browne W, Mellows S, et al. Comparison of chiropractic and outpatient management of low back pain: A feasibility study. J Epidemiol Commun Health 1986;40:12–17.

111. Meenan RF, Gertman PM, Mason JH. Measuring health status in arthritis: The arthritis impact measurement scales. Arthritis Rheum 1980;23:146–151.

112. Meenan RF, Gertman PM, Mason JH, Dunaif R. The arthritis impact measurement scales: Further investigations of a health status measure. Arthritis Rheum 1982;25:1048–1053.

113. Melzack R. The McGill Pain Questionnaire. In: Melzack R, ed. Pain Measurement and Assessment. New York: Raven, 1975:41–47.

114. Melzack R. The McGill Pain Questionnaire. Major properties and scoring methods. Pain 1975;1:277–299.

115. Million R, Hall W, Nilsen KH, Baker RD, Jayson MIV. Assessment of the progress of the back pain patient. Spine 1982;7:204–212.

116. Mooney V, Matheson LN. Objective measurement of soft tissue injury: Feasibility study examiner's manual. Industrial Medical Council, State of California, 1994.

117. Morley S, Pallin V. Scaling the affective domain of pain: A study of the dimensionality of verbal descriptors. Pain 1995;63:39–49.

118. Nelson EC, Landgraf JM, Hays RD, et al. The COOP function charts: A system to measure patient function in physicians' offices. In: Lipkin M Jr, ed. Functional Status Measurement in Primary Care: Frontiers of Primary Care. New York: Springer-Verlag, 1990:97–131.

119. Ohlund C, Eek C, Palmblad S, Areskoug B, Nachemson A. Quantified pain drawing in subacute low back pain: Validation in a non-selected outpatient industrial sample. Spine 1996;21:1021–1031.

120. Parker H, Wood PLR, Main CJ. The uses of the pain drawing as a screening measure to predict psychological distress in chronic low back pain. Spine 1995;20:236–243.

121. Patrick D, Deyo R, Atlas S, et al. Assessing health-related quality of life in patients with sciatica. Spine 1995;20:1899–1909.

122. Pengel LHM, Refshauge KM, Maher CG. Responsiveness of pain, disability, and physical impairment outcomes in patients with low back pain. Spine 2004;29:879–883.

123. Pincus T, Vlaeyen JWS, Kendall NAS, Von Korff MR, Kalauokalani DA, Reis S. Cognitive-behavioral therapy and psychosocial factors in low back pain. Spine 2002;27:E133–E138.

124. Pinfold M, Nierre KR, O'Leary EF, Hoving JL, Green S, Buchbinder R. Validity and internal consistency of a whiplash-specific disability measure. Spine 2004;29:263–268.

125. Pope DP, Croft PR, Pritchard CM, Silman AJ. Prevalence of shoulder pain in the community: The influence of case definition. Ann Rheum Dis 1997;56:308–312.

126. Pransky G, Feuerstein M, Himmelstein J, Katz JN, Vickers-Lahti M. Measuring functional outcomes in work-related upper extremity disorders: Development and validation of the Upper Extremity Function Scales. J Occup Environ Med 1997;39:1195–1202.

127. Price DD, Harkins SW, Baker C. Sensory-affective relationships among different types of clinical and experimental pain. Pain 1987;28:297–307.

128. Ransford HV, Cairns D, Mooney V. The pain drawing as an aid to psychological evaluation of patients with low back pain. Spine 1976;1:127.

129. Reid DC. Sports injury assessment and rehabilitation. New York: Churchill Livingstone, 1992.

130. Riddle DL, Stratford PW, Binkley JM. Sensitivity to change of the Roland-Morris back pain questionnaire: Part 2. Phys Ther 1998;78:1197–1207.

131. Rissanen A, Alarant H, Sainio P, Harkonen H. Isokinetic and non-dynametric tests in low back pain patients related to pain and disability index. Spine 1994;19:1963–1967.

132. Roach KE, Budiman-Mak E, Songsirdej N, Lertratanakul Y. Development of a shoulder pain and disability index. Arthritis Care Res 1991;4:143–149.

133. Roland M, Fairbank J. The Roland-Morris Disability Questionnaire and the Oswestry Disability Questionnaire. Spine 2000;25:3115–3124.

134. Roland M, Morris R. A study of the natural history of back pain: Part I: Development of a reliable and sensitive measure of disability in low back pain. Spine 1983;8:141–144.

135. Rosenfeld RM. Meaningful outcomes research. In: Isenberg SF, ed. Managed Care: Outcomes and Quality. A practical guide. New York: Thieme, 1998:99–115.

136. Rowe CR. Evaluation of the shoulder. In: Rowe CR, ed. The Shoulder. New York, NY: Churchill Livingstone, 1987:633.

137. Rozzi SL, Lephart SM, Sterner R, Kuligowski L. Balance training for persons with functionally unstable ankles. J Orthop Sp Phys Ther 1999;29: 478–486.

138. Ruta DA, Garratt AM, Wardlaw D, Russell IT. Developing a valid and reliable measure of health outcome for patients with low back pain. Spine 1994; 19:1887–1896.

139. Scrimshaw SV, Maher C. Responsiveness of visual analog and McGill pain scale measures. J Manipulative Physiol Ther 2001;24:501–504.

140. Smilkstein G. The family APGAR: A proposal for family function test and its use by physicians. J Fam Pract 1978;6:1231–1235.

141. Stewart WF, Lipton RB, Simon D, et al. Validity of an illness severity measure for headache in a population sample of migraine sufferers. Pain 1999;79:291–301.

142. Stratford PW, Binkley J, Solomon P, Gill C, Finch E. Assessing change over time in patients with low back pain. Physical Ther 1994;74:528–533.

143. Stratford P, Gill C, Westaway M and Binkley J. Assessing disability and change on individual patients: A report of a patient specific measure. Physiother Can 1995;47:258–263.

144. Stratford PW, Binkley J, Solomon P, et al. Defining the minimum level of detectable change for the Roland-Morris questionnaire. Phys Ther 1996;76:359–365.

145. Stratford PW, Binkley J. Measurement properties of the RM18: A modified version of the Roland-Morris disability scale. Spine 1997;22:2416–2421.

146. Stratford PW, Binkely JM, Riddle DL, Guyatt GH. Sensitivity to change of the Roland-Morris Back Pain Questionnaire: Part 1. Phys Ther 1998;78: 1186–1196.

147. Stratford PW, Riddle DL, Binkely JM, Spadoni G, Westaway MD, Padfield B. Using the Neck Disability Index to make decisions concerning individual patients. Physiother Can 1999;50:107–119.

148. Stratford PW, Binkley J. Applying the results of self-report measures to individual patients: An example using the Roland-Morris Questionnaire. J Orthop Sports Phys Ther 1999;29:232–239.

149. Stratford PW, Binkley JM, Watson J, Heath-Jones T. Validation of the LEFS on patients with total joint arthroplasty. Physiother Can 2000;52:97–105.

150. Stratford PW, Binkley JM, Stratford DM. Development and initial validation of the upper extremity functional index. Physiother Can 2001;53:259–266.

151. Streiner DL, Norman GR. Health measurement scales: A practical guide to their development and use, 2nd ed. New York: Oxford University Press, 1995.

152. Stroud MW, McKnight PE, Jensen MP. Assessment of self-reported physical activity in patients with chronic pain: Development of an abbreviated Roland-Morris Disability Scale. J Pain 2004;5: 257–263.

153. Stucki G, Lian M, Fossel A, et al. Relative responsiveness of condition-specific and generic health status measures in degenerative lumbar spine stenosis. J Clin Epidemiol 1995;48:1369–1378.

154. Stucki G, Daltroy L, Liang MH, Lipson SJ, Fossel AH, Katz JN. Measurement properties of a self-administered outcome measure in lumbar spinal stenosis. Spine 1996;21:796–803.

155. Tait RC, Chibnall JT, Margolis RB. Pain extent: Relations with psychological state, pain severity, pain history and disability. Pain 1990;41:295–301.

156. Taylor SJ, Taylor AE, Foy MA, Fogg AJB. Responsiveness of common outcome measures for patients with low back pain. Spine 1999;24:1805–1812.

157. Thomas E, Silman AJ, Croft PR, Papageorgiou AC, Jayson MIV, Macfarlane GJ. Predicting who develops chronic low back pain in primary care: A prospective study. BMJ 1999;318:1662–1667.

158. Turk DC. Editorial: Here we go again: Outcomes, outcomes, outcomes. Clin J Pain 1999;15:241–243.

159. Turner JA, Robinson J, McCreary CP. Chronic low back pain: Predicting response to non-surgical treatment. Arch Phys Med Rehabil 1983;64: 560–563.

160. Turner JA, Franklin G, Haegerty PJ, et al. The association between pain and disability. Pain 2004;112:307–314.

161. Uden A, Astrom M, Bergenudd H. Pain drawings in chronic low back pain. Spine 1988;13:389–392.

162. Vernon HT, Mior S. The Neck Disability Index: A study of reliability and validity. J Manipula Physiol Ther 1991;14:409–415.

163. Vernon HT, Aker P, Aramenko M, Battershill D, Alepin A, Penner T. Evaluation of neck muscle strength with a modified sphygmomanometer dynamometer: Reliability and validity. J Manipula Physiol Ther 1992;15:343–349.

164. Vernon HT, Piccininni J, Kopansky-Giles D, Hagino C, Fuligni S. Chiropractic rehabilitation of spinal pain patients: Principles, practices and outcome data. J Can Chiropr Assoc 1995;39:147–153.

165. Vernon H. The Neck Disability Index: Patient assessment and outcome monitoring in whiplash. In: Allen ME, ed. Musculoskeletal Pain Emanating from the Head and Neck: Current Concepts in Diagnosis, Management and Cost Containment. Binghamton, NY: The Haworth Medical Press, an imprint of The Haworth Press, Inc, 1996:905–104.

166. Vernon H. Correlations among ratings of pain, disability and impairment in chronic whiplash-associated disorder. Pain Res Manage 1997;4: 207–213.

167. Vernon H. Assessment of self-rated disability, impairment, and sincerity of effort in whiplash-associated disorder. J Musculoskel Pain 2000;8: 155–167.

168. Von Korff M, Ormel J, Keefe F, et al. Grading the severity of chronic pain. Pain 1992;50:133–149.

169. Von Korff M, Jensen MP, Karoly P. Assessing global pain severity by self-report in clinical and health services research. Spine 2000;25:3140–3151.

170. Waddell G, Main CJ. Assessment of severity in low back disorders. Spine 1984;9:204–208.

171. Waddell G, Somerville D, Henderson I, Newton M. Objective clinical evaluation of physical impairment in chronic low back pain. Spine 1992;17:617–628.

172. Ware JE, Sherbourne CD. The MOS 36-item Short Form Health Survey (SF-36). Med Care 1992;30:473–483.

173. Ware Jr. JE, Snow K, Kosinski M, et al. SF36 physical and mental health summary scales: A user's manual. Boston, MA: The Health Institute, New England Medical Center, 1993a.

174. Ware JE. SF-36 Health Survey: Manual and Interpretation Guide. Boston, MA: The Health Institute, New England Medical Center, 1993b.

175. Ware Jr. JE, Kosinski M, Keller SD. SF-12: How to Score the SF-12 Physical the Mental Health Summary Scales. second ed. Boston, MA: The Health Institute, New England Medical Center, 1995.

176. Ware Jr. JE. SF-36 Health survey update. Spine 2000;23:3130–3139.

177. Wegener L, Kisner C, Nichols D. Static and dynamic balance responses in persons with bilateral knee osteoarthritis. J Orthop Sports Phys Ther 1997;25: 13–18.

178. Westaway M, Stratford PW, Binkley J. The Patient Specific Functional Scale: Validation of its use in persons with neck dysfunction. J Orthop Sports Phys Ther 1998;27:331–338.

179. Wheeler AH, Goolkasian P, Baird AC, Darden BV. Development of the neck pain and disability scale. Spine 1999;24:1290–1294.

180. Williams JW Jr, Holleman DR Jr, Simel DL. Measuring shoulder function with the Shoulder Pain and Disability Index. J Rheumatol 1995;22:727–732.

181. Williams RM, Myers AM. A new approach to measuring recovery in injured workers with acute low back pain: Resumption of activities of daily living scale. Phys Ther 1998;78:613–623.

182. World Health Organization. International Classification of Human Functioning, Disability and Health: ICF. Geneva: WHO, 2001.

183. Wright JG, Young NL. The patient-specific index: Asking patients what they want. J Bone Joint Surg (Am) 1997;79:974–983.

184. Yeomans SG. The Clinical Application of Outcomes Assessment. Stamford, CT: Appleton & Lange, 2000.

185. Yeomans SG. Chiropractic and Managed Care. ACA/FYI, June/July 1992:29–31.

GLOBAL IMPRESSION OF CHANGE

Since the start of my care, my overall status is:

1. ☐ Very Much Improved

2. ☐ Much Improved

3. ☐ Minimally Improved

4. ☐ No Change

5. ☐ Minimally Worse

6. ☐ Much Worse

7. ☐ Very Much Worse

Farra JT, Young JP, LaMoureauz L, Werth JL, Poole RM. Clinical importance of changes in chronic pain intensity measured on an 11-point numerical pain rating scale. Pain 2001;94:149–158.

Hagg O, Fritzell P, Nordwall A. The clinical importance of changes in outcome scores after treatment for chronic low back pain. Eur Spine J 2003;12:12–20.

Name _____ Signature _____

Date _____

Form 1 (48,61)
Global Impression of Change.

REVISED OSWESTRY DISABILITY QUESTIONNAIRE

Name _____ **Date** _____

This questionnaire has been designed to give us information as to how your back or leg pain is affecting your ability to manage in every day life. Please answer by checking **one box in each section** for the statement that best applies to you. We realize you may consider that two or more statements in any one section apply, but please just shade the spot that indicates the statement *that most clearly describes your problem.*

Section 1: Pain Intensity
A. I have no pain at the moment
B. The pain is very mild at the moment
C. The pain is moderate at the moment
D. The pain is fairly severe at the moment
E. The pain is very severe at the moment
F. The pain is the worst imaginable at the moment

Section 2: Personal Care (Washing, Dressing, etc.)
A. I can look after myself normally without causing extra pain
B. I can look after myself normally but it causes extra pain
C. It is painful to look after myself and I am slow and careful
D. I need some help but can manage most of my personal care
E. I need help every day in most aspects of self care
F. do not get dressed, wash with difficulty and stay in bed

Section 3: Lifting
A. I can lift heavy weights without extra pain
B. I can lift heavy weights but it gives me extra pain
C. Pain prevents me lifting heavy weights off the floor but I can manage if they are conveniently placed, e.g., on a table
D. Pain prevents me lifting heavy weights but I can manage light to medium weights if they are conveniently positioned
E. I can only lift very light weights
F. I cannot lift or carry anything

Section 4: Walking
A. Pain does not prevent me walking any distance
B. Pain prevents me from walking more than 2 kilometers
C. Pain prevents me from walking more than 1 kilometer
D. Pain prevents me from walking more than 500 meters
E. I can only walk using a stick or crutches
F. I am in bed most of the time

Section 5: Sitting
A. I can sit in any chair as long as I like
B. I can only sit in my favorite chair as long as I like
C. Pain prevents me sitting more than one hour
D. Pain prevents me from sitting more than 30 minutes
E. Pain prevents me from sitting more than 10 minutes
F. Pain prevents me from sitting at all

Section 6: Standing
A. I can stand as long as I want without extra pain
B. I can stand as long as I want but it gives me extra pain
C. Pain prevents me from standing for more than 1 hour
D. Pain prevents me from standing for more than 30 minutes
E. Pain prevents me from standing for more than 10 minutes
F. Pain prevents me from standing at all

Section 7: Sleeping
A. My sleep is never disturbed by pain
B. My sleep is occasionally disturbed by pain
C. Because of pain I have less than 6 hours sleep
D. Because of pain I have less than 4 hours sleep
E. Because of pain I have less than 2 hours sleep
F. Pain prevents me from sleeping at all

Section 8: Social Life
A. My social life is normal and gives me no extra pain
B. My social life is normal but increases the degree of pain
C. Pain has no significant effect on my social life apart from limiting my more energetic interests, e.g., sport
D. Pain has restricted my social life and I do not go out as often
E. Pain has restricted my social life to my home
F. I have no social life because of pain

REVISED OSWESTRY DISABILITY QUESTIONNAIRE (*Continued*)

Section 9: Traveling	**Section 10: Employment/Homemaking**
A. I can travel anywhere without pain	A. My normal homemaking/job activities do not cause pain.
B. I can travel anywhere but it gives me extra pain	B. My normal homemaking/job activities increase my pain, but I can still perform all that is required of me.
C. Pain is bad but I manage journeys more than 2 hours	C. I can perform most of my homemaking/job activities, but pain prevents me from performing more physically stressful activities (e.g., lifting, vacuuming).
D. Pain restricts me to journeys of less than 1 hour	D. Pain prevents me from doing anything but light duties
E. Pain restricts me to short necessary journeys less than 30 minutes	E. Pain prevents me from doing even light duties
F. Pain prevents me from traveling except to receive treatment	F. Pain prevents me from performing any job or homemaking chores

Minimum Detectable Change (90% confidence): 15 points
Minimum Clinically Important Difference (90% confidence): 6 points

Form 2 (52)
Oswestry Low Back Pain Disability Index. Form reproduced with permission from Fritz JM, Irrgang JJ. A comparison of a modified Oswestry Low Back Pain Disability Questionnaire and the Quebec Back Pain Disability Scale. Physical Ther 2001;81:776–788.

ROLAND-MORRIS LOW BACK PAIN AND DISABILITY QUESTIONNAIRE

When your back hurts, you may find if difficult to do some of the things you normally do. Mark only the sentences that describe you today.

1. ☐ I stay at home most of the time because of my back.

2. ☐ I change position frequently to try and get my back comfortable.

3. ☐ I walk more slowly than usual because of my back.

4. ☐ Because of my back, I am not doing any jobs that I usually do around the house.

5. ☐ Because of my back, I use a handrail to get upstairs.

6. ☐ Because of my back, I lie down to rest more often.

7. ☐ Because of my back, I have to hold on to something to get out of an easy chair.

8. ☐ Because of my back, I try to get other people to do things for me.

9. ☐ I get dressed more slowly than usual because of my back.

10. ☐ I stand up only for short periods of time because of my back.

11. ☐ Because of my back, I try not to bend or kneel down.

12. ☐ I find it difficult to get out of a chair because of my back.

13. ☐ My back is painful almost all of the time.

14. ☐ I find it difficult to turn over in bed because of my back.

15. ☐ My appetite is not very good because of my back pain.

16. ☐ I have trouble putting on my socks (or stockings) because of pain in my back.

17. ☐ I walk only short distances because of my back pain.

18. ☐ I sleep less well because of my back.

19. ☐ Because of back pain, I get dressed with help from someone else.

20. ☐ I sit down for most of the day because of my back.

21. ☐ I avoid heavy jobs around the house because of my back.

22. ☐ Because of back pain, I am more irritable and bad tempered with people than usual.

23. ☐ Because of my back, I go upstairs more slowly than usual.

24. ☐ I stay in bed most of the time because of my back.

Patient name _____ Patient signature _____ Date _____

Form 3 (134)
Roland-Morris Low Back Pain and Disability Form reprinted with permission from Roland M, Morris R. A study of the natural history of back pain: Part I: Development of a reliable and sensitive measure of disability in low-back pain. Spine 1983;8:141–144.

NECK PAIN DISABILITY INDEX QUESTIONNAIRE

PLEASE READ: This questionnaire is designed to enable us to understand how much your neck pain has affected your ability to manage your every day activities. Please answer each section by circling the ONE CHOICE that most applies to you. We realize that you may feel that more than one statement may relate to you, but *PLEASE JUST CIRCLE THE ONE CHOICE THAT MOST CLOSELY DESCRIBES YOUR PROBLEM RIGHT NOW.*

SECTION 1—Pain Intensity
A I have no pain at the moment.
B The pain is very mild at the moment.
C The pain is moderate at the moment.
D The pain is fairly severe at the moment.
E The pain is very severe at the moment.
F The pain is the worst imaginable at the moment.

SECTION 2—Personal Care (Washing, Dressing, etc.)
A I can look after myself normally without causing extra pain.
B I can look after myself normally, but it causes extra pain.
C It is painful to look after myself and I am slow and careful.
D I need some help, but manage most of my personal care.
E I need help every day in most aspects of self care.
F I do not get dressed, I wash with difficulty, and I stay in bed.

SECTION 3—Lifting
A I can lift heavy weights without extra pain.
B I can lift heavy weights, but it gives extra pain.
C Pain prevents me from lifting heavy weights off the floor, but I can manage if they are conveniently positioned, for example, on a table.
D Pain prevents me from lifting heavy weights, but I can manage light to medium weights if they are conveniently positioned.
E I can lift very light weights.
F I cannot lift or carry anything at all.

SECTION 4—Reading
A I can read as much as I want to with no pain in my neck.
B I can read as much as I want to with slight pain in my neck.
C I can read as much as I want to with moderate pain in my neck.
D I cannot read as much as I want because of moderate pain in my neck.
E I cannot read as much as I want because of severe pain in my neck.
F I cannot read at all.

SECTION 5—Headaches
A I have no headaches at all.
B I have slight headaches which come infrequently.
C I have moderate headaches which come infrequently.
D I have moderate headaches which come frequently.
E I have severe headaches which come frequently.
F I have headaches almost all the time.

SECTION 6—Concentration
A I can concentrate fully when I want to with no difficulty.
B I can concentrate fully when I want to with slight difficulty.
C I have a fair degree of difficulty in concentrating when I want to.
D I have a lot of difficulty in concentrating when I want to.
E I have a great deal of difficulty in concentrating when I want to.
F I cannot concentrate at all.

SECTION 7—Work
A I can do as much work as I want to.
B I can only do my usual work, but no more.
C I can do most of my usual work, but no more.
D I cannot do my usual work.
E I can hardly do any work at all.
F I cannot do any work at all.

SECTION 8—Driving
A I can drive my car without any neck pain.
B I can drive my car as long as I want with slight pain in my neck.
C I can drive my car as long as I want with moderate pain in my neck.
D I cannot drive my car as long as I want because of moderate pain in my neck.
E I can hardly drive at all because of severe pain in my neck.
F I cannot drive my car at all.

NECK PAIN DISABILITY INDEX QUESTIONNAIRE (*Continued*)

SECTION 9—Sleeping	*SECTION 10—Recreation*
A I have no trouble sleeping.	A I am able to engage in all of my recreational activities with no neck pain at all.
B My sleep is slightly disturbed (less than 1 hour sleepless).	B I am able to engage in all of my recreational activities with some pain in my neck.
C My sleep is mildly disturbed (1–2 hours sleepless).	C I am able to engage in most, but not all of my recreational activities because of pain in my neck.
D My sleep is moderately disturbed (2–3 hours sleepless).	D I am able to engage in a few of my recreational activities because of pain in my neck.
E My sleep is greatly disturbed (3–5 hours sleepless).	E I can hardly do any recreational activities because of pain in my neck.
F My sleep is completely disturbed (5–7 hours)	F I cannot do any recreational activities at all.

Patient name _____ Patient signature _____ Date _____

Form 4 (162)

Neck Disability Index reprinted with permission from Vernon H, Mior S. The Neck Disability Index: A study of reliability and validity. J Manipulative Physiol Ther 1991;14:409–415.

UPPER EXTREMITY FUNCTION SCALE QUESTIONNAIRE

Please indicate which of the following things you have difficulty in doing because of your symptoms. Circle the number that indicates how much difficulty you have with each activity.

	NO PROBLEM									MAJOR PROBLEM (Cannot do it at all)
1. Sleeping	0	1	2	3	4	5	6	7	8	9	10
2. Writing	0	1	2	3	4	5	6	7	8	9	10
3. Opening jars	0	1	2	3	4	5	6	7	8	9	10
4. Picking up small objects with fingers	0	1	2	3	4	5	6	7	8	9	10
5. Driving a car more than 30 minutes	0	1	2	3	4	5	6	7	8	9	10
6. Opening a door	0	1	2	3	4	5	6	7	8	9	10
7. Carrying milk jug from the refrigerator	0	1	2	3	4	5	6	7	8	9	10
8. Washing dishes	0	1	2	3	4	5	6	7	8	9	10

COMMENTS _____

_____

_____

_____

_____

_____

_____

Patient name _____ Patient signature _____ Date _____

Form 5 (126)

Upper Extremity Function Scale reprinted with permission from Pransky G, Feuerstein M, Himmelstein J, Katz JN, Vickers-Lahti M. Measuring functional outcomes in work-related upper extremity disorders: Development and validation of the Upper Extremity Function Scales. J Occup Environ Med 1997;39: 1195–1202.

UPPER EXTREMITY FUNCTIONAL INDEX

We are interested in knowing whether you are having any difficulty at all with the activities listed below because of your upper limb problem for which you are currently seeking attention.
Please check (✓) an answer for **each** activity.

Today, <u>do you</u> or <u>would you</u> have any difficulty at all with:

Activities	Extreme Difficulty Or Unable to Perform Activity	Quite a Bit of Difficulty	Moderate Difficulty	A Little Bit of Difficulty	No Difficulty
Any of your usual work, household, or school activities					
Your usual hobbies, recreational or sporting activities					
Lifting a bag of groceries to waist level					
Lifting a bag of groceries above your head					
Grooming your hair					
Pushing up on your hands (e.g., from bathtub or chair)					
Preparing food (e.g., peeling, cutting)					
Driving					
Vacuuming, sweeping, or raking					
Dressing					
Doing up buttons					
Using tools or appliances					
Opening doors					
Cleaning					
Tying or lacing shoes					
Sleeping					
Laundering clothes (e.g., washing, ironing, folding)					
Opening a jar					
Throwing a ball					
Carrying a small suitcase with your affected limb)					

Patient name: _____ Signature: _____ Date: _____

Score _____ /80   MDC (minimum detectable change) = 9 points   Error +/– 5 scale points

Form 6 (16)
Upper Extremity Functional Index reprinted with permission from Stratford PW, Binkley JM, Stratford DM. Development and initial validation of the upper extremity functional index. Physiother Can 2001;53:259–266.

FUNCTIONAL ASSESSMENT SCALE (FAS)

Please respond to the following questions, circling only one answer that best describes your abilities.

1. PAIN: How much pain do you have?
a. No pain during walking
b. Occasional ache, does not stop you from walking
c. Mild pain after walking a long time, may take aspirin
d. Moderate pain with normal walking. May take medication stronger than aspirin or Tylenol® after excessive activities that cause considerable pain.
e. Severe pain, but able to walk. May need regular medication stronger than aspirin.
f. Totally disabled with pain, unable to walk

2. WALKING DISTANCE: How far can you walk?
a. Unlimited distance
b. 6 blocks
c. 2 or 3 blocks
d. Indoors, around the house only
e. Bed to chair, unable to walk

3. WALKING AIDS: How much support do you need to walk?
a. No support needed to walk comfortably
b. One cane needed for long walks
c. One crutch needed most of the time
d. Two canes needed most of the time
e. Two crutches or walker needed most of the time

4. STANDING: How long can you stand?
a. Comfortable standing without support for 45 minutes
b. Comfortable standing without support for 30 minutes
c. Comfortable standing without support for 15 minutes
d. Not able to stand without support for 15 minutes

5. STAIRS: How do you climb steps?
a. Foot over foot without a banister
b. Foot over foot with a banister
c. Using stairs with banister and outside support (example: cane)
d. Unable to climb stairs

Patient name _____ Patient signature _____ Date _____

Form 7 (177)
Functional Assessment Score reprinted with permission from Wegener L, Kisner C, Nichols D. Static and dynamic balance responses in persons with bilateral knee osteoarthritis. J Orthop Sports Phys Ther 1997;25:13–18.

LOWER EXTREMITY FUNCTIONAL SCALE

We are interested in knowing whether you are having any difficulty at all with the activities listed below because of your lower limb problem for which you are currently seeking attention.
Please check (✓) an answer for **each** activity.

Today, <u>do you</u> or <u>would you</u> have any difficulty at all with:

Activities	Extreme Difficulty Or Unable to Perform Activity	Quite a Bit of Difficulty	Moderate Difficulty	A Little Bit of Difficulty	No Difficulty
Any of your usual work, household, or school activities					
Your usual hobbies, recreational or sporting activities					
Getting into or out of the bath					
Walking between rooms					
Putting on your shoes or socks					
Squatting					
Lifting an object, like a bag of groceries from the floor					
Performing light activities around your home					
Performing heavy activities around your home					
Getting into or out of a car					
Walking 2 blocks					
Walking a mile					
Going up or down 10 stairs (approximately 1 flight of stairs)					
Standing for 1 hour					
Sitting for 1 hour					
Running on even ground					
Running on uneven ground					
Making sharp turns while running fast					
Hopping					
Rolling over in bed					

Patient name _____ Patient signature _____ Date _____
Score _____/80   MDC (minimum detectable change) = 9 points   Error +/− 5 scale points

Form 8 (16)

Lower Extremity Functional Scale reprinted with permission from Binkley JM, Stratford POW, Lott SA, Riddle DL. The lower extremity functional scale (LEFS): Scale development, measurement properties, and clinical application. Phys Ther 1999;79:371–383.

PATIENT SPECIFIC FUNCTIONAL AND PAIN SCALES (PSFS)

Name _____ **Date**_____

Clinician: Complete after the history and before the physical examination

Initial Assessment:
In your visits here we want to know what <u>3 activities</u> in your life you are unable to do or are having the most difficulty with as a result of your chief problem. Please list and score at least 3 activities you are unable to perform or having the most difficulty with because of your chief problem.

<u>**Follow-up Assessment:**</u>
When you were assessed on _____, you told us that you had difficulty with the following activities. Please score the activities you told us previously you were unable to perform or having the most difficulty with because of your chief problem.

Patient Specific Activity Scoring scheme (Point to one number):

0	1	2	3	4	5	6	7	8	9	10

Unable
to perform
activity

Able to perform
activity at same
level as before
injury or problem

Date and Score

Activity					
1.					
2.					
3.					
4.					
5.					

Total score = sum of activity scores divided by number of activities
MDC for average score = 2 points
MDC for single activity = 3 points

Form 9
Patient Specific Functional Scale reprinted with permission from Stratford P, Gill C, Westaway M, Binkley J. Assessing disability and change on individual patients: A report of a patient specific measure. Physiother Can 1995;47:258–263.

PATIENT SATISFACTION SCALE

Here are some questions about the treatment you have been receiving. In terms of your satisfaction, how would you rate each of the following? Choose one response on each line.

	Strongly agree	Agree	Neither agree nor disagree	Disagree	Strongly disagree
1. The doctor gave me enough information about the cause of my back pain.					
2. The doctor did NOT give me a clear explanation of the cause of my pain.					
3. The doctor told me what to do to prevent future back problems.					
4. The doctor seemed to believe that my pain was real.					
5. The doctor did NOT understand the concerns I had about my back problem.					
6. The doctor did NOT seem comfortable dealing with my back pain.					
7. The doctor was NOT concerned about what happened with my pain after I left the office.					
8. The treatment the doctor prescribed for my back pain was effective.					
9. The doctor seemed confident that the treatment she/he recommended would work.					
10. The doctor gave me a clear idea of how long it might take for my back to get better.					

Patient name _____ Patient signature _____ Date _____

Form 10 (29)
Patient Satisfaction Scale reprinted with permission from Cherkin D, Deyo RA, Berg AO. Evaluation of a physician education intervention to improve primary care for low-back pain: II. Impact on patients. Spine 1991;16:1173–1178.

THE BACK BOURNEMOUTH QUESTIONNAIRE

The following scales have been designed to find out about your back pain and how it is affecting you. Please answer ALL the scales by circling ONE number on EACH scale that best describes how you feel:

1. Over the past week, on average, how would you rate your back pain?
    No pain   Worst pain possible
    0   1   2   3   4   5   6   7   8   9   10

2. Over the past week, how much has your back pain interfered with your daily activities (housework, washing, dressing, walking, climbing stairs, getting in/out of bed/chair)?
    No interference   Unable to perform activity
    0   1   2   3   4   5   6   7   8   9   10

3. Over the past week, how much has your back pain interfered with your ability to take part in recreational, social, and family activities?
    No interference   Unable to perform activity
    0   1   2   3   4   5   6   7   8   9   10

4. Over the past week, how anxious (tense, uptight, irritable, difficulty in concentrating/relaxing) have your been feeling?
    Not at all anxious   Extremely anxious
    0   1   2   3   4   5   6   7   8   9   10

5. Over the past week, how depressed (down-in-the-dumps, sad, in low spirits, pessimistic, unhappy) have you been feeling?
    Not at all depressed   Extremely depressed
    0   1   2   3   4   5   6   7   8   9   10

6. Over the past week, how have you felt your work (both inside and outside the home) has affected (or would affect) your back pain?
    Have made it no worse   Have made it much worse
    0   1   2   3   4   5   6   7   8   9   10

7. Over the past week, how much have you been able to control (reduce/help) your back pain on your own?
    Completely control it   No control whatsoever
    0   1   2   3   4   5   6   7   8   9   10

Patient name _____ Patient signature _____ Date _____

Form 11 (21)

Bournemouth Back Questionnaire reprinted with permission from Bolton JE, Breen AC. The Bournemouth Questionnaire: A short-form comprehensive outcome measure. I. Psychometric properties in back pain patients. J Manipula Physiol Ther 1999;22:503–510.

THE NECK BOURNEMOUTH QUESTIONNAIRE

The following scales have been designed to find out about your back pain and how it is affecting you. Please answer ALL the scales by circling ONE number on EACH scale that best describes how you feel:

1. Over the past week, on average, how would you rate your neck pain?
    No pain   Worst pain possible
      0   1   2   3   4   5   6   7   8   9   10

2. Over the past week, how much has your neck pain interfered with your daily activities (housework, washing, dressing, lifting, reading, driving)?
    No interference   Unable to perform activity
      0   1   2   3   4   5   6   7   8   9   10

3. Over the past week, how much has your neck pain interfered with your ability to take part in recreational, social, and family activities?
    No interference   Unable to perform activity
      0   1   2   3   4   5   6   7   8   9   10

4. Over the past week, how anxious (tense, uptight, irritable, difficulty in concentrating/relaxing) have you been feeling?
    Not at all anxious   Extremely anxious
      0   1   2   3   4   5   6   7   8   9   10

5. Over the past week, how depressed (down-in-the-dumps, sad, in low spirits, pessimistic, unhappy) have you been feeling?
    Not at all depressed   Extremely depressed
      0   1   2   3   4   5   6   7   8   9   10

6. Over the past week, how have you felt your work (both inside and outside the home) has affected (or would affect) your neck pain?
    Have made it no worse   Have made it much worse
      0   1   2   3   4   5   6   7   8   9   10

7. Over the past week, how much have you been able to control (reduce/help) your neck pain on your own?
    Completely control it   No control whatsoever
      0   1   2   3   4   5   6   7   8   9   10

Patient name _____ Patient signature _____ Date _____

Form 12 (22)

Bournemouth Neck Questionnaire reprinted with permission from Bolton JE, Humphreys BK. The Bournemouth Questionnaire : A short-form comprehensive outcome measure. II. Psychometric properties in neck pain patients. J Manipula Physiol Ther 2002;25:141–148.

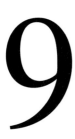

9

Assessment of Psychosocial Risk Factors of Chronicity—"Yellow Flags"

Craig Liebenson and Steven Yeomans

Learning Objectives

After reading this chapter you should be able to understand:

- The prognosis for acute low back pain becoming chronic
- What prognostic factors have been identified to predict the risk of acute back or neck pain becoming chronic
- How to capture a "yellow flags" score reliably and efficiently
- Which prognostic risk factors are amenable to intervention and what type of intervention is appropriate

Introduction

> **Practice-Based Problem**
>
> Is it possible to increase the quality and efficiency of care by stratifying acute or subacute patients into groups that are either more or less likely to recover, and thus match them to more or less aggressive management?

It is a commonly held belief that acute low back pain (LBP) resolves within 4 to 6 weeks for most individuals (75%–90%) (45,107). This is primarily based on insurance surveillance data concerning disability. Such an optimistic picture has led to false confidence in a passive management philosophy involving symptomatic approaches (bed rest and medication) or a non-management approach of leaving it alone to let "nature run its course." However, there are two problems with this perspective. First, the view that most acute episodes resolve quickly and completely is disputed by a number of studies of primary care patients (13,22,117). Second, there is a growing body of evidence that it is more cost-effective to prevent chronicity in those at risk for it rather than waiting to treat only those in whom it becomes fully apparent.

Von Korff et al demonstrated in a non-occupational setting that after 1 month only 30% of neck and low back pain patients had achieved pain-free status, and after 1 year 50% still reported recurrent or persistent pain (117). Most recent studies show that the majority of acute episodes tend to improve rapidly, although not completely, and then run an intermittent chronic course with less severe "flare-ups." The original episode frequently lasts for as long as 3 months—not 4 to 6 weeks—before it can even be said to have remitted (13,22). The "flare-ups," which are predictable in the majority of cases 1 year later, are mild to moderately activity-limiting and painful and lead to general dissatisfaction with the symptoms (13,21,22,117). Thus, back problems typically run recurrent or chronic remitting courses with occasional acute self-limiting episodes.

Even though only a small percentage (7%) of individuals with acute LBP have chronic unremitting pain and disability, this group accounts for the majority of the costs (11,107). More specifically, 7.4% of patients account for approximately 75% of all the costs and 85% of the disability days (50,107). Thus, identifying potential risk factors for acute pain becoming chronic has become a "holy grail" of LBP research (1).

Risk Factors of Chronicity

Assessment of spine patients has traditionally focused on finding the physical cause of the pain. Imaging techniques have figured prominently in this endeavor.

Unfortunately, this has been an inefficient use of resources because of the poor specificity of this expensive screening approach (4,5,7,54,57,58,64,111,124). Clinical scientists have summarized that the following measurable outcomes are representative criteria of patient recovery: pain, function (disability), well-being, work status, and satisfaction (6,25). According to Pinchus et al, the risk of long-term LBP-related activity limitations (disability) and work loss (participation) arises from four main sources that interact with each other (Table 9.1) (94). Individual factors have been referred to as psychosocial "yellow flags" (63). "Yellow flags" are analogous to the concept of "red flags" in that they both influence the management and prognosis of the patient. Whereas "red flags" are indications for biomedical laboratory or imaging investigations and possibly specialist referral, "yellow flags" are indications for investigating the cognitive, affective, and behavioral aspects of LBP.

Most yellow flags pertain to individual or work related factors, yet the effect the treatment provider has on outcome is also important (23,99). Reis et al evaluated both the patients' and clinicians' perceptions of worry, coping, limitations, expectation of pain relief, and pain interference. When evaluated individually, both patients' and clinicians' perceptions were found to predict outcome at 2, 4, 8, and 12 months. Because many patient characteristics are stable and thus non-responsive to change (such as premorbidity, high levels of depression, and catastrophizing), other risk factors that may be amenable to change such as patients' or clinicians' perceptions and expectations should receive greater attention.

The influence of perception on outcome is highlighted by Kalauokalani et al.'s study of 135 patients with chronic LBP who were allocated randomly to receive either massage or acupuncture (61). Patient expectations regarding the potential helpfulness of each treatment correlated more than other variables with subsequent functional outcomes as assessed at 10 weeks using the modified Roland Score.

Phase of Care

Because the majority of acute patients have a very good prognosis overly aggressive early management

---

Table 9.1 Four Main Factors that Influence Chronic Disability [from Pinchus et al (94)]

- Individual
- Treatment provider
- Compensation or health care system
- Workplace or home environment

is an inefficient use of limited health care resources. However, the same cannot be said for patients who are still symptomatic in the subacute phase. Thus, the subacute phase, beginning at the end of the first month, has now been recognized as a critical period when more aggressive management strategies can potentially have a large impact on preventing chronic pain and disability and thus reducing costs (32).

Frank has presented the concept of the "number needed to treat" to determine the cutoff for when it would be more efficient and cost-effective to substitute more aggressive treatment for less aggressive approach. He states that it is possible to show that "the number (of individuals) needed to treat" to prevent a single case from passing into chronicity at 6 months off work declines swiftly over the first month and then remains rather stable" (32).

According to Frank, there are three distinct stages in terms of risk of an acute episode becoming chronic (Fig. 9.1) (32). In the acute stage (first 4 weeks), the risk of chronicity is low. In the subacute stage (weeks 4–12), the risk is high "ipso facto" and the survival curve suggests aggressive treatment will be cost-effective here. In the chronic stage (after 12 weeks) recovery halts.

This is borne out by a recent study of worker's compensation claimants, in which it was found that the most robust predictors of future status (recurrence likelihood) were preadmission health care visits and more previous back-related claims (43).

Psycho-Social and Other Factors

Psychological variables have been demonstrated to account for 26% of self-reported pain and 36% of self-reported disability (Roland-Morris scale) (87). Six separate review papers of varying methodologic rigor all agreed that psychological characteristics such as coping strategies, self-efficacy beliefs, fear–avoidance behavior, and distress are examples of relevant factors than can be identified (31,55,73,76,94,114). Thus, the presence of psychosocial "yellow flags" indicative of a decreased likelihood of recovery has been proposed as a technique for early identification and matched appropriate management of those with a poorer prognosis (63,77,79,81,100,118).

Do Structural or Psychologic Factors Predict Future Disabling LBP?

A prospective, longitudinal study of 100 subjects with mild persistent low back pain and a predisposition to disc degenerative disease was performed. The development of disabling LBP over a 5-year period was strongly predicted by baseline psychosocial variables ($p<0.0001$–0.004). Structural variables on both MRI and discography testing at baseline had only weak association with back pain episodes and no association with disability or future medical care. Of the structural findings measured only moderate or severe Modic changes of the vertebral end plate were weakly associated with an adverse outcome.

The primary outcome measures at testing during each 6-month interval:

- Episodes of serious back pain (visual analogue scale score of 6)

- Episodes of occupational disability less than 1 week

- Episodes of occupational disability for 1 week

(continued)

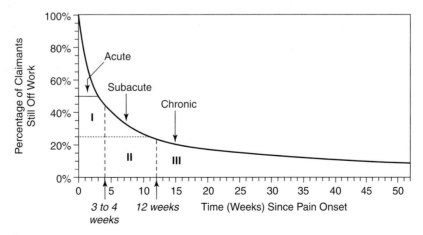

Figure 9.1 Three-phase model of low back pain natural history (32). From Frank JW, Kerr MS, Brooker AS, et al. Disability resulting from occupational low back pain. Part 2: What do we know about secondary prevention? Spine 1996;21:2918–2929.

Gatchel et al. generated a statistical algorithm to identify acute patients at risk for chronic pain/disability (40). By including factors such as gender, self-reported pain, and disability scores, scores on Scale 3 (hysteria) of the Minnesota Multiphasic Personality Inventory (MMPI), and workers' compensation and personal injury status, 90.7% of cases could be correctly classified as high or low risk for chronic pain/disability. The hysteria subscale of the MMPI had an odds ratio of 1.5 for predicting return to work. Thus, individuals with high hysteria scores on the MMPI are 1.5-times more likely to have chronic LBP than those without such scores. The large Boeing prospective trial also found this scale was predictive of future work-related injury (3). However, this is considered to be of minimal utility because it reflects personality, which is considered a trait measure that is not sensitive to change (94).

Further validation of this model showed that a number of other factors also correlate with high risk (98). A less positive temperament identified with the Schedule for Nonadaptive and Adaptive Personality (SNAP), high workaholism (SNAP), an avoidant coping style, and an axis I (psychiatric) disorder were found to predict with 80.8% accuracy (80% sensitivity and 81.5% specificity) whether a person was at high or low risk for chronic LBP (98).

Fransen et al. also showed that early identification of risk factors can predict time off work because of back pain (33). This theoretically should lead to targeted interventions to those individuals at greatest risk for future disability. It was found if workers, at the time they make their initial claim for workman's compensation, report any of the following that the odds that they will still be receiving compensation 3 months later will be significantly increased:

• severe radiating lower limb pain

• at least moderate physical disability (Oswestry)

• psychological distress

• the need to lift for at least three-fourths of the day

• a workplace unable to provide light duties on return to work

The authors concluded, "Importantly, these determinants each retained significant associations with chronic occupational back pain, even when statistical adjustments were made for age, gender, and the other significant individual, psychosocial, or workplace risk factors" (33).

Schultz et al. found that cognitive factors were the most predictive of time off work for low back pain over a 3-month period (102). Cognitive beliefs relating to perceptions of current health, physical status, and expectations of recovery were most relevant. Another very important predictor was sciatica. The overall correct prediction rate was 77.6%.

Thomas and colleagues performed a prospective study that followed 5000 asymptomatic individuals for 18 months and correlated pre-morbid and clinical factors with development of chronic LBP (112). Ten percent of these individuals had LBP, with 34% of these reporting persistent, disabling LBP at 1 week, 3 months, and 12 months after onset. The premorbid features which correlated with persistent, disabling LBP were: sex (female), age (increasing), high psychosocial distress, below average self-rated health, low level of physical activity, history of LBP, and job dissatisfaction. Each of these had a 2- to 5-fold effect on the odds of being associated with persistent symptoms.

The episode specific factors that correlated with the development of persistent disabling LBP were the presence of widespread pain, long duration of symptoms before consultation, leg pain, and significant restrictions in spinal movement. Widespread pain was the most highly correlating item with an odds ratio of 6.4. The other factors were associated with a 2- to 5-fold increased chance of poor outcome. Only 6% of patients with a poor outcome were missed if a minimum of three factors were used to identify risk!!!

Shaw et al. showed that low back disability was related to the following problem-solving approaches: problem avoidance, lack of positive problem-solving orientation, and impulsive decision-making (104).

Fear–Avoidance Beliefs

One of the major goals of care is to reduce activity intolerances associated with pain (2,81). Thus, the cognitive association of activity with pain or anticipation of pain is an important psychological construct (14,24,95,101). In fact, the belief that an activity will be painful has been shown to be more predictive of physical performance than purely nociceptive factors (68,69). Anxious patients predict pain sooner during the performance of physical tasks such as range of motion (ROM) or straight leg raise tests (14,15,24). Council et al. documented substantial correlations between pain expectancies and self-rated physical disability with the performance of simple motor tasks (22).

It is important to distinguish those factors that are associated with chronic pain from those that predict it. For instance, Ciccione showed that depression, somatization, and current pain ratings combined to explain 34% of the variance in work disability in a chronic group (15). However, these factors explained only 8% of the variance in an acute sample! More significant is the finding that pain expectancies accounted for 33% of the variance in acute subjects ($P < 0.001$) (15). Fritz et al. has also confirmed that initial fear–avoidance beliefs were significant predictors of subacute status at 4 weeks independent of pain intensity, physical impairment, disability, or therapy received (34,35). Thus, fear–avoidance beliefs such as pain expectancies begin in acute pain and precede other psychosocial problems that develop as acute pain becomes chronic.

Linton and colleagues found that fear–avoidance beliefs were even prospectively related to the development of acute pain and dysfunction in asymptomatic individuals (75). Those with scores above the median had twice the risk for acute LBP (odds ratio 2.4). Catastrophizing was also evaluated, but its predictive power was more limited (odds ratio 1.5).

Although numerous studies demonstrate the effectiveness of cognitive–behavioral strategies (30,36,65, 74,80,95) simpler re-activation approaches may be all that is needed. Mannion reported that three different active care approaches, none of which consisted of psychological or cognitive–behavioral approaches,

all improved psychological variables related to self-report of pain and disability (87).

Abnormal illness behavior contributes to a slower or inadequate recovery (92,97). Patients who equate hurt with harm develop a disabling form of thinking. They develop fear–avoidance behavior that promotes deconditioning (Fig. 1.9) (81,116). It is important to identify the patient who is fearful and avoid encouraging them to take on a "sick role." According to Troup (113), "If fear of pain persists, unless it is specifically recognized and treated, it leads inexorably to pain-avoidance and thence to disuse."

Cervical and Upper Quarter Risk Factors

Tenenbaum et al. has shown that whiplash-associated disorders classification II patients with neuropsychologic problems have a worse prognosis over a 3-year follow-up period (110). Confidence in one's ability to work after 2 years is correlated with 3-year outcome ($P < 0.0001$) for neck pain caused by whiplash (91). Carroll et al. have demonstrated that high levels of passive coping are associated with disabling cervical or lumbar spine pain (10). These patients have difficulty functioning with pain, are less likely to take responsibility for care, and have lower self-rated health.

Macfarlane et al. performed a prospective study aimed at determining the relative contributions of psychological and work-related factors in the onset of forearm pain (82); 1953 individuals were followed-up for 1 year and 105 (8.3%) developed forearm pain. Increased risks for forearm pain were associated with a number of factors. Psychological distress had a relative risk (RR) of 2.4 (95% confidence interval 1.5–3.8). Multiple areas of pain had a RR of 1.7 (95% confidence interval 0.95–3.0). Repetitive movements of the arm had a RR of 4.1 (95% confidence interval 1.7–10), whereas that of the wrist was 3.4 (95% confidence interval 1.3–8.7). Dissatisfaction with a colleague or supervisor support had a RR of 4.7 (95% confidence interval 2.2–10).

Hill et al. recently reported that the most important factors related to persistent neck pain were age (51–68), concomitant LBP, and regular cycling (53). Age was by far the most significant factor. Both age older than 40 and concomitant LBP were also found to be accurate predictors by Hoving et al. (56). Other authors have has reported that concomitant LBP was a significant prognostic factor for chronic neck pain (20,72,86,93).

Feuerstein (29) followed acute (<6 weeks from onset) cervical and upper quarter pain patients for up to 1 year to ascertain what factors were predictive of 1-month, 3-month, and 12-month outcomes. The findings are summarized in Tables 9.2 and 9.3.

Table 9.2 Risk Factors for Prolonged Cervical and Upper Quarter Pain (29)

1 month
- Upper extremity co-morbidity (RR 1.58)
- Pain severity (RR 1.45)
- Ergonomic risk factor (RR 1.07)
- Low job support (RR 1.03)
- Catastrophizing pain coping style (RR 1.54)

3 months
- Pain severity (RR 10.46)
- Job stress (RR 1.20)
- Catastrophizing pain coping style (RR 1.98)

12 months
- Number of pain treatment episodes (RR 1.77)
- Past recommendations for surgery (RR 6.43)
- Catastrophizing pain coping style (RR 1.87)

Assessment

Linton reviewed psychological risk factors in back and neck pain with the objective to summarize current knowledge concerning the role psychological factors play in the cause and development of back and neck pain (76). In doing so, 913 potentially relevant articles were located and 37 studies consisting of only those with prospective designs to ensure quality. The review procedure resulted in the reporting of the main predictor variables and the outcome criteria. If a statistically significant relation was determined, a plus (+) or minus (–) was used to indicate a positive or negative association, respectively. If no statistical significant relationship was found, a zero (0) was used. The conclusions include a grading system similar to that used for meta-analysis review and guidelines preparation (78). These grades include the following:

Level A: Evidence is supported from two or more good-quality prospective studies

Level B: Evidence is supported from at least one good-quality prospective study

Table 9.3 The Sensitivity and Specificity of Cervical and Upper Quarter Pain Predictors (29)

Duration	Sensitivity	Specificity
1 month	77.4%	71.8%
3 months	80.6%	82.4%
12 months	80.6%	83.3%

Level C: Inconclusive data exist

Level D: No studies were found to meet the criteria utilized

Table 9.4 offers a summary of the conclusions drawn from this review of prospective studies.

What follows is a list of those specific risk factors—called "yellow flags"—for acute LBP pain becoming chronic. These have been identified primarily from an assortment of prospective longitudinal studies. Few cross-sectional studies were used as sources for the "yellow flags." They are divided into those related to symptoms, examination, psychosocial, functional, and work-related factors (Table 9.5). "Yellow flags" are primarily subjective and have a significant psychosocial predominance. Whereas "red flags" such as cauda equina syndrome, cancer, fracture, and infection require urgent attention, further testing, and possibly specialist referral, "yellow flags" only require a shift in the focus of care. These risk factors have been reported to predict future chronic pain or disability in the United States (13,51,83,84), New Zealand (63,77,79), and in England (8).

Subjective psychologic screening through the history taking has low sensitivity and predictive value for identifying distressed or disabled patients, thus formal screening of some sort such as with a questionnaire is recommended (42,46). A 2-item screening test for depression taken from the Primary Care Evaluation of Mental Disorders Procedure (PRIME-MD) was found to be more accurate in screening for depressive symptoms than a physical therapist's own subjective ratings, even for individuals with severe depression (46). Many of these factors can be captured with a simple easy-to-administer form (see appendix).

Linton has suggested the ideal cutoff for considering one definitely at risk is a score of 50% or more, or 65 or more points out of 130 points (77,79,81).

- At this level, the specificity is 75% (people with lower scores who are correctly predicted not to develop chronic disability) and sensitivity is 86% to 88% (people with higher scores who are correctly predicted to develop chronic disability).
- If the cutoff is higher, specificity may increase, even up to 88%, but sensitivity can be compromised down to 34%.
- If the cutoff is lower, sensitivity may increase to more than 90%, but specificity can be compromised down to less than 50%.
- Therefore, the utility of the YF screen depends on the need to know the patients who are at risk versus the need to avoid mislabeling people at risk.

Table 9.4 Grading System for Evaluating Prospective Psychological Risk Factors of Neck and Low Back Pain Chronicity

Risk Factor	Evidence Level
1. Psychosocial variables are clearly linked to the transition from acute to chronic pain disability.	Level A
2. Psychological factors are associated with reported onset of back and neck pain	Level A
3. Psychosocial variables generally have more impact than biomedical or biomechanical factors on back pain disability	Level A
4. No evidence exists to support the idea of a "pain-prone" personality link	Level D
5. Results are mixed with regard to whether personality and traits are risk factors	Level C

6. Cognitive factors (attitudes, cognitive style, fear–avoidance beliefs) are related to the development of pain and disability
   a. Passive coping is related to pain and disability
   b. Pain cognitions (e.g., catastrophizing) are related to pain and disability
   c. Fear–avoidance beliefs are related to pain and disability
	Level A

7. Depression, anxiety, distress, and related emotions are related to pain and disability	Level A
8. Sexual and/or physical abuse may be related to chronic pain and disability	Level D
9. Self-perceived poor health is related to chronic pain and disability	Level A
10. Psychosocial factors may be used as predictors of the risk for developing long-term pain and disability	Level A

Reproduced with permission from Linton SJ. A review of psychological risk factors in back and neck pain. Spine 2000; 9:1148–1156.

Clinical Pearl

It is recommended that a screen of "yellow flags" be performed on the first visit for all spine pain patients.

If the "yellow flags" screen is delayed, then it certainly should be performed as part of the biopsychosocial re-evaluation of a patient who is not recovering satisfactorily at the 4- to 6-week mark. Many of the variables are also worthwhile outcomes of care and can be reassessed at regular intervals (every 4–6 weeks) in the same way as other outcome measurement tools such as the Oswestry or Neck Disability Index questionnaires are utilized.

Two simple questionnaires, the Tampa Scale for kinesiophobia (17 items) and the fear–avoidance beliefs (16 items), were shown to have good internal consistency, test–retest reliability, and concurrent validity for assessing pain-related fear in acute LBP patients (108). All patients had LBP for no more than 4 weeks. This study demonstrates that patients can be classified early as having a psychosocial component to their pain. The implication is that such patients would be suitable for a more cognitive–behaviorally oriented treatment program coupled with functional rehabilitation aimed at reducing activity intolerances and physiologic impairments.

The Waddell Nonorganic Low Back Pain Signs

Introduction

The Waddell non-organic signs are used as objective measures for evaluating abnormal psychosocial issues in patients with low back pain (118). Contrary to the premise behind provocative orthopedic tests in which pain reproduction to identify the specific pain generator is the goal, the objective when performing the non-organic tests is to purposely not try to provoke pain. It can sometimes be difficult to discriminate between patients with a physiological or organic explanation for the test response; therefore, repeating the test a few times to assure evaluator reliability is recommended. Hence, these tests must be performed and interpreted carefully, because applying the test too vigorously can result in a false-positive result.

Table 9.5 Yellow Flags Risk Factors for Acute LBP Becoming Chronic

History and Symptoms
- Duration of symptoms 4–12 weeks (112)
- Sciatica (8,13,33,70,90,103,112)
- History of previous episodes of back pain requiring treatment (8,13)
- Severe pain intensity at 3 weeks (8); at 4 weeks (26); at 6 weeks (41); and at 8 weeks (28)
- Delaying treatment at least 7 days (90,115)
- Widespread pain (112)

Examination
- Positive straight leg raise test (8,19,66,71)
- Positive neurological examination (motor, sensory, reflex) (47,66,52)
- Positive range of motion (ROM) or orthopedic findings (47,52,68,109,112)
- Lack of centralization of peripheral symptoms with repetitive ROM testing (123)

Psychosocial
- 3 or more Waddell signs of illness behavior (70,90,122); no (33)
- Self-rated health as poor (10,112) [(26) at 4 weeks]
- Symptom satisfaction (13)
- Fear–avoidance beliefs (3 questions) [(26) at 4 weeks] (34,49,66,77–79)
  - belief that physical activity makes pain worse
  - belief that if person has pain with activity they should cease the activity
  - belief that person with pain should not perform normal activities with pain
- Anxiety (14,79,80,94)
- Coping (praying, hoping, catastrophizing) (8,70) [large effect sizes (94)]
- Distress/depression (22,27,77,108) [odds ratio approximately 3 and medium magnitude effect size (94)]
- Poor locus of control (yes: 47,70,77–79) (no: 8,88)
- Low expectation of recovery (51,77–79)
- Blaming others (90)
- Negative family or workplace social situation (90)
- Increased number of children being cared for (47)
- Anticipation of future disability or ability to return to work (51,77,78)

Work-Related
- Receiving compensation (90)
- Litigation (90)
- Physically demanding job (or perception of) (47,51,33)
- Job dissatisfaction (3,12,13,19,112,125) (no: 77–79)
- Subjective work-related ability (47)
- Prior disability in the prior 12 months (77–79)
- A workplace unable to provide light duties on return to work (33)
- Low job control or low supervisor support (60)

Functional
- Light work tolerance (77–79)
- Sleep (77–79,90)
- At least moderate physical disability (score of 20/100 or higher with the Oswestry) (33)

The Prognostic Value of the Waddell Signs

The Waddell signs for low back pain have been widely utilized because they have been reported to help identify patients with underlying significant psychologi-

cal distress (118,122). Many studies have identified non-organic behavior using the Waddell signs as predictors of suboptimal surgical and rehabilitation outcomes (16–18,27,62,118,119). Gaines and Hegmann (39) reported in LBP subjects that the presence of even only one sign delayed the median time to return to work by almost four times (58.5 vs. 15 days) and was associated with an increased use of physical therapy and CT scanning.

Fritz and colleagues used the non-organic signs as a screening tool to determine when it was safe to return acute low back pain patients to work (34). The best cutoff values were two or more signs (negative likelihood ratio = 0.75), three or more symptoms (0.62), and an index score of three or more (0.59). The authors reported that even with optimal cutoff values, none of the nonorganic tests served as effective screening tools for early identification of acute LBP patients at increased risk for delay in returning to work. Similarly, Polatin and colleagues reported no significant associations between Waddell total positive score or changes in score and therapeutic success as measured by any of the behavioral outcomes such as return to work in a cohort of patients with chronic, long-term low back pain (96).

The relationship of Waddell signs and the Minnesota Multiphasic Personality Inventory (MMPI) has also been reported (89). Waddell's original article reported that a low but consistent correlation existed between non-organic physical signs and the first three MMPI scales (hypochondriasis, Hs; depression, D; hysteria, Hy) (118). Maruta et al. found that among male patients, MMPI scales 1 (Hs), 3 (Hy), and 8 (schizophrenia, Sc) and high Waddell signs (3–5 signs) were found to correlate with statistically significance, but among the female patients, none of the first three scales correlated, only MMPI scale 8.

In a work-disabled population, non-organic signs were compared to the centralization phenomenon of McKenzie as predictors of the return to work rate (62). The authors reported that the Waddell score was more predictive of the work return outcome compared to the centralization of symptoms.

In 1998, Main and Waddell (85) published a "reappraisal" of the way the non-organic signs should be interpreted. They stressed that isolated signs should not be over-interpreted and that multiple signs suggest that the patient does not have a straightforward physical problem. Psychological factors that coexist with physical conditions may require both physical management of the structural pathology and a psychosocial and behavioral management of their illness. They also stress that the signs are not by themselves, a test of credibility or faking.

Evaluation

There are five signs that are evaluated. The presence of three out of five of these signs is significantly correlated with disability (118). The signs are:

1) Superficial or nonanatomic tenderness—widespread sensitivity to light touch in the lumbar region and pain referred to other areas such as thoracic, sacrum, or pelvis.

2) Simulation—axial loading (light pressure to the skull should not significantly increase low back pain. Passive rotation of the shoulders and pelvis together in a standing patient should not reproduce low back pain.

3) Distractions—difference of 40 to 45 degrees between the supine and seated straight leg raising tests.

4) Regional disturbances—sensory or motor disturbance ("giving way") that is not neurologically correlated.

5) Overreaction—inappropriate overreaction such as guarding, limping, rubbing the affected area, bracing oneself, grimacing, or sighing are all signs of illness behavior.

Because three of the five signs include two separate tests, there are a total of eight tests that make up the five Waddell signs. For those signs that include two tests, if either of the two tests is positive, a positive sign is reported. In other words, it is not necessary for both tests to be positive to result in a positive sign, but rather only one of the two tests. The final score is documented as the total number of positive signs over five (e.g., 2/5). Non-organic LBP must be considered and the psychosocial issues clinically addressed when three or more of the five signs are positive. Wernecke et al. found that these behavioral signs could be improved by a physical rehabilitation program (122).

Waddell's signs were shown to be an integral component of a broader assessment of risk for non-return to work in chronic LBP individuals (67). The full assessment also included measurement of pain intensity, a step test, and a pseudo-strength test. If two of the four tests were positive, correct prediction of risk occurred with a positive predictive value of 0.97 and sensitivity of 0.45. Pain intensity was positive if the Numeric Rating Scale (0–10) score was 9 or 10. The step test was performed for 3 minutes and was positive if the patient stopped it prematurely (see Chapter 12). The pseudo-strength test involved the patient holding two 3-kg weight with straight arms against gravity for 2 minutes. The test was positive if the test was stopped prematurely.

According to Waddell this examination should not be performed on acute patients (118).

1) Tenderness

a) Superficial: Superficial tenderness is defined as widespread sensitivity to light touch of the skin over the lumbar spine. This is evaluated by applying light touch over the lumbar skin

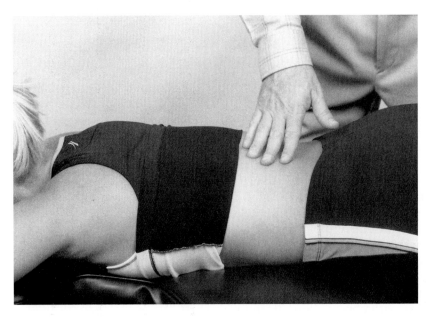

Figure 9.2 Waddell sign—superficial tenderness.

in a manner that should NOT normally pro-voke pain (Fig. 9.2).

b) Non-anatomic: Non-anatomic is defined as bone tenderness over a wide area, often extend-ing to the thoracic spine, sacrum, or pelvis. This is characterized by a non-anatomical, wide area of pain, not localized to one struc-ture or anatomical region.

2) Simulation

a) Axial compression: apply light downward pressure on the head in the direction of the floor (Fig. 9.3). A modification of applying the pressure to the shoulders is suggested to avoid cervical spine symptoms.

b) Trunk rotation: do not turn the shoulders more than the pelvis when trunk rotation is applied (Fig. 9.4).

3) Distraction: Sitting Versus Supine Straight Leg Raise (SLR)

- Sitting distracted SLR (simultaneous testing of the plantar reflex) and supine undistracted SLR (Figs. 9.5A and B)

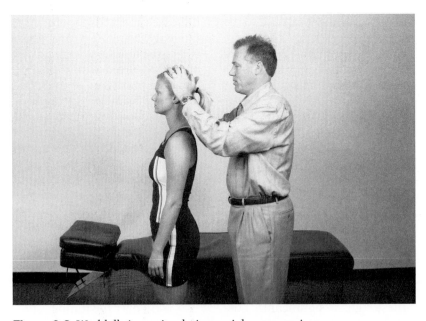

Figure 9.3 Waddell sign—simulation, axial compression.

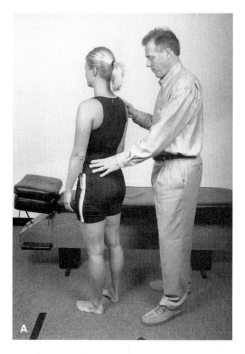
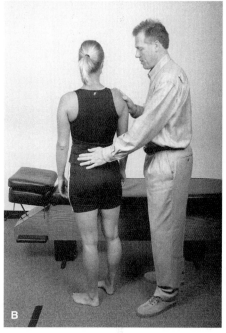

Figure 9.4 **(A)** and **(B)** Waddell sign—simulation, trunk rotation.

- More than a 40-degree difference was defined as significant

This is sometimes referred to as a positive "flip" sign as the patient is "flipped" from supine to sitting (or vise versa).

4) Regional Disturbance

   a) Motor (Fig. 9.6A)

   b) Sensory (Fig. 9.6B)

- Positive test: non-anatomical neurological loss and/or inconsistency on repeated testing
- Findings may include (but are not limited to): breakaway weakness, multiple weakness in an extremity (rule out pain-induced vs. fear-induced weakness), global or patchy altered sensory findings

5) Exaggeration/overreaction

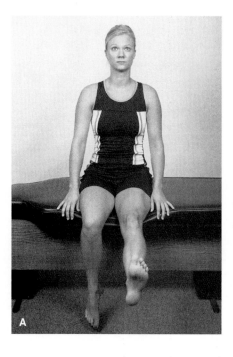
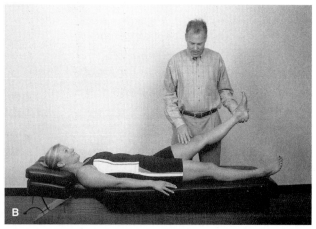

Figure 9.5 **(A)** and **(B)** Waddell sign—distraction: sitting versus supine straight leg raise.

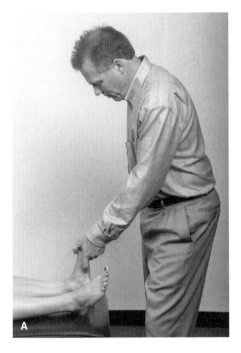

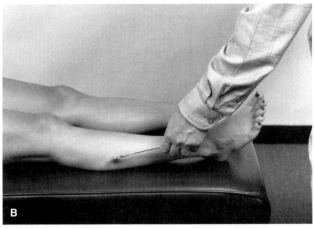

Figure 9.6 (A) Waddell sign—regional disturbance, motor. **(B)** Waddell sign—regional disturbance, sensory.

This sign includes an inappropriate response at any time during the entire physical examination when exaggeration, overreaction, or a disproportionate response such as a tremor, outcry, or collapse occurs (Fig. 9.7). A list of descriptors includes the following:

- Assisted movement (cane, walker, furniture)
- Rigid or slow movement
- Bracing: both limbs supporting weight while seated
- Rubbing the affected area for more than 3 seconds
- Clutching, grasping affected area for more than 3 seconds
- Grimacing
- Sighing with shoulders rising and falling

Nonorganic Neck Pain Signs

Sobel and colleagues developed and assessed the reliability of a group of non-organic signs applicable to neck pain patients (106). Twenty-six consecutive patients with neck pain histories of more than 4 months were evaluated by two health care providers for the presence of cervical nonorganic signs. As patterned after the low back pain signs of Waddell, the five signs consist of seven tests as follows:

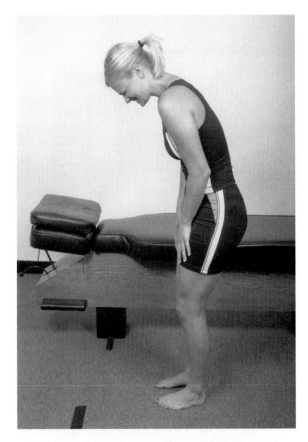

Figure 9.7 Waddell sign—exaggeration/over-reaction.

1. Tenderness
   a. Superficial: patient reports pain with light touch or pinching
   b. Non-anatomical: widespread tenderness outside of the cervical/upper thoracic region to deep palpation

2. Simulation

   Rotation of the head/shoulders/trunk/pelvis while standing

3. Range of motion

   Patient rotates neck right and left as far as possible (positive if >50% deficit in either direction)

4. Regional disturbance
   a. Sensory loss: light touch or pinprick decrease that is non-anatomical
   b. Motor loss: manual muscle testing with non-anatomical weakness with "giveway weakness" or observed normal strength but weakness when formal tests are performed

5. Overreaction

   At any time during the examination, any of the following are observed:
   - Moderate to extremely stiff, rigid, or slow movements
   - Rubbing the affected area for more than 3 seconds
   - Clutching, grasping, or squeezing the area for more than 3 seconds
   - Grimacing because of pain
   - Sighing
   - Disproportionate verbalization
   - Muscle tension

The percent of agreement between the two raters ranged between 68% and 100% with simulation (seated test) being the lowest (68%) and regional sensory disturbance being the highest (100%). The average agreement was 84.6% and the kappa coefficients ranged from 1.00 to 0.16. As the number of positive signs increased, so did the percentage of agreement. This ranged from 77% agreement with a kappa of 0.44 for one sign to 92% agreement (kappa 0.76 for five signs). The test is considered positive if three of five signs are present (106).

Similar to Waddell in his description of the low back pain tests, the authors discussed the importance of care being taken when assessing for over-reaction. This is because over-reaction is very subjective given the cultural variations in response to painful maneuvers as well as the evaluator's own emotional feelings about the patient.

Weaver et al. reported that Waddell signs are an efficient way to identify chronic LBP patients that may be either depressed or anxious (121). The study also suggested that the presence of even just two signs is correlated with more depressive and anxiety symptoms.

Treatment for Patients with High "Yellow Flags" Scores

The results of the "yellow flags" scoring instrument should be used for three purposes: first, to make an informed comment on prognosis; second, to steer care toward the most appropriate interventions; and third, to document patient progress with reliable outcomes.

A patient with a high "yellow flags" score is either experiencing abnormal illness behavior or is at risk for this. Management should be oriented toward reducing dependency on medication and other passive forms of treatment and encourage the development of self-treatment skills. Such a patient is at increased risk for treatment failure with medication, manipulation, exercise, and surgery unless a biobehavorial approach is used. In certain cases, specialist referral for behavorial medicine counseling regarding affective and cognitive issues is required. It is important to realize that "yellow flags" are not the patient's fault, but they suggest management strategies need to be altered to maximize the likelihood of recovery (see Chapters 14 and 31).

Treatments incorporating cognitive–behavioral strategies have been shown to be effective for acute, subacute, and chronic patients (see Chapter 1) (44, 81). Chronically disabled workers have been shown to respond to a light multidisciplinary program that incorporated exercise, activity modification, and fear–avoidance beliefs advice (37,38,48,105). Workers with poor prognoses because of the presence of substantial psychosocial "yellow flags" have responded to extensive multidisciplinary programs that incorporate a structured cognitive–behavioral approach (48,105). A mainstay of these approaches was that return to activity was quota-based, rather than being contingent on absence of symptoms. Such graded activity or "graded exposures" is performed for a specific duration or frequency independent of symptoms.

Another aspect of successful programs is the emphasis on reduction of back-related worry. Reactivation advice included reassurance regarding the safety of gradually resuming activities. These approaches de-emphasize labels suggesting a purely biomedical diagnosis such as herniated disc, arthritis, or injury as the sole cause of pain.

Patient Beliefs About the Nature and Treatment of Their Pain can Change with Cognitive–Behavioral Therapy

Patients with chronic LBP who believed their pain was caused by structural pathology had more disability at baseline and demonstrated greater reductions in disability after a cognitive–behavioral intervention. In all patients, as biomedical/pathology beliefs were reduced, reported disability also decreased.

Walsh DA, Radcliffe JC. Pain beliefs and perceived physical disability of patients with chronic low back pain. Pain 2002; 97:23–31.

■ CONCLUSION

The acute phase of patient care is best served by a minimalist approach. Either excessive diagnostic testing or treatment can be iatrogenic (32). But waiting for pain to become chronic before instituting more aggressive measures is also ineffectual because it is easier to prevent than to treat chronic pain. The key time frame for more focused aggressive management is between 4 and 12 weeks. In particular, those with "yellow flags" should be more aggressively managed as early as possible. The 1-month mark may appear to be a reasonable "decision point" for such evaluation (if it has not already occurred).

The "yellow flags" screen is the ideal re-evaluation tool for a patient not recovering as well as hoped for. It adds little if anything to the cost of the re-evaluation modality of choice—advanced imaging (magnetic resonance imaging)—and is much more likely to reveal clinically useful information that can guide care (9).

A positive "yellow flags" screen does not necessitate cognitive–behavioral therapy (87). But at a minimum, care must shift from primarily passive to active approaches. When these fail, then psychosocial counseling, specifically cognitive–behavioral therapy, is indicated not necessarily because these issues caused acute pain, but because they are interfering with the normal recovery process (78). Framing patient care in this manner takes away the stigma associated with the determination that psychological factors are clinically relevant.

Pain is always a "mind–body" problem. Although physical factors may be involved in the condition's cause, once pain becomes persistent, frustration and even anger are normal reactions. Evaluating "yellow flags" is part of the biopsychosocial approach to managing activity limiting disorders of the spine. It is easy to incorporate into management pathways and will allow customization of appropriate care to each individual patient.

Audit Process
Self-Check of the Chapter's Learning Objectives

- What is the prognosis for acute low back pain becoming chronic?
- What prognostic factors can be used to predict the risk of acute back or neck pain becoming chronic?
  ○ Symptom factors
  ○ Physical examination factors
  ○ Psychosocial factors
  ○ Work-related factors
  ○ Functional factors
- Have a few patients fill out the "yellow flags" questionnaire and score it.
  ○ Was it an administrative challenge?
  ○ Do certain items on the questionnaire stand out?
- Would your "report of findings" be different for a patient with a high level of fear–avoidance beliefs than someone without these?

■ REFERENCES

1. Beurskens AJ, Bombardier C, Croft P, et al. Outcome measures for low back pain research. Spine 1998;23:2003–2013.
2. Bigos S. Agency for Health Care Policy and Research (AHCPR). Acute low-back problems in adults. Clinical Practice Guideline Number 14. Washington, DC: US Government Printing, 1994.
3. Bigos SJ, Battie MC, Spengler DM, et al. A prospective study of work perceptions: Psychosocial factors affecting the report of back injury. Spine 1991;16:1–6.
4. Boden SD, Davis DO, Dina TS, et al. Abnormal magnetic-resonance scans of the lumbar spine in asymptomatic subjects. J Bone Joint Surg [Am] 1990;72:403.
5. Boden SD, McCowin PR, Davis Do, Dina TS, Mark AS, Wiesel S. Abnormal magnetic-resonance scans of the cervical spine in asymptomatic subjects. J Bone Joint Surg 1990;72A:1178–1184.
6. Bombardier C. Outcome assessments in the evaluation of treatment of spinal disorders: Summary and general recommendations. Spine 2000;25: 3100–3103.
7. Brandt-Zawadzki MN, Jensen MC, Obuchowski N, et al. Interobserver and intraobserver variability in interpretation of lumbar disc abnormalities: A comparison of two nomenclatures. Spine 1995;20: 1257–1263.
8. Burton AK, Tillotson K, Main C, Hollis M. Psychosocial predictors of outcome in acute and sub-acute low back trouble. Spine 1995;20:722–728.
9. Carragee EJ, Alamin TF, Miller JL, Carragee JM. Discographic, MRI and psychosocial determinants

of low back pain disability and remission: A prospective study in subjects with benign persistent back pain. Spine J 2005;5:24–35.

10. Carroll L, Mercado AC, Cassidy JD, Cote P. A population-based study of factors associated with combinations of active and passive coping with neck and low back pain. J Rehabil Med 2002;34: 67–72.

11. Cats-Baril WL, Frymoyer JW. Demographic factors associated with the prevalence of disability in the general population: Analysis of the NHANES I database. Spine 1991;16:671–674.

12. Cats-Baril WL, Frymoyer JW. Identifying patients at risk of becoming disabled because of low-back pain. The Vermont Rehabilitation Engineering Center predictive model. Spine 1991;16:605–607.

13. Cherkin DC, Deyo RA, Street JH, Barlow W. Predicting poor outcomes for back pain seen in primary care using patients' own criteria. Spine 1996; 21:2900–2907.

14. Ciccione DS, Just N. Pain expectancy and work disability in patients with acute and chronic pain: A test of the fear avoidance hypothesis. J Pain 2001;2: 181–194.

15. Ciccone DS, Just N, Bandilla EB. Non-organic symptom reporting in patients with chronic non-malignant pain. Pain 1996;68:329–341.

16. Connally GH, Sanders SH. Predicting low back pain patients' response to lumbar sympathetic nerve blocks and interdisciplinary rehabilitation: The role of pretreatment overt pain behavior and cognitive coping strategies. Pain 1991;44:139–146.

17. Cooke C, Menard MR, Beach GN, Locke SR, Hirsch GH. Serial lumbar dynamometry in low back pain. Spine 1992;17:653–662.

18. Cooke C, Dusik LA, Menard MR, Fairburn SM, Feach GN. Relationship of performance on the ERGOS work simulator to illness behavior in a workers' compensation population with low back versus limb injury. J Occup Med 1994;36:757–762.

19. Coste J, Delecoeuillerie G, Cohen DE, Lara A, Le Parc JM, Paolaggi J. Clinical course and prognostic factors in acute low back pain: An inception cohort study in primary care practice. BMJ 1994;308: 577–580.

20. Coté P, Cassidy JD, Carroll L. The factors associated with neck pain and its related disability in the Saskatchewan population. Spine 2000;25: 1109–1117.

21. Council JR, Ahern DK, Follick MJ, Kline CL. Expectancies and functional impairment in chronic low back pain. Pain 1988;33:323–331.

22. Croft PR, Macfarlane GJ, Papageorgiou AC, Thomas E, Silman AJ. Outcome of low back pain in general practice: A prospective study. BMJ 1998;316: 1356–1359.

23. Croft PR, Papageorgiou AC, Ferry S, et al. Psychologic distress and low back pain. Evidence from a prospective study in the general population. Spine 1995;20:2731–2737.

24. Crombez G, Vlaeyen JW, Heuts PH, et al. Pain-related fear is more disabling than pain itself: Evidence on the role of pain-related fear in chronic back pain disability. Pain 1999;80:329–339.

25. Deyo RA, Battie M, Beurskens AJ, et al. Outcome measures for low back pain research. Spine 1998;23:2003–2013.

26. Dionne CE, Koepsell TD, Von Korff M et al. Predicting long-term functional limitations amount back pain patients in primary care settings. J Clin Epidemiol 1997;30:31–43.

27. Dzioba RB, Doxey NC. A prospective investigation into the orthopedic and psychologic predictors of outcome of first lumbar surgery following industrial injury. Spine 1984;9:614–623.

28. Epping-Jordan JE, Wahlgren DR, Williams RA, et al. Transition to chronic pain in men with low-back pain: Predictive relationships among pain intensity, disability, and depressive symptoms. Health Psychol 1998;17:421–427.

29. Feuerstein M, Huang GD, Miller J, Haufler AJ. Development of a screen for predicting clinical outcomes in patients with work-related upper extremity disorders. J Occup Environ Med 2000;42:749–761.

30. Fordyce WE, Brochway JA, Bergman JA, et al. Acute back pain: A control-group comparison of behavioral vs. traditional management methods. J Behav Med 1986;9:127.

31. Frank J, Sinclair S, Hogg-Johnson S, et al. Preventing disability from work-related low-back pain. New evidence gives new hope—if we can just get all the players onside. Can Med Assoc J 1998;158: 1625–1631.

32. Frank JW, Kerr MS, Brooker AS, et al. Disability resulting from occupational low back pain. Part 2: What do we know about secondary prevention? Spine 1996;21:2918–2929.

33. Fransen M, Woodward M, Norton R, Coggan C, Dawe M, Sheridan N. Risk factors associated with the transition from acute to chronic occupational back pain. Spine 2002;27:92–98.

34. Fritz JM, Wainner RS, Hicks GE. The use of non-organic signs and symptoms as a screening tool for return-to-work in patients with acute low back pain. Spine 2000;25:1925–1931.

35. Fritz JM, George SZ, Delitto A. The role of fear-avoidance beliefs in acute low back pain: Relationships with current and future disability and work status. Pain 2001;94:7–15.

36. Frost H, Lamb SE, Shackleton CH. A functional restoration program for chronic low back pain: A prospective outcome study. Physiother 2000;86: 285–293.

37. Frost H, Lamb S, Klaber Moffett JA, Faribank JCT, Moser JS. A fitness program for patients with chronic low back pain: Two-year follow-up of a randomized controlled trial. Pain 1998;75:273–279.

38. Frost H, Klaber Moffett JA, Moser JS, Faribank JCT. Randomized controlled trial for evaluation of fitness programmed for patients with chronic low back pain. Br Med J 1995;310:151–154.

39. Gaines WG, Hegmann KT. Effectiveness of Waddell's nonorganic signs in predicting a delayed return to regular work in patients experiencing acute occupational low back pain. Spine 1999;24: 396–401.

40. Gatchel RJ, Polatin PB, Mayer TG. The dominant role of psychosocial risk factors in the development

of chronic low back pain disability. Spine 1995;20: 2702–2709.

41. Gatchel R. Polatin PB, Kinney RK. Predicting outcome of chronic back pain using clinical predictors of psychopathology: A prospective analysis. Health Psychol 1995;14:415–420.

42. Grevitt M, Pande K, O'Dowd J, Webb J. Do first impressions count? A comparison of subjective and psychologic assessment of spinal patients. Eur Spine J 1998;7:218–223.

43. Gross DP, Battie MC. Predicting timely recovery and recurrence following multidisciplinary rehabilitation in patients with compensated low back pain. Spine 2005;30:235–240.

44. Guzman J, Esmail R, Karjalainen K, Malmivaara A, Irvin E, Bombardier C. Multidisciplinary bio-psycho-social rehabilitation for chronic low back pain (Cochrane Review). In: Cochrane Library, Issue 2. Oxford: Update Software, 2003.

45. Hadler NM. Regional back pain. N Engl J Med 1986;315:1090–1092.

46. Haggman S, Maher CG, Refshauge KM. Screening for symptoms of depression by physical therapists managing low back pain. Phys Ther 2004;84:1157–1166.

47. Haldorsen EMH, Inhalhl A, Ursin H. Patients with low-back pain not returning to work. A 12-month follow-up study. Spine 1998;23:1202–1208.

48. Haldorsen EMH, Grasada AL, Skouen JS, et al. Is there a right treatment for a particular patient group? Comparison of ordinary treatment, light multidisciplinary treatment, and extensive multidisciplinary treatment for long-term sick-listed employees with musculoskeletal pain. Pain 2002:95:49–63.

49. Hasenbring M, Marienfeld G, Kuhlendahl D, Soyka D. Risk Factors of chronicity in lumbar disc patients: A prospective investigation of biologic, psychologic, and social predictors of therapy outcome. Spine 1994;19:2759–2765.

50. Hashemi L, Webster BS, Clancy EA, Volinn E. Length of disability and cost of workers' compensation low back pain claims. J Occup Environ Med 1998;40:261–269.

51. Hazard RG, Haugh LD, Reid S, Preble JB, MacDonald L. Early prediction of chronic disability after occupational low back injury. Spine 1996;21: 945–951.

52. Hellsing AL, Linton SJ, Kalvemark M. A prospective study of patients with acute back and neck pain in Sweden. Phys Ther 1994;74:116–128.

53. Hill J, Lewis M, Papageorgiou AC, Dziedzic K, Croft P. Predicting persistent neck pain. Spine 2004;29: 1648–1654.

54. Hitselberger WE, Witten RM. Abnormal myelograms in asymptomatic patients. J Neurosurg 1968;28:204.

55. Hoogendoorn WE, van Poppel MN, Bongers PM, et al. Systematic review of psychosocial factors at work and private life as risk factors for back pain. Spine 2000;25:2114–2125.

56. Hoving JL, de Vet HCW, Twisk JWR, et al. Prognostic factors for neck pain in general practice. Pain 2004;110:639–645.

57. Jarvik JG, Deyo RA. Imaging of lumbar intervertebral disc degeneration and aging, excluding disc herniations. Radiol Clin North Am 2000;38: 1255–1266.

58. Jensel MC, Brant-Zawadzki MN, Obuchowki N, et al. Magnetic resonance imaging of the lumbar spine in people without back pain. N Engl J Med 1994;2:69.

59. Junge A, Dvorak J, Ahern S. Predictors of bad and good outcomes of lumbar disc surgery: A prospective clinical study with recommendations for screening to avoid bad outcomes. Spine 1995;20: 4600–4608.

60. Kaila-Kangas L, Kivimaki M, Riihimaki H, Luukkonen R, Kirjonen J, Leino-Arjas P. Psychosocial factors at work as predictors of hospitalization for back disorders. A 28-year follow-up of industrial employees. Spine 2004;29:1823–1830.

61. Kalauokalani D, Cherkin DC, Sherman KJ, et al. Patient expectations and treatment effects: Lessons from a trial of acupuncture and massage for low back pain. Spine 2001;26:1418–1424.

62. Karas R, McIntosh G, Hall H, Wilson L, Melles T. The relationship between nonorganic signs and centralization of symptoms in the prediction of return to work for patients with low back pain. Phys Ther 1997;77:354–368.

63. Kendall, NAS, Linton, SJ, Main, CJ. Guide to assessing psychosocial yellow flags in acute low back pain: Risk factors for long-term disability and work loss. Wellington, NZ: Accident Rehabilitation & Compensation Insurance Corporation of New Zealand and the National Health Committee, 1997:1–22.

64. Kendrick D, Fielding K, Bentler E, Kerslake R, Miller P, Pringle M. Radiography of the lumbar spine in primary care patients with low back pain: Randomized controlled trial. BMJ 2001;322:400–405.

65. Klaber Moffet J, Torgerson D, Bell-Syer S, et al. A randomized trial of exercise for primary care back pain patients: Clinical outcomes, costs, and preferences. Br Med J 1999;319:279–283.

66. Klenerman L, Slade P, Stanley I, et al. The prediction of chronicity in patients with an acute attack of low back pain in a general practice setting. Spine 1995;20:478–484.

67. Kook JP, Oesch PR, De Bie RA. Predictive tests for non-return to work in patients with chronic low back pain. Eur Spine J 2002;11:258–266.

68. Lackner JM, Carosella AM. The relative influence of perceived pain control, anxiety, and functional self-efficacy on spinal function among patients with chronic low back pain. Spine 1999;24:2254–2261.

69. Lackner JM, Carosella AM, Feuerstein M. Pain expectancies, pain, and functional self-efficacy expectancies as determinants of disability in patients with chronic low back disorders. J Consult Clin Psych 1996;64:212–220.

70. Lancourt J, Ketteljut M. Predicting return to work for lower back pain patients receiving worker's compensation. Spine 1992;17:629–640.

71. Lanier DC, Stockton P. Clinical predictors of outcome of acute episodes of low-back pain. J Fam Pract 1988;27:483–489.

72. Leino P, Magni G. Depressive and distress symptoms as predictors of low back pain, neck-shoulder pain, and other musculoskeletal morbidity: A 10-year follow-up of metal industry employees. Pain 1993;53:89–94.

73. Liebenson CS, Yeomans SG. Yellow Flags: Early identification of risk factors of chronicity in acute patients. J Rehabil Outcomes Meas 2000;4:31–40.

74. Lindstrom A, Ohlund C, Eek C, et al. Activation of subacute low back patients. Phys Ther 1992;4:279–293.

75. Linton SJ, Buer N, Vlaeyen J, Hellsing AL. Are fear-avoidance beliefs related to a new episode of back pain? A prospective study. Psychol Health 2000;14:1051–1059.

76. Linton SJ. A review of psychological risk factors in back and neck pain. Spine 2000;9:1148–1156.

77. Linton SJ, Hallden BH. Can we screen for problematic back pain? A screening questionnaire for predicting outcome in acute and subacute back pain. Clin J Pain 1998;14:1–7.

78. Linton SJ, Andersson T. Can chronic disability be prevented? A randomized trial of a cognitive-behavioral intervention for spinal pain patients. Spine 2000;25:2825–2831.

79. Linton SJ, Hallden K. Risk factors and the natural course of acute and recurrent musculoskeletal pain: Developing a screening instrument. In: Jensen TS, Turner JA, Wiesenfeld-Hallin Z, eds. Proceedings of the 8th World Congress on Pain, Progress in Pain Research and Management, Vol 8. Seattle: IASP Press, 1997.

80. Linton SL, Hellsing AL, Andersson D. A controlled study of the effects of an early active intervention on acute musculoskeletal pain problems. Pain 1993;54:353–359.

81. Linton SL. New avenues for the prevention of chronic musculoskeletal pain and disability. Amsterdam: Elsevier, 2002.

82. Macfarlane GJ, Hunt IM, Silman AJ. Role of mechanical and psychosocial factors in the onset of forearm pain: prospective population based study. BMJ 2000;321:676—679.

83. Magni G, Moreschi C, Rigatti-Luchini S, Merskey H. Prospective study on the relationship between depressive symptoms and chronic musculoskeletal pain. Pain 1994;56:289–297.

84. Magni G, Marchitti M, Moreschi C, Merskey H, Luchini SR. Chronic musculoskeletal pain and depressive symptoms in the National Health and Nutrition Examination: I. Epidemiological follow-up study. Pain 1993;53:161–168.

85. Main CJ, Waddell G. Behavioral responses to examination: a reappraisal of the interpretation of "nonorganic signs." Spine 1998;23:2367–2371.

86. Mäkelä M, Heliövaara M, Sievers K, Impivaara O, Knekt P, Aromaa A. Prevalence, determinants, and consequences of chronic neck pain in Finland. Am J Epidemiol 1991;134:1356–1367.

87. Mannion AF, Junge A, Taimela S, Muntener M, Lorenzo K, Dvorak J. Active therapy for chronic low back pain. Part 3. Factors influencing self-rated disability and its change following therapy. Spine 2001;26:920–929.

88. Mannion AF, Dolan P, Adams MA. Psychological questionnaires: Do "abnormal" scores precede or follow first-time low back pain? Spine 1996;21:2603–2611.

89. Maruta T, Goldman S, Chan CW, Ilstrup DM, Kunselman AR, Colligan RC. Waddell's nonorganic signs and Minnesota Multiphasic Personality Inventory profiles in patients with chronic low back pain. Spine 1997;22:72–75.

90. McIntosh G, Frank J, Hogg-Johnson S, Bombardier C, Hall H. Prognostic factors for time receiving workers' compensation benefits in a cohort of patients with low back pain. Spine 2000;25:147–157.

91. Miettinen T, Leino E, Airaksinen O, Lindgren KA. The possibility to use simple validated questionnaires to predict long-term health problems after whiplash injury. Spine 2004;29:E47–E51.

92. Philips HC, Grant L. The evolution of chronic back pain problems. Behav Res Ther 1991;29:435–441.

93. Pietri-Taleb F, Riihimaki H, Viikari-Juntura E, Lindstrom K. Longitudinal study o the role of personality characteristics and psychological distress in neck trouble among working men. Pain 1994;58:261–267.

94. Pincus T, Burton A, Vogel S, Field AP. A systematic review of psychological factors as predictors of chronicity/disability in prospective cohorts of low back pain. Spine 2002;27:E109–E120.

95. Pincus T, Vlaeyen JWS, Kendall NAS, Von Korff MR, Kalauokalani DA, Reis S. Cognitive-behavioral therapy and psychosocial factors in low back pain: Directions for the future. Spine 2002;27:E133–E138.

96. Polatin PB, Cox B, Gatchel RJ, Mayer TG. A prospective study of Waddell Signs in patients with chronic low back pain: When they may not be predictive. Spine 1997;22:1618–1621.

97. Potter R, Jones JM. The evolution of chronic pain among patients with musculoskeletal problems: A pillow study in primary care. Br J Gen Pract 1992;42:462–464.

98. Pulliam CB, Gatchel RJ, Gardea MA. Psychosocial differences in high risk versus low risk acute low-back pain patients. J Occupat Rehab 2001;11:43–52.

99. Reis S, Hermoni D, Borkan J, et al. The RAMBAM–Israeli Sentinel Practice Network The LBP Patient Perception Scale. A new predictor of chronicity and other episode outcomes among primary care patients. (In Preparation).

100. Royal College of General Practitioners (RCGP). The development and implementation of clinical guidelines. Report of the Clinical Guidelines Working Group. London: Royal College of General Practitioners, 1995:1–31.

101. Royal College of General Practitioners (RCGP). Clinical Guidelines for the Management of Acute Low Back Pain. London, Royal College of General Practitioners (www.rcgp.org.uk), 1999.

102. Schultz IZ, Crook JM, Berkowitz J, et al. Biopsychosocial multivariate model of occupational low back disability. Spine 2002;27:2720–2725.

103. Selim AJ, Xinhua SR, Graeme F, et al. The importance of radiating leg pain in assessing health outcomes among patients with low back pain. Spine 1998;23:470–474.

104. Shaw WS, Feuerstein M, Haufler AJ, Berkowitz SM, Lopez MS. Working with low back pain: Problem-solving orientation and function. Pain 2001;93:129–137.

105. Skouen JS, Grasdal AL, Haldorsen EMH, et al. Relative cost-effectiveness of extensive and light multidisciplinary treatment programs versus treatment as usual for patients with chronic low back pain on long-term sick leave. Spine 2002;27:901–910.

106. Sobel JB, Sollenberger P, Robinson R, Polatin PB, Gatchel RJ. Cervical nonorganic signs: A new clinical tool to assess abnormal illness behavior in neck pain patients: A plot study. Arch Phys Med Rehabil 2000;81:170–175.

107. Spitzer WO, Le Blanc FE, Dupuis M, et al. Scientific approach to the assessment and management of activity-related spinal disorders: A monograph for clinicians. Report of the Quebec Task Force on Spinal Disorders. Spine 1987;12(suppl 7):S1–S59.

108. Swinkels-Meewisse EJCM, Swinkesl RAHM, Verbeek ALM, Vlaeyen JWS, Oostendorp RAB. Psychometric properties of the Tampa Scale for kinesiophobia and the fear-avoidance beliefs questionnaire for acute low back pain. Man Ther 2003;8:29–36.

109. Takala EP, Vikari-Juntura E. Do functional tests predict low back pain. Spine 2000;25(16):2126–2132.

110. Tenenbaum A, Rivano-Fischer M, Tjell C, Edblom M, Sunnerhagen KS. The Quebec Classification and a new Swedish classification for whiplash-associated disorders in relation to life satisfaction in patients at high risk of chronic functional impairment and disability. J Rehabil Med 2002;34:114–118.

111. Teresi LM, Lufkin RB, Reicher MA, et al. Asymptomatic degenerative disk disease and spondylosis of the cervical spine: MR Imaging. Radiol 1987;164:83–88.

112. Thomas E, Silman AJ, Croft PR, Papageorgiou AC, Jayson MIV, Macfarlane GJ. Predicting who develops chronic low back pain in primary care: A prospective study. BMJ 1999;318:1662–1667.

113. Troup JDG. The perception of pain and incapacity for work: Prevention and early treatment. Physiother 1988;74:435.

114. Truchon M, Fillion L. Biopsychosocial determinants of chronic disability and low-back pain: A review. J Occup Rehabil 2000;10:117–142.

115. van den Hoogen HJM, Koes BW, Deville W, van Eijk JTM, Bouter LM. The prognosis of low back pain in general practice. Spine 1997;22:1515–1521.

116. Vlaeyen JWS, Linton S. Fear-avoidance and its consequences in chronic musculoskeletal pain. A state of the art. Pain 2000;85:317–332.

117. Von Korff M, Deyo RA, Cherkin D, Barlow W. Back pain in primary care: Outcomes at 1 year. Spine 1993;18:855–862.

118. Waddell G, McCulloch JA, Kimmel E, Venner RM. Nonorganic physical signs in low back pain. Spine 1980;5:117–125.

119. Waddell G, Morris EW, Di Paola MP, Bicher M, Finlayson DA. Concept of illness tested as an improved basis for surgical decisions in low back disorders. Spine 1986;11:712–719.

120. Walsh DA, Radcliffe JC. Pain beliefs and perceived physical disability of patients with chronic low back pain. Pain 2002;97:23–31.

121. Weaver CS, Kvaal SA, McCracken L. Waddell signs as behavioral indicators of depression and anxiety in chronic pain. J Back Musculoskel Rehabil 2003/2004;17:21–26.

122. Werneke MW, Harris EX, Di Paloa MP, Bicher M, Finlayson D. Clinical effectiveness of behavioral signs for screening chronic low-back pain patients in a work-oriented physical rehabilitation program. Spine 1993;18:2412–2418.

123. Werneke M, Hart DL. Centralization phenomenon as a prognostic factor for chronic low back pain and disability. Spine 2001;26:758–765.

124. Wiesel SE, Tsourmans N, Feffer HL, et al. A study of computer-assisted tomography. I. The incidence of positive CAT scans in an asymptomatic group of patients. Spine 1984;9:549.

125. Williams DA, Feuerstein M, Durbin D, Pezzulo J. Healthcare and indemnity costs across the natural history of disability in occupational low back pain. Spine 1998;23:2329–2336.

YELLOW FLAG FORM

Name _____ Primary complaint-_____

1. Please indicate your usual level of pain during **the past week**
    No pain   **Worst pain possible**
    0   1   2   3   4   5   6   7   8   9   10

2. Does pain, numbness, tingling or weakness <u>extend</u> into your leg (from the low back) &/or arm (from the neck)?
    None of the time   **All of the time**
    0   1   2   3   4   5   6   7   8   9   10

3. How would you **rate your general health?**   (10-x)
    Poor   **Excellent**
    0   1   2   3   4   5   6   7   8   9   10

4. If you had to spend the rest of your life with your <u>condition as it is right now</u>, how would you feel about it?
    Delighted   **Terrible**
    0   1   2   3   4   5   6   7   8   9   10

5. How anxious (eg. tense, uptight, irritable, fearful, difficulty in concentrating / relaxing) you have been feeling during **the past week:**
    Not at all   **Extremely anxious**
    0   1   2   3   4   5   6   7   8   9   10

6. How much you have been able to control (i.e., reduce/help) your pain/complaint on your own during **the past week:**
    I can reduce it   **I can't reduce it at all**
    0   1   2   3   4   5   6   7   8   9   10

7. Please indicate how depressed (eg. Down-in-the-dumps, sad, downhearted, in low spirits, pessimistic, feelings of hopelessness) you have been feeling in **the past week:**
    Not depressed at all   **Extremely depressed**
    0   1   2   3   4   5   6   7   8   9   10

8. On a scale of 0 to 10, how certain are you that you will be doing normal activities or working in <u>**six months?**</u>
    Very certain   **Not certain at all**
    0   1   2   3   4   5   6   7   8   9   10

9. I can do light work for an hour?
    Completely agree   **Completely disagree**
    0   1   2   3   4   5   6   7   8   9   10

10. I can sleep at night
    Completely agree   **Completely disagree**
      0   1   2   3   4   5   6   7   8   9   **10**

11. An increase in pain is an indication that I should stop what I am doing until the pain decreases.
    Completely disagree   **Completely agree**
      0   1   2   3   4   5   6   7   8   9   **10**

12. Physical activity makes my pain worse?
    Completely disagree   **Completely agree**
      0   1   2   3   4   5   6   7   8   9   **10**

13. I should not do my normal activities including work with my present pain.
    Completely disagree   **Completely agree**
      0   1   2   3   4   5   6   7   8   9   **10**

Please sign your name _____ Date _____

SCORING & RISK:

Low risk of chronic disability – under 55 points
Moderate risk of chronic disability – 55 to 65 points
High risk of chronic pain and disability – over 65 points

10

Evaluation of Muscular Imbalance

Vladimír Janda, Clare Frank, and
Craig Liebenson

Learning Objectives
After reading this chapter you should be able to understand:

- The etiology of muscle imbalance
- How to evaluate muscles for tightness or inhibition
- The interplay of different synergist and antagonist muscles during basic movement patterns
- How to evaluate posture for signs of muscle imbalance
- The basic elements of gait analysis

This chapter is dedicated to the memory of Pr. Vladimír Janda (1928–2002) who passed away on November 25, 2002.

Introduction

The primary basis of the functional approach to musculoskeletal pain syndromes is the interdependence of all structures from both the central nervous and musculoskeletal system in the production and control of motion. Movement of non-contractile and contractile elements is produced and controlled by muscle activity. Ultimately, it is the central nervous system in response to various stimuli that controls the activity of muscles and consequently, the pattern of motion in an individual's musculoskeletal system. The muscular system lies at a functional crossroad because it is influenced by stimuli from both the central nervous system and musculoskeletal system. Dysfunction in any component of these systems is ultimately reflected in the muscular system in the form of altered muscle tone, muscle contraction, muscle balance, coordination, and performance. Therefore, a strictly localized lesion does not exist. Muscle imbalance is a systemic change in the quality of muscle dysfunction that results in altered joint mechanics leading to pain, dysfunction, and eventually degeneration. Muscle imbalance is the altered relationship and balance between muscles that are prone to inhibition or weakness and those that prone to tightness or shortness. Moderately tight muscles are usually stronger than normal. However, in the presence of pronounced tightness, some decrease of muscle strength occurs. This weakness is called "tightness weakness" (1) to express the closed association between muscle weakness and altered viscoelasticity of the muscle. Therefore, when diagnosing muscle weakness, careful differential diagnoses have to be made. The treatment of tightness weakness is not in strengthening, which would increase tightness and possibly result in a more pronounced weakness, but in stretching, oriented toward influencing the viscoelastic property of the muscle, i.e., the noncontractile but retractile connective tissue. Stretching of tight muscles also results in improved strength of inhibited antagonistic muscles, probably mediated via Sherrington's law of reciprocal innervation.

The etiology and terminology of muscle tone is full of controversies, partly because various authors' definitions of muscle tone differ. Therefore, a detailed differential diagnosis has to be made among others because each condition requires a different type of treatment (2). Unfortunately, a precise and adequate analysis is often neglected. An imprecise diagnosis results in disappointing therapeutic results. Unfortunately, the detailed physiology of muscle tone is unknown and studies of muscle tone changes caused by altered or impaired function have not been studied sufficiently in the laboratory or in the clinic.

In principle it is necessary to differentiate whether the main changes occur in the connective tissue of the muscle (viscoelastic properties) or in over-activation of the contractile components of the muscle (contractile properties). According to Mense and Simons, "Muscle tension depends physiologically on 2 factors: the basic viscoelastic properties of the soft tissues associated with the muscle, and/or the degree of activation the contractile apparatus of the muscle" (9). In the former, we speak about muscle tightness, stiffness, loss of flexibility, or extensibility (length), and in the latter, it is a real increase of muscle contractile activity such as in spasmodic torticollis or trismus. In principle, with respect to viscoelastic changes, the muscle gets shorter at rest (decreased extensibility), either because of shortening of contractile muscle fibers or because of retraction of the connective tissue within the muscle and the adjacent fascia. With respect to contractile changes, the increased muscle tone may involve the majority of muscle fibers of the muscles or only a limited number as found as "taut bands" in trigger points.

Clinically, resting muscle tone presents a combination of both situations (contractile and viscoelastic properties), and it is the role of the clinician to establish an appropriate diagnosis (9). However, measuring muscle tone objectively presents a dilemma. Tests of viscoelasticity involve measurements of the velocity of motion, viscosity, thixotropy, and resonant frequency when load is gradually applied (9). Tests of contractile activity are simpler in that EMG can be used; however, this is not without inherent difficulties, as in trigger points where only small loci in the muscle show increased electrical activity (9).

A detailed differential diagnosis of muscle tone is necessary for the proper treatment approach, and this can be accomplished by a combination of inspection and palpation (Table 10.1). Layer palpation of the skin, subcutaneous tissue, fascia, fat, and any other structure in the area concerned, although purely subjective is a practical clinical tool and with much practice and experience, detecting the type of muscle tone present in the concerned area can be skillfully achieved. Inspection of posture, movement patterns, and gait also yields invaluable clinical information about the underlying source of increased muscle tension.

Muscle imbalance should be considered a systemic reaction of the striated muscles. It is therefore a general reaction of the whole muscle system and not just an isolated response of an individual muscle (4). This view is strongly supported by the recent findings of neurodevelopmental kinesiology, which show developmental movement patterns corresponding to the muscle imbalance found in children when their motor system is fully myelinized (at the age of 6 to 7 years) or in adults (7,8,12). The basis from a neurodevelopmental viewpoint is that neonatal and early infant posture is maintained by a "tonic" muscle system. Subsequent neurodevelopment of the upright pos-

Table 10.1 Functional Types of Muscular Hypertonicity (from Janda) (2)

Types	Anatomically Distributed*	Spontaneously Painful**	Other Signs
Limbic	no	no	stress i.e., tension headache
Segmental	yes	yes	antagonist weak, painful to stretch
Reflex "spasm"	not always	yes ↑ E.M.G. at rest	:Defense Musculare" i.e. wry neck
Trigger Points (partial "muscle spasm")		part of active TP—yes muscle latent TP—no	parts of muscle hyperirritable, neighboring muscle fibers inhibited
Muscle Tightness	yes	no	↑ irritability, ↓ extensibility

*Anatomically distributed = hypertonicity is present in specific anatomically defined muscles and not in parts of different muscles in the same area.
**Spontaneously painful = a muscle is a source of pain at rest and not merely painful on palpation.
Reproduced with permission from Liebenson CS. Active Muscular Relaxation Techniques, Part One: Basic Principles and Methods. J Manipulative Physiol Ther 1989;12:6 (Table 2).

ture occurs with the co-activation of a "phasic" muscle system with the "tonic" muscle system. Failure of this co-activation between the tonic and phasic muscle system results in a muscle imbalance and is clearly evident in children with cerebral palsy in which the "tonic" muscle system prevails. In addition, the typical muscle responses seen in chronic low back patients are observed to be identical or very similar to those that are seen in some structural lesions of the central nervous system. For example, in spasticity seen in a cerebrovascular accident or cerebral palsy, muscles that develop spasticity or even spastic contractures are those that commonly respond by tightness in musculoskeletal conditions. It is proposed that these typical muscle responses observed in the typical hemiplegic posture may be an extreme expression of the imbalance between the muscular chains that exist to some extent under normal physiologic conditions. Thus, the tendency for some muscles to develop weakness or tightness does not occur randomly but rather in typical "muscle imbalance patterns" (3). Furthermore, the development of these patterns can be predicted clinically and preventative measures should be taken because muscle imbalance does not remain limited to a certain part of the body, but gradually involves the whole striated muscular system (6). A thorough evaluation is necessary to introduce preventive measures because muscle imbalance usually precedes the appearance of pain syndromes.

Muscle imbalance develops mainly between predominantly "tonic" muscles, that is, muscles that are prone to develop tightness and predominantly "phasic" muscles, that is, muscles that are prone to develop inhibition (Table 10.2). Muscle imbalance involves muscles of the whole body; however, if the imbalance is more evident or starts to develop gradually and predictably in the pelvic region, we speak about the pelvic or distal crossed syndrome, and if it is more evident or starts in the shoulder girdle/neck region, we term it as a proximal or shoulder girdle crossed syndrome (5).

The proximal (upper, shoulder–neck) crossed syndrome is characterized by the development of tightness in the upper trapezius, levator scapulae, and pectoralis major, and inhibition in the deep neck flexors and lower stabilizers of the scapula. Topographically, when the inhibited and tight muscles are connected, they form a cross (Fig. 10.1). This pattern of muscle imbalance produces typical changes in posture and motion. In standing, elevation and protraction of the shoulders are evident, as are also rotation and abduction of the scapula, a variable degree of winging, and a push-forward head position. This altered posture is likely to stress the cervicocranial and the cervicothoracic junctions. In addition, the stability of the shoulder blades is decreased, because of the altered angle of the glenoid fossa, and, as a consequence, all movement patterns of the upper extremity are altered.

The distal (lower, hip–pelvic) crossed syndrome is characterized by tightness of the hip flexors and spinal erectors and inhibition and weakness of the gluteal and abdominal muscles. As in the upper crossed syndrome, a line connecting the tight and inhibited muscles forms a cross (Fig. 10.2). This imbalance results in an anterior tilt of the pelvis, increased flexion of the hips, and a compensatory hyperlordosis in the lumbar spine. This imbalance tends to over-stress both hip joints as well as the lower back.

Table 10.2   Muscle Imbalances

Muscle that have a tendency to develop: Tightness/Shortness	Weakness/Inhibition
Gastrocsoleus	Tibialis anterior
Hip flexors	
Rectus femori	Vasti (in particular, the vastus medialis obliquus)
Iliopsoas	Gluteus maximus
Tensor fascia lata	Gluteus medius and minimus
Adductors	Abdominal wall
Hamstrings	Lower and middle trapezius
Erector spinae	Serratus anterior
Quadratus lumborum	Deep neck flexors (longus colli and capitis)
Piriformis	Scalenes
Upper trapezius/levator scapulae	Upper extremity extensors
Pectorals	
Sternocleidomastoid	
Short deep cervical extensors	
Upper extremity flexors	

A combination of these two syndromes is expressed in a layer (stratification) syndrome (Fig. 10.3). When a layer syndrome is observed in a patient, it is a sign of a poorer prognosis in terms of rehabilitation because of the fixed muscle imbalance patterns at the central nervous system level.

Examination of joints must precede muscle evaluation of muscles to exclude any anatomical barrier. In clinical practice, it is advisable to begin muscle

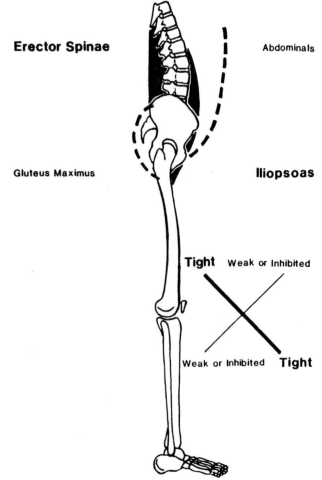

Figure 10.2 Lower crossed syndrome.

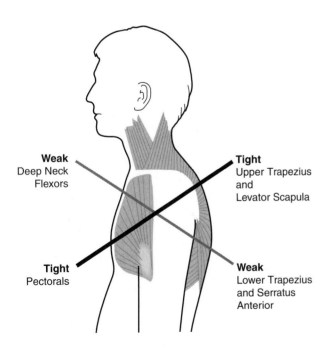

Figure 10.1 Upper crossed syndrome.

Muscle Hypotrophy   **Muscle Hypertrophy**

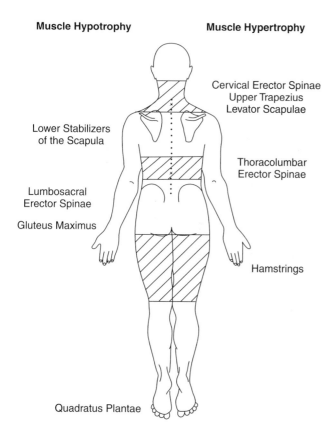

Cervical Erector Spinae
Upper Trapezius
Levator Scapulae

Lower Stabilizers
of the Scapula

Thoracolumbar
Erector Spinae

Lumbosacral
Erector Spinae

Gluteus Maximus

Hamstrings

Quadratus Plantae

Figure 10.3 Layer (stratification) syndrome.

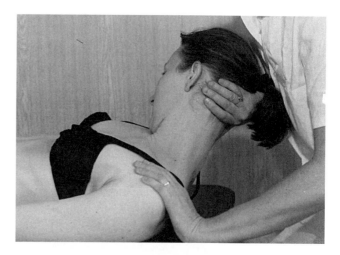

Figure 10.4 Upper trapezius.

evaluation by analyzing erect standing posture and gait. This analysis requires experience and keen observational skill. In addition, it serves as a screening tool by providing quick and reliable information to direct the clinician the necessary tests that need to be performed in detail and those that can be omitted. The clinician is given an overall view of the patient's muscle function through posture and gait analysis and is challenged to look comprehensively at the patient's entire motor system and not to limit attention to the local level of the lesion. Evaluation of muscle imbalance in a patient with an acute pain syndrome, however, is unreliable and must be undertaken with precaution. A precise evaluation of tight muscles and movement patterns can be performed only if the patient is pain-free or almost pain-free. Its usefulness is greatest in the chronic phase or in patients with recurrent pain after the acute episode has subsided.

Evaluation Of Tight Muscles

Upper trapezius (Fig. 10.4) is tested with the patient supine, with the head passively flexed and side-bent to the contralateral side. Once the slack is taken up, the shoulder girdle is pushed distally. Normally, a soft barrier is felt at the end of the push; however,

when the movement is restricted, the barrier has an abrupt firm to hard end-feel.

Levator scapulae (Fig. 10.5) is examined in a similar manner, except that the head is also rotated to the contralateral side.

Pectoralis major (Fig. 10.6) is tested with the patient supine. The trunk must be stabilized before the arm is placed into abduction because a possible twist of the trunk might mimic the normal range of movement. The arm should reach the horizontal level. To estimate the clavicular portion, the arm is allowed to hang down loosely and the examiner applies a posterior glide to the shoulder. Normally, only a slight soft barrier is felt.

Deep posterior neck muscles can be tested only by thorough palpation. Evaluation of the sternocleidomastoid is not reliable because it crosses too many segments (Fig. 10.7).

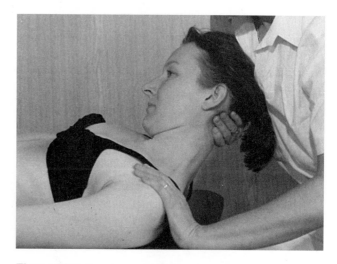

Figure 10.5 Levator scapulae.

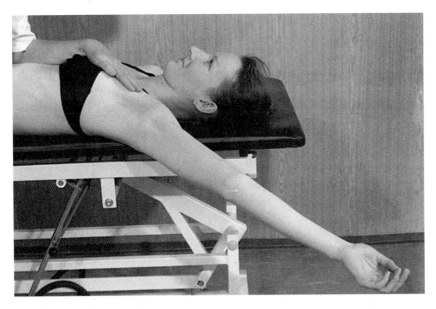

Figure 10.6 Pectoralis major.

Hip flexors (iliopsoas [Fig. 10.8] and rectus femoris [Fig. 10.9]) are tested with the patient in a modified Thomas position. The presented modification also allows for a screening examination of the short thigh adductors and the tensor fascia latae.

The patient is supine with the torso on the plinth and the tested leg loosely hanging. The non-tested leg is maximally flexed to stabilize the pelvis and flatten the lumbar spine. A flexed position of the hip joint indicates tightness of the iliopsoas, whereas the oblique position of the lower leg indicates tightness of the rectus. The inability to achieve passive hyperextension in the hip joint and passive full flexion of the knee (135 degrees) confirms the tightness of the iliopsoas and the rectus, respectively. Limitation of passive hip adduction to 15 degrees or less indicates the tightness of the tensor fascia lata (Fig. 10.10); abduction less than 25 degrees indicates shortness of the one-joint thigh adductors. This test can be influenced by the stretch of the joint capsule and thus more specific test should be performed to confirm the tightness of the adductors (Fig. 10.11).

Confirmation of tightness is clear when excessive soft tissue resistance and decreased range of motion are encountered on application of pressure in the following directions:

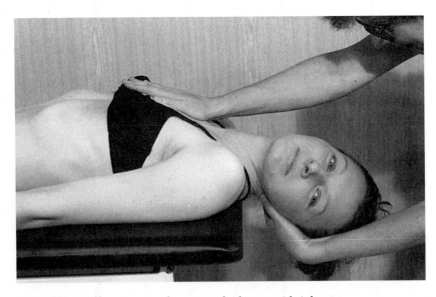

Figure 10.7 Screening test for sternocleidomastoid tightness.

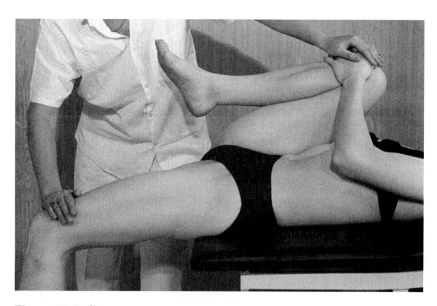

Figure 10.8 Iliopsoas.

- Hip extension less than 10 to 15 degrees—iliopsoas. A simultaneous extension of the knee joint points to the shortening of the rectus femoris.

- Knee flexion less than 100 to 105 degrees—rectus femoris. Compensatory hip flexion may occur during the test.

- Hip adduction less than 15 to 20 degrees—tensor fascia lata and the iliotibial band. An

associated deepening of the groove on the outside of the thigh is also noted In the presence of tightness.

- Hip abduction less than 15 to 20 degrees—short hip adductors. The tendency toward compensatory hip flexion should be controlled during the test.

Hamstrings (Fig. 10.12) tightness is evaluated by the straight leg raise test. To avoid the influence of

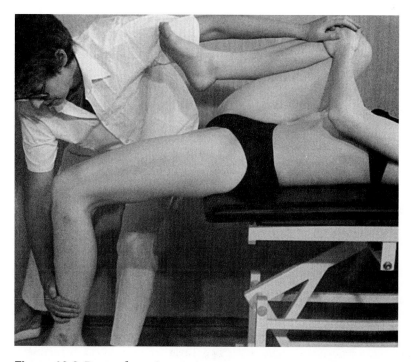

Figure 10.9 Rectus femoris.

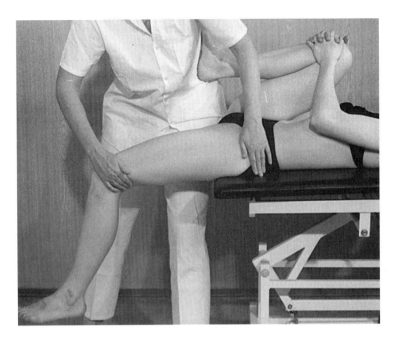

Figure 10.10 A screening test for tensor fascia lata tightness.

tight iliopsoas on the position of the pelvis and consequently on the range of hip flexion, the non-tested leg should be in placed in flexion. Under these circumstances, the normal range of motion is 90 degrees.

Thigh adductors are tested with the patient lying supine at the edge of the plinth (Fig. 10.13). The passive abduction in the hip joint should be at least 45 degrees. Tight hamstrings may contribute to the range limitation. If this situation occurs, bending the knee should increase the range of movement.

The piriformis muscle is tested with the patient in a supine position. The tested leg is placed with the hip joint in flexion not more than 60 degrees and in maximal adduction. The pelvis is stabilized by applying a force on the hip through the long axis of the femur (Fig. 10.14). Then, the adduction and internal rotation of the hip is performed. Normally, a soft, gradually increasing resistance is noted at the end of the range of motion. If the muscle is tight, the end feel is hard and may be associated with pain deep in the buttocks.

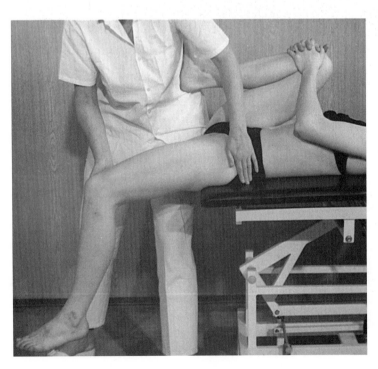

Figure 10.11 Screening test for the short hip adductors.

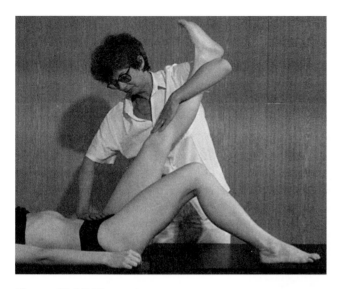

Figure 10.12 Hamstrings.

Quadratus lumborum is difficult to examine because this muscle spans many spinal segments. In principle, passive trunk side bending is tested while the patient assumes a side-lying position (Fig. 10.15). The reference point is the level of the inferior angle of the scapula, which should be raised approximately 2 inches from the floor. A simpler screening test entails observation of the spinal curve during active lateral flexion of the trunk.

Spinal erectors are also difficult to examine for the same reason as the quadratus lumborum. As a screening test, forward bending in a short sit allows observation of the gradual curvature of the spine (Fig. 10.16). A more reliable test, however, is the dual inclinometer test for lumbar flexion mobility shown in Chapter 12.

Triceps surae are tested by performing passive dorsiflexion of the foot. Normally, the therapist should

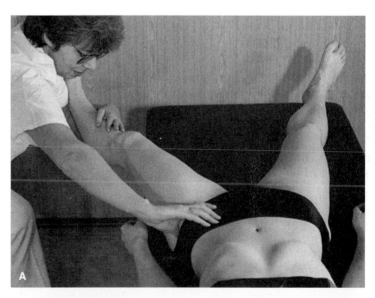

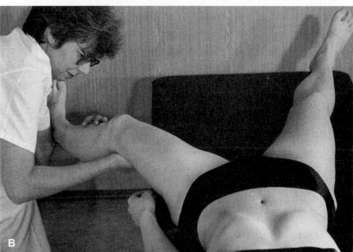

Figure 10.13 Thigh adductors **(A)**; test if hamstrings are tight **(B)**.

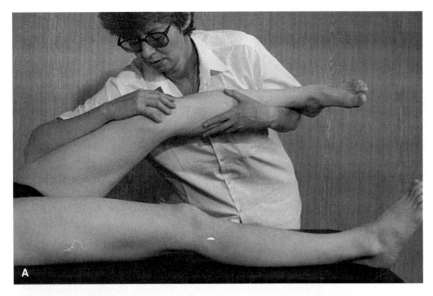

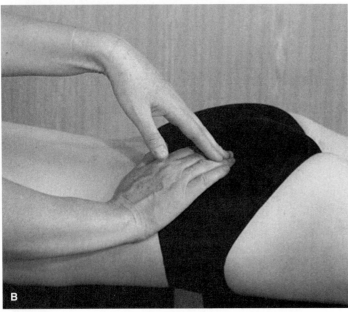

Figure 10.14 Screening test for piriformis tightness **(A)**; palpation test for piriformis tension or irritability **(B)**.

be able to achieve passive dorsiflexion to 90 degrees (Figs. 10.17 and 10.18).

More detailed description of the tests is available elsewhere (3).

Evaluation Of Inhibited Muscles

Classic muscle strength testing involves resistance of a movement in the direction characteristic for the specific muscle or muscle groups being tested. The production of a movement is in actuality, a series of muscles acting as prime movers, synergists, or stabilizers that combine together to produce a movement (3). Therefore, classic muscle strength testing does not provide sufficient nor reliable infor-

mation. The quality of performance of the movement is of greater importance than the test for strength. This type of evaluation is less focused on the strength of the particular movement, but more focused on the sequencing and degree of activation of the prime movers and their synergists. In this respect, the initiation of the movement is more important than the end of the movement. Poor quality and control of movement can produce and/or perpetuate adverse stresses on joints and muscle mechanics. Although movement patterns are individualized, the typical normal and abnormal patterns can be recognized.

In principle, six basic movement patterns provide overall information about the movement quality of the particular subject: hip (hyper)extension, hip

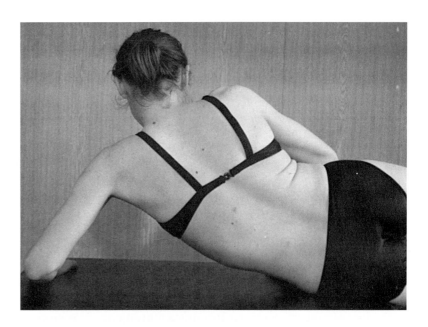

Figure 10.15 Screening test for quadratus lumborum tightness.

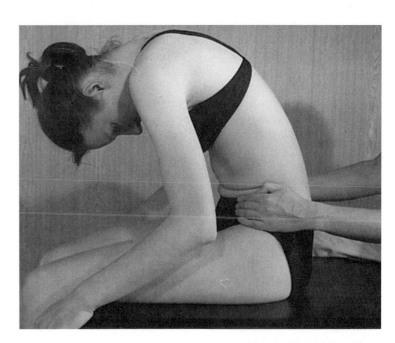

Figure 10.16 Screening test for erector spinae tightness.

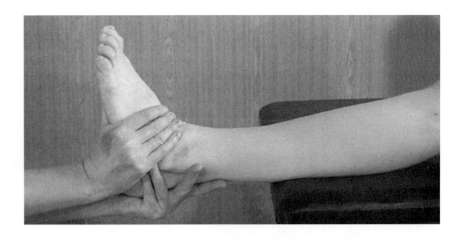

Figure 10.17 Gastrocnemius.

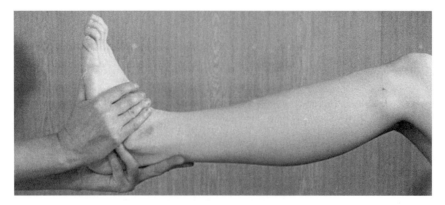

Figure 10.18 Soleus.

abduction, curl up, push up, neck flexion, and shoulder abduction. During movement pattern testing, minimal verbal cues should be used which test an individual's habitual way of performing a movement. If the cues are too "leading," then the test will be of the subject's ability to learn how to perform the movement correctly, rather than how the subject is habitually performing it.

The hip (hyper)extension movement test (Fig. 10.19) is examined to analyze one of the most important phases of the gait cycle—i.e., hyperextension of the hip at the terminal stance phase of gait (10,11). This test is performed with the patient lying prone. During straight leg lifting into extension, the sequencing and degree of activation of the hamstrings, gluteus maximus, spinal extensors, and shoulder girdle muscles are observed. The first sign of altered pattern is when the hamstrings and erector spinae are readily activated during the movement, whereas contraction of the gluteus maximus is delayed, decreased, or absent. The poorest pattern occurs when the erector spinae on the ipsilateral side or even the shoulder girdle muscles initiate the movement and activation of the gluteus maximus is weak and substantially delayed. In this situation, the entire motor performance is changed. Little if any extension in the hip

joint is noted and the leg lift is achieved through pelvic anterior tilt resulting in hyperlordosis of the lumbar spine, which undoubtedly over-stresses this region. Knee flexion should be noted because it indicates the hamstrings are predominating over the gluteus maximus.

Hip abduction (Fig. 10.20) gives information about the quality of the lateral muscular pelvic brace and thus indirectly about the stabilization of the pelvis in walking. It is tested with the patient in the side-lying position. The gluteus medius and minimus together with the tensor fascia lata act as prime movers while the quadratus lumborum acts as a pelvic stabilizer. The first sign of an altered abduction pattern is a tensor mechanism of hip abduction, when compensatory hip flexion is observed instead of pure abduction The poorest pattern of hip abduction occurs when the quadratus lumborum, in addition to stabilizing the pelvis, initiates the movement through elevation of the pelvis. This altered pattern can cause excessive stress to the lumbar and lumbosacral segments during walking.

Trunk curl-up (Fig. 10.21) is tested to estimate the interplay between the usually strong iliopsoas and the abdominal muscles. Initially, the examiner observes the patient's spontaneous pattern of sitting

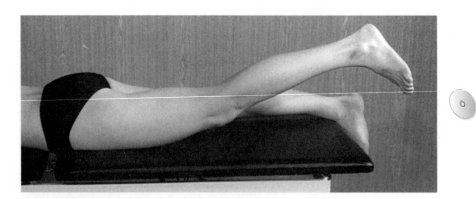

Figure 10.19 Hip extension.

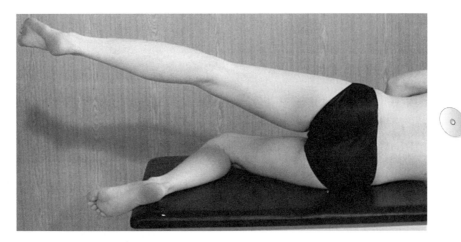

Figure 10.20 Hip abduction.

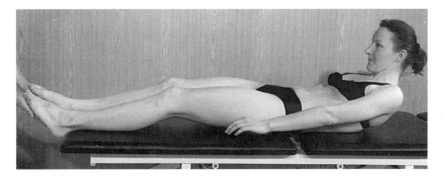

Figure 10.21 Trunk curl-up.

up. In the presence of weak abdominals and strong dominant iliopsoas, the curling movement of the trunk is minimal and the movement will be performed with an almost straight back and anterior tilting of the pelvis. The movement is thus performed mostly in the hip joint rather than by kyphosis of the trunk. Another way to detect if the iliopsoas is the dominant mover during the curl-up is for the clinician to place his hands under the patient's heels. The iliopsoas is predominant over the abdominals when the pressure of the patient's heels on the clinician's hands is lost.

Push-up (Fig. 10.22) from the prone position provides information about the quality of the stabilization of the scapula. During the push-up, and particularly in the beginning phase of lowering the body from

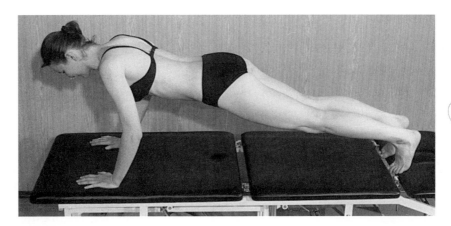

Figure 10.22 Push-up.

maximum push-up, excessive scapular rotation, elevation, adduction, or abduction are noted. The type of motion depends on what muscles are dominant. If levator scapulae are dominant, then one might see an elevation and downward rotation of the scapulae. If the serratus anterior is not functioning adequately, winging of the scapula will be observed.

Head flexion (Fig. 10.23) provides information about the interplay between the sternocleidomastoideus and the deep neck flexors. This information is essential in estimating the dynamics of the cervical spine and is tested with the patient supine. The subject is asked to raise the head slowly in the habitual way. When the deep neck flexors are inhibited and the sternocleidomastoideus is overactive, the jaw juts forward at the beginning of the movement with hyperextension in the cervicocranial junction. If the pattern is unclear, slight resistance of approximately one to two finger weights against the forehead may be applied. This slight resistance may exaggerate the hyperextension even more, indicating a weakness of the deep neck flexors.

Shoulder abduction (Fig. 10.24) provides information about the coordination of muscles of the shoulder girdle. It is tested while the patient is sitting, with the elbow flexed to control undesired rotation.

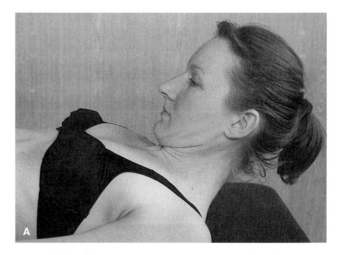

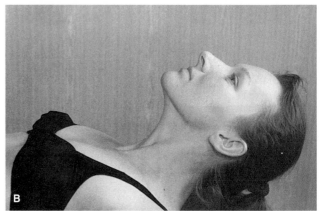

Figure 10.23 Head flexion "correct" **(A)** and "incorrect" **(B)**.

Clinical Pearl
Stretch Before Strengthening

If a movement pattern is faulty, the general rule of thumb is to initiate rehabilitation by treating tight muscles related to the faulty pattern. Once tight muscles are addressed then facilitation and training of the "weak link" can proceed. The reason for this is if muscle tightness is present, then strength training will typically reinforce "trick" movements, thus perpetuating the muscle incoordination. For instance, if the trunk curl-up test is positive, then treatment commences with releasing the iliopsoas first and then commencing an abdominal training program. With the tight hip flexors relaxed and lengthened, abdominal training will proceed with less joint stress and easier isolation of the target muscles.

The exception to this general rule of stretching tight muscles before strengthening "weak" muscles is if length testing shows that the iliopsoas is not actually tight. In this case, facilitation of the inhibited muscle can begin right away. However, because the movement pattern is faulty, a training position and range must be found that allows isolation of the agonist muscle without excessive substitution of synergist or antagonist muscles.

Shoulder abduction is a result of three components: abduction in the glenohumeral joint, rotation of the scapula, and elevation of the shoulder girdle. Movement is stopped at the point at which shoulder girdle elevation commences. This usually occurs at approximately 60 degrees of abduction at the glenohumeral joint. In an individual with shoulder dysfunction, shoulder girdle elevation starts earlier or may even initiate the movement.

Analysis Of Muscular Imbalance in Standing

In an analysis of standing, an attempt is made to differentiate between possible provocative causes, including structural variations, age, altered joint mechanics, and residual effects of pathologic processes. In this chapter, only muscular changes are described, although all biomechanical deviations, such as scoliosis, leg length difference, and all other

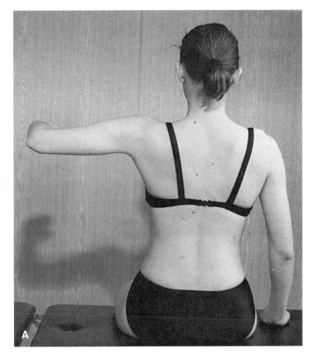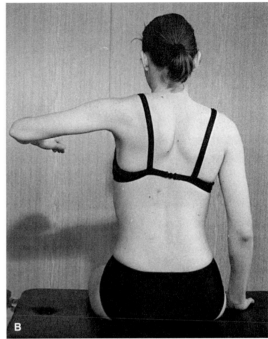

Figure 10.24 Shoulder abduction "correct" (**A**) and "incorrect" (**B**).

orthopedic deviations are taken into consideration. In muscular analysis, the main concern is with size, shape, and tone of the superficial muscles known to react by hyperactivity and tightness or by weakness and inhibition. The role of deeper muscles may need to be confirmed or negated in subsequent muscle length tests.

The patient is first observed from behind and an overall impression of posture is determined. Attention is then directed toward the position of the pelvis, because abnormalities of other structures such as the lumbar spine, sacroiliac joints, and lower limbs are, as a rule, reflected in the pelvis. An increase or decrease in sagittal tilt (posterior or anterior pelvic tilt), a lateral shift, an oblique position (pelvic un-leveling), rotation (transverse plane), and torsion (multiplanar distortion) should be noted. The pelvic crossed syndrome may be responsible for the increased anterior tilt of the pelvis. This condition is usually associated with increased lumbar lordosis. The pelvic rotation is usually associated with shortness of the piriformis and/or iliopsoas; an oblique position of the pelvis is associated mostly with leg length asymmetry. Tightness of thigh adductors, quadratus lumborum, and iliopsoas tend to shorten the leg, whereas tightness of the piriformis tends to lengthen the leg.

Next, the shape, size, and tone of the buttock are observed. Observation of the gluteus maximus is directed to the upper half of the muscle where contour and tone is noted. The general appearance of the gluteus, whether one is bulkier or sagging, gives the clinician a clue on the motor function of the muscle. Usually, the gluteus is hypotonic and inhibited on the side where the sacroiliac joint is blocked. The hamstrings are usually well developed, but it is important to look at their bulk relative to that of the glutei, because when the latter is inhibited, the hamstrings often become predominant. This change is readily evident if the impairment is unilateral. The shape of the line of the medial aspect of the thigh gives important information about the thigh adductors. In individuals with adductor tightness, the one-joint adductors form a distinct bulk in the upper one third of the thigh. The one-joint adductors are, as a rule, short and tender on palpation in patients with painful hip joint afflictions. On the calf, differentiation must be made between the gastrocnemius and the soleus. If the whole triceps surae is short, the Achilles tendon seems broader, and if the soleus is tight, in addition, the lower leg becomes cylindrical (Fig. 10.25).

Careful examination of the back muscles is warranted. The bulk of the erector spinae should be compared from side to side, as well as from the lumbar to the thoracolumbar region. There should be no evident difference between sides and regions. Prevalence or hypertrophy of the thoracolumbar spinal erectors may be indicative of poor muscle stabilization in the lumbosacral region (Fig. 10.26).

The interscapular space and the position of the shoulder blades give information about the quality of the lower stabilizers of the scapula. If these muscles are weak and/or inhibited, slight abduction, elevation, and winging of the shoulder blade are observed (Fig. 10.27). Tightness of the upper trapezius and levator scapulae (Fig. 10.28) can be seen on the neck shoulder line. In areas of tightness, the contour straightens. If tightness of the levator predominates, the contour of the neckline appears as a double wave in the area of insertion of the muscle on the scapula. This straightening of the neck shoulder line is sometimes described as a "Gothic shoulder" in that it is reminiscent of the form of Gothic church windows.

Viewing the patient from the front, the quality of the abdominals is observed first. Ideally, the abdominal wall is flat. A sagging and protruded abdomen may reflect generalized weakness of the abdominals. When the obliques are dominant, a distinct groove is apparent on the lateral side of the recti. This finding indicates a possible decrease in the stabilizing func-

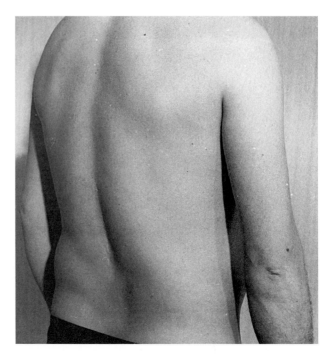

Figure 10.26 Right thoracolumbar erector spinae hypertrophy.

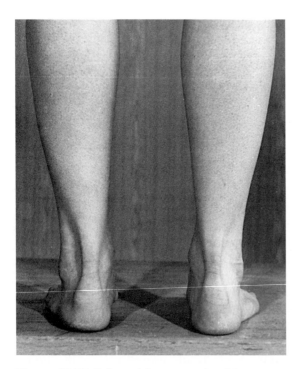

Figure 10.25 Soleus tightness on the right.

tion of the abdominal wall in the anteroposterior direction, an important factor for stabilization of the spine (Fig. 10.29).

The two anterior thigh muscles that can influence the lumbopelvic posture are the tensor fasciae lata and the rectus femoris. Normally, the bulk of the tensor is not distinct. Its visibility, coupled with the appearance of a groove on the lateral side of the thigh, usually indicates that this muscle is overused and short. When the rectus femoris is tight, the position of the patella shifts slightly upward and also laterally in the case of concurrent tightness of the iliotibial tract.

Tightness of the pectoralis major is characterized by a more prominent muscle belly and thickness of the anterior axillary fold. Typical imbalance will lead to rounded and protracted shoulders. Much information can be obtained from observation of the anterior aspect of the neck and throat. Normally, the sternocleidomastoid muscle is just slightly visible. Prominence of the insertion of the muscle, particularly its clavicular (proximal) portion, is a sign of tightness. A groove along this muscle is an early sign of weakness of the deep neck flexors. Straightening of the throat line (this is the angle made between the chin and throat line—

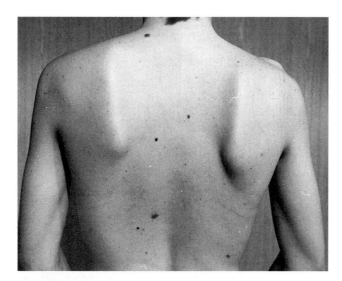

Figure 10.27 Abduction and winging of the right scapula.

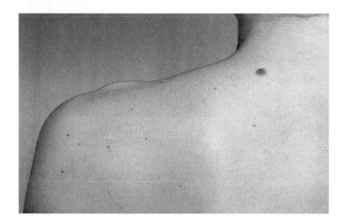

Figure 10.28 Tightness of the levator scapulae.

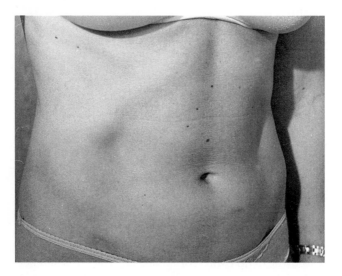

Figure 10.29 Oblique abdominal dominance.

normal is usually approximately 90 degrees) is usually a sign of increased tone of the suprahyoid muscles, which may be the underlying cause of a temporomandibular joint dysfunction. Palpation of the suprahyoids often reveals trigger points. Additionally, head posture should be observed. From a muscular point of view, a forward head posture is linked to weakness of the deep neck flexors and dominance or even tightness of the sternocleidomastoid.

From this brief description, it is evident that neglecting the analysis of the muscular system in standing leads to a loss of a substantial amount of information. Only the main changes or most frequent findings are mentioned in this chapter; however, other less common or subtle signs will provide additional valuable information.

Gait Assessment

Gait is the most automatized movement. The basic gait reflexes are regulated on a spinal cord level; however, the more complex reflexes are regulated on the subcortical or even cortical level. The variety of the gait patterns is remarkable. In fact, there are no two people on the world who would have the same gait. This fact has lead to a proposal to use the gait pattern to identify individuals in criminology. The gait pattern is so deeply fixed that it can be changed only with greatest difficulties, if at all. Thus the individual subject maintains his/her gait pattern during the whole adult lifetime. Only a severe injury that requires adaptation of the whole motor system results into changes of the gait pattern, although even in this case some basic qualities will remain unchanged.

For these reasons it is very difficult, if not impossible, to estimate norms. Therefore, statistical data regarding gait are of a very limited value in the clinics and for an individual patient. Despite all these difficulties and diagnostic limitations, the visual gait analysis is of a paramount importance as it provides important information about possible over-stresses of critical segments of the human body in the individual patient. In addition, skilled observation of gait helps the clinician toward a more detailed diagnosis and rational of treatment.

In principle, two general types of gait can be recognized:

The proximal type: The body is propelled forward mainly by pronounced hip and knee flexion, followed by hip extension beyond the midline. The center of gravity remains relatively level with minimal stress on the ankle joints and possibly greater over-stress on the hip joint.

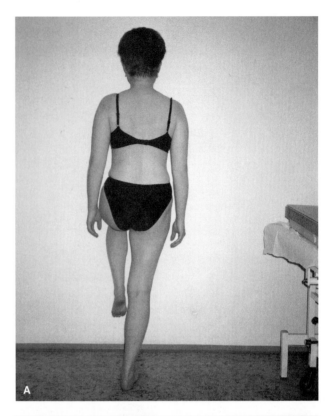

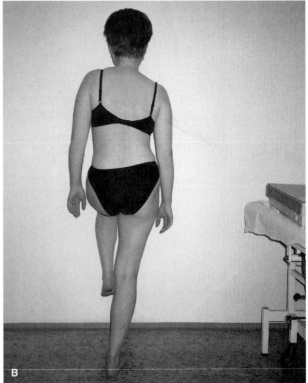

Figure 10.30 One-leg standing test. **(A)** Normal one-leg stance, pelvis and shoulders level, minimum of lateral pelvic shift. **(B)** Positive Trendelenburg sign. Lateral shift and oblique position of the pelvis, contralateral shoulders elevated.

In the distal type, the body is propelled forward virtually by plantar flexion of the feet with minimal motion at the hip and knee joint. The center of gravity is elevated with each step. This type of gait is seen as "bouncy" or similar to gait observed in children with muscular dystrophy who walk on their toes.

After estimating the type of gait, length, and symmetry of the length of the step, the movements of the pelvis are observed. There are five basic movements that we should look at: 1.) anterior and 2.) posterior pelvic tilt in the sagittal plane, 3.) lateral and oblique shift, 4.) pelvic rotation, and 5.) the "butterfly" movement of the pelvis, which is an "opening" and "closing" of the pelvis as a result of movement in the sacroiliac joint.

Anterior pelvic tilt has to be correlated with the lumbar lordosis and thus stability of the whole torso. The easiest way to estimate this clinically is to compare the position of the pelvis with the position of the shoulders. If the trunk stability is good, the whole body—particularly in two critical areas, the pelvis and shoulders—will move forward in one line. If trunk stability is insufficient, the shoulder movements will lag behind. Pelvic movements are associated with the range of hip extension and lateral muscular pelvic brace, which is important during one leg stance. It has to be noted that approximately 85% of gait cycle involves standing on one leg A quick test to check on the lateral brace is to have the patient perform a single leg stance with his eyes open (Fig. 10.30). The clinician observes for the amount of pre-shift to the stance leg and un-leveling of the pelvis and/or shoulders. The normal pre-shift to the stance leg should not be more than 1 inch and the patient should be able to perform the single leg stance for approximately 15 seconds without any compensatory movements.

Arm movements during gait are another source of valuable information. Symmetry of arm movements is observed, with particular attention to whether the movement is predominantly initiated by movement in the shoulders (which is ideal), or by a pronounced elbow flexion. The third type of arm movement observed is movement initiated predominantly by rotation of the trunk. The latter is often the result of increased stresses on the whole spine.

Clinical Pearl

Differentiating Muscle Weakness from Inhibition for the Gluteus Maximus

Muscle strengthening programs are often time-consuming. In many instances of supposed muscle weakness, detailed analysis reveals that the muscle is not actually weak, but only inhibited. In such cases the correct management is facilitation, not strength training. Identifying the specific nature of the muscle dysfunction is a "time-saver" in the clinic.

Hip Extension/Gluteus Maximus

The gluteus maximus is an important hyper-extensor of the hip. The hip (hyper)extension test is a simple screen showing the interplay of gluteus maximus, hamstrings, erector spinae, and hip flexor muscles. The importance of this movement is that it is an essential phase of the gait cycle. Neither faulty gait during "toe off" nor a faulty hip extension movement pattern tells us if the gluteus maximus is weak or inhibited. However, a simple test involving backward walking will make this differentiation.

During backward walking, the gluteus maximus is normally facilitated. Thus, incoordinated backward walking as evidenced by increased lumbar lordosis or an anterior pelvic tilt indicates that the gluteus maximus is truly weak and not merely inhibited. This is particularly striking if the dysfunction is unilateral. This suggests that longer-term training will be required to improve function. In contrast, an improved lumbo-pelvic posture during backward walking in comparison to standing posture, forward walking, or during the prone hip (hyper)extension test suggests that the gluteus maximus is only inhibited and probably can be trained easily.

If inhibition is present, treatment may involve postisometric relaxation (PIR), facilitation (PNF diagonals, Sister Kenny methods), or joint manipulation. If weakness is present, then progressive resistance training (e.g., bridges, squats, lunges, and single leg reaches) will also be required. A goal-oriented continuum of care might look like this:

Continuum of Care

- Inhibit—hip flexors

- Facilitate—gluteus maximus

- Mobilize—lower quarter and lumbo-pelvic joints

Clinical Pearl
Differentiating Muscle Weakness from Inhibition for the Gluteus Medius

The gluteus medius is the most important lateral stabilizer of the hip and pelvis. During gait an insufficiency of the lateral brace on the stance leg will lead to pelvic un-leveling (i.e., Trendelenburg) and difficulty achieving clearance of the toes from the ground on the contralateral swing leg. The person may not trip, but an uneconomical gait will result. The hip abduction test is a simple screen showing the interplay of gluteus medius, tensor fascia lata, quadratus lumborum, and hip adductors. Unfortunately, neither pelvic un-leveling during gait nor a faulty hip abduction movement pattern will tell us if the gluteus medius is weak or only inhibited. However, a simple test involving walking while holding a light object in the hands overhead will make this differentiation.

During this test the gluteus medius is normally facilitated. Thus, incoordination as evidenced by increased lateral sway or pelvic un-leveling indicates muscle weakness not inhibition is involved. This is most notable if the dysfunction is unilateral. In contrast, an improvement in lateral pelvic stability or pelvic obliquity when compared to normal walking or standing posture suggests gluteus medius inhibition not weakness is present.

If weakness is present, then progressive resistance training (clam shell, single leg bridge, wall ball, and single leg reaches) will also be required. A goal-oriented continuum of care might look like this:

Continuum of Care

- Inhibit—adductors, Piriformis, TFL, quadratus lumborum, psoas
- Facilitate—gluteus medius
- Mobilize—lower quarter and lumbo-pelvic joints

Hypermobility

Muscles can be involved in many other afflictions. One of the most common situations is constitutional hypermobility. This vague non-progressive clinical syndrome of unknown origin is not really a disease. It is characterized by a general laxity of connective tissues, muscles, and, in particular, ligaments. Muscle strength in affected individuals usually is low, and even a vigorous strengthening exercise does not lead to evident hypertrophy. The muscle tone is decreased when assessed by palpation and the range of movement in joints is comparatively increased. Despite joint instability, it has not been confirmed that "hypermobile" subjects are more prone to musculoskeletal pain syndromes.

Constitutional hypermobility involves the entire body, although all areas may not be affected to the same extent and slight asymmetry can be observed. This syndrome is noted more frequently in women and it typically involves the upper part of the body. With aging, hypermobility decreases. Patients with constitutional hypermobility may develop muscle tightness as well, although it is never so evident. Mostly, this tightness is considered a compensatory mechanism to stabilize, in particular, the weight-bearing joints. Therefore, stretching, if necessary, should be performed gently and only in key muscles that are supposed to be decisive in a particular syndrome. Because the muscles generally are weak, they may be easily overused and, therefore, trigger points in muscles and ligaments develop easily. There is no effective treatment of the syndrome of constitutional hypermobility. However, reasonably prolonged strengthening and sensorimotor programs are usually helpful.

Assessment of hypermobility is in principle based on estimation of muscle tone by palpation and range of motion of the joints. In clinical practice, orientation tests usually are sufficient. In the upper part of the body, the most useful tests are head rotation, high arm cross (Fig. 10.31), touching the hands behind the neck (Fig. 10.32), extension of the elbows (Fig. 10.33), and hyperextension of the thumb (Fig. 10.34). In the lower part of the body, the best choices are the forward bending test (Fig. 10.35), lateral flexion test, leg raising test, and dorsiflexion of the foot (Fig. 10.36).

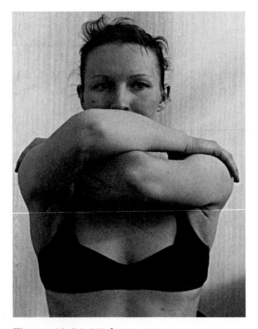

Figure 10.31 High arm cross.

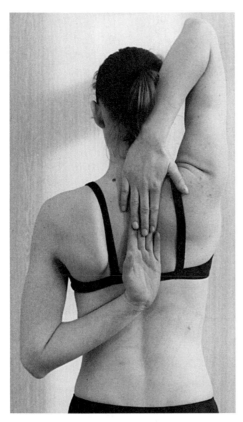

Figure 10.32 Touching the hands behind the neck.

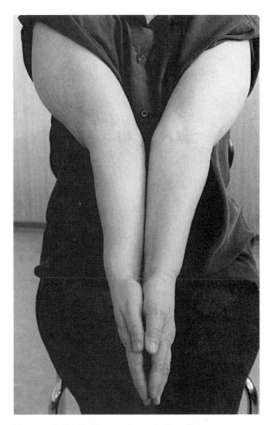

Figure 10.33 Extension of the elbows.

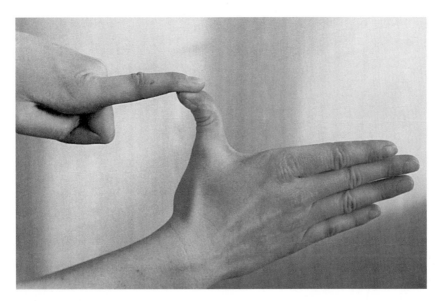

Figure 10.34 Hyperextension of the thumb.

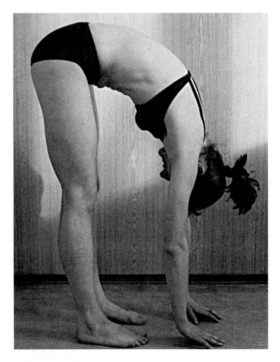

Figure 10.35 The forward bending test.

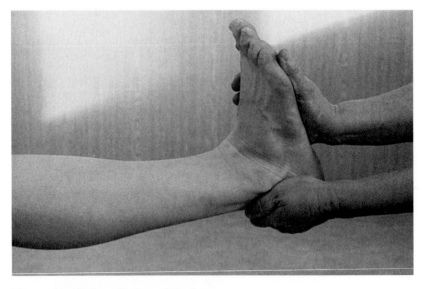

Figure 10.36 Dorsiflexion of the foot.

■ CONCLUSION

Muscle imbalance is an essential component of dysfunction syndromes of the musculoskeletal system. Important approaches in the overall therapeutic program lie in the recognition of factors that perpetuate the dysfunction and normalization. This fact is true regardless of whether muscle imbalance is considered to cause the joint dysfunction or to occur parallel to it.

Audit Process
Self-Check of the Chapter's Learning Objectives

- Can you evaluate the length of each of the muscles which have a tendency to become tight?

- Can you perform and interpret the six basic movement patterns described in this chapter?

- Can you identify signs of muscle imbalance from postural or gait analysis?

■ REFERENCES

1. Janda V. Muscle strength in relation to muscle length, pain and muscle imbalance. In: Harms-Rindahl K, ed. Muscle Strength. New York: Churchill Livingstone, 1993.
2. Janda V. Muscle spasm—a proposed procedure for differential diagnosis. J Manual Med 1991;6:136.
3. Janda V. Muscle Function Testing. London: Butterworths, 1983.
4. Janda V. On the concept of postural muscles and posture. Austr J Physiother 1983;29:S83–S84.
5. Janda V. Die Muskulären Hauptsyndrome bei vertebragenen Beschwerden. In: Neumann HD, Wolff HD, eds. Theoretische Fortschritte und praktische Erfahrungen der Manuellen Medizin. Konkordia, Bühl 1978:61–65.
6. Janda V. Muscles, central nervous regulation and back problems. In: Korr I, ed. Neurobiologic mechanisms in Manipulative Therapy. New York: Plenum Press, 1978:27–41.
7. Kolář P. Systematization of muscle imbalances from the viewpoint of developmental kinesiology. Rehabilitace Fys Lék 2001;8:152–164.
8. Kolář P. The sensomotor nature of postural functions. Its fundamental role in rehabilitation. J Orthop Med 1999;21:40–45.
9. Mense S, Simons DG. Muscle pain: Understanding its nature, diagnosis, and treatment. Pain associated with increased muscle tension. Baltimore: Lippincott Williams & Wilkins, 2001: 99–130.
10. Vogt L, Banzer W. Dynamic testing of the motorial stereotype in prone hip extension from the neutral position. Clin Biomechan 1997;12:122–127.
11. Vogt L, Pfeifer K, Banzer W. Neuromuscular control of walking with chronic low-back pain. Man Ther 2003;8:21–28.
12. Vojta V, Peters A. Das Vojta-Prinzip. Berlin: Springer Verlag, 1992.

11

Quantification of Physical Performance Ability

Craig Liebenson and
Steven Yeomans

Learning Objectives
After reading this chapter you should be able to understand:

- How to evaluate physical performance tests based on their reliability, validity, and practicality.
- How to administer quantifiable tests of physical impairment that relate to spinal disorders.

Introduction

Functional capacity and physical performance evaluations have become an important part of the physical examination of work-injured and chronic pain patients (96,100). This unique evaluation is needed because traditional examination methods such as orthopedic, neurologic, and imaging tests are able to accurately diagnose the cause of pain in only approximately 10% of patients (148). When advanced imaging modalities are used, an excessive amount of coincidental findings (high false-positive rate) unrelated to the patients condition or prognosis are uncovered (12,24,59,60,61,66). Amazingly, most tests used in the physical examination of musculoskeletal patients are unreliable. For instance, orthopedic tests such as Kemp's or Patrick Fabere's have not been shown to be reliable or to have predictive validity (102,140,141). To avoid basing treatment decisions on often-misleading imaging procedures, unreliable orthopedic tests, or merely on the patient's subjective self-report of symptoms, the focus of evaluation has gradually been shifting toward identification of functional or physical performance deficits (93–101).

One exception is that with the use of diagnostic injections at least 50% of chronic spine pain patients presenting to specialist diagnostic centers can have the pain generator successfully identified (see chapter 6) (8,140,141). However, the cause of the tissue's sensitivity may not be revealed and therein lies the added value of both physical performance and functional testing in such patients.

Psychosocial factors are also very important in caring for chronic pain patients and predicting which acute patients are most likely to have chronic pain (see Chapter 9). However, physical performance testing may reveal salient impairments that were at least partially responsible for the pain in the first place (87). This can help to focus the patient on the important goal of reactivation and functional restoration.

The physical examination can be used for diagnostic, prescriptive, and outcome purposes. The examination of physical performance ability (PPA) is a key part of the physical examination because it can help identify specific impairments responsible for biomechanical overload of various pain generators (67). Additionally, it can identify impairments related to specific functional limitations that affect an individual in performing their daily tasks at home, work, or sport (41,91). This chapter discusses the rationale (why), indications (when), methods (what), and implementation (how) related to performing a PPA assessment.

Rationale—Why

The World Health Organization (WHO) has operationally defined function in its International Classification of Impairments, Disabilities, and Handicaps (ICDH) document (57). Most significantly, the ICDH document distinguishes between general functional ability and specific functional deficits. General functional ability relates to activity level or disability, whereas specific functional ability is related to impairment in body function. General functional ability or disability is what the patients can or cannot do (or perceive they can do!) in their daily life. This is assessed with activity intolerance questionnaires (i.e., Oswestry, Matheson's activity sorts) (see Chapter 8) or tests of actual patient's general functional abilities such as walking, reaching, carrying, etc. (see Chapter 12). In contrast, specific functional deficits are found only on clinical examination and may or may not be related to the patient's symptoms or functional abilities (18,34). In this case it is the clinician's perception that influences the significance of the findings. The PPA testing in this chapter is mainly tests of such impairments or specific functional deficits. Because the relationship between specific functional impairments and disability is indirect, the PPA evaluation is but one tool in the evaluation of patients.

Evaluation of PPA does not substitute for the traditional history and examination of orthopaedic, neurologic, or vital signs. Diagnostic triage to identify patients with "red flags" of serious disease and nerve root compression syndromes is a first step in evaluation and requires a focused approach (see Chapter 8) (6) when "red flags" are present imaging or laboratory investigations are indicated. If imaging tests are ordered in the absence of "red flags," they can be misleading because of their high false-positive rates for clinically insignificant age-related degenerative findings (9,12,59,60,66).

Because less than 10% of acute patients can receive an accurate, specific diagnosis, most recent guidelines label the remaining 90% as having "non-specific" low back pain (LBP) (6,138,142,148). This failure to more accurately diagnose or classify 90% of LBP has not been deemed a limitation because the condition's favorable natural history has been touted. Recent epidemiological studies show that the course of these "non-specific" low back pain (LBP) cases is longer-lasting and more recurrent than previously supposed (23). The use of the "non-specific" label has been interpreted to mean that the majority of patients are a homogenous group who share a uniform clinical picture and prognosis. However, what it more likely indicates is that we are not very good at subclassifying a heterogenous group into discreet groups requiring individualized care (70,71). Current attempts at providing better care for LBP patients have emphasized improving our ability to diagnose or classify patients into meaningful subgroups (see Chapter 34) (36,38,88,109,150,160–162,169).

The most important reasons for performing a PPA evaluation are to identify treatment targets—prescriptive—and establish baseline levels of functional impairment from which to judge future progress by—outcomes. Establishing a "functional diagnosis" is an invaluable clinical guide that can influence treatment decisions and steer care toward meaningful end points of care. The PPA evaluation should focus on relevant functions that can be safely and reliably measured. Where normative data bases exist, this is most helpful and, whenever possible, using tests that include quantification is ideal for outcomes-based reporting. The most valid tests are those that most closely resemble the actual way we use our bodies in performing activities of daily living (ADLs). The most valued characteristic of a functional measure is its utility. The utility or usefulness of the procedure is the degree to which it meets the needs of the patient, referrer, and payer. Five issues pertaining to a test's utility have been described in hierarchical order (Table 11.1) (50,92).

High-tech instrumentation and dynametric assessment of the low back have been considered the "gold standard" of lumbar spine functional assessment. This is largely because of their reliability and reproducibility. However, the validity of some of the high-tech testing approaches has become a source of controversy (45,120,135). Matheson says, "the interpretation of the test score should be able to predict or reflect the evaluee's performance in a target task" (90). If an effort factor can be measured, this will help

---

Table 11.1 Key Features of Functional/Performance Tests Utility (50, 90)

---

1. Safety: Given the known characteristics of the patient, the procedure should not be expected to lead to injury
2. Reliability: The test score should be dependable across the evaluators, patients, and the date or time of administration
3. Responsiveness: The test should detect clinically meaningful change in a condition or attribute over time over and above random improvement
4. Validity: The interpretation of the test score should be able to predict or reflect the patient's performance in a target work setting
5. Practicality: The test should be easy to administer and interpret. The cost of the test procedure should be reasonable. Cost is measured in terms of the direct expense of the test procedure plus the amount of time required of the patient, plus the delay in providing the information derived from the procedure to the referral source

---

unmask a malingerer. However, as Dvir has pointed out, this is very difficult to accomplish, especially with strength testing (29).

Grabiner et al. has demonstrated that normal strength measurements from a high-tech approach do not necessarily correlate with normal human function (45). In this study, electromyography (EMG) was used during isometric trunk extension. The results revealed decoupling, or asymmetric lumbar paraspinal muscle activity, was present in low back pain subjects who were considered normal on high-tech dynametric testing. This decoupling phenomenon was able to differentiate between pain and non-pain subjects. This study suggests that musculoskeletal function involves not only strength but also coordination during the performance of a specified task. Because spinal movement and coordination use complex neuromuscular functions, simple strength assessment by high-tech dynamometer does not necessarily correlate with assessment of spinal function.

As Lewit puts it, ". . . in many fields of medicine the importance of changes in function is now well recognized, whereas in the motor system, where function is paramount, this fundamental aspect is rarely considered. However, the functioning of the locomotor system is extremely complex, . . . and diagnosis of disturbed function is a highly sophisticated proceeding carried out, as it were in a clinical no man's land" (78).

LaRocca in a Presidential Address to the Cervical Spine Research Society Annual Meeting in December of 1991 criticizes his colleagues for jumping to a psychological diagnosis when they cannot find a structural cause for a patient's persistent pain, ". . . The error here is the automatic leap to psychology. It assumes that all organic factors have been considered, when in reality the clinician's appreciation of the complexity of such factors in often severely limited" (73). Newton and Waddell said, "There is no convincing evidence that isokinetic or any other iso-measure has greater clinical utility in the patient with low back pain than either clinical evaluation of physical impairment, isometric strength, simple isoinertial lifting or psychophysical testing" (56,120).

At the present time, the quality of high-tech tests is not demonstrated sufficiently to lead to the abandonment of lower-tech qualifiable tests of spinal function. Many reliable low-tech ways to identify functional pathology have been identified. The inclinometer is an example of a very simple tool that can safely provide a great amount of valid and reliable information. Often a patient's musculoskeletal function cannot be quantified. However, qualifiable tests may be performed that give insight into clinically relevant muscle imbalances, joint stiffness, postural dysfunctions, and movement incoordination (38,109, 110,160).

Many chiropractors, osteopaths, and manual therapists use tools that lack reliability such as motion palpation of the accessory movement of joints—commonly called "end feel." Lack of reliability may be caused by a multiplicity of factors (79) and is not a sufficient reason to abandon a test that is simple, time-efficient, and theoretically able to test something in a way not possible with more accurate or sophisticated means. However, such tests must at least be targeted for research into their reliability and validity or their users risk being considered "cultists" (125).

Rissanen et al. found that non-dynamometric tests correlated better with pain and disability than did isokinetic tests (88,135). They concluded, "The non-dynamometric tests are still useful in clinical practice in spite of the development of more accurate muscle strength evaluation methods."

Reliability has been reported in several low-tech tests that do not provide numerical quantification results. For example, the NIOSH Low Back Atlas identified 19 tests with significant reliability (<0.74 Cohen's Kappa and >0.79 coefficient for interclass correlation, coefficient [ICC]) (117,118). Moffroid et al. studied the ability of the 53 NIOSH tests to discriminate between low back pain and non-painful subjects (90,109). It was found that 23 of the 53 tests could not discriminate adequately between the two groups and when the seven strongest tests were grouped together, a sensitivity of 87% and specificity of 93% were obtained. Interestingly, the most important measurements were those that assessed passive mobility, dynamic mobility, strength, and symmetry. Harding et al., as well as others, reported a group of low-tech tests were determined safe, reliable, and valid for assessment of physical dysfunction in chronic pain subjects (49,93). A series of simple trunk and lower extremity endurance tests have been shown be reliable (1,103,106). A normative database segregated by age, gender, and vocation (blue collar versus white collar) were determined for some of these tests on more than 500 individuals (1).

Indications—When

According to Mooney, a PPA evaluation is recommended 2 weeks after injury to identify the "weak functional link" (112). Triano suggests 4 weeks as an appropriate time to begin testing (159). Functional testing is not terribly helpful in the acute stage and, in fact, may be contraindicated. However, as soon as the patient is out of the acute "guarding" stage, a PPA evaluation can provide ideal outcomes as well as help

identify key functional pathologies that should be addressed with reactivation care. Mooney reports that the functional capacity evaluation should be mandatory for any patient still experiencing pain after 6 to 7 weeks (112).

Are Functional Tests Predictive of Short-Term Outcome?

- Fritz et al. reported that a Physical Impairment Index performed on acute patients (<3 weeks duration) was predictive of outcome 4 weeks later (39).
- The tests were found to be reliable and responsive to change (although less responsive than the Oswestry disability index)
  - Flexion ROM (single inclinometer at T12/L1)
  - Extension ROM (single inclinometer at T12/L1)
  - Lateral flexion ROM (average of each side—single inclinometer at T9-T12)
  - Straight leg raise ROM (average of each side—inclinometer at superior tibial crest with the knee held in extension)
  - Spinal tenderness (any superficial or deep tenderness is noted)
  - Bilateral active straight leg raise (raised 6 inches up and held for 5 seconds)
  - Active sit-up (knees flexed 90 degrees and feet held flat by the examiner. Patient sits up until fingers touch the knees and holds for 5 seconds)

Are Functional Tests Predictive of Long-Term Outcome?

- Enthoven et al. reported that functional tests are not predictive of 12-month outcome if performed in the early acute phase (35).
- However, if performed at the 4-week mark they are significant predictor of future pain and disability.
- The best predictors were thoraco-lumbar ROM, isometric trunk extensor endurance, and finger tip to floor distance.

Hart et al., report indications for functional testing include the following (50):

1. Plateau of treatment progress
2. Discrepancy between subjective and objective findings

3. Difficulty in returning the patient to gainful employment

4. Vocational planning or medical–legal case settlement

The PPA assessment will allow objective confirmation of patient status to complement the patient's subjective self-report of their symptoms. It also allows the health care provider to document patient progress over time. It will help to motivate the patient to pursue reactivation after injury. Prolonged passive care (e.g., hot packs, massage, ultrasound) directed at providing symptomatic relief may only achieve short-term results. When symptomatic not functional outcomes are the patient's only goal, dependency on palliative treatments rather than reactivation advice can result (86,138).

The "sports medicine" approach that measures functional impairment and uses reactivation advice and active exercise to rehabilitate injured tissues is recognized as the "standard of care" for soft tissue injuries (21,47,86,138,149,164). This active approach is better suited to alleviating pain, completing soft tissue healing, and preventing reoccurrences.

Physical Performance Ability Test Methods—What

A number of sophisticated high-tech measurement devices have been developed to enhance patient evaluation (MedX, Cybex, Iso B-200, IsoTrak, EMG). Research is driven by the use of such devices (19, 82–101,124,126,129,130,137,143,158). However, evaluation of PPA can be performed with minimal if any special equipment or high cost. Though high-tech testing equipment is always an option, it is not necessary and in many instances may actually correlate less well with actual functional disability than simpler low-tech approaches (120,135). Simple, low-tech tests have evolved to a point at which many are reliable (1,5,103,117,118,135,152).

The best tests are quantifiable and have established normative databases that allow comparison by sex, age, occupation, and history of back pain (1,49,103, 106,145). Ideally, maximal performance (sincerity of effort) can be differentiated from feigned performance although this is usually not possible especially with strength testing (30,48).

Flexibility/Mobility

Introduction

Evaluation of mobility and flexibility is a common practice for most musculoskeletal medicine practitioners. Range of motion (ROM) is usually restricted in acute situations and is one of the primary objective outcomes that can be tracked to show progress over time. However, in chronic patients ROM testing may be of less value.

Sincerity of effort is an important consideration during ROM testing. In the *Guides to the Evaluation of Permanent Impairment* the validity of a patient's effort is based on the repeatability of scores obtained over a series of measures (25). For instance in the *Guides* each measure must be within 5 degrees of the average of at least three measures that are less than 50 degrees. If the average is more than 50 degrees, then each measure must be within 10% of that average. Thus, each measure must be within a certain standard deviation (SD) from the mean. Another measure of validity called the coefficient of variation (CV) has been shown to be even more useful. The CV is obtained by dividing the SD by the mean of the scores. The CV range for intraobserver goniometric measurements in the extremities has been shown to be between 4% and 10% (11,33, 146,147). The CVs for lumbar motion are in the range of 6% to 14% (101,102), with patients having a greater range than asymptomatic individuals (107). CVs for the cervical spine range are reported to be up to 5% (29,30,72).

Dvir has shown that in healthy individuals sincerity of effort for cervical ROM may be judged from the CV (29). Using the AMA Guides protocol for determining insincere effort in lumbar spine ROM assessment, an unacceptable rate of false-positives was reported. The AMA guides recommendation regarding using ROM for determining impairment is considered invalid (173).

Gilford showed that the circadian rhythm influenced flexibility, with muscle length or joint ROM measures are more reliable in the afternoon (42). Others have verified this diurnal variation in lumbar spinal ROM (36,170). Similarly, Porter reported similar variance with orthopedic testing such as the straight leg raise (SLR) orthopedic test in which the SLR was found to be tighter in the morning (127).

When performing ROM tests, it is important to perform each test as precisely as possible. For example, Ekstrand, et al. observed an improvement in the CV from 7.5 ± 2.9 to 1.9 ± -0.7 after using the tests for 2 months and subsequent refinement, paying attention to the details regarding (33):

1. Standardized inclinometer placement and make sure the pendulum of the gravity type swings freely

2. Stiffening up the examination table (plywood with Velcro bands)

3. Identify bony anatomical landmarks (mark on skin)

4. The examination bench height was standardized for each visit

The quantity of motion is perhaps of less importance than its quality (85,88,105,108). Velocity and symmetry of motion characteristics can be reliably identified with a simple and inexpensive triaxial goniometer system called a B Tracker (Isotechnologies, Hillsborough, NC) (85). Marras' (88) more sophisticated and expensive system utilizing the lumbar motion monitor to monitor three-dimensional kinematics of the lumbar spine during performance of industrial tasks has been shown to predict future industrial back injury claim. A novel technique for evaluating relative motion at C7-T1 and T1-T2 segments has found that a synchronous pattern of greater mobility at the higher segment is normal and that a non-synchronous or inverse pattern with greater mobility at the lower segment is predictive of future of neck–shoulder pain in a 2-year prospective follow-up study (122). This low-tech method utilizes skin markings and a flexible tape measure.

Table 11.2 shows the ROM tests that will be described in detail.

Ankle Dorsiflexion Mobility/ Gastrocnemius Length

Tightness of the gastrosoleus has been shown to be correlated with increased knee injury risk in male college athletes (33,68). This test evaluates the length or tension of the gastrocnemius muscle and/or the articulation of the ankle joint (Fig. 11.1).

Patient Position

• Patient stands upright, feet parallel, and knees straight

Table 11.2 Mobility Tests

1. Ankle dorsiflexion mobility/gastrocnemius and soleus length
2. Knee flexion mobility/quadriceps length (Nachlas test)
3. Hip flexion mobility/hamstring length (Straight leg raise test)
4. Hip extension mobility (modified Thomas test/psoas-rectus femoris length)
5. Hip rotation mobility (internal and external)
6. Lumbar spine mobility
7. Cervical spine mobility

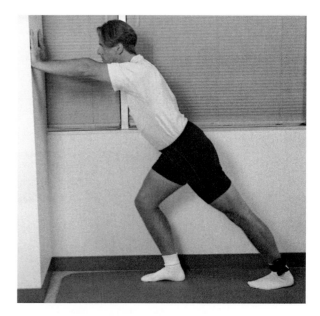

Figure 11.1 Ankle dorsiflexion mobility/gastrocnemius length.

Test

• The inclinometer is positioned above the lateral malleolus and "zeroed" in upright standing position

• The patient leans forward, placing the hands on a wall

• The tested leg is moved backwards until a lunge position is assumed and the heel begins to lift from the floor; the front knee will be in a flexed position.

• The subject pushes the heel down or slides slightly forward until the heel is flat on the floor; when the of maximum ankle dorsiflexion is achieved, the angle is recorded

Quantification

• The normative data reveals 22.5 degrees

• Standard deviation (SD) 0.7

• Intra-assay CV 2.2%

• Inter-assay CV 2.5% (33).

Soleus length/Ankle Dorsiflexion Test

This soleus length/ankle dorsiflexion test (33) evaluates the length or tension of the soleus muscle and/or the articulation of the ankle joint (Fig. 11.2).

Patient Position

• The patient position in this test is prone.

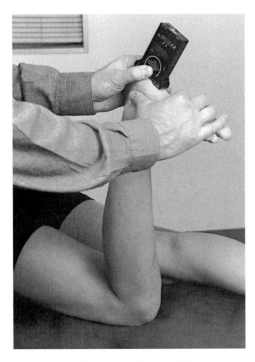

Figure 11.2 Soleus length/ankle dorsiflexion test.

Test

- The knee is flexed and the ankle is dorsiflexed to a maximum angle maintaining heel-to-floor contact
- Alternatively, the patient may stand on the non-tested leg and place the tested foot on a bench and the ankle is dorsiflexed to a maximum angle maintaining heel-to-bench contact
- The inclinometer position is the same as the first test (see Fig. 11.1)

Quantification

- The normative data reveals 24.9 degrees
- SD 0.8

- Intra-assay CV 2.2%
- Inter-assay CV 2.6% (33).

Knee Flexion Mobility/Quadriceps Length (Nachlas Test)

The knee flexion mobility/quadriceps length (Nachlas test) (33) evaluates the length or tension of the quadriceps femoris muscle and/or the articulation of the knee joint (Fig. 11.3).

Patient Position

- The patient is prone on table
- The inclinometer is positioned at the posterior aspect of the mid-calf and zeroed (alternate position is on anterior shin after being zeroed to bottom of table or desk)
- The pelvis is stabilized

Test

- Patient's knee is passively flexed (approximate heel to buttock)
- The angle is measured at point just before lumbar spine begins to extend or hip raises up

Quantification

- The normal angle equals 147.9 degrees
- Standard deviation of 1.6
- Intra-assay CV (%) 0.5%
- Inter-assay CV (%) 1.1 (33)

Hip Flexion Mobility/Hamstring Length— Straight Leg Raise Test (SLR)

The hip flexion mobility/hamstring length—straight leg raise test (SLR) (33,40,165) evaluates the length or tension of the hamstring muscle and/or the articulation of the hip joint (Fig. 11.4).

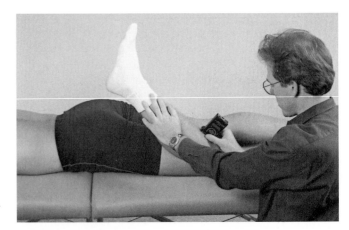

Figure 11.3 Knee flexion mobility/quadriceps length (Nachlas test).

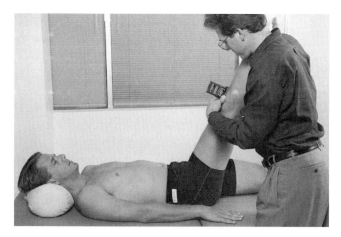

Figure 11.4 Hip flexion mobility/hamstring length. Straight leg raise test (SLR).

Patient Position

- The patient lies supine on a firm table and the inclinometer is placed just superior to the patellae (or alternatively on mid-tibia or strapped to lower leg with Velcro) and then zeroed

Test

- The patient's calf is placed in the crook of the doctor's elbow or rests in the doctor's hand
- The patient's hip is flexed without permitting any knee flexion to occur
- The angle is recorded just before pelvic movement or knee flexion

Quantification

- Normal ROM is 70 to 90 degrees (use 80 degrees as the mean for patient comparison)

Hip Extension Mobility/Psoas-Rectus Femoris Length (Modified Thomas Test)

This tests tightness in the iliopsoas (33, 165), which has been shown to be correlated with increased knee injury risk in male college athletes (68). Reduced ROM in hip extension has been reported frequently in LBP subjects (69,161,165). Preliminary data from McGill suggest that decreased hip extension mobility may be predictive of disabling LBP (104). Van Dillon reported that chronic LBP subjects had less passive hip extension ROM than asymptomatic subjects (161). Studies in adolescents have documented that future episodes of LBP are correlated with decreased hip extension ROM (69,161). Some controversy exists, however, because Nadler reported that hypermobility in the lower ex-

tremity was correlated with future LBP in college athletes (113,114).

The modified Thomas test evaluates the range of motion of the hip and/or the length or tension of the hip flexor muscle group (iliopsoas muscle) (Fig. 11.5).

Patient Position

- The patient perches at the end of bench in a manner where the ischial tuberosities are supported on the end of the table's edge
- The knee and hip are flexed and the knee is drawn up tight to the chest to eliminate lumbar lordosis and the patient is lowered to a supine position maintaining the knee-to-chest position

Test

- The inclinometer is zeroed to the horizontal of the table top
- The leg being tested is allowed to extend towards the floor and hang freely fully relaxed
- The knee should be brought to the chest to fully remove the slack and flatten the lumbar lordosis firmly to the table
- Place the inclinometer on the anterior thigh just below the ASIS. Record the angle when tested leg is fully relaxed, hip extended, and the lumbar lordosis is removed

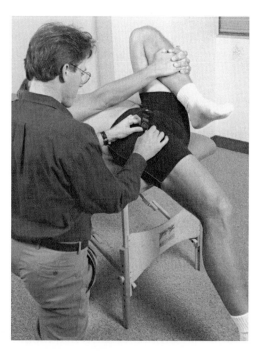

Figure 11.5 Hip extension mobility/psoas-rectus femoris length (modified Thomas test).

Quantification

- The normative data is 6.5 degrees
- SD 1.1
- Intra-assay CV 0.7%
- Inter-assay CV 1.2% (165)

Alternatively, Ekstrand published the following method (33).

Patient Position

- Patient lies supine with the knees straight on the bench

Test

- Place the inclinometer 5 cm above the patella on the lateral thigh and set to zero
- The leg being tested is passively flexed to 90 degrees using the initial inclinometer 0 degrees reading and the inclinometer reset to zero
- The rest of the test is the same as the last three steps described previously

Quantification

- The normative data is 83.5 degrees
- SD 1.1
- Intrassay CV 0.7%
- Interassay CV 1.2% (33)

Note

A qualitative screen for the hip flexors can also be performed to differentiate muscle tightness in the iliopsoas from the rectus femoris (RF) (see chapter 11) (14).

- Hip flexor muscle group tightness exists if the extended leg fails to reach horizontal (has <0 degrees hip extension ROM)
- RF is tight if knee has <90 degrees flexion passively or <110 degrees flexion with over-pressure when the hip is maintained in 0 degrees extension
- Iliopsoas is tight if hip does not achieve 0 degrees extension when leg is tested with RF slackened by extending the knee
- Tensor fascia lata (TFL) is tight if thigh abducts from a neutral position when being tested

Hip Rotation (Internal and External) Mobility

Decreases in hip internal rotation have shown correlation to LBP (20,32,33,117,118,132). Cibulka reported that bilateral loss of hip internal rotation is associated with LBP, whereas a unilateral restriction is associated with signs of sacro-iliac involvement (20) (Fig. 11.6).

Patient Position

- The patient lies prone with non tested leg in 30 degrees abduction and tested leg at 0 degrees abduction
- The pelvis is firmly stabilized
- The patient's knee is placed in 90 degrees flexion so that sole faces the ceiling

Test

- The inclinometer is placed on the distal tibia in the frontal plane and zeroed
- The hip is passively internally/externally rotated until opposite pelvis starts to move (usually rises upwards)
- The measurement is taken just before the opposite pelvis rising upwards and the angle is recorded

Quantification

- The normal range is 38 to 45 degrees internal rotation
- The normal range is 35 to 45 degrees external rotation

Note

- The AMA *Guides to the Evaluation of Permanent Impairment* test hip rotation supine, with knee extension and no pelvic stabilization (25)
- The hip ROM may also be tested in seated position
- A supine test with the hip and knee flexed at 90 degrees may be used to estimate mobility
  - This will also allow for testing of hip capsule integrity (capsular dysfunction presents with pain in internal rotation in this position)

Lumbar Spine Mobility

With lumbar spine mobility (93,98,101), there is controversy over the accuracy of spinal range of motion because of intrinsic and extrinsic operator error (100,101). Thus far, the most accepted "low-tech" assessment method for measuring spinal range of motion is the use of dual inclinometric ROM assessment (100). The clinical significance in non-acute

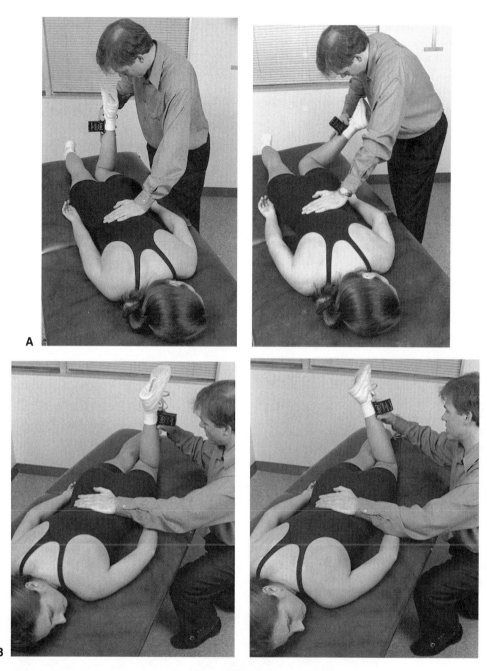

Figure 11.6 Hip rotation ([**A**] internal and [**B**] external) mobility.

patients of reduced mobility is controversial. Gronblad found that there was a lack of significant correlation between spinal mobility and either self-report of activity intolerances (Oswestry) or pain intensity (46). This was particularly true for sagittal plane motions such as trunk flexion. However, asymmetry in lateral flexion may be correlated (46). Biering-Sorenson found that increased trunk flexion mobility not hypomobility predicted future LBP in men (5). It has also been recently reported that patients with spondylolisthesis tended to be hypermobile, whereas those with spinal stenosis, disc prolapse, or degenerative disc disease tended to be hypomobile (105).

Lumbar ROM and Functional Ability are not Correlated in LBP Individuals

Subjects: chronic LBP patients

Methods: a three-dimensional lumbar motion monitor and 4-hour functional battery including isometric and dynamic pull/pull, carry, and lifting assessments.

Results: Weak or nonexistent correlation between ROM and functional ability

Parks KA, Crichton KS, Goldford RF, McGill SM. A comparison of lumbar range of motion and functional ability scores in patients with low back pain. Spine 2003;28:380–384.

Moffroid demonstrated that if patients are clustered into subgroups, an inflexibility group can be identified (109). A problem with many scientific studies is that non-specific back pain patients are considered one large homogenous group. This leads to the incorrect conclusion based on statistical evidence that parameters such as mobility are not relevant. However, it has been pointed out that such large groups should be considered heterogenous with many small subgroups within them (70). If subgroups are not studied independently then a clinical variable such as decreased mobility will be mistakenly concluded to be unimportant.

Flexion (erector spinae flexibility) (Fig. 11.7A)

Patient Position

- The patient stands with the knees straight and feet slightly apart.

Test

- A "warm-up" of several repetitions in each direction is recommended after which time the measurements can be calculated
- The inclinometers are placed on the sacral apex and T12 spinous process (use skin marking pencil) and are oriented vertically
- The inclinometers are zeroed and patient is requested to flex maximally and the new angle is recorded

- If the hamstrings are tight patient may bend knees

*Note: If the tightest SLR exceeds the sum of the sacral hip motion measured in flexion and extension by more than 15 degrees, the lumbosacral flexion test is invalid (25).

Extension (Fig. 11.7B)

Patient Position

- The starting position is the same as for flexion

Test

- The patient is requested to extend maximally, and the angle is recorded

Lateral Flexion (Fig. 11.7C)

Patient Position

- The starting position is the same as for flexion
- The inclinometers are oriented horizontally

Test

- The patient is requested to side bend maximally to the right/left
- To minimize rotation patient is instructed to slide fingers along the side of their leg
- The angle is recorded

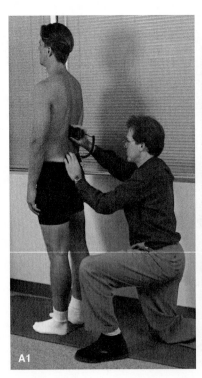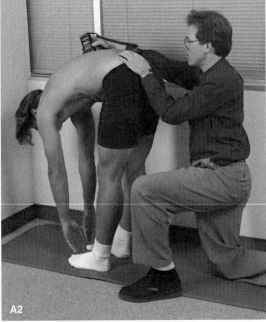

Figure 11.7 Lumbar spine mobility.
(A) Flexion (erector spinae flexibility).
(B) Extension.
(C) Lateral flexion.

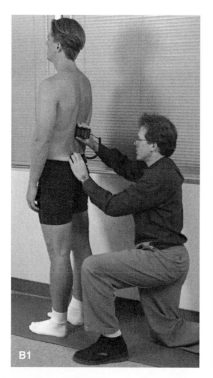

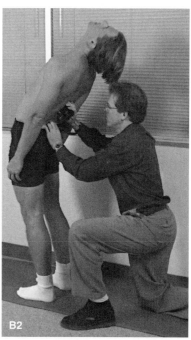

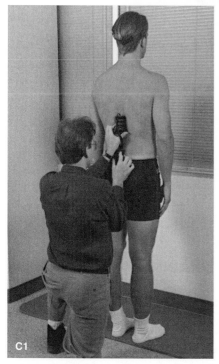

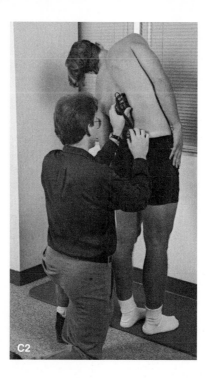

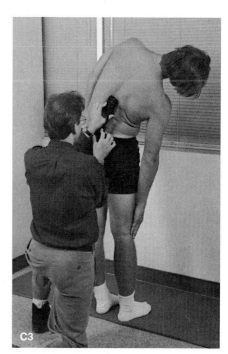

Figure 11.7 (*Continued*)

Quantification (93, 98)

The normal range is as follows:

- Trunk flexion 65 degrees
- Trunk extension 30 degrees
- Trunk lateral flexion 25 degrees

Cervical spine mobility (97, 171)

Flexion/Extension (Fig. 11.8A)

Patient Position

- The patient sits erect into the chair back
- The inclinometers are placed at T1 and the other on the occiput (or strap to head with Velcro strap)

Test

- The patient is requested to flex neck maximally and angle the is recorded

- The patient is requested to extend neck maximally and the angle is recorded

Lateral Flexion (Fig. 11.8B)

Patient Position

- The patient position same as flexion/extension and the inclinometers are placed in the frontal plane at the same bony landmarks, occiput, and T1

Test

- The patient is instructed to side-bend maximally to the left and right and the angles are recorded

Rotation (61) (Fig. 11.8C)

Position

- According to the AMA protocol, this is tested this supine with only one gravity inclinometer

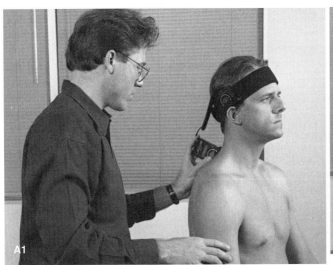

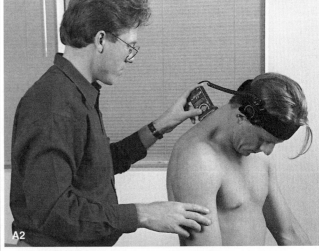

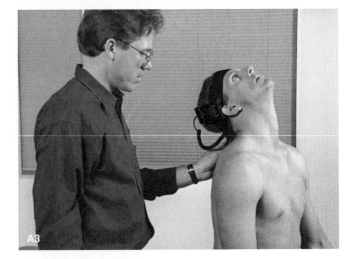

Figure 11.8 Cervical spine mobility.
(A) Flexion/extension.
(B) Lateral flexion.
(C) Rotation.

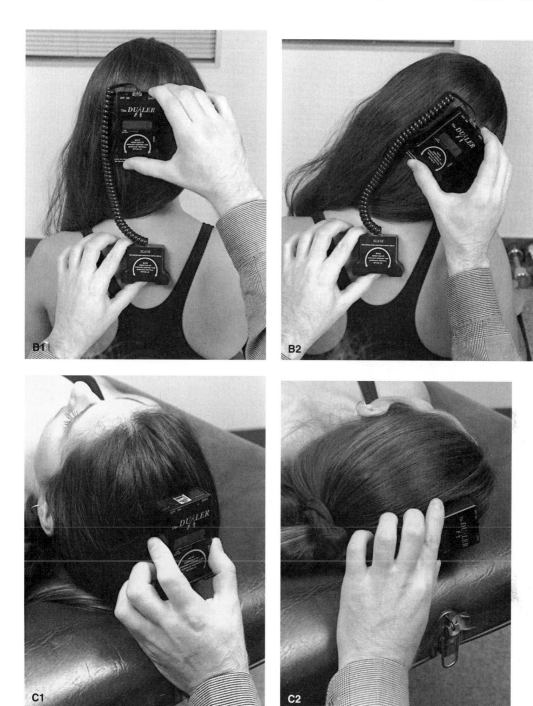

Figure 11.8 (*Continued*)

Test

- The supine patient rotates head fully and angle is recorded

Quantification (98)

The normal range is as follows:

- Cervical flexion 50 degrees
- Cervical extension 63 degrees
- Cervical lateral flexion 45 degrees
- Cervical rotation 85 degrees

Shoulder Mobility

Reliability of upper quarter ROM tests has not been studied as extensively as it has in the spine or lower quarter. However, it is a necessary part of the clinical examination to check for asymmetrical ROM, obvious limitations, and mechanical sensitivities there. In particular arm abduction, flexion, internal rotation, and external rotation ROMs are important to observe. Goniometric assessment of shoulder flexion and abduction has been shown to be reliable for both passive and active ROM testing in either the sitting upright or supine positions (139).

Strength/Endurance

Introduction

Gronblad reported that there is a higher correlation between strength/endurance tests and activity intolerance or pain intensity than with mobility tests (46). Endurance testing in particular has been shown to be promising. Decreased endurance of the trunk extensors has been shown not only to correlate with pain (5,74,121) but also to predict recurrences (5) and chronicity (35), as well as first-time onset of episodes in healthy individuals (81). One study has disputed that this test correlates with low back trouble (156). The test, if performed in the manner described by Biering-Sorensen, has been shown to be reliable in various populations—asymptomatic (74), symptomatic (110), and those with a history of LBP (74). One study claimed the test was unreliable, but a small sample (12 subjects) and a different procedure using a Roman Chair was utilized (99).

It has also been found that reduced endurance of the deep neck flexors has been correlated with neck pain after whiplash or concussion (4,63,144,157,167).

Normal ratios of trunk flexor, extensor, and side support muscles have been established (103). A reduced ratio of trunk extensor to flexor strength/ endurance discriminates between LBP patients and control subjects. The normal ratio is approximately 1.3:1, with the extensors being stronger (94,95).

Nadler et al. demonstrated that hip muscle imbalance is associated both retrospectively and prospectively with LBP in female athletes (114, 115). In particular, asymmetric hip extensor strength was significantly correlated with LBP incidence. Those with LBP had a 15% strength imbalance compared with only a 5.3% imbalance in those without LBP. This same asymmetry was not found in male athletes, but it is interesting to note that National Collegiate Athletic Association Injury Surveillance Data from 1997 to 1998 showed that female athletes were almost twice as likely as males to have LBP develop (National Collegiate 1997–1998). Other consistent findings include increased fatigability of the gluteus maximus in individuals with chronic LBP (65,75).

It is known that trunk strength is related to effort. It has been suggested that preferential motion that is submaximal is a preferred mode of testing (7). The extent to which strength measurements can differentiate maximal (sincere) performance from feigned performance has been studied extensively. Consistency of effort as determined by the CV is significantly higher in feigned weakness as opposed to maximal performance; however, the sensitivity and specificity of the measures have not been shown to be high enough be considered medico-legally valid (26–28,48, 77,146).

Two studies compared the performance of physical capacity tests to the nonorganic signs (22,52). Using lumbar dynamometry to measure strength, Cooke and colleagues demonstrated that patients with three or more Waddell Signs had lower performance values than those with two or less. Similarly, Hirsch et al reported in a 5-week or greater LBP sample of 85 men aged between 18 and 60 years old, physical performance was significantly poorer when three or more Waddell signs were present.

Table 11.3 shows the strength/endurance tests that are described in detail.

Squat Endurance Tests

Repetitive Squat Test (1) (Fig. 11.9)

Patient Position

- Standing with feet 15 cm apart.

Test

- The patient squats until thighs are horizontal and returns to upright position
- The speed is approximately 2 to 3 seconds/repetition

Table 11.3 Strength/Endurance Tests

1. Squat endurance test
   a. Repetitive
   b. Static
2. Trunk flexor endurance tests
   a. Repetitive sit-up endurance test
   b. Static quarter sit-up endurance test
   c. Isometric trunk flexor endurance
3. Side bridge tests
4. Static trunk extensor endurance test
   a) Sorensen
   b) Back Strong
   c) Ito variation
5. Grip strength

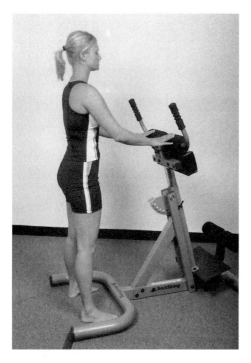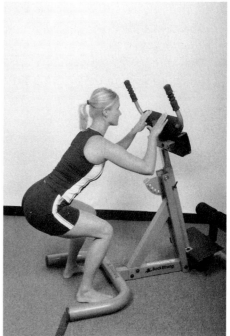

Figure 11.9 Repetitive squat endurance test.

Termination Criteria

- The patient continues until unable, pain in knee or back becomes significant, or 50 repetitions are achieved

Quantification (1)

Count number of repetition

Normals: The following chart is used to determine the normal for the subject being evaluated (Table 11.4).

Static Squat Test (106)

Patient Position

- Head, shoulders, and buttocks against a 90-degree wall
- Feet far enough away from the wall to allow hips, knees, and ankles to flex to 90 degrees with the knees not passing in front of the toes.

Table 11.4 Repetitive Squat Test Normative Data (1)

| Age | Males (n=242) | | | | | | Females (n=233) | | | | | |
| | Blue Collar | | White Collar | | All | | Blue Collar | | White Collar | | All | |
	X	SD	X	SD	X	SD	X	SD	X	SD	X	SD
35–39	39	13	46	8	42	12	24	11	27	12	26	12
40–44	34	14	45	9	38	13	22	13	18	8	20	12
45–49	30	12	40	11	33	13	19	12	26	13	22	13
50–54	28	14	41	11	33	14	13	10	18	14	14	11
35–54	33	14	43	10	37	13	20	12	23	12	21	12

X = Average
SD = Standard deviation
Note: The last row represents the average of all the ages (35–54)

Test

- Instruct the subject to slide down the wall until the hips, knees, and ankles are flexed at 90 degrees.
- Instruct the subject to sustain the position for as long as possible.
- Instruct the subject to breathe normally during the test.
- Record the duration in seconds that the subject is able to sustain the wall squat position.
- Normative data are shown in Table 11.5.

Termination Criteria

- Subject is unable to assume the starting position.
- Subject is no longer able to maintain the wall squat position.
- Subject terminates the test.
- Subject refuses to attempt the test

Table 11.5 Static Squat Test Normative Data (106)

Age	Males	Females
19–29	Mean 99.454 N = 98 SD 45.201	Mean 92.607 N = 97 SD 64.202
30–39	Mean 103.51 N = 75 SD 72.179	Mean 87.646 N = 69 SD 63.621
40–49	Mean 94.855 N = 42 SD 64.071	Mean 55.653 N = 43 SD 44.891
50–59	Mean 96.226 N = 34 SD 104.30	Mean 47.392 N = 38 SD 47.261
60+	Mean 45.204 N = 23 SD 27.081	Mean 39.059 N = 29 SD 35.830

Trunk Flexor Tests

Repetitive Sit-Up Test (1) (Fig. 11.10)

Patient Position

- Supine, knees flexed 90 degrees, ankles fixed.

Test

- The patient sits up until the thenar pad of the hand touches the superior pole of the patella, and then curls back down to the supine position at 2 to 3 seconds/repetition

Termination Criteria

- Count the total number of repetitions achieved up to a maximum of 50

The normative data for trunk strength segregated by age, sex, and occupation are in Table 11.6 (1).

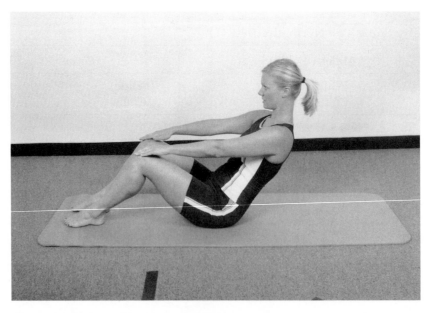

Figure 11.10 Repetitive sit-up endurance test.

Table 11.6   Repetitive Sit-Up Test Normative Data (1)

Age	Males (n=242)						Females (n=233)					
	Blue Collar		White Collar		All		Blue Collar		White Collar		All	
	X	SD	X	SD	X	SD	X	SD	X	SD	X	SD
35–39	29	13	35	13	32	13	24	12	30	16	27	14
40–44	22	11	34	12	27	13	18	12	19	13	19	12
45–49	19	11	33	15	24	14	17	14	22	15	19	14
50–54	17	13	36	16	23	16	9	10	20	13	11	11
35–54	23	13	35	13	27	14	17	13	24	15	19	14

X = AVERAGE
SD = Standard deviation

Static Quarter Sit-Up (106)

Patient Position

- Supine lying on an exercise mat, with knees flexed at approximately 90 degrees and heels in contact with the floor.
- Arm straight and parallel to spine, palms of hands in contact with the mat
- Head in contact with the mat

Test

- Measure a distance of 12 cm (8 cm if the subject is older than 40) from the caudal edge of the mat. At the fingertips of the subjects, attach two strips of tape to the mat at right angles to the trunk.
- Instruct the subject to raise the head and shoulders by sliding the palms forward from the tape until the fingertips touch the end of the mat.
- Instruct the subject to maintain the partial sit-up position for as long as possible.
- Instruct the subject to breathe normally during the test.
- Record the duration in seconds that the subject is able to sustain the partial sit-up position.
- The normative data are shown in Table 11.7.

Termination Criteria

- Subject is unable to reach the end of the mat.
- Subject is unable to sustain the partial sit-up position.
- Subject's feet do not maintain contact with the floor.
- Subject terminates the test.

Isometric Trunk Flexor Endurance Test (103)

McGill and colleagues established normative data for a healthy, young group of males and females for a simple curl-up test (Table 11.8). This test requires a wedged piece of wood or thick foam to support the patient at a fixed angle of 50 degrees. (see Fig. 32.17)

Table 11.7   Static Quarter Sit-Up Normative Data (in seconds) (106)

Age	Males	Females
19–29	Mean 72.6 N = 98 SD 67.3	Mean 66.9 N = 97 SD 54.7
30–39	Mean 73.2 N = 75 SD 73.1	Mean 68.9 N = 69 SD 66.0
40–49	Mean 77.8 N = 42 SD 89.3	Mean 70.0 N = 43 SD 86.3
50–59	Mean 94.1 N = 34 SD 129.4	Mean 55.0 N = 38 SD 57.1
60+	Mean 54.9 N = 23 SD 75.6	Mean 55.0 N = 29 SD 97.9

Table 11.8 McGill's Side Bridge, Trunk Flexor, and Trunk Extensor Endurance Normative Data (103)

Task	Men			Women			All		
	Mean	SD	Ratio	Mean	SD	Ratio	Mean	SD	Ratio
Extensor	146	51	1.0	189	60	1.0	177	60	1.0
Flexor	144	76	0.99	149	99	0.79	147	90	0.86
Side bridge, right	94	34	0.64	72	31	0.38	81	34	0.47
Side bridge, left	97	35	0.66	77	35	0.40	85	36	0.5

Patient Position

- Both knees and hips are flexed 90 degrees
- Arms are folded across chest
- Toes are anchored either with a strap or by the tester

Test

- The support is pulled back 10 cm (4 inches)
- The subject holds the isometric posture as long as possible

Termination Criteria

- When any part of the subjects back touches the support

The mean endurance for young healthy men and women is 134 seconds, with standard deviation (SD) of 76 (Table 11.8). The ratio of trunk flexor to extensor endurance is 0.77 normally (0.84 in young males and 0.72 in young females).

Side Bridge (103)

The side bridge endurance test is illustrated in Figure 11.11.

Patient Position

- The subject lays on one side supported by the pelvis, lower extremity, and forearm (elbow bent with hand facing forward)
- The top leg is placed in front of the lower leg with both feet on the floor
- The upper arm is placed against the chest with the hand touching the anterior lower shoulder

Test

- The pelvis is raised off the table as high as possible so long as the spine is not side-bending. It should be held in a line with a long axis of the body supporting the weight between the feet and elbow.
- Subject statically maintains this elevated position
- If the subject is fatigued and drops part-way, give one additional cue to raise the spine back up

Termination Criteria

- Subject is unable to lift body up from the floor
- Subjects thigh touches the floor
- The second time the subject drops the pelvis or thigh part way from the starting height
- Significant LBP causes the test to be stopped

Quantification

The mean endurance for young healthy men and women is 84.5 seconds, with a SD of 34.5 (103). The ratio of right side bridge to left side bridge endurance is normally 0.96 (103). According to McGill, a side to side difference of greater than 0.05 suggests unbalanced endurance (104). The side bridge-to-extensor endurance ratio is normally 0.49 (103). See Table 11.8 for these comparative data.

Static Trunk Extensor Endurance Test

Sorensen Test (1,5) (Fig. 11.12)

Patient Position

- Prone with the inguinal region/anterior superior iliac spine (ASIS) at the end of the table.
- Arms at sides, ankles fixed (by strap or hands), holding horizontal position.
  - Plump line can be used to ensure horizontal position

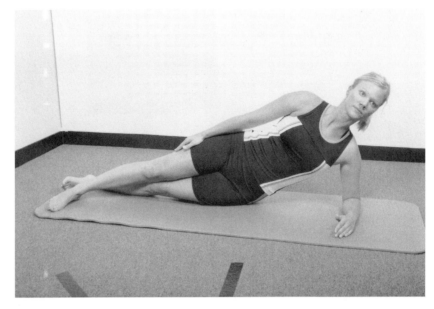

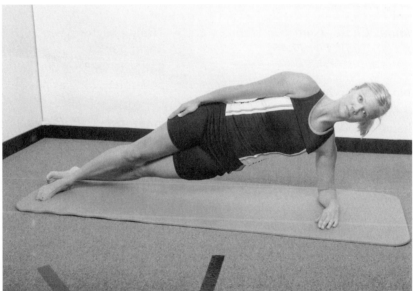

Figure 11.11 Side bridge endurance test.

Technique

- The patient maintains the horizontal position as long as possible
- Timing begins when horizontal and unsupported
- Subjects are verbally encouraged to hold this position as long as possible

Termination Criteria

- Time the duration the position can be held, up to a maximum of 240 seconds
- If patient drops below the horizontal position, give one additional chance to regain it. But on dropping below horizontal a second time, the duration is recorded
- If the patient reports low back pain or cramping in the legs, the test may be stopped and the time recorded

Quantification

See Table 11.9. A dynamic variation on this test is the repetitive arch-up test (1). In a prospective study of Finnish workers between the ages of 30 and 65 years, reduced repetitive trunk extensor endurance strongly correlated with an increased risk of work disability caused by chronic back disorders over a 12-year period (136).

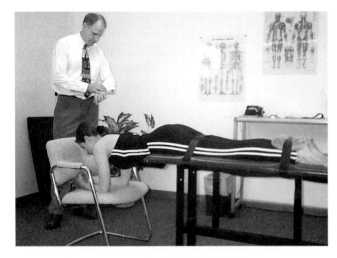 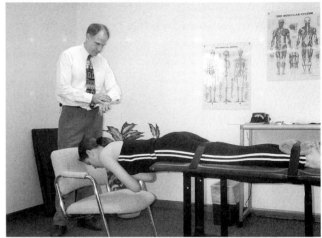

Figure 11.12 Static trunk extensor endurance. Sorensen test. Reproduced with permission from Yeomans S. Clinical Application of Outcomes Assessment. In: Yeomans S, ed. Stamford, CT: Appleton and Lange, 1999.

Variable Angle Roman Chair Isometric Trunk Extensor Endurance Test (163) (Fig. 11.13)

Patient Position

- Angle on variable angle Roman chair (Back Strong) unit set at 0 degrees (horizontal)
- Subject keeps hands at sides
- Positioned with ASIS aligned to the superior edge of the pelvic restraint pad
- Subject's ankles are positioned under the ankle pad
- Legs held as straight as possible

Test

- Instructed to elevate torso to a position horizontal to the floor

- Timing begins when horizontal and unsupported
- Subjects are verbally encouraged to hold this position as long as possible

Termination Criteria

- When torso drops 10 degrees below horizontal, the time is recorded in seconds

Ito's Trunk Extensor Endurance Test (58):
Ito et al. reported a reliable assessment of the low back extensor endurance strength that can be used as an alternative to the static back endurance (58). The Ito test is a timed test performed by instructing the prone subject lying on a pelvic pillow to fully flex the cervical spine and contract the gluteal muscles to

Table 11.9   Static Trunk Extensor Endurance—Sorensen Test Normative Data (1)

	Males (n=242)						Females (n=233)					
	Blue Collar		White Collar		All		Blue Collar		White Collar		All	
Age	mean	SD	mean	SD	mean	SD	mean	SD	mean	SD	mean	SD
35–39	87	38	113	47	97	43	91	61	95	48	93	55
40–44	83	51	129	57	101	57	89	57	67	51	80	55
45–49	81	45	131	64	99	58	90	55	122	73	102	64
50–54	73	47	121	56	89	55	62	55	99	78	69	60
35–54	82	45	123	55	97	53	82	58	94	62	87	59

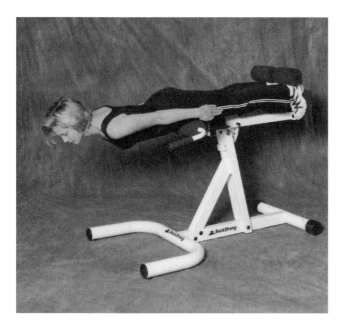

Figure 11.13 Stack trunk extensor endurance. Back Strong Sorensen adaptation photo, permission of Back Strong International.

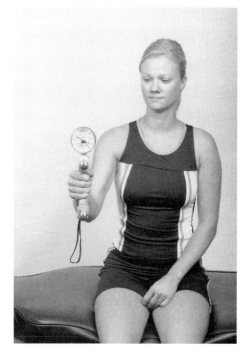

Figure 11.14 Grip strength.

stabilize the spine, and extend the trunk so that it is in line with the pelvis. Like the Sorenson test, the Ito test has been reported to be able to discriminate between subjects with and without low back pain (58,109). The normative data for the Ito test is shown in Table 11.10.

Grip Strength

Grip strength (153) dynamometry is primarily used to evaluate upper extremity strength of the grip (Fig. 11.14). It can be used to evaluate motor function in cervical nerve root compression or carpal tunnel syndrome or as a general evaluation for fitness. In healthy 45- to 68-year-old men studied in the Honolulu Heart Program, grip strength was found to independently predict future functional independence at a 25-year follow-up (131). Classically, this test is performed in a sitting or standing position with the test elbow flexed 90 degrees. However, allowing the patient to locate a pain-free arm position if the 90-degree elbow-flexed position is painful can avoid a "false-positive" test caused by pain-induced weakness. A Jamar hand dynamometer was used in the normative data study (153). Therefore, it is important to evaluate and calibrate non-Jamar dynamometers to a Jamar standard if the normative data tables are needed.

Patient Position

- Seated
- There are five handle positions on a Jamar grip dynamometer, of which the second

Table 11.10 Ito's Prone Trunk Extensor Endurance Test Normative Data (58)

	Healthy		CLBP	
	Males	Females	Males	Females
Extensor Endurance	208.2 66.2 (.97)*	128.4 53.0 (.94)*	85.1 55.6 (.93)*	70.1 51.8 (.95)*

*The test–retest correlation (r).
CLBP = chronic low back pain
The mean endurance strength of the flexor and extensor trunk muscles are reported with the corresponding test-retest correlation (r) values. All test–retest correlations for both groups for the corresponding endurance measurements were significantly high (p < 0.01).

(4 cm) or third position (6 cm) is the strongest and, therefore, most often used, depending on hand size.

Test

- The patient is instructed to squeeze the grip as hard as possible
- This is repeated two additional times with verbal encouragement to make a maximum effort

Quantification (153)

- The average of three readings are taken and considered normal if the scores are within 20% of each other, usually switching between the left and right hands for each of the three repetitions.
- If there is a 20% or greater variation in the three readings, differentiation between full effort (i.e., psychosocial issues) versus pain-induced weakness is necessary (153).
- Most commonly, the normal upper extremity is compared to the abnormal and, therefore, there is no reason to use normative data unless bilateral upper extremity problems exist (25,153).

Balance/Motor Control

Introduction

Motor control is considered to be essential to spine stability. It is believed to be more important than strength. Mannion suggests new aspects of physical function relating to motor control should be investigated as a possible cause of the approximately 50% of disabling pain that is unaccounted for by psychological, structural, or voluntary performance measures (87). These include those involved in non-voluntary reflex control of movement such as position sense, delayed reaction times, and balance tests (87,104).

Kinesthetic awareness of position sense (13,43, 119,155) has been shown to be compromised in LBP individuals and neck pain patients (51,80,133). This is the ability to reproduce positions in space and is called repositioning ability or error. Altered reaction times of muscles has been correlated with LBP (53,54,82,84,129,130,154,168). Work at Yale University demonstrated a slow reaction time, increased activation, and slow relaxation after unexpected perturbations (129,130). Finnish researchers have reported that anticipated loads to the arms in unsupported standing result in delayed reaction times in patients with chronic sciatica but not in healthy control subjects (76). Australian researchers have

reported that a delayed activation of the transverse abdominus muscle during arm or leg movements has been found to distinguish LBP patients from normal subjects (53,54). Finnish scientists have reported that reaction times to visual stimuli have been shown to be slower in chronic LBP patients than in asymptomatic individuals (83,84).

Incoordination is correlated with LBP (2,55,56, 45,124) and neck pain (31,62,63,116). O'Sullivan found that an increased ratio of rectus abdominus to transverse abdominus/oblique abdominal activation is correlated with LBP (123). Control subjects were able to preferentially activate internal oblique and transverse abdominus muscles without significant rectus abdominus activation. LBP patients could not do this. Nedherhand found that a decreased ability to relax the upper trapezius muscles during static tasks and after exercise distinguished between chronic whiplash-associated disorder (WAD) classification II patients and healthy control subjects (116).

Sterling et al reported that WAD II or III patients evaluated within 1 month of injury had increased EMG activity of superficial neck flexors (SCM) during performance of the cervico-cranial flexion test than asymptomatic control subjects (151). Jull et al has reported similar results in both WAD and insidious onset neck patients (64).

Balance deficits have been demonstrated to be related to LBP (15,83,111,156). Byl showed that excessive anterior to posterior body sway on an unstable surface or poor single leg standing balance ability is correlated with LBP (15). Mok et al demonstrated that LBP patients had poorer balance than age- and gender-matched controls when vision was removed or a smaller base of support was used (111). Poor balance was correlated with future LBP by Takala (156).

Table 11.11 shows the motor control tests that are described in detail.

One-Leg Standing Balance Test

The one-leg standing balance test (3,10,15,16,17) is illustrated in Fig. 11.15.

Patient Position
- Standing

Table 11.11 Balance/Motor Control Tests

1. One-leg standing balance
2. Prone abdominal hollowing cuff test
3. Cervico-cranial flexion test of Jull

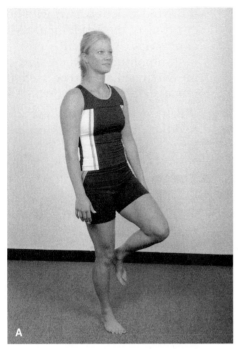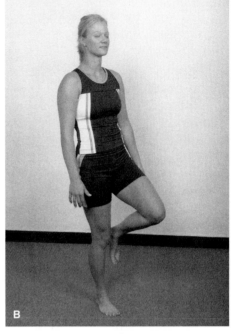

Figure 11.15 One-leg standing balance test.
(A) Eyes open—preparation
(B) Eyes closed—test

Test

- The patient stands on one leg with the opposite leg flexed at the hip and knee.
- The patient should be instructed to fix their gaze at a point on the wall directly in front of them.
- The patient should practice with eyes open once for up to 10 seconds.
- They should then attempt to balance as long as possible on one leg with eyes closed for up to 30 seconds.
- The subject may repeat the test up to a maximum of five times in an attempt to reach the 30-second target successfully. If the subject can stand for 30 seconds on the first eyes-closed attempt, they may discontinue the test.

Termination Criteria

- Reaching out
- Hopping
- Putting foot down
- Touching foot to weight-bearing leg

Quantification

- The best score with eyes closed for each leg should be recorded.
- The normative data are shown in Table 11.12.

Abdominal Hollowing (Cuff Test)

The Prone Abdominal Drawing-In Test or Abdominal Hollowing Test (134) is Shown in Figure 11.16.

Patient Position

- Prone
- Feedback unit is placed under abdomen with navel in the center and distal edge of the pad in line with right and left anterior superior iliac spines
- Pad inflated to 70 mm Hg

Test

- Breathe in and out, and then without breathing in to slowly draw the abdomen in so

Table 11.12 Single-Leg Stance Eyes Closed Normative Data (10)

Age (years)	Eyes Open (seconds)	Eyes Closed (seconds)
20–59	29–30	21–28.8
60–69	22.5	10
70–79	14.2	4.3

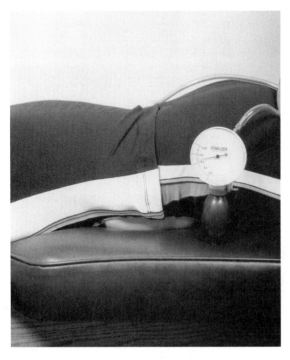

Figure 11.16 Prone abdominal hollowing test. Drawing-in from 70 mm Hg to 66 mm Hg

it lifts off the pad (draw abdomen away from waistband of pants)
- Don't change spinal position
- Then breath normally without losing the drawing in maneuver
- Try for a few repetitions to be sure the patient has given it their best shot
- Perform 10 times

Quantification
- Fail if more than 10-mm Hg decline in cuff pressure or less than 4-mm Hg drop in cuff pressure during 10-second hold (a 4–10-mm Hg range is acceptable)
- Fail if thoraco-lumbar hypertonus, lumbar extension, posterior pelvic tilt, or breath holding occurs

Cervico-Cranial Flexion Test of Jull

This test (62,63) is illustrated in Figure 11.17.

Pre-Test Routine
- Supine patient with knees bent and feet flat (crook lying)
- Ask patient to move their head as if nodding "yes" (cervico-cranial flexion)

- If the movement occurs with head retraction or lifting of the head, then passively model the appropriate movement. Active assistance, large amplitude movements, or eye movements may also be used. If the pattern is inadequate, then delay formal testing.
- When the patient can actively perform the nodding movement with cervico-cranial flexion they can proceed to the test.

Patient Position
- Supine with head in "neutral" position so that head is not extended on the neck or chin jutting forward
  - Use a small folded towel to align head if necessary
  - The towel should be placed under the occiput and leave the cervical spine free
- Place an inflatable cushion (Stabilizer™, Chattanooga South Pacific) under the neck suboccipitally to support it without pushing it up
- Inflate the bag to 20 mm Hg
- Gently squeeze the sides of the bag to distribute the air—the pressure should decrease
- Re-inflate and repeat the gentle squeezing a few times until the pressure stabilizes at 20 mm Hg

Test

1st phase
- The pressure cuff dial is turned towards the patient and the patient should confirm that that they can see that the dial is set to 20 mm Hg.
- The patient is instructed to place the tongue on the roof of the mouth (just behind the front teeth), lips together but teeth slightly separated (this inhibits the jaw depressors, hyoid or platysma).
- The patient is asked to gently nod to a target of 22 mm Hg on the cuff and to hold the needle steady for 5 seconds while breathing normally
- If successful, the patient is instructed to relax back to 20 mm Hg again and then perform the chin nod movement to 24 mm Hg
  - If the patient does not return to 20 mm Hg, the clinician can reposition the head to achieve the 20 mm Hg starting point.
- This is repeated until a maximum of 30 mm Hg is achieved

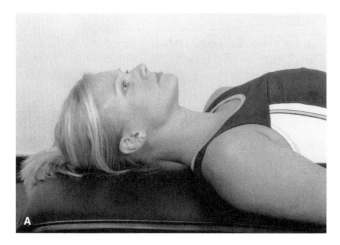
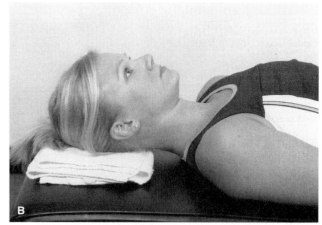
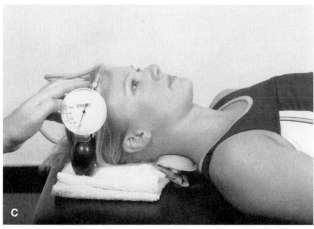
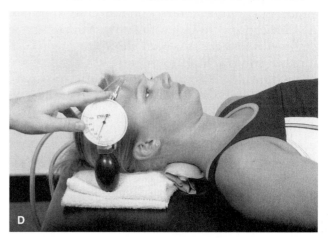

Figure 11.17 Cervico-cranial flexion test of Jull.
(A) Incorrect head/neck alignment
(B) Correct head/neck alignment
(C) Beginning position with stabilizer cuff inflated to 20 mm Hg
(D) Successful nodding motion to 28 mm Hg

Quantification

- The ability to target and hold the position steady (based on the pressure recording) is measured while observing activity in the superficial neck flexor mm (SCM, anterior scalenes)
- Failure occurs if any of the following occurs
  - Inability to reach target pressure
  - Inability to hold target pressure steady for 5 seconds (e.g., if stabilizer pressure needle oscillates)
  - Superficial muscle substitution is observed

2nd phase

- The maximum pressure that the patient can hold steady, without superficial muscle activity is then tested for endurance (i.e., their ability to maintain the pressure for 10 seconds for 10 repetitions)

Pain-free subjects on average can successfully target and hold pressure steady at 26 mm Hg without superficial muscle activity (62,63). Chronic headache or neck pain WAD patients can usually only target 22 to 24 mm Hg and cannot hold the dial steady at any pressure level (62,63). Ideal performance is to be able to hold pressure steady for 10 seconds at 28 or 30 mm Hg. Kinesthetic awareness of head/neck position is also measured by the patient's ability to return to 20 mm Hg of pressure in between repetitions. Both insidious onset neck pain and whiplash patient were shown to have significantly greater SCM activity (with EMG) than control subjects at each test level (*P*<0.05) regardless of whether the pain was acute or chronic (64).

Falla et al have shown that reduced performance in this test is associated with dysfunction of the deep neck flexor muscles (37).

Aerobic Fitness

Introduction

Cardiovascular or aerobic fitness is extremely important to measure to establish fitness baselines. Healthy aging and good aerobic fitness go hand in hand. Patients with heart disease, depression, chronic pain, chronic fatigue syndrome, or fibromyalgia may need aerobic fitness more than strength, endurance, motor control, or flexibility training. Aerobic capacity testing with a submaximal bicycle ergometer test has not been shown to predict future outcome (128). However, the test results have been shown to improve with a multidisciplinary rehabilitation program for work-related back problems (128).

Ideally, direct measures of maximum oxygen uptake would be performed. However, this requires expensive, specialized equipment and is risky for certain elderly groups and cardiac patients. Thus, other indirect measures have been developed for large-scale screening of cardiovascular fitness and/or prediction of maximal oxygen uptake. Both maximal and submaximal exercise protocols are used. Maximal procedures provide a better estimation of VO_2 and are of particular value with younger populations or individuals without risk factors for heart disease. Submaximal procedures are safer for elderly populations, symptomatic individuals, or those with cardiac risk factors.

Most submaximal tests are based on the measurement of heart rate (HR). There are a few limitations of this approach. HR can vary independently of VO_2 because of levels of excitement or emotional state. This section will present a few examples of submaximal tests. HR is not a linear function of VO_2 relative to submaximal workloads up to maximum loads. Table 11.13 shows the aerobic fitness tests that are described in detail.

Table 11.13 Aerobic Fitness Tests

1. Step tests
   a. YMCA 3-minute bench step test
   b. Harvard step test
2. Bicycle test
3. Treadmill test

Step Tests

The Harvard Method (166)

This 5-minute step test is a simple, inexpensive, reliable method for assessing cardiovascular fitness. This is an excellent test for a relatively fit population. However, it may be too strenuous for an older or less fit population. Also, the 20-inch step height required may lead to leg fatigue before aerobic fatigue in shorter or heavier individuals. The equipment required is:

- 20-inch step
- Metronome
- Timer

Patient Position

- Standing in front of step

Test

- Set the metronome at 120 beats per minute (BPM) to elicit a stepping rate of 30 steps/minute
- Stepping cycle
  - A four-count beat
  - Count 1—one foot on step
  - Count 2—other leg lifted on step and subject straightens both the back and legs
  - Count 3—first foot is brought back down
  - Count 4—second foot is brought back down

Termination Criteria

- Maximum of 5 minutes or until exhaustion.
- Subject is considered exhausted when he or she cannot maintain the pace for 15 seconds.

Quantification

- At completion of test the subject sits down and the pulse is counted from 1 to 1.5, 2 to 2.5, and 3 to 3.5 minutes into recovery. The number of heartbeats during the three 30-second periods is recorded.
- Calculation

Index = 100 × duration in seconds ÷ 2 × sum of pulses

Example: subject steps for 3 minutes and 10 seconds (190 seconds) with pulses of 82, 80, and 70 beats for the three recovery periods.

$100 \times 190 \div (2 \times 232) = 41$. This subject is thus "poor."

Index	Classification
>90	Excellent
80–89	Good
65–79	High average
55–64	Low average
<55	Poor

YMCA 3-Minute Bench Step Test (44)

This alternative to the Harvard method is shown in Figure 11.18. This test uses a shorter 12-inch bench and a metronome set at 96 bpm (24 steps/minute). The test duration is also shorter—3 minutes. At the end of the 3 minutes of stepping, the patient immediately sits down and the recovery heart rate is counted for a full minute. It is important that the recovery heart rate be counted within 5 seconds of ending the 3 minutes of exercise. An estimated VO_2 max can be estimated from the 3-minute step test (44,172).

A 2- to 3-minute bike test very similar to step tests can also be used (44,172), i.e., the cycle ergometer test. A disadvantage of this test is that not all adults are familiar with cycling.

A third option for aerobic fitness evaluation uses a treadmill (172). An advantage of treadmill testing is that most individuals can walk comfortably. A disadvantage is that the equipment is more expensive. Before beginning, the patient should receive instructions describing the test. Walking or running shoes should be worn. The treadmill should have rails for the patient to use if needed (especially at first) and there should be an emergency stop button or switch mechanism. The patient should initially straddle the belt and start "pawing" or "pedaling" the belt using one foot as it begins to move. Patients will often look down at the belt, walk with a very short stride, and drift to the rear of the belt at first. They should be encouraged to look forward, walk with a more lengthened normal stride, and walk in the center of the belt.

The patient's heart rate will need to be measured while exercising. Relatively inexpensive accurate heart rate monitors made by companies such as Polar (1-800-227-1314 or http://www.polar.fi/sampola/) are recommended.

Implementation—How

Functional assessments yield relevant targets for treatment and thus are prescriptive. This is of particular value because most diagnostic procedures identify only pathoanatomy or the pain generators, not physiological information about the patient's source of "instability" or mechanical overload. Assessing impairment, functional capacity, or PPA is also invaluable as an outcome to objectively show progress, document the need for further treatment, and determine appropriate end points of care. The quantifiable assessment of function complements the use of other outcome tools such as subjective questionnaires that identify self-report of activity intolerances (see Chapter 9).

The PPA should be used in conjunction with functional assessments such as of actual activities performed (see Chapters 13 and 14), movement sensitivity (Chapter 16), muscle imbalances (Chapter 11), and joint play (Chapter 22) help complete the patient's clinical picture. Such a functional assessment yields a "functional diagnosis" that is of value in the clinical management of patients, especially those slow to recover from acute pain or those with chronic pain.

Many quantitative tests of function suffer from having very large standard deviations for their ranges of normal responses. For example, when assessing abdominal strength using the repetitive sit-up test (1), the normative data for a blue-collar, 46-year-old man is a mean of 19 repetitions with a standard deviation of 11. To deal with this wide range, using a cutoff of 85% of the normative mean, such as 16 repetitive sit-ups of the 19 mean, results in a more sensitive approach (by increasing the number of true-positives in a LBP population). Using a 95% confidence interval, a range of normal between 19 plus or minus 10.45 or 8.55 to 29.45 repetitions can be expected when testing 95% of 46-year-old, blue-collar males. The 95%

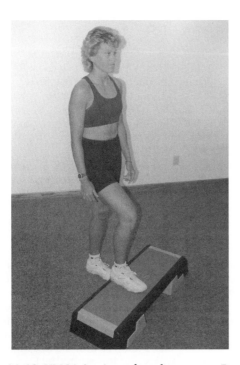

Figure 11.18 YMCA 3-minute bench step test. Reproduced with permission from Yeomans S. Clinical Application of Outcomes Assessment. Stamford, CT: Appleton and Lange, 1999.

confidence interval illustrates the expected variation in scores caused by biovariability (i.e., ectomorphic, mesomorphic, and endomorphic).

This approach will reduce the specificity (number of true-negatives in a normal population) of the tests but it adds to the utility and practicality. The balance between sensitivity, specificity, practicality, and utility allows for use of a method by adjusting the mean normative data so it can be applied in a clinical setting. Other methods have been reported such as using a percentile of the mean (106) or breaking the normative data into five categories ranging from extremely poor to extremely good (172).

In a clinical setting, certain tests that minimally stress injured or painful tissues can be used to quantify dysfunction from the beginning of acute care. These include ROM/muscle length tests and balance tests. Other tests such as endurance tests involve moderate levels of biomechanical load and thus should NOT be used during the acute phase.

Although it is common to perform a comprehensive PPA evaluation to profile patients in many circumstances, individual tests or small clusters of tests can also be used. For instance, concern about lower quarter function in a lumbar spine patient might lead to squatting and balance tests being performed. In another instance, a construction worker might benefit from a test battery that might include trunk flexor, extensor, and side bridge tests, along with a squatting test to unmask a "weak link." An athlete who is very strong might be unaware of motor control issues and therefore can be a candidate for balance and abdominal coordination tests (abdominal hollowing). A subacute LBP patient may NOT be a candidate for strength testing, but the abdominal hollowing test may be particular useful.

Asymptomatic individuals are starting to present to musculoskeletal health care clinics seeking preventive advice. In such cases, a performance evaluation using the PPA can give a risk assessment or stability profile that can result in some preventive prescriptive exercise advice.

Tests that are positive should lead to a specific prescription of exercises matched to the functional deficits identified. Re-evaluation at regular intervals (4–6 weeks) should then be performed to re-assess progress toward established goals. Thus the identification of functional deficits is an ideal way to establish goals for care or endpoints of care.

■ CONCLUSION

PPA tests are proving to be valuable tools for both identifying functional limitations and establishing realistic goals in the management of LBP patients.

They can complement the other evaluation benchmarks such as orthopedic/neurological findings, imaging results, self-report of activity intolerances, and diagnostic anaesthetic blocks. The unique value of these tests is that they measure functional ability that is clinically relevant because the goal of care is restoration of function!

Audit Process
Self-Check of the Chapter's Learning Objectives

- What is the normal range in seconds for endurance in different populations for the trunk extensor and side bridge tests?

- What is the normal range in seconds for the single leg standing balance test in different age groups and sexes?

- What is the normal range for pressure on the feedback cuff during the cervico-cranial flexion and prone abdominal hollowing tests?

- During what stage of patient care should strength/endurance testing be performed and why?

- During what stage of patient care should motor control testing be performed and why?

■ REFERENCES

1. Alaranta H, Hurri H, Heliovaara M, et al. Non-dynamometric trunk performance tests: Reliability and normative data. Scand J Rehab Med 1994;26:211–215.
2. Arendt-Nielson L, Graven-Nielson T, Svarrer H, Svensson P. The influence of low back pain on muscle activity and coordination during gait. Pain 1995;64:231–240.
3. Atwater SW, Crowe TR, Deitz JC, et al. Interrater and test retest reliability of two pediatric balance tests. Phys Ther 1990;20:79–87.
4. Barton PM, Hayes KC. Neck flexor muscle strength, and relaxation times in normal subjects and subjects with unilateral neck pain and headache. Arch Phys Med Rehabil 1996;77:680–687.
5. Biering-Sorensen F. Physical measurements as risk indicators for low-back trouble over a one-year period. Spine 1984;9:106–119.
6. Bigos S, Bowyer O, Braen G, et al. Acute low-back problems in adults. Clinical Practice Guideline. Rockville, Md: U.S. Department of Health and Human Services, Public Health Service, Agency for Health Care Policy and Research, 1994.
7. Bishop JB, Szpalaski M, Ananthraman SK, McIntyre DR, Pope MH. Classification of low back pain from dynamic motion characteristics using an artificial neural network. Spine 1997;22:2991–2998.

8. Bogduk N, Lord SM. Cervical zygapophysial joint pain. Neurosurg Q 1998;8:107–117.

9. Bogduk N. What's in a name? The labeling of back pain. Med J Aust 2000;173:400–401.

10. Bohannon RW, Larkin PA, Cook AC, Gear J, Singer J. Decrease in timed balance test scores with aging. Phys Ther 1984;64:1067–1070.

11. Boone DC, Azen SP, Lin CM, et al. Reliability of goniometric measurements. Phys Ther 1978;58: 1355–1360.

12. Brandt-Zawadzki MN, Jensen MC, Obuchowski N, et al. Interobserver and intraobserver variability in interpretation of lumbar disc abnormalities: A comparison of two nomenclatures. Spine 1995;20: 1257–1263.

13. Brumagne S, Cordo P, Lysens R, Verschueren S, Swinnen S. The role of paraspinal muscle spindles in lumbosacral position sense in individuals with and without low back pain. Spine 2000;25:989–994.

14. Bullock-Saxton JE, Bullock MI. Repeatability of muscle length measures around the hip. Physiother Can 1994;46:105–109.

15. Byl N, Sinnot PL. Variations in balance and body sway in middle-aged adults: Subjects with healthy backs compared with subjects with low-back dysfunction. Spine 1991;16:325–330.

16. Byl N. Spatial orientation to gravity and implication for balance training. Orthop Phys Ther Clin North Am 1992;1:207–236.

17. Chandler JM, Duncan PW, Studenski SA. Balance performance on the postural stress test: Comparison of young adults, healthy elderly and fallers. Phys Ther 1990;70:410–415.

18. Cholewicki J, McGill SM. Mechanical stability of the in vivo lumbar spine: Implications for injury and chronic low back pain. Clin Biomech 1996; 11(1):1–15.

19. Cholewicki J, Simons APD, Radebold A. Effects of external loads on lumbar spine stability. J Biomechan 2000;33:1377–1385.

20. Cibulka MT, Sinacore DR, Cromer GS, Delitto A. Unilateral hip rotation range of motion asymmetry in patients with sacroiliac joint regional pain. Spine 1998;23:1009–1015.

21. Colledge AL, Hunter SJ. Using functional improvements to promote active therapy and determine the length of treatment of workers' compensation patients, a 3-year analyzes of 63,000 claims. J Occip Med Submitted.

22. Cooke C, Menard MR, Beach GN, Locke SR, Hirsch GH. Serial lumbar dynamometry in low back pain. Spine 1992;17:653–662.

23. Croft PR, Macfarlane GJ, Papageorgiou AC, Thomas E, Silman AJ. Outcome of low back pain in general practice: A prospective study. BMJ 1998;316:1356–1359.

24. Deyo RA. Imaging of lumbar intervertebral disc degeneration and aging, excluding disc herniations. Radiol Clin North Am 2000;38:1255–1266.

25. Doege TC, ed. Guides to the Evaluation of Permanent Impairment, 4th ed. Chicago: AMA, 1993:3–112.

26. Dvir Z, David G. Suboptimal muscle performance: Measuring isokinetic strength with a new testing protocol. Arch Phys Med Rehabil 1996;77:578–581.

27. Dvir Z. Differentiation of submaximal from maximal trunk extension effort: An isokinetic study using a new testing protocol. Spine 1997;22:2672–2676.

28. Dvir Z. Coefficient of variation in maximal and feigned static and dynamic grip effort. Am J Phys Med Rehabil 1999;78:216–221.

29. Dvir Z, Keating J. Identifying Feigned Isokinetic Trunk Extension Effort in Normal Subjects: An Efficiency Study of the DEC. Spine 2001;26: 1046–1051.

30. Dvorak J, Antinnes JA, Panjabi M, et al. Age- and gender-related normal motion of the cervical spine. Spine 1992;17:S393–S398.

31. Edgerton VR, Wolf SL, Levendowski DJ, Roy RR. Theoretical basis for patterning EMG amplitudes to assess muscle dysfunction. Med Sci Sp Exer 1996;28:744–751.

32. Ellison JB, Rose SJ, Sahrmann SA. Patterns of rotation range of motion: A comparison between healthy subjects and patients with low back pain. Phys Ther 1990;70:537–541.

33. Ekstrand J, Wiktorsson M, Oberg B, Gillquist J. Lower extremity goniometric measurements: A study to determine their reliability. Arch Phys Med Rehab 1982;63:171–175.

34. Ensink F-BM, Saur PMM, Frese K, Seeger D, Hildebrandt J. Lumbar range of motion: Influence of time of day and individual factors on measurements. Spine 1996;21:1339–1343.

35. Enthoven P, Skargren E, Kjellman G, Oberg B. Course of back pain in primary care: A prospective study of physical measures. J Rehabil Med 2003;35:168–173.

36. Erhard RE, Delitto A. Relative effectiveness of an extension program and a combined program of manipulation and flexion and extension exercises in patients with acute low back syndrome. Phys Ther 1994;74:1093–1100.

37. Falla DL, Jull GA, Hodges PW. Patients with neck pain demonstrated reduced electromyographic activity of the deep cervical flexor muscles during performance of the craniocervical flexion test. Spine 2004;29:2108–2114.

38. Fritz JM, George S. The use of a classification approach to identify subgroups of patients with acute low back pain. Spine 2000;1:106–114.

39. Fritz JM, Piva SR. Physical impairment index: Reliability, validity, and responsiveness in patients with acute low back pain. Spine 2003;28:1189–1194.

40. Gajdosik RL, Rieck MA, Sullivan DK, et al. Comparison of four clinical tests for assessing hamstring muscle length. J Orthop Sports Phys Ther 1993;18: 614–618.

41. Gaudino WA, Matheson LM, Mael F. Development of the functional assessment taxonomy. J Occup Rehab 2001;11:155–175.

42. Gilford LS. Circadian variability in human flexibility and grip strength. Aust J Physiol 1987;33:3–9.

43. Gill KP, Callaghan MJ. The measurement of lumbar proprioception in individuals with and without low back pain. Spine 1998;23(3):371–377.

44. Golding LA, Myers CR, Sinning WE, eds. Y's Way to Physical Fitness, Third Edition. Champaign, IL: Human Kinetics, 1989.

45. Grabiner MD, Koh TJ, Ghazawi AE. Decoupling of bilateral paraspinal excitation in subjects with low back pain. Spine 1992;17:1219–1223.

46. Gronblad M, Hurri H, Jouri JP. Relationships between spinal mobility, physical performance tests, pain intensity and disability assessments in chronic low back pain patients. Scand J Rehab Med 1997;29:17–24.

47. Hagins M, Adler K, Cash M, Daugherty J, Mitrani G. Effects of practice on the ability to perform lumbar stabilization exercises. J Orthop Sports Phys Ther 1999;(9):546–555.

48. Hamilton-Fairfax A, Balnave R, Adams RD. Review of sincerity of effort testing. Safety Sci 1997;25: 237–245.

49. Harding VR, Williams AC de C, Richardson PH, et al. The development of a battery of measures for assessing physical functioning of chromic pain patients. Pain 1994;58:367–375.

50. Hart DL, Isernhagen SJ, Matheson LN. Guidelines for functional capacity evaluation of people with medical conditions. J Orthop Sports Phys Ther 1993;18:682–686.

51. Heikkila H, Astrom PG. Cervicocephalic kinesthetic sensibility in patients with whiplash injury. Scand J Rehab Med 1996;28:133–138.

52. Hirsch G, Beach GN, Cooke C, Menard MR, Locke S. Relationship between performance on lumbar dynamometry and Waddell score in a population with low back pain. Spine 1991;16:1039–1043.

53. Hodges PW, Richardson CA. Delayed postural contraction of transversus abdominis in low back pain associated with movement of the lower limb. J Spinal Disord 1998;11(1):46–56.

54. Hodges PW, Richardson CA. Altered trunk muscle recruitment in people with low back pain with upper limb movement at different speeds. Arch Phys Med Rehabil 1999;80(9):1005–1012.

55. Hussein TM, Simmonds MJ, Olson SL, et al. Kinematics of gait in normal and low back pain subjects. Boston, MA: American Congress of Sports Medicine 45th Annual Meeting, 1998.

56. Hussein TM, Simmonds MJ, Etnyre B, et al. Kinematics of gait in subjects with low back pain with and without leg pain. Washington, DC: Scientific Meeting & Exposition of the American Physical Therapy Association, 1999.

57. ICDH-2. International Classification of Functioning and Disability. Beta-2 Draft. Full Version, World Health Organization, Geneva, 1999.

58. Ito T, Shirado O, Suzuki H, Takahashi M, Kaneda K, Strax TE. Lumbar trunk muscle endurance testing: An inexpensive alternative to a machine for evaluation. Arch Phys Med Rehabil 1996;77:75–79.

59. Jarvik JG, Hollingworth W, Heagerty P, Haynor DR, Deyo RA. The longitudinal assessment of imaging and disability of the back (LAIDBack) study. Spine 2001;26:1158–1166.

60. Jarvik JG. Editorial. Don't duck the evidence. Spine 2001;26:1306–1307.

61. Jensel MC, Brant-Zawadzki MN, Obuchowski N, et al. Magnetic resonance imaging of the lumbar spine in people without back pain. N Engl J Med 1994;2:69.

62. Jull G, Barret C, Magee R, Ho P. Further clinical clarification of the muscle dysfunction in cervical headache. Cephalgia 1999;19:179–185.

63. Jull GA. Deep cervical flexor muscle dysfunction in whiplash. J Musculoskel Pain 2000;8:143–154.

64. Jull G, Kristjansson E, Dalll'Alba P. Impairment in the cervical flexors: A comparison of whiplash and insidious onset neck pain patients. Man Ther 2004;9:89–94.

65. Kankaapaa M, Taimela S, Laaksonen D, et al. Back and hip extensor fatigability in chronic low back pain patients and controls. Arch Phys Med Rehabil 1998;79:412–417.

66. Kendrick D, Fielding K, Bentler E, Kerslake R, Miller P, Pringle M. Radiography of the lumbar spine in primary care patients with low back pain: Randomized controlled trial. BMJ 2001;322:400–405.

67. Kibler WB, Herring SA, Press JM. Functional Rehabilitation of Sports and Musculoskeletal Injuries. Aspen, 1998.

68. Krivickas LS, Feinberg JH. Lower extremity injuries in college athletes: Relation between ligamentous laxity and lower extremity muscle tightness. Arch Phys Med Rehabil 1996;77:1139–1143.

69. Kujala UM, Taimela S, Salminen JJ, Oksanen A. Baseline anthropometry, flexibility and strength characteristics and future low-back-pain in adolescent athletes and nonathletes. A prospective, one-year, follow-up study. Scand J Med Sci Sports 1994;4:200–205.

70. Laboeuf-Yde C, Lauritsen JM, Lauritzen T. Why has the search for causes of low back pain largely been nonconclusive? Spine 1997;22:877–881.

71. Laboeuf-Yde C, Manniche C. Low back pain: Time to get off the treadmill. J Manipulative Physiol Ther 2001;24:63–65.

72. Lantz CA, Chen J, Buch D. Clinical validity and stability of active and passive cervical range of motion with regard to total and unilateral uniplanar motion. Spine 1999;24:1082–1089.

73. LaRocca H. A taxonomy of chronic pain syndromes. 1991 Presidential Address, Cervical Spine Research Society Annual Meeting, December 5, 1991. Spine 1992;10S:S344–S355.

74. Latimer J, Maher CG, Refshauge K, Colaco I. The reliability and validity of the Biering-Sorensen test in asymptomatic subjection and subjects reporting current or previous non-specific low back pain. Spine 1999;24:2085–2090.

75. Leinonen V, Kankaanpaa M, Airaksinen O, et al. Back and hip flexion/extension: Effects of low back pain and rehabilitation. Arch Phys Med Rehabil 2000;81:32–37.

76. Leinonen V, Kankaanpää M, Luukkonen M, Hänninen O, Airaksinen O, Taimela S. Disc herniation-related back pain impairs feed-forward control of paraspinal muscles. Spine 2001;26:E367–E372.

77. Lemastra M, Olszynsi WP, Enright W. The sensitivity and specificity of functional capacity evaluations in determining maximal effort. Spine 2004;29:953–959.

78. Lewit K. Manipulative therapy in rehabilitation of the motor system, 2nd Edition. London: Butterworths, 1991.

79. Lewit K, Liebenson C. Palpation—problems and implications. J Manipulative Physiol Ther 1993;16:586–590.

80. Loudon JK, Ruhl M, Field E. Ability to reproduce head position after whiplash injury. Spine 1997;22:865–868.

81. Luoto S, Heliovaara M, Hurri H, Alaranta H. Static back endurance and the risk of low-back pain. Clin Biomech 1995;10:323–324.

82. Luoto S, Taimela S, Hurri H, et al. Psychomotor speed and postural control in chronic low-back pain patients: A controlled follow-up study. Spine 1996;21:2621–2627.

83. Luoto S, Aalto H, Taimela S, et al. One-footed and externally disturbed two-footed postural control in chronic low-back pain patients and healthy controls: A controlled study with follow-up. Spine 1998;23:2081–2090.

84. Luoto S, Taimela S, Hurri H, et al. Mechanisms explaining the association between low back trouble and deficits in information processing. A controlled study with follow-up. Spine 1999;24(3):255–261.

85. Magnusson ML, Bishop JB, Hasselquist L, Spratt KF, Szpalski M, Pope MH. Range of motion and motion patterns in patients with low back pain before and after rehabilitation. Spine 1998;23:1631–2639.

86. Manniche C, et al. Danish Health Technology Assessment (DIHTA). Low back pain: Frequency Management and Prevention from an HAD Perspective, 1999.

87. Mannion AF, Junge A, Taimela S, Muntener M, Lorenzo K, Dvorak J. Active therapy for chronic low back pain. Part 3. Factors influencing self-rated disability and its change following therapy. Spine 2001;26:920–929.

88. Marras WS, Ferguson SA, Gupta P, et al. The quantification of low back disorder using motion measures. Methodology and validation. Spine 1999;24(20):2091–2100.

89. Matheson L. An introduction to lift capacity testing as a component of functional capacity evaluation. IRG, 1991.

90. Matheson L. Basic requirements for utility in the assessment of physical disability. American Pain Society 1994;3:195.

91. Matheson LM, Gaudino WA, Mael F, Hesse BW. Improving the validity of the impairment evaluation process: A proposed theoretical framework. J Occup Rehabil 2000;10:311–320.

92. Matheson L, Kaskuta VK, Mada D. Development and construct validation of the hand function sort. J Occup Rehabil 2001;11:75–86.

93. Mayer TG, Tencer AF, Kristoferson S, Mooney V. Use of noninvasive techniques for quantification of spinal range-of-motion in normal subjects and chronic low-back dysfunction patients. Spine 1984;9:588–595.

94. Mayer T, Gatchel R, Kishino N, et al. Objective assessment of spine function following industrial injury: A prospective study with comparison group and one-year follow-up. Spine 1985;10:482–493.

95. Mayer TG, Smith S, Keeley J, Mooney V. Quantification of lumbar function part 2: Sagittal plane trunk strength in chronic low back patients. Spine 1985;10:765–772.

96. Mayer TG, Gatchel RJ, Mayer H, et al. A prospective two-year study of functional restoration in industrial low back injury. JAMA 1987;258:1763–1767.

97. Mayer T, Brady S, Bovasso E, et al. Noninvasive measurement of cervical tri-planar motion in normal subjects. Spine 1994;18:2191–2195.

98. Mayer TG, Gatchel RJ, Keeley J, Mayer H, Richling D. A male incumbent worker industrial database. Spine 1994;19:755–761.

99. Mayer TG, Gatchel R, Betancur J, Bovasso E. Trunk muscle endurance measurement: Isometric contrasted to isokinetic testing in normal subjects. Spine 1995;20:920–927.

100. Mayer RS, Chen I-H, Lavender SA, Trafimow JH, Andersson GBJ. Variance in the measurement of sagittal lumbar spine range of motion among examiners, subjects, and instruments. Spine 1995;20:1489–1493.

101. Mayer T, Kondraske G, Beals S, Gatchel R. Spinal Range of Motion. Accuracy and sources of error with inclinometric measurement. Spine 1997;22:1976–1984.

102. McCombe PF, Fairbank JCT, Cockersole BC, Pynsent PB. Reproducibility of physical signs in low back pain. Spine 1989;14:908–918.

103. McGill SM, Childs A, Liebenson C. Endurance times for stabilization exercises: Clinical targets for testing and training from a normal database. Arch Phys Med Rehabil 1999;80:941–944.

104. McGill SM. Low Back Disorders: Evidence-based Prevention and Rehabilitation. Champaign, IL: Human Kinetics, 2002.

105. McGregor AH, McCarthy ID, Dore CJ, et al. Quantitative assessment of the motion of the lumbar spine in the low back pain population and the effect of different spinal pathologies of this motion. Eur Spine J 1997;6(5):308–315.

106. McIntosh G, Wilson L, Affleck M, Hall H. Trunk and lower extremity muscle endurance: Normative data for adults. J Rehabil Outcomes Measure 1998;2:20–39.

107. McIntyre DR, Glover LH, Seeds RH, et al. The characteristics of preferred low back motion. J Spinal Disord 1990;3:147–155.

108. McIntyre DR, Glover LH, Candance-Conino M, et al. A comparison of the characteristics of preferred low back motion of normal subjects and low back pain patients. J Spinal Disord 1991;4:90–95.

109. Moffroid MT. Distinguishable groups of musculoskeletal low back pain patients and asymptomatic control subjects based on physical measures of the NIOSH low back atlas. Spine 1994;19:1350–1358.

110. Moffroid MT, Reid S, Henry S, Haugh LD, Ricamato A. Some endurance measures in persons with chronic low back pain. J Orthop Sports Phys Ther 1994;20:81–87.

111. Mok NW, Brauer S, Hodges PW. Hip strategy for balance control in quiet standing is reduced in people with low back pain. Spine 2004;29:E107–E112.

112. Mooney V. The place of active care in disability prevention. In: Liebenson CL, ed. Rehabilitation of the Spine: A practitioner's manual. Baltimore: Williams & Wilkins, 1996.

113. Nadler SF, Wu KD, Galsi T, Feinberg JH. Low back pain in college athletes: A prospective study correlating lower extremity overuse or acquired ligamentous laxity with low back pain. Spine 1998;23: 828–833.

114. Nadler SF, Malanga GA, DePrince ML, Stitik TP, Feinberg JH. The relationship between lower extremity injury, low back pain, and hip muscle strength in male and female collegiate athletes. Clin J Sports Med 2000;10:89–97.

115. Nadler SF, Malanga GA, Feinberg JH, Prybicien M, Stitik TP, DeFrince M. Relationship between hip muscle imbalance and occurrence of low back pain in collegiate athletes: A prospective study. Am J Phys Med Rehabil 2001;80:572–577.

116. Nederhand MJ, Ijzerman MJ, Hermens HK, Baten CTM, Zilvold G. Cervical muscle dysfunction in the chronic whiplash associated disorder Grade II (WAD-II). Spine 2000;15:1938–1943.

117. Nelson RM, Nestor DE. Standardized assessment of industrial low-back injuries: Development of the NIOSH low-back atlas. Top Trauma Acute Care Rehabil 1988;2:16–30.

118. Nelson RM. NIOSH low back atlas of standardized tests/measures. U.S. Department of Health and Human Services, National Institute for Occupational Safety and Health, December 1988.

119. Newcomer KL, Laskowski ER, Yu B, Johnson JC, An KN. Differences in repositioning error among patients with low back pain compared with control subjects. Spine 2000;25:2488–2493.

120. Newton M, Thow M, Somerville D, et al. Trunk strength testing with iso-machines: Part 2: Experimental evaluation of the Cybex II Back Testing System in normal subjects and patients with chronic low back pain. Spine 1993;18(7):812–824.

121. Nicolaisen T, Joregnesen K. Trunk strength, back muscle endurance and low back trouble. Scand J Rehabil Med 1985;17:121–127.

122. Norlander S, Gustavsson BA, Lindell J, Nordgren B. Reduced mobility in the cervico-thoracic motion segment—a risk factor for musculoskeletal neck-shoulder pain: A two-year prospective follow-up study. Scand J Rehab Med 1997;29:167–174.

123. O'Sullivan P, Twomey L, Allison G. Evaluation of specific stabilizing exercise in the treatment of chronic low back pain with radiologic diagnosis of spondylolysis or spondylolisthesis. Spine 1997;24: 2959–2967.

124. Paarnianpour M, Nordin M, Kahanovitz N, Frank V. The triaxial coupling of torque generation of trunk muscles during isometric exertions and the effect of fatiguing isoinertial movements on the motor output and movement patterns. Spine 1998;13:982–992.

125. Patajin J, Ellis R. Low back pain: Reproducibility of diagnostic procedures in manual/musculoskeletal medicine. J Orthop Med 2001;23:36–42.

126. Peach JP, McGill SM. Classification of low back pain with the use of spectral electromyogram parameters. Spine 1998;23:1117–1123.

127. Porter RW, Trailescu IF. Diurnal changes in straight leg raising. Spine 1990;15:103–106.

128. Protas EJ, Mayer TJ, Dersh J, Keeley J, Gatchel RJ, McGeary D. Relevance of aerobic capacity measurements in the treatment of chronic work-related spinal disorders. Spine 2004;29:2158–2166.

129. Radebold A, Cholewicki J, Panjabi MM, Patel TC. Muscle response pattern to sudden trunk loading in healthy individuals and in patients with chronic low back pain. Spine 2000;25:947–954.

130. Radebold A, Cholewicki J, Polzhofer BA, Greene HS. Impaired postural control of the lumbar spine is associated with delayed muscle response times in patients with chronic idiopathic low back pain. Spine 2001;26:724–730.

131. Rantanan T, Guralink JM, Foley D, et al. Midlife grip strength as a predictor of old age disability. JAMA 1999;281:558–560.

132. Reid DC, Burnham RS, Saboe LA, Kushner SF. Lower extremity flexibility patterns in classical ballet dancers and their correlation to lateral hip and knee injuries. Am J Sports Med 1987;15:347–352.

133. Revel M, Minguet M, Gergoy P, VAillant J, Manuel JL. Changes in cervicocephalic kinesthesia after a proprioceptive rehabilitation program in neck pain: A randomized controlled study. Arch Phys Med Rehabil 1994;75:895–899.

134. Richardson C, Jull G, Hodges P, Hide J. Therapeutic Exercise for Spinal Segmental Stabilization in Low Back Pain. Edinburgh: Churchill Livingstone, 1999.

135. Rissanen A, Alaranta H, Sainio P, Harkonen H. Isokinetic and non-dynamometric tests in low back pain patients related to pain and disability index. Spine 1994;19:1963–1967.

136. Rissanen A, Heliovaara M, Alaranta H, et al. Does good trunk extensor performance protect against back-related work disability. J Rehabil Med 2002;34:62–66.

137. Roy SH, DeLuca CJ, Emley M, et al. Spectral electromyographic assessment of back muscles in patients with low back pain undergoing rehabilitation. Spine 1995;20:38–48.

138. Royal College of General Practitioners (RCGP). Clinical Guidelines for the Management of Acute Low Back Pain. London: Royal College of General Practitioners (www.rcgp.org.uk), 1999.

139. Sabari JS, Matzev I, Lubarsky D, Liskay E, Homel P. Goniometric assessment of shoulder range of motion: Comparison of testing in supine and sitting positions. Arch Phys Med Rehabil 1998;79: 647–651.

140. Schwarzer AC, Aprill CN, Derby R, Fortin J, Kine G, Bogduk N. The relative contributions of the disc and zygapophyseal joint in chronic low back pain. Spine 1994;19:801–806.

141. Schwarzer AC, Aprill CN, Derby R, Fortin J, Kine G, Bogduk N. Clinical features of patients with pain stemming from the lumbar zygapophysial joints. Is the lumbar facet syndrome a clinical entity? Spine 1994;19:1132–1137.

142. Schwarzer AC, Aprill CN, Bogduk N. The sacroiliac joint in chronic low back pain. Spine 1995;20:31–37.

143. Shirado O, Ito T, Kaneda K, et al. Flexion-relaxation phenomenon in the back muscles: A comparative

study between healthy subjects and patients with chronic low back pain. Am J Phys Med Rehabil 1995;74:139–144.

144. Silverman JL, Rodriguez AA, Agre JC. Quantitative cervical flexor strength in healthy subjects and in subjects with mechanical neck pain. Arch Phys Med Rehabil 1991;72:679–681.

145. Simmonds MJ, Olson SL, Jones S, et al. Psychometric characteristics and clinical usefulness of physical performance tests in patients with low back pain. Spine 1998;23(22):2412–2421.

146. Simonsen JC. Coefficient of variation as a measure of subject effort. Arch Phys Med Rehabil 1995;76:516–520.

147. Solgaard S, Carlsen A, Kramhoft M. Reproducibility of goniometry of the wrist. Scand J Rehabil Med 1986;18:5–7.

148. Spitzer WO, Le Blanc FE, Dupuis M, et al. Scientific approach to the assessment and management of activity-related spinal disorders: A monograph for clinicians. Report of the Quebec Task Force on Spinal Disorders. Spine 1987;12(suppl 7): S1–S59.

149. Spitzer WO, Skovron ML, Salmi LIR, et al. Scientific monograph of the Quebec Task Force on Whiplash-Associated Disorders: Redefining "Whiplash" and its management. Spine 1995;20(Suppl):S1–S73.

150. Stankovic R, Johnell O. Conservative treatment of acute low-back pain. A prospective randomized trial. McKenzie method of treatment versus patient education in "mini back school." Spine 1990;15: 120–123.

151. Sterling M, Jull G, Vicenzino B, Kenardy J. Characterization of acute whiplash-associated disorders. Spine 2004;29:182–188.

152. Strender LE, Sjoblom A, Sundell K, Ludwig R, Taube A. Interexaminer reliability in physical examination of patients with low back pain. Spine 1997;7: 814–820.

153. Swanson AB, Matex IB, de Groot Swanson G. The strength of the hand. Bull Prosthet Res Fall 1970; 145–153.

154. Taimela S, Österman K, Alaranta H, et al. Long psychomotor reaction time in patients with chronic low-back pain—preliminary report. Arch Phys Med Rehab 1993;74:1161–1164.

155. Taimela S, Kankaanpää M, Luoto S. The effect of lumbar fatigue on the ability to sense a change in lumbar position. A controlled study. Spine 1999; 24(13):1322–1327.

156. Takala EP, Vikari-Juntura E. Do functional tests predict low back pain? Spine 2000;25(16):2126–2132.

157. Treleavan J, Jull G, Atkinson L. Cervical musculoskeletal dysfunction in post-concussion headache. Cephalalgia 1994;14:273–279.

158. Triano JJ, Schultz AB. Correlation of objective measure of trunk motion and muscle function with low-back disability ratings. Spine 1987;12:561–565.

159. Triano J. Personal communication. 1994.

160. Van Dillen LR, Sahrmann SA, Norton BJ, et al. Reliability of physical examination items used for classification of patients with low back pain. Phys Ther 1998;78:979–988.

161. Van Dillen LR, McDonnell MK, Fleming DA, Sahrmann SA. The effect of hip and knee position on hip extension range of motion measures in individuals with and without low back pain. J Orthop Sports Physical Ther 2000;30(6):307–316.

162. Van Dillen LR, Sahrmann SA, Norton BJ, et al. The effect of active limb movements on symptoms in patients with low back pain. J Orthop Sports Phys Ther 2001;31(8):402–413.

163. Verna JL, Mayer JM, Mooney V, Pierra EA, Robertson VL, Graves JE. Back extension endurance and strength: The effect of variable-angle roman chair exercise training. Spine 2002;27:1772–1777.

164. Waddell G, Burton AK. Occupational health guidelines for the management of low back pain at work—evidence review. London: Faculty of Occupational Medicine, 2000.

165. Wang S, Whitney SL, Burdett RG, et al. Lower extremity muscular flexibility in long distance runners. J Orthop Sports Phys Ther 1993;2:102–107.

166. Ward, A, Ebbeling C, Ahlquist LE. Indirect methods for estimation of aerobic power. In: Foster C, ed. Physiologic Assessment of Human Fitness. Champaign, IL: Human Kinetics, 1995.

167. Watson DH, Trott PH. Cervical Headache: An investigation of natural head posture and cervical flexor muscle performance. Cephalgia 1993;13:272–284.

168. Wilder DG, Aleksiev AR, Magnusson ML, Pope MH, Spratt KF, Goel VK. Muscular response to sudden load. A tool to evaluate fatigue and rehabilitation. Spine 1996;21:2628–2639.

169. Wilson L, Hall H, McIntosh G, Melles T. Intertester reliability of a low back pain classification system. Spine 1999;24:248–254.

170. Wing P, Tsang I, Gabnon F, Susak L, Gagnon R. Diurnal changes in the profile shape and range of motion of the back. Spine 1992;17:761–766.

171. Youdas J, Carey J, Garret T. Reliability of measurements of cervical spine range of motion—comparison of three methods. Phys Ther 1991;71:98–106.

172. Yeomans SG. The Clinical Correlation of Outcomes Assessment. Stamford, CT: McGraw-Hill, 2000.

173. Zuberbier OA, Hunt DG, Kozlowski AJ, et al. Commentary on the American Medical Association Guides' lumbar impairment validity checks. Spine 2001;26:2735–2737.

12

Physical Performance Tests: An Expanded Model of Assessment and Outcome

Maureen J. Simmonds
and Ellen Lee

Introduction
Functional Assessment Methods
  Patient Self-Reports
  Clinician-Measured Tests of Function
Physical Performance Test Battery
  Psychometric Properties
  Factors That Influence Task Performance
  Biomechanical and Electromyographic
  Task Analysis

Learning Objectives
After reading this chapter you should be able to understand:

- That impairment tests and functional ability are not equivalent.
- How to perform a standardized battery of quantifiable functional tests.
- The influence of back pain versus leg symptoms on task performance, including gait.

Introduction

Traditionally standard clinical assessments were largely based on a narrow biomedical model. In patients with low back pain (LBP), clinical tests focused on physical impairment. Impairment tests such as spinal range of motion, strength, and specific joint movements are described in great detail (20), entrenched in current practice, and have apparent clinical usefulness. Yet many are unreliable (10,18) and the constrained manner of testing may have little to do with the patient's problem of pain and dysfunction, especially when the problem is chronic or recurrent. In the case of spinal problems recurrence is the norm (19). Unfortunately, the functional ability of patients with LBP has often been inferred from the results of these tests. The incongruence between impairment test results and functional ability of patients can confuse and frustrate both clinicians and patients.

Treatment plans are guided by clinical assessments. A narrow focus biomedical assessment framework will inevitably lead to a narrowly focused treatment. It is, therefore, not surprising that the outcomes of back-specific exercise treatment regimes in patients with chronic LBP are often inconclusive (14). The problem of back pain, especially disabling back pain, is greater than a problem of the spine, its muscles, and its range of motion; therefore, assessment rationale and tests should be expanded.

Recognition of the importance of function and the limitations of the narrow biomedical/biomechanical model has led to a shift towards an expanded bio-psychosocial model of assessment. This conceptual model recognizes salient factors beyond the anatomical and biomechanical aspects of the spine that can affect the functional ability of the person as a whole. It takes into account psychosocial factors in addition to physical factors. These factors have intricate and interwoven relationships that ultimately influence the function of a whole person. For example, psychosocial factors such as depressed mood, negative or passive coping, fear of pain and reinjury with consequent avoidance of activity, stress or anxiety, low educational level, medicolegal compensation claims, and substance abuse are predictive of chronic physical disability (27). The actual level of spinal impairment can play a minimal role in predicting disability.

This assessment and management model focuses on the integration and consideration of functional activity, physical pathology/impairment, and psychosocial factors (49).

Functional Assessment Methods

There are two major approaches in assessing physical function: patient self-reports and clinician-measured tests.

Patient Self-Reports

Patient self-reports of physical function are commonly used in clinical settings because they are relatively quick, simple, and practical to administer and score (see Chapter 8). This method uses questionnaires that are generic, disease-specific, or patient-specific. The Medical Outcomes Study 36-item Short Form Health Survey (SF-36) (52) is an example of a generic questionnaire that is widely used and has established psychometric properties (30,31). It can be used in a variety of disease groups including LBP. However, the degree of validity varies across the different disease groups (31). Disease-specific questionnaires tend to be more relevant to the target disease group. Roland Morris Disability Questionnaire (RMDQ) (38) and Oswestry Disability Questionnaire (15) are examples of such disease-specific questionnaires. They sample a range of different activities, including self-care, mobility, the performance of household chores, and other work-related activities that are relevant to LBP. They have accepted norms and established reliability and validity (2,3). However, patients' needs and normal functional level are idiosyncratic. Therefore, patient-specific questionnaires have also been developed. The Patient-Specific Questionnaire (PSQ) is an example. This questionnaire samples up to five important activities that patients identify they are unable to do or have difficulty doing because of their problem. The patient then scores each activity on a scale of 0 to 10. Moderate to excellent reliability, validity, and sensitivity to change have been established in patients with knee dysfunction (5) and LBP (42,48).

Although patient self-reports using standardized questionnaires of physical function have clinical usefulness, they still may not be a valid reflection of a patient's actual functional status (17), especially when an external reference is unavailable. Self-report measures are more closely associated with other self-report measures than with physical capabilities observed or measured by clinicians (9). Even with psychometrically sound patient self-reports and clinician-measured tests of the same functions, the test measures are moderately correlated at best (16, 26). This can be partly explained by findings that show patients and clinicians or normal subjects often misjudge estimates of distance walked or the time that an activity takes (40,41). Likewise, estimates of the time that an activity or static position can be tolerated is influenced by so many factors that the accuracy or validity of the estimates must be seriously challenged. Reporting bias may also vary with situational demands, memory, and verbal ability (6). Therefore, it is evident that complementation of patient self-report of function with clinician-measured tests of physical function is necessary. Each method of measurement taps a different aspect of physical performance.

Self-report measures of function are important to use as assessment tests to help identify functional difficulties and as outcome measures to determine the effectiveness of the intervention. Self-report measures that assess why an activity is limited are also essential. It is beyond the scope of this chapter to address the many different constructs that can influence physical function or are a consequence of physical dysfunction. However, a couple of points are noteworthy. For example, measures of pain (intensity, quality and location) must be obtained through the patient's self-report. Practitioners' estimates of a patient's pain are known to be inaccurate and are generally underestimated. Pain behavior is usually more indicative of a patient's distress and culture than their pain per se. It is also helpful to find out about the patient's beliefs (and false beliefs) about their spine and the anticipated effect of physical activity. The beliefs of the patient and the impact of the physical dysfunction help to identify problems and direct treatment. For example, fear of injury or activity (50,51) is a problem relevant to rehabilitation that can be assessed using the Tampa Scale of Kinesphobia (50,51). Clearly, a different treatment approach is necessary for those patients who are unable to complete an activity because of fear of pain or fear of re-injury, rather than a physical impairment.

Clinician-Measured Tests of Function

Clinician-measured tests of physical function provide a useful, quick, simple, quantitative method of determining a patient's physical function. This method involves the use of a range of tasks or a standardized battery of tasks that essentially sample the construct of physical function. The tests are simple, everyday tasks that are easy for the patient to perform and easy for the clinician to measure and interpret. In the next section of the chapter, we describe a simple clinical performance task battery that can be used to assess physical function in individuals with LBP. We then summarize the experimental evidence that supports the reliability and validity of the test battery. Secondly, based on the premise that optimum management of physical function is based on optimum understanding of how LBP impacts task performance, we present the results of biomechanical experiments that have characterized physical performance on specific tasks.

Physical Performance Test Battery

Recently, Simmonds and colleagues developed, tested, and refined a comprehensive but simple and standardized battery of performance tests for indi-

viduals with LBP. The battery includes tasks that are fundamental components of day-to-day activities commonly compromised by LBP. For example, most individuals with LBP have difficulty withstanding compressive and shear spinal loads, and generally move more slowly than pain-free individuals (28,29,39,43). Therefore, performance on the task battery is mostly based on how quickly a task can be performed or how far a subject can reach forward (an indirect test of spinal load). The only equipment needed for these simple clinical tests is a stopwatch, a tape measure or meter rule, and a few 1-kilogram/2-kilogram weights. The tasks are outlined in Table 12.1 and shown in Figures 12.1 through 12.5.

Psychometric Properties

Reliability

The psychometric properties and clinical usefulness of these performance tests are established (47). Test–retest, inter-rater reliability, day-to-day stability, and validity were tested in 48 healthy pain-free control subjects and 44 subjects with LBP. All tests have excellent inter-rater reliability. Intraclass correlation coefficients (ICC $_{1,1}$) were all equal or greater than 0.95. The simplicity of the tasks and the method of testing (stopwatch or tape measure) probably contribute to the excellent level of inter-rater reliability. Test–retest (within session) and day-to-day stability is also adequate to excellent for all tests. Examination of the reliability results revealed an interesting phenomenon. The two tasks that involved repeated movements (repeated flexion and sit-to-stand) have relatively lower levels of stability, suggesting that performance changes during the task. Reduced fear of the activity and/or physiological warm-up are the most likely explanations because the speed of performance increased with repetitions, and the change was much more marked in the LBP group.

The lower level of stability of the two tasks that require fast dynamic performance is an interesting observation and important point. Some authors and many clinicians have asserted that within subject variability of task performance is indicative of insincerity of effort. Despite the dearth of credible evidence supporting this simplistic view and some evidence that refutes the notion (32), the search for the physical performance "lie detector" has remained a popular quest. Our results suggest that variability in task performance is not a "lie detector." Variability in performance during a repeated movement is a characteristic of the task itself, and thus is not an indication of questionable patient motivation. None of the patients in our study was involved in litigation

Table 12.1 Simmonds Physical Performance Battery for Patients with Low Back Pain

Task	Procedure	Measure
Repeated sit-to-stand (see Fig. 12.1)	Subjects rise to standing and return to sitting as quickly as possible five times; after a brief pause, the task is repeated	The average of the two task times is recorded
Repeated trunk flexion (see Fig. 12.2)	The subjects are timed as they bend forward to the limit of their range and return to the upright position as fast as tolerated five times; after a brief pause, the task is repeated	The average of the two task times is recorded
Loaded reach (see Fig. 12.3)	Subjects stand next to a wall on which a meter rule is mounted horizontally at shoulder height; they hold a weight that is 5% of their body weight (up to maximum of 5 kg) at shoulder height and close to the body and then reach forward	Maximum distance reached in centimeter is recorded
50-Foot walk	Subjects walk 25 feet, turn around, and walk back to start as fast as they can	Time taken is recorded
5-Minute walk	Subjects walk as far and as fast as they can for 5 minutes	Distance walked is recorded
360-Degree rollover (see Fig. 12.4A to 12.4D)	Subjects lie supine on a treatment bed and they roll over 360 degrees as fast as they can; after a brief pause, they roll 360 degrees in the opposite direction	The time to complete a rollover in both directions is summed and recorded
Sorensen fatigue test (see Fig. 12.5) (for patients with minimal dysfunction)	Subjects lay prone on a standard treatment table with thighs and calves stabilized; they lift their upper body and hold the position for as long as possible	Time taken to fatigue is recorded

or was receiving workers compensation payments. Also, it seems unlikely that patients would have purposefully exerted a less consistent effort during the repeated flexion and sit-to-stand task but performed consistently for the other tasks. Thus, variability in task performance must be judged within the context of the task itself.

Responsiveness

Responsiveness of the task battery was measured and compared with the RMDQ and PSQ. Twenty-eight patients attending physical therapy were assessed initially and after 4 to 6 weeks of physical therapy. Standardized response means (SRM) were 1.39 to 1.98 for each of the five activities identified by the patient. Three performance tasks were comparable to the RMDQ in regards to responsiveness.

The SRM of the RMDQ was 0.81. The SRMs of the 5-minute distance walk, loaded reach, and timed repeated flexion task were 0.81, 0.73, and 0.73, respectively (42).

Validities

The importance of reliability of the tests becomes moot if the tests are not valid. Therefore, face validity of the tasks was evaluated by examining group differences. A multivariate analysis of variance revealed that pain-free subjects outperformed subjects with LBP on all the tasks in this battery ($F_{10,65} = 3.52$, $p < 0.0001$). Validity was further established through the examination of correlational patterns between the performance and external (impairment and pain) tests. High correlations between tests provide evidence of convergent validity suggesting that

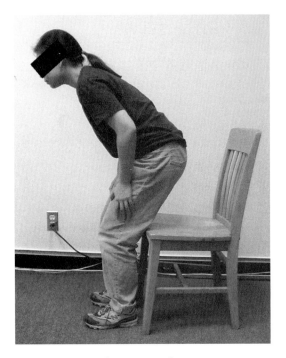

Figure 12.1 Repeated sit-to-stand.

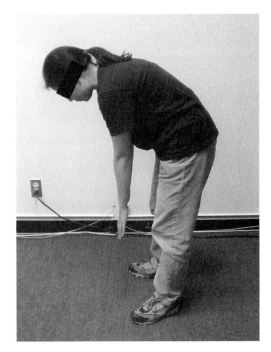

Figure 12.2 Repeated trunk flexion.

the tests are assessing a similar construct. However, low correlations between tests show discriminant validity suggesting the tests are assessing dissimilar constructs. The task battery shows good convergent and discriminant validity through stronger correlational patterns among the performance tests (r=.41 to 0.89) and weaker correlations between performance and external tests (r=0.12 to r=0.36). Tasks that comprised similar performance characteristics correlated most strongly. For example, tasks that involved walking were most highly correlated (r=0.89). In contrast, tasks that comprised dissimilar performance characteristics were less strongly correlated. For example, the correlation between the loaded reach task that is performed relatively slowly and the repeated flexion task that is performed relatively

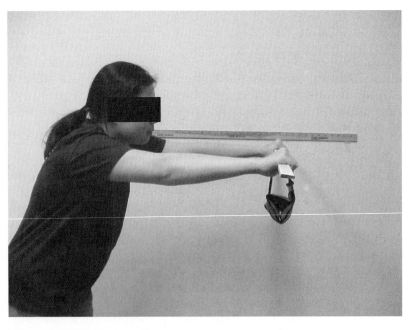

Figure 12.3 Loaded reach.

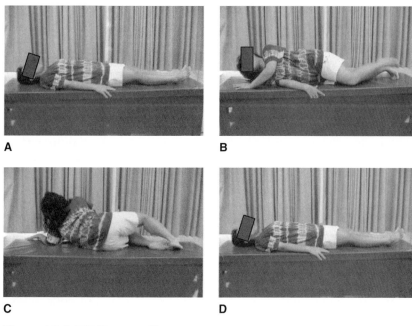

Figure 12.4 360-Degree rollover.
(A) Starting position.
(B) Roll from back to right side.
(C) Roll from front to left side.
(D) End position.

quickly was r=–0.53. Both tasks involve different stresses on the trunk but clearly the speed of postural adjustment to those stresses is differentially challenging. Finally, pain and performance tests were better predictors of disability (r^2=0.61) than pain and impairment tests (r^2=0.47) (46).

Further validation of the task battery was investigated through factor analysis. This statistical technique examines the number of underlying constructs measured by the task battery. Novy and colleagues (33) examined the factor structure of the task battery in 103 patients with back pain. They derived two factors, namely speed/coordination and endurance/strength that underlie the Simmonds battery of physical performance tasks. The speed/coordination factor was identified by 50-foot speed walk, repeated trunk flexion, sit to stand, and rollover. The rollover task had a 0.86 loading on this factor and appears to be a strong

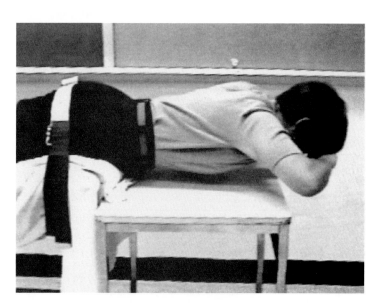

Figure 12.5 Sorensen fatigue test.

indicator of speed/coordination. The second factor, endurance/strength, was identified by 5-minute walk and loaded reach task. In contrast to the other tasks tested here, the Sorensen fatigue test was not associated with salient loadings on either factor and is discussed further.

The two derived factors are not only meaningful but also may be helpful in guiding rehabilitation. When scores of physical performance tasks indicate patients are compromised in speed/coordination of movement, clinicians could design exercise protocols to target the underlying factor (Table 12.2). Likewise, patients who demonstrate a poor performance on indicators of endurance/strength may benefit from a training protocol that targets and enhances these deficits (Table 12.2). DeLooze and colleagues have shown that reduced strength compromises the capability of the spine to withstand a mechanical load (7). Therefore, patients may have better endurance in withstanding spinal loading in both the 5-minute walk and loaded reach tasks after the training.

The Sorensen test has been removed from the standard test battery for a few reasons. First, it is the least "functional" test. Second, it is a physically challenging test that pain-free healthy controls find difficult. Third, based on its statistical properties on the factor analysis, the Sorensen test can be removed without compromising the factor structure.

Finally, we also question the validity of the test as one of back muscle endurance. Kankaanpaa et al. suggest that there is load-sharing between back and hip extensors during the test because both muscle groups fatigue significantly in pain-free individuals during the test (25). Although short hold times (low performance) of the Sorensen test are related to poor muscle endurance and are predictive of future LBP in normals (4,8,24), these results cannot be generalized to individuals who already have LBP. We have found that although the majority of pain-free individuals (80.5%) stop the test because of fatigue/weakness,

only 29.6% of individuals with LBP stop for this reason. Rather, most individuals with LBP (63%) stop the test because of pain. Thus, we suggest the Sorensen test for individuals with back problems as a test of pain tolerance, not back muscle endurance (44).

Factors That Influence Task Performance

A variety of factors influence task performance we have examined a non-modifiable factor, gender, and a modifiable factor, pain location.

Gender

Although men outperform women on most physical tasks, LBP changes performance ability. The potentially differential impact of LBP on the physical performance of men and women has received little scrutiny. Novy and colleagues (34) examined performance differences in men and women with and without low back pain. They examined performance on the task battery of 33 men and 46 women with non-specific mechanical LBP, and 21 men and 25 healthy control subjects. They used a discriminant function analysis and found that the four groups of subjects performed the physical tasks significantly differently in two major ways. The first difference irrespective of gender was that the healthy control subjects outperformed the patients with LBP on tasks (sit-to-stand, repeated trunk flexion, Sorenson fatigue test, 50-foot speed walk) that involve trunk control, coordination, and stability while withstanding heavy or quickly changing loads on the spine (i.e., healthy men outperform healthy women, LBP men, and LBP women, respectively). The second difference irrespective of patient or non-patient status was that men outperform women on tasks involving anthropometric features of limb length (distance walk and loaded reach), i.e., healthy men outperform LBP men, healthy women, and

Table 12.2 Physical Performance Battery Normative Database

Test	Mean	SD	Minimum	Maximum
Repeated sit-to-stand (seconds)	7.35	1.42	4.45	11.54
Repeated trunk flexion (seconds)	7.44	1.04	5.17	9.59
Loaded reach (cm)	67.62	6.43	55.50	84.03
50-Foot fast walk (seconds)	8.30	0.85	6.80	10.78
5-Minute distance walk (m)	514.10	70.25	284.68	683.97
360-degree Roll-over (seconds)	6.33	1.24	4.15	10.08

LBP women, respectively. Thus, expectation of treatment outcome must consider the specific demands of the task as well as gender.

Location of Pain

Physical performance is also influenced by location of pain. Patients with radiating or referred leg pain are generally outperformed on physical performance tasks by patients with back pain only. However, performance differences are again task-specific (45). We tested a total of 60 patients with LBP on the physical performance battery. Twenty-nine patients had back pain and 31 patients had leg pain. Patients with back pain outperformed those with leg pain on the 50-foot speed walk, repeated trunk flexion, 360-degree roll-over, and the loaded reach. There was no performance difference between groups on the 5-minute walk, sit-to-stand, or Sorenson test. Thus, it appears that individuals with leg pain have much greater difficulties with tasks that involve high compressive spinal loads or high-velocity movements.

Biomechanical and Electromyographic Task Analysis

Physical performance tasks are complex movements. A better understanding of all performance task components and the manner in which they operate may ultimately lead to simple mathematical rules that explain the complex movement patterns. At present these rules are still elusive. It is axiomatic that the optimal management of task performance difficulties requires a sound understanding of the physical demands of the task and the physiological (neuromuscular and biomechanical) requirements of task performance. Walking, rising from sitting, bending, and reaching are dynamic tasks that are frequently compromised for patients with LBP. However, there has been little systematic, quantitative study on functional movement patterns, especially in the context of clinical rehabilitation. This final section of this chapter will focus specifically on movement characteristics during task performance.

The general dearth of empirically derived data on normal and altered motor performance and the stability and the short-term and long-term implications of altered motor performance have led to the use of treatment approaches that frequently lack a scientific rationale. For example, many treatment regimens (especially orthopedic regimens) are designed to "normalize" movement and obtain symmetry in posture and performance. However, normal movement in the presence of impairment may be neither possible nor desirable, and asymmetry of posture and movement is the norm. So it is unreasonable to

assume asymmetry is a problem or that it warrants "normalizing," except in extreme cases.

It is plausible that many altered movement strategies expressed by patients with impairments are actually the most efficient and effective for that patient. For some patients, it may be more important for them to be able to complete a task than to be concerned with how they complete it. Other patients may lack flexibility in motor patterns and be unable to modify a movement pattern enough to accommodate their impairment and still complete the task.

Patients with LBP tend to move slower and with less force compared to pain-free individuals. The decrease in performance speed can be a useful strategy if it results in tasks being performed and being performed with less pain. However, if a task is performed too slowly it becomes very costly and burdensome in terms of time taken. Thus it a less useful strategy and an alternative one should be sought. Improved knowledge of task demands and of normal and altered motor performance patterns in patients with different etiologies can help therapists identify task difficulties and the component of the task that is specifically difficult. Therapy can then focus more appropriately on modifying the task, modifying the patient's task performance, or modifying the patient's impairment, attitude, and/or beliefs toward disability.

Some research on motor performance patterns has been performed. However, most research has been descriptive and cross-sectional and has characterized and compared motion and muscle performance characteristics in subjects with and without LBP during specific task performance. For example, movement patterns differ between subjects with and without LBP as tasks are performed, e.g., walking (1,22,23), wheel turning (39), symmetric and asymmetric trunk flexion (28), reaching (37), and rising from sitting (11–13). Altered postural control and muscle reaction times may be some of the factors that contribute to the alteration of movement patterns in individuals with LBP. Radebold et al. demonstrated these phenomena in patients with chronic LBP during unexpected movement perturbations in sitting (36). However, further systematic investigation of the mechanisms, the factors that influence changes in motor pattern, and the stability of altered patterns during dynamic movements (e.g., walking, trunk flexion, reaching, and rising from sitting) is necessary.

Marras and colleagues (28) measured angular position, velocity, and acceleration of the trunk as 171 subjects with LBP and 339 healthy control subjects wore a triaxial goniometer and flexed and extended their trunk in five different planes. The tests correctly classified 94% of subjects into LBP or control groups. The authors suggested that motion signatures differed among patients with LBP of different etiology.

Although validation is clearly necessary, the work is intriguing given the diagnostic conundrum of LBP.

Arendt-Nielsen et al. (1) conducted a series of gait studies and examined electromorphic (EMG) activity in the erector spinae in subjects with clinical and experimentally induced LBP. They found differences in amount and timing of EMG activity between patients and control subjects during all phases of gait. Most importantly they showed that experimentally induced muscle pain modulated EMG activity and gait patterns in a similar manner to that of clinical LBP.

In our laboratory, we are conducting integrated, biomechanical, and EMG analyses of the walk, sit-to-stand, and loaded reach tasks in an effort to understand the effect of LBP on physical performance.

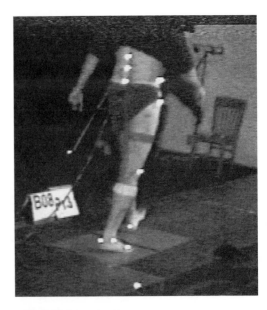

Figure 12.6 Gait analysis.

Walking—Temporal and Spatial Parameters

We have compared the gait characteristics of 44 subjects with LBP and 47 healthy control subjects walking at their preferred and fastest speed (23). Patients walked significantly slower at both preferred and fastest speed. The velocity of the fastest walking speed of the patients was similar to the preferred speed of the control group. It was also interesting to note that patients increased their walking speed by increasing their cadence, whereas control subjects increased their speed by increasing stride length. The difficulty associated with stride extension may account for patient's inability to walk as fast as their pain-free counterparts. However, LBP does not result from a single etiology. The altered gait strategy appears to be related to pain and especially to the location of pain. Location of pain can of course contribute to diagnostic decisions. Hussein et al. (22) examined the effect of pain location on gait patterns in individuals with LBP. He measured and analyzed the gait of 60 subjects with LBP grouped according to the presence of back pain (BP) or leg pain (LP) (21). Significant group differences were revealed. Patients with LP had an asymmetrical gait pattern (i.e., different step lengths) and were outperformed by those with BP only in terms of walking speed and stride length. They were particularly limited in step length on the affected side. Limitation in step length and walking speed would of course be related. However, whether the limitation in walking speed was caused by anticipated pain or actual pain is not clear. A variety of factors could account for these gait difficulties. Impairment level problems include limitations in range of spinal rotation, tight hamstrings, and sensitivity of the sciatic nerve to stretch. Further investigations are clearly indicated and are ongoing.

Walking—Ground Reaction Force, Muscle Control, and Motion Parameters

A more detailed and comprehensive analysis of gait (Fig. 12.6) in patients with BP, LP, and an age-matched and gender-matched control group is ongoing. In this experiment, subjects walk at their preferred and fastest speeds. A force platform is used to measure the ground reactions forces (GRF). Electromyographic activity is recorded from the paraspinal, glutei, hamstrings, quadriceps, gastrocnemius, and pretibial muscles during one gait cycle (i.e., from the first initial contact at the force platform to the second initial contact of the test leg). And the Ariel Performance Analysis System (APAS) is used to quantify motion parameters (angular displacement of lumbar spine, unilateral hip, knee, and ankle). The preliminary data from one subject in each group are presented.

Preliminary GRF data revealed that the normal subject had the highest before/after (Fig. 12.7) and vertical GRF (Fig. 12.8), followed by BP and LP subjects, respectively. This was expected because faster walking speed produces more GRF (35). Interestingly, the LP patient seemed to have somewhat different GRF patterns. The LP patient had slightly more backward force at preferred speed walking (Fig. 12.7A) and also more vertical GRF at loading response (F1) at preferred and fastest speed walking (Fig. 12.8A and 12.8B) than the BP patient despite having the slowest walking speed (Fig. 12.9). This may have been partly caused by altered sensory input at the lower limb and step length asymmetry in the LP patient (step length difference between non-test and test leg at preferred speed: normal = 0.97 cm,

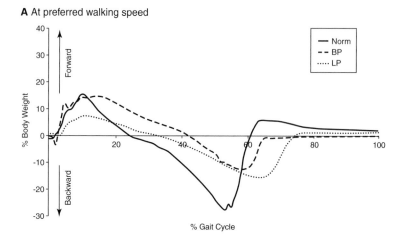

A At preferred walking speed

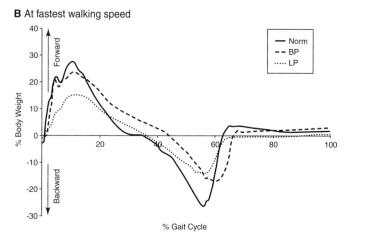

B At fastest walking speed

Figure 12.7 Before/after ground reaction forces during a gait cycle.
(A) At preferred walking speed.
(B) At fastest walking speed.

BP = 0.12 cm, LP = 2.33 cm; and at fastest speed: normal = 1.24 cm, BP = 4.34 cm, LP = 3.52 cm).

In general, both patients had more average muscle activity than the normal subject in most muscle groups at both preferred and fastest walk speeds (Fig. 12.10A and 12.10B). However, between patient differences were observed. The patient with BP had higher average muscle activities than the LP patient. Specifically, the BP patient recruited more contralateral paraspinal and hamstrings muscles of the test leg during preferred speed walking and more ipsilateral paraspinal and pretibial muscles during fastest speed walking.

Despite having lower levels of EMG activity in the paraspinals compared to the subjects with spinal problems, the normal subject still exhibited a greater magnitude of spinal motion at both preferred and fastest walk speeds (Fig. 12.11A and 12.11B). The preliminary results are intriguing, but it needs to be established whether these individual differences are representative of group differences (i.e., BP, LP, and normal).

Sit-to-Stand

The sit-to-stand (Fig. 12.12A–D) and loaded reach tasks (Fig. 12.13A–B) are also being investigated in pain-free individuals and among patients with LBP with and without a history of surgery. Preliminary findings from the biomechanical analyses have revealed some interesting insights into movement differences and/or compensations in the presence of LBP. For example, during rising from sitting, patients with LBP use less hip (flexion/extension) motion compared to control subjects and appear to compensate through an increase in the motion of the knee (13). Further, patients with a history of spinal fusion

A At preferred walking speed

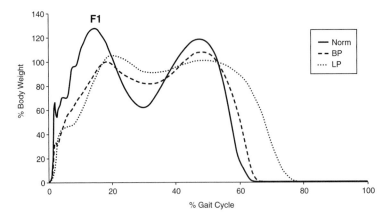

B At fastest walking speed

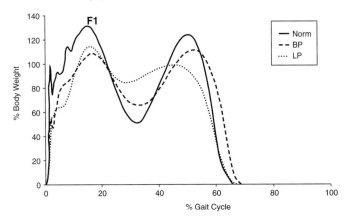

Figure 12.8 Vertical ground reaction forces during a gait cycle. **(A)** At preferred walking speed. **(B)** At fastest walking speed.

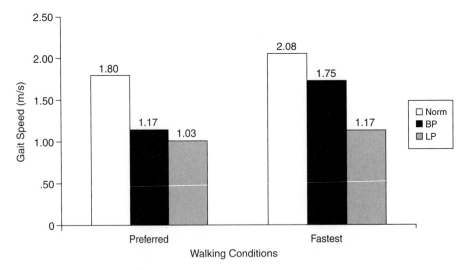

Figure 12.9 Gait speed.

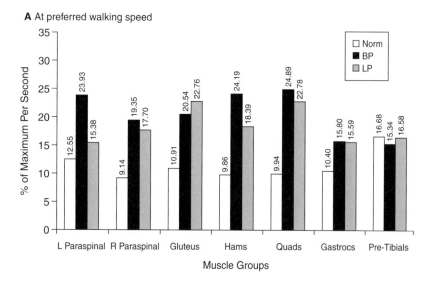

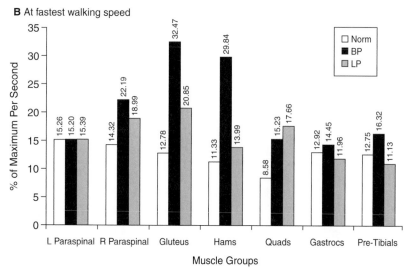

Figure 12.10 Average EMG activities during a gait cycle. **(A)** At preferred walking speed. **(B)** At fastest walking speed.

(>6 months postoperative status) exhibit restrictions in center of gravity displacement during this task, possibly because of limited trunk mobility. They compensate by increasing the displacement of their head to achieve standing (11). It is worth noting that all subjects (with and without LBP) were asymmetrical regarding their performance of the task (12).

In the loaded reach task, we have found that pain-free subjects reach further forward and withstand a greater magnitude of spinal load than patients with LBP regardless of surgical status (37). Not surprisingly, patients with lumbar fusion compensate for spinal restriction by increasing motion at the hip, knee, and ankle motions compared with the other two groups. They also exhibit relatively lower EMG activity in paraspinal and rectus femoris muscles but greater EMG activity in gluteus and hamstrings mus-

cles compared with control subjects or with non-surgical patients.

The interdependency in the relationship between movement and EMG activity makes it difficult to determine whether differences in EMG activity between groups are causes, correlates, or consequences of altered movement patterns. More importantly, the adaptive strategies distant from the trunk (e.g., between group differences in ankle movements) emphasize the need for "whole person" assessment rather than spinal assessment.

Interestingly, non-surgical patients with LBP exhibit significantly greater lateral sway as they move forward (22.36 cm, compared to 10.88 cm and 11.11 cm for spinal fusion and control groups). It is possible that this increased lateral sway is pain related because of the relatively high level of pain in

A At preferred walking speed

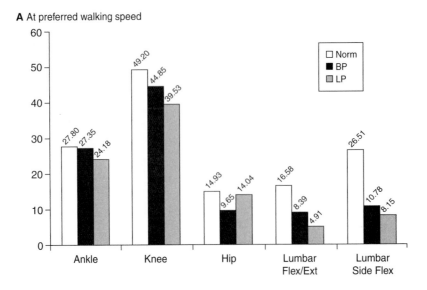

B At fastest walking speed

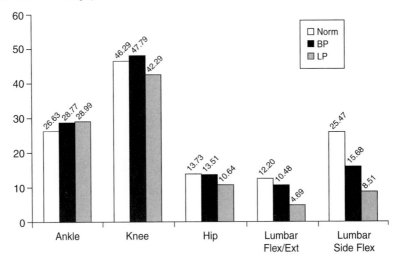

Figure 12.11 Total range of motion during a gait cycle. **(A)** At preferred walking speed. **(B)** At fastest walking speed.

the non-surgical patients. It could also be caused by the relatively slow rate of forward movement in the LBP group resulted in greater lateral sway (similar to riding a bicycle slowly). The fact that this study was cross-sectional in design limits the interpretation of these findings.

■ CONCLUSION

Physical performance and LBP are complex multi-dimensional constructs. They can be influenced by physical, cognitive, emotional, social, task, and environmental factors. The physical performance task battery appears to provide a psychometrically sound and meaningful basis for physical therapy assessment, treatment, and outcome measurement. It is plausible that physical performance tests will also provide a reasonable basis by which patients are divided into homogenous subgroups. Thus, individual treatment protocols for the subgroups can be developed based on a theoretically credible and testable foundation. Monitoring physical performance over time may ultimately facilitate clinical decisions regarding optimum timing and duration of physical therapy interventions. Another advantage of using physical performance tests for assessment is that clinical decisions can be driven into a mode that is more holistic, that focuses on physical function and activity, that identifies movement difficulties, and that has a credible, theoretical basis.

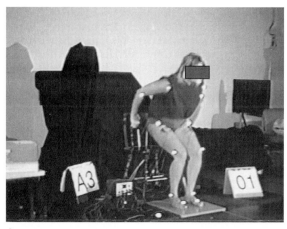

A

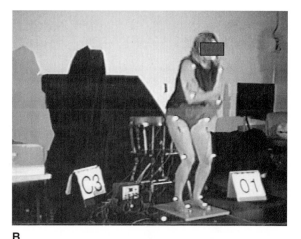

B

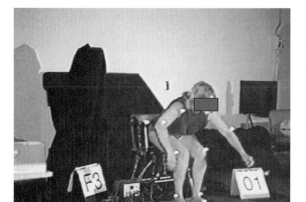

C

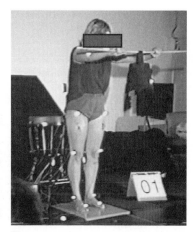

D

Figure 12.12 Biomechanical analysis of sit-to-stand task.
(A) Condition 1: Arms pushing from chair.
(B) Condition 2: Arms crossed.
(C) Condition 3: Arms free.
(D) Condition 4: Arms pushing knees.

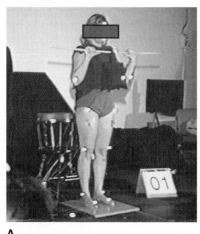

A

B

Figure 12.13 Biomechanical analysis of loaded reach task.
(A) Starting position.
(B) End position.

■ REFERENCES

1. Arendt-Nielsen L, Graven-Nielsen T, Svarrer H, et al. The influence of low back pain on muscle activity and coordination during gait: a clinical and experimental study. Pain 1996;64:231–240.

2. Beurskens AJ, de Vet HC, Koke AJ. Responsiveness of functional status in low back pain: A comparison of different instruments. Pain 1996;65:71–76.

3. Beurskens AJ, de Vet HC, Koke AJ, et al. Measuring the functional status of patients with low back pain. Assessment of the quality of four disease-specific questionnaires. Spine 1995;20:1017–1028.

4. Biering-Sorensen F, Thomsen CE, Hilden J. Risk indicators for low back trouble. Scand J Rehabil Med 1989;21:151–157.

5. Chatman AB, Hyams SP, Neel JM, et al. The Patient-Specific Functional Scale: measurement properties in patients with knee dysfunction. Phys Ther 1997;77:820–829.

6. Craig KD, Prkachin KM, Grunau RVE. The facial expression of pain. In: Turk DC, Melzack R, eds. The facial expression of pain. Guilford Press, 1992:257–276.

7. de Looze MP, Zinzen E, Caboor D, et al. Muscle strength, task performance and low back load in nurses. Ergonomics 1998;41:1095–1104.

8. Dedering A, Nemeth G, Harms-Ringdahl K. Correlation between electromyographic spectral changes and subjective assessment of lumbar muscle fatigue in subjects without pain from the lower back. Clin Biomech (Bristol, Avon) 1999;14:103–111.

9. Deyo RA, Centor RM. Assessing the responsiveness of functional scales to clinical change: An analogy to diagnostic test performance. J Chronic Dis 1986;39:897–906.

10. Donahue MS, Riddle DL, Sullivan MS. Intertester reliability of the modified version of McKenzie's lateral shift assessments obtained in patients with low back pain. Phys Ther 1996;76:706–716.

11. Etnyre BR, Simmonds MJ, Lee CE, et al. Head and center of gravity motion during sit-to-stand between back pain patients and a control group. 13th International Congress of World Confederation for Physical Therapy. Yokohama, Japan, 1999.

12. Etnyre BR, Simmonds MJ, Radwan H. Comparison of electromyographic duration and frequency characteristics between low back pain patients and a control group. Third Interdisciplinary World Congress on Low Back and Pelvis Pain. Vienna, Austria, 1998.

13. Etnyre BR, Simmonds MJ, Radwan H, et al. Hip and knee displacements during sit-to-stand movements between low back pain patients and a control group. 13th International Congress of World Confederation for Physical Therapy. Yokohama, Japan, 1999.

14. Faas A. Exercises: Which ones are worth trying, for which patients, and when? Spine 1996;21:2874–287; discussion 288–289.

15. Fairbank JC, Couper J, Davies JB, et al. The Oswestry low back pain disability questionnaire. Physiotherapy. 1980;66:271–273.

16. Fisher K, Johnston M. Validation of the Oswestry Low Back Pain Disability Questionnaire, its sensitivity as a measure of change following treatment and its relationship with other aspects of the chronic pain experience. Physiother Theory Pract 1997;13:67–80.

17. Fordyce WE, Lansky D, Calsyn DA, et al. Pain measurement and pain behavior. Pain 1984;18:53–69.

18. Freburger JK, Riddle DL. Using published evidence to guide the examination of the sacroiliac joint region. Phys Ther 2001;81:1135–1143.

19. Gatchel RJ, Polatin PB, Mayer TG. The dominant role of psychosocial risk factors in the development of chronic low back pain disability. Spine 1995;20:2702–2709.

20. Grieve GP. Mobilization of the Spine, 4th ed. New York, NY: Churchill Livingstone, 1984.

21. Hussein TM. Kinematic gait characteristics: A comparison of patients with chronic low back pain with and without referred leg pain (Dissertation). Houston, TX: Texas Woman's University, 1999.

22. Hussein TM, Simmonds MJ, Etnyre B, et al. Kinematics of gait in subjects with low back pain with and without leg pain. Washington, DC: Scientific Meeting & Exposition of the American Physical Therapy Association, 1999.

23. Hussein TM, Simmonds MJ, Olson SL, et al. Kinematics of gait in normal and low back pain subjects. Boston, MA: American Congress of Sports Medicine 45th Annual Meeting, 1998.

24. Ito T, Shirado O, Suzuki H, et al. Lumbar trunk muscle endurance testing: An inexpensive alternative to a machine for evaluation. Arch Phys Med Rehabil 1996;77:75–79.

25. Kankaanpaa M, Laaksonen D, Taimela S, et al. Age, sex, and body mass index as determinants of back and hip extensor fatigue in the isometric Sorensen back endurance test. Arch Phys Med Rehabil 1998;79:1069–1075.

26. Lee CE, Simmonds MJ, Novy DM, et al. Self-reports and clinician-measured physical performance among patients with low back pain: A comparison. Arch Phys Med Rehabil 2001;82:In press.

27. Main CJ, Watson PJ. Screening for patients at risk of developing chronic incapacity. J Occup Rehabil 1995;5:207–217.

28. Marras WS, Parnianpour M, Ferguson SA, et al. The classification of anatomic- and symptom-based low

back disorders using motion measure models. Spine 1995;20:2531–2546.

29. Marras WS, Wongsam PE. Flexibility and velocity of the normal and impaired lumbar spine. Arch Phys Med Rehabil 1986;67:213–217.

30. McHorney CA, Ware JE Jr, Lu JF, et al. The MOS 36-item Short-Form Health Survey (SF-36): III. Tests of data quality, scaling assumptions, and reliability across diverse patient groups. Med Care 1994;32:40–66.

31. McHorney CA, Ware JE Jr, Raczek AE. The MOS 36-Item Short-Form Health Survey (SF-36): II. Psychometric and clinical tests of validity in measuring physical and mental health constructs. Med Care 1993;31:247–263.

32. Newton M, Thow M, Somerville D, et al. Trunk strength testing with iso-machines. Part 2: Experimental evaluation of the Cybex II Back Testing System in normal subjects and patients with chronic low back pain. Spine 1993;18:812–824.

33. Novy DM Simmonds MJ, Lee CE Physical Performance Tasks: What are the Underlying Constructs? Arch Phys Med Rehabil 2002;83(1):44–47.

34. Novy DM, Simmonds MJ, Olson SL, et al. Physical performance: differences in men and women with and without low back pain. Arch Phys Med Rehabil 1999;80:195–198.

35. Perry J. Gait Analysis: Normal and Pathological Function. Thorofare, NJ: SLACK Inc, 1992.

36. Radebold A, Cholewicki J, Polzhofer GK, et al. Impaired postural control of the lumbar spine is associated with delayed muscle response times in patients with chronic idiopathic low back pain. Spine 2001;26:724–730.

37. Radwan HA. Motion patterns, electromyographic activity, and ground reaction forces during a loaded functional reach task: A comparison among subjects with low back pain, subjects with lumbar spine fusion and a control group (Dissertation). Houston, TX: Texas Woman's University, 1999.

38. Roland M, Morris R. A study of the natural history of back pain. Part I: Development of a reliable and sensitive measure of disability in low-back pain. Spine 1983;8:141–144.

39. Rudy TE, Boston JR, Lieber SJ, et al. Body motion patterns during a novel repetitive wheel-rotation task. A comparative study of healthy subjects and patients with low back pain. Spine 1995;20:2547–2554.

40. Sanders SH. Automated versus self-monitoring of 'up-time' in chronic low-back pain patients: A comparative study. Pain 1983;15:399–405.

41. Sharrack B, Hughes RAC. Reliability of distance estimation by doctors and patients: Cross sectional study. BMJ 1997;315:1652–1654.

42. Simmonds MJ, Campbell A, Wang WT. Assessing functional change in patients with low back pain: A comparison of measures. Yokohama, Japan: 13th International Congress of the World Confederation for Physical Therapy, 1999.

43. Simmonds MJ, Claveau Y. Measures of pain and physical function in patients with low back pain. Physiother Theory Pract 1997;13:53–65.

44. Simmonds MJ, Lee CE. The Sorensen endurance test: a test of fatigue or pain? Phoenix, AZ: American Pain Society, 2001.

45. Simmonds MJ, Lee CE, Jones SC. Pain distribution and physical function in patients with low back pain. Yokohama, Japan: 13th International Congress of the World Confederation for Physical Therapy, 1999.

46. Simmonds MJ, Olson S, Novy DM, et al. Disability prediction in patients with back pain using performance based models. Charleston, SC: North American Spine Society/American Pain Society Meeting, 1998.

47. Simmonds MJ, Olson SL, Jones S, et al. Psychometric characteristics and clinical usefulness of physical performance tests in patients with low back pain. Spine 1998;23:2412–2421.

48. Stratford P, Gill C, Westaway M, et al. Assessing disability and change on individual patients: A report of a patient specific measure. Physiother Can 1995;47:258–263.

49. Turk DC, Rudy TE, Stieg RL. The disability determination dilemma: Toward a multiaxial solution. Pain 1988;34:217–229.

50. Vlaeyen JW, Kole-Snijders AM, Boeren RG, et al. Fear of movement/(re)injury in chronic low back pain and its relation to behavioral performance. Pain 1995;62:363–372.

51. Waddell G, Newton M, Henderson I, et al. A Fear-Avoidance Beliefs Questionnaire (FABQ) and the role of fear-avoidance beliefs in chronic low back pain and disability. Pain 1993;52:157–168.

52. Ware JE Jr, Sherbourne CD. The MOS 36-item short-form health survey (SF-36). I. Conceptual framework and item selection. Med Care 1992;30:473–483.

13

Employment Screening and Functional Capacity Evaluation to Determine Safe Return to Work

Leonard Matheson and
Vert Mooney

Learning Objectives
On completion of this chapter you should be able to:

- Assess the validity of pre-employment and pre-placement screening.
- Define fitness for duty evaluation.
- Explain the American and Disabilities Act restrictions and protections.
- Define the roles of the treating physician versus the evaluating physician.
- Assess the validity of a Functional Capacity Evaluation and be aware of what it can tell about job capacity.
- Assess the appropriate physical therapy and the expectations of physical therapy reporting.

Introduction

This chapter describes the historical background of employment screening from a health care perspective, beginning with the use of spinal x-rays to screen for risk of injury. Medical examination is less useful and justified for employee selection than it is for baseline comparisons. The use of technologies such as spinal MRI procedures may provide a basis for avoiding expensive and needless surgery when a problem such as an asymptomatic degenerative spine is found to be present before employment. The use of functional capacity evaluation is more often justified, both to identify applicants for employment who will be the most productive workers and to assist the physician and plant manager to properly place a worker returning from sick leave.

Validity of Pre-Employment Pre-Placement Screening

It is self-evident that an employer would like to avoid hiring those who have greater liability of injury than the average. Recent estimates of direct costs of work related injuries and illnesses in the United States are in excess of $65 billion. In addition, the indemnity costs are $106 billion to American Industry (48). What can be done at the onset of employment to reduce the incidents of the employed? This chapter addresses employment screening for new employees and those who are returning to work after experiencing lost time because of injury or illness.

The earliest form of pre-employment testing was the use of back x-rays. In early years it was felt that abnormal findings could predict those who would have injuries at work. However, when scientific studies were initiated, it was found that in asymptomatic people, 10% had disc degeneration, spondylolysis, or spondylolisthesis (25). Actually, when studied, it turned out that people with "normal" radiographs actually had a higher rate of injury compared to those who showed radiographic abnormalities (43). In another study in a steel plant where the workers were performing heavy work, abnormalities seen in x-ray did not predict a higher incidence of low back injuries (13). This is to be expected of course. The incidence of spondylolysis is approximately 5% in the U.S. general population, but the rate of significant disabling back pain in Americans with spondylolysis is only approximately 0.5% (2). Thus, because of the lack of predictive validity, and with the additional awareness of the threats of radiation, pre-employment radiographs have not been demonstrated to be cost-effective.

Of course the more modern imaging technique is the MRI. This is extremely sensitive to soft tissue changes in the disc, but no study has showed that abnormalities noted in MRI are predictive of later pain symptoms. There is, however, a possible rationale that can be applied to a lumbar MRI if it could be performed cheaply enough. It is well-recognized that degenerative changes in the spine increase in a rate approximately correlated with age. Currently, when a worker is injured, the MRI shows a significant degenerative change and the individual does not respond to undefined physical therapy, a justification is made for fusion, whether there is causal evidence for impairment. If it can be demonstrated that the degenerative changes that are suggesting the need for fusion were actually found in the MRI when the worker was hired (and the worker had been successfully employed in the interim), the enthusiasm for surgery is decreased. This strategy apparently has been successful in reducing the incidence of the very expensive spinal fusions at the Steelcase company (39). It is not clear whether in the future that the safer, but the more expensive, imaging tool MRI compared to plain x-rays will be more helpful than the now discarded x-ray screening.

If imaging studies are not predictive of spinal disease, then how about physical strength testing? There only has been one study that purports to demonstrate that strength testing could predict an incidence of back injuries (24). The workers studied in this group performed extremely demanding physical work in the tire manufacturing business. They had to lift heavy tires off of workplaces, twist, and put them down in a constant repetitive manner. The heavy job demands facing that group of workers is somewhat unique. Using essentially the same testing method, a more recent study of pre-employment testing of aircraft workers for Boeing indicated that isometric testing of total body lift function could not predict of incidence of back injury (3).

Selection for employment on the basis of lifting tests is not possible unless the specific demands of the job are being tested. In another recent study, careful strength testing using isokinetic technology was performed on 33 experienced warehouse workers to measure back strength. The pre-placement individuals had to meet that minimum standard before they were hired in that job category. There was a significant reduction in back pain claims as a result of this strategy (44), but such a study may bring up another aspect of pre-placement testing. An applicant for the job, when it is recognized that specific testing is being performed, may not persist with the application for that job if he/she feels physically poorly qualified or has a history of workers' compensation claims. Pre-placement strength testing can give a baseline that would question the validity of an individual's claim for injury later.

Is there evidence that back strength is a predictor for back injury? We conducted a study to investigate that proposition (35). Using specific isometric testing over 7 points of range, we tested 152 shipyard workers as to their lumbar extensor strength. These individuals were all veterans in their job, had not had back claims for at least 3 years, and were followed-up for an additional 2 years. Nine percent of that study group had a back claim over the next 2 years. It was noteworthy that all but two of these injured workers had higher strengths than the average. Thus, back strength itself was not a predictor of injury. These workers were classified also regarding PDC levels of medium, heavy, and very heavy work. Even though they performed various types of work with varying physical demands, the back strengths did not vary among these three groups. Thus, even the demands of the job did not apparently affect back strength.

Are there factors that can predict work injury? Chaffin and Clark found a threefold increase of injuries and the risk of back problems in subjects with a history of back pain (8). Sciatica is a predictor of back pain (38,4). A prospective study by Lloyd and Troop (27) found four historical factors to be predictive of recurrent low back pain. These were residual leg pain on work placement, history of sickness absence of 5 weeks or more, falls as a cause of back pain, and a history of two or more previous episodes of back pain.

Thus, we do have some predictors of who might get industrial back pain. With this knowledge, is it possible to discriminate in hiring practices? In 1984 the American Medical Association summarized the objectives for pre-placement examinations as follows (15):

- To evaluate the medical fitness of individuals to perform their duties without hazard to themselves or fellow workers.
- To assist employees in maintaining maintenance or improvement of their health.
- To detect the effects of harmful working conditions and to advise corrective measures.
- To establish a record of the medical condition of the employee at the time of each examination.

However, there was a considerable question as to whether the employees or the employer benefited from medical evaluation programs at all (16). Actually, there never has been a scientific study demonstrating the levels of success or risk of avoidance accomplished by medical evaluations in the past. In fact, the case was being made that even evaluation was discriminating in preventing people with disabilities from entering the workplace. Thus, the American with Disabilities Act (ADA) passed in 1990. It prohibits disability-based discrimination in all aspects of employment and mandates that medical examinations be conducted only after an offer of employment is made to an applicant. An employer cannot reject a candidate because of medical concerns about insignificant or uncertain future risks or inability to perform non-essential job functions. Employers are required to maintain the confidentiality of medical information and to provide reasonable accommodations for qualified applicants who have disabilities.

In the past it was possible for physicians to recommend to employers that they do not hire applicants because of speculative risks of injury or costs of accommodation. Under the ADA, the incorrect medical advice can result in significant and costly litigation. Thus, any medical advice has to be specifically based on appropriate evidence.

Employers may require an applicant to undergo the physical examination before beginning employment, but only after a job has been offered. The reason for conducting such an evaluation may include medical determination of the ability to meet job performance requirements or medical standards. The ADA allows an employer to reject a person only after stringent criteria are met. An applicant may be rejected if he poses a direct threat to himself or others in the workplace. He may be rejected if a disability prevents performance of essential job functions or when accommodations cannot be made without undue hardship. This phase of the legislation may result in litigation as to what is accommodation that would create undue hardship to the employer. Specifically, also, the ADA prohibits employers to inquire about a history of back problems, which the job applicant may choose not to disclose, before a job offer. The Equal Employment Opportunity Commission (EEOC) notes that 46% of back impairment charges have come from discharged employees versus 15% in the hiring process (22). Let's take a closer look at the laws and guidelines surrounding health care practice in employment screening.

Pre-Placement and Fitness for Duty Screening

Increasingly, health care professionals are being asked to provide pre-placement screening and fitness for duty screening services. It is important to recognize that these services must be provided within the context of the laws that govern employee placement and selection. This legal context is quite different from that in which all other laws based on the English Common Law heritage are found. That is, the laws governing employee placement and selection are frequently concerned with establishing parity for disadvantaged individuals. The Equal Employment Opportunity (EEO) laws in the United States, and similar laws in Canada and most industrialized countries, are intended to precipitate social change. As such, the laws and the rules governing those laws have developed so that they favor the employee or potential employee who chooses to use them. In all other aspects of the law, the individual against whom an action is brought (the defendant) does not have the burden of proof. The plaintiff or applicant who brings the action maintains the burden of proof and, if the plaintiff is not able to establish beyond a reasonable doubt that the defendant is at fault, the defendant will win the lawsuit. The difference in the EEO arena is that the burden of proof is on the defendant. In an EEO action, the defendant must demonstrate that there was no unfair discrimination in the defendant's hiring, placement, or promotional procedures. The EEO laws have been developed in recognition of the fact that discrimination exists within society based on factors other than ability. The basic tenet of these laws is that one must not unfairly discriminate.

Discrimination in selection for employment and for placement after hiring is only acceptable as long as it is fair and appropriate to the situation. If a selection procedure is used and decisions for placement are made based on the results of the selection procedure, it must be able to be demonstrated that the selection procedure is relevant to the decision that was made. For example, it is entirely appropriate to use a test of typing speed and accuracy to select individuals to be placed in a job in which typing is a necessary and important job function. However, this same test would not be appropriate for individuals applying for a job as a warehouse worker if typing is not a necessary part of that job. To use another example, a test of infrequent lifting from floor to eye level would be appropriate as long as the evaluation task can be demonstrated to predict subsequent competence and/or safety in the warehouse worker's job. It would only be appropriate to use that same test of lifting with a secretary if the secretarial job description required lifting as a usual and necessary job function. In either case, the test must be such that the individual's performance can be shown to be related to subsequent performance on the job.

It is important to appreciate that the applicant's competence in performance of job functions must be considered separately from the applicant's safety in the job. Although in most health care professionals' minds these are linked, competence and safety are separate issues and must be considered separately. The important point here is that assessment of competency is much easier to perform and defend than assessment of safety. The health care professional

who is providing pre-placement evaluation services probably will be best able to provide tests of competency rather than tests of safety when one considers the legal context within which all of the testing must be conducted. Stated another way, the evaluator must be prepared to defend his or her recommendations against a challenge based on one or another (or perhaps several) of the EEO laws. It is much easier a priori to develop an effective defense if the recommendation for placement is based on competence than if the recommendation is based on safety. In addition, if, for some reason, an a priori defense has not been developed and the evaluator is unprepared, a defense based on competence will be possible to reconstruct, whereas a defense based on safety will be impossible to put together after the fact. The defense that an employer will use has to do with:

1. Whether the individual is a member of a protected group.
2. Whether the use of the selection device brought about an adverse impact.
3. Whether the use of the selection device can be demonstrated to be based on a business necessity.

If an individual is not from a protected group, and/or there is no adverse impact, and there is a business necessity for use of the test, then the employer will prevail. However, if an individual is a member of a protected group and there is adverse impact without business necessity, the plaintiff will prevail.

Even if the employer puts forth an adequate defense, individuals in the United States who are members of the disabled protected group have still another set of protections based on the legal requirement that the employer provide reasonable accommodation. That is, the employer must demonstrate that it is not reasonable to make changes in the work place or manner of work that would sufficiently accommodate the handicap presented by the prospective employee so that job performance would not be affected.

Because each of the States in the United States can develop laws that extend beyond the basic requirements of the federal EEO laws, various definitions have come up that are relevant in certain states. For example, the definition of "handicapped worker" includes individuals who are hypertensive in California but does not apply in any other states, includes individuals who are alcoholics in Wisconsin but does not apply in any other states, and includes individuals with glaucoma in North Carolina but does not apply in any other states. Conversely, certain states have delimited the term. The important point to appreciate is that there is great variability.

The laws briefly outlined should be considered basic. The protections that are described for workers may have been expanded by a particular state or municipal government.

Title VII of the Civil Rights Act of 1964 prohibits discrimination on the basis of race, color, national origin, sex, or religion. This Act is enforced by the Equal Employment Opportunity Commission. Title VII includes employers that have 15 or more employees that are engaged in "an industry affecting commerce," all state and local governments and schools, almost all unions, and almost all employment agencies.

Executive Order 11246 (1965) amended by Executive Order 11375 (1968) prohibits discrimination on the basis of race, color, religion, or national origin by contractors doing business with the federal government. This is administered by the Secretary of Labor through the Office of Federal Contract Compliance Programs. Any employer who has a contract of $10,000 or more or who does business with the federal government worth $50,000 or more is covered.

The Age Discrimination and Employment Act of 1967 (ADEA) was amended in 1978 and protects employees and applicants for employment between the ages of 40 and 70 years. Employers with 20 or more employees for 20 or more weeks of the year are included. Enforcement of the ADEA is vested with the Equal Employment Opportunity Commission.

The Equal Pay Act of 1963 is an amendment to the Fair Labor Standards Act of 1938 and is the basis behind the "Equal Pay for Equal Work" movement, which requires that employers provide wages to employees at a rate that is not gender-specific. This is currently under the jurisdiction of the Equal Employment Opportunity Commission.

The Health Care Act of 1973 is similar to Executive Order 11246 and Executive Order 11375 but extends the protection to individuals who are handicapped and expands the threshold for coverage to any contractor who has more than $2,500 of business with the federal government. A handicapped person is covered if he or she has a physical or mental impairment that substantially limits one or more major life activities or has a record of such impairment or is regarded by others as having such an impairment, even though the person may not, in fact, have such an impairment. Under Section 504 of the Act, an employer may not inquire about whether the applicant is handicapped or about the nature or severity of a handicap unless two criteria are met:

1. A pre-employment medical examination is required of all applicants.
2. The information sought is relevant to the applicant's ability to perform job-related functions.

Although, originally, individuals with alcohol or drug abuse problems were considered handicapped, subsequent amendments by Congress have excluded this as a handicapping condition. The Health Care Act is administered by the Office of Federal Contract Compliance Programs. The OFCCP has administratively expanded the concept of handicap to include, for instance, obesity and epilepsy. In addition, the concept of reasonable accommodation has been developed by the OFCCP. The Health Care Act itself does not require the employer to make reasonable accommodation.

The Vietnam Veterans Readjustment Act of 1974 covers disabled veterans and non-disabled veterans of the Vietnam era and is similar to the Health Care Act of 1973 and the Executive Orders 11246 and 11375 in that it covers contractors with the federal government wherein the value of the contract is $10,000 or greater. This is also under the jurisdiction of the Department of Labor, administered through the Office of Federal Contract Compliance Programs.

Americans With Disabilities Act

The Americans with Disabilities Act was signed into law by President George Bush on July 26, 1990. The Act states that:

> No covered entity shall discriminate against a qualified individual with a disability because of the disability of such individual in regard to job application procedures, the hiring, advancement, or discharge of employees, employee compensation, job training, and other terms, conditions, and privileges of employment.

Purpose of the ADA

In the ADA, Congress attempted to address several important issues that had been introduced and less effectively addressed in the Health Care Act of 1973. These include:

1. To provide a clear and comprehensive national mandate for the elimination of discrimination against individuals with disabilities.
2. Provide clear, strong, consistent, and enforceable standards that address discrimination against individuals with disabilities.
3. To insure that the federal government plays a central role in enforcing the standards in the Americans with Disabilities Act on behalf of individuals with disabilities.
4. Invoke Congressional authority, including the power to enforce the 14th Amendment and to regulate commerce to address the major areas

of discrimination faced by individuals with disabilities.

Types of Discrimination Targeted by the ADA
Congress recognized that discrimination against individuals with disabilities takes several forms and exists in a number of areas. Discrimination limits individuals with disabilities in areas of employment, housing, access to public facilities, and access to public transportation and communication. With regard to discrimination against individuals with disabilities in the area of employment, Congress specifically identified the following as covered by the Act:

1. Limiting, segregating, or classifying the disabled.
2. Participating in a contractual relationship that has the effect of subjecting employees to discrimination prohibited by the Act.
3. Utilizing standards that have the effect of discrimination based on disability.
4. Basing employment decisions for a qualified individual on the known disability of the person with whom the qualified individual is known to have a relationship.
5. Not making reasonable accommodations to the limitations of the qualified individual unless the covered entity can demonstrate that this would pose undue hardship on the operation of the business.
6. Using qualification standards that screen out or tend to screen out individuals with disabilities, unless the standard is shown to be job-related and is consistent with business necessity.
7. Using employment tests that reflect the individual's impairment rather than providing a valid measure of the job's demands.

Definitions Provided by the ADA
As is necessary with every law, certain definitions are developed and provided by Congress to be used by agencies enforcing the law. Those that relate specifically to the employment aspects of the Act include:

Disability—A physical or mental impairment that substantially limits one or more major life activities; a record of such impairment; or being regarded as having such impairment.

Covered entity—An employer, employment agency, labor organization, or joint labor action committee.

Employer—A person engaged in an industry affecting commerce who has 15 or more employees in each of 20 or more calendar weeks in the current or preceding year. For 2 years after

the effective date, "employer" is a person engaged in an industry affecting commerce who has 25 or more employees in each of 20 or more calendar weeks in the current or preceding year. The effective date for the legislation is July 26, 1990. Therefore, employers with 25 or more employees are covered as of July 26, 1992, and employers with 15 or more employees are covered as of July 26, 1994.

Qualified Individual with a Disability
An individual with a disability who, with or without reasonable accommodation, can perform the essential functions of the job that he/she holds or desires. The Act provides a non-exhaustive set of conditions or disorders that are specifically excluded from the definition, including homosexuality, bisexuality, transvestitism, pedophilia, transsexualism, exhibitionism, voyeurism, gender identity disorders not resulting from physical impairment, other sexual behavior disorders, compulsive gambling, kleptomania, pyromania, and psychoactive substance abuse disorders resulting from current illegal use of drugs. In addition, an amendment to the Health Care Act of 1973 states that "individual with handicaps" does not include an alcoholic whose current use of alcohol prevents performance of job duties or constitutes a direct threat to property or to the safety of others.

Direct threat—As part of a qualification standard, an employer may exclude a qualified individual from employment if that individual can be shown to pose a direct threat to the health and safety of others in the work place. This must be a significant and identifiable risk, not merely an elevated risk. The employer must demonstrate that the individual poses a direct threat. The plaintiff is not required to prove an absence of risk.

Essential functions of the job—Consideration shall be given to the employer's judgment as to what functions of the job are essential. A written job description, prepared before advertising or interviewing, shall be considered evidence of the essential function. However, there is no presumption in favor of the employer's judgment. The weight that evidence based on job description will be given will depend directly on how closely it is tailored to the essential duties of the actual job.

Reasonable accommodation—This is not specifically defined. As was the practice with the Health Care Act of 1973, reasonable accommodation takes many forms and is dependent on the employee, job, covered entity's facility, and covered entity. Reasonable accommodation is based on procedures that have been developed to implement the Health Care Act of 1973. The Americans with Disabilities Act introduces reasonable accommodation with the phrase, "the term 'reasonable accommodation' may include. . . ." The act provides specific examples, including making existing facilities readily accessible to and usable by individuals with disabilities. In addition, other methods of restructuring include job restructuring, part-time or modified work schedules, reassignment to a vacant position, acquisition or modification of equipment, modification of examinations, training materials, or policies, provision of readers or interpreters, or other similar accommodations.

Undue hardship—An action requiring significant difficulty or expense. This is considered in light of the accommodations and how they are to be implemented, involving both the direct cost and net cost of the accommodations. In addition, the facility's financial resources, number of persons employed, and impact on operations is taken into account. Beyond the individual facility, the covered entity's resources are considered based on the financial resources of the entity, the number of persons employed, and the impact on operations of the entity. Finally, the composition, structure, and function of the work force at the entity and the facility's geographic separateness from administrative control, along with the physical relationship of the facility to the covered entity will be taken into account. Determination of undue hardship is factual and is made on a case-by-case basis. The burden of proof is on the employer.

Fitness for Duty Evaluation

As the disabled individual concludes his treatment program and is released by his physician, determination regarding return to work at the usual and customary employment, requirement of reasonable accommodation, or a decision of no return to employment despite accommodation, is based on a fitness for duty evaluation (FFDE). The FFDE is a content-valid functional capacity evaluation based on the previously conducted physical demands job analysis. The FFDE is conducted by a health care professional with proper education, training, and experience. The FFDE is based on the critical job tasks of the target job. These are identified by reviewing the physical demands job analysis in light of the employee's impairment. The FFDE process follows these steps:

1. Physical demands job analysis review—The fitness for duty evaluation begins with review and confirmation of the physical demands job analysis in consultation with the supervisor, employee, and treating physician to identify the critical job tasks that will be the focus of the evaluation.

2. Medical records review—A review of pertinent medical records is undertaken, facilitated by contact with the evaluee's physician if the evaluee is in active treatment. Confirmation that the impairment is stable and identification of work restrictions that may affect subsequent testing are the focus of these activities.

3. Structured interview—A structured interview between the evaluator and evaluee is confidential and focuses on the evaluee's injury and medical history. In addition, the evaluee's perception of current functional limits is reviewed. The purpose of the interview is to begin screening out individuals who cannot be tested safely and to identify performance limits that may not be apparent.

4. General health questionnaire—The evaluee must complete a general health questionnaire and injury history. A questionnaire such as the Cornell Medical Index or the EPIC Health Questionnaire (12) provides a broad overview of health status. The questionnaire is reviewed by the evaluator to identify problems that may underlie performance in the testing situation.

5. Perceived functional limits test—Whereas most of the critical job tasks have been identified by interaction between the treating physician and evaluator, it is necessary to screen for tasks that have been missed through the use of a test of perceived functional limits. The Spinal Function Sort and Hand Function Sort are used effectively to perform this task (Figs. 13.1 and 13.2).

6. Screening examination—Depending on the evaluee, his or her impairment, and the specific demands of the job, pre-evaluation screening should review active or passive range of motion, sensibility, muscular spasm, local swelling, cognitive function, resting blood pressure and heart rate, or other pertinent musculoskeletal, neurologic, or physiologic function.

7. Progressive functional testing—A protocol based on progressive functional testing of the evaluee's ability to perform critical job tasks is designed based on the physical demands job analysis, physician's prophylactic restrictions, evaluee's health, evaluee's perception of his or her limits,

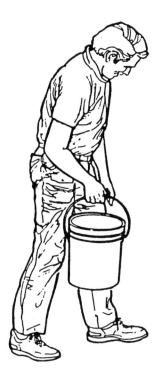

Figure 13.1 Spinal function sort—carrying a 30-lb bucket 30 feet. With permission from Matheson L, Matheson, M. Spinal Function Sort. Wildwood, MO: Employment Potential Improvement Corporation, 1989.

Pre-Placement Screening

Pre-placement screening has attracted substantial attention from employers in recent years because of its value in assisting employers to maintain a cost-effective work force by assuring that workers are selected who are likely to perform job tasks in a safe and productive manner. The Americans with Disabilities Act allows pre-placement screening as long as it is job-related, conducted after a conditional offer of employment is made to the applicant, is universally applied, is a valid indicator of essential function, and is a business necessity.

Pre-placement screening is conducted by properly trained evaluators who use simulations of essential work demands that are content-valid or validated performance tests that have been statistically demonstrated to predict performance in these work simulations.

Pre-placement screening is conducted using a protocol based on a physical demands job analysis. A content-valid test is used or a testing protocol is developed and a validation study conducted to demonstrate that the protocol is statistically related to the essential job demands. A scientific validation study is necessary to objectively establish the statistical relationship between test demands and essential job

and the results of the screening examination. The most conservative of these parameters is used as a performance target and may be exceeded only with the utmost consideration given to the evaluee's safety.

8. Next-day follow-up—A telephone or in-person follow-up must be conducted the day after the evaluation to elicit the evaluee's symptomatic response to the activity of the examination. This becomes a formal record that is added to the evaluee's file. This addresses the evaluee's readiness to return to work.

9. Report preparation—The evaluator prepares a formal report that describes the Fitness for Duty Evaluation. This report is maintained in the confidential file. A synopsis that includes recommendations for the employee, employer, and treating physician is excerpted and provided to the employer for distribution. If the evaluation results in a recommendation against returning to the previous employment, reasonable accommodation options must then be addressed. If viable options do not exist or are insufficient, the evaluator must provide rationale for a recommendation of no return to employment.

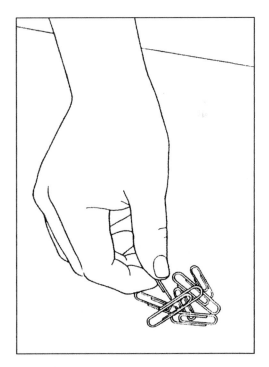

Figure 13.2 Hand function sort—pick out one large paper clip from a group of small paper clips. With permission from Matheson L, Matheson M, Grant J. Hand Function Sort. Wildwood, MO: Employment Potential Improvement Corporation, 1995.

demands. Additionally, the validation study sets standards that minimize disparate impact for identified groups, including, but not limited to, individuals with disabilities, minority groups, females, and older workers.

The validation study is conducted by a team that is composed of professionals such as an industrial psychologist, physiologist, ergonomist, and job analyst. Additionally, with proper training, an occupational therapist, physical therapist, or vocational evaluator can provide a validation study.

Development of Testing Procedures

Employee selection procedures must be developed within the context of the Uniform Guidelines on Employee Selection Procedures (18). The Guidelines provide several important definitions. These include:

> Selection procedure—Any standard that is used as a basis for any employment decision is considered a selection procedure. The exact quote from the Uniform Guidelines is:
>> . . . any measure, combination of measures, or procedure used as a basis for any employment decision. Selection procedures include the full range of assessment techniques from traditional paper and pencil tests, performance tests, training programs or probationary periods, and physical, educational, and work experience requirement through informal or casual interviews and unscored application forms. (12 [page 215])

Adverse impact—There is no adverse impact if the worst performing group is achieving at a rate 80% as well as the best performing group, the groups defined as blacks, Native Americans, Asians, Hispanics, females, and males. Adverse impact is usually based on review of the mix of employees who are successfully hired. That is, it is not usually a question of one or another selection criterion, but the selection process as a whole.

> Content validity—This has to do with the concept that the test is a "piece of the job." As such, the test may be considered content valid. Content validity cannot be used for issues such as personality or intelligence but can be used when the test sample focuses on the necessary knowledge, skill, or ability to successfully complete the job. The EPIC Lift Capacity Test (30,21) can be used as a content-valid test. The Uniform Guidelines list these nine factors that must be considered in the use of a content valid test:

1. Appropriateness of content validity studies—If a test is a representative and fair sample of job tasks or demands, it will be considered appropri-

ate. Generally speaking, this means that the test bears an easily observable relationship to necessary job demands.

2. Job analysis for content validity—A formal job analysis that identifies important work behaviors must be conducted. The job analysis must demonstrate that the worker characteristics are necessary for successful job performance.

3. Development of selection procedures—Although the employer may utilize a standard "off the shelf" selection procedure, the employer has the burden of demonstrating the relevance of that test procedure to the particular circumstance. It is often less troublesome to develop a selection procedure specifically based on the employer's situation.

4. Standards for demonstrating content validity—The test user must demonstrate that behavior measured in the test constitutes a representative and fair sample of that which is required to successfully perform the job and that the knowledge, skill, and ability that is measured is that which is minimally necessary for successful job performance and that the test actually measures these factors.

5. Reliability—One of the advantages of the content valid approach is that validation tests based on statistical significance are not necessary. However, the Uniform Guidelines require that "whenever feasible, appropriate statistical estimates should be made of the reliability of the selection."

6. Previous training or experience—This simply has to do with the need for the employer to demonstrate that any requirement for previous training or experience is justified by demonstrating the relationship between this experience and the content of the job.

7. Content validity of training success—This has to do with the use of a training program as a selection device and simply means that the content of the training program must be demonstrated to have relationship to the content of the job.

8. Operational use—The selection device must be a measure of usual and customary duties.

9. Ranking based on content validity studies—Uniform guidelines require that employers not use a ranking system unless the ranking system can be demonstrated to relate to job performance. That is, if a ranking system is used, higher-ranked employees must be shown to do better in terms of job performance than lower-ranked employees.

Screening by Health Care Professionals

Pre-placement screening that is performed by health care professionals will usually be based on content validity using a careful and well-documented job analysis to establish the business necessity of the test. The business necessity defense rests on five issues:

1. The examination, test, or procedure on which the employment decision is based is found to be job-related.

2. The examination, test, or procedure has a high predictive value and is the most accurate test that is feasible to use. This will often not be possible to establish initially and will require a longitudinal study if the employer is to have confidence that a subsequent EEO action will be defensible. Reliance on a cross-sectional study is to be discouraged in that if adverse impact is already current, the cross-sectional study will be confounded.

3. The examination, test, or procedure indicates that the applicant has a strong likelihood for the development of a serious injury or illness in the foreseeable future and the likelihood of injury or illness represents a significant variation from the general worker population, or discriminates effectively between individuals of varying degrees of productivity. Because the former, having to do with job safety, is so difficult to establish, the latter, having to do with job competency, is more frequently used. When a test is being used to predict successful job performance, the length of time that is required to pass before the individual is judged to have been successful or unsuccessful on the job is finite and predictable. However, when the test is being used to screen for potential injury, considerably more time must pass before an individual is judged to be free from injury. This length of time is open to wide variance and interpretation.

4. The disqualification or other adverse personnel action is based on an individualized determination of fitness. Use of a simple cutpoint is not acceptable. This requires that each personnel decision involve a multifaceted review of the employee. Professional judgment must be exercised.

5. No reasonable accommodation will permit the disabled individual to perform the necessary job function. If the applicant qualifies as a disabled individual, the employer must be prepared to demonstrate that reasonable accommodation is not possible and/or sufficient. This, of course, does not hold when the applicant does not qualify as a handicapped individual.

Role of the Treating Physician

The treating physician should be aware of predictors of back injuries and recurrence once the individual was employed. Even though there is no evidence that back strength alone is a predictor of back injury, there remains the question as to the role of diminished back strength in recurrence of back pain. In a recent study we investigated the role of strength training to reduce incidence of back injury in an industrial setting (36). The strip mining company had an average 9-year history of 2.94 injuries per 200,000 employee hours. This was devastating with their insurance rates. They initiated a once per week back-strengthening program. The participants in the program were asked to volunteer. Eventually approximately half of the 400 employees volunteered. Ninety percent (90%) of those who did volunteer stated that they had some history of back problems, although they had no current workers' compensation claims.

After the 20-week lumbar extensor strengthening program, they increased their strength an average of 54% in flexion and an average of 104% in extension. At the 1-year follow-up, those who did not participate in the once per week 5-minute exercise program had an incidence of injuries of 2.55 per 200,000 employee hours, whereas those who did participate had one short injury, which came out to 0.52 injuries per 200,000 employee hours. The insurance liability dropped precipitously.

A more recent study using similar back strengthening protocols in the airline industry demonstrated similar results (11). In this report, 622 participants in the exercise group were compared to a non-exercise group of 2,937. The back injuries in the exercise group analyzed were 5.7 per year and non-exercise group were 179 per year. Put another way, there were nine injuries per 1,000 in the exercise group, and 61 per 1,000 in the non-exercise group. The cost of back injuries in the exercise group was $206 participants per year, whereas the cost of back injuries in the non-exercising group was $4,883 for non-participants. The exercises were once per week lumbar extensor strengthening for 5 minutes on MedX equipment, which isolates the appropriate muscles (Fig. 13.3).

Obviously it is apparent that there is a relationship between strength and back injury prevention. Thus, a rational treatment program has been developed by several preferred provider organizations in the Southern California area (Table 13.1).

One aspect of the treating physician's role is to encourage speed of initiating appropriate treatment.

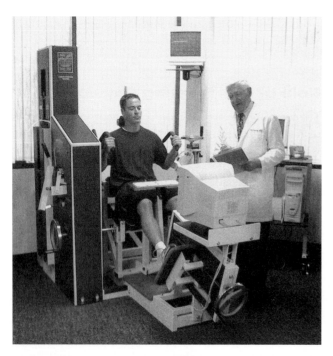

Figure 13.3 MedX Lumbar Extension Machine.

Of course many doctors interweave decisions as to how rapidly a person can resolve their back problem and how long they remain on disability with how soon they get to see the patient. A recent extensive study by McIntosh et al. has tried to clarify the predictive issues (34). In this study, 2,007 workers in Ontario were analyzed from onset of claim to 1 year after the accident. Prolonged disability and delay in return to work was found to be predicted by several factors. Three or more positive Waddell signs and pain referral to the leg were physical examination predictors. Older age groups and working in the construction industry were also predictors of prolonged disability. Interestingly, however, one of the most significant predictors was lag time from injury to treatment initiation. Even though it is recognized that many back problems are self-limiting, initiation of an active program certainly can place the patient into a framework of being able to control his pain. Along with the recurrence history, duration of current symptoms increases the fear that the problem will not resolve.

A recent study clearly documents the psychological barriers to an affective active treatment program (28). Marras et al. performed a fascinating study on normal subjects, which has significant implications concerning the respect of for psychological barriers necessary in evaluating the efficacy of an active exercise program in its potential to return workers to the workplace. In this particular study, students were being tested as to lifting performance under very specific evaluation conditions. Their muscle activity, spinal range, and speed were evaluated by specialized testing. Two tests were performed. The first test the students were encouraged and supported in their exercise. On the second round of tests, the students

Table 13.1 Treatment of Medical Back Problems

- A program of progressive exercise should be initiated after no more than 2 to 3 days of bed rest. Passive methods (either ice or hot packs) are only useful as an adjunct to exercise. Other techniques are not appropriate.
- An objective, reproducible functional assessment should occur if more than 2 weeks of treatment are required.
- Most patients need instruction on appropriate exercise but do not need a formal program of physical therapy. When physical therapy is indicated, duration should not exceed 6 weeks and frequency should not exceed three treatments weekly.
- Diagnostic radiographs are seldom appropriate initially and, with rare exceptions, are not appropriate at intervals during treatment.
- Unless neurologic function has deteriorated or progressive exercise has failed, specific diagnostic techniques (e.g., CT scan, magnetic resonance imaging, bone scan, EMG, nerve conduction studies) are not appropriate.
- More than 7% of employed patients with medical back problems return to work within 4 weeks of onset. Careful re-evaluation of the treatment plan is warranted if the patient has not progressed significantly in 4 weeks.
- If treatment lasts 6 weeks, the patient should be evaluated by an appropriate medical specialist. The evaluation should include objective measurement of functional status, reassessment of treatment goals, and confirmation of appropriateness of treatment.
- If the patient has not returned to work within 3 months, the patient should be referred to a specialized center for computerized reassessment and care planning.

were criticized and psychologically stressed. All the students were psychologically tested before the lifting tests. It turns out that those who on testing earlier were introverts showed significantly more co-activity of muscle function and thus had additional spinal loading compared to the extroverts who did not internalize the criticisms and lifted more efficiently. These findings may explain why people with psychological barriers, such as demonstrated with positive Waddell findings in the McIntosh study, have delay in returning to work.

Few treatment programs have expert psychologists and psychotherapists associated with them. Although certainly it would be an asset, that addition greatly increases the costs and certainly is not appropriate for every chronic and subacute patient. Generally, programs that have a comprehensive physical, as well as psychological, approach to management of chronic musculoskeletal problems are known as tertiary care centers. They may have an inpatient component to create an environment that is conducive to controlling psychological factors.

The simpler alternative for treating individuals with fear, anxiety, and insecurity is the recognition that providing objective unbiased feedback of performance is an asset to treating their anxiety. Thus, treatment programs that use specific equipment, which can measure performance such as resistance training, offer a concrete maneuver to assist patients in recognizing that they can take control of their chronic pain problems. This equipment at least will provide feedback baselines in terms of range of motion, amount of resistance being used, and number of repetitions. By scoring performance on each occasion, the individual can document their progress without any extraneous factors. In addition, with the use of equipment that isolates various muscle groups and joints, the extraneous muscle activity, again noticed in the Marras study, can be blocked out to allow more efficient effective exercise programs. This can document progress in a measurable manner.

Thus, the treating physician has the responsibility to keep focused on objective measures of improving performance and the rate of improvement. If the treatment program plateaus, then some change has to occur. Here the individual is ranked as having reached maximum medical improvement or another strategy has to be initiated. This strategy might be injection procedures, consideration of surgical intervention, or a complete change in format for the treatment program.

Although the treating physician generally does not control the physical treatment program being performed by physical therapists and exercise science people, he/she must expect these treatment programs to offer sufficient information on which to make a judgment as to progress or alternative strategies. The report must be crisp and offer sufficient information on which to make judgments. It should give information that would assist the treating physician or the evaluating physician criteria on which to make judgments in terms of function. It also should include total number of visits, the type of treatment, and the subjective and objective findings. Finally, a brief note as to assessment and future plans should be available. An example of such a report is in Figure 13.4.

A recent study clearly documents the role of objective testing in modifying physical therapy practice (9). This study notes the change in physical therapy practice after the State Labor Commission in Utah requested a report from therapists before more treatment would be authorized. After every six visits, a report identifying changes in at least three essential physical functions, such as lifting, carrying, range of motion, sitting tolerance, etc., was requested. If no improvement is noted, restorative services will not be continued to be authorized. There were approximately 30,000 claims in 1997 and approximately 33,000 claims in 1999 after the initiation of the new report form. Associated with the institution of this form, the frequency of treatments decreased 34% from 17 in 1997 to 11.4 in 1999. Hot pack usage decreased 45%, electrical stimulation decreased 22%, and massage decreased 38%. However, therapeutic

Spine & Sport™
Functional Capacity Evaluation
Summary Page

Patient: John Doe   Date: 05/01/01

The information contained in this report is intended to be used in conjunction with the physician's assessment of the patient when determining return to work status. Please call if you have any questions or need additional information regarding the Functional Capacity Test.

Subjective Complaints	Usual pain severity: slight / Worst pain severity: severe Usual pain frequency: constant / Worst pain frequency: intermittent
Perceived Ability	Medium
Waddell's	2/5
Cardiovascular Rating	Excellent
Reliability	Reliable global effort
Objective PDC	Medium Work
Functional Occupation Duty Simulation	Restricted to Unable
% Loss of Lift Capacity	-37%

*Note: The % Loss of Lift Capacity, Disability Category determinations, and Work Restrictions outlined in this report are based entirely on FCE objective measurements and do not take into consideration subjective factors of disability, other factors of disability or the primary treating physician's clinical opinions.

Please refer to narrative report pages 1 to 7 for complete explanation and details of the Functional Capacity Test.

Figure 13.4 Report form.

exercise increased 31% and joint mobilization increased 27%. The carriers' cost-savings were approximately $1.1 million per year. No attempt from the State Labor Commission was made to control physical therapy practice, just the request that objective measures be incorporated in their report form. More efficient treatment was encouraged by focus on functional measurement.

One final responsibility of the treating physician is to define the return to work status. Certainly the sooner the person returns to work, the more likely a successful completion of the health care process can be expected. The probability of return to work decreases as length of time off increases (45). One strategy to return the worker to work sooner is to return them to modified duty. Trying to make a judgment regarding whether the worker can perform full duty or modified duty is difficult. It must be recognized that a correlation does not always exist between the patient's ability to accomplish physical activities and the pain (42).

Moreover, there is no conclusive evidence that early return to work causes additional harm to the back. In fact, the patients absorbed in work gain considerable periods of pain relief (49). Also, if a treating physician does not focus on return to work, the patient's view of himself begins to become one of dependency and incapability (7). Disabilities are considered to be a learning behavior; thus, the shorter time the individuals have to learn, the less that they might become disabled (10).

The problem still remains concerning modified work versus regular work. Hall et al. performed a study that did focus on that problem (17). In this study, 1,438 consecutive workers with back pain and undergoing treatment were in the study group. In the control group, after an active treatment program, patients were returned to work according to the estimate of their pain. Modified work is recommended when the patients had pain symptoms. In the experimental group, pain was not allowed to be a restriction to regular work. The persistence of pain in the absence of any objective findings was not judged as an acceptable reason for suggesting a limited return. Only objective findings such as nerve root irritation, sciatic scoliosis, and objective reduction in range of motion below job requirements, were recognized as a cause for restriction. In follow-up, a significantly larger number of patients returning to unrestricted work in the experimental group compared to the control group of usual care. The probability of successful outcome decreased with age in the study group. Other studies have shown that age is an additional deterrent to rapid return to work. The study, however, did demonstrate the problem of using pain alone as the definition of work status. It demon-

strated also that the expectation of normal activity was a positive ingredient in returning the individual to non-restricted work.

Thus, in summary, the treating physician has the responsibility to initiate rational treatment as soon as possible. He has the responsibility to expect feedback of progress from the treatment program to which he has referred the patient. He must continually focus on return to normal activity as the expectation for the soft tissue injury. Psychological support with feedback of progress is a reasonable "carrot" for the anxious patient.

Role of the Evaluating Physician

The evaluating physician and the treating physician may on occasion be the same. However, in many jurisdictions, especially when litigation is involved, the treating physician is thought to be biased. After all, that clinician is receiving compensation for the care of the patient and continuing requests for treatment can be interpreted as self-serving. Also, of necessity, that physician has sought to achieve good communication with the patient and, therefore, has never acted in an adversarial manner. Obviously, the testing physician would be a patient advocate and may be willing to overlook significant history or symptom magnification.

The Independent Medical Evaluator specifically is restrained from performing medical treatment. In the report, it is more important to refer to the individual being examined as the examinee or the applicant, rather than the patient. Usually the report is quite a bit more detailed and expansive than a typical report from the treating physician, even on the occasion of declaration of maximum medical benefit (or P&S in California terms). The job skills of the Independent Medical Evaluator (IME) have been outlined by the American Board of Independent Medical Examiners (ABIME) (40). Often the IMEs are performed to provide information for case management and for evidence in hearings and other legal proceedings (6). They are common components of all workers' compensation statues, but they may vary from state to state (47).

In that the evaluation is often being performed for disability, a thorough description of the patient's past and current job with its physical demands is necessary. A significant amount of social history is necessary to offer some insight into psychophysiologic problems. A review of medical records is also quite necessary. The treating physician seldom takes into account the past medical records in that they usually do not assist in the current treatment plan. However, the evaluating physician is assembling data on which to make a definitive statement regarding diagnosis and prognosis. All past medical information, therefore, is valuable. In addition to the usual physical examination, ideally a functional capacity test is performed.

It must be recognized that especially in the spine, the physical examination is seldom helpful in clarifying impairment and disability. The only functional examination advocated in the AMA Guidelines (14) is a test for range of motion. The accuracy of this test is often questioned. Recently, a far more accurate range test using Optoelectric Motion Analysis System performed by the same technician (far more accurate than the inclinometer method advocated in the JAMA Guidelines) was not predictive. This test, when applied to 111 patients with work-related back pain, at the beginning and conclusion of treatment, was not predictive of the disability at follow-up (41). Obviously, if objective evaluation of function is necessary, a far more comprehensive system needs to be developed.

The evaluating physician ultimately has to identify the impairment with associated causation issues. The evaluator also has to identify the functional deficits, especially as related to job, and identify whether alternative work is possible and if vocational health care is necessary. In most jurisdictions, the clinician is paid more for this type of evaluation than is the treating physician who is expected to present similar information. Thus, the specialty of evaluating physicians has grown. Up to this point, however, the specialty has not placed emphasizes on standardized functional testing but rather prefers to rely more on history and typical physical examination.

This is a significant problem. In a study from Washington, they found that only 5% of their compensation claims were from individuals with non-verifiable muscle and back symptoms (46). Unfortunately, these accounted for 84% of the cost. There certainly is a place for objective functional capacity evaluation.

Functional Capacity Evaluation

Information from functional capacity evaluation (FCE) has been used in the return to work decision-making process for persons with medical impairment for many years (19,31). FCE information is used to translate the effect of the impairment in terms of ability to perform work tasks. FCE is a "detailed examination and evaluation that objectively measures the client's current level of function in terms of the demands of competitive employment" (1). In this context, the primary purpose of the FCE is to compare a client's safe functional abilities to the demands of work (1 [page 47]) to facilitate the return-to-work decision (18,19).

One example of a standardized functional capacity evaluation that is designed to be time-efficient is the "California Functional Capacity Protocol" (Cal-FCP) (37). The Cal-FCP is a 120-minute, 11-part test of functional capacity designed to develop an estimate of lost work capacity to be used in a case-management process and to address disability rating. The Cal FCP allows measurement of the injured worker's work capacity by the treating physician or by other health care practitioners. It is administered 30 days after the injury if the injured worker either has not returned to work or continues in active treatment. Frequently, because of its low cost, it is administered on a serial basis, every 3 weeks, to measure response to treatment. This pattern of use addresses a concern of the treating physician to maintain case control. Additionally, the involvement of the treating physician to interpret the results of the Cal-FCP recognizes that he or she is the best professional to consider the test results in light of issues such as the injured worker's motivation, fears, and goals, and to integrate other medical findings. The information derived from the Cal-FCP is presented to the treating physician as a recommendation, along with all of the data collected during the examination.

Once the Cal-FCP test protocol was developed, training of experienced health care clinicians was undertaken at five centers in various parts of California. A demonstration project was designed to evaluate the feasibility of implementation of the protocol across a broad spectrum (33). The duration of the Cal-FCP protocol in hands other than its developers, the internal consistency of the protocol, and its usefulness in measurement of work capacity were addressed. Sixty-four subjects (32 females and 32 males) were studied. Subjects in the study included adults who were undergoing treatment for work-related soft tissue musculoskeletal injuries as part of the California workers' compensation program. Lumbar spine patients predominated (n=46), with knee (n=5) and cervical patients (n=4) also represented. The remaining subjects had a variety of soft tissue injuries. Subjects reported onset of symptoms 1 month to 10 years before program entry, with a mean (SD) of 1.82 (2.1) years. Only two of the subjects were tested within 30 days of injury onset, whereas 23 subjects were tested within 1 year of injury. The Cal-FCP test battery was administered by exercise physiologists, a registered nurse, physical therapists, and occupational therapists who had participated in a special 2-day training program that included a knowledge test and required demonstration of reliability on the EPIC lift capacity test (ELC) (Fig. 13.5) (32). This study 33 found no new injuries or exacerbation of current impairment. The mean duration of test administration was 84 minutes. This sample demonstrated a mean loss of lift capacity of

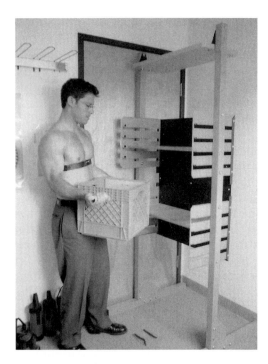

Figure 13.5 EPIC lifting capacity.

41%, with no significant difference between men and women. Seven of the subjects (four men and three women) had no loss of lift capacity. An additional 11 subjects (six men and five women) had a loss of lift capacity that was less than 25%, which is interpreted by the California disability determination model as indicating no residual disability. Thus, 18 of the subjects were found to not qualify for disability benefits! Because of the protection of human subjects' rights guidelines under which the study was conducted, this information was not revealed to their employers or insurance carriers or physicians. Twelve of the 64 subjects had effort ratings by the evaluator that were less than full effort. There were no significant differences between groups based on age, time since injury, duration of testing, pinch, or grip. Significant differences were found between the full effort and less than full effort groups for Spinal Function Sort (29) score and loss of lift capacity. Interestingly, SFS score predicted absolute lift capacity and capacity considered as a percent of body weight on ELC test 3. The SFS score also predicted lost work capacity. This study demonstrated the usefulness of the Cal-FCP in evaluating injured workers. There are several other functional capacity evaluation protocols that are useful (5,20,23,26).

■ CONCLUSION

Employment selection and placement is an important service area for health care professionals and is becoming increasingly complex. This chapter has described the historical background of employment screening from a health care perspective, beginning with the use of spinal x-rays to screen for risk of injury. As we have noted, medical examination is less useful and justified for employee selection than it is for baseline comparisons. The use of technologies such as spinal MRI procedures may provide a basis for avoiding expensive and needless surgery when a problem such as an asymptomatic degenerative spine is found to be present before employment. The use of functional capacity evaluation is more often justified, both to identify applicants for employment who will be the most productive workers and to assist the physician and plant manager to properly place a worker returning from sick leave. Although these methods are promising, peer-reviewed studies are needed to provide scientific justification. In the interim, individually conducted validation studies that focus of the use of FCE to select workers based on productivity will suffice, although the expense of such studies is likely to limit their use to large companies with expensive self-insured workers' compensation systems.

Audit Process
Self-Check of the Chapter's Learning Objectives

- What are the criteria for assessing the validity of pre-employment and pre-placement screening procedures?

- Can you describe what the fitness for duty evaluation is?

- Explain the American and Disabilities Act restrictions and protections.

- Define the roles of the treating physician versus the evaluating physician.

- What tests are involved in the Functional Capacity Evaluation presented in this chapter and what is its relevance to job capacity?

- What are realistic expectations for reporting on the delivery of conservative care approaches for managing spinal problems?

■ REFERENCES

1. APTA. Occupational health guidelines: Evaluating functional capacity. Alexandria, VA: American Physical Therapy Association, 1997.
2. Bailey W. Observation on the etiology and frequency of spondylolisthesis and its precursors. Radiology 1947;48:107–112.

3. Battie MC, Bigos SJ, Fischer LD, et al. Isometric lifting strength as a predictor of industrial back pain reports. Spine 1989;14:851–856.

4. Biering-Sorensen F, Thomsen CE, Hilden J. Risk indicators for low back trouble. Scand J Rehabil Med 1989;23:151–157.

5. Blankenship K. The Blankenship system functional capacity evaluation procedure manual. Macon, GA: The Blankenship Corporation, 1994.

6. Brigham CR, Babitsky S, Mangraviti JJ. The Independent Medical Evaluation Report: A Step-by-Step Guide with Models. Falmouth, MA: SEAK, Inc, 1996.

7. Catchlove R, Cohen K. Effects of a directive return to work approach in the treatment of workman's compensation patients with chronic pain. Pain 1982;14:181–191.

8. Chaffin DB, Park KYS. A longitudinal study of low-back pain as associated with occupational weight lifting factors. Am Ind Hyg Assoc J 1973;34:513–525.

9. Colledge AL, Hunter SJ. Using functional improvements to promote active therapy and determine the length of treatment of workers' compensation patients, a 3-year analyzes of 63,000 claims. J Occup Med (Submitted).

10. Derebery VJ, Tullis WH. Delayed recovery in the patient with a work compensable injury. J Occup Med 1983;25:829–835.

11. Driesinger TE. Does prevention work. San Diego, CA: San Diego Comprehensive Care Symposium, July 2000.

12. EEOC. Uniform guidelines on employee selection procedures (1978). Federal Register 1993;July 1:212–239.

13. Gibson ES, Martin RH, Terry CW. Incidence of low back pain and pre-placement x-ray screening. J Occup Environ Med 1980;22:515–519.

14. The Guides to the Evaluation of Permanent Impairment, 4th ed. Chicago, IL: American Medical Association, 1993.

15. Guiding principles for medical examinations in industry. Chicago, IL: American Medical Association, 1984:1.

16. Hainer BL. Pre-placement evaluations [review]. Prim Care Clin Office Pract 1994;23:237–247.

17. Hall H, McIntosh G, Melles T, Holowachuk B, Wai E. Effect of discharge recommendations on outcome. Spine 1994;19(18):2033–2037.

18. Hart D, Berlin S, Brager P, et al. Standards for performing functional capacity evaluations, work conditioning and work hardening programs state of Maryland. Annapolis, MD: Joint Committee on Industrial Services, 1993.

19. Hart D, Iserhagen S, Matheson L. Guidelines for functional capacity evaluation of people with medical conditions. J Orthop Sports Phys Ther 1993;18(6):682–686.

20. Isernhagen SJ. Functional capacity evaluation. In: Isernhagen SJ, ed. Work injury: Management and prevention. Rockville, MD: Aspen, 1988.

21. Jay M, Lamb J, Watson R, et al. Sensitivity and specificity of the indicators of sincere effort of the EPIC Lift Capacity test on a previously injured population. Spine 2000;25(11):1405–1412.

22. Johns RE, Bloswick DS, Elegante JM, Colledge AL. Chronic, recurrent low back pain: A methodology for analyzing fitness for duty and managing risk under the Americans with Disabilities Act. 1994;36(5):537–547.

23. Key G. Key functional assessment procedures manual. Minneapolis, MN: Key Functional Assessment, Inc, 1986.

24. Keyserling WM, Herrin GD, Chaffin DB. Isometric strength testing as a means of controlling medical incidents on strenuous jobs. J Occup Med 1980;22:332–336.

25. Lawrence JS. Disc degeneration: Its frequency and relationship to symptoms. Ann Rheum Dis 1969;28:123–127.

26. Lechner D, Jackson J, Roth D, Straaton K. Reliability and validity of a newly developed test of physical work performance. J Occup Med 1994;36(9):997–1004.

27. Lloyd DCEF, Troup JDG. Recurrent back pain and its prediction. J Soc Occup Med 1983;33:66–74.

28. Marras WS, Davis KG, Heaney CA, Maronitis AB, Allread GW. The influence of psychosocial stress, gender, and personality on mechanical loading of the lumbar spine. Spine 2000;25(23):3045–3054.

29. Matheson L. Development of a measure of perceived functional ability. J Occup Rehabil 1993;3(1):15–30.

30. Matheson L. EPIC Lift Capacity Test Examiner's Manual. Fort Bragg, CA: Work Evaluation Systems Technology, 1994.

31. Matheson L, Ogden L. Work tolerance screening. Trabuco Canyon, CA: Rehabilitation Institute of Southern California, 1983.

32. Matheson L, Mooney V, Grant J, et al. A test to measure lift capacity of physically impaired adults (part 1): Development and reliability testing. Spine 1995;20(19):2119–2129.

33. Matheson LN, Mooney V, Grant JE, Leggett S, Kenny K. Standardized evaluation of work capacity. J Back Musculoskel Rehabil 1996;6:249–264.

34. McIntosh G, Frank J, Hogg-Johnson S, Bombardier C, Hall H. 1999 Young investigator research award winner: Prognostic factors for time receiving workers' compensation benefits in a cohort of patients with low back pain. Spine 2000;25(2):147–157.

35. Mooney V, Kenney D, Leggett S, Holmes B. Relationship of lumbar strength in shipyard workers to workplace injury claims. Spine 1996;23(17):2001–2005.

36. Mooney V, Kron M, Rummerfield P, Holmes B. The effect of workplace based strengthening on low back injury rates: A case study in the strip mining industry. J Occ Rehab 1995;5(3):157–167.

37. Mooney V, Matheson L. California Functional Capacity Protocol (Cal-FCP) Examiner's Manual. San Diego, CA: OrthoMed Foundation, 1994.

38. Pedersen PA. Prognostic indicators in low back pain. J R Coll Gen Pract 1981;31:209–236.

39. Personal communication. Dr. Lester Sachs, Medical Director.

40. Peterson KW, et al. The American Board of Independent Medical Examiners. J Occup Environ Med 1997;39(6):509–514.

41. Poitras S, Loisel P, Prince F, Lemaire J. Disability measurement in persons with back pain: A validity study of spinal range of motion and velocity. Arch Phys Med Rehabil 2000;81:1394–1400.

42. Rainville J, Ahern DK, Phalen L, Childs LA, Sutherland R. The association of pain with physical activities in chronic low back pain. Spine 1992;17:1060–1064.

43. Redfield JT. The low back x-ray as a pre-employment screening tool in the forest products industry. J Occup Environ Med 1971;13:239–226.

44. Reimer DS, Halbrook BD, Dreyfuss PH, Tibiletti C. A novel approach to pre-employment worker fitness evaluations in a material-handling industry. Spine 1994;19:2026–2032.

45. Spitzer WO, LeBlanc FE, Dupuis M. Scientific approach to the assessment and management of activity-related spinal disorders. Spine 1987; 12(suppl):S1–S59.

46. State of Washington Department of Labor and Industries. Attending Doctor's Handbook. 1996:4.

47. Tompkins N. Independent medical examination: The how, when and why of this useful process. OSHA Compliance Advisor. 1992;235:7–12.

48. Walton M. The Demming Management Method. New York: Putnam, 1986.

49. Wynn Parry CB. Pain in avulsion lesions of the brachial plexus. Pain 1980;9:41–53.

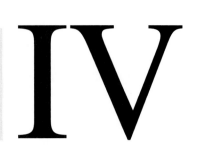
Acute Care Management (first 4 weeks)

Editor's Note

While acute patients recover quickly with minimal or no care, the minority who become chronic are notoriously difficult to treat. Therefore, modern approaches attempt to prevent chronicity BEFORE it is established without over-treating the majority of acutes who would get better on their own. Therefore, the current "state of the art" in spine care is to encourage early patient reactivation. This is both a cognitive–behavioral and physical approach. This involves reassuring patients that they are not injured or damaged, providing them with simple pain relieving modalities, and focusing them on the safety and value of gradual reactivation and self-management.

This section introduces a model that begins from the patient's mind and emotions. The clinician should make a concerted effort to educate the patient that their back problem is more of an illness like a cold than an actual disease process. Then a gradual re-activation process guided by symptoms as in the McKenzie model is commenced. The patient's first steps in returning to activities includes simple spine sparing activity modifications. No model of acute spine care would be complete without the sure anchor of manipulative therapy. Its role in pain relief and functional reactivation is far from controversial. Not only joint manipulation but also soft tissue, muscle, and nerve mobilizations are all integrated into the conservative care of patients in this section. However, as with all passive modalities these should be offered in a time-limited manner as adjuncts to self-management.

14

Active Self-Care: Functional Reactivation for Spine Pain Patients

Craig Liebenson

Learning Objectives

After reading this chapter you should be able to:

- Understand the value of self-care in managing spinal conditions.
- Understand the behavioral psychology underpinning motivating patients to change their lifestyle.
- Identify faulty biomechanics during activities of daily living.
- Understand the difference between a biomedical and biopsychosocial report of findings.

Introduction

Activity is effective therapy for a large variety of health care conditions (e.g., heart disease, arthritis, low back pain, osteoporosis, depression, etc.) (19,36, 40,84,178). Physical inactivity is an independent risk factor for cardiovascular and other diseases (124). When patients are in pain, they typically worry that they will cause more harm than good if they are active (171). Physicians typically prescribe overly restrictive activity restrictions, which are responsible for interfering with the recovery process and promoting chronic pain behaviors (26,27,80,114). Frequently, advice to "let pain be your guide" is given, which only reinforces attitudes and beliefs that foster pain–avoidance behavior and deconditioning (83).

In contrast, the idea that "hurt doesn't necessarily equal harm" and that rest is bad for tissues has not received as much attention. Such reactivation advice has been shown to be more effective than traditional, more passive advice for low back pain (LBP) (26,27,83,114) and for neck pain (23,120,143). Active self-management coping styles have been shown to be superior to passive coping styles for back and neck pain as well as other chronic pains (20,35). A stepped-care approach involving incrementally more structured and comprehensive patient education is required to influence a patient's belief systems and concerns about activity. The clinician's goal is to modify the patient's health behavior in the direct of reactivation.

Back pain has traditionally been viewed as primarily an acute, self-limiting condition. However, it is now recognized to involve frequent recurrences or even a chronic course (44). Biomedicine is better suited for acute than chronic conditions. Research has emphasized the value of self-management skills for management of chronic illnesses (20,78,79,112, 125,152). This involves such things as exercise, minimization of activities of daily living limitations, monitoring of illness, and managing flare-ups. Holman and Lorig (28,79,111,112) found that a self-management approach decreased pain and reduced the use of medical services by 43%. Self-care has also been recommended for both acute and chronic low back pain (127,154).

Unfortunately, most management approaches for back problems are concerned only with diagnostic triage and pain management. Borkan called for research on whether "educating and empowering patients to treat their own problems would counteract the negative impact that medicalization of the problem has had on individuals and society" (25). Today, a swell of research validates that such pre-emptive patient education is effective for low back pain (26,27,83,114).

Turner points out that interventions encouraging resumption of normal activities have been more successful than those that only taught improved body mechanics and lifting techniques (e.g., traditional back school) (163). Von Korff has reported that an intervention that addressed patient worries about back pain, enhanced self-care confidence, and encouraged an active problem-solving approach was successful in reducing activity limitations (173). Whereas pain-relief modalities will always be in vogue, patient education about self-care through gradual reactivation is rapidly gaining scientific traction as the standard of care for prevention of disability associated with LBP.

Fear–Avoidance Beliefs and Chronic Disabling Pain

Patients who are at the greatest risk for chronic, disabling pain often have poorly developed coping skills (94). They may tend to catastrophize their illness and feel powerless to help themselves. When patients fear pain, or catastrophize by fearing the worst possible outcome, they are less likely to resume activity or perform exercise (167). It is easy for them to become dependent on short-term symptom-relieving approaches such as manipulation, massage, medication, and various physical therapy modalities. A key to getting a patient to become active in their own self-care program is to shift them from being a pain avoider to a pain manager (100,102, 141,162).

Fear–avoidance behavior leads to deconditioning. Two-thirds of acute LBP patients believe that a wrong movement will cause serious harm (123,173). An individual who perceives that an activity will be painful will have a reduced physical capacity (98). In fact, the cognitive association of activity with pain or anticipation of pain has been shown to be more predictive of physical performance than purely nociceptive factors (4). Council asked patients to anticipate how much pain they would expect to have when performing 10 simple tasks (42). Substantial correlations between expectancies and performance were found. Crombez used a standard exercise task and found that injury expectancies explained 16% of the variance in work disability in chronic patients and 33% in acute subjects (45).

Heuts et al. reported that patients' pain intensity and pain-related fear accounted for 40% of the variance in functional limitations (75). Two aspects of pain-related fear were most relevant—activity avoidance—"the belief that activity may result in (re)injury or increased pain," and somatic focus—the belief in an underlying somatic medical problem. Flynn et al. also found that fear–avoidance beliefs predict return to work in patients with acute LBP (51). The risk of prolonged work restriction increased from 29% to 58% with a score more than 34 on the Fear–Avoidance Beliefs Questionnaire. For a score of less than 30, the risk of prolonged work restriction decreased from 29% to 3%.

Equating hurt with harm is a disabling form of thinking for a back pain patient (113,166,167). It promotes deconditioning and thus leads to less stability. It is important to identify the patient who is fearful and to avoid encouraging them to take on a "sick role." According to Troup, "If fear of pain persists, unless it is specifically recognized and treated, it leads inexorably to pain–avoidance and thence to disuse" (162).

The goal with the fearful patient is to increase confidence in normal activities and/or exercises (51,96). Certain activities should be avoided, such as early morning flexion (153). But other activities such as brisk walking and McKenzie centralization maneuvers or gradual stabilization training are safe and effective (54,77,83,110,157). In chronic patients, the target of treatment may be the stiffness and atrophy caused by the patient overprotecting himself or herself during the acute phase. Muscles and joints, which lose their mobility while the patient restricts their activities during acute pain, should be expected to cause discomfort and re-mobilizing them may hurt but certainly won't harm. It is useful to reassure patients by explaining that their pain is caused by dysfunction, not tissue damage or pathology (i.e., herniated disc or arthritis) (22,178).

Alongside the individual's attitude toward pain (e.g., catastrophizing), external influences such as the transmission of beliefs by the health care provider are crucial (138). Sullivan has shown that if pain is viewed as a sign of danger, it is perceived as more intense (161). Ostelo developed a screening questionnaire for clinicians to determine their orientation (biomedical versus biopsychosocial) (135). The biomedical orientation is in line with persistent back pain myths, which Deyo has unmasked (48). These include the need for an accurate diagnosis of the structural cause of pain, the need to rest until pain is gone, and the belief that back pain leads to chronic disability. Houben et al. recently used this screening tool and found that clinician orientation predicts both the clinicians harmfulness ratings of physical activities and their recommendations for physical activity that they give their patients (80,170).

Step 1: Reassurance and Reactivation Advice

What: Brief educational approaches including advice to gradually increase activity from a cognitive–behavioral (CB) perspective.

Who: Patients in the acute phase of a painful episode.

It has been shown how valuable appropriate patient advice can be (30). In particular, when that advice is given in a biopsychosocial context, which reduces pain-related anxiety and encourages patients to gradually resume normal activities (56,95,101,103,114). Such advice focuses on the consequences of pain—such as activity limitations, rather than the pain itself.

There are six fundamental things that patients want reassurance about that should be addressed in the initial report of findings (ROF) (Table 14.1).

Identify Back-Related Worries and Fears As Well As the Patient's Goals

Back-related worries and fears are perhaps the most important thing to identify in acute patients. Patients typically worry how long their pain may persist and what its impact will be on their activities. Most patients recover, but those with significant worries require a unique approach to prevent disabling disuse atrophy. According to Balderson and Von Korff (13), simple, brief educational approaches are needed to address fear–avoidance beliefs and assure resumption of normal activities:

- Identify and address patient worries and support self-care (123,173)

Table 14.1 Six Key Points in the Initial Report of Findings

---

1. What are the patient's concerns/goals? Identify back-related worries and fears
2. Is it serious? Assurance that there is no serious disease.
3. What is the cause? Injuries and degenerative processes can precipitate pain, but pain persists because of controllable factors.
4. What should the patient avoid and what should they do? Specific activity modification and reactivation advice.
5. What can make the patient more comfortable? Pain relief options.
6. How long will it last? Recovery expectations.

- Two-thirds of patients have concerns that a wrong movement might cause a serious problem
- Half believe avoiding certain movements is the safest way to prevent LBP from getting worse
- To solicit patient worries, ask open-ended questions about the pain or activity concerns
- Explore these so you have a better understanding of your patient's concerns and motivations for avoidance behavior
- Then patient is evaluated for common concerns
- Then patient is given relevant information, individualized to the unique needs
- Further discussion is encouraged to promote understanding and integration into the patient's personal belief system.
- Patient is given written information to take home—this can be shared with family members

Goal Setting

According to Bandura, health promotion should begin with goals, not means. Goal setting should be mutual and related to activities deemed important to the patient (15). It works best when patient is in pain and the goal is to reduce pain (62,148,149). According to a study by Turner et al, patients seeking care for back pain apparently have two major goals: to receive information about how to manage their symptoms and to receive advice about how to resume normal activities (163). The primary goal in pain management is to reduce any pain-related disability the patient has (18,179,180). In the AHCPR guidelines, it was stated that "the main goal for treatment of back pain has shifted from treatment of pain to treatment of activity intolerances related to pain" (18). In acute LBP disorders in which an exact cause of symptoms can only be identified 15% of the time, the patient's participation in the treatment program is absolutely essential (176,178). Specific activity modification advice aimed at reducing exposure to repetitive strain is one aspect of patient education (18,43,116,155,158).

Assurance That There Is No Serious Disease—Doesn't Severe Pain Signify Serious Damage?

A powerful myth in modern back pain culture is that structural pathology is responsible for pain. Cartesian thinking promoted the view that the pain one experiences is directly related to tissue damage or injury. However, Melzack and Wall's gate control theory of pain led to the discovery that there are descending influences on the nociceptive pathways that directly influence pain perception (121,140). Pain not only is the result of ascending nociception but also is a result of a dynamic process of perception whereby some painful stimuli are interpreted as potentially harmful and some are not. The Cartesian approach can be summed up in the adage "let pain be your guide." This is now considered to be responsible for promoting unnecessary fear and functional limitations.

Most patients who have chronic back pain or are experiencing a stubborn acute episode have had some imaging of their spine. They usually come into our offices with their films and courageously bear their label of having a serious problem such as a herniated disc, spinal stenosis, or degenerative arthritis (22). They have found the cause of their pain and now they want us to "fix" them.

What they have usually not been told is that such structural pathology is present in an unusually large percentage of asymptomatic individuals (Fig. 14.1) (34). Also, it does not even predict future problems when found in younger people (24). Therefore, it may be a coincidental finding. Whereas it is bad news that the cause of pain may still be a mystery, the good news is that surgery is likely NOT indicated and the long-term disabling potential of their condition is significantly lessened.

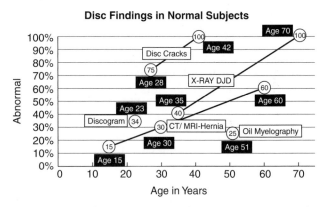

Figure 14.1 False-positive rates for disc herniation with various imaging modalities. Imaging findings of disc abnormalities increase in frequency with age in patients without symptoms. (CT, computed tomography; DJD, degenerative joint disease; MRI, magnetic resonance imaging.) From Bigos S, Müller G. Primary care approach to acute and chronic back problems: definitions and care. In: Loeser JD, ed. Bonica's Management of Pain, third edition. Philadelphia: Lippincott, Williams & Wilkins, 2001.

If Pain Is Not Caused by Serious Disease, Then What Is Causing My Pain? (Doesn't Severe Pain Signify Serious Damage?)

Most patients are reassured when told that structural pathology is more related to age—like graying hair or wrinkling skin—than to symptoms, or that people with pristine spines often have symptoms whereas some with horrible spines are pain-free! It is helpful to reassure them that the difference between people whose structural pathology is causing symptoms and those in whom it is not has to do with their ability to adapt to the changes, and this ability can be trained. Therefore, instead of the negative message that they need to either learn to live with their problem by compromising their lifestyle or resort to surgery, patients learn that there are things that they can do to control the symptoms by modifying their activities and training improved fitness.

All patients want to know the cause of their pain. Fortunately, serious problems are easy to identify. Tumors and infections are extremely rare, and nerve root disorders occur less than 10% of the time (see Chapter 7). Although most problems are not as serious, it is not always possible to pin-point an exact cause of the pain. However, we can conclude that the problem is a simple, uncomplicated mechanical one and reassure them that we do know what factors prolong pain (e.g., distress, deconditioning) and what treatments help resolve the problem.

Most patients are overly concerned with doing the wrong thing or doing too much. However, too little motion is just as deleterious as too much (119)! One of the only factors that has been shown to predict future back problems is reduced endurance of the back muscles (17). One of the most potent predictors of recurrent back problems is atrophy of those same muscles that occurs when an acute episode strikes (77). Studies have shown that those who train the back muscles with gentle exercises actually reduced the likelihood of such recurrences (77).

Similarly, neck pain patients after a whiplash or those with chronic headache have both been found to have a weakness of their deep anterior neck muscles (90). When these muscles are trained, improvement ensues (91,92).

The most common cause for persistent pain is when external load repeatedly exceeds physical capacity or tolerance (Fig. 14.2). This is typically caused by deconditioning or lack of fitness, NOT injury or structural pathology. Educating patients about the role and value of fitness for prevention or treatment of chronic symptoms is very simple. Evidence clearly shows the strong relationship between dysfunction and pain (see Chapter 1). The same cannot be said for a relationship between most pathology and pain (see Chapter 4).

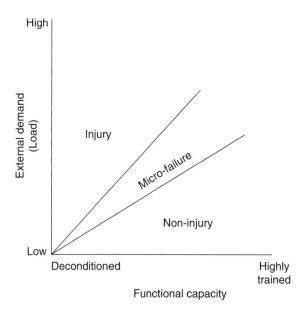

Figure 14.2 Relationship between external demand and functional capacity.

Specific Reactivation Advice— "What Should and Shouldn't I Do?"

Specific activity modification and reactivation advice is one of the most important aspects of patient education. As Karel Lewit says, "the first advice is to teach the patient how to avoid what harms him." Rest is not best, nor is prolonged sitting, or improper bending, lifting, and twisting (BLT), especially first thing in the morning. Simple ergonomic advice or spine sparing strategies are at least as important in spine care as palliative or stabilizing measures.

Reactivation should be gradual. Pain is not a good guide because appropriate activities may be uncomfortable. Allowing pain to be a guide leads to activity avoidance and deconditioning. "No pain no gain" is also inappropriate and will lead to overstrain. Many patients who have trouble recovering either avoid activity entirely or jump back in too aggressively leading to a "boom or bust" cycle (31).

Whereas some people catastrophize pain and avoid activities, others with positive moods may try to ignore pain and overexert (71). People use different "stop rules" with activities. The "as many as can" (AMAC) leads to persistence until the task is completed (171). The "feel like discontinuing" (FLD) leads to termination when the task is not enjoyable. Negative mood has different effects depending on a person's stop rules. If AMAC then negative mood leads to continuation, if FLD then negative mood leads to stopping.

Instead of AMAC or FLD, the preferred approach incorporates pacing (68,105). This is a "quota-based" or "graded exposure" approach (68,69,105). Quota-based consists of the patient's activity levels being gradually increased in a step-wise manner limited by quota, not pain. Graded exposures consists of the patient gradually encountering feared stimuli in a supervised setting involving safe, low-load maneuvers. The goal of these methods is to enhance the patient's confidence or self-efficacy.

Reactivation advice is designed to assure patients of the safety and value of activity. Emphasizing the benefits of nourishing tissues through movement and the dangers of deconditioning are emphasized. Specific topics discussed include:

a. Benefits and risks of rest versus activity

b. Micro-breaks and ergonomic workstation advice

c. Morning tasks and household chores

d. Lifting

e. Safety and benefits of general light activity such as walking or swimming

Rest Versus Activity

Deyo performed a controlled clinical trial that compared 2 days of bed rest against 2 weeks. Two days of bed rest was found to be as effective as 2 weeks while limiting the negative effects of prolonged immobilization (47). A Cochrane Collaboration review concluded that bed rest (65):

• Has no positive effect for LBP

• May have slightly harmful effects

• Yields no improvement with 7 days compared with 2 to 3 days in LBP or sciatica

A day or two of bed rest may be appropriate for acute low back pain. But it is important to reinforce that the rest is because of the pain not for the pain (1). The patient is resting because the pain is so severe that they cannot do anything, but rest will only stiffen and weaken them and as soon as possible they should start gentle movements (Fig. 14.3).

Patients are informed that prolonged rest reduces blood supply and thus slows healing and recovery. The health care provider's (HCP) role is therefore to assure patients that early, gradual reactivation is both safe and effective and to instruct the patient in how to accomplish this. Additionally, a very "hot" low back may require a stronger pain-management approach guided by patient preferences (manipulation, modalities, medication) to enable the patient to resume near-normal activities sooner.

If one does rest for severe, acute low back pain, resting in a semi-traction position is often pain-relieving (Fig. 14.4).

Micro-Breaks and Ergonomic Workstation Advice

When one thinks about activities "bad" for the back, strenuous things such as BLT or certain sports that combine all three usually come to mind. However, prolonged static postures such as in sitting are extremely deleterious for the back. Both, too little or too much strain is harmful (Fig. 14.5). Stauber reported that the keys to preventing repetitive strain injuries are appropriate rest times, job rotation, and self-pacing (158).

Prolonged sitting is one of the most deleterious activities most people engage in. After only 3 minutes of full flexion of the spine, ligamentous creep or laxity occurs that persists even after 30 minutes of rest (63,116)! Even if the static posture is not strenuous, if just 4% of maximum voluntary contraction ability (MVC) is encountered, a negative metabolic state is established (11,144). Other researchers have found that very low levels of muscle contractions during static work loads involving the neck resulted in fatigue and pain (67,85,168). Jensen suggested that any sustained static work load of more than 10 minutes should not exceed 2% of MVC (85).

Adams and Hutton (3) believe that prolonged full flexion renders the spine susceptible to flexion over-

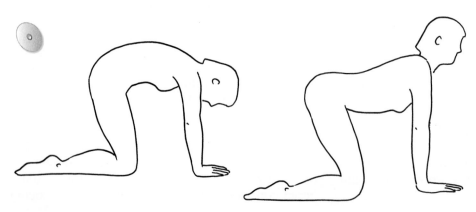

Figure 14.3 Cat camel.

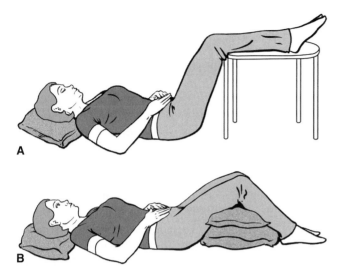

Figure 14.4 (A, B) Semi-traction position for severe, acute low back pain.

and increased discharges when irregular load is handled (sustained elevated muscle tension) (183). Prolonged sitting was shown to further disturb these variables and a brief walking break was shown to improve them again.

Solomonow et al. have demonstrated that the creep reaction may be much more stubborn than previously believed (155). Creep develops in ligaments after just 10 minutes of static flexion. Reduced muscle activity with spasms was found during static flexion periods during a 7-hour recovery period. Multifidus spasm and acute inflammation of ligaments were noted. The dysfunction was reported to outlast the period over which strain occurred by 60 times. The chief three components of cumulative trauma disorders noted were:

1. Magnitude of load
2. Duration of load
3. Frequency of such loads

Acute patients should not sit for more than 20 minutes without taking a "micro-break." The slouched posture leads to overload in the neck, mid back, and lower back, as well as negatively affecting respiration (Fig. 14.7). Regular "micro-breaks" help to centrate the overall posture for better gravity tolerance. The Brügger relief position (Fig. 14.8 A,B) is performed by

load during lifting. According to Bogduk and Twomney (21), "After prolonged strain ligaments, capsules, and IV discs of the lumbar spine may creep, and they may be liable to injury if sudden forces are unexpectedly applied during the vulnerable recovery phase." Once a tissue is strained, it has difficulty returning to its original length. The energy lost after prolonged or repetitive loading is called hysteresis and is represented by the difference between the new and old stress/strain curves (Fig. 14.6).

Wilder showed that the motor control signature associated with low back pain involves a slow reaction time, decreased peak torque output (power),

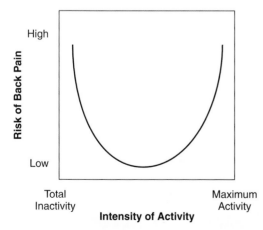

Figure 14.5 Relationship between activity history and injury. From Abenheim L, Rossignol M, Valat JP, Nordin M, Avouac B, Blotman F, Charlot J, et al. The role of activity in the therapeutic management of back pain: Report of the International Paris Task Force on Back Pain. Spine 2000;25:1S–33S.

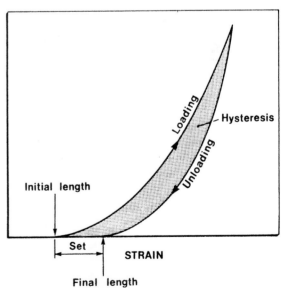

Figure 14.6 Stress–strain curve illustrating hysteresis. When unloaded, a structure regains shape at a rate different to that at which it deformed. Any difference between the initial and final shape is the "set." From Bogduk N, Twomey LT. Clinical Anatomy of the Lumbar Spine. 2nd ed. Melbourne: Churchill Livingstone, 1991.

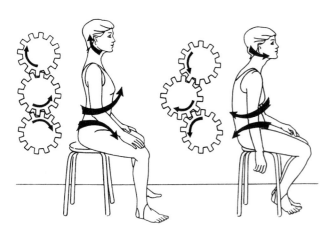

Figure 14.7 Cog wheel model of joint centration in upright posture. Reproduced with permission from: Brügger A. Lehrbuch der funktionellen Störungen des Bewegungssystems. Zollikon/Benglen: Brügger-Verlag, 2000:150.

relaxing the arms at the side, supinating the forearms fully, abducting the fingers fully, and then exhaling actively as if trying to make a candle flame flicker but not go out. The standing overhead arm reach (Fig. 14.8 C,D) is performed by reaching the arms overhead gently, taking a big breathe in and holding it, then reaching the arms up all the way and holding.

Erect sitting involves disc pressures significantly higher than that of normal standing. Sitting slumped forward (anterior sitting) increases disc pressure

even more, whereas slumping backwards (posterior sitting) increases pressure the most (8,10). Using a lumbar support or back rest reduces disc pressures (145). A seat–backrest angle of 95 to 105 degrees reduces both erector spinae EMG and disc pressure (9,145).

The chair seat should have certain characteristics to provide a stable base and yet not be too constraining (133). The height of the chair is very important. Too low a seat height will place too much strain on the ischial tuberosities. Too high a seat will increase pressure on the thighs. Chairs lacking variable height adjustments may need to be complemented by a footrest. The seat edge should not press into the popliteal fossa or this will lead to too rigid a sitting posture. A slight depression for the buttocks is beneficial for stability. A concave seat increases weight-bearing through the greater trochanters and internally rotates the femur again restricting movement of the legs. A saddle type seat is thus preferred. Seat angle is controversial, although it is apparent that a forward-sloping seat will increase lumbar lordosis during sitting and maintain the erect sitting position.

The proper desk height is normally approximately 27 to 30 cm. above the seat (60). The shoulders should be able to relax with the elbows bent 90 degrees and the hands relaxed on the desk surface. A slanted desk (10 to 20 degrees) and/or arm rests may also be helpful for reducing neck and shoulder girdle strain. Figures 14.9 through 14.11 show correct and incorrect sitting positions and workstations. Table 14.2 is an

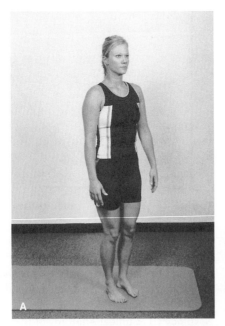
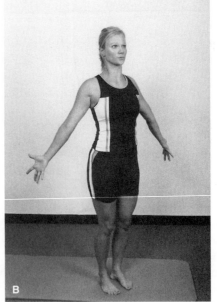
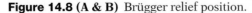

Figure 14.8 (A & B) Brügger relief position.

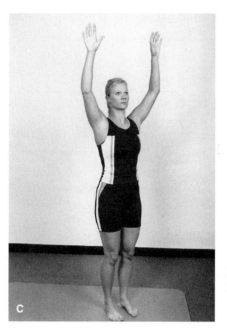 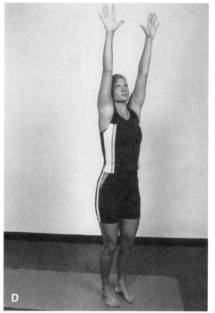

Figure 14.8 (C & D) Standing overhead arm reach

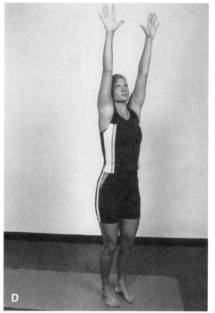

Figure 14.9 Typical slouched desk posture.

ergonomic checklist that can be given to patients or used during the history/evaluation.

Sleep

When resting or sleeping, it is advisable to sleep with pillows under or between the knees (Fig. 14.12). The neck can be easily irritated by improper sleep positions. Maintaining cervical lordosis is a key. Either too firm or too soft of a pillow is to be avoided (Fig. 14.13).

Daily Activities

The problems of prolonged flexion are not limited to sitting and are particular magnified in the morning. The morning is recognized as a dangerous time for the spine. Reilly et al. showed that 54% of the loss of disc height (water content) occurs in the first 30 minutes after arising (139). Disc bending stresses are increased by 300% and ligaments by 80% in the morning (3). Avoidance of early morning flexion has been shown to be a wise strategy when recovering from acute LBP (153). Therefore, avoidance of high-risk activities (BLT) early in the morning, after sitting, or stooping in full flexion is crucial to injury prevention.

Simply getting out of a bed can be a disaster waiting to happen. Most people perform a sit-up to get out of bed, but rolling onto the side and avoiding

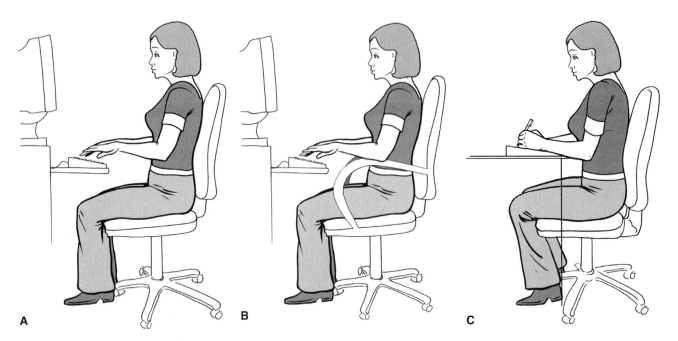

Figure 14.10 (A–C) Correct desk posture.

spine twisting or bending motions is preferable (Fig. 14.14).

Many daily activities involve bending and are thus potentially dangerous if performed incorrectly, for instance, getting in and out of a chair, car, or bed. It is important to spare the spine by hinging with the hips instead of the spine. This entails maintaining mild

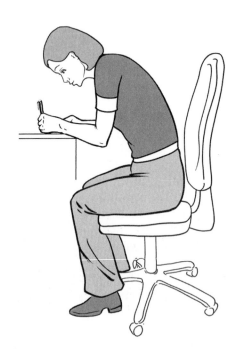

Figure 14.11 Incorrect desk posture caused by chair too low or desk too high.

lordosis—the position of "static elastic equilibrium"—when getting in/out of chairs; lifting and bending; squatting, stooping, or kneeling; and stretches (e.g., hamstring).

To perform the hip-hinge while rising up from a chair or sitting back down (Fig. 14.15):

- Start by perching at edge of a chair
- Maintain lordosis
- Stand up and then return to perch position
- This can be progressed by using the seat of a normal height chair

Key errors to watch for are:

- Flexion of the lumbo-pelvic spine (bending forward from waist instead of hips) (Fig. 14.15A)
- Thoraco-lumbar hyperextension

Troubleshooting:

- Use a high bench, bar stool, arm rest of a chair or couch, or top of the backrest on a chair turned backwards (Fig. 14.16)
- Use a dowel to demonstrate to the patient the difference between squatting with a hip hinge versus squatting with a stooped posture (Fig. 14.17)

Common daily activities can often overload the spine and perpetuate painful syndromes. Simple biomechanical corrections can reduce spine load

Table 14.2   Workstation Ergonomic Checklist

Chair	Y/N
Seat height adjustable	
Feet should be on floor and knees no higher than hips	
Arm rests	
Good lumbar support	
Seat back should be able to recline (95 to 105 degrees)	
Tiltable seat pan	
Tilt seat forward for desk work	
Tilt seat backward for reclining work	
Computer	
Center of monitor nose level	
No glare on monitor	
Keyboard height so that wrists are not bent, elbows at a 90-degree angle, and shoulders relaxed (not shrugged)	
Other	
Document holder	
Head set	

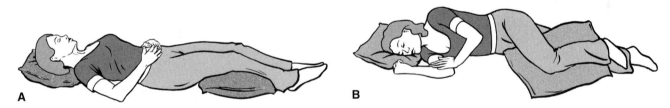

Figure 14.12 (A & B) Spine sparing sleep postures.

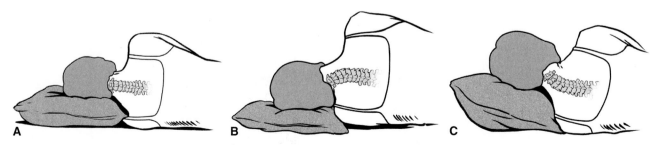

Figure 14.13 Pillows and the neck **(A)** ideal, **(B)** too thin or soft, or **(C)** too hard or firm.

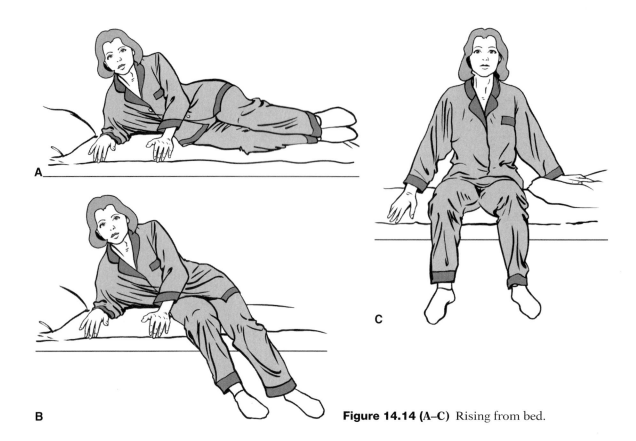

Figure 14.14 (A–C) Rising from bed.

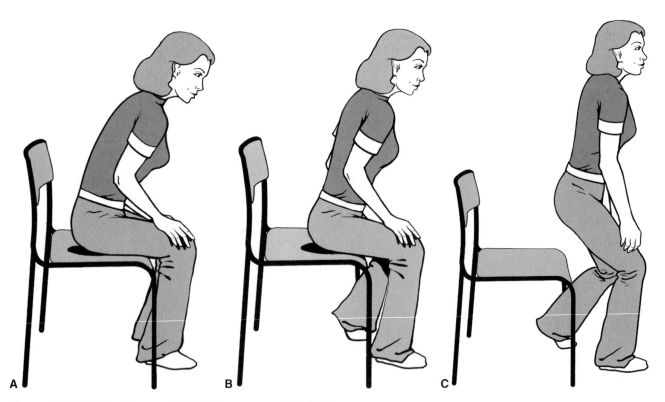

Figure 14.15 Rising from a chair (**A**) incorrect and (**B & C**) correct.

considerably. Low back strain when brushing teeth can be reduced by placing a hand on the counter top or by using a foot stool (Fig. 14.18). Strain is increased by bending forward from the waist.

When washing one's face it is important to squat by hinging from the hips instead of stooping forward from the waist (Fig. 14.19).

When putting on socks or tieing shoes, it is ideal to bring the foot up to a higher surface and then hinge from the hips. If the foot cannot be raised it is still possible to hip hinge rather than rounding the back by scooting to the edge of a stool or chair (Fig. 14.20).

When changing a baby, the most important thing is to have a changing area of proper height. If it is too low, stooping will be unavoidable (Fig. 14.21).

When carrying objects, always hold them as close to the chest as possible to reduce the objects mass (Fig. 14.22). When picking up a bag with a handle, avoid shrugging your shoulder and leaning to side by allowing your gripping muscles in the fingers to hold the bag (Fig. 14.23). This will reduce neck, shoulder, and lower back strain.

Pushing a stroller or cart can lead to lower back, upper back, or neck strain if the handles are too low (Fig. 14.24).

When moving an object on wheels like a cart, it is easier to maintain a good upright spine posture

(*text continues on page 311*)

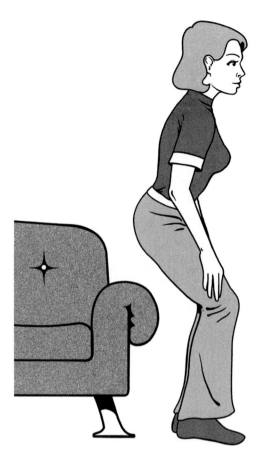

Figure 14.16 Learning to squat with a hip hinge.

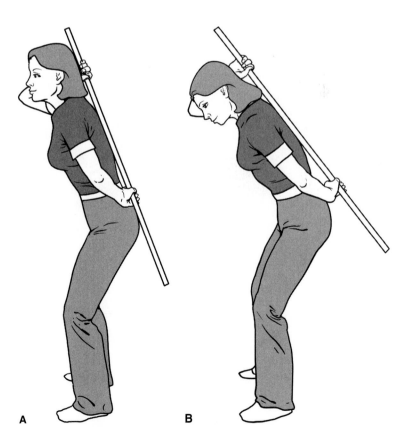

Figure 14.17 Hip hinge **(A)** correct and **(B)** incorrect.

A   B

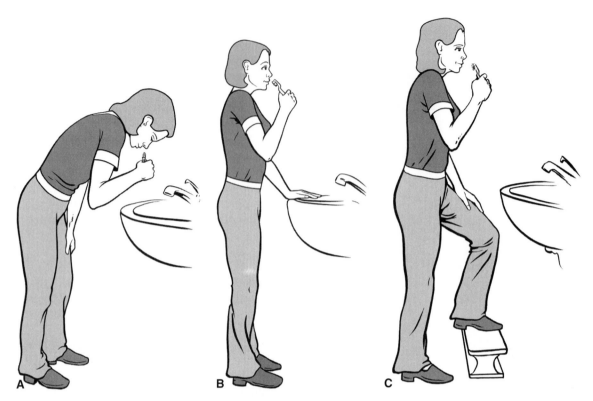

Figure 14.18 Brushing teeth **(A)** incorrect and **(B & C)** correct.

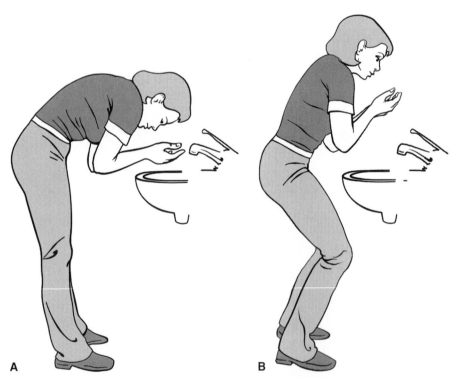

Figure 14.19 Face washing **(A)** incorrect and **(B)** correct.

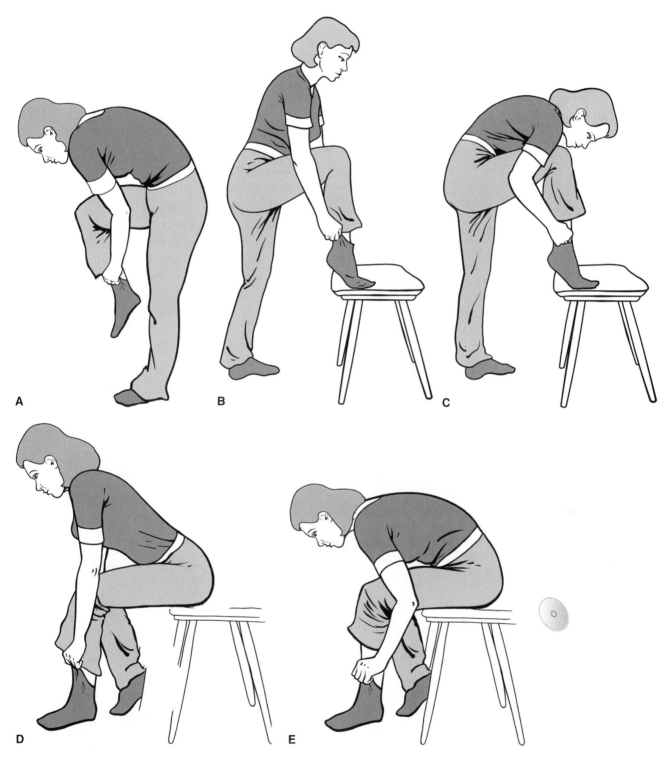

Figure 14.20 Putting on socks **(A)** incorrect, **(B)** raising foot up correctly, **(C)** raising foot up incorrectly, **(D)** leaning forward correctly, and **(E)** leaning forward incorrectly.

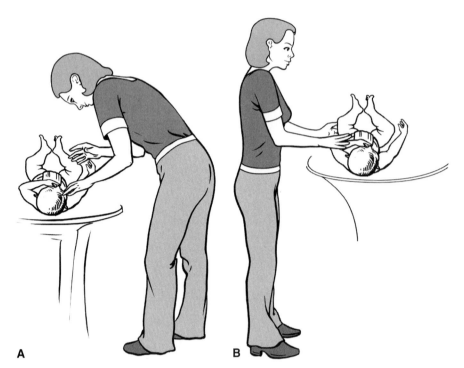

Figure 14.21 Changing a baby with **(A)** changing table too low and **(B)** correct height.

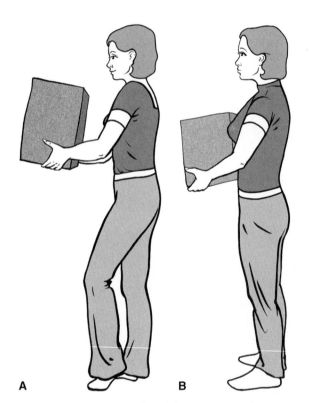

Figure 14.22 Carrying a box **(A)** incorrect and **(B)** correct.

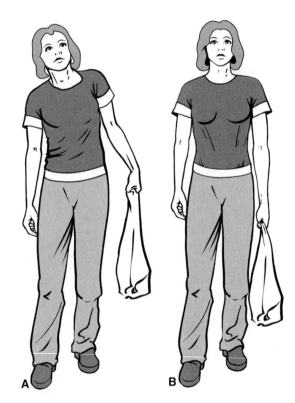

Figure 14.23 Carrying a bag **(A)** incorrect and **(B)** correct.

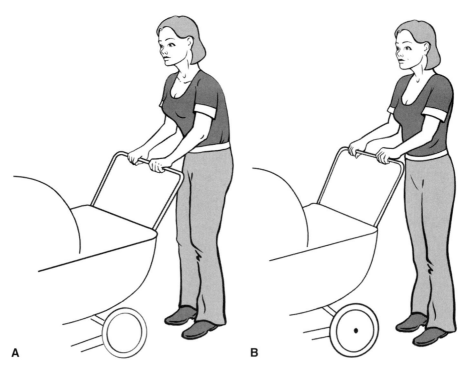

Figure 14.24 Pushing a stroller **(A)** incorrect with handles too low and **(B)** correct height.

and generate power when pushing rather than when pulling (Fig. 14.25).

Placing a child's car seat in the back of a car is a potentially deleterious biomechanical challenge. The key is to avoid full flexion of the spine and keep the load as close as possible (Fig. 14.26). When reaching in to place the baby into the car seat even when the load can't be kept close, it is still possible to maintain lordosis.

Sitting in a car can overload the neck or low back. The key is to maintain slight lordosis. A good lumbar support and/or a sitting wedge are both helpful to facilitate lordosis (Fig. 14.27).

Lifting

Lifting is a common activity of daily living (ADL) and work demand. It places high levels of load on the back and can be dangerous to perform. However, there is specific activity modification advice that can reduce the risk of back strain when lifting. Some traditional advice such as to lift with your legs not your back has been updated in light of a growing body of biomechanical research (117). Modern lifting advice centers on two components.

1. Maintaining slight lumbar lordosis when lifting.
2. Avoiding lifting at certain times of day such as on arising in the morning or after sitting for a prolonged period of time (e.g., 30 minutes) (3).

There has been much debate as to the safest methods of lifting. Squatting is typically recommended in preference to stooping. Unfortunately, most workers fail to follow this advice if repetitive lifts are required. Garg and Herrin point out the increased energy expenditure with squatting versus stooping (57). Increased end range flexion loading of the spine has been shown to occur as a result of a fatiguing repetitive task such as lifting (156).

Most low back injuries are not the result of a single exposure to a high magnitude load, but instead are the result of cumulative trauma from sub-failure magnitude loads. For instance, repeated small loads (e.g., bending) or a sustained load (e.g., sitting). According to McGill, it is usually a result of "a history of excessive loading which gradually, but progressively, reduces the tissue failure tolerance" (118).

In particular, low back injury has been shown to result from repetitive motion at end range (see chapter 5). Disc herniation has been shown to be related to repeated flexion motion (33), especially if coupled with lateral bending and twisting (2,58).

What appears to be an attainable goal is the maintaining of lordosis, independent of thigh and trunk angles (118). Adams and Hutton reported that compressive loads on a fully flexed lumbar disc (i.e., stooped posture) cause posterior herniation of nuclear material with less load than would cause end plate fracture in the upright position (3). According to McGill "Because ligaments are not recruited when

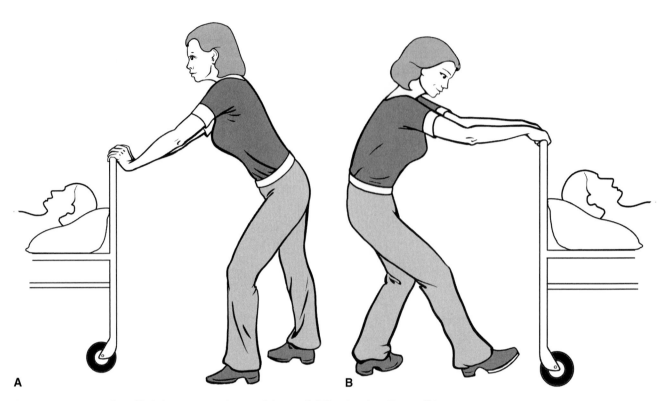

Figure 14.25 Push/pull: **(A)** spine-sparing pushing and **(B)** spine-loading pulling.

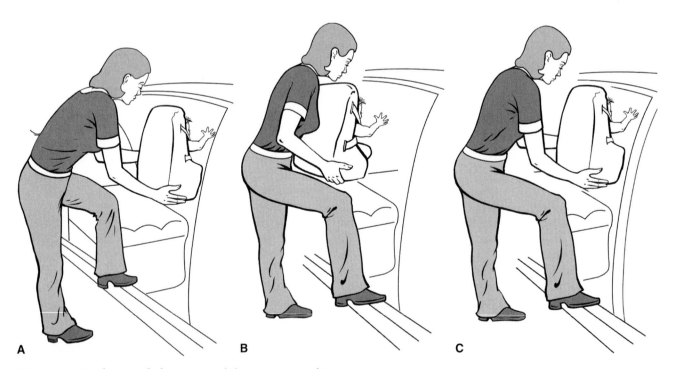

Figure 14.26 Placing a baby in a car: **(A)** incorrect reaching position, **(B)** correct holding position, and **(C)** correct reaching position.

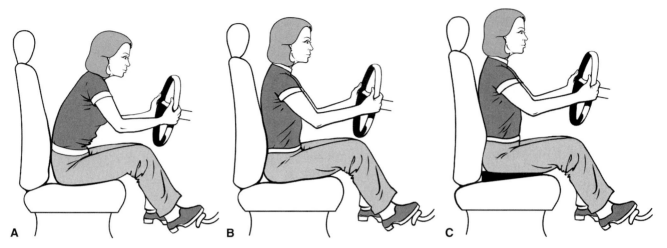

Figure 14.27 Driving (**A**) incorrect and slouched, (**B**) correct and upright, and (**C**) correct with a wedge support.

lordosis is preserved, nor is the disc bent, it appears that the annulus is at low risk for failure" (118). This was supported by the work of Hickey and Hukins (76). Lifting with lordosis allows the further benefit of activating the musculature and thus providing for neuromuscular control to protect ligamentous tissues.

Lifting technique is important, but what may be even more significant is when lifting is performed. The risk of injury during forward bending activities is increased in the early morning (153).

Prolonged flexion such as in sitting can render the back very vulnerable to lifting. McGill and Brown found that after just 3 minutes of full flexion, subjects

lost half their stability (e.g., stiffness) (116). Adams and Hutton believe that prolonged full flexion may cause ligamentous creep and render the spine susceptible to flexion overload during lifting (2). According to McGill, a brief course of extension exercises before lifting may be preventive of injury (118).

Co-contraction of the lumbar erector spinae muscles during lifting appears to redistribute compressive forces on the spine in a similar way to adding guide wires to a flexible rod or rigging on a ship's mast (see Chapter 5) (Fig. 14.28) (118). The increase in compressive loading on the spine is substantial if even a small amount of torsion is required during lifting

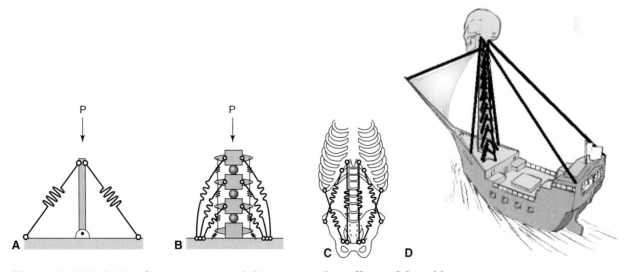

Figure 14.28 A–D Muscle co-contraction (**A**) Increasing the stiffness of the cables (muscles) increases the stability. (**B**) Spine stiffness (and stability) is achieved by a complex interaction of stiffening structures along the spine and (**C**) those forming the torso wall. (**D**) Stability system requires 360 degrees of support. (**D**) is reproduced with permission of Liebenson CS. Advice for the clinician and patient: Spinal stabilization—an update. Part 1—biomechanics. J Bodywork Movement Ther 2004;8:81.

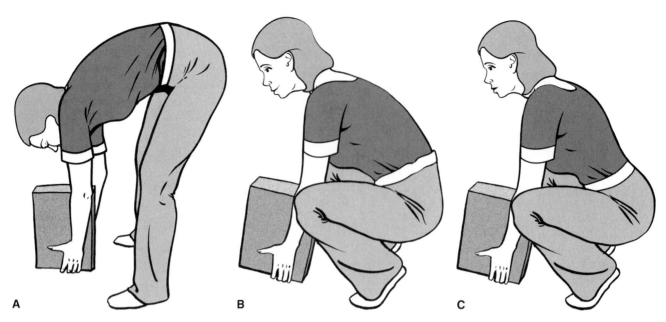

Figure 14.29 Lifting **(A & B)** incorrect and **(C)** correct.

(118). To prevent injury, objects should not be lifted if they are awkwardly placed. To reduce the extensor moment, the load should be held as close as possible to the trunk and lifted smoothly (Fig. 14.29) (117). A jerky lift is only appropriate for highly trained individuals who are required to lift awkwardly placed light objects. The purpose of such a lift is to avoid loading the spine in flexion for any longer than absolutely necessary (117). Table 14.3 summarizes the present state of knowledge regarding lifting advice.

General Light Activity

Information and advice emphasizing the value of fitness and the safety of resuming activities achieved superior outcomes to advice that reinforced rest, activity restrictions, and the notion that the spine was injured or damaged (arthritis, herniated disc) (30). Reassuring workers and encouraging resumption of ordinary activities was superior to medication, bed rest, or mobilization exercises (114).

Table 14.3 McGill's Rules for Lifting (117,119)

---

1. Maintain normal lordosis
2. Do not lift immediately after prolonged flexion or rising from bed
3. Lightly co-contract the back muscles before and during lifting
4. Keep the load as close as possible, as long as lordosis is maintained
5. Avoid twisting

Callaghan and colleagues (32) found that walking without flexibility increases spinal load. Specifically, slow walking with restricted arm swing increased "static" spine loads, whereas fast walking produced more cyclic loading patterns. It was determined that fast walking could be used as a "safe" back exercise. Other researchers have consistently reported that back pain patients have a much stiffer and "guarded" gait pattern than asymptomatic individuals. Hussein and colleagues (81,82) have reported that stride length is decreased during the gait of LBP individuals compared to normal subjects. Lamoth and colleagues (99) recently found that pelvis–thorax coordination in the LBP group differed significantly from that in the control group. Specifically, they reported that the gait of LBP patients was characterized by a more rigid, less flexible pelvis–thorax coordination and slower gait velocity than in asymptomatics. In asymptomatic individuals at gait velocities more than 3.0 km/h, coupled transverse plane rotation of the pelvis and thoracic regions becomes uncoupled because of counter-rotation. However, in LBP subjects this uncoupling did not occur. Indahl has reported that even if it hurts, somewhat that flexible walking is a safe and effective exercise for low back pain patients (83).

Pain Relief Options

Though there are no magic bullets for eliminating pain, there are a number of pain relief options. If the pain can be softened, then it will be easier to encourage the patient to resume activities. The main goal is to avoid the debilitation of rest and build activity tolerance through safe conditioning. According to the Danish guidelines, over-the-counter pain medication, prescription NSAIDS, and manipulation are all recommended for pain relief (46). Physical therapy modalities, muscle relaxants, McKenzie exercises, acupuncture, and epidural injections (for sciatica) are optional. Sedatives, epidurals for back pain, and surgery in the acute phase (except in cauda equina syndrome) are all recommended against. The recent American Occupational guidelines recommend offering the patient a choice or recommended options and letting their preference guide the selection of which one (70).

Occasionally, a brief period of restricted activity or even rest is necessary for severe, acute low back disorders. It should be explained that rest is being prescribed because of the pain, rather than for the pain. In other words, the rest is recommended because most other movements are aggravating the pain, not because the rest is healing. In fact, as soon as possible the patient should begin resuming light activities such as walking, knees to chest, or cat-camels. Relative rest positions and simple light exercises often relieving in acute disorders are shown in Figures 14.3 and 14.4. Generally, if the patient is extension-biased, then the sphinx will be pain centralizing or relieving (Chapter 15) (Fig. 14.30A). If the patient is flexion-biased, then the knee to chest exercise will be pain-relieving (Fig. 14.30B and 14.30C).

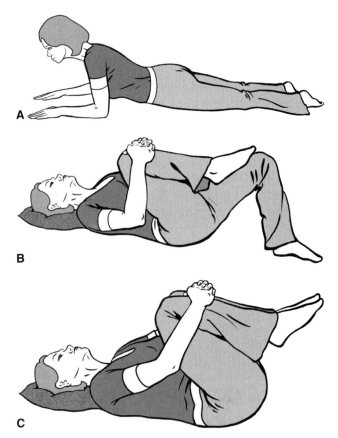

Figure 14.30 Light exercises for certain acute back pain patients (**A**) the sphinx, (**B**) single knee to chest, and (**C**) double knee to chest.

How Long Will It Last?— Recovery Expectations

Most patients want to know how long to expect their pain to last. Giving an accurate prognosis to patients is an important role of the physician (see Chapter 9). The natural history is generally very positive in the short-term, but symptoms and activity intolerances tend to linger and recur. If an overly optimistic prognosis is given, this risks frustrating the patient who does not recover quickly (38). In contrast, an overly pessimistic prognosis may increase fear and anxiety in someone who would otherwise recover more quickly (38).

Practice-Based Problem
• Patients want to know how long it will take for them to recover.   • What is the natural history for spinal conditions?   • What are the main prognostic indicators of a prolonged or speedy recovery from the patient's history and examination?

Linton found that FABs in asymptomatic individuals are related to future onset of LBP 1 year later (106). Fritz and George found that FABs are significantly present in acute LBP patients and they are a predictor of 1 month disability (53). Klenerman found the same predictive pattern (97). Waddell found that FABs were predictive of disability in a chronic LBP group (177). Buer and Linton studied a large of group of 35- to 45-year-olds in the general population (exclusion criteria—chronic pain) and found a step-wise relationship between FABs and disability with those in the highest quartile of FABs having more than double the chance of having reduced ADLs (odds ratio [OR] of 2.5) (28). FABs were more closely related to an increase in disability than pain (2.5 versus 1.25 Ors). Catastrophizing was related to ADL with an OR of 1.8 and to pain by OR 1.75.

Patients who have unrealistic expectations about recovery are at an increased risk for being disappointed. Thus, besides identifying which patients have higher yellow flags scores or increased FABs, an important area of inquiry is how to determine which patients respond best to manipulation, medication, or exercise. Flynn et al. (2002) demonstrated a "clinical prediction rule" for identification of patients most likely to respond to spinal manipulation (51). Not surprisingly, low FABs are one of the chief findings correlating with a speedy recovery.

Stig et al. studied patients with an episode that has lasted at least 2 weeks, as well as a minimum of 4 weeks of pain in the previous 12 months (159). Fully 50% of patients were found to be significantly better within four visits or 2 weeks of starting chiropractic care; 75% were much better by 12 visits. Such statistics can be very important for sharing with patients so they can have a clear idea of what to expect regarding the speed of their recovery.

According to Axen et al. certain criteria were present in a sub-group who had a 84% chance of improving by the fourth chiropractic visit (12). These criteria are:

- Decreased pain immediately after visit one
- Decreased pain reported at visit two
- Decreased disability reported at visit two
- Common reaction (local pain or fatigue lasting 24 hours) or no reaction to first treatment

All of the criteria had to be present.

In contrast, if all of the following criteria were present, the chance of being recovered by the fourth visit was only 30%:

- No immediate improvement immediately after visit one
- No decreased pain at visit two
- No decreased disability reported at visit two
- An uncommon reaction (local pain or fatigue lasting more than 24 hours; new radiating pain, other reactions) to the first treatment

Of particular note is that local pain or fatigue lasting 24 hours after spinal manipulation is a common reaction and is consistent with a positive prognosis.

Echoing Axen's emphasis on the prognostic power, an improvement in patient symptoms by the conclusion of the first visit Hahne et al. identified that within-session improvement in range of motion after treatment predicted future outcome (66). Linear regression analysis shows that within-session changes predicted 12% to 64% of between-session improvement in ROM and pain. Therefore, the clinician is encouraged to audit the response to treatment and empirically search for those treatments (preferably self-care) that result in within-session improvement.

Clinical Pearl

An immediate improvement in symptoms or function in the first visit predicts a faster recovery for the patient (12,66)

- Therefore, always identify the patients mechanical sensitivity (MS) to provocative maneuvers (range of motion and orthopedic tests).
- Audit the patients MS after treatment.
- Based on the audit, offer prognostic information to the patient regarding the likelihood of a quick or slower recovery.

Fortunately, pain typically runs a course—like a common cold or flu. However, if there is excessive emphasis on pain relief instead of reactivation this can actually reinforce avoidance behaviors (126). The most important factors that determine recovery are related to how a person copes with their pain. If all the focus on care is on pain relief, then avoidance behavior will be promoted with the result being that physical and psychological deconditioning will ensue. Patients should be informed that light activities, while uncomfortable, are not harmful. If patients are overly concerned about pain and fearful of activities, then a "stepped up" approach including exercise and supervised exposure to feared activities is needed (13).

Summary

Once a patient has been given a proper report of findings (ROF), most patients' back-related worries are reduced. This ROF would include the material discussed. In summary, it includes:

- They are reassured that their pain is not caused by a serious disease process
- The positive relationship of activity and recovery is described
- Specific activity modification advice and reactivation activities are shown
- It is explained that "flare-ups" are common but are not signs of re-injury.
  - Use first-aid approach
  - Just a "spasm," not serious even if uncomfortable
- Stress it is explained can heighten tension and lower pain thresholds and tolerances

Patients learn that care involves three basic aspects—palliative, spine sparing, and spine stabilizing. Palliative care is what most people want, but it only addresses the symptoms and not the cause of the trouble. Motivating patients to reduce their exposure to harmful habits (e.g., prolonged sitting or improper lifting technique) via spine-sparing strategies is the most efficient self-care approach for both acute and chronic problems. Generally, spine stabilizing strategies are recommended as a preventive/conditioning tool and most patients will only elect to adhere to a modest stability regime.

Those patients with entrenched activity related fears or who have numerous barriers to engaging in sparing and stabilizing self-care methods require a more structured cognitive behavior (CB) approach.

Step 2: Cognitive Behavioral Approach

What: More structured approach involving cognitive behavioral (CB) classes or sessions addressing patient's worries and fears and teaching simple, safe, and effective methods to reduce these apprehensions.

Who: Subacute patients at heightened risk for chronic pain (i.e., high yellow flags score) or those in the chronic phase (94).

Subacute patients at risk for chronicity are typically reducing activities because of the belief that their vulnerable tissues need more rest or are in danger of being harmed. At 2 months, 23% to 45% of LBP subjects report performing no or less housework, decreased sexual activity, and difficulty standing or walking for short periods (123).

The most common worries subacute back pain patients have about their condition are:

- Concern about serious disease
- Fear that severe pain indicates a serious problem
- Anxiety about long-term disability or chronic pain
- Worry that movement or activity will worsen the problem

According to Balderson and Von Korff care may need to be "stepped up" for those patients who continue to have residual activity intolerances or have substantial fears and worries as evidence by a high yellow flags score (13). Such patients need a more structured intervention that incorporates CB principles at each phase of patient care.

Fears About Specific (work) Activities are Correlated with Work Capacity Independent of Pain or General Fears About Activity (175)

- An individual's belief that participating in work-related activities is potentially harmful is related to actual physical capacity for work.

- Work-specific fears are more highly correlated with work capacity than fears about general physical activity or pain severity.

- A treatment approach combining cognitive behavioral and physical therapy approaches for chronic pain patient was able to decrease FABs, pain severity, and increase physical work capacity.

- It is not clear whether changes in distress lead to improved physical capacity or the other way around.

Clinical Pearl

Patient Beliefs About the Nature and Treatment of Their Pain Can Change with Cognitive-Behavioral Therapy (181)

Patients with chronic LBP who believed their pain was caused by structural pathology had more disability at baseline and demonstrated greater reductions in disability after a cognitive behavioral intervention. In all patients as biomedical/pathology beliefs were reduced, reported disability also declined.

Social Cognitive Theory and Behavioral Change

Bandura has summarized the core determinants of social cognitive theory that are essential for achieving a change in behavior (15):

- Knowledge of health risks and benefits of health practices/behaviors
- Perceived self-efficacy that one can exercise control over health habits
- Outcome expectations about costs/benefits of different health habits
- Health goals and concrete plans/strategies for achieving them
- Perceived facilitators and impediments to the changes being sought

Perceived self-efficacy governs if individuals translate perceived risks into a search for health information as well as if they translate health information into healthy behavior. According to Bandura, surprisingly self-changers are the majority for alcohol, smoking, and heroin abuse (15).

For each risk factor people are given a detailed guide on how to improve their health functioning

- Monitor health habits
- Set short-term goals
- Report changes being made

According to Jensen et al., how well patients with chronic pain do depends more on what they do than what is done to them (87). Thus, behavioral change and maintenance are the keys. For example,

- Remain active
- Exercise regularly
- Increase activity tolerance

Specific pain coping skills include activity pacing, relaxation, and cognitive restructuring. This requires motivation. Two factors are decisive to motivation, which in turn influences behavior.

- The perceived importance of behavior change
- The belief that behavior change is possible (self-efficacy)

Motivation or "readiness to change" is deemed a state amenable to change, rather than a trait that is constant. When applying motivational principles to improve patient adherence to pain self-management clinicians have a significant influence on patients knowledge, skills, and beliefs (128). Motivational interviewing (MI) is designed to address and resolve ambivalence about behavioral change. There are three key components: importance, confidence, and readiness. A meta-analysis of 26 controlled studies of MI showed its efficacy (29).

Patient-centered counseling that was developed by Ockene et al. and Rosal et al. involves a brief 5- to 10-minute physician patient contact with the following goals (128,142):

- Increase patient's awareness of risks of problem behavior
- Increase patient's knowledge of health problem
- Increase self-efficacy regarding ability to change health behavior
- Enhance skill for long-term adherence

It has proven efficacy for alcohol consumption (131), diet (73,132), and smoking (129, 130).

There are two primary variables to all behavioral change models: (1) the importance of engaging versus not engaging in self-management behaviors (outcome expectancy, value, importance); and (2) self-efficacy and confidence. Bandura's Social Cognitive Theory is the most thorough approach to promoting self-efficacy (14). The three things that influence it are personal experience, modeling, and verbal persuasion. Personal experience may be the most important. The more the patients see themselves performing a behavior, the better, for instance, with graded exposure training (GET) via quota-based exercise. It is also helpful to see others do it, as in group settings.

Clinicians can increase a patient's perception of the importance of self-management by encouraging positive outcome expectancies while encouraging acceptance of costs of not engaging in self-treatment (90). Identify and incorporate contingencies or reinforcers for self-management coping behaviors. Providing reinforcement for gradual change to self-management coping styles (step by step).

The construct of readiness to change comes from the transtheoretical model of behavioral change (137):

- Precontemplation—belief that health care behavior is responsible
- Contemplation—consideration of self-management approach
- Action—beginning self-management
- Maintenance—commitment to ongoing self-management

The Pain Stages of Change Questionnaire (PSOCQ) measures these constructs, has good internal consistency, and is valid (88). Motivation to self-manage pain directly influences pain self-management behaviors. This is in turn influenced by the following factors (89):

- Information concerning the costs/benefits of self-management
- Manner in which information is communicated
- Barriers to the use of coping strategies
- Self-efficacy concerning ability to engage in self-mgmt behaviors

PSOCQ changes were associated with changes in pain self-management coping strategies. Depression decreased as the precontemplation score decreased or the action maintenance scores increased. Decreases in precontemplation score were correlated with decreases in disability in patients with fibromyalgia, but not in pain clinic patients. Pain intensity decreased as the precontemplation score decreased or the action maintenance scores went up. Pretreatment and posttreatment and 6-month follow-up were evaluated.

Graded Exposure Training

GET involves a combination of behavioral and physical reconditioning. Operant models were the first to be used and they emphasized rewarding well behaviors while ignoring illness behaviors as individuals exercised to a time contingent quota rather than to pain tolerance (52,101).

GET starts with baseline testing to identify feared activities (perceptual activity intolerances) and pain tolerance. Then patients are gradually exposed to their feared stimuli so they can experience that it is safe to do so. A lecture on fear–avoidance behavior is not as effective as direct evidence (14). "Graded exposures" should be specific to the feared activity (170). Goubert et al. showed this was necessary because effects of exposures to one movement don't necessarily translate to other dissimilar movements (59). In GET the patient should be involved in establishing their own goals for exposure to feared stimuli. Then quotas are agreed on, which are systematically increased until the goal is achieved. Initial quotas should be set to sub-threshold levels to assure success. They are time-contingent, rather than pain-contingent. This enhances motivation and is a form of positive reinforcement. Patients' progress is documented and audited at each treatment session.

Cognitive Intervention Plus Exercise has Superior Functional Outcome to Lumbar Fusion for Chronic LBP Patients (93)

Patients

- At least 1 year of low back pain. Nearly half of them had previous lumbar surgery and nearly half of the patients were previous lumbar fusion patients.

Interventions

- Cognitive intervention plus stabilization exercises or lumbar fusion

1-year Outcomes

- Sorensen trunk extensor endurance reduced from a mean of 68 seconds to 48 seconds in the fusion group, unchanged in the exercise group.
- Isokinetic trunk muscle strength reduced nearly 25% in the fusion group and improved 30% in the exercise group.
- Density of back muscles decreased significantly in the fusion group and was unchanged in the exercise group.

Graded Exposures Training Not More Successful than Usual Care for Lumbar Disc Surgery Patients (134)

Patients

- First time lumbar disc surgery after persisting pain or sciatica

Interventions

- Graded exposure therapy versus Usual care

1-year Outcomes

- No clinically significant differences between the groups as measured by Roland Morris disability score, range of motion, pain catastrophizing, and fear of movement.

Cognitive Behavioral Therapy

This CB approach is introduced with an explanation of the *fear–avoidance model* using the patient's own symptoms, beliefs, and behaviors to illustrate the viscous circle. Reassurance by itself is not sufficient to help patients overcome their fears (69). Self-reassurance is required so individually tailored practice tasks are designed. Patients select the activity they want to work on. They are given education and reassurance regarding that activity. Together clinician and patient explore what is feared about the activity. Healthy behaviors are reinforced, whereas pain behaviors (i.e., sighing, grimacing) are not (52). Reinforcement includes such things as attention or praise (52). The specific reactivation goals that the patient has helped to select are reviewed weekly. When progress is noted it is important that it is not attributed to the clinician's intervention, but to the patient's efforts (69). Anderson suggested that supporting self-care of chronic illness through patient-centered approaches was more successful than physician-centered directive ones (7).

Highly specialized programs including rehabilitative exercises and psychologically oriented classes have been developed (105) (see Chapter 31). The classes involve education about the psychology and neurophysiology of pain followed by quota based "graded-exposures" to their own feared movements or activities. The desired outcome is that the patient develops a personalized coping program. The program includes six 2-hour sessions (once per week) with a clinical psychologist along with rehabilitation. The class size is from six to 10 people and covers material summarized in Table 14.4. Linton and Andersson and Linton and Ryberg found that non-

Table 14.4 Cognitive Behavioral Class Topics/Skills (106)

1. Causes of pain and prevention of chronic problems—problem solving, applied relaxation, learning, and pain
2. Managing your pain—activities, maintain daily routines; scheduling activities; relaxation training
3. Promoting good health, controlling stress at home and at work—warning signals; cognitive appraisal; beliefs
4. Adapting for leisure and work—communication skills; assertiveness; risk situations; applying relaxation
5. Controlling flare-ups—plan for coping with flare-up; coping skills review; applied relaxation; own program
6. Maintaining and improving results—risk analysis; plan for adherence; own program finalized

responsive patients at 6 months respond to such programs and the effects are still present at 1-year follow-ups (104,107).

A key component of each CB class involves problem-solving. The classes are not "passive schools," but require active engagement (108). According to Shaw et al., it is important to address a chronic patient's problem-solving style, which has been shown to be correlated with increased disability (147,148). This involves:

- problem avoidance
- lack of positive problem solving orientation
- impulsive decision making

Van den Haut and others describe the following strategies for improving a patient's problem solving ability—a record of coping attempts tool, brainstorming (the more solutions the better), and to focus on the consequences of pain not pain itself (6,167,168).

Von Korff et al. emphasized a classroom approach similar to Linton's (173). The program included four 2-hour classes held once per week for 10 to 15 patients. Lay leaders were used who themselves were recurrent or chronic back pain patients and had received 2 days of formal training.

The classes used flip charts to present standardized information on the following topics:

- "red flags" indicating a serious condition
- more common and less worrisome sources of back pain

- factors that increase or decrease pain
- appropriate pacing of exercise and activity
- posture and body mechanics
- role of positive and negative attitudes
- how to handle flare-ups
- co-management with your health care provider

The lay leaders used action planning or problem-solving techniques to collaborate with the patients. The goals were to:

- identify activity limitations related to back pain
- set personal goals to overcome those limitations
- brainstorm possible steps to achieve these goals
- develop a specific plan of action
- implement the plan

On subsequent sessions, patients reviewed their action plans, evaluated their progress toward agreed on goals, and attempted to problem solve difficulties that arose implementing the plan. Most action plans focused on increasing exercise.

Recently, Von Korff et al. reported a brief fear-reducing and activating intervention (one to four sessions) produced sustained benefits in chronic back pain patients (174).

Intervention:

- Session 1: 90-minute visit with psychologist

  identifying and addressing fears about back pain relationship between resuming normal activities and quality of life

  Set activity and exercise goals

  Develop and action plan
- Session 2: 60-minute visit with physical therapist (7 to 10 days later)

  Standardized physical examination

  Discussed unresolved patient concerns

  Taught stretches/exercises relevant to action plan

  Offered guidance in overcoming barriers the patient had encountered
- Session 3: 30 minutes with physical therapist (10 days later)

  Action plan

  Exercises relevant to the action plan
- Session 4: 30 minutes with psychologist (2 weeks later)

  Reviewed progress

Encouraged use of relaxation techniques

Developed plans for sustaining progress, managing flare-ups, and resuming activities when a flare-up occurred.

Key point: flare-ups are common but manageable

Control group received usual care (primary care visits, physical therapy, and prescription and non-prescription medicine). A 2–year follow-up showed that the intervention led to significant reduction in:

- pain-related fear
- average pain
- activity limitations caused by pain

Neurophysiologic Aspects

It is essential to validate chronic patients' pain experience. Even if structural pathology or injury does not explain the patient's pain, the pain is still real. Modern neurophysiology helps us explain our patients' chronic pain. A simple metaphor for discomfort in deconditioned tissues is to compare persistent pain in underused tissues to gardening after the winter or hiking for the first time in years. "Rusty" tissues are expected to be uncomfortable but not hazardous; therefore, reactivation is safe even if uncomfortable.

It is often difficult for chronic pain patients to understand that their spine is not damaged. One very simple explanation is that they have central sensitization. This is what causes phantom limb pain and is caused by pain memory not tissue damage. Basically, the nervous system has become habituated to pain so that its threshold and tolerance has dropped and now it responds to non-noxious stimuli as if it were injurious. The logical treatment is graded exposures to re-habituate those pathways. Janet Travell, the White House physician to John F. Kennedy, said, "Tissues heal, but muscles learn. They readily develop habits of guarding that long outlast the source of the pain." When pain persists longer than it takes for an injury to heal (e.g., 8 to 12 weeks for a bone fracture) the pain threshold drops (allodynia) so that even non-noxious stimuli can elicit painful perceptions. Understanding this is essential to realizing that pain can be present that is not caused by injured or damaged tissues and thus that hurt may not equal harm.

Step 3: Multidisciplinary Biopsychosocial Approach

What: A comprehensive, multidisciplinary biopsychosocial approach involving this CB model along with strategies that address return-to-work obstacles (employer, compensation system, etc.), as well as co-morbid psychological illness.

Who: For chronic cases if steps 1 and 2 fail.

Multidisciplinary care (psychologist, pain management specialist, physical therapist) and workplace involvement are keys to success in these most complex cases. Step three is a comprehensive, multidisciplinary biopsychosocial approach involving this CB model along with strategies that address return to work obstacles (employer, compensation system, etc.), as well as co-morbid psychological illness (13). Patients with chronic problems over 1 year can respond to a more expensive and comprehensive multidisciplinary approach (64,184).

Marhold et al. looked at the effects of CB therapy on return to work (RTW) in those already on sick leave (115). This program involved six CB sessions plus six more on RTW issues. The 1-year follow-up showed less days off work for those with short-term sick leave, but no improvement for those with long-term sick leave. Thus, it is better to prevent than treat chronic disability! Fortunately, only 10% of patient report ongoing work disability. Unfortunately, this group accounts for the majority of costs, and treatments are not as effective as for subacute or acute patients.

Motivation Issues

Communication problems in medicine are important and common (149). Patient anxiety, distress, and dissatisfaction are related to lack of information or a suitable explanation. According to Deyo, 20% to 25% of patients are dissatisfied with their care for back and neck pain. (47). Chiropractors have been more successful than their medical counterparts in providing helpful advice for spinal trouble largely because they offer an explanation of what is causing the pain and they offer simple steps to deal with it (37).

However, there is evidence that patient education is certainly not always effective (37,39,72). In particular, in a health maintenance organization, clinic patient education was unsuccessful (39). Also, in a worker's compensation setting in Vermont, patient education very similar to a successful program in Great Britain was ineffective (72). Therefore, written education material is a weak intervention by itself. Little et al. found that a mismatch between verbal and written information resulted in the combination being less effective than either alone (109). It may be easier to educate patients who then change the HCP's behavior than vice versa (26,27,146).

Table 14.5 describes an overview of techniques for motivating patients to resume activity.

A coordinated approach in which all caregivers give the same advice and use reinforcing educational material is more powerful (61). The key factors related to motivating patients to resume or increase activity are typically missed when HCPs focus on cure of symptoms rather than control of them. Acute back pain is an illness like a cold that responds best to advice that reassures and reactivates the patient. Chronic back pain, like asthma or diabetes, does not have a cure, but with lifestyle adjustments and appropriate self-management control of symptoms it can be achieved (172).

Such patient-centered approaches are dramatically different from the traditional way many patients are assessed and treated. Typically, a biomedical approach is taken that emphasizes a disease approach. Patients receive various labels describing what is wrong with their backs (subluxation, herniated disc) and are either given proposed treatments to fix the problem (months of adjustments, spinal surgery) or are told to learn to live with it (activity avoidance or anti-inflammatory medicine).

Clinicians and patients should negotiate their roles, responsibilities, and expectations. Without agreed-on goals, patient participation is unlikely. What this ROF does is shift the model from a biomedical physician-centered fix/cure one to a biopsychosocial patient-centered cope/adapt one. From this platform realistic expectations, specific activity modification advice, and self-treatment exercises can be laid out in a "shared decision-making" environment (182).

If physical performance rehabilitation is being proposed to the patient, then the rationale for developing a higher level of musculoskeletal function needs to be explained to the patient. If their muscles are too tight or weak, then it is explained that this is what leads to instability, irritation, and thus pain with activity. Restoration of function prevents pain or irritation from arising in the first place. Such rehabilitation may be somewhat more painful in the short-term, but improving function is explained as the preventive key to long-term pain relief. The chronic pain patient learns that always seeking temporary pain relief will do nothing to prevent the problem from starting again. Only improving function and modifying activities in biomechanically appropriate ways will prevent the pain from beginning over and over again. Flare-ups are not failures to manage the pain, but challenges to learning how to better self-manage their back condition (68,69).

Counseling Patients in General Medical Practice on Exercise is Effective in Increasing Physical Activity at 1 Year (50)

The green prescription:

- Primary care doctors were given 4 hours of training in how to use motivational techniques
- Screening test were used to identify "less active" patients
- Goals were collaboratively determined (walking, home exercise) and put on a green card
- Exercise specialists made three follow-up calls (10 to 20 minutes each) over the following 3 months to encourage and support patients
- A quarterly newsletter was sent to patients from the exercise specialists about physical activity
- As a result of this approach physical activity in "less active" patients was significantly increased from baseline at 1-year follow-up

---

Table 14.5 Enhancing Patient Motivation to Resume Activity

- Collaboratively establish functional goals
- Reassurance that the spine is not damaged
- Education that gradual reactivation will enhance recovery whereas excessive rest will interfere with recovery
- Consistent verbal and written messages
- Make exercises simple enough to be performed at home without significant equipment needs
- Establish realistic expectations such as "flare-ups" are not unexpected nor do they suggest failure

Compliance With Ongoing Active Treatment

One of the greatest stumbling blocks to prescription of home exercise is the belief by the HCP that the patient won't comply. Many issues are related to poor compliance such as a patient's recent history of activities, type of goals that are established, ease of utilization, lack of confidence in the exercise, fear of pain, boredom with the prescription, and if the patient is only motivated to achieve pain relief rather than prevent recurrences. Acquisition of self-management skills also depends on readiness to change (49).

Converting a pain patient from a passive recipient of care to an active partner in their own care involves a paradigm shift from seeing the doctor as healer to seeing him or her as a helper (100,176,178). When health care providers promise to fix or cure a pain problem, they only perpetuate the idea that something is wrong that can be fixed (i.e., put back in place). In pain medicine, the likelihood of recurrence is high (more than 70%) and therefore it is important to show a patient how to care for oneself in addition to offering palliative care (176). Simple advice regarding activity is often better than more sophisticated forms of conservative care including mobilization or ergonomics (43,114). Promoting a positive state of mind and avoiding the disabling attitudes, which accompany pain, is crucial to recovery (100,178).

Patients at the greatest risk for chronic pain often have poorly developed coping skills (94). Patients who fear pain or catastrophize by fearing an inevitable poor outcome are also less likely to perform exercise (30,113,169,179). A key to getting a patient to become active in their own rehabilitation program is to shift them from being a pain avoider to a pain manager (100,102,141,162,176,178).

It appears that fewer exercises, which are customized for the patient and targeted to achieve collaboratively agreed-on goals, have the greatest likelihood of achieving compliance (16,96). An important point to remember is that as complexity increases compliance decreases. The patients should always feel as if the program is being individually tailored to meet their needs (74). Whereas fearful patients require regular reassurance of an exercise's safety to improve confidence and self-efficacy, less fearful patients need exercises to be moderately challenging to maintain interest (96,136). This can be used to identify entry level exercises as well as determine when it is appropriate to progress a patient. It is important to keep the less fearful patient sufficiently challenged to avoid boring the patients while at the same time being sure they are performing exercises with the necessary control to isolate the "deep" stabilizer muscles.

Objectification of functional deficits and activity intolerances is a key tool in motivating patients (5,100,122,136,150,151). Simple, reliable, low-tech tests of muscular endurance are ideal for quantifying the patient's percent normal of various physical capacities such as squatting, trunk flexion, or trunk extension endurance. Because there is such a large normal range with these tests, they are more appropriate for getting a patient started than actually monitoring their progress. Functional disability or activity intolerances questionnaires are preferable for monitoring progress over time because they are not only reliable but also responsive to clinically significant change over time (160).

Focusing patients on function rather than pain is an important first step. Then, baseline levels of functional impairment, pain distribution, and intensity, and level of disability should be quantified. These quantifiable baselines can be used to track the patient's progress objectively. Treatment should be guided by the results of the objective, functional capacity evaluation. Progress can be monitored at regular intervals (every 2 to 4 weeks) to give the patient accurate feedback of how they are improving. As the patient sees their walking and sitting tolerance go up along with, for instance, their number of trunk curls, this will serve as positive reinforcement. Pretreatment and posttreatment checks of painful maneuvers (i.e., Kemp's test or lumbar flexion) or measurable functional deficits (i.e., strength, flexibility) is an excellent way to enhance compliance (Table 14.6).

Turk has suggested that 25% of patients fail to maintain exercise programs (160). Building confidence in the value of the exercises, keeping them challenging, customization, making them short and simple, and reinforcing the long-term goals to be achieved all contribute to consistency (41,86). Simple programs established collaboratively have the best chance of success. The goals should be oriented functionally and quota-based. Whenever possible, quantifiable feedback of progress should be used to motivate the patient to form new habits.

■ CONCLUSION

It is not easy getting patients to exercise, but the psychological literature suggests that biobehavioral reeducation can improve adherence, compliance, and motivation (86,164,165). In fact, evidence from controlled clinical trials has shown that biobehavioral strategies when combined with exercise programs improve compliance and outcomes (30,41,52, 55,56,83,95,101,103).

Establishing appropriate goals is a key to recovery from disability and prevention of chronic pain.

Table 14.6 Tips for Enhancing Compliance

- Education that hurt does not necessarily equal harm
- Education that fitness is key to prevention
- Make exercises simple enough to be done at home without significant equipment needs
- Link exercises to specific functional deficits/goals
- Encourage patients to work at an exercise level which is "somewhat hard" for them
- Establish realistic expectations such as "flare-ups" are not unexpected nor do they suggest failure

Appropriate goals include: controlling pain, learning how to modify activities (i.e., sitting or lifting advice), reducing activity limitations (i.e., sitting, standing, walking intolerances), return to work, and beginning an exercise program. These goals once collaberatively established should lead to discussion of the means to reach those goals. This is a form of contract negotiation and the patient should realize that to achieve the goals requires adherence to a certain regimen. Additionally, relapse is something to expect and thus not be viewed as a failure of the program, but rather another opportunity to learn self-management techniques.

A report of findings that is patient-centered involves giving promising advice about how to return individuals to their chosen activities. Most patients who are prone to chronicity have significant fears and worries about their future capabilities. Such patients concerns should be identified early on and addressed through ongoing reassuring reactivation advice. Unfortunately, treatments which create physician dependency and do not promote self-management skills undermine this goal.

Audit Process
Self-Check of the Chapter's Learning Objectives

- What are patient's expecting on the first visit?

- Can you prescribe activity modification advice that is spine sparing?

- Can you incorporate the core determinants of social cognitive theory into your approach to motivating patients to engage in active self-care?

- Can you give a report of findings that emphasizes the patient's role in recovery?

■ REFERENCES

1. Abenheim L, Rossignol M, Valat JP, et al. The role of activity in the therapeutic management of back pain: Report of the International Paris Task Force on Back Pain. Spine 2000;25:1S–33S.

2. Adams MA, Hutton WC. Gradual disc prolapse. Spine 1985;10:524–531.

3. Adams MA, Dolan P, Hutton WC. Diurnal variations in the stresses on the lumbar spine. Spine 1987;12:130.

4. Al-Obaidi SM, Nelson RM, Al-Awadhi S, Al-Shuwaie N. The role of anticipation and fear of pain in the persistence of avoidance behavior in patients with chronic low back pain. Spine 2000;25:1126–1131.

5. Alaranta H, Hurri H, Heliovaara M, et al. Non-dynamometric trunk performance tests: Reliability and normative data. Scand J Rehab Med 1994;26:211–215.

6. Aldrich S, Eccleston C, Crombez G. Worrying about chronic pain: Vigilance to threat and mis-directed problem solving. Behav Res Ther 2000;38:457–470.

7. Anderson RM. Patient empowerment and the traditional medical model: A case of irreconcilable differences? Diabetes Care 1995;18:412–415.

8. Andersson GB, Jonsson B, Ortengren R. Myoelectric activity in individual lumbar erector spinae muscles in sitting. A study with surface and wire electrodes. Scand J Rehabil Med 1974;3(suppl):19–108.

9. Andersson GB, Ortengren R, Nachemson AL, et al. The sitting posture: An electromyographic and discometric study. Orthop Clin North Am 1975;6:105–120.

10. Andersson GB, Murphy RW, Ortengren R, Nachemson AL. The influence of back rest inclination and lumbar support on lumbar lordosis. Spine 1979;4:52–58.

11. Andersson GBJ. Occupational Biomechanics. In: Wienstein JN, Wiesel SW, eds. The Lumbar Spine: The International Society for The Study of The Lumbar Spine. Philadelphia: WB Saunders, 1990:213.

12. Axen I, Rosenbarum A, Robech R, Wren T, Leboeuf-Yde C. Can patient reactions to the first chiropractic treatment predict early favorable treatment outcome in persistent low back pain? J Manipulative Physiol Ther 2002;25:450–454.

13. Balderson BHK, Von Korff M. The Stepped Care Approach to Chronic Back Pain. In: Linton SL, ed. New Avenues for The Prevention of Chronic Musculoskeletal Pain and Disability. Amsterdam: Elsevier, 2002.

14. Bandura A. The anatomy of stages of change. Am J Health Prom 1997;12:8–10.

15. Bandura A. Health promotion by social cognitive means. Health Education & Behavior 2004;31:143–164.

16. Bassett SF, Petrir KJ. The effect of treatment goals on patient compliance with physiotherapy exercise programs. Physiother 1999;85:130–137.

17. Biering-Sorensen F. Physical measurements as risk indicators for low-back trouble over a one-year period. Spine 1984;9:106–119.

18. Bigos S, Bowyer O, Braen G, et al. Acute low back problems in adults. Clinical Practice Guideline. Rockville, MD: U.S. Department of Health and Human Services, Public Health Service, Agency for Health Care Policy and Research, 1994.

19. Blair SN, et al. Influences of cardiorespiratory fitness and other precursors on cardiovascular disease and all-cause mortality in men and women. JAMA 1996;276:205–210.

20. Blyth FM, March LM, Nicholas MK, Cousins MJ. Self-management of chronic pain: A population-based study. Pain 2005;113:285–292.

21. Bogduk N, Twomney L. Clinical Anatomy of the Lumbar Spine and Sacrum, 3rd ed. Edinburgh: Churchill Livingston, 1997.

22. Bogduk N. What's in a name? The labeling of back pain. Med J Austral 2000;173:400–401.

23. Borchgrevink GE, Kaasa A, McDonoagh D, et al. Acute treatment of whiplash neck sprain injuries. Spine 1998;23:25–31.

24. Borenstein DG, O'Mara JW, Boden SD, et al. The value of magnetic resonance imaging of the lumbar spine to predict low-back pain in asymptomatic subjects. J Bone and Joint Surg 2001;83-A:1306–1311.

25. Borkan JM, Cherkin DC. An agenda for primary care research on low back pain. Spine 1986;21:2880–2884.

26. Buchbinder R, Jolley D, Wyatt M. 2001 Volvo Award Winner in Clinical Studies: Effects of a media campaign on back pain beliefs and its potential influence on management of low back pain in general practice. Spine 2001;26:2535–2542.

27. Buchbinder R, Jolley D. Population based intervention to change back pain beliefs: Three-year follow-up population survey. Br Med J 2004;328: 321–323.

28. Buer N, Linton SJ. Fear-avoidance beliefs and catastrophizing: Occurrence and risk factor in back pain and ADL in the general population. Pain 2002;99: 485–491.

29. Burke B, Arkowitz H, Dunn C. The Efficacy of Motivational Interviewing and Its Adaptions: What We Know So Far. In: Miller W, Rollnick S, eds. Motivational Interviewing: Preparing People to Change, 2nd ed. New York: Guilford Press, 2002:217–250.

30. Burton K, Waddell G. Information and advice to patients with back pain can have a positive effect. Spine 1999;24:2484–2491.

31. Butler D, Moseley L. Explain Pain. Adelaide, Australia: Noigroup Publications, 2003.

32. Callaghan JP, Patla AE, McGill SM. Low back three-dimensional joint forces, kinematics and kinetics during walking. Clin Biomech 1999;14:203–216.

33. Callaghan J, McGill SM. Intervertebral disc herniation: Studies on a porcine spine exposed to highly repetitive flexion/extension motion with compressive force. Clin Biomech 2001;16:28–37.

34. Carragee EJ, Barcohana B, Alamin T, van den Haak E. Prospective controlled study of the development of lower back pain in previously asymptomatic subjects undergoing experimental discography. Spine 2004;29:1112–1117.

35. Carroll L, Mercado AC, Cassidy JD, Cote P. A population-based study of factors associated with combinations of active and passive coping with neck and low back pain. J Rehabil Med 2002;34:67–72.

36. Casper J, Berg K. Effects of exercise on osteoarthritis: A review. J Strength Condition Res 1998; 12:120–125.

37. Cherkin DC, Deyo RA, Berg AO. Evaluation of a physician education intervention to improve primary care for low back pain: 2 Impact on patients. Spine 1991;16:1173–1178.

38. Cherkin DC, Deyo RA, Street JH, Barlow W. Predicting poor outcomes for back pain seen in primary care using patients' own criteria. Spine 1996;21: 2900–2907.

39. Cherkin DC, Deyo RA, Street JH, Hunt M, Barlow W. Pitfalls of patient education. Limited success of a program for back pain in primary care. Spine 1996;21:345–355.

40. Christmas C, Andersen RA. Exercise and older patients: Guidelines for the clinician. J Am Geriatr Soc 2000;48:318–324.

41. Cook FM, Hassenkamp AM. Active rehabilitation for chronic low back pain: The patient's perspective. Physiother 2000;86:61–68.

42. Council JR, Ahern DK, Follick MJ, Kline CL. Expectancies and functional impairment in chronic low back pain. Pain 1988;33:323–331.

43. Coury HJCG. Self-administered preventive program for sedentary workers: Reducing musculoskeletal symptoms or increasing awareness? Applied Ergonomics 1998;29:415–421.

44. Croft PR, Macfarlane GJ, Papageorgiou AC, Thomas E, Silman AJ. Outcome of low back pain in general practice: a prospective study. Br Med J 1998;316: 1356–1359.

45. Crombez G, Vlaeyen JW, Heuts PH, et al. Pain-related fear is more disabling than pain itself: Evidence on the role of pain-related fear in chronic back pain disability. Pain 1999;80:329–339.

46. Danish Health Technology Assessment (DIHTA). Manniche C, et al. Low back pain: Frequency Management and Prevention from an HAD Perspective, 1999.

47. Deyo RA, Diehl AK, Rosenthal M: How many days of bed rest for acute low back pain? N Engl J Med 1986;315:1064.

48. Deyo RA. Low-back pain. Sci Am 1998;279:48–53.

49. Djijkdstra A, Vlaeyen JWS, Rijnen H, Nielson W. Readiness to adopt the self-management approach to cope with chronic pain in fibromyalgic patients. Pain 2001;90:37–46.

50. Elley CR, Kerse N, Arroll B, Robinson E. Effectiveness of counseling patients on physical activity in general practice: Cluster randomized controlled trial. BMJ 2003;326:793.

51. Flynn T, Fritz, J, Whitman J, et al. A clinical prediction rule for classifying patients with low back pain who demonstrate short-term improvement with spinal manipulation [Exercise Physiology and Physical Exam]. Spine 2002;27:2835–2843.

52. Fordyce WE, Brockway JA, Bergman JA, Spengler D. Acute back pain: A control-group comparison of behavioral vs traditional management methods. J Behav Med 1986;9:127–140.

53. Fritz JM, George SZ. Identifying psychosocial variables in patients with acute work-related low back pain: The importance of fear-avoidance beliefs. Phys Ther 2002;82:973–983.

54. Fritz JM, Delitto A, Erhard RE. Comparison of classification-based physical therapy with therapy based on clinical practice guidelines for patients with acute low back pain: A randomized clinical trial. Spine 2003;28:1363–1371.

55. Frost H, Lamb S, Klaber Moffett JA, Faribank JCT, Moser JS. A fitness program for patients with chronic low back pain: Two-year follow-up of a randomized controlled trial. Pain 1998;75:273–279.

56. Frost H, Lamb SE, Shackleton CH. A functional restoration program for chronic low back pain: A prospective outcome study. Physiother 2000;86: 285–293.

57. Garg A, Herrin G. Stoop or squat: A biomechanical and metabolic evaluation. Am Inst Indus Eng Trans 1979;11:293–302.

58. Gordon SJ, Yang KH, Mayer PJ, et al. Mechanism of disc rupture-a preliminary report. Spine 1991;16:450–456.

59. Goubert L, Francken G, Crombez G, Vansteenwegen D, Lysens R. Exposure to physical movement in chronic back pain patients: No evidence for generalization across different movements. Behav Res Ther 2002;40:415–429.

60. Grandjean E. Fitting The Task to The Man, 4th ed. London: Taylor and Francis, 1988.

61. Grimshaw JM, Russell IT. Effect of clinical guidelines on medical practice: A systematic review of rigorous evaluations. Lancet 1993;342:1317–1322.

62. Groth GN, Wulf MB. Compliance with hand rehabilitation: Health beliefs and strategies. J Hand Ther 1995;8:18–22.

63. Gunning J, Callaghan JP, McGill SM. The role of prior loading history and spinal posture on the compressive tolerance and type of failure in the spine using a porcine trauma model. Clin Biomech 2001;16:471–480.

64. Guzman J, Esmail R, Karjaleinan K, Malmivaara A, Irvin E, Bombardier C. Multidisciplinary rehabilitation for chronic low back pain: A systematic review. Br Med J 2001;322:1511–1515.

65. Hagen KB, Hilde G, Jamtvedt G, Winnem MF. The Cochrane review of bed rest for acute low back pain and sciatica. Spine 2000;25:2932–2939.

66. Hahne A, Keating JL, Wilson S. Do within-session changes in pain intensity and range of motion predict between-session changes in patients with low back pain. Aust J Physiother 2004;50:17–23.

67. Hamilton N. Source document position as it affects head position and neck muscle tension. Ergonomics 1996;39:593–610.

68. Harding V, Williams AC. Extending physiotherapy skills using a psychological approach: Cognitive-Behavioural management of chronic pain. Physiother 1995;81:681–687.

69. Harding VR, Simmonds MJ, Watson PJ. Physical therapy for chronic pain. Pain—Clinical Updates. Int Assoc Study Pain 1998;6:1–4.

70. Harris JS, Glass LS. Occupational Medicine Practice Guidelines: Evaluation and Management of Common Health Problems and Functional Recovery in Workers, 2nd ed. Beverly Farms, MA: OEM Press, 2003.

71. Hasenbring M. Attentional Control of Pain and The Process of Chronification. Progress in Brain Research. Amsterdam: Elsevier, 2000;129:525–534.

72. Hazard RG, Reid S, Haugh LD, McFarlane G. A controlled trial of an educational pamphlet to prevent disability after occupational low back injury. Spine 2000;25:1419–1423.

73. Hebert J, Ebbeling C, Ockene I, et al. A dietitian-delivered group nutrition program leads to reductions in dietary fat, serum cholesterol, and body weight: The Worcester Area Trial for Counseling in Hyperlipidemia (WATCH). J Am Diet Assoc 1999;99:544–552.

74. Henry KD, Rosemond C, Eckert LB. Effect of number of home exercises on compliance and performance in adults over 65 years of age. Phys Ther 1999;79:270–277.

75. Heuts PHTG, Vlaeyen JWS, Roelofs J, et al. Pain-related fear and daily functioning in patients with osteoarthritis. Pain 2004;110:228–235.

76. Hickey DS, Hukins DWL. Relation between the structure of the annulus fibrosis and the function and failure of the intervertebral disc. Spine 1980;5:106–116.

77. Hides JA, Jull GA, Richardson CA. Long-term effects of specific stabilizing exercises for first-episode low back pain. Spine 2001;26:e243–e248.

78. Holman H, Lorig K. Patient self-management: A key to effectiveness and efficiency in care of chronic disease. Public Health Rep 2004;119:239–243.

79. Holman H. Chronic disease—the need for a new clinical education. JAMA 2004;292:1057–1059.

80. Houben RMA, Ostelo RWJG, Vlaeyen JWS, Wolters PMJC, Peters M, Stom-van den Berg SGM. Health care providers' orientations towards common low back pain predict perceived harmfulness of physical activities and recommendations regarding return to normal activity. Eur J Pain 2005;9:175–183.

81. Hussein TM, Simmonds MJ, Olson SL, et al. Kinematics of gait in normal and low back pain subjects. Boston, MA: American Congress of Sports Medicine 45th Annual Meeting, 1998.

82. Hussein TM, Simmonds MJ, Etnyre B, et al. Kinematics of gait in subjects with low back pain with and without leg pain. Washington, DC: Scientific Meeting & Exposition of the American Physical Therapy Association, 1999.

83. Indahl A, Velund L, Eikeraas O. Good prognosis for low back pain when left untampered: A randomized clinical trial. Spine 1995;20:473–477.

84. Itoi E, Sinaki M. Effect of back-strengthening exercise on posture in healthy women 49 to 65 years of age. Mayo Clin Proc 1994;69:1054–1059.

85. Jensen BR, Schibye B, Sogaard K, Simonsen EB, Sjogarrd G. Shoulder muscle load and muscle fatigue among industrial sewing machine operators. Eur J Applied Physiol 1993;6:467–475.

86. Jensen GM, Lorish CD. Promoting patient co-operation with exercise programs: Linking research, theory and practice. Arthritis Care and Research 1994;7:181–189.

87. Jensen MP, Nielson WR, Kerns RD. Toward the development of a motivational model of pain self-management. J Pain 2003;4;477–492.

88. Jensen MP, Nielson WR, Turner JA, Romano JM, Hill ML. Readiness to self-manage pain is associated with coping and with psychological and physical functioning among patients with chronic pain. Pain 2003;104:529–537.

89. Jensen MP, Nielson WR, Kerns RD. Toward the development of a motivational model of pain self-management. J Pain 2003;4:477–492.

90. Jensen MP, Nielson WR, Turner JA, Romano JM, Hill ML. Changes in readiness to self-manage pain are associated with improvement in multidiscipli-

nary pain treatment and pain coping. Pain 2004;111: 84–95.

91. Jull GA. Deep cervical flexor muscle dysfunction in whiplash. J Musculoskel Pain 2000;8:143–154.

92. Jull G, Trott P, Potter H, et al. A randomized control trial of physiotherapy management of cervicogenic headache. Spine 2002;27:1835–1843.

93. Keller A, Brox JI, Gunderson R, Holm I, Friss A, Reikeras O. Trunk muscle strength, cross-sectional area, and density in patients with chronic low back pain randomized to lumbar fusion or cognitive intervention and exercises. Spine 2003;29:3–8.

94. Kendall NAS, Linton SJ, Main CJ. Guide to assessing psychosocial yellow flags in acute low back pain: Risk factors for long-term disability and work loss. Wellington, NZ: Accident Rehabilitation & Compensation Insurance Corporation of New Zealand and the National Health Committee, 1997. Available at http://www.nhc.govt.nz.

95. Klaber Moffet J, Torgerson D, Bell-Syer S, et al. A randomized trial of exercise for primary care back pain patients: Clinical outcomes, costs and preferences. Br Med J 1999;319:279–283.

96. Klaber Moffett J. Pain: Perception and Attitudes in Topical Issues in Pain 2: Biopsychosocial Assessment and Management—Relationships and Pain. In: Gifford L, ed. Cornwall: CNS Press, 2000.

97. Klenerman L, Slade P, Stanley I, et al. The prediction of chronicity in patients with an acute attack of low back pain in a general practice setting. Spine 1995;20:478–484.

98. Lackner JM, Carosella AM, Feuerstein M. Pain expectancies, pain, and functional self-efficacy expectancies as determinants of disability in patients with chronic low back disorders. J Consult Clin Psych 1996;64:212–220.

99. Lamoth CJC, Meijer OG, Wuisman PIJM, van Dieën J H, Levin MF, Beek PJ. Pelvis-thorax coordination in the transverse plane during walking in persons with nonspecific low back pain. Spine 2002;27: E92–E99.

100. Liebenson CS. Improving activity tolerance in pain patients: A cognitive-behavioral approach to reactivation. Top Clin Chiropr 2000;7:6–14.

101. Lindstrom A, Ohlund C, Eek C, et al. Activation of subacute low back patients. Phys Ther 1992;4: 279–293.

102. Linton SJ. The relationship between activity and chronic back pain. Pain 1985;21:289–294.

103. Linton SL, Hellsing AL, Andersson D. A controlled study of the effects of an early active intervention on acute musculoskeletal pain problems. Pain 1993;54:353–359.

104. Linton SJ, Andersson T. Can chronic disability be prevented? A randomized trial of a cognitive-behavioral intervention for spinal pain patients. Spine 2000;25:2825–2831.

105. Linton SJ. Cognitive-behavioral therapy in the early treatment and prevention of chronic pain: A therapist's manual for groups. Örebro: 2000.

106. Linton SJ, Buer N, Vlaeyen J, Hellsing AL. Are fear-avoidance beliefs related to a new episode of back pain? A prospective study. Psychol Health 2000;14: 1051–1059.

107. Linton SJ, Ryberg M. A cognitive-behavioral group intervention as prevention for persistent neck and back pain in a non-patient population: A randomized controlled trial. Pain 2001;90:83–90.

108. Linton SJ. Cognitive Behavioral Therapy in The Prevention of Musculoskeletal Pain: Description of a Program. In: Linton SL, ed. New Avenues for The Prevention of Chronic Musculoskeletal Pain and Disability. Amsterdam: Elsevier, 2002.

109. Little P, Roberts L, Blowers H, et al. Should we give detailed advice and information booklets to patients with back pain? A randomized controlled factorial trial of a self-management booklet and doctor advice to take exercise for back pain. Spine 2001;26: 2065–2072.

110. Long A, Donelson R, Fung T. Does it matter which exercise? Spine 2004;29:2593–2602.

111. Lorig KR, Mazonson PD, Holman HR. Evidence suggesting that health education for self-management in patients with chronic arthritis has sustained health benefits while reducing health care costs. Arthritis and Rheumatism 1993;36:439–446.

112. Lorig KR, Holman H. Self-management education: History, definition, outcomes, and mechanisms. Ann Behav Med. 2003;26:1–7.

113. Main CJ, Watson PJ. Psychological aspects of pain. Man Ther 1999;4:203–215.

114. Malmivaara A, Hakkinen U, Aro T, et al. The treatment of acute low back pain—bed rest, exercises, or ordinary activity? N Engl J Med 1995;332:351–355.

115. Marhold C, Linton SJ, Melin L. Cognitive behavioral return-to-work program: Effects on pain patients with a history of long-term versus short-term sick leave. Pain 2001;91:155–163.

116. McGill SM, Brown. Creep response of the lumbar spine to prolonged full flexion. Clin Biomech 1992;7: 43–46.

117. McGill SM, Norman RW. Low Back Biomechanics in Industry: The Prevention of Injury Through Safer Lifting. In: Grabiner M, ed. Current Issues in Biomechanics. Champaign, IL: Human Kinetics, 1993.

118. McGill SM. Low Back Exercises: Prescription for The Healthy Back and When Recovering From Injury. Resources Manual for Guidelines for Exercise Testing and Prescription, 3rd ed. Lippincott, Williams & Wilkins: Indianapolis, 1998.

119. McGill SM. Low Back Disorders: The Scientific Foundation for Prevention and Rehabilitation. Champaign, IL: Human Kinetics, 2002.

120. McKinney LA. Early mobilization and outcome in acute sprains of the neck. BMJ 1989;299:1006.

121. Melzack R, Wall PD. Pain mechanisms: A new theory. Science 1965;150:978.

122. Moffett JK, Frost H. Back to fitness program: The manual for physiotherapists to set up classes. Physiother 2000;86:295–305.

123. Moore JE, Von Korff M, Cherkin D, et al. A randomized trial of a cognitive-behavioral program for enhancing back pain self-care in a primary care setting. Pain 2000;88:145–153.

124. NIH. Physical activity and cardiovascular health. NIH Consensus Development Panel on Physical

Activity and Cardiovascular Health. JAMA. 1996;276:241–246.

125. Newman S, Steed L, Mulligan K. Self-management interventions for chronic illness. Lancet 2004;364: 1523–1537.

126. Nicholas MK. Reducing Disability in Injured Workers: The Importance of Collaborative Management. In: Linton SL, ed. New Avenues for The Prevention of Chronic Musculoskeletal Pain and D. Amsterdam: Elsevier, 2002.

127. Nordin M. Self-care techniques for acute episodes of low back pain. Best Practice & Research. Clin Rheumatol 2002;16:89–104.

128. Ockene J, Quirk M, Goldberg R, et al. A residents' training program for the development of smoking intervention skills. Arch Intern Med 1988;148: 1039–1045.

129. Ockene J, Kristeller J, Goldberg R, et al. Increasing the efficacy of physician-delivered smoking interventions: A randomized clinical trial. J Gen Intern Med 1991;6:1–8.

130. Ockene J, Zapka J. Physician-based smoking intervention: A rededication to a five-step strategy to smoking research. Addict Behav 1997;22:835–848.

131. Ockene J, Adams A, Hurley T, Wheeler E, Hebert J. Brief physician- and nurse practitioner-delivered counseling for high-risk drinkers: Does it work? Arch Intern Med 1999;159:2198–2205.

132. Ockene J, Hebert J, Ockene G, et al. Effect of physician-delivered nutrition counseling training and an office-support program on saturated fat intake, weight, and serum lipid measurements in a hyperlipidemic population: Worcester Area Trial for Counseling in Hyperlipidemia (WATCH). Arch Intern Med 1999;159:725–731.

133. Ortiz D, Smith R. Ergonomic Considerations in Rational Manual Therapies Ed. Basmajian JV, Nyberg R. Baltimore, MD: Williams and Wilkins, 1993:441–450.

134. Ostelo RWJG, de Vet JCW, Vlaeyen JWS, et al. Behavioral graded activity following first-time lumbar disc surgery. Spine 2003;28:1757–1765.

135. Ostelo RWJG, Stomp-van den berg SGM, Vlaeyen JWS, Wolters PMJC, de Vet HCW. Health care providers' attitudes and beliefs towards chronic low back pain: the development of a questionnaire. Man Ther 2003;8:214–222.

136. Paley C. A way forward for determining optimal aerobic exercise intensity? Physiother 1997;83: 620–624.

137. Prochaska J, DiClemente C. The Transtheoretical Approach: Crossing Traditional Boundaries of Therapy. Homewood, IL: Dow Jones Irwin, 1984.

138. Rainville J, Carlson N, Polatin P, Gatchel RJ, Indahl, A. Exploration of physicians' recommendations for activities in chronic low back pain. Spine 2000;25:2210–2220.

139. Reilly T, Tynell A, Troup JDG. Circadian variation in the human stature. Chronobiology It 1984;1:121.

140. Ren K, Dubner R. Descending modulation in persistent pain: An update. Pain 2002;100:1–6.

141. Roland M, Waddell G, Moffett JK, Burton K, Main C, Cantrell T. The Back Book. London: The Stationary Office, 1996.

142. Rosal M, Ebbeling C, Lofgren I, Ockene I, Hebert J. Facilitating dietary change: The patient-centered counseling model. J Am Diet Assoc 2001;101: 332–341.

143. Rosenfeld M, Gunnarsson R, Borenstein P. Early intervention in whiplash-associated disorders: A comparison of two treatment protocols. Spine 2000;25:1782–1787.

144. Sato H, Ohashi J, Owanga K, et al. Endurance time and fatigue in static contractions. J Human Ergol 1984;3:147–154.

145. Schuldt K, Ekholm J, Harms-Ringdahl K, et al. Effects of changes in sitting work posture on static neck and shoulder muscle activity. Ergonomics 1986;29:1525–1537.

146. Scotland's Working Backs Partnership. Working Backs Scotland, www.workingbacksscotland.com, 2000.

147. Shaw WS, Pransky G, Fitzgerald TE. Early prognosis for low back disability: Intervention strategies for health care providers. Disabil Rehabil 2001;23: 815–828.

148. Shaw WS, Feuerstein M, Huang GD. Secondary Prevention in The Workplace. In: Linton SL, ed. New Avenues for The Prevention of Chronic Musculoskeletal Pain and Disability. Amsterdam: Elsevier, 2002.

149. Simpson M, Buckman R, Stewart M, et al. Doctor-patient communication: The Toronto consensus statement. Br Med J 1991;303:1385–1387.

150. Slujis EM, Knibbe JJ. Patient compliance with exercise. Patient Education Counseling 1991;17:191–204.

151. Slujis EM, Kik GJ, van de Zee J. Correlates of exercise compliance in physical therapy. Phys Ther 1993;73:771–782.

152. Smith BH, Elliot AM. Active self-management of chronic pain in the community. Editorial. Pain 2005;113:249–250.

153. Snook SH, Webster BS, McGorry RW, Fogleman MT, McCann KB. The reduction of chronic non-specific low back pain through the control of early morning lumbar flexion. Spine 1998;23: 2601–2607.

154. Snook SH. Self-care guidelines for the management of non-specific low back pain. J Occup Rehab 2004;14:243–253.

155. Solomonow M, Hatipkarasulu S, Zhou B, Baratta RV, Aghazadeh F. Biomechanics and EMG of a common idiopathic low back disorder. Spine 2003:28:1235–1248.

156. Sparto PJ, Paarnianpour M, Reinsel TE, Simon S. The effect of fatigue on multijoing kinematics and load sharing during a repetitive lifting test. Spine 1997;22:2647–2654.

157. Stankovic R, Johnell O. Conservative treatment of acute low-back pain. A prospective randomized trial. McKenzie method of treatment versus patient education in "mini back school." Spine 1990;15: 120–123.

158. Stauber WT. Factors involved in strain-induced injury in skeletal muscles and outcomes of prolonged exposures. J Electromyography 2004;14:61–70.

159. Stig LC, Nilsson O, Lefoeuf-Yde C. Recovery pattern of patients treated with chiropractic spinal manipu-

lative therapy for long lasting or recurrent low back pain. J Manipulative Physiol Ther 2001;24:288–291.

160. Stratford PW, Binkley J. Applying the results of self-report measures to individual patients: An example using the Roland-Morris Questionnaire. J Orthop Sports Phys Ther 1999;29:232–239.

161. Sullivan MD. Finding pain between minds and bodies. Clin J Pain 2001;17:146–156.

162. Troup JDG. The perception of musculoskeletal pain and incapacity for work: Prevention and early treatment. Physiother 1988;74:435–439.

163. Turner JA. Educational and behavioral interventions for back pain in primary care. Spine 1996;21:2851–2859.

164. Turk DC, Rudy TE. Neglected topics in the treatment of chronic pain patients—relapse, noncompliance, and adherence enhancement. Pain 1991;44:5–28.

165. Turk DC. Commentary on correlates of exercise compliance in physical therapy. 1993;73:783–784.

166. Van den Hout JHC, Vlaeyen JWS, Kole-Snijders AMJ, Heuts PHTG, Willen JEHL, Sillen WJT. Graded activity and problem solving therapy in sub-acute non-specific low back pain. Physiother 1998;84:167.

167. Van den Haut JHC, Vlaeyen JWS. Problem-Solving Therapy and Behavioral Graded Activity in The Prevention of Chronic Pain Disability. In: Linton SL, ed. New Avenues for The Prevention of Chronic Musculoskeletal Pain and Disability. Amsterdam: Elsevier, 2002.

168. Veiersted KB, Westgaard RH, Andersen P. Pattern of muscle activity during stereotyped work and its relation to muscle pain. Internat Arch Occup Environ Health 1990;62:31–41.

169. Vlaeyen JWS, Crombez G. Fear of movement/(re)injury, avoidance and pain disability in chronic low back pain patients. Man Ther 1999;4:187–195.

170. Vlaeyen JWS, De Jong J, Geilen M, Heuts PHTG, Van Breukelen G. Graded exposure in the treatment of pain-related fear: A replicated single case experimental design in four patients with chronic low back pain. Behav Res Ther 2001;39:151–166.

171. Vlaeyen JWS, Morley S. Active despite pain: The putative role of stop-rules and current mood. Pain 2004;110:512–516.

172. Von Korff M. Collaborative care. Ann Intern Med 1997;127:187–195.

173. Von Korff M, Moore JE, Lorig K, et al. A randomized trial of a lay-led self-management group intervention for back pain patients in primary care. Spine 1998;23:2608–2615.

174. Von Korff, Balderson BHK, Saunders K, et al. A trial of an activating intervention for chronic back pain in primary care and physical therapy settings. Pain 2005;1113:323–330.

175. Vowles KE, Gross RT. Work-related beliefs about injury and physical capability for work in individuals with chronic pain. Pain 2003;101:291–298.

176. Waddell G. A new clinical model for the treatment of low back pain. Spine 1987;12:634.

177. Waddell G, Newton M, Henderson I, et al. A fear-avoidance beliefs questionnaire (FABQ) and the role of fear-avoidance beliefs in chronic low back pain and disability. Pain 1993;52:157–168.

178. Waddell G. The Back Pain Revolution, 2nd ed. Edinburgh: Churchill Livingstone, 2004.

179. Waddell G, McIntosh A, Hutchinson A, Feder G, Lewis M. Low back Pain Evidence Review. London: Royal College of General Practitioners (www.rcgp.org.uk), 1999.

180. Waddell G, Burton AK. Occupational health guidelines for the management of low back pain at work—evidence review. London: Faculty of Occupational Medicine, 2000.

181. Walsh DA, Radcliffe JC. Pain beliefs and perceived physical disability of patients with chronic low back pain. Pain 2002;97:23–31.

182. Weinstein JN. The missing piece: Embracing shared decision making to reform health care. Spine 2000;25:1–4.

183. Wilder DG, Aleksiev AR, Magnusson ML, Pope MH, Spratt KF, Goel VK. Muscular response to sudden load. A tool to evaluate fatigue and rehabilitation. Spine 1996;21:2628–2639.

184. Williams ACdeC, Nicholas MK, Richardson PH, Pither CE, Fernandes J. Generalizing from a controlled trial: The effects of patient preference versus randomization on the outcome of inpatient versus outpatient chronic pain management. Pain 1999;83:57–65.

15

McKenzie Spinal Rehabilitation Methods

Gary Jacob, Robin McKenzie, and Steve Heffner

Introduction

The Three Syndrome Patterns and Explanations

Postural Syndrome

Dysfunction Syndrome

Derangement Syndrome

Acute Spinal Antalgia Paradigms of McKenzie Method Derangement Management

Kyphotic Antalgia Management—Extension Principle—Posterior Derangement

Acute Coronal Antalgia Management: Lateral-Then-Extension Principle—Relevant Postero-Lateral Derangement

Acute Lordotic Antalgic Management—Flexion Principle—Anterior Derangement

Learning Objectives

After reading this chapter you should be able to understand

- McKenzie Method descriptions of patterns of mechanical and symptomatic responses to movement and positioning
- McKenzie Method classification of mechanical and symptomatic response patterns into three syndromes: the postural, dysfunction, and derangement syndromes
- McKenzie Method pathoanatomical explanations of the syndrome patterns
- Management of the postural, dysfunction, and derangement syndromes

Introduction

The goal of rehabilitation is independence in self-care. To serve that purpose, spinal rehabilitation promotes self-efficacy. However, such efforts are often delayed when clinicians provide passive, palliative comfort care while waiting for things to "calm down" before the "good stuff" (rehabilitation) is introduced. The combined fears of patient and practitioner may be roadblocks to the exploration of patient self-generated movements for therapeutic purposes. The specter of dependency and deconditioning of physique and psyche is raised when patients are passive receptacles of care. Any delay in patient active participation is a delay in developing patient empowerment through self-management skills, the ultimate goal of rehabilitation.

This chapter introduces McKenzie Method management of common lower cervical and lower lumbar spinal symptoms, which uses patient-generated movements for acute and chronic symptoms. Whether acute or chronic, McKenzie Method concepts and skills promote independence in self-care from day one, without passive therapy detours on the rehabilitation road to recovery. The McKenzie Method educates patients regarding movement and positioning strategies that have the potential to rapidly ameliorate complaints if the practitioner and patient choose to make self-generated movement and positioning the centerpiece of care.

This chapter attempts to enrich the reader's appreciation of the conceptual foundations of the McKenzie Method to promote facility with its practical applications. Our consideration of McKenzie Method management of common lower cervical and lower lumbar symptoms is but a slice of the McKenzie Method "pie" and does not include appropriate McKenzie Method management of headaches, the extremities, adherent nerve root (epidural fibrosis), nerve root entrapment, and other conditions. Further study is encouraged by means of the texts authored by Robin McKenzie (5–7) and postgraduate study within the McKenzie Institute International (1). We close the chapter with only a brief consideration of the research literature and the reader is directed to the Literature Relevant to the McKenzie Method on the McKenzie Institute International web site (2) to peruse the expansive literature regarding the McKenzie Method.

The Three Syndrome Patterns and Explanations

The McKenzie Method recognizes three clinical patterns (syndromes) of mechanical and symptomatic responses to loading that are amenable to mechanical (movement and positioning) therapies. The constructs of these three syndromes occur on two levels. The first level is the description of phenomenological patterns of mechanical and symptomatic responses to spinal loading. The second level is the pathoanatomical explanations of those phenomenological patterns. The syndromes are named after the pathoanatomical explanations, but this should not detract from the phenomenological observations on which those explanations are based.

We first consider the phenomenological patterns (the what) of the syndromes, after which we consider the pathoanatomical models proposed to make sense of what occurs (the why). Phenomenology gives equal importance to subjective and objective data and resists temptations to conjecture what the pathoanatomical underpinnings are. A phenomenological accounting for mechanical and symptomatic responses to loading includes a meticulous description of objective phenomena that can be observed and measured by clinicians (ranges of motion, antalgic posturing, etc.) and subjective phenomenon reported by the patient (symptom location, frequency, quality, duration, provocations/palliations, etc.). Considering phenomenology before pathoanatomy permits a better appreciation of phenomena, permits the reader to posit his or her own pathoanatomical explanations to explain the why of what's going, and enables one to appreciate how McKenzie Method pathoanatomical explanations account for phenomenon.

The three syndrome patterns of mechanical and symptomatic responses to loading for which therapeutic movement and positioning strategies may be used are as follows.

1. The Postural Syndrome
2. The Dysfunction Syndrome
3. The Derangement Syndrome

Although the syndromes are named according to McKenzie Method pathoanatomical explanations, we will, for each syndrome, first consider how the patterns behave and then consider the explanation for those behaviors.

Postural Syndrome

Postural Syndrome: Phenomenological Pattern

Examination of the postural syndrome patient reveals full and pain-free range of motion. Symptoms are only elicited with sustained end range loading, a "finding" typically obtained from history versus the examination.

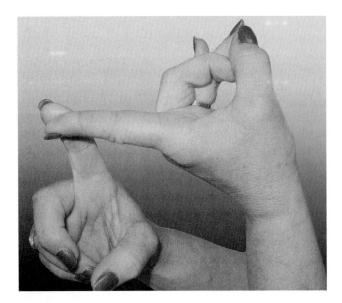

Figure 15.1 The bent finger.

Symptoms are intermittent because they only occur with sustained end range loading, a position typically only assumed intermittently. There are no responses at beginning or middle range. There is no practitioner-observed or patient-perceived range of motion loss or deviation from intended movement plane directions. There is no particular "curative" direction to load in.

It takes time for the end range loading to be provocative, i.e., the end range loading must be prolonged and static. The symptoms at the mechanically unimpeded end range are in response to an abnormal amount or (more commonly) duration of load at that end range.

Symptoms cease once the end range loading ceases. The reaction occurs only at the end range being loaded. Loading in other movement plane directions has no effect on the reaction at the mechanically unimpeded end range, nor does loading at the mechanically unimpeded end range affect other movement plane directions.

The remedy is to avoid loading at the provocative mechanically unimpeded end range, which eventually results in resolution of its symptomatic effects.

Although the postural syndrome can occur in any movement plane direction, the movement plane direction most commonly culpable for lower cervical and lower lumbar postural syndrome symptoms is flexion.

Postural Syndrome: Pathoanatomical Explanation

Postural syndrome patterns are the result of an excessive amount or duration of end range loading of normal articular containing or restraining elements. The solution is to avoid the excessive end range loading, i.e., to adopt new postural habits that do not challenge restraining or containing elements. Normal tissue can be symptomatic in response to abnormal forces without there having to be something wrong with the tissue. If the tissue is normal but the load is "wrong" (i.e., abnormal), symptoms may result.

The McKenzie Method uses the "bent finger" as a tool to educate about the postural syndrome (Fig. 15.1).

If a healthy finger is hyperextended far enough, an abnormal amount of force is brought to bear on normal structures, causing discomfort. If the finger were hyperextended to the point of pain and then backed off to the first point of no pain, sustaining that position over time would result in discomfort caused by the abnormal *duration* of force brought to bear on normal structures.

Postural Syndrome: Clinical Intervention

The most common postural syndrome provocateur for the lower cervical and lower lumbar spine is sustained flexion. For many, flexion is the most frequent posture assumed throughout the day as it is promoted with sitting slouched and other activities (Fig. 15.2).

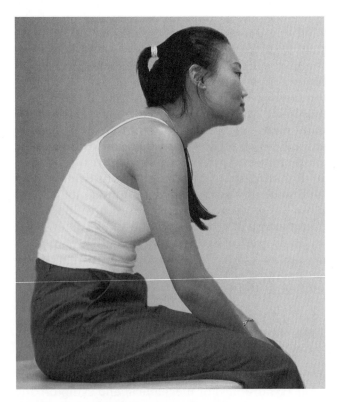

Figure 15.2 Slouched posture when sitting.

Sitting is frequently reported by patients to be causing, perpetuating, or aggravating lower cervical and lower lumbar symptoms. Reports of aggravation from sitting should raise suspicions that correction of sitting posture has clinical relevance. As a result of common relaxed slouched sitting, the upper cervical spine is at extension end range, whereas inferior spinal levels (i.e., the rest of the spine) are at as much flexion end range as slouched sitting position permits.

For the lower cervical and lower lumbar spine, aggravation from sustained flexion would cause one to consider the maintenance of lordosis (beginning range extension positioning) as a remedy. Considering the amount of time people spend sitting symptomatically slouched, McKenzie Method postural correction most often concerns correction of the slouched sitting posture. The McKenzie Method uses the slouch-overcorrect-relax strategy to help patients find appropriate lordotic sitting posture. The patient begins from the slouched, provocative sitting posture and then "overcorrects" by simultaneously hyper-extending the lumbar spine and hyper-retracting the head and neck. The patient then "lets go 10%" to find the neutral sitting posture (Fig. 15.3).

Postural syndrome principles are consistent with stabilization philosophies of avoiding excessive end range loading and remaining safe within a neutral zone. The postural syndrome theme may therefore be characterized as end range loathing.

Dysfunction Syndrome

Dysfunction Syndrome: Phenomenological Pattern

There is loss of range of motion with a new, premature, limited symptomatic end range being established. Loading at the premature, limited symptomatic end range results in a beneficial reaction at that end range only.

Repetitive loading at that end range results in no significant changes during the examination, other than a temporary increase in discomfort every time loading at the limited mechanically impeded end range occurs. It takes days, weeks, or months of repetitive mechanically impeded end range loading to achieve a beneficial effect. Benefit is not derived from avoiding any movement plane direction in particular.

The dysfunction syndrome pattern is one wherein loading at a mechanically impeded end range results in symptoms at that end range only, with symptoms ceasing once the end range loading ceases. The behavior (symptoms, range of motion) of the mechanically impeded end range does not substantially change in response to repetitive loading during the course of the examination. The reaction occurs at the same end range that is loaded. Movements in other movement plane directions have no effect on the reaction that occurs from loading at the mechanically impeded end range, nor does loading at the mechanically impeded end range affect the behavior of other movement plane directions.

Symptoms occur as soon as the mechanically impeded end range is reached. They are intermittent as they only occur at end range without responses to loading within the beginning or middle range in the same or other movement plane directions. Correction is achieved by loading at the mechanically impeded end range on a frequent basis.

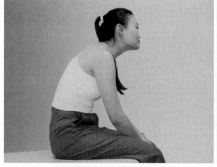
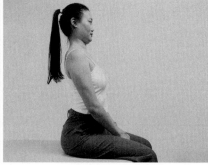
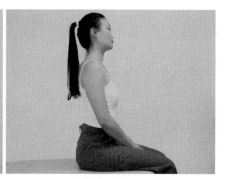

A   B   C

Figure 15.3 Slouched (**A**), overcorrect (**B**), let go 10% to neutral lordotic sitting (**C**).

Dysfunctions are named after the movement plane direction within which the mechanically impeded end range occurs.

Dysfunction Syndrome: Pathoanatomical Explanation

The model for the dysfunction syndrome is that of "short" tissue," i.e., tissue resistant to flexibility demands. It involves the adverse reaction of normal loads on abnormal tissue. The solution is to promote flexibility by means of frequent end range loading to remodel tissue. Improvement is increased flexibility, congruent with strategies to "stretch" or remodel short tissue.

Clinical Pearl

For the postural syndrome, the motto "if it hurts don't do it" applies; the remedy is to avoid loading at the symptomatic mechanically unimpeded end range. The principal is one of end range loathing. For the dysfunction syndrome, the motto "no pain no gain" applies; the remedy is to pursue loading at the symptomatic mechanically impeded end range. The principal is one of end range loading.

Dysfunction Syndrome: Clinical Intervention

Treatment of the dysfunction syndrome uses the remedy of "stretching."

For the McKenzie Method, an appreciation of how short tissue behaves is important to avoid treating short tissue that does not exist and to permit one to have greater success in identifying and treating short tissue when it does exist. Shortened muscular tissue is often the target of treatment when mechanical and symptomatic response patterns do not support the existence of the short tissue claimed. If the muscle is not "short," laboring toward making it long may not be prudent.

Clinical Pearl

Shortened tissue is often erroneously assumed to be the cause of symptoms. A careful evaluation often fails to demonstrate the expected painful loss of motion.

There are various terms used to describe muscle shortening, one of the most extreme being "spasm." Medically defined, spasm is the violent involuntary

sustained contraction of muscle that prohibits joint motion in the direction opposite the afflicted muscle's action. Therefore, if a particular muscle were claimed to be in spasm, that claim would predict a specific painful range of motion loss. Detection of the painful preclusion predicted by a specific spasm claimed would confirm that claim. When range of motion patterns fail to support the existence of the spasms claimed, or are the opposite of what is predicted, the clinical relevance of the claim can no longer be entertained.

Spinal antalgias are good examples of how spasm is inappropriately claimed. Consider the patient who presents with an acute lumbar kyphotic (Fig. 15.4) or the patient who presents with an acute lumbar scoliotic antalgia away from the side of pain (Fig. 15.5). It is not uncommon for these antalgias to be explained away as being caused by paravertebral muscle spasm despite the fact that the explanations predict antalgias opposite of the patient presentations.

Regarding kyphotic antalgia, paravertebral muscle spasm would result in fixed hyperextension of the spine, not the fixed flexion of kyphotic antalgia. Flexion positioning of the spine could not be attributed to spasms of muscles that extend the spine. For the acute left lumbar scoliotic antalgia away from a painful right side, right paravertebral muscle spasm is often blamed for the situation. Spasm of muscles to the right side of the spine would not permit an antalgia to the left but would result in an antalgia to the right. As these two cases demonstrate, discomfort localized to a muscle does not a spasm make.

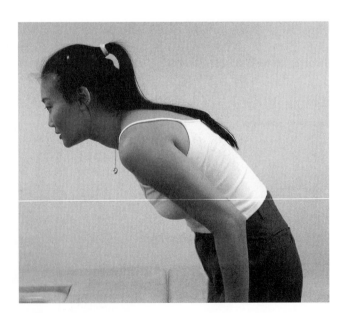

Figure 15.4 Lumbar kyphotic antalgia.

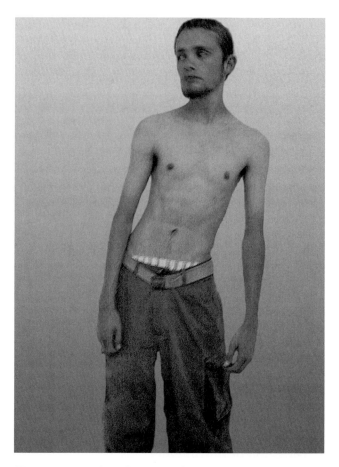

Figure 15.5 Left scoliotic antalgia.

Is the location of symptoms or palpation findings adequate to determine the presence of shortened muscular tissue? What other information might be important?

Other terms, such as hypertonicity, hyperactivity, contracture, scar, myofascitis, etc., are used to describe muscle shortening. These terms imply a lesser degree of shortening than spasm. With spasm, motion restriction is so great that the spine is "held" in the direction of the muscle action (pull) and neutral positioning cannot be achieved towards the movement plane direction opposite the muscles action (pull). With muscle shortening less severe than spasm, movement may be permitted beyond neutral, into the movement plane direction opposite the shortened muscle's pull, but a painful restriction is still predicted in that opposite direction. In summary, if a shortened muscle is culpable for symptoms, a specific painful range of motion restriction is predicted. Interventions designed to lengthen tissue have better outcomes when the short tissue targeted is really there.

Table 15.1 indicates the painful range of motion losses predicted if particular muscles were "short." One could not conclude that any of the listed muscles were short if the painful motion restrictions predicted did not exist or were the opposite of what is predicted.

When Dysfunction Syndrome patterns are identified, procedures are instituted to improve flexibility, i.e., a stretching routine is instituted. There are numerous ways to "stretch" inflexible spinal joint complexes and most conservative spinal care specialists have expertise regarding stretching instruction. The McKenzie Method uses "stretches" for dysfunctions that are the same end range movements used to "compress" derangements.

Derangement Syndrome

Derangement Syndrome: Phenomenological Pattern

A mechanically unimpeded end range is an end range of motion that is not restricted by mechanical factors.

Table 15.1   Predicted Painful Motion Restrictions Based on Particular Muscles Being Short

Muscle Shortened	Motion Painfully Restricted
Paravertebral	Flexion
Suboccipital	Cervical flexion and lateral flexion to opposite side
Upper trapezius	Cervical flexion, rotation to opposite side
SCM	Cervical extension, rotation to same side
Levator scapulae	Cervical flexion, rotation to opposite side
Rhomboids	Raising of the arm on the same side
QL	Lumbar flexion, lateral flexion to opposite side
Psoas	Thoracolumbar and hip extension
Piriformis	Hip adduction and internal rotation
Gluteus maximus	Hip flexion and internal rotation

Any loss of motion toward that end range would be caused by symptoms or factors other than mechanical factors. A mechanically impeded end range is a premature, early end range, before normal end range, caused by mechanical factors versus symptoms, and may be perceived by the patient to be a mechanical limitation (stiffness or obstruction) with or without pain.

For the Derangement Syndrome, excessive loading toward, or at a mechanically unimpeded end range increases symptoms and promotes a mechanically impeded end range in another direction. The promotion of instability in one direction promotes rigidity in another. Conversely, loading in the direction of rigidity diminishes that rigidity and also diminishes the provocative power of the direction without restriction. The reduction of rigidity in one direction decreases the instability in another. These are some of the most important McKenzie Method observations.

The Derangement Syndrome patterns are complex co-reactions between movement plane directions precipitated by loading at beginning range, middle range, and/or end range (the latter being mechanically impeded or not). Treatment strategies involve avoiding a detrimental mechanically unimpeded end range direction (end range loathing) while pursuing a beneficial mechanically impeded end range (end range "loading"). Symptoms may be intermittent or constant. Changes may be slow and temporary or rapid and maintained, i.e., there is a high degree of reactivity to loading.

Unique to derangements are constant symptoms and adverse mechanical and symptomatic responses during motion occurring in the direction of a detrimental mechanically unimpeded end range. Not only do adverse responses occur at the mechanically unimpeded end range, as with the postural syndrome, but they also occur during motion in the same movement plane direction as the mechanically unimpeded end range. In addition, symptoms may centralize (retreat toward the center of the body) or peripheralize (away from the center towards the periphery, often into the extremities). Centralization is an optimistic prognosticator even when it is associated with increased central symptoms. Peripheralization is a dire prognosticator even when it is associated with a relative diminution of the level of symptom intensity.

There are three derangement syndrome subtypes, each with a unique pattern of potential mechanical and symptomatic responses to loading. The difference between the three subtypes concerns the movement plane directions within which the responses occur. What they have in common is that they all involve at least one potential "direction of detriment" and one "direction of correction," the former being a mechanically unimpeded, the latter a mechanically impeded, end range. The term potential signifies that there are multiple possible mechanical and symptomatic responses to loading for each derangement syndrome subtype and that all of the potential responses may or may not be present. In other words, partial patterns may exist.

Practice-Based Problem:

When a patient presents acute, how does one determine the appropriateness or inappropriateness of movement and positioning therapies, including which end ranges to load at and which end ranges to avoid?

The full palette of potential derangement phenomena is described, below, concerning what can occur when loading in the direction of detriment and in the direction of correction. Two qualifiers must be mentioned. The patterns, as described, represent cases that are amenable to mechanical therapy. Cases not amenable to mechanical therapy would evidence a different pattern. In addition, the patterns, as described, may require a few repetitions of movement to become established and clearly displayed.

Direction of Detriment

- A mechanically unimpeded end range (MUER) movement plane direction
- Adverse mechanical and/or symptomatic responses during motion towards and/or at the MUER
  - Increased symptoms in the same movement plane direction
  - Promotion of a mechanically impeded end range in another movement plane direction.

Direction of Correction

- A mechanically impeded end range (MIER) movement plane direction
- No mechanical and/or symptomatic responses during motion
- Beneficial mechanical and symptomatic responses at the MIER only
  - Diminution of the MIER in the same movement plane direction
  - Diminution of the provocative power of the MUER direction of detriment

The three derangement subtypes are named according to conclusions about the pathoanatomical mechanism, i.e., according to the direction of movement of intradiscal nuclear Derangement that best explains the patient's mechanical and symptomatic responses to loading as follows.

1. Posterior derangements
2. Relevant posterolateral derangements
3. Anterior derangements

The examples considered for the three subtypes of derangements will be three spinal antalgias, which serve as excellent examples of derangements because all of the potential derangement features are present in these "extreme" cases.

An acute kyphotic antalgia (Fig. 15.4) would be an extreme example of a posterior derangement. An acute coronal antalgia (lumbar scoliosis or acute cervical torticollis) (Figs. 15.5 and 15.21) would be extreme example of a relevant posterolateral derangement. An acute lordotic antalgia (Fig. 15.24) would be an extreme example of an anterior derangement.

Derangement Syndrome: Pathoanatomical Explanation

Intradiscal nuclear derangement is the model used to explain the dramatic and long-lasting detrimental or beneficial responses to movement and positioning exhibited by lower cervical and lower lumbar derangement syndrome patterns.

The intradiscal nuclear derangement model considers compression rather than stretching forces to explain mechanical and symptomatic responses. Habitual loading in one movement plane direction compresses and displaces intradiscal nuclear material in another, often opposite, movement plane direction. Loading in directions that promote intradiscal derangement of nuclear material may cause adverse mechanical and symptomatic responses in the beginning, middle, and end range of that movement plane direction as the derangement progresses as movement progresses. The end range of the detrimental direction is mechanically unimpeded as intervertebral disc material has been displaced or "pushed out of the way," thus offering less resistance to compression of the intervertebral disc (approximation of vertebral end plates) in that direction.

The accumulation of displaced/deranged intradiscal nuclear material causes a painful obstruction to end range loading (mechanically impeded end range) in the movement plane direction it has deranged into. An example would be flexion causing derangement of intradiscal nuclear material posterior, which then obstructs (get in the way of) extension. The accumulated intradiscal nuclear material offers a

greater resistance to compressive forces (approximation of vertebral end plates). Mechanical and symptomatic responses in the movement plane direction within which the accumulated intradiscal nuclear material has deranged are not realized until the obstruction offered by that material is met, i.e., at the mechanically impeded end range. Mechanical and/or symptomatic responses do not occur *during motion* in the direction of the obstructed end range—the movement that caused the nuclear displacement is being avoided and the accumulated deranged nuclear material has yet to be encountered.

The remedy is to compress the accumulated deranged nuclear material (the obstruction to movement), to reduce the derangement, i.e., to send displaced nuclear material back from whence it came, i.e., to a more "central" intervertebral disc location.

As nuclear material migrates through posterior, lateral, or anterior annular tears, symptoms migrate in similar directions. If loading strategies cause nuclear material to migrate to a more central or peripheral location, the topography of symptoms follows suit. Changes in symptom location may be referred to as centralization and peripheralization, respectively. A response to loading involving an increase of central symptoms with diminution of peripheral symptoms (centralization) has a positive prognosis and is appreciated as reflecting the return of deranged intradiscal nuclear material to a more central location. As intradiscal nuclear material returns to a more central location, so do symptoms. As intradiscal nuclear material returns to a central, more confined, more highly pressurized environment, an increase of the intensity of central symptoms (at times, a pressure-type pain) may occur. A response to loading causing an increase of peripheral symptoms (peripheralization) has a negative prognosis, even if symptom intensity lessens, and is appreciated as reflecting intradiscal nuclear material deranging peripheral from its normal, central location.

The positing of the intervertebral disc nuclear derangement model fleshes out phenomenological observations, as follows.

Posterior Derangement Pathoanatomical Explanation

Posterior Derangement Direction of Detriment: Flexion

- Flexion is the mechanically unimpeded movement plane direction. Loading in flexion displaces intradiscal nuclear material posterior resulting in less intradiscal resistance to flexion. If flexion is not possible, it is because of increased symptoms of, not mechanical resistance from, deranged intradiscal nuclear material.

- Flexion loading has adverse mechanical and/or symptomatic responses at beginning, middle, and end range (including peripheralization) as nuclear material is progressively deranged posterior.

- Flexion loading promotes an obstruction to extension caused by the accumulation of deranged intradiscal nuclear material in that direction.

Posterior Derangement Direction of Correction: Extension

- Extension is mechanically impeded because of the accumulation of, and resistance to compression from, deranged intradiscal nuclear material.

- Extension loading has no responses during motion because it does not promote the derangement and has yet to meet the obstruction to movement from the derangement.

- Extension loading has beneficial mechanical and/or symptomatic responses at the mechanically impeded end range only (including centralization), the point at which the accumulated intradiscal nuclear material is compressed and returned to a more central location.

- Extension mechanically impeded end range loading results in flexion becoming less provocative. As nuclear derangement is reduced to a more central location, more flexion would be required to achieve the degree of posterior intradiscal nuclear derangement that existed before extension loading.

Clinical Pearl

In a posterior derangement, mechanically restricted extension is increased by flexion loading. Extension loading diminishes the provocative effect of flexion.

Relevant Posterolateral Derangement Pathoanatomical Explanation

A lateral component is "relevant" or not depending on whether loading outside the sagittal plane (i.e., loading laterally) is necessary to reduce the derangement. "Relevance" refers to the relevance of a lateral loading strategy. If there are symptoms that

are "lateral" but the derangement is reduced with loading in the sagittal plane, any lateral component to the intradiscal derangement is not considered relevant (to loading strategies).

Unilateral symptoms, including sciatica, are often adequately addressed with sagittal extension motions without having to resort to lateral techniques. A relevant lateral component is, therefore, not exhibited for these cases despite MRI that may demonstrate lateral intradiscal derangement. If symptoms are central and a lateral loading strategy is required for resolution, a relevant lateral component is considered to exist even though unilateral symptoms did not.

With relevant posterolateral derangement, extension loading is initially detrimental but after a course of coronal loading becomes beneficial. The initial phase of treatment, wherein lateral loading was required, represents a relevant lateral component. After lateral loading is successfully used, the relevant lateral component no longer exists.

A relevant posterolateral derangement may be thought of as a posterior derangement that has progressed to develop a relevant lateral derangement component as well. In the presence of a relevant lateral derangement, extension strategies fail to capture and return the lateral derangement to a more central location and, to the contrary, often promote the lateral component of the derangement. Treatment of the relevant posterolateral derangement is a two-step process. The first step reduces the lateral derangement with coronal (non-sagittal) loading strategies. The second step is to proceed with posterior derangement management, already considered above. The relevant lateral derangement must first be reduced to a more central location by means of lateral techniques, after which extension is transformed from being detrimental to being beneficial by reducing the posterior derangement that remains after the relevant lateral derangement is reduced (eliminated). We will now consider the case of an individual whose spinal symptoms are right-sided and whose mechanical and symptomatic responses are consistent with a relevant right posterolateral derangement.

Relevant Right Posterolateral Derangement Directions of Detriment: Flexion, Left Lateral, Extension

- Flexion and left lateral movements are the mechanically unimpeded movement plane directions. Loading in flexion and left lateral movements derange intradiscal nuclear material posterior and right lateral (i.e., right posterolateral) resulting in less intradiscal resistance to flexion and left lateral movements. If flexion or left lateral movements are not possible, it is because of increased symptoms of, and not the mechanical resistance from, deranged intradiscal nuclear material.

- Flexion and left lateral loading have adverse mechanical and or symptomatic responses at beginning, middle, and end range (including peripheralization) as nuclear material is progressively deranged right posterolateral.

- Flexion and left lateral loading promote an obstruction to extension and right lateral movements caused by the accumulation of deranged intradiscal nuclear material in those directions.

- Extension is a mechanically impeded movement plane direction that is initially detrimental to load at end range. Although extension is mechanically impeded because of accumulation of intradiscal nuclear material, intradiscal nuclear material has accumulated both posterior and right lateral. Extension end range loading fails to capture and return the relevant right lateral component to a more central location and promotes right lateral derangement of intradiscal nuclear material. It is the failure of extension to reduce the derangement that causes this type of derangement to be classified as relevant posterolateral.

Relevant Right Posterolateral Derangement Direction of Correction: Right Lateral Loading

- Right lateral loading is mechanically impeded because of the accumulation of, and resistance to compression from, deranged intradiscal nuclear material.

- Right lateral loading has no responses during motion because it does not promote the derangement and has yet to meet the obstruction to movement from the derangement.

- Right lateral loading has beneficial mechanical and/or symptomatic responses at end range only (including centralization); the point at which the accumulated deranged intradiscal nuclear material is compressed and returned to a more central location.

- Right lateral loading results in flexion, left lateral, and extension loading becoming less provocative as a result of a reduction of right lateral derangement of nuclear material. Because nuclear derangement is reduced to a more central location, a greater degree of

flexion, left lateral, and/or extension loading would be required to achieve the degree of lateral intradiscal nuclear derangement that existed before right lateral loading reduction of derangement.

- After right lateral loading is recovered, extension is no longer detrimental, but is transformed into something beneficial after the relevant lateral component is reduced, i.e., once the "lateral" component is taken out of the posterolateral derangement. Extension loading no longer promotes lateral derangement because there is no lateral derangement to promote. From this point on, the progression is as for posterior derangement, which essentially is what is left without the relevant lateral component. Extension results in further improvement as the remaining posterior component is reduced.

Anterior Derangement Pathoanatomical Explanation

Anterior Derangement Direction of Detriment: Extension

- Extension is the mechanically unimpeded movement plane direction. Loading in extension deranges intradiscal nuclear material anterior resulting in less intradiscal resistance to extension. If extension is not possible it is because of increased symptoms of, and not the mechanical resistance from, deranged intradiscal nuclear material.

- Extension loading has adverse mechanical and/or symptomatic responses at beginning, middle, and end range (including peripheralization) as nuclear material is progressively deranged anterior.

- Extension loading promotes an obstruction to flexion because of the accumulation of deranged intradiscal nuclear material in that direction.

Anterior Derangement Direction of Correction: Flexion

- Flexion is mechanically impeded because of the accumulation of, and resistance to, compression from deranged intradiscal nuclear material.

- Flexion loading has no responses during motion as it does not promote the derangement and has yet to meet the obstruction to movement from the derangement.

- Flexion loading has beneficial mechanical and/or symptomatic responses at the mechanically impeded end range only (including centralization), the point at which the accumulated intradiscal nuclear material is compressed and returned to a more central location.

- Flexion mechanically impeded end range loading results in extension becoming less provocative. As nuclear derangement is reduced to a more central location, more extension would be required to achieve the degree of anterior intradiscal nuclear derangement that existed before flexion loading.

Acute Spinal Antalgia Paradigms of McKenzie Method Derangement Management

With the McKenzie Method, antalgia is typically resolved within a few visits with self-generated movement initiated as the centerpiece of care beginning with the first visit. A prudent progression of forces is used to reverse the antalgia while being mindful of centralization and peripheralization phenomena to judge the appropriateness of the strategy.

Delay of movement therapy for spinal antalgia often results from the misconception that acute spinal antalgia represents the "wisdom" of the body avoiding a position that is deleterious. The situation, so conceived, precludes the exploration of movements to reverse the antalgia. Antalgia is rarely caused by neural or other pernicious pathological processes; standard history and examination procedures rule out these infrequent contributors.

Patients presenting with acute spinal deformities are unable to achieve neutral spinal positioning in the movement plane direction opposite the antalgia. It is as if the precluded movement plane direction has "collapsed" into the opposite movement plane direction within which the patient is "trapped." The McKenzie Method management strategy is to first achieve neutral spine positioning and then to "recover" the precluded movement plane direction, guided all the time by centralization and peripheralization phenomena.

The criteria for the preferred loading strategy are not only centralization phenomena but also the degree to which adverse mechanical responses resolve. Although the McKenzie Method is known for being mindful of symptomatic responses, mechanical responses are equally important and may, at times, be the only sign that a positive response to loading has occurred. For some patients, the presenting symptom may be perception of a mechanical restriction to motion, perceived as a stiffness limitation versus significant pain.

For introductory educational purposes, the McKenzie Method management of spinal antalgias offers excellent examples of derangement management because the derangement subtype is easy to identify as opposed to the significant investigative efforts required when antalgia is absent. Appreciation of the presentation and management of the three acute spinal antalgias informs the process of learning how to detect, evaluate, and manage derangements when there is no antalgia, because most derangement presentations can be construed as partial patterns of the full antalgia patterns.

Kyphotic Antalgia Management—Extension Principle—Posterior Derangement

Lumbar Kyphotic Antalgia Management—Extension Principle—Posterior Derangement

The patient presenting with a lumbar kyphotic antalgia (Fig. 15.6) typically has symptoms that are central or symmetrical and do not radiate beyond the knee, consistent with a central, posterior derangement that does not affect more lateral articular or neurologic structures.

There are detrimental responses within the mechanically unimpeded flexion movement plane direction, both during motion and at end range. For extension there are responses at that mechanically impeded end range only. There are no responses "during motion" for extension because extension motion is not possible

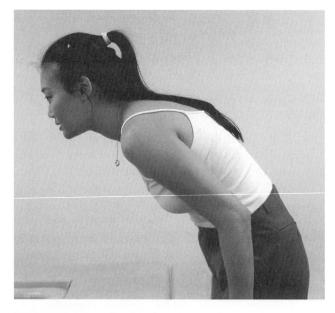

Figure 15.6 Lumbar kyphotic antalgia.

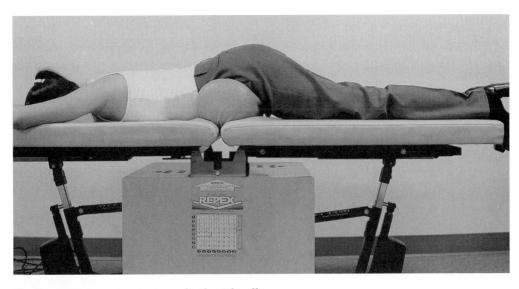

Figure 15.7 Prone patient on plinth with pillow.

(there is no extension); the mechanically impeded extension end range is met in the flexed position. As the patient improves, extension movements become possible but still evidence a mechanically impeded end range with responses continuing to occur at the mechanically impeded extension end range only.

When a patient presents with a lumbar kyphotic antalgia, the first step is to achieve neutral (0 degrees of flexion) positioning of the spine, which is difficult to accomplish in the erect standing posture. The patient is placed prone on the plinth with a bolster pillow under the abdomen (Fig. 15.7) to relax in a position accommodating the antalgia.

After some time, the pillow is removed and the patient is flat prone (Fig. 15.8) and may experience centralization discomfort as a result.

After achieving prone 0-degree flexion (neutral positioning), the next step is to recover extension. The patient is asked to rise up on elbows (Fig. 15.9) and to rest in that position for a few moments; again, an increase of centralization discomfort may be experienced.

Next, the patient is asked to perform a prone extension (Fig. 15.10).

From what may be described as a push-up position, the elbows are extended in an attempt to passively extend the trunk over the pelvis. Instruction is given to relax the buttocks because contraction of the gluteus maximus flexes the lumbar spine, a roadblock to extension. For patients having difficulty relaxing the buttocks, it is useful to assume a knocked-kneed, pigeon-toed positioning of the lower extremities to

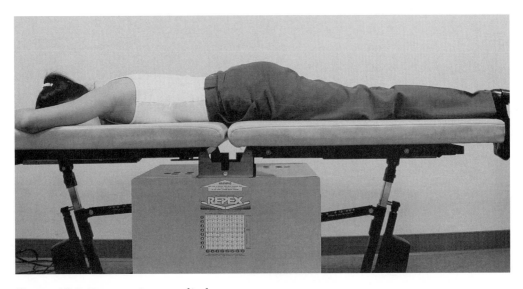

Figure 15.8 Prone patient on plinth.

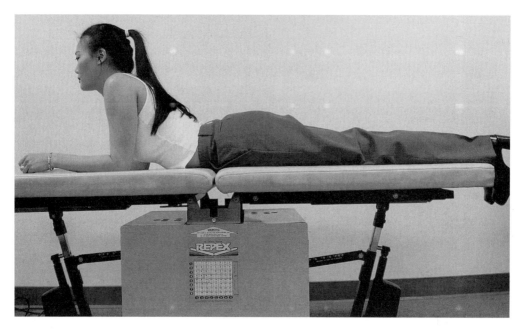

Figure 15.9 Prone on elbows.

stretch–relax the gluteus maximus. The patient is given the verbal cue to let the pelvis "sag" to the table. There is a momentary rest/pause at extension end range and then again at the starting position. The exercise is performed approximately 10 times.

When performing any end range loading exercise or mobilization, patients are asked to report when discomfort is perceived to change in any fashion. The clinician monitors whether these changes occur dur-

ing motion or at end range. Although the most important criteria is patient status subsequent to the performance of any exercise, during the exercise there is special interest as to what is occurring *at* the moment of end range loading and whether symptoms centralize or peripheralize *at* the moment of end range loading. Centralization and/or peripheralization reactions *at* the mechanically impeded extension end range herald whether benefit or detriment

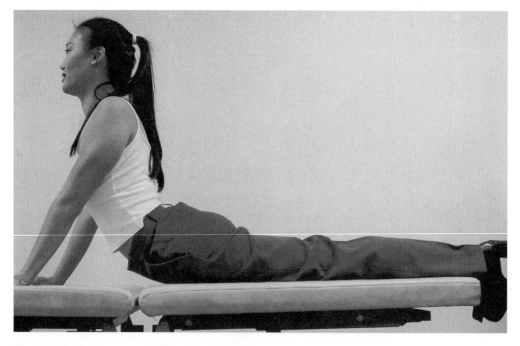

Figure 15.10 Prone extension.

will be experienced after end range loading ceases. It is an optimistic prognosticator if symptoms become more central or diminish *at* each extension end range loading. If radiation to the extremity occurs every time loading *at* end range is achieved, this would raise concerns that loading at that end range may not be the most prudent strategy.

After the patient is able to achieve extension from the prone position they should, within 1 or 2 days, be able to tolerate and benefit from extension in standing (Fig. 15.11) as an alternative self-treatment, in addition to prone extension.

Flexion postural syndrome principles of avoiding deleterious flexion end range and maintaining lumbar lordosis are used. Self-treatment for the posterior derangement centers on avoiding flexion, maintaining lumbar lordosis while sitting (and making transitions between postures) and periodically pursuing extension end range loading, either prone or standing (the former usually being more effec-

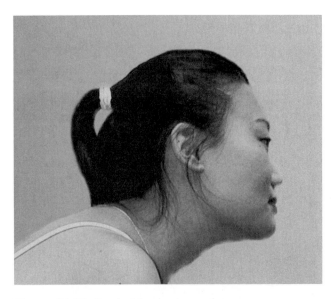

Figure 15.12 Cervical kyphotic antalgia.

tive). Education would be conducted concerning centralization and peripheralization phenomena.

One of the goals of care is the achievement of full pain-free extension, appreciated to represent the reduction of the posterior derangement. Subsequent to this, flexion would be revisited for two reasons. The first would be to confirm that flexion is no longer provokes derangement; the second is to explore whether a flexion dysfunction developed due to formation of scar tissue or avoidance of flexion during the course of care. Flexion would continue to be avoided if it was determined that it still had the power to promote posterior derangement. Flexion would be pursued if the pattern of reaction was consistent with flexion dysfunction. Flexion loading to remodel dysfunction would be followed by extension as a prophylactic measure to ensure that the recent reduction of the posterior derangement stayed that way.

Cervical Acute Kyphotic Antalgia Management—Extension Principle— Posterior Derangement

For cervical kyphotic antalgia (Fig. 15.12), the patient is unloaded in a supine position with additional unloading introduced by means of manual axial traction. Even though this requires "hands-on," patients are soon able to self-treat with techniques that resemble, and can replace, clinician manual methods used to get them "going."

The patient is initially made comfortable in the antalgic position. The supine patient's head rests on a pillow supporting the flexed antalgic position.

To achieve 0 degrees of flexion, manual axial traction is used (Fig. 15.13).

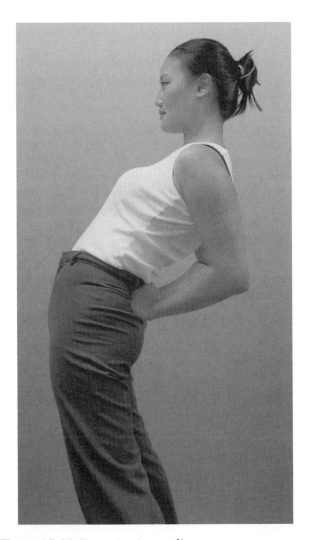

Figure 15.11 Extension in standing.

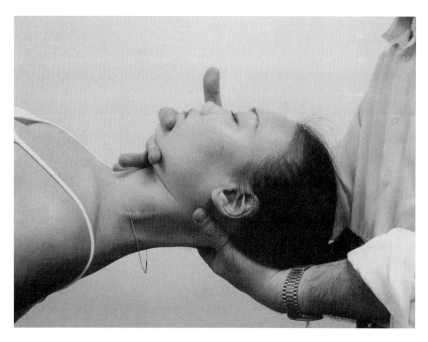

Figure 15.13 Manual supine cervical traction.

The therapist places the index and middle finger of one hand anterior and inferior to the chin, respectively. The thumb and index finger of the other hand abuts the inferior border of the occiput. The patient is asked to occlude (not clench) the teeth to avoid biting the tongue or disturbing the TMJ. Axial traction is then applied along the vector of the flexion antalgia. While maintaining the axial traction, cervical retractions are performed in a slow, gentle, repetitive manner to achieve beginning range lower cervical extension (lordosis) and neutral head and neck positioning (Fig. 15.14).

A momentary rest occurs at end range retraction and at the starting point for each repetition. Appropriateness is monitored by means of centralization and peripheralization.

Next, extension is introduced from the retracted position. As soon as extension is initiated, retraction forces are withdrawn, with axial traction forces maintained throughout (Fig. 15.15).

As always, centralization and peripheralization phenomena judge appropriateness. The head and neck are extended within tolerance. With each repetition further extension is attempted. At extension

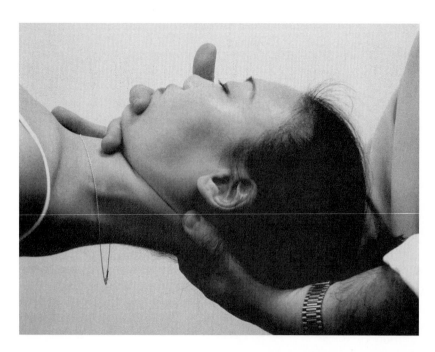

Figure 15.14 Manual supine cervical traction–retraction to introduce lordosis.

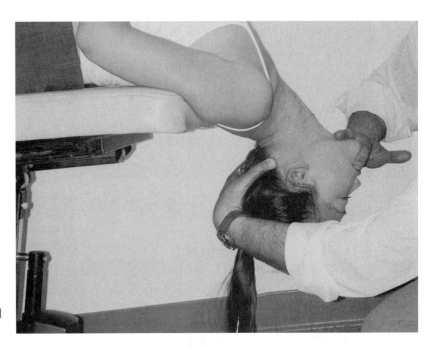

Figure 15.15 Manual supine cervical traction–retraction–extension.

end range, gentle very small rotations of the head are performed to facilitate further extension. As always, feedback from the patient is essential to evaluate what is occurring during motion and at end range. Responses at end range are of particular interest.

Patients are shown how to perform self-treatment exercises to the degree they are capable. Options include sitting retractions followed by sitting retraction–extension (Fig. 15.16).

For sitting cervical retractions, instruction to keep the head level to avoid nodding is helpful. Maintenance of lumbar lordosis is essential to achieve maximum cervical retraction or extension end range loading in the sitting position. Sitting extension is

performed from the retracted position to achieve maximum extension end range. Once extension is introduced, the retraction is not maintained (the retraction is "lost"). Gentle mini-rotations are performed at end range to permit further extension.

As with lumbar Kyphotic antalgia, self-treatment involves the flexion postural syndrome treatment principles of avoiding flexion and maintaining lumbar and cervical lordosis (the former required for the latter) while sitting and making transitions between postures. Periodically throughout the day, cervical retraction extensions are performed. Education regarding centralization and peripheralization would be conducted.

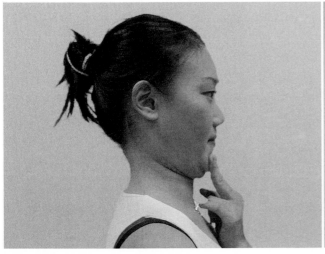

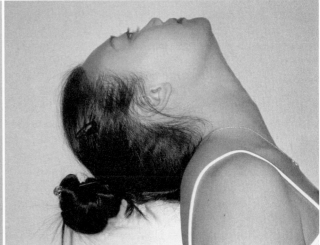

A

B

Figure 15.16 Sitting cervical retraction and sitting retraction–extension.

As with the lumbar spine, subsequent to the achievement of full pain-free extension, flexion would be revisited to confirm whether flexion is still provoked derangement or if a flexion dysfunction developed because of avoidance of flexion. Flexion would continue to be avoided if it was determined that it still promoted posterior derangement. Flexion would be pursued if the pattern of reaction was consistent with flexion dysfunction and would be followed by extension as a prophylactic measure to ensure the recent reduction of posterior derangement stayed that way.

Acute Coronal Antalgia Management: Lateral-Then-Extension Principle— Relevant Postero-Lateral Derangement

Unilateral and extremity symptoms are more common with coronal antalgia than with sagittal antalgias.

As with kyphotic lumbar and cervical antalgias, unloading tactics are used to initiate treatment for cervical coronal antalgia (acute torticollis) but may or may not be necessary for lumbar coronal antalgia (acute scoliosis). Acute lumbar scoliosis can often be corrected in the loaded standing position with strategies that may prove more effective than unloaded alternatives.

As with the kyphotic antalgias, the acute coronal antalgias can be visually identified. The coronal antalgias (lumbar scoliosis or cervical torticollis) may be associated with a kyphotic antalgia or not. Whether a kyphotic component is visualized or not, the treatment progression for coronal antalgia involves the two-step progression of recovering motion in the coronal plane opposite the antalgia (the relevant lateral component) followed by recovery of motion in the extension (sagittal) plane. The progression is the lateral-then-extension principle.

With coronal antalgia, if extension end range loading is performed before recovery of the coronal movement in the direction opposite the antalgia (i.e., reduction of the relevant lateral component), the patient may worsen. However, after recovery of motion in the coronal movement plane direction opposite the antalgia, extension end range loading is transformed from detrimental to beneficial. In fact, the tolerance of, and/or benefit from, extension is a sign of progress.

For our examples of lumbar and cervical coronal antalgias, we will consider a patient with right-sided symptoms and a coronal antalgia to the left, interpreted as a right posterolateral derangement. The goal is to first recover movement in the right coronal movement plane direction (i.e., to reduce the right lateral component of the derangement) and then to recover extension (to reduce the posterior derangement that remains).

Lumbar Acute Scoliosis Antalgia Management

When considering acute lumbar scoliosis, two terms are useful, those being *lateral shift* and *side gliding*. The term "lateral shift" is equivalent to antalgia and is referenced as right or left depending on the direction of the coronal deviation of the trunk over the pelvis. Someone with a left antalgia has a left lateral shift (Fig. 15.17).

If lateral shift refers to a position in the coronal plane, side gliding is the *movement* that gets you to, or away, from that position. Side gliding is movement of the trunk relative to the pelvis in the coronal plane with the shoulders kept level.

For our patient with a left lateral shift, the first intervention to explore is side gliding against the wall, which permits self-correction in the loaded standing posture without need to visit the plinth (Fig. 15.18).

Our left lateral shift patient is positioned with the left side of the body toward the wall. The medial epicondyle of the left elbow remains in contact with the left rib cage on the axillary line. The patient leans the lateral aspect of the left arm against the wall. The feet are placed together a few feet away from the wall. The patient places the right hand on the superior aspect of

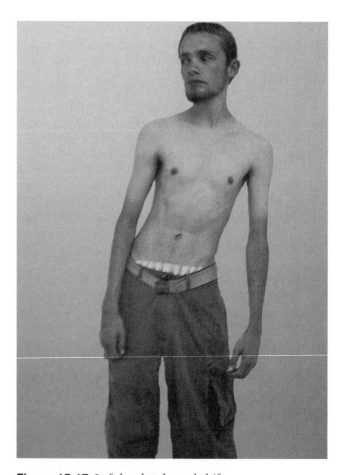

Figure 15.17 Left lumbar lateral shift.

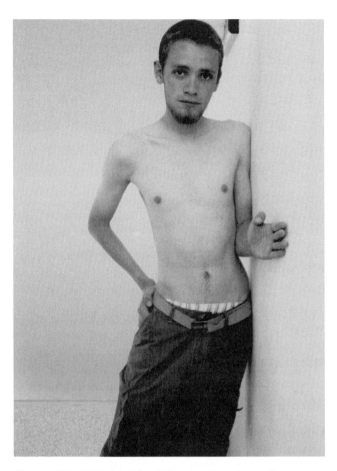

Figure 15.18 Right side-gliding against the wall to correct a left lateral shift.

the lateral right ilium and pushes the pelvis toward the wall until the painful obstruction is met; this end range loading is maintained for a moment. The pelvis is then backed off to the first point of tolerable discomfort; there is a moment of rest and the procedure is repeated. With each repetition, further progression to the wall should be achieved. If the feet are placed a proper distance from the wall, contact between the pelvis/hip and the wall should not occur, even as side gliding improves. The appropriateness of the intervention, as always, is judged by centralization and peripheralization phenomena.

If considerable improvement is noted, extension may be performed at the end range of the coronal movement opposite the antalgia; however some, patients do not benefit from extension until some days have passed. Should side gliding not be well-tolerated, the introduction of a slight degree (e.g., 10 degrees) of flexion may transform the maneuver into something of benefit. As the patient progresses, the need to flex should resolve and tolerance and benefit from extension should evolve.

If the patient cannot adequately achieve coronal end range movements with side gliding against the

wall, therapist overpressure may be required. If this does not turn out well, the therapist may have to offer even more assistance by manually inducing side gliding maneuvers absent benefit of the wall. In essence, the therapist becomes a wall with arms (Fig. 15.19).

The patient stands with feet shoulder width apart with the left arm positioned as it would be to lean against the wall. The therapist is on the patient's left-side, oriented in the patient's coronal plane and adopting a three-point stance with the forward foot behind the patient. The angle of the therapist's neck/shoulder girdle contacts the patient's left arm just above the elbow. The therapist reaches around the patient, interlacing fingers just below the crest of the right ilium. Therapist mobilizations are then applied by simultaneously pulling the pelvis (with the interlaced hands) and pushing the trunk (with the angle of neck/shoulder girdle against the patient's arm) in the coronal movement plane. Use of a mirror helps ensure that the patient's shoulders remain level so that side gliding correction is used as opposed to lateral flexion. As with the wall side gliding, adverse reactions often indicate the need for a slight degree of flexion. As with wall side gliding, if significant benefit is experienced, extension can be added at the point of coronal end range in the direction opposite the antalgia. To do this, our patient's right hand would be placed on the therapist's right wrist (behind the patient) and used as a fulcrum to lean back on.

Should standing side gliding strategies prove futile, prone extensions from a lateral shift position may be explored. For our patient with a left lateral shift, this

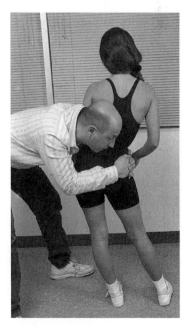

Figure 15.19 Therapist-assisted right side-gliding to correct a left lateral shift.

would be prone extensions from a right lateral shift position (Fig. 15.20).

In the prone position, the pelvis is positioned at coronal end range in the direction opposite the presenting coronal antalgia. Our patient places the pelvis to the left (essentially performing a right lateral shift as the trunk is now to the right of the pelvis) and prone extensions are performed from the right lateral shift position. Benefit is monitored by centralization as well as the ability of the exercise to diminish the antalgia, once performed.

Self-care would include use of flexion postural syndrome principles (avoiding flexion and maintaining lumbar lordosis while sitting and making transitions between postures) with the periodic performance of the preferred coronal end range loading strategy. Although extension end range loading initially fails to benefit, or is of detriment, maintenance of a minimal lordosis (beginning range extension positioning) is usually tolerated and avoids the deleterious effects of flexion. Education regarding centralization and peripheralization would be conducted.

After recovery of movement in the coronal movement plane direction opposite the presenting coronal antalgia, self-treatment continues by using the extension principle for the posterior derangement that remains once the relevant lateral component

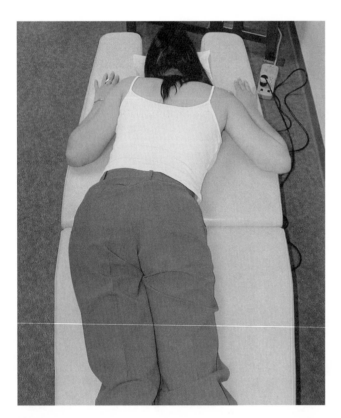

Figure 15.20 Prone extension from a right lateral shift position to correct a left lateral shift.

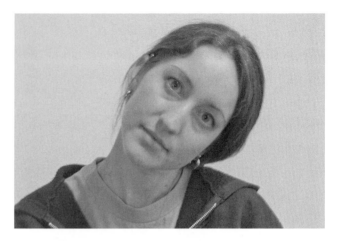

Figure 15.21 Torticollis: left coronal antalgia demonstrated.

of the postero-lateral derangement is reduced/eliminated.

Cervical Acute Torticolis Antalgia Management

As with lumbar scoliosis, cervical antalgia in the coronal plane (i.e., torticollis) (Fig. 15.21) may or may not be associated with kyphotic antalgia. As with lumbar scoliosis, whether a kyphotic component is visible or not, after the coronal movement plane direction opposite the antalgia is recovered, the extension principle is explored. As with cervical acute kyphotic antalgia, manual axial traction is required to get things going. Soon thereafter, the responsibility of treatment is transferred to the patient using techniques resembling what the clinician used.

The patient is placed supine with the head comfortably placed on a pillow in a manner that does not challenge the antalgia. The therapist's manual contacts are the same as were used with the cervical kyphotic antalgia. Axial traction is applied, at first in the direction of the antalgia. While maintaining axial traction, a lateral flexion mobilization is conducted in the direction opposite the antalgia until the painful obstruction is met at which point there is a momentary pause (Fig. 15.22). The therapist then backs off to the first point of tolerable discomfort, pauses a moment (traction maintained throughout), and repeats the procedure, gaining lateral flexion in the direction opposite the antalgia with each repetition. If lateral flexion fails, the coupled motion of rotation may be attempted in its place, using the same protocols.

As with the lumbar spine, premature attempts to recover extension may be detrimental. Unlike the lumbar spine, combined lateral and extension movements are not used. As is occasionally the case with the lumbar spine, cervical coronal antalgia more often requires a degree of flexion be maintained when recovering lateral movements. As with the lumbar spine,

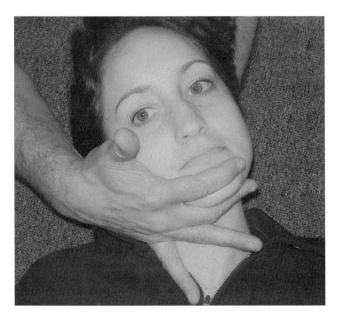

Figure 15.22 Correction of left torticollis.

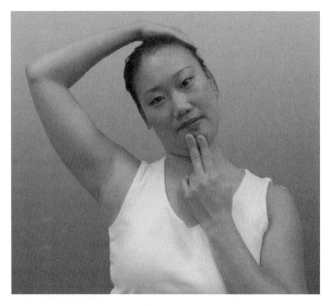

Figure 15.23 Sitting cervical retraction/lateral flexion to recover coronal motion.

subsequent to the recovery of coronal movement in the direction opposite the antalgia, extension end range loading is transformed from detrimental to beneficial. As always, the appropriateness of any loading strategy is audited by centralization and peripheralization.

Patient self-care includes the employment of flexion postural syndrome principles as well as self-generated lateral flexion mobilizations in the direction opposite the coronal antalgia. Education regarding centralization and peripheralization is provided. At first, lateral flexions may only be possible supine with the head on a pillow. As the patient progresses, the ability to perform and benefit from lateral flexion mobilizations in a seated, retracted head and neck position (which promotes lower cervical lordotic extension) is of benefit (Fig. 15.23).

Subsequent to the achievement of end range in the coronal movement plane direction opposite the coronal antalgia, treatment progress is to the extension principle whether there is a visible acute kyphotic antalgic component or not.

Acute Lordotic Antalgic Management— Flexion Principle—Anterior Derangement

Clinical Pearl

Considering the lower cervical and lower lumbar flexion stressors in everyday life (e.g., prolonged sitting, bending), one would predict that flexion as a treatment of lower cervical and lower lumbar symptoms would be the exception rather than the rule. It has been our experience that conditions requiring flexion are less common than those requiring extension.

Regarding the kyphotic and coronal antalgias, a similar mechanical "deformity" occurs in both the lumbar and cervical areas. Lordotic antalgia differs inasmuch as it occurs for the lumbar spine but not for the cervical spine. Nonetheless, patients presenting with cervical symptoms amenable to flexion end range loading strategies have many of the same mechanical and symptomatic responses to loading as those presenting with an acute lumbar lordotic antalgia except, of course, for the lack of an antalgia that can be visualized.

In addition, the lumbar lordotic antalgia has a unique feature. Whereas most low backs that respond to the extension principle do not present with an acute lumbar kyphosis, most low backs that respond to the flexion principle present with an acute lordotic antalgia (Fig. 15.24).

Manual therapists are usually more adept at promoting flexion end range loading than they are at promoting extension end range loading strategies. Typically these skills have been acquired and used according to the notion that short posterior muscular structures are culpable for symptoms and need to be stretched. The McKenzie Method more often uses flexion loading strategies to compress deranged intradiscal nuclear material that has accumulated within the anterior intervertebral disc space to return that material to a more central location as opposed to promoting the flexibility of posterior extra-articular structures. Figs. 15.25 and 15.26 demonstrate lumbar and cervical flexion strategies.

Self-treatment involves education regarding centralization and peripheralization but there would be

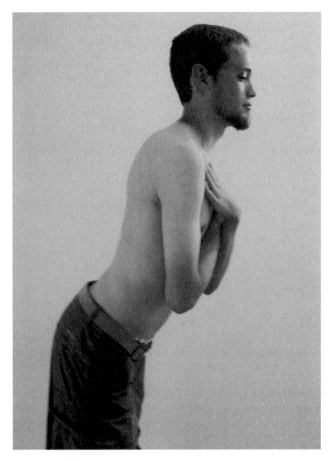

Figure 15.24 Lumbar acute lordosis antalgia: attempting flexion.

no education regarding flexion postural syndrome treatment principles, because flexion is not of detriment. The patient would be dissuaded from any extension end range loading postural habits or any

extension end range loading for that matter, including "McKenzie prone extensions!"

■ CONCLUSION

McKenzie Method clinical reasoning would predict that a majority of individuals with spinal symptoms would benefit from minimizing flexion and periodically pursuing extension, considering the amount of time we spend flexed in everyday life. The McKenzie Method predicts that loading in one movement plane direction may be more beneficial than loading in other movement plane directions whether symptoms are acute or chronic. These predictions have been verified within the recent peer-reviewed evidence-based literature.

Snook (8) demonstrated how controlling lumbar flexion in the early morning serves as a form of self-care for reducing pain and costs associated with chronic, non-specific low back pain. The McKenzie Method predicts that avoiding flexion would minimize low back pain for most patients. Early morning flexion is perceived to be particularly provocative because of imbibition of fluid by intradiscal nuclear material over a night of unloading. Theoretically, if the patient has posterior derangement of nuclear material, the imbibition of fluid makes intradiscal nuclear pressures and the risk of debilitating derangements even greater.

Larsen, Weidick and Leboeuf-Yde (3) demonstrated it may be possible to reduce the prevalence of back problems and use of health care services during military service, at a low cost, using lumbar prone extensions with a back/ergonomic school including McKenzie Method disc theories. Military recruits

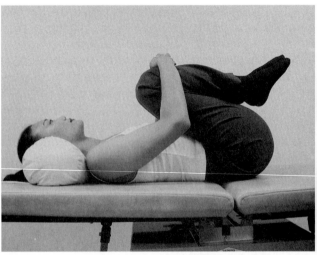

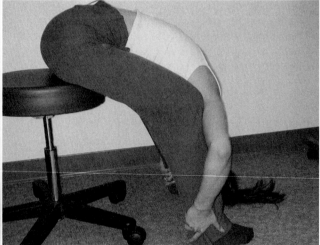

A   B

Figure 15.25 Promotion of lumbar flexion.

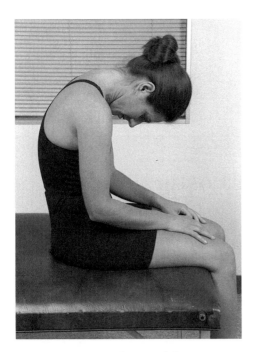

Figure 15.26 Promotion of cervical flexion.

were taught McKenzie Method extension principles (including lumbar lordotic body mechanics and prone extensions were performed periodically throughout the day) resulting in the favorable outcomes noted.

Long, Donelson, and Fung (4) showed that a McKenzie assessment could identify a large subgroup of acute, subacute, and chronic low back patients with a direction of preference ("an immediate, lasting improvement in pain from performing either repeated lumbar flexion, extension or side glides/rotation tests"). Regardless of the direction of preference, "the response to contrasting exercise prescriptions was significantly different." Exercises matching the patient's direction of preference significantly and rapidly decreased pain and medication use and improved disability, degree of recovery, depression, and work interference outcomes. Of the original 312 subjects who underwent assessment, 53.5% demonstrated a directional preference for pure sagittal extension, the remainder required prone extensions from a lateral shift position or movements in other planes. The majority of subjects, therefore, required

an extension component to their preferred loading strategy.

Audit Process
Self-Check of the Chapter's Learning Objectives

- What are the three syndromes as defined by the McKenzie Method?

- What are the responses during motion and at end range for each syndrome?

- What is the role of pursuing or avoiding end range loading for each syndrome?

- According to the McKenzie Method, what are the possible reasons a patient might experience increased discomfort with sitting versus standing and vice versa? Consider each syndrome and subtypes to account for the phenomena.

■ REFERENCES

1. McKenzie Institute International home page http://www.mckenziemdt.org. Accessed May 9, 2005.
2. Literature Relevant to the McKenzie Method® http://www.mckenziemdt.org/libResearchList.cfm?pSection=int. Accessed May 9, 2005.
3. Larsen K, Weidick F, Leboeuf-Yde C. Can passive prone extensions of the back prevent back problems? A randomized, controlled intervention trial of 314 military conscripts. Spine 2002;27(24):2747–2752.
4. Long A, Donelson R, Fung T. Does it matter which exercise? A randomized control trial of exercise for low back pain. Spine 2004;29(23):2593–2602.
5. McKenzie R. The Cervical and Thoracic Spine Mechanical Diagnosis and Therapy. Waikanae, New Zealand: Spinal Publications, 1990.
6. McKenzie R, May S. The Lumbar Spine Mechanical Diagnosis & Therapy, volume one and volume two. Waikanae, New Zealand: Spinal Publications, 2003.
7. McKenzie R, May S. The Human Extremities Diagnosis & Therapy. Waikanae, New Zealand: Spinal Publications, 2000.
8. Snook SH, Webster BS, McGorry RW. The reduction of chronic, nonspecific low back pain through the control of early morning lumbar flexion: 3-year follow-up. J Occup Rehabil 2002;12(1):13–19.

16

Brügger Methods for Postural Correction

Dagmar Pavlu,
Sibyle Petak-Krueger,
and Vladimír Janda

Learning Objectives
After reading this chapter, you should be able to understand:

- The relationship between faulty posture and impaired muscle coordination
- Simple clinical techniques for improving upright and balancing antagonist muscles
- Simple self-treatments for improving posture and balancing antagonist muscles

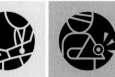

Introduction

Alois Brügger (1920–2001), the Swiss neurologist, developed his concept in early 1950s, almost at the same time when Kabat (5) published his concept on proprioceptive neuromuscular facilitation. Brügger thus belongs to those pioneers who started to introduce in a systematic way and functional approach to the clinical management of musculoskeletal disorders. His approach is widely used in Europe, particularly in German-speaking countries. Brügger is known as an "expert" clinician, particularly for his keen ability to observe changes in function in patients. The modern emphasis on evidence-based practice does not diminish the value of his observations, but clearly there exists a need to test his hypothesis.

Many of the principles of Brügger's work are now considered part of the modern "standard of care." For instance, an emphasis on early patient reactivation and on functional goals are signatures of the modern approach. The milestones of Brügger's concept can be summarized as follows:

1. He introduced the concept of central motor regulation as the main cause of the impaired function of the musculoskeletal system. The trigger of the motor dysregulation may be located anywhere in the body, even in the viscera. In fact, the greater neural density in an area, the greater response. The nociceptive stimulation from the periphery provokes an adaptive reaction on the spinal level and later on a subcortical level. According to Brügger, adaptive changes in the subcortex are decisive to changes in motor behavior. Brügger uses the term "nociceptive somatomotor blocking effect," under which the fundamental principle of development of functional motor impairment is understood. Because of this effect, movements and posture are altered and will be fixed on a higher regulatory level. At this stage the patient can be still pain-free. Brügger considers the changes in the motor program as a protective mechanism, and the stimulus will be perceived as painful only if these regulatory mechanisms become insufficient. This concept is currently becoming more popular and accepted as part of motor control theory.

2. Brügger understands any movement as a complex that, again, provokes a response of the whole body. He speaks about a global body response. In this relation he understands the muscle synergy in loops and does not consider as very significant the activity of an isolated muscle. This concept of functional muscle loops is becoming more well-appreciated today. As a matter of fact, the concept of diagonals or Bennighoff (1) and Tittels (9) loops, although different from Brügger's concept, correspond to the same philosophy. As an example, the great diagonal muscle loop can be used (Fig. 16.1).

3. The concept of global movements and interplay between body segments is demonstrated in the example of the cog wheel model (Fig. 16.2).

4. The basic principle of the assessment is an attempt to find out the trigger factors and their overlay. The goal of treatment is the recognition and amelioration of these trigger factors. This is the basic starting point in any steps to improve the motor patterns or programs. The ultimate aim is to achieve improved movement performance on an automatic basis, particularly those that are associated with activities of daily living. All effort is oriented to improving posture. According to Brügger's definition of ideal posture, the most common cause of the triggering factors is considered overuse or faulty use of the motor system. The typical faulty and ideal sitting and standing posture is evident from Figure 16.3.

Brügger described and analyzed posture and proposed a mechanism for its improvement. He emphasized a holistic concept of neuromusculoskeletal disorders and stressed strongly that impairment of function always involves the whole body. Before the concept of trigger points came into fashion, he developed his concept of painful muscle spots and used the term "tendomyosis" (2,3,6).

To better understand the terminology used by Brügger, here are some definitions.

Activities of Daily Living This term does not correspond exactly to the ADL term used in occupational therapy. Brügger means all activities performed during the day without any other specification. Performing these activities with good posture requires a specific task-oriented program with the goal being to integrate improved postural biomechanics into all activities during the day (4).

Agist From Latin, agree. This refers to muscles that receive the command "to act" either eccentrically against the resistance of the therapist or concentrically without external resistance.

Contracture According to Brügger, this is a loss of eccentric as well as concentric contraction ability of the muscle.

Disturbing Factor Triggers that impair function. There are two types:
   a. persistent, such as contractures, OGE effect (Obolenskaja-Goljanitzki effect), scars
   b. transient, such as inappropriate footwear, furniture, lightening, climatic changes, etc.

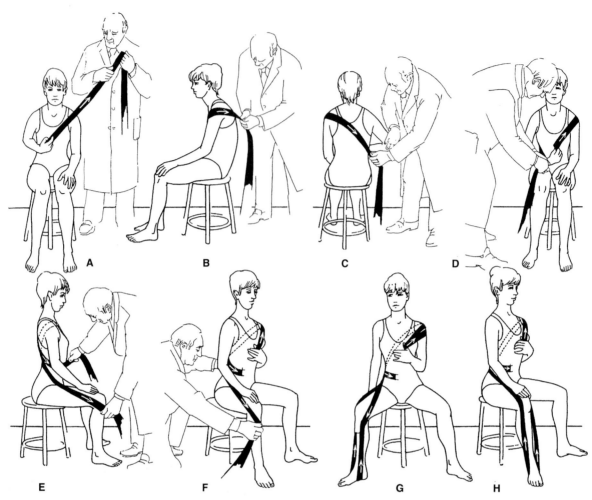

Figure 16.1 Great diagonal muscle loop (pectoralis major, infraspinatus, trapezius, transversus abdominis, sartoriuus, tensor fastiae latae, peronei, tibialis posterior, and tibialis anterior). With permission from Brügger A. Lehrbuch der funktionellen Störungen des Bewegungssystems. Zollikon/Benglen: Brügger-Verlag, 2000:197.

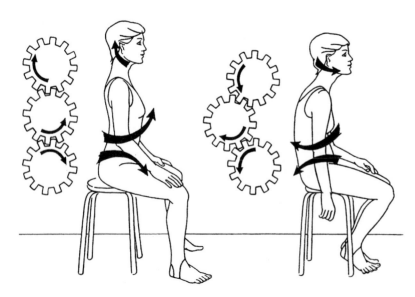

Figure 16.2 Cog wheel model. With permission from Brügger A. Lehrbuch der funktionellen Störungen des Bewegungssystems. Zollikon/Benglen: Brügger-Verlag, 2000:150.

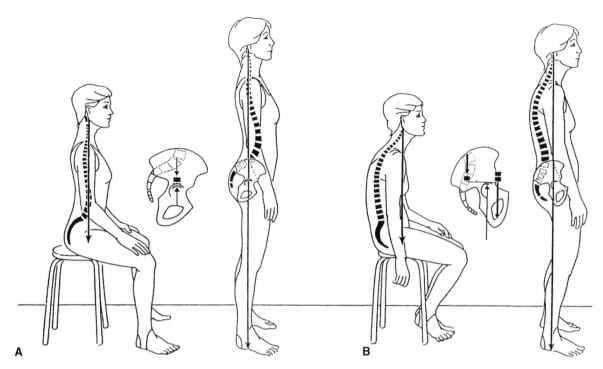

Figure 16.3 Sitting and standing postures
(A) ideal
(B) faulty
With permission from Brügger A Lehrbuch der funktionellen Störungen des Bewegungs-
systems. Zollikon/Benglen: Brügger-Verlag, 2000:404.

Nociceptive Somatomotor Blocking Effect A term under which Brügger understands the fundamental principle of development of functional motor impairment. Because of this effect, movements and posture are altered and will be fixed at a higher regulatory level.

OGE Effect Described in 1927 and is characterized by edema in the interstitial tissue caused by either repetitive long-lasting strain or maximum short-term overuse.

Primary Movements There are three primary movements: anterior pelvic tilt, elevation of the chest, and elongation of the neck.

Springing Test of D5 (dorsal 5) is considered a fundamental test to estimate treatment efficiency. It is not understood not only as a localized evaluation but also as a screen for mobility of the whole body. By means of passive extension of the spine, not only the three primary movements of the axial system are evaluated but also the movements of the extremities are evaluated.

Tendomyosis A reflex status of the muscle associated either with increased or with decreased muscle tone. It has a protective function for the whole body.

Examination of the Patient

Brügger worked out a specific sequence of examination of the patient:

1. Evaluation of habitual, uncorrected posture. This is performed in that posture in which the subject spends most of the working hours. This postural analysis in particular notices not only the deviation from the "ideal" norm but also especially areas that are prone to overuse. Next is the examination of the "primary" movements, such as tilting of the pelvis, elevation of the rib cage, and elongation of the neck.

2. Evaluation of the corrected posture. Clinician performs the correction in a way that is for the given patient at the given time possible. Again, the primary movements are evaluated and the difference is noticed in comparison to the ideal posture. The comparison between the corrected and habitual posture allows an estimation of the degree of dysfunction as well as the prognosis for recovery.

3. Springing test of D5. This is an essential standard test (Fig. 16.4). The test preferably is performed in a corrected sitting posture; however, if the patient cannot sit, this test can be performed in standing position. It is considered as a diagnostic test and

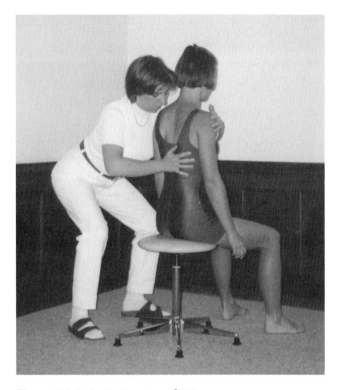

Figure 16.4 Springing test of D5.

is also performed after each treatment session to control the effect of therapy by comparison to the results at baseline. Decrease of the springing motion is an important sign that the therapeutic procedure was not appropriate.

4. Other tests. These include the straight leg raise, shoulder blade protraction, pelvic rotation, external shoulder rotation, and rotation of the head. Surprisingly enough, Brügger does not consider palpation as an important examination as according to him changes in muscle tone are secondary to changes in posture.

5. Estimation of the working hypothesis. Based on the patient's history, visual observation and evaluation of function the individual disturbing factors and their possible interplay are estimated. The overlap of the disturbing factors estimates the sequence of the treatment. The working hypothesis is not rigid but modified for each treatment session.

The Treatment Program

The main goal is to attempt to influence the disturbing factors to achieve optimal posture and movement patterns.

The main treatment approaches include, among others:

- Instruction and motivation to maintain an adequate erect posture

- Positioning in the horizontal position
- Hot pack
- Agistic–eccentric contractions (7)
- Exercise with Thera-Band (8)
- ADL
- Application of the retrocapital support
- Shaking
- Six basic exercises and gait

Instruction and Motivation to Maintain Erect Posture

The main idea is that deviations of posture represent for the body a situation that is associated with disuse or more accurately overuse, not only of the musculoskeletal system also but of the viscera. This is then a source of increased nociceptive afferentation. Therefore, every patient from the very beginning is taught how to stand properly, how to achieve it, and how to maintain it.

As a teaching device, the cog wheel model is used (Fig. 16.2).

The proper correction of posture is performed in two phases, namely:

- An approximate or verbal correction. In sitting, this includes adaptation of the height of the chair and correction of the sitting posture. In standing, it is mainly the correction of the position of the feet and graceful erect posture.

- The fine or tactile correction. The therapist corrects by positioning the patient to achieve the optimum degree of thoracolumbar lordosis, which should run from the sacrum up to D5. The therapist supports the critical segment whose correction results in the optimal improvement. The contact areas are the pelvis, rib cage, and the neck.

Positioning in the Supine Position

Positioning is considered as a preparatory procedure. The patient is usually supine and lower extremities are slightly abducted and externally rotated. Upper extremities are elevated, and the hands and fingers are relaxed. The lumbar spine is supported by a special pillow, the size of which is chosen according to the extension ability of the spine. The patient is placed in this position for approximately 30 minutes. If for some reason it is not possible to achieve this starting position, an adaptive position is used to achieve a comfortable position (Fig. 16.5). Usually positioning is combined with heat therapy such as a fango. This is usually placed on areas that are mostly overused, such as over the neck extensors and upper

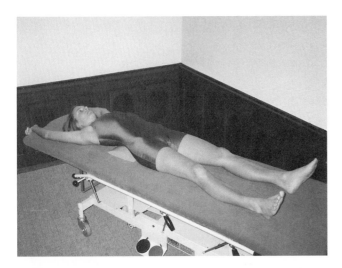

Figure 16.5 Preparatory procedure: positioning in the supine position.

trapezius, the symphysis and thigh adductors area, lumbar spine and the area of the iliac crest, the area of sternum, and the sternocostal junction.

This type of positioning is also recommended as a self-treatment. The patient should spend approximately 30 minutes per day in the recommended position.

The Hot Roll

The most used passive procedures are hot rolls (Fig. 16.6). They are applied at the beginning of the treatment when the disturbing elements are most evident. The passive procedures are applied for the shortest possible time and the active procedures should be started as soon as possible. The application of a hot roll is combined with a deep transverse manual massage. The hot roll is applied in particular to influence the OGE changes, such as edema that occurred because of repetitive movements. The goal of application of the hot rolls is to influence the lymphatic system and to achieve manual muscle relaxation.

To make a hot roll, a spin frote towel is used, in the hollow of which hot water is poured. During application the towel is unwound and the massage is performed.

Agistic–Eccentric Contraction Approach

The agistic–eccentric contraction is one of the basic approaches of Brügger's method in which alternating concentric and eccentric muscle contractions of antagonistic muscle groups are performed. Its goal is to achieve the functional synergism or reduce the functional antagonism. In this way, muscle length and/or hypertonicity is influenced. As a consequence, the global movement patterns improve. By no means is it just a localized exercise.

The technique is always applied in the erect position and can be divided into two phases:

1. Active movement without resistance performed by shortened antagonistic muscle groups (antagonists to muscles which are shortened). During this movement the shortened muscle is elongated.

2. Eccentric contraction against manually applied resistance to the antagonists of the shortened muscle group.

Application of agistic–eccentric procedures is controlled by the therapist (regulates and influences the parameters). Parameters are either positive, i.e., increase of range of movement, increase of muscle strength, decrease of tremor, or improvement of an uncoordinated movement, and negative, i.e., decrease of muscle strength, increase of tremor, or uncoordinated movement. Agistic–eccentric procedures are applied as long as either the negative parameters appear or the positive parameters increase.

Examples

Agistic–eccentric contraction procedure to influence the shortened muscle length or hypertonicity of finger flexors in standing (Fig. 16.7):

Starting Position Erect corrected standing. Therapist stabilizes with one hand the wrist in a slight dor-

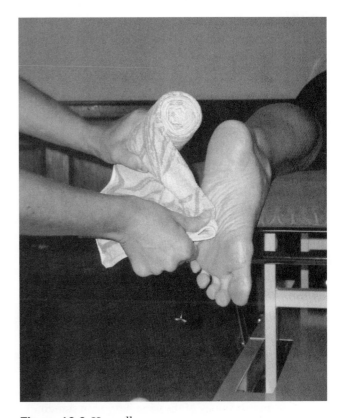

Figure 16.6 Hot roll.

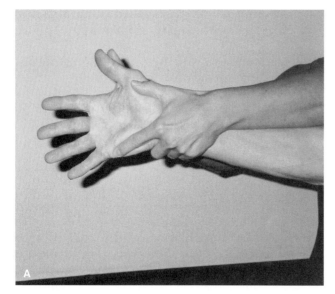

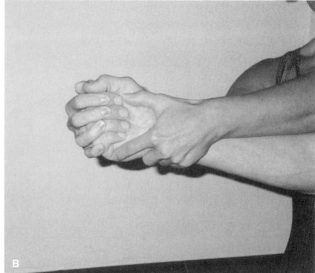

Figure 16.7 Agistic–eccentric contraction procedure to influence the shortened muscle length or hypertonicity of finger flexors (in standing). **(A)** Phase 1. **(B)** Phase 2.

siflexion, and the therapist's second hand is placed on the dorsal aspect of the patients fingers.

Phase 1 The patient performs, actively (without external resistance), extension and abduction of the fingers (Fig. 16.7A).

Phase 2 The therapist performs flexion of the fingers, which the patient hampers. Thus the eccentric contraction of the finger extensors occurs (Fig. 16.7B)

Agistic–eccentric contraction procedure to influence shortened muscle length or hypertonicity of the wrist flexors in standing (Fig. 16.8):

Starting Position Erect corrected standing. The therapist supports with one hand the patient's forearm, and the second hand is placed on the dorsal aspect of the hand.

Phase 1 The patient performs, actively (without external resistance), extension of the wrist (Fig. 16.8A).

Phase 2 The therapist performs wrist flexion, which the patient hampers. Thus the eccentric contraction of wrist extensors occurs (Fig. 16.8B).

Agistic–eccentric contraction procedure to influence shortened muscle length or hypertonicity of the trunk flexors in a supine position (Fig. 16.9):

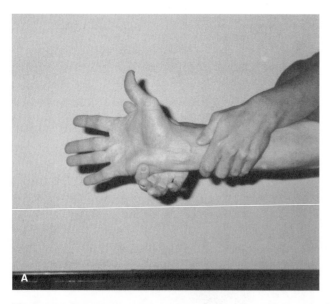

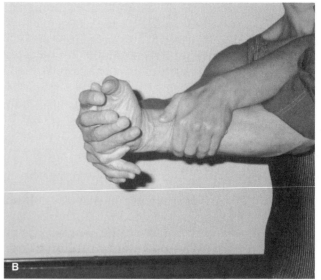

Figure 16.8 Agistic–eccentric contraction procedure to influence shortened muscle length or hypertonicity of the wrist flexors (in standing). **(A)** Phase 1. **(B)** Phase 2.

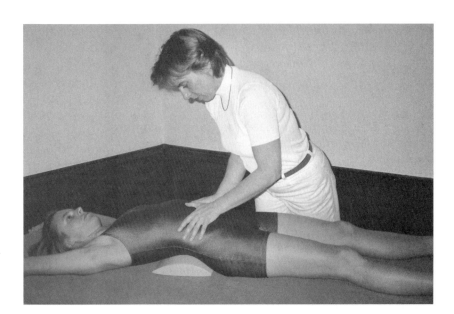

Figure 16.9 Agistic–eccentric contraction procedure to influence shortened muscle length or hypertonicity of the trunk flexors in a supine position.

Starting Position Supine, in an ideally corrected position with the pillow in the thoracolumbar region.

Phase 1 The therapist places his hands flat on the abdominal wall and the patient inhales "into the abdomen" so that the abdominal wall bulges. The patient breathes superficially.

Phase 2 The therapist "travels" with his hands on the abdominal wall in the direction of the muscle fibers.

Do not forget the dorsal aspect of the trunk because of the insertions of the abdominals.

Agistic–eccentric contraction procedure to influence shortened muscle length or hypertonicity of trunk rotators in sitting. This example is for the rotation to the left (Fig. 16.10):

Starting Position Erect corrected sitting posture. Externally rotated upper extremities help to stabilize

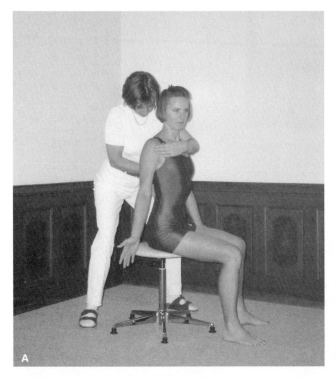
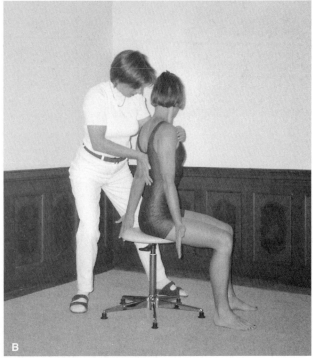

Figure 16.10 Agistic–eccentric contraction procedure to influence shortened muscle length or hypertonicity of trunk rotators in sitting. (This example is for the rotation to the left.) **(A)** Phase 1. **(B)** Phase 2.

the trunk. One forearm of the therapist is placed transversally on the upper chest and the other stabilizes between the shoulder blades.

Phase 1 The patient performs, actively (without external resistance), rotation to the right side.

Phase 2 The therapist rotates the patient's trunk to the left side and the patient tries to hamper this movement.

Agistic–eccentric contraction procedure to influence shortened muscle length or hypertonicity of the internal rotators of the hip supine (Fig. 16.11):

Starting Position Supine in an ideally corrected position. The thoracolumbar area is supported by a pillow. The treated lower extremity is in 90-degree hip and knee flexion and the heel is supported. The

patient holds his foot actively in the zero position. The other hand stabilizes the distal part of the thigh.

Phase 1 Active external hip rotation without resistance (Fig. 16.11A).

Phase 2 The therapist performs internal hip rotation against the patient's resistance (Fig. 16.11B).

Agistic–eccentric contraction procedure to influence shortened muscle length or hypertonicity of the plantar flexors of the foot in sitting position (Fig. 16.12):

Starting Position Erect corrected sitting. Upper extremities are in external rotation to help to stabilize the trunk. The heel is slightly shifted forwards. One hand of the therapist is placed on the dorsal aspect of the foot and the other controls the position of the lower extremity in the knee area.

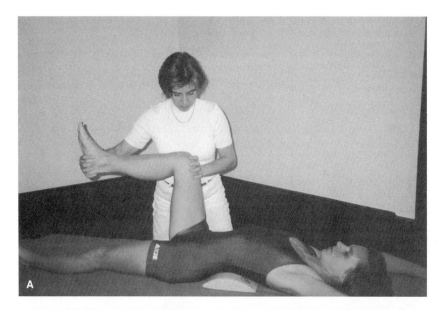

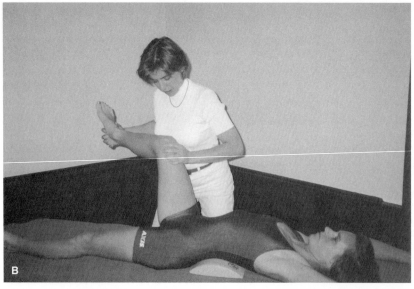

Figure 16.11 Agistic eccentric contraction procedure to influence shortened muscle length or hypertonicity of the internal rotators of the hip supine. **(A)** Phase 1. **(B)** Phase 2.

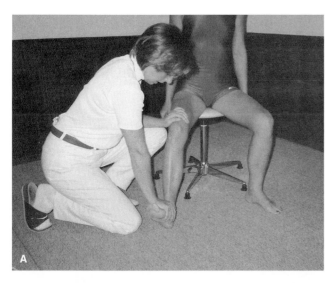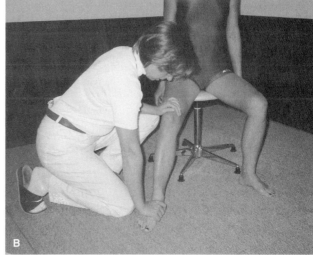

Figure 16.12 Agistic–eccentric contraction procedure to influence shortened muscle length or hypertonicity of the plantar flexors of the foot in sitting. **(A)** Phase 1. **(B)** Phase 2.

Phase 1 Active dorsiflexion of the foot (without external resistance) (Fig. 16.12A).

Phase 2 The therapist performs the plantar flexion and supination of the foot, and the patient tries to hamper this (Fig. 16.12B).

Regarding Phases

The starting positions for the agistic–eccentric contraction procedures should be considered as examples only. The agistic–eccentric procedures can be performed from any position; however, whenever it is possible, the vertical position is preferred because this position is the closest to the most frequent postures.

Exercises With Thera-Band

In Brügger's concept, the Thera-Band exercises are considered as an integrative part of the comprehensive program, particularly as self exercises. The Thera-Band is an elastic band that enables alternating eccentric and concentric contractions of the given muscle groups. There are several different types of elastic bands giving different resistance. For practical reasons, they are differently colored.

The main goals of the Thera-Band exercises are:

- Improvement of coordination achieved by alternation of eccentric and concentric muscle contraction, adjusted by different degree of resistance of the band

- Reduction of functional shortening of overused muscles
- Improvement of kinesthetic sense
- Dynamic muscle strengthening
- Helping to start an early self-treatment program

Mostly "light-resistance bands" (white and yellow) are used.

The performance of an exercise can be divided in two phases:

1. Active resisted movement to activate muscle groups that are anatomical antagonists to muscles that are shortened. During this movement, the shortened muscle is elongated.

2. Eccentric contraction resisted by the Thera-Band of that muscle group that is an anatomical antagonist of the shortened muscles. Performing this movement, the patient resists the movement against the direction of the tension of Thera-Band. The speed of this second phase should be half the speed of the first phase.

The Thera-Band exercises are adapted and corrected according to the results of the functional tests. As an example, we show some exercises to improve function of the internal rotators of the shoulder (Fig. 16.13), trunk flexors (Fig. 16.14), finger flexors (Fig. 16.15), hip internal rotators (Fig. 16.16), and thigh adductors and plantar flexors/supinators of the foot (Fig. 16.17), and a "great" combined exercise (Fig. 16.18). The pictures are self-explanatory.

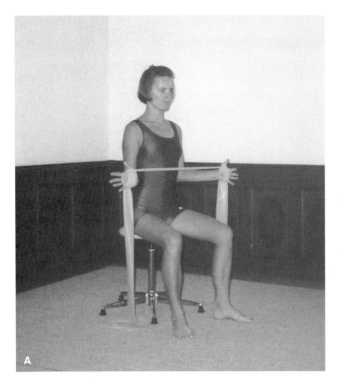
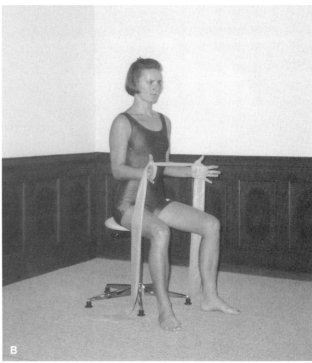

Figure 16.13 Thera-Band exercise to improve function of the internal rotators of the shoulder. **(A)** Phase 1. **(B)** Phase 2.

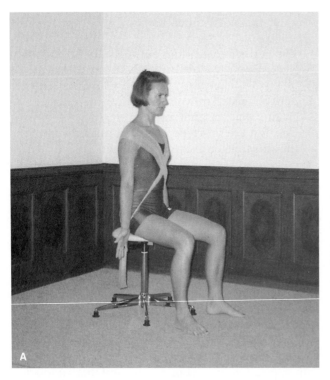
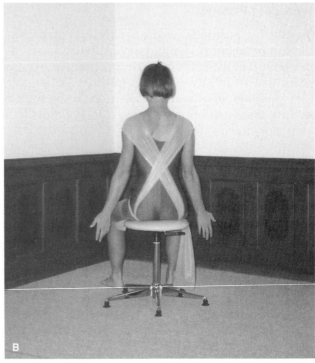

Figure 16.14 Thera-Band exercise to improve function of the trunk flexors. **(A)** Phase 1. **(B)** View from behind.

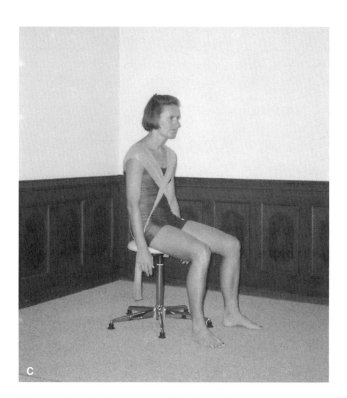

Figure 16.14 *(Continued)* **(C)** Phase 2.

Regarding Thera-Band Exercises

The starting positions for the exercises with Thera-Band should be considered as examples only. The exercises with Thera-Band can be performed from any position; however, whenever it is possible, the vertical position is preferred because this position is the closest to the most frequent postures.

ADL Training

Achievement of good movement patterns during activities of daily living represents an essential part of Brügger's concept. They are the most important but at the same time the most difficult procedures. Therefore, they are incorporated into each therapeutic lesson from the very beginning of the therapeutic program. The main goal is to achieve an automatic control of the learned erect postures (standing, sitting, forward bending, etc.) in various postural situations. Therefore, they are taught as much as possible in real situations and not just as a laboratory model. The proportion of the ADL training gradually increases so that finally they represent the largest proportion of the program. The use of

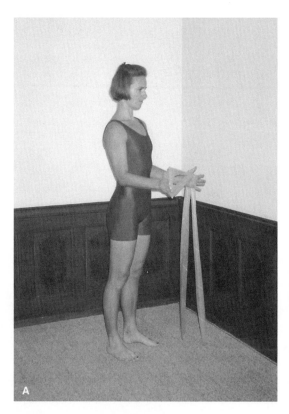

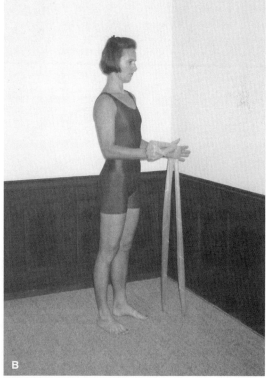

Figure 16.15 Thera-Band exercise to improve function of the finger flexors.
(A) Phase 1. **(B)** Phase 2.

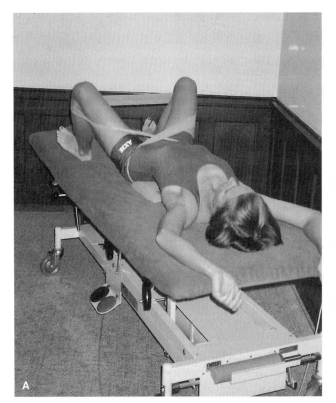
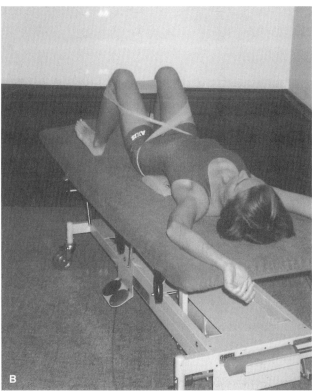

Figure 16.16 Thera-Band exercise to improve function of the hip internal rotators.
(A) Phase 1. **(B)** Phase 2.

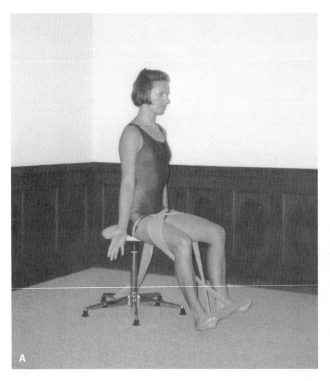
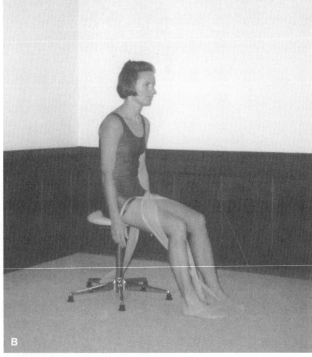

Figure 16.17 Thera-Band exercise to improve function of the thigh adductors and plantar flexors/supinators of the foot in sitting. **(A)** Phase 1. **(B)** Phase 2.

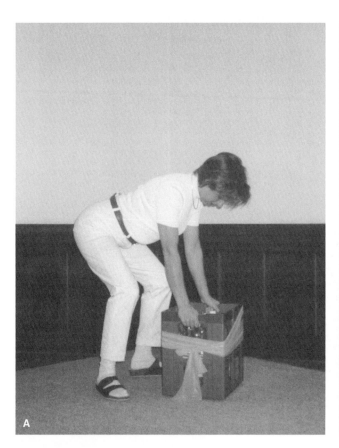

Figure 16.18 "Great" combined exercise with Thera-Band.

Thera-Band increases the demands on the exercise. For example, to lift a weight from the standing position apart from achieving a stable starting position on a relatively broader basis first, Brügger stresses the stabilization of the thoracolumbar lordosis. (Fig. 16.19)

"Retrocapital" Support of the Foot

The retrocapital support (Fig. 16.20) is a small cushion specifically designed to facilitate the functional stirrup of the foot. It is placed usually under the second metatarsal bone. Before placement of the retrocapital support, the foot has to be pretreated by a hot roll, manipulative procedures, etc., to decrease eventual swelling or muscle shortening. It is presumed that the cushion does not only function mechanically but also provokes a chain of reflexes regulating posture. This original concept was later approved because it is understood that the facilitation of foot proprioceptors plays the most important role in regulation of erect posture. As the functional stirrup is understood, a muscle loop consisted of the tibialis posterior and peroneus longus. This subloop is a part of the great diagonal sling (Fig. 16.1) that runs up to

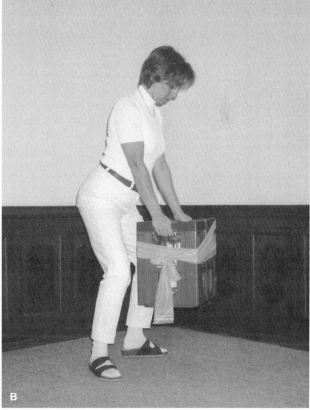

Figure 16.19 ADL exercise: lifting a weight from the standing position (with stabilization of the thoracolumbar lordosis). **(A)** Phase 1. **(B)** Phase 2.

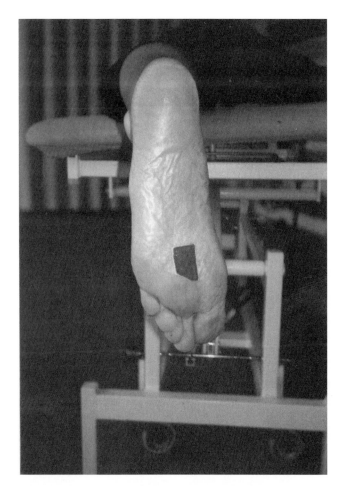

Figure 16.20 Retrocapital support of the foot.

m. peroneus longus. Functional tapes in the foot region are very useful, particularly in acute situations such as in ankle sprains, in habitual unstable ankle or to correct some evidently unfavorable foot positions.

The purpose of taping should support the exteroceptive and proprioceptive input to improve kinesthesia and function as a feedback mechanism. For example, if the tape is applied on the paraspinal area, it can be indicated as a reminder to maintain a corrected erect standing. Brügger calls it "memory tape." Application of tapes is particularly useful at the beginning of the ADL training program.

Other Therapeutic Procedures

Other procedures that have characteristics of the global movements are the therapeutic gait, called Brügger body walking, and six basic Brügger exercises.

Brügger Body Walking

Brügger body walking or therapeutic gait is particularly appropriate as a functional training, with the

the contralateral shoulder. The response to the support may be quite individual. However, in general, it should be used for several months to achieve reprogramming of movement.

Functional Taping

Usually the circular taping is used to stabilize the joint or to fix it in a desired position. The reason for taping in Brügger's concept is to achieve a dynamic stability, not to limit the mobility but on the contrary to optimize the movement in the right direction.

Example To support the muscle sling the tape is applied in the course of the tibialis anterior and peroneus longus muscles, which act as a functional stirrup from their crossing on the planta in an oblique direction beyond the ankles (Fig. 16.21).

Other tapes in the foot region that can be applied are, for example, the functional support of the transverse foot arch. In this case, the tape is applied along the both heads of the m. adductor hallucis (l). To stabilize the calcaneus in a neutral position, the tape follows the loop from m. flexor hallucis longus and

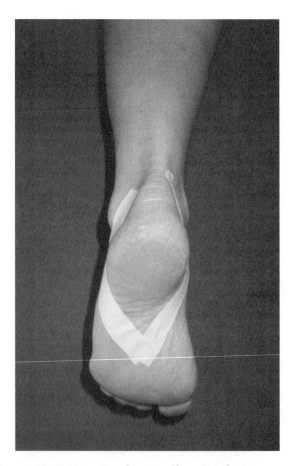

Figure 16.21 Functional taping (functional stirrup: m. tibialis posterion and m. peronaeus longus).

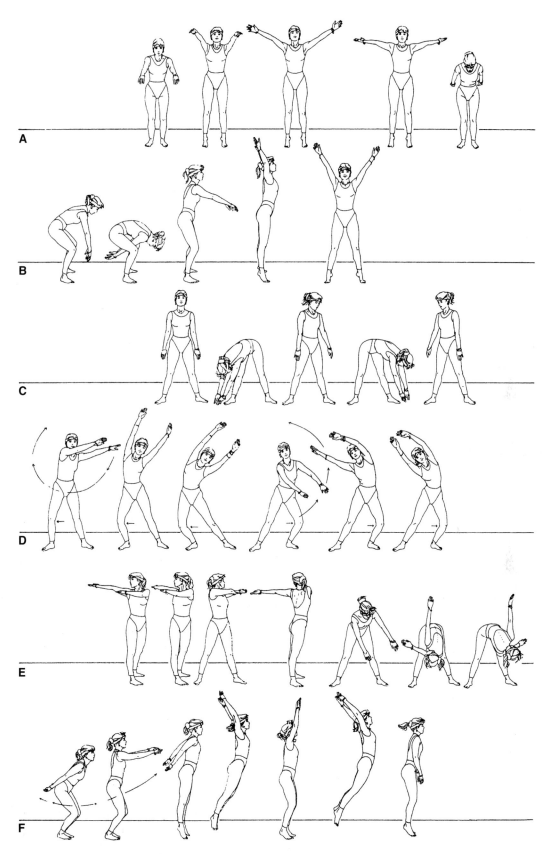

Figure 16.22 (A–F) Basic exercises, numbers 1 to 6. With permission from Brügger A. Lehrbuch der funktionellen Störungen des Bewegungssystems. Zollikon/Benglen: Brügger-Verlag, 2000:432.

goal to improve the movement patterns of the whole body. Speed of the gait should be reasonably fast but should never influence the rhythmic breathing. The compensatory arm movements should be initiated in the shoulder joints and not in the elbows. The duration of the gait training depends on the abilities of the patient. In principle, it is recommended to start with short periods and to prolong them gradually up to 30 minutes. It is useful to integrate short training units into the activities of daily living (for example, during walking in longer corridors, etc.).

Therapeutic gait can be combined with the Thera-Band, which is wound on the body. This gives an ideal resistance to guide the desired movement.

Brügger's Six Basic Exercises

Brügger's six basic exercises are very simple basic exercises to teach the ideal body posture and movement. They are compiled to exercise all body segments in all planes and to reinforce the awareness of correct movements and postures. In principle, these exercises should function against the constrained movements and postures that often prevail in daily activities.

Example Exercise to improve erect posture (Fig. 16.22A).

Slight repetitive squats combined with relaxed swinging arm movements. Through abduction, the arms reach in the final position extension and external rotation. The feet alternate from full-standing tip-toe stance.

Other exercises are more complex and involve all parts of the body (Fig. 16.22B to 16.22F).

Audit Process
Self-Check of the Chapter's Learning Objectives

- Describe how movements of the pelvis, rib cage, and head on neck influence posture.

- Why is the standing position ideal for therapeutic procedures such as agistic eccentric contraction, Thera-Band self-treatment, or the six basic exercises?

- How is the test of the fifth dorsal segment performed and intrepreted?

■ REFERENCES

1. Benninghoff A, Goertler K. Lehrbuch der Anatomie des Menschen. München. Vienna, Austria: Urban und Schwarzenberg, 1968.
2. Brügger A. Die Erkrankungen des Bewegungsapparates und seines Nervensystems. Stuttgart, New York: G. Fischer-Verlag, 1980.
3. Brügger A. Lehrbuch der funktionellen Störungen des Bewegungssystems. Zollikon/Benglen: Brügger-Verlag, 2000.
4. Brügger A. Gesunde Körperhaltung im Alltag. Zürich: Brügger-Verlag, 1990.
5. Kabat H. Studies on neuromuscular dysfunktion XII: New concepts and techniques of neuromuscular re-education for paralysis. Perm Found Med Bull 1950;8: 121–143.
6. Pavlů D. Co je skutečně Brüggerův sed? Rehabil fyz lék 2000;7:166–169.
7. Rock CM, Petak S. Agisticko-excentrické kontrakční postupy. Benglen/Zürich: Brügger-Verlag. 2000.
8. Rock CM, Petak S: Základní cvičení s Thera-Bandem. Zürich: Brügger-Institut, 1999.
9. Tittel K. Funktionelle Anatomie. Leipzig: Ambrosius Barth, 1999.

17

Rehabilitation of Breathing Pattern Disorders

Maria Perri

Learning Objectives
After reading this chapter you should be able to understand:

- The key role of respiration in spinal stability and in general health
- How to assess the motor patterns of respiration
- How to correct faulty patterns of respiration
- The relationship between respiration and abdominal bracing

In many instances, altered breathing patterns, whatever their origins, are maintained by nothing more sinister than pure habit.

Lum 1994 (27)

Introduction

Breathing with normal respiratory mechanics has a potent role in the neuromusculoskeletal system. Respiratory mechanics play a key role in both posture and spinal stabilization. Far beyond simply breathing correctly while performing a stabilization exercise, respiratory mechanics must be intact for both normal posture and spinal stabilization to be possible. In essence, the dynamic interaction between the key muscles of respiration must be functioning normally and, most importantly, a normal motor program for respiration must be subcortically "set" in the nervous system.

Chaitow, Bradley, and Gilbert state, "Nowhere in the body is the axiom of structure governing function more apparent than in its relation to respiration. Ultimately, the self-perpetuating cycle of functional change—creating structural modification—leading to reinforced dysfunctional tendencies can become complete, from whichever direction dysfunction arrives" (7).

Breathing mechanics are influenced directly by:

- biomechanical factors such as rib head fixations or classical upper/lower crossed patterns of muscle imbalance
- biochemical factors involving anything that effects the body's delicate pH balance including allergy, infection, poor diet, hormonal influences or kidney dysfunction
- psychosocial factors such as chronic anxiety, anger or depression

The evaluation of respiratory mechanics should be a routine part of every physical examination, especially for patients with chronic cervical symptoms, stress-related conditions (including high blood pressure), and delayed response to previous treatment. The goal of this chapter is to provide the practitioner with practical means of assessing respiration, identifying faulty patterns of breathing, and correcting them. This commonly requires three things:

1. Treatment of underlying causative factors
2. Breathing re-training with correct mechanics
3. Practice until this new program becomes "subcortical" and functionally integrated

Correction of faulty respiratory mechanics is integral to the success of any rehabilitation program of the locomotor system.

"If breathing is not normalized—no other movement pattern can be."

Karel Lewit (25)

Respiration

Correcting Faulty Breathing Mechanics

We are hardly aware of our breathing under normal circumstances. The rate and volume of our breath is influenced by physical, chemical, or emotional demands and then returned to normal relaxed abdominal breath once the demand is over. All of this is regulated and coordinated efficiently by our autonomic nervous system, without our ever having to think about it. That is, as long as the system is functioning normally.

Most of the time, faulty breathing patterns develop subcortically, often in compensation for injury or pain, or to maintain the blood pH, when other factors (stress, high altitude, infection, kidney disease, etc.) have altered the pH. A problem develops when an automatic response becomes an ingrained motor program, especially when the initial trigger no longer exists. This is often seen in chronic hyperventilation syndrome (11). In fact, the faulty pattern often becomes self-perpetuating. Once a pattern of overbreathing is established, it can be maintained by only a 10% increase in minute volume, which could be achieved by a combination of 10% deeper breaths, 10% faster breathing, or an occasional sigh (30).

The importance of addressing the underlying biomechanical, biochemical, and psychosocial factors in the ultimate success of any respiratory training program cannot be overstated. A shift in our thinking and in our evaluation of the patient must occur. We must move away from an examination of only the "hardware" (i.e., structural pathology) to one that also assesses key causative factors, including metabolic dysfunction as well as programs (i.e., "software") of movement, control, and coordination. And most importantly, our treatment must address these issues and work to restore normal subcortical motor programs. Motor training is possible because the cerebral cortex via the corticospinal tract allows for full voluntary control of respiratory patterns. For respiratory training to be effective, the conscious mind, ultimately, must be taken out of the loop. The new motor program must be practiced till accessed as the program of choice, automatically, in functional activities.

The Role of Respiratory Mechanics

Normal Respiration (1,7,13,21,22,25,26)

At its most basic level, respiration allows us to take oxygen (O_2) from inhaled air and excrete carbon dioxide (CO_2) with exhaled air. Changes in CO_2 (the body converts CO_2 to carbonic acid for transport in the blood) regulate the moment-to-moment concentration of pH in the bloodstream, whereas the kidneys regulate long-term levels of pH. The drive to breathe is regulated by the concentration of CO_2 (not O_2) in the blood. During exercise, as the body needs more O_2, it produces more CO_2 (high acidity), which immediately stimulates more breathing. The converse is also true; reduced exertion reduces the need for oxygen, decreases CO_2 production (low acidity), and lessens the drive to breathe (35).

The primary muscles responsible for respiration are the diaphragm, intercostal muscles, scalenes, transverse abdominus, muscles of pelvic floor, and the deep intrinsic muscles of the spine (1,19). Each of these muscles, in addition to respiration, serves a dual role in postural function as stabilizer (see the following box). The scalene muscles lift and expand the rib cage during inspiration and are active at a low level during every inspiratory effort and are therefore considered a primary, not an accessory muscle (9,10).

Postural Function of Respiratory Muscles

In 1976, Skladal et al. first described the diaphragm as "a respiratory muscle with a postural function" after observing that the diaphragm contracts when the patient stands on his toes (32). According to Kendall, McCreary and Provance, of the more than 20 primary and accessory muscles associated with respiration, almost all of them have a postural function (22).

Minor activity of the scalenes occurs with even a light breath, but more obvious visual and palpable activity occurs when demand is increased (10). The scalenes along with the accessory muscles including the sternocleidomastoid (SCM) and upper trapezius musculature are activated normally on high levels of ventilatory demand or at high lung volumes such as in hyperinflation (13).

The diaphragm is the primary muscle of respiration. It is basically a dome-shaped flat muscle that forms the floor of the thoracic cavity. Most anatomists divide it anatomically into three sections: sternal, costal, and lumbar, named for their origins. All sections insert into the central tendon, a thin strong aponeurosis with no bony attachment. The diaphragm attaches to the inner surface of the lower six ribs and their costal cartilages, posterior surface of xiphoid process, the body of lumbar vertebra 1–4 and their vertebral discs, and arcuate ligaments. It forms a circular attachment around the entire inner surface of the thorax.

During inspiration, the diaphragm contracts, the central tendon becomes more fixed as the dome flattens and moves downwards. This increases the volume and decreases the pressure of the thoracic cavity. At the same time, this increases the pressure in the abdominal cavity while decreasing its volume and causes the vaulting "outward" of the abdominal wall. The transverse abdominis and the pelvic floor muscles work in concert with the diaphragm to raise intra-abdominal pressure. The rectus abdominus must be relaxed for the vaulting outward to occur.

With continued contraction, the vertical fibers attached to the lower ribs expand them "open" in a horizontal direction commonly termed "bucket handle" motion (Figs. 17.1 and 17.2). The dimensions of the thorax are enlarged in all directions as in the filling up of a balloon (see the following box). With each normal (resting) breath, this bucket handle movement occurs at every rib level, which has a gentle micro-massaging effect that maintains healthy spinal movement along with circulation and nutritional flow to the musculoskeletal structures.

Cylindrical Breathing

It is important to note that the motion of the abdomen and rib cage during respiration is not only in the anterior–posterior plane. It is cylindrical, resembling a balloon being filled and expanding in all directions.

Movement of the upper ribs develops in the last phase of inspiration and is commonly known as "pump handle" motion (Fig. 17.3). The parasternal and scalene muscles play an important stabilizing role during inspiration to counteract the expiratory action of the diaphragm on the upper rib cage. As the diaphragm descends, it decreases the pleural pressure necessary for inspiration. The decrease in pleural pressure is greatest in the cephalad regions around the apex of the lung. If unopposed by the contraction of the parasternals and scalenes, the upper rib cage moves inward in the direction that is reflexive of expiration (10). As a result of their function in maintaining rib cage integrity, the scalenes are now categorized as core stabilizers not as accessory muscles as they have been in the past.

Normal movement in the upper ribs is an integral part of normal respiration and varies in response to the intensity of imposed physical demand. Recruiting the accessory muscles is normal as physical demand increases. Upper chest "lifting" is not normal during relaxed breathing, in which a "fanning open" motion should be observed. The faulty pattern of lifting "up" of the sternum vertically during

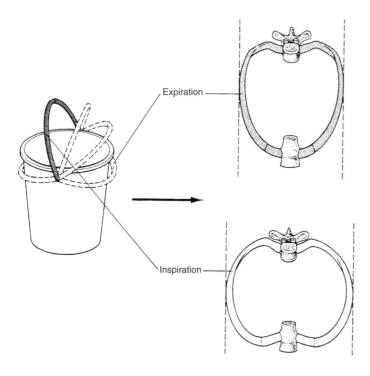

Figure 17.1 Bucket handle motion of ribs. Reproduced with permission from Iyengar BKS, Light on Pranayama, The Yogic Art of Breathing. New York: Crossroads Publishing, 1996:22.

inspiration, instead of widening in the horizontal plane, occurs because of over-activity in the scalene, trapezius and levator scapulae muscles. This faulty pattern commonly termed "chest breathing" (Fig. 17.4) is the most important fault in respiration and can impact the emotional as well as physical well being of a person. Chronic cervical overstrain, diminished activity of inter-costal muscles, and reduced rib motion is commonly seen. Deep clavicular grooves (Fig. 17.5) can be seen when this becomes a chronic pattern (26).

During expiration, the reverse occurs as in inspiration. In quiet respiration, expiration is produced

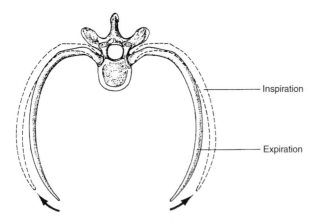

Figure 17.2 Bucket handle motion of ribs. Reproduced with permission from Iyengar BKS, Light on Pranayama, The Yogic Art of Breathing. New York: Crossroads Publishing, 1996:22.

passively by elastic forces from the abdominal wall, costal cartilages, and lungs. The diaphragm relaxes and ascends. The abdominal wall is "drawn in" toward the spine and the ribs and thorax move down and "in." Expiration is faulty when the breath is held and not fully exhaled, rib motion is reduced, or paradoxical breathing occurs, and the abdomen expands instead of being pulled in during exhalation.

Forced or active expiration results from muscle activity. The internal intercostal muscles contract and move the ribs and sternum downward and backward, whereas the muscles of the anterior abdominal wall increase the pressure in the abdominal cavity and force the diaphragm upward (1).

The moment one breathes against resistance, as during speech, the abdominal muscles come into play.

(Lewit)

The ability to maintain an abdominal brace while continuing to breathe is a normal mechanism that increases stability in times of need. It occurs subcortically in response to the need for increased stability during demanding activities, i.e., throwing a punch, lifting a weight, or performing a short sprint, but often needs to be trained in those with a history of back problems (28). This differs from Valsalva maneuver, produced by holding the breath usually after inspiration, but it can occur without regard to the phase of respiration when stability is required

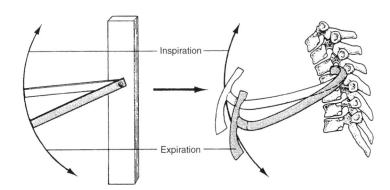

Figure 17.3 Pump handle motion of the upper ribs. Reproduced with permission from Iyengar BKS, Light on Pranayama, The Yogic Art of Breathing. New York: Crossroads Publishing, 1996:22.

in an emergency situation, i.e., a car accident (26). Breath-holding during quiet respiration or bracing is pathological.

When breathing is relaxed, both phases of respiration should occur through the nose. Mouth breathing occurs as the demand for oxygen increases, as in athletics. Mouth breathing during normal, relaxed breathing is pathological. The rhythm of the breath is equal (inspiration and expiration) during normal breathing and slows as relaxation occurs (see the following box). The torso should remain relaxed; no excess effort should be seen in the abdominal or scalene muscles. No excess yawns or tension should be seen in the face, lips, jaw, or tongue, and no excess noises or sighs should be audible.

Breathing Rhythm

The rhythm of the breath should be equal in both phases of respiration. As diaphragmatic breathing predominates, the breath rate can usually decline from 14 to 15 breaths per minute to 8 to 12 breathes per minute. The exhalation phase can become twice as long as the inhalation (7).

As clinicians, we must begin to view respiratory movements not only as a secondary automatic process of gas exchange but also as an exact motor process driven by a motor program that we can enter and influence.

The Relationship Between Dysfunction and Common Pain Syndromes

The diaphragm plays a vital role in spinal stability (see the following boxes). When its function is compromised, the spine is inevitably affected. And of course, the reverse is also true. When there is muscle dysfunction, as in neck and back pain, it is very common to also find abnormal breathing patterns. The following findings are commonly found when dysfunction occurs and the spine is compromised:

Respiration and Spinal Stability

When postural stability is required during an aerobic challenge and when the physiological demand for O_2 is high, the nervous system will naturally select maintenance of respiration over spine stability. An example of this occurs during repetitive bending or lifting activities when the back becomes vulnerable because of poor aerobic fitness, even if the motor control system is well-trained (28).

(continued)

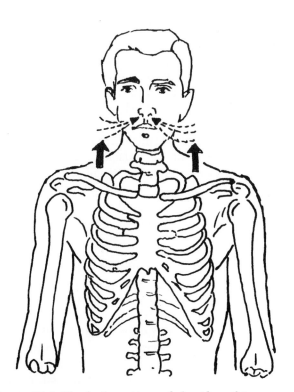

Figure 17.4 The faulty pattern of chest breathing.

Respiration and Spinal Stability (*continued*)

A simple exercise to train the respiratory and stability functions of the diaphragm can be incorporated into the side-bridge exercise. Once heart rate is increased with sufficient aerobic activity, isometrically hold the side-bridge position while performing a 360-degree brace and simultaneously breathing in and out deeply. It is normal to feel a more intense "burn" than when performing the side-bridge without an increased heart rate and breathing.

Stability and Aerobic Activity

Studies have shown during a mildly aerobic challenge, such as repetitive limb movements, that tonic activity of the diaphragm and transverse abdominus muscles can be maintained (15,16).

It has also been shown that good abdominal strength without proper coordination between the abdominals and diaphragm will lead to spine instability during challenging aerobic activities (17,18).

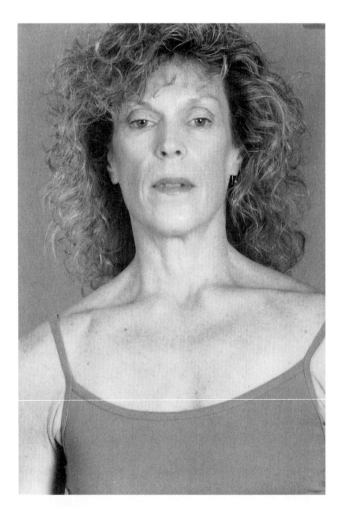

Figure 17.5 Deep clavicular grooves.

The most important fault in respiration of lifting the thorax with the accessory muscles of respiration instead of widening it in the horizontal plane is over-straining the cervical spine and musculature, contributing to recurrent cervical syndromes (25).

Although the pectoralis major, pectoralis minor, latissimus dorsi, serratus anterior, and trapezius are not typically considered accessory respiratory muscles, they assume a more respiratory than postural function in the dysfunctional or paradoxical breather and contribute to the faulty pattern of lifting the ribcage up during inspiration. This can lead to overuse syndromes in these muscles (19).

Lifting the thorax is part of a reflexive reaction to a sudden, intense stimulus that occurs during the "startle reflex." The head juts forward during this reaction as the person raises the shoulders in a complex pattern of flexion, which begins in the head and passes down the entire body (5,20). This pattern may become chronic and ingrained in the motor program, even when the initial stressful trigger no longer exists.

The most severe dysfunction is paradoxical breathing, in which the abdomen is drawn in during inhalation and out during exhalation. It may occur as a temporary reaction when bracing for anticipated action. The chronic pattern may be related to stress, severe chronic obstructive pulmonary disease, or simply result from the habit of holding the abdomen rigid in an attempt to have the appearance of a flat stomach.

Faulty respiration can contribute to low back dysfunction in a number of ways. The diaphragm, transverse abdominis (TrA), pelvic floor, and deep spinal intrinsics work in harmony such that dysfunction in one affects the others and inevitably effects spinal stabilization. When the diaphragm is inhibited, normal rib motion is altered or lost, as is the ability of the core muscles to stabilize the low back.

In particular, poor coordination of respiration and abdominal bracing during increased demand can inhibit the abdominal wall muscles. McGill found that poor cardiovascular endurance will lead to the nervous system selecting maintenance of respiration over spinal stability during an exertional challenge (Respiration and Spinal Stability box). An example would be a deconditioned middle-aged man shoveling snow. When breathing becomes labored, to maintain respiration, abdominal muscle effort will be reduced and the ability to maintain an abdominal brace is diminished, thus compromising spinal stability (28).

It has been theorized that increased tonic tone of the cervical accessory muscles and the diaphragm occurs as a result of decreased antagonistic tonic activity of the abdominal musculature. Hruska found this, especially in patients with forward head postures, temporomandibular dysfunction, and chronic sinus problems. Clinically, he has reported that hemi-diaphragm hypertonicity occurs with ipsilateral abdominal and oblique muscle weakness. This dysfunctional muscle chain is correlated with contralateral neck pain (19).

Forward head posture can develop as a postural compensation of living in the electronic age of computers and video games, as well as in relieving chronic dyspnea and shortness of breath seen in chronic respiratory disease. Patients with chronic airflow limitation (CAL) seen in emphysema, chronic bronchitis, and asthma often revert to an oral breathing strategy. "Mouth breathing" reduces the pharyngeal air space by decreasing suprahyoid tension, which allows the hyoid bone to fall down and back. The compensated forward head position that results helps to restore normal air space dimension at the expense of creating biomechanical stress that can perpetuate dysfunction in the musculoskeletal system (12).

To improve respiration, these patients commonly use the accessory muscles of respiration, lean forward while standing, look down with the head poked forward, and sigh with pursed lips (24).

Shoulder girdle mechanics are compromised in faulty respiration when chest breathing predominates and forward head posture results. The cumulative factors of hypertonic upper trapezius and levator scapulae, forward migration and internal rotation of the glenohumeral joint, compression of the sterno-clavicular and acromio-clavicular joints, and concomitant shortening of the pectoralis lead to shoulder impingement and neurovascular compression syndromes.

Faulty respiratory mechanics can contribute to recurrent mid thoracic pain from the lack of the mobilizing effect of normal rib motion. The loss of the bucket handle motion of the lower ribs and its gentle micro-massaging effect that promotes healthy spinal motion and circulation can adversely affect the entire thoraco-lumbar spine.

Shallow breathing leads to decreased expiration and decreased mobilization of the rib cage into extension. When this occurs, extension restrictions are commonly found at the T4-T6 levels. An increased kyphosis results that can become a fixed thoracic kyphosis if the faulty pattern becomes chronic. This, in turn, contributes to both the forward head and anterior shoulder postures.

Static over-contraction of the diaphragm can also change the rib cage dimension and anatomic arrangement of the ribs. As a result of ongoing external rotation of the mid to lower thoracic ribs, secondary to diaphragmatic hypertonicity, the posterior mediastinum is lengthened or stretched, and the mid thoracic spine becomes flatter. Compensatory increase of the lumbar lordosis (leading to dysfunction in the low back) and posterior rotation of the cranium also occur (19).

The Metabolic Function of Respiration

The rehabilitative power of the breath has been understood in ancient cultures for thousands of years. Breathing exercises are known to have a powerful healing effect on digestion, circulation, insomnia, and in the regulation of high blood pressure, anxiety, and mental states (34). According to one medical researcher, poor breathing plays a role in more than 75% of the ills people bring to their doctors (14). According to another researcher, there is a female preponderance in hyperventilation syndrome/breathing pattern disorder that ranges from 2:1 to 7:1 (8). The incidence of breathing pattern disorders as a primary diagnosis in general internal medicine practice is reported to be up to 10% of all patients (7), but why?

The important link respiration has on health lies in its role as a "doorway to the autonomic nervous system." One explanation is the essential function CO_2 has in maintaining the body's acid–base balance. "If you hold your breath, your blood, your entire body, really starts to become more acidic. If you breathe more than your body needs, your body begins to turn alkaline" (7). Subtle changes in the acid/base balance can have tremendous effects on the endocrine and immune systems, muscle function, pain perception, and emotional lability.

The body compensates for changes in pH by increasing or decreasing respiration. For example, keto-acidosis, a byproduct of a very popular diet that promotes high protein/low carbohydrate intake, increases the acidic state of the blood, which will promote deeper, faster breathing (the higher CO_2 content stimulates the breathing drive). Corrective overbreathing is also commonly seen after the acidosis that results from prolonged diarrhea. Use of steroids and diuretics as well as excessive vomiting causes alkalosis, which suppresses the breathing drive in an attempt to bring the pH back to a normal level (7).

Influences of Respiratory Dysfunction on General Health

Stresses in the modern world have lead to a widespread loss of normal breathing mechanics. Normal respiratory patterns are too often the exception rather than the rule. In a recent textbook, Leon Chaitow describes the health impact that may result: "Breathing dysfunction is seen to be at least an associated factor in most chronically fatigued and anxious people and almost all people subject to panic attacks and phobic behavior, many of whom also display multiple musculoskeletal symptoms" (6,7).

According to Chaitow, habitual chronic overbreathing (hyperventilation) increases the amount of carbon dioxide (CO_2) exhaled, leading to respiratory alkalosis. Alkalosis produces a sense of apprehension and anxiety that frequently leads to panic attacks and phobic behavior that results from a decrease in the threshold of peripheral nerve firing and an increase in muscular tension, muscle spasm, spinal reflexes, and significantly heightened perception of pain, light, and sound. It is no coincidence that this pattern duplicates the scenario of chronic pain conditions and can also result in emotional lability (6,7).

Unfortunately, normal patterns of breathing are the exception rather than the rule. In 2003, we performed a pilot study of 96 people to assess the incidence of faulty breathing in the general public. Only 25% of those studied exhibited normal breathing mechanics. When taking a normal breath, 53% of those tested were chest breathers, 56% lacked normal movement of the lower rib cage, and 19% had deep clavicular grooves. When asked to take a deep breath, the number of chest breathers increased to 74%. The study showed a significant correlation between neck pain, especially pain rated high on a visual analogue scale and breathing pattern disorders (29).

Chronic upper chest breathing and over-breathing result in dysfunction, which has a devastating effect on the entire organism well beyond the havoc it reaps with spinal stability, motor control, and the postural program. Chaitow reiterates and supports our opinion that "recovery is possible only when breathing is normalized."

Assessment of Respiration

Introduction

The average clinician can very easily and accurately assess respiration using the tools outlined.

It is important to take a thorough history to assess underlying factors that may influence respiration, including:

- History of cardiac, pulmonary, renal, or other organic disease
- Medications
- Menstrual cycle (progesterone tends to increase respiratory rate)
- Hormonal imbalance
- Diet
- Stress levels
- History of anxiety or panic attacks
- Chronic emotional state such as anxiety, anger, or fear
- Recent history of vomiting or diarrhea

Respiratory patterns should be included as an integral part of every functional examination but can also pro-

vide valuable information quickly and easily during an average treatment visit. It is important to note that respiration can be best assessed by observing the patient's movements while he is unaware that breathing is being examined. As soon as our awareness shifts to our breath; breathing mechanics are instantly shifted. Also, many patients will revert to a faulty chest breathing when asked to take a "deep breath" in. This false-positive can be avoided by asking the patient to take an "a slow, relaxed, full breath in" rather than "a deep breath in." The most accurate information is gleaned when the patient's cortical mind is kept out of it altogether by assessing respiration when they are focused on other tasks.

Assessing Respiratory Movement

It is important to note that a patient's ability to breathe normally may alter in different positions or situations. Some patients show relatively normal patterns when relaxed and in the supine position but change to "chest breathers" when they are challenged by a functional position or activity; like driving, working at a computer, or addressing a golf ball. Be sure to assess respiration in different positions, especially those that increase pain or are frequent during activities of daily living.

Respiratory movements are assessed in the following positions:

1. Seated or standing
2. Supine
3. Prone
4. In functional activities

There are several basic things to look for (in every position) while assessing respiration (Table 17.1):

1. Is the breath initiated in the abdomen or in the chest?
2. Does the rib cage widen in a horizontal plane during inspiration?
3. Is the upper chest movement normal or vertical?

Normally, movement from breathing should initiate in the abdomen, not the chest (Fig. 17.6). (It is very common for an abdominal breather to revert to a chest-breathing strategy when asked to take a deep breath in and the cortex dominates the movement.)

As the inspiration continues, the normal movement of the lower ribcage is to widen in a horizontal plane. Movement of the ribs can best be assessed by palpation in the seated or standing positions. Absence of movement in the lower ribcage is a common faulty finding (Fig. 17.7).

Table 17.1 Primary and Secondary Respiratory Faults

Primary Respiratory Faults

a. There is a lifting "up" motion of the entire ribcage (most obvious in the upper chest) during inspiration
b. Chest movements predominate over abdominal breathing
c. There is no lateral excursion of the lower ribs
d. Abdominal movement is paradoxical:
    The abdomen moves "in" during inhalation and "out" during exhalation
e. There is inability to maintain an abdominal brace and breathe normally

Secondary Respiratory Faults

a. Breathing is shallow with little to no motion in the abdomen or rib cage
d. Asymmetrical motion is seen in the abdomen or rib cage
e. The sequence from lower abdomen to middle chest to upper chest is altered
f. The rhythm is abrupt or "over-effort" is seen
g. Inhalation and exhalation are rapid or uneven in duration
h. Excess tension is seen in the face, lips, jaw, or tongue
i. Sighs or yawns are frequent

The final stage of inspiration includes a normal fanning open of the upper ribs. The most common and key respiratory fault is lifting the upper ribs up in a vertical plane (see the next box and Fig. 17.4).

Chest Breathing

The most common fault is substitution of the scalenes and upper trapezius for an inhibited diaphragm, resulting in the upper ribs rising "up" in a vertical direction during inspiration and the chest, rather than the abdomen, initiating and dominating the movement. When this pattern of chest breathing occurs, shrugged shoulders, frequent sighing, and failure of the lower ribs to widen in the horizontal plane are also seen.

As the practitioner becomes more skilled in respiratory assessment, the following "refinements" in observation can be made:

Abdominal breathing can be further categorized by the area of the abdomen that moves:

1. Just below the rib cage
2. At the umbilical level
3. Below the umbilicus

The deeper and more relaxed the breath, the lower in the abdomen it occurs. It has been our clinical experience that even those who have practiced breathing exercises for years do not always know how to breathe from very low in the abdomen. People, who are naturally relaxed, without any training, often automatically breathe from the lowest part of their abdomen. Patients prone to anxiety or in acute pain rarely have the ability to breathe naturally from below their navel and can benefit greatly from a daily practice of breathing exercises (Fig. 17.11).

The basic pattern of movement is the abdomen expanding outward during inhalation and being drawn toward the spine during exhalation. In paradoxical breathing, the exact opposite pattern occurs; the abdomen is drawn inward during inspiration and expands outward during exhalation (see the following box).

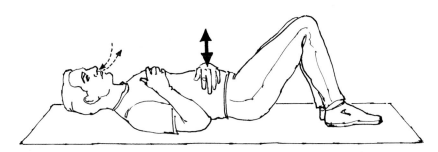

Figure 17.6 Movement in the abdomen during normal respiration.

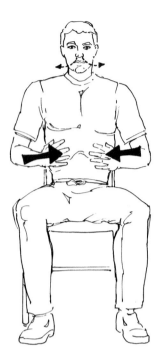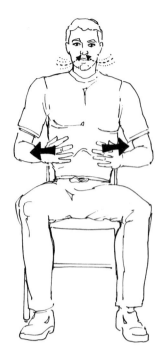

Figure 17.7 Assessing lateral rib motion (seated).

Paradoxical Breathing

Paradoxical breathing is a dysfunction in which the abdomen is drawn in during inhalation and out during exhalation. This pattern may relate to stress and a chronic firing of the startle reflex, or simply may be from the habit of holding the abdomen rigid in an attempt to have the appearance of a flat stomach. To correct this dysfunction, the patient must learn how to relax the rectus abdominis and use the diaphragm.

A more advanced observation is the direction of the movement. It is important to note that it is not in the anterior–posterior plane where the abdomen moves "up and down," but rather a cylindrical opening up (much like the filling up of a balloon). Many traditions that teach breathing exercises fail to emphasize this vital point and many exercises are performed only in the plane. Encouraging patients to practice exercises in a more cylindrical orientation will greatly improve the benefit they derive from them.

Asymmetrical movement on the right and left is an abnormal but common finding, especially in scoliosis and chronic pain. The side of chronic pain usually exhibits diminished motion.

Assessing Respiratory Movement Seated and Standing

Assessing respiration in the seated or standing position gives the clinician a more functional perspective and is the position of choice for the skilled practitioner. Palpation, in addition to observation, of the lower ribs is encouraged for the therapist as well as the patient when assessing (and treating) lower rib motion.

(Figs. 17.7 and 17.10) It is more ideal to assess lateral rib motion in the seated or standing position because the rib cage can move more freely than in the supine or prone positions.

It is normal in upright positions for widening of the thorax to be more prominent than abdominal movement. In upright positions, the abdominal's postural role is switched "on" and less movement is visible than in the supine position. Still, vertical motion of the upper ribcage should be absent, the lower ribs should expand laterally, and movement should initiate in the abdomen, not in the chest.

When asked to perform an abdominal brace, normal but slightly reduced respiratory motion should continue. The brace should be maintained also during an aerobic challenge.

Assessing Respiratory Movement Supine

The supine position is the easiest position for the practitioner to learn assessment and to begin treatment (Fig. 17.6). Abdominal and chest movement as well as paradoxical breathing are most easily seen in this position. Although limited, lateral rib motion is also easy to assess in the supine position (Fig. 17.8). In this position, abdominal motion should predominate over lateral rib motion and no lifting of the upper ribs should be visible. A normal pattern of respiration should be maintained when an abdominal brace

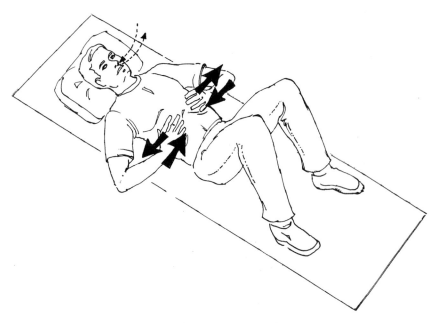

Figure 17.8 Assessing lateral rib motion (supine).

is performed. In severe dysfunction, the vertical lifting of the chest can be seen in the supine position with relaxed breathing.

Supine is less functional than other positions and it is advised that assessment and training progress to functional positions that duplicate activities of daily living.

Assessing Respiratory Movement Prone

Respiration in the prone position should be assessed with the skin of the back visible. The spinous processes subtly separate on inhalation and move closer together on exhalation. The respiratory wave begins in the lumbar spine and moves cephalward in both inhalation and exhalation. In the lumbar region, the circumference of the waist appears as if it were increasing in belt size. Movement in the lower ribs is posterio-lateral. The opening and closing motion of the ribs can also be seen into the upper thoracic spine.

Faulty breathing, as in the supine position, occurs when the spine and upper rib cage is lifted "up" during inhalation without sufficient expansion of the ribs or when the respiratory sequence is altered.

Fixation at a specific spinal level can easily be observed as respiratory movement is often absent at that level, whereas movement in the segments above and below is normal. It is very common to see an absence of spinal process and rib motion at the same level that is painful. It is fundamental in correcting the functional disturbances in the area of the symptom to train the patient to bring the breath to that area and facilitate movement in the ribs while breath-

ing. Often areas with absent respiratory movement must be manipulated before the patient's attempt to mobilize it with the breath can be successful. The converse is also true; if the patient does not learn to mobilize the area with the breath, the chronic patterns of fixation are very difficult to correct.

Assessing Respiratory Movement in Functional Activities

The end goal of respiratory assessment is to make it functional and reflect the specific daily activities of each patient. Ask the patient to perform a movement that they do frequently throughout the day or that gives them pain.

It is not enough to know how the patient breathes when resting or when static. The most significant point is whether the patient can breathe with normal mechanics during functional activities, specifically those that require an abdominal brace or increased respiratory function. The coordination between respiratory mechanics and abdominal bracing is more difficult to assess during functional activity but gives the most valuable information and must not be overlooked.

"Thinking of breathing, one naturally has in mind the respiratory system. Yet it is the motor system that makes the lungs work and coordinate the specific respiratory movements with the other motor activity. This task is so complex that it would take a miracle if disturbances did not occur."

Karel Lewit

Respiratory Training

Continuum of Care

Key Advice: Avoid slumped posture, tight clothing, and holding tension in the abdominals, and be mindful of signs of stress such as sighing and raising the shoulders

Key Manipulation: ribs 1-4, and C3, C4, T2-T9 (autonomic supply/pulmonary reflex)

Key Facilitation Exercises: Respiratory training/bracing, yoga, qi gong/tai chi

Key Relaxation Exercises: scalenes, upper trapezius, and levator scapulae

Rehabilitation Strategies

The approach to correction of faulty breathing patterns can be summarized in two steps:

1. Correction of underlying causative factors

2. Motor control training

When making a treatment plan, it is important to discuss the patient's goals and commitment to the lifestyle changes that may be required (e.g., reducing caffeine intake or seeing a therapist to resolve emotional upsets). For change to be lasting, the underlying factors that trigger the faulty breathing must be addressed. The most effective treatment plans begin with what the patient CAN do, progress by "attacking success," and have an element of fun for the patient. Practice times must be realistic for each individual and instructions as simple as possible for the patient to follow. Most importantly, it is essential for the patient to be motivated to take the time every day to do the exercises; it helps if the patient understands the huge impact regular breathing practice can have on physical and mental health (Table 17.2).

It is essential to treat underlying functional imbalances so that respiratory therapy can have lasting benefits. Initial treatment must include ergonomic advise, postural retraining, correction of muscle imbalance including hypertonic and inhibited mus-

Table 17.2 Benefits of Respiratory Motor Retraining

- Improved core stability and loco-motor function
- Muscle relaxation
- Release of stress and tension
- Improved pain management
- Enhanced physical performance
- Increased energy and endurance

cles, manipulation/mobilization of joint/rib head fixation, correction of faulty movement patterns and improved proprioception (see the following box). Addressing underlying bio-chemical and stress factors is also essential for a lasting change to occur (see the following box). Referral to a nutritionist, medication or yoga class or to a therapist who specializes in stress management may be indicated.

Diaphragmatic trigger points

The diaphragm has a dual postural and respiratory function. Faulty breathing and the presence of diaphragmatic trigger points may be an indication of deficiency in the local stabilizing system (i.e. transverse abdominis or pelvic floor dysfunction). In this situation, the underlying dysfunction must be corrected and stability to the area re-established BEFORE the diaphragm can be treated directly and breath re-training begun. This is similar to NOT treating tight hamstrings until lumbo-pelvic stability is restored.

CAUTION before beginning respiratory training

ALL organic, metabolic disease must be ruled out BEFORE respiratory therapy begins. Co-management with the patient's MD is essential especially when the patient presents with chest pain, breathlessness or dizziness. Breath re-training can have a potent effect on the blood pH; patients on prescription medication should be instructed to report any "changes" they may experience after practice.

Motor Training of Respiration

There are three basic principles of motor training that apply in restoring normal breathing mechanics (31):

1. Kinesthetic (cognitive) awareness of faulty breathing patterns.

2. Re-training of diaphragmatic breathing motor pattern and coordination with abdominal bracing (neuro-muscular coordination).

3. Automatizing and functionally integrating the new motor program of normal breathing both at rest and during activity.

Before respiratory training can begin, it is essential that the patient have a cognitive awareness of his/her habitual pattern of breathing and an understanding of what normal is. As with many functional imbalances, even after the patient has a mental understanding of what is expected, he may not have the motor control that allows his body to perform the correct movement.

It is important initially, especially in patients who have habitual patterns of upper chest breathing, to first relax the overactive synergists (scalenes, upper trapezius) and to avoid instructions that focus on inhalation. Tasking the patient's conscious mind to "try" to relax the chest and breathe into the abdomen often just re-enforces tension and faulty mechanics. A focus on exhalation, "emptying the lungs," allows an automatic fuller, deeper inhalation to follow (7).

So, although the goal is improved mechanics, especially during inhalation, initially, the focus is kept on exhalation with little instruction and subcortical facilitation of diaphragmatic activity. In reality, the mind is kept occupied while the real changes are being made (see the following box).

Focus of Respiratory Training

It is important for the patient to practice a "low, slow" steady rhythm and to avoid deep breaths and sighs. The therapist is encouraged to facilitate the abdomen and lateral ribs with slight overpressure during inhalation while the cortical mind is kept preoccupied with exhalation. As training progresses, the patient is encouraged to lengthen the exhalation phase so that it is twice as long as inhalation.

When fatigued and stressed, patients often revert to old, inefficient breathing patterns. Daily practice and awareness is recommended. If dizziness, tension, or discomfort arises during practice, the patient should stop and relax for several minutes and then resume practice with NORMAL, not deep, breaths. If symptoms continue, a peel-back or evaluation and treatment of underlying imbalances are in order.

Patients are encouraged to focus on their breath at least once an hour by creating "reminders" in their home and work environments; a small red dot on a computer screen, a timer, a ritual of practice every time they do a certain activity, i.e., stop at a red light, etc. The time it takes for a new motor program to automatize is variable for each person. Several weeks to months of daily practice is required for most motor programs to automatize a new "subcortical" program.

The exercises presented are simple and straightforward. Their goal is to teach correct patterns of movement with minimal cortical involvement and to have these new patterns become habit.

The Basics of Respiratory Retraining

The main goal of respiratory training is to move from a chest-breathing to a "belly-breathing" strategy that allows for horizontal motion of the lower ribs and

then to coordinate normal mechanics with the ability to stabilize the spine, as during abdominal bracing. Respiratory training is best begun in the supine position with the knees bent but can be performed in any position. It is important that the environment is conducive to relaxation and both the doctor and patient do not feel rushed. As in all motor training, patience and peel-backs are important for patients who lack the motor skills to perform the movements easily.

1. Kinesthetic Awareness

A. Belly Breathing Versus Chest Breathing Patients are asked to place one hand on their abdomen and one hand on their chest while relaxing and to notice their breath (Fig. 17.6). They are then given the simple instruction to notice which moves more, the abdomen or the chest?

If the abdomen movement predominates, tell the patients that they are breathing in a normal pattern and proceed to 1B—lateral rib motion.

If chest movement predominates, proceed to 1C—basic awareness training.

B. Lateral Rib Motion Patients are asked to place one hand on each side of the lower ribs while they relax and notice their breath (Figs. 17.7 and 17.8). This awareness can be performed in the seated or supine position. They are then given the instruction to notice if there is motion in the lateral ribs during inspiration and expiration.

If the lateral ribs move normally, give the patients feedback and proceed to 2C—training normal rhythm.

If there is no lower rib motion, proceed to 1C—basic awareness training.

C. Basic Awareness Training Goal: To be able to differentiate "normal" and faulty breathing mechanics.

The patient is shown normal mechanics using a verbal explanation and visual examples and guided to experience the motion of:

a. How the abdomen moves "inward" during exhalation, especially forced exhalation and "outward" during inhalation.

b. How the lower ribs "close" in the horizontal plane during exhalation and widen during inspiration.

It is a revelation to many patients that their lower ribcage can move in a horizontal plane. It is important to demonstrate horizontal movement of the ribs to patients who simply have no reference point or idea of how that movement is even possible.

c. How the upper ribs close and open during breathing without "lifting up." It is valuable to have the patient experience an exaggerated chest breath during inspiration. (Often it is easier to correct upper chest breathing when the patient has a clear idea of "what NOT to do.")

The therapist asks the patient to assess his own pattern of breathing and gives accurate feedback so that the patient has a realistic understanding of their starting point:

- If the patient continues to have difficulty breathing from the abdomen, proceed to 2A—facilitating deep diaphragmatic breathing.
- If the patient has difficulty with lateral rib excursion, proceed to 2B—facilitating lateral rib motion.
- If movement in the abdomen, ribs, and upper chest is normal, proceed to 2C—training normal rhythm.

2. Respiratory Motor Program Retraining

For exercises 2A, 2B, and 2C, the patients are guided to relax and "do nothing" but observe their exhalation. They are encouraged to slowly "empty the lungs" with pursed lips "until the first sense of a need to inhale" (NO STRAIN), pause for a moment, and then breathe in through the nose.

A. Facilitating Deep Diaphragmatic Breathing Training position: The therapist puts one hand on the patient's back at the T9 level and one hand below the xiphoid process and instructs the patient to relax and breathe normally.

Without verbal instruction, the therapist relaxes the pressure during exhalation and gently applies a slight pressure during inhalation, bringing both hands toward midline, to facilitate the diaphragm and discourage over-activity of the abdominals (Fig. 17.9). The therapist encourages the patient to keep focus on a low, slow exhalation and to feel the breath being moved from deep in the abdomen. After several breaths, the upper chest and abdomen begin to relax and the diaphragm begins to activate and initiate the breath (see the following box).

> ### Deep Diaphragmatic Breathing
>
> You will note a distinct difference between this type of deep diaphragmatic breath and breathing that is generated superficially by the abdominal muscles pushing "out" on inhalation and being pulled "in" on exhalation. It takes only minutes to facilitate this relaxed breathing and is essential for the patient (and therapist!) to experience so that real diaphragmatic activation is experienced and hopefully, duplicated in training.

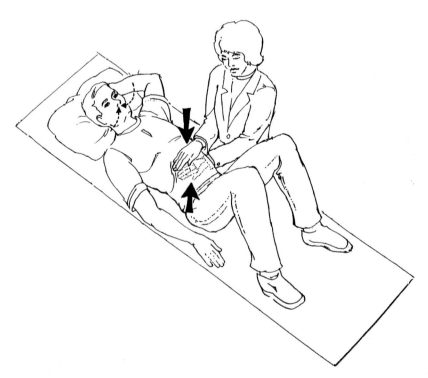

Figure 17.9 Supine facilitation of diaphragmatic breathing.

Clinical Pearl

Occupational therapists are able to effectively re-train breathing of severely handicapped children by facilitating the diaphragm and avoiding instructions that bring in the conscious mind.

B. Facilitating Lateral Rib Motion Training position: The therapist puts one hand on either side of the lower ribs and instructs the patient to relax and breathe normally (Fig. 17.10).

Without verbal instruction, the therapist relaxes the pressure during exhalation and gently applies a slight pressure during inhalation, bringing both hands toward midline to facilitate lateral motion of the lower ribs. The therapist encourages the patient to keep focus on a low, slow exhalation and to feel their rib cage contract and expand with each breath.

If the ribs DO NOT MOVE after several cycles of breath with lateral rib facilitation, return to section 1C—basic awareness training.

C. Training Normal Rhythm Once normal mechanics in the abdomen, lateral ribs, and upper chest have been achieved, the patient's attention is drawn to the rhythm of the breath. The patient is asked to "lengthen" the exhalation and told that as the breath relaxes and deepens, over time, the exhalation will take approximately twice as much time as the inhalation (see the following box).

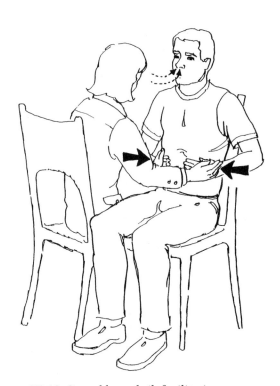

Figure 17.10 Seated lateral rib facilitation.

The Ideal Goal of Respiratory Training

The "ideal" end goal is to relax the breath to six to eight cycles per minute with a 7- to 8-second exhalation and a 2- to 3-second inhalation (7). Initially, the goal is simply to lengthen the exhalation and to exhale completely without strain.

Try to avoid exhaling to an excessive, forced degree, which might provoke a large, gasping inhalation subsequently. If exhalation has been complete, inhalation will automatically be deeper.

Leon Chaitow

D. Coordinating Breathing with Bracing Now that normal mechanics are in place, ask the patient to place his hands on the abdominal obliques and perform an abdominal brace with 10% maximum effort (see Chapter 26 for more specific instruction on abdominal bracing) while maintaining a normal pattern of breathing. Once this ability is achieved, increase the demand by inducing a simultaneous increased aerobic and stability challenge: Have the patient increase the heart rate (several minutes on a treadmill or step will do) and then perform a side-bridge while attempting to maintain an abdominal brace. It is vital that the patient learn to maintain an abdominal brace during exertional challenges.

Automatization and Functional Integration

It may take several days of practice for some patients to be able to perform this movement and rhythm with ease. If unable to relax the upper chest, lifting the arms over head and resting the head on clasped hands (beach posture; Fig. 17.11) often helps. Relaxing more and "doing" less is often the key to success.

Respiratory training is a motor skill that is best practiced frequently throughout the day. Patients are instructed to practice "low, slow breathing" twice per day:

1. Twice per day (morning and afternoon or evening) for 10 to 20 breaths
2. Once per hour for two to three breaths

For most patients, it is easiest to learn to breathe normally in the supine position and to link breathing with bracing in the standing position. Once an efficient new pattern is learned, patients are asked to bring attention to their breath during activities of daily living and finally during exertional challenges. As in all motor training, 3 months of daily training is required to create a new "habit" (23).

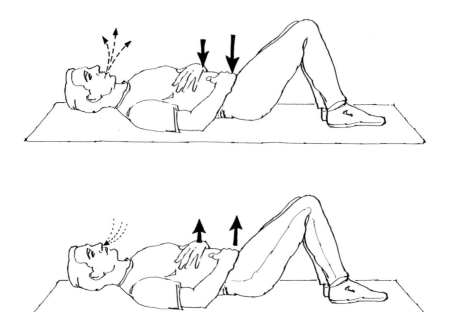

Figure 17.11 Exercise to deepen abdominal breathing (three levels).

Respiratory Training: Prone

Some patients who have difficulty with abdominal breathing are better facilitated in the prone position. Patients who have difficulty breaking the pattern of chronically lifting the upper chest "up" during inhalation can gain valuable and immediate feedback from training prone, especially over a gym ball.

It is very common for patients to "stop breathing" in areas of acute or chronic pain, even after the pain is no longer present. Guiding the patient to feel the area that lacks movement and restore movement to it is vital in the restoration of normal motor function. The therapist can gently touch the back in areas that lack normal movement and help the patient focus on bringing the breath to that area.

Respiratory Training: Facilitation Techniques

The following techniques can enhance respiratory training in all of the training positions:

1. The best facilitation is the doctor's or patient's hand over the desired area of movement with slight overpressure.
2. Facilitate abdominal breathing from as low as possible by moving the facilitating hand lower on the abdomen as relaxation progresses until it is just above the pubic bone. (Fig. 17.11).
3. Pursing the lips or blowing out of a straw is helpful to facilitate a low, slow exhalation.

4. Placing the tongue on the hard palate just behind the front teeth (the "resting tongue position") is a technique that is effective in all training positions.
5. Bringing the arms overhead with hands clasped behind the head (beach position) helps to inhibit the upper chest and encourage abdominal breathing (Fig. 17.12).
6. For those patients who simply cannot inhale and expand the abdomen:

    a. Instruct the patient to blow up a balloon a few times per day.

    b. Ask the patient to squeeze a ball between his knees or push his hands into the table while inhaling (Facilitating the pelvic floor or TrA will activate the diaphragm subcortically.).
7. For those patients who cannot co ordinate breathing and bracing, it is suggested that you train breathing mechanics and bracing separately first and then blend the two skills together. Standing is often the best training position.

Respiratory Training: The Buteyko Control Pause

The Buteyko Control Pause, just like the slow exhalation phase of the breathing exercises, acclimates people to tolerate more normal levels of CO_2. It is an effective exercise to balance the alkalosis that results from chronic "over-breathing" (hyperventilation) and has reported remarkable results reducing, and often eliminating, the symptoms of asthma (2,4,7,33).

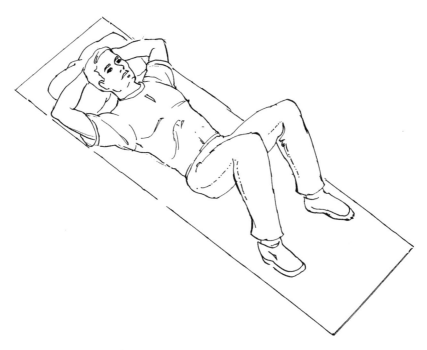

Figure 17.12 Beach position.

The patient is asked to sit in a relaxed position and breathe gently through the nose for 20 to 30 seconds. After a NORMAL inhalation, the patient is instructed to gently exhale most of the air through the nose and then HOLD the breath out until the first sign of discomfort. The hold time is measured.

- Normal holding time is 30 to 35 seconds
- Ideal holding time is 45 to 60 seconds
- A typical asthmatic pattern is 13 to 20 seconds
- Severe asthmatics will hold less than 10 seconds
- Over time, the comfortable holding time should improve

Although books and videos are available, patients are encouraged to learn this technique from a trained Buteyko teacher and to practice the Buteyko Control Pause under expert supervision.

Respiratory Training: In Activities of Daily Living

It is especially important to train respiration and bracing in the position that increases a patient's symptoms (driving, sitting at a computer, etc.) and those they are required to maintain during activities of daily living. Do not assume practicing normal respiratory mechanics and bracing in the supine position will correct patterns of coordination and faulty breathing in the seated or standing position. Two positions that facili-

tate the postural program and promote normal respiratory mechanics are the Brügger relief position and simply sitting upright with the hands clasped behind the back. For those challenged by prolonged sitting, these "relief" positions are suggested every 20 minutes.

It is not unusual for a patient to revert to faulty patterns in situations that are new or stressful. Many a golfer who has had breathing/bracing training still holds his breath or reverts to a faulty pattern when addressing the ball or when challenged with a difficult putt. The key in training normal respiratory mechanics is to transition the new motor skill to functional activities. This transition must be part of the training; most patients cannot make that leap on their own.

Training in activities of daily living follows the same basic principles as outlined here.

Exercise Prescription

Home Exercises to Enhance Proper Breathing

A. Supine, seated, and standing belly breathing with and without bracing in front of a mirror to facilitate coordination and monitor excessive upper chest motion.

B. Low, slow breathing focused on:
   - Lengthening the exhalation
   - Relaxation, so that movement occurs from the lowest possible part of the abdomen (Fig. 17.11)

• Relaxation, so that lateral rib motion is enhanced (Figs. 17.7 and 17.8)
C. The Buteyko Controlled Pause breathing.
D. Sitting on a chair with armrests, press elbows down into arm rests during deep inhalation (Fig. 17.13) (25).
E. Other exercises can also be found in chapter 24 on yoga.

Troubleshooting

If progress is slow and there is difficulty training normal breathing, the following should be addressed:

• Underlying biomechanical dysfunction must be corrected including:
  1. Hypertonicity in the scalenes, upper trapezius, and levator scapulae musculature
  2. Fixations in ribs 1-4 and the thoraco-lumbar spine
  3. Soft tissue restrictions and trigger points in the diaphragm
  4. Elimination of tight clothing
  5. Weight loss
• Underlying biochemical factors should be explored:
  1. Underlying metabolic disease
  2. Poor diet, nutritional deficiency
  3. Caffeine intake reduction
• Underlying stress factors needs to be resolved:
  1. Program of yoga or stress reduction
  2. Lifestyle change

3. Referral to a therapist to resolve emotional issues
4. Proper referral to handle sleep disturbances

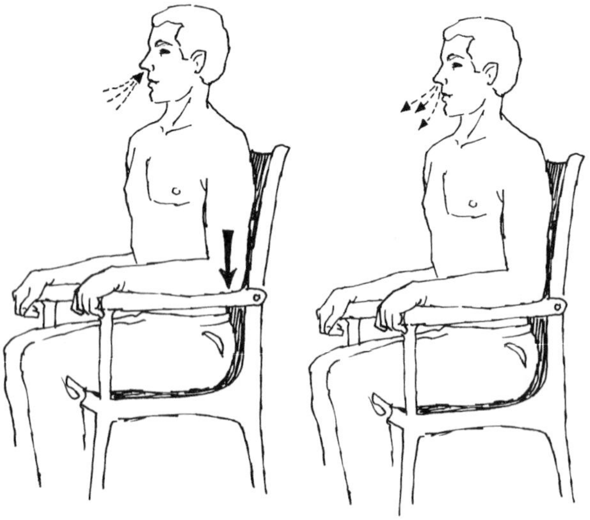

■ CONCLUSION

Normal respiratory mechanics are a foundational key to spinal stability and good health. Assessing respiration and treating faulty patterns of breathing is vital for core stability to be normalized. The end goal is to restore a normal motor program of breathing coordinated with the ability to abdominal brace that is subcortical and becomes the movement pattern of choice in a patient's activities of daily living.

Our breath is an open door to our autonomic nervous system. Every thought and movement easily and constantly influences breathing mechanics. Truly, the state of one's breathing is often a reflection of their state of well being. The importance of restoring normal respiratory mechanics for good health and for successful rehabilitation cannot be understated. Breath work, like brushing one's teeth, is recommended for daily hygiene. Even 2 minutes of daily practice can ensure that normal patterns are reinforced in the motor program, which can have a profound effect on treatment outcomes and on a patient's experience of life.

"To our ordinary consciousness, breathing only serves to maintain our body. But if we go beyond our mind, breathing can open up a completely new foundation for our life."

Ilsa Meddendor

Figure 17.13 Self-exercise for inhibiting chest-lifting during inspiration.

Audit Process
Self-Check of the Chapter's Learning Objectives

• How does a respiratory challenge interfere with spinal stability?

• Describe how you would assess for normal diaphragmatic function.

• How can diaphragmatic breathing be trained?

■ REFERENCES

1. Acland R. The video atlas of human anatomy. Tape 3. The trunk. Baltimore, MD: Williams & Wilkins, 1998.
2. Ameisen P. Every breath you take. New Zealand: Tandem Press, 1997.
3. Bowler S, et al. Buteyko breathing in asthma: a controlled trial. South Brisbane, Queensland: Mater Hospital, 1995.

4. Bradley D. Hyperventilation syndrome/breathing pattern disorders. Auckland, NZ: Tandem Press, 1998

5. Brown D, et al. New observations on the normal auditory startle reflex in man. Brain 1991;114:1891–1902.

6. Chaitow L. Clinical Application of Neuromuscular Techniques, vol 1. The Upper Body. London: Churchill Livingstone, 2000:50–52.

7. Chaitow L, Bradley D, Gilbert C. Multidisciplinary Approaches to Breathing Pattern Disorders. London: Churchhill Livingstone, 2002.

8. Damas-Mora J, Davies L, Taylor W, Jenner F. Menstrual respiratory changes and symptoms. Br J Psych 1980;136:492–497.

9. De Troyer A, Estennne M. Coordination between rib cage muscles and diaphragm during quiet breathing in humans. J Appl Physiol 1984;57:899.

10. De Troyer A, Estenne M. Functional Anatomy of The Respiratory Muscles. In: Belmen M, ed. Respiratory Muscles: Function in Health and Disease. Philadelphia: WB Saunders, 1985:175–195.

11. Gardener WN. The pathophysiology of hyperventilation disorders. Chest 1996;109:516–534.

12. Gonzalez H, et al. Forward head posture: It's structural and functional influence on the stomatognathic system, a conceptual study. J Craniomandib Pract 1996;14:71–80.

13. Williams, P ed. Gray's Anatomy, 38th ed. Edinburgh: Churchill Livingstone, 1995.

14. Hendricks G. Conscious Breathing. New York: Bantam Books, 1995:17–45.

15. Hodges P, Gandevia S. Activation of the human diaphragm during a repetitive postural task. J Physiol London 2000;522:165–175.

16. Hodges P, Gandevia S. Changes in intra-abdominal pressure during postural and respiratory activation of the human diaphragm. J Appl Physiol 2000;89: 967–976.

17. Hodges PW, Butler JE, McKenzie D, Gandevia SC. Contraction of the human diaphragm during postural adjustments. J Physiol London 1997;505: 239–248.

18. Hodges PW, McKenzie DK, Heijnen I, Gandevia SC. Reduced contribution of the diaphragm to postural control in patients with severe chronic airflow limitation. Melbourne, Australia: Proceedings of the Thoracic Society of Australia and New Zealand, 2000.

19. Hruska J. Influences of dysfunctional respiratory mechanics on orofacial pain. J Orofacial Pain Related Dis 1997;41:21–27.

20. Jones F, Kennedy J. An electromyographic technique for recording the startle pattern. J Psychol 1951;32: 63–68.

21. Kapandji LA. The Physiology of the Joints, vol. 3. The Trunk. Edinburgh: Livingston, 1974.

22. Peterson Kendall F, Kendall McCreary E, Geise Provance P. Muscles Testing and Function, 4th ed. Baltimore: Williams & Wilkins, 1993:325–329.

23. Kotke FJ. From reflex to skill: The training of coordination. Arch Phys Med Rehabil 1980;61:551–561.

24. Lareau S, Larson J. Ineffective breathing pattern related to airflow limitation. Nurs Clin North Am 1987;22:179–191.

25. Lewit K. Manipulative Therapy in Rehabilitation of the Locomotor System, 3rd ed. Oxford: Butterworth, 1999:26–29.

26. Lewit K. Relation of Faulty Respiration to Posture, with clinical implications. J Amer Osteopath Assoc 1980;8:525.

27. Lum L. Hyperventilation Syndromes: Physiological Considerations in Clinical Management. In: Timmons B, ed. Behavioral and Psychological Approaches to Breathing Disorders. New York: Plenus Press, 1994.

28. McGill SM, Sharratt MT, Seguin JP. Loads on the spinal tissues during simultaneous lifting and ventilatory challenge. Ergonomics 1995;38:1772–1792.

29. Perri M, Halford L. Pain and faulty breathing: a pilot study. J Bodywork Movement Ther 2004;8:237–312.

30. Saltzman HA, Heyman A, Sieker HO. Correlation of clinical and physiologic manifestations of sustained hyperventilation. N Engl J Med 1963;268:1431–1436.

31. Shumway-Cook A, Woollacott M. Motor control-Theory and practical applications. Baltimore: Lippincott Williams & Wilkins, 1995.

32. Skládal J, et al. Bránice člověka ve světle normalní a klinické fysiologie (The human diaphragm in normal and clinical physiology). Prague: Academia No 14, 1976.

33. Stalmatsky A. Freedom from asthma—Buteyko's revolutionary treatment. Great Britain: Kyle Cathie Ltd, 1997.

34. Weil A. Breathing. Boulder: Sounds True, 1999.

35. West JB. Respiratory physiology: The essentials. Philadelphia: Lippincott Williams & Wilkins, 2000.

18

Soft Tissue Manipulation

Karel Lewit and Alena Kobesová

Learning Objectives

After reading this chapter you should be able to understand:

- The barrier phenomenon, as an essential element in palpation for diagnosis and treatment.
- How to distinguish normal from the pathological barrier when stretching, shifting, or exerting pressure on soft tissues, and how to obtain release for therapy.
- That the barrier principle has to be applied to the skin, the connective tissues, the muscles, the fascias and the subperiosteal tissues.
- The close relationship of the pathological barrier with increased resistance, tension and pain, and the significance of release, i.e., the normalization of tension and the relief of pain.
- That the art of palpation is essential. To have learned palpation is to be able to feel the painful lesions in the soft tissues.

Introduction

By definition it is understood that soft tissues comprise all structures surrounding bones and joints relating to the motor system; i.e., skin, subcutaneous connective tissue, the superficial and deep fascia, and the muscles between them. Unlike the other structures mentioned, muscles are contractile and constitute the driving force of the motor system; nevertheless, they are part of the soft tissues and can be treated by soft tissue techniques, as will be shown in this chapter.

Although soft tissues are mainly passive structures like bones and joints, they have to move whenever muscles contract. But unlike bones and joints where mobility has been studied in detail, mobility of soft tissues has been neglected to a large extent. Yet, if our muscles contract to move bones and joints, all the surrounding tissues have to move as well. The range of these movements is considerable and quite in keeping with joint mobility (7).

There are two types of movement: one is stretching, which is most obvious at the body surface, i.e., the skin. That this movement can be considerable can be easily measured if we compare the distance between the head and the buttocks when stooping and then in back bending, or if we measure the distance between the fingers and the wrist during palmar and dorsal flexion. It is therefore no coincidence that the skin stretches much more easily in a cranio-caudal or proximo-distal direction than in a transverse direction.

The second type of movement is shifting of one soft tissue layer against the underlying one. This is particularly vital in relation to the contractile element, the muscles. Whenever muscles contract, they have to move freely against the surrounding tissues, in particular against bone. This must happen without friction, although the muscle may shorten even to a fraction of its length.

These are no doubt very complex movements that up to now have been largely neglected, very little studied, and therefore poorly understood. They are, however, essential for the normal functioning of the motor system. Being "only soft," one might believe that they could be no serious mechanical obstacle to our powerful muscles: they interfere mainly by very powerful reflex mechanisms.

Although shifting and stretching of soft tissues has been little studied and we know hardly any norms, we have to diagnose soft tissue lesions first and then treat them. Our main tool for both diagnosis and treatment is the barrier phenomenon and it is precisely this key phenomenon that differentiates soft tissue manipulation techniques from massage.

The Barrier Phenomenon (Concept), Palpation, and Pain

When shifting or stretching, there is always, like in joints, a free range but soon resistance is met. The first resistance is where we define the barrier. It normally easily gives and springs. The pathological barrier restricts the free range and is abrupt. We therefore have to first diagnose a pathological barrier and then obtain release, i.e., soft tissue manipulation.

This was described for joints. Examining joint motion there is a free range where resistance is practically nil. Resistance then starts to increase, up to a point at which no further excursion is possible under normal conditions. As the range of maximum passive motion surpasses active motion, chiropractors define the barrier as the end of passive movement (12). Osteopaths, however, define the barrier as the end of active movement (4). In our opinion, both these definitions are flawed.

Engaging the barrier at maximum passive range for any type of manipulation (thrust or springing mobilization) is incompatible with gentle, physiological techniques. The barrier has a protective function, which is to resist maximum range. Therefore, the stretch reflex is elicited at this point so that the patient's muscular forces are overcome.

Engaging the barrier at the end of active movement makes no sense for whether we are mobilizing joints or treating soft tissues, and we first examine and then produce passive motion (mobilization or thrust).

Therefore, we define the physiological barrier as the point where the first (slight) resistance is met, no matter whether we are moving joints or stretching soft tissue or shifting soft tissues one against the other: there is always a free range up to the barrier (Fig. 18.1). In our diagram, we distinguish the anatomical barrier (A), the physiological barrier (Ph), the pathological barrier (Pat), and the neutral point N0. N1 stands for a changed neutral point caused by a pathological barrier in joint dysfunction. The physiological barrier springs and gives easily; the pathological barrier restricts motion, is abrupt, and springs very little. Although this definition is essential for the

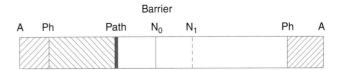

Figure 18.1 The barrier phenomenon. The anatomical, physiological, and pathological barriers and the neutral points.

technique of (soft tissue) manipulation, it is not without problems. Not every therapist will sense the first resistance at exactly the same point. A subjective element cannot be ruled out. The reason for this is that every manual technique relies on palpation. Palpation is an extremely sophisticated procedure in the hands of the expert. Unlike vision or hearing, it cannot be reproduced by any instrument. The reason is that our hands have receptors not only for touch and pressure but also for motion, position, and qualities like temperature, moisture, and friction. In addition, the hands produce a reaction in the patient, establishing a feedback situation. There is no single instrument that can supply a comparable amount of information as the hands of a trained examiner processed by the brain.

The basic soft tissue technique, like a common denominator, is as follows: first, for diagnosis, we engage the barrier or, in other words "take up the slack," to decide whether there is a normal physiological barrier or a restrictive abrupt pathological barrier. We also speak of the normal or pathological "end feel."

If we diagnose abnormality, we wait at the barrier and without our substantially changing force or direction, release will take place; this we have to sense. Release may take from a few seconds to up to half a minute or more, and has to be sensed right up to the very end; the longer the better. During the process of release, we may change force and/or direction very slightly. Even eye movements and the phase of breathing can be incorporated to enhance the release of tissue tension (see Chapter 19) (9). This is termed respiratory or visual synkinesis. The great advantage of this method is the feedback situation; sensing release to the very end, we know that the job has been done.

There is a close relationship between the pathological barrier, release, and relief from pain. It can be said in a nutshell that the structure at which release has been achieved ceases to be painful. In other words, a pathological barrier goes hand-in-hand with increased tension, and whenever release sets in, we feel that tension diminishes and we know that we have relieved pain. Those who know how to palpate can sense where the patient feels the pain and also when pain (at least locally) subsides. Therefore, in this chapter, we present mainly techniques based on the barrier phenomenon. In our view, this is the principal difference between massage and soft tissue techniques, although the former is frequently presented as such. Our approach is based on the barrier phenomena and its precise diagnosis and release. We feel justified to call it "soft tissue manipulation."

The Clinical Paradox: Palpation is subjective, yet it is our only tool to objectify the patient's pain. All soft tissue structures react to painful (nociceptive) stimulation: the muscle by spasm, most frequently with trigger points (TrPs), the skin and the subcutaneous tissues by increased resistance to stretching and folding (skin rolling), and the fascias by resisting both stretch and shifting against other tissue layers, particularly bone. A very rich clinical symptomatology indeed, it should be called the "clinical objectivisation of pain," except that it can only be detected by palpation, and this is considered purely "subjective." This paradox could be put as "not understanding what we comprehend and what is manifest" (1,8).

Skin

In painful lesions, the skin is tender in the segment where pain (nociceptive stimulation) originates. This used to be called a "Head's zone," particularly if the origin of pain was an internal organ; we usually call it a hyperalgesic (skin) zone (HAZ). We can easily diagnose such a zone by palpation: the skin fold there is thicker, i.e., the skin resists folding and on stretching we find a restrictive barrier that hardly springs (compared with the other side; Fig. 18.2). For treatment, we engage the barrier very gently and wait for release. Once release sets in, it continues without our increasing the initial force, until we reach the normal barrier. After this, there should be symmetry on both sides.

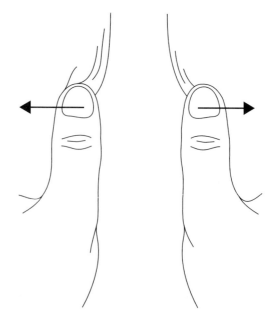

Figure 18.2 Skin stretch.

Stretching should be tested in the direction in which the skin is stretched under physiological conditions: at the trunk in a cranio-caudal and at the extremities in a proximo-distal direction.

Skin folding and particularly skin rolling are certainly quite popular procedures; they can, however, be very unpleasant and painful and have no advantage over skin stretching. However, there is a screening procedure, which does not make use of the barrier phenomenon and which is most elegant and rapid for detecting HAZs. This is skin drag, and it is usually the first technique we apply for diagnosis. We make a light, not too fast stroking movement over the skin, most typically over the patient's back, in a cranio-caudal direction; we sense friction. In the HAZs, friction is increased because of hyperhydrosis in the HAZ. The area in which we find increased skin drag corresponds to the HAZ and should be stretched. Small areas can be stretched between two fingers, larger areas between both thumbs, and very large areas between the ulnar aspects of our crossed hands. Once the normal barrier is re-established, skin dragm will be normal, the same as on the other unaffected side.

There is a very specific HAZ with diagnosis and treatment that is of special interest. This is found at the interdigital folds on hands and feet. It is found mainly in root syndromes if the patient feels pain and/or numbness radiating to fingers or toes. Normally the interdigital fold springs very easily, as can not only be felt but also be seen. Lack of springing here is a true neurological sign of a root lesion. At the hand, the interdigital fold between the second and third and between the third and fourth finger correspond to the C7 root, and the fold between the fourth and fifth finger to the C8 root. The fold between the first and second and between the second and third toe correspond to the L5, and the folds between the third and fourth and the fourth and fifth toe correspond to the S1 root.

If there is stiffness in one of the interdigital folds, we engage the barrier very gently and just wait for release. Normalization of the barrier at this location can have a surprisingly favorable effect in root syndromes radiating to the toes or fingers.

Connective Tissue

If subcutaneous tissue or connective tissue in muscles is at fault, we produce a fold between the fingers of both hands and stretch it (Fig. 18.3). With a very gentle stretch, we engage the barrier and wait for release. During release the S-shaped fold deepens. It is most important never to squeeze the tissue between our fingers, only to stretch it, i.e., so that the curves of the "S" deepen.

In clinical practice we use connective tissue folds most frequently to treat active scars and for stretching short muscles (not TrPs!). This is our favorite technique when treating short muscles and should be applied to all muscles accessible to folding. This is because the technique avoids the stretch reflex, which is necessarily provoked by stretching a muscle in its length. We may perform folding between our fingers and in very large muscles (e.g., hamstrings) between the palms of both hands. The muscles that are most frequently treated in this way are the upper trapezius, the pectoralis, the biceps, the hamstrings, the adductors, and the soleus.

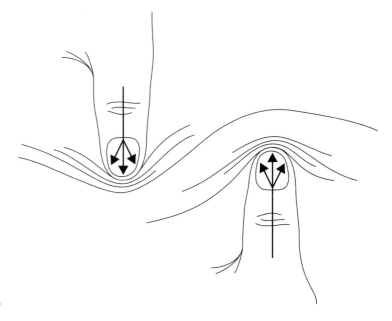

Figure 18.3 Stretching a soft tissue fold.

Using Slight Pressure Mainly on Muscles

Very slight pressure to reach the barrier and then waiting at the barrier until release takes place is a most effective method to treat TrPs that are accessible to our fingers (Fig. 18.4) after being diagnosed by "snapping palpation" (11). It is therefore a useful alternative to relaxation methods. This method uses such slight pressure that the patient barely feels it. The therapist simply waits until he (she) senses the resistance of the TrP "melting" under the fingers. The patient either feels nothing or experiences a sensation of warmth.

It should be pointed out that "schemic" (forceful) pressure (2), which can be very painful, is necessary in cases in which the TrP is no longer entirely reversible. This is the case if pain has been for a long period at one point, which is not part of a typical chain, or which does not react to postisometric relaxation or reciprocal inhibition and/or remains unchanged after treatment of a typical chain with all the rest of the TrPs responding to treatment. In such cases, dry needling is the best alternative.

Muscles like the spinal erectors are treated by the tip of a finger or thumb; wherever it is possible to place the muscle between our thumb and forefinger (the SCM, the upper trapezius, even the pectoralis, biceps, triceps, etc.), this is preferable. In very deep muscles like the iliopsoas, the subscapularis, the pterygoids, and the pelvic floor, even very slight pressure is painful; therefore, relaxation methods are preferable. Once release has been followed to the end, no TrP should be felt either by the examiner or by the patient.

In very large muscles like the gluteus maximus, we may sense full release by pressure in one direction, but on changing the direction of pressure we find there is still a pathological barrier in another direction; this must be treated by changing the direction of pressure. Normalization of pressure is fully accomplished if on changing direction no more resistance can be sensed.

Even deeply situated connective tissue structures, where making a fold is technically impossible, can be treated by mere pressure. This is quite frequently the case in the deeper layers of scars (the alternative being needling or local anaesthesia.). However, the noninvasive gentle pressure should be our first choice, because it also has the advantage of a feedback situation: when we sense the release, we know the job has been done.

The Fascias (13)

The function the of fascias is in general to enable contracting muscle to move smoothly against all neighboring structures. But there are also fascias into which muscles insert, such as the lumbodorsal fascia. In these circumstances, muscle fibers and fibers of the fascia are closely interconnected. If several muscles insert into a large fascia, it integrates the action of these muscles.

It is mainly in cases of chronic myofascial pain that fascia becomes dysfunctional; this severely affects muscles so that some neurologists (10) speak of "dystrophy." Muscles can be both hypertonic and atrophic. On examination, the fascia does not shift (glide) against neighboring structures, most obviously against bone.

For diagnosis, we shift the fascia to engage the barrier. By continuing slight pressure against a pathological barrier, release sets in after the usual latency period and should continue until the normal barrier is reached. It is important to know that on the back the painful side is not necessarily the restricted side. The characteristic finding is what has been called the "tight–loose complex," i.e., there is restriction on one side and laxity on the other (13). Treatment is, of course, given to the restricted side; the effect is, however, that not only does the restricted side become more mobile but also does the loose side get firmer. As in other instances, normalization does not necessarily imply increased mobility, but primarily restored symmetry.

Fascia on the Back

We find movement restriction in the back fascias, most frequently in chronic back pain, particularly in root syndromes. For diagnosis, the patient lies prone with the head in a neutral position and the arms alongside the trunk. We examine the mobility of soft tissues against bone, first in a cranial direction, then take up the slack and spring the barrier, comparing the two sides.

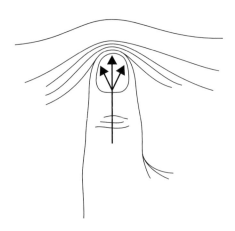

Figure 18.4 Exerting pressure.

For treatment, the patient turns her head to the restricted side; the arm on the same side is fully extended and so are the fingers of that hand. The toes of the foot of the same side press against the end of the table. The therapist stands at the side of the table, facing the patient's head, and fixes the soft tissues with one hand in the thoracolumbar area while mobilizing with the other hand over the shoulder blades in a cranial direction, engaging the barrier (Fig. 18.5).

The patient is told to breathe in, to hold her breath, and then to breathe out. During inhalation, resistance increases, whereas during exhalation, release is obtained and the therapist's hand moves the soft tissues in a cranial direction, slightly rotating his hand medially. This is usually repeated two or three times. It is helpful if the patient is told to cough once or twice.

Diagnosis in a caudal direction is very similar—examination of mobility of the buttocks in a caudal direction. For treatment, the patient is in exactly the same position as described. The therapist now faces the patient's buttocks. One hand fixes the soft tissues in the thoracic region, the other takes up the slack by slight pressure to the buttock in a caudal direction (Fig. 18.6).

The main difference between the the two cases is that now the therapist tells the patient to breathe out slowly, because here resistance increases during exhalation; he then slowly breathes in. It is during inhalation that release is obtained and the therapist's hand moves in a caudal and slightly medial direction.

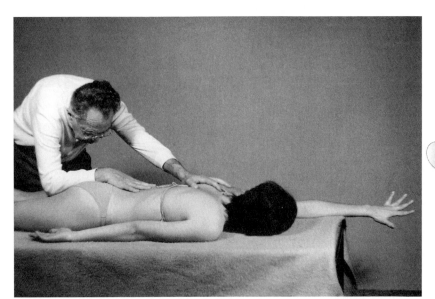

Figure 18.5 Shifting and stretching fascias on the back in a cranial direction.

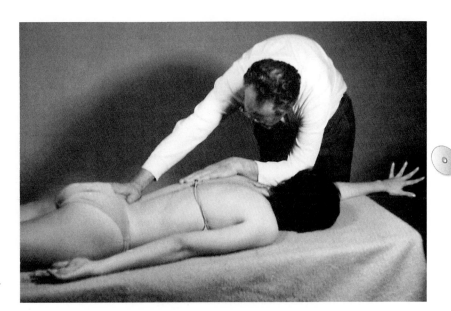

Figure 18.6 Shifting and stretching fascias on the back in a caudal direction.

In this case, as we have pointed out, resistance increases during exhalation. This is caused by a respiratory synkinesis: the spinal erector trunci contracts in lordotic posture during deep exhalation (10). After treatment, we always check for symmetry.

The Buttocks

In the preceding paragraph, the buttocks were mobilized in a caudal direction. Quite frequently the opposite direction is restricted. In such cases there is hypertonus at the buttocks, frequently caused by a deep TrP in the gluteal muscles. This can also be treated by gentle pressure, as we have seen. Restriction of cranial motion is examined by comparing the two sides. On the side of restriction (hypertonus), we find a most striking palpatory illusion if we examine the position of the ischial tuberosities: on the side of increased tonus it appears to be lower than on the other, with the difference being quite considerable (1 to 2 cm) (Fig. 18.7). After soft tissue treatment, symmetry is restored (8).

For treatment, the barrier is engaged in a cranial direction, and after a short latency release is obtained and the buttock moves up. We see this lesion most frequently in connection with a forward-drawn posture caused by TrPs in the straight abdominal muscles.

Thoracic Fascia

There is considerable mobility of soft tissue around the thorax in a circular direction. Normal mobility here seems to be of great clinical importance. We see restriction frequently in thoracic and breast pain, particularly with TrPs in the subscapularis and the diaphragm. Restriction of soft tissue mobility is of major importance in such cases.

For examination, the therapist stands or sits at the side of the patient, moving the soft tissues at the level of the breast in a ventro-medial direction around the axis of the thorax. His thumb and forefinger are stretched apart as he compares mobility on the two sides (Fig. 18.8).

For treatment, we wait at the barrier to obtain release taking up the same position. We may also work from the opposite side of the table and move the soft tissue with the wrist. This is the technique that the patient uses for self-treatment (supine) (Fig. 18.9).

Fascia on the Neck and the Cervicothoracic Junction

The clinically relevant movement of all soft tissue layers in the cervical region is around the long axis of the neck. It is examined by placing our palm with the fingers and thumb around the neck from the dorsal aspect (Fig. 18.10) and producing a rotatory movement around the neck. First engage the barrier in the direction of the thumb, and then spring it for diagnosis; if we find a pathological barrier, we engage it and wait for release. Moving in the direction of the thumb, we mobilize a narrower section of soft tissue than in the direction of the fingers; therefore, if we find a pathological barrier only in a smaller area of the neck, mobilization in this direction may be more appropriate (more specific). If, however, the entire length of the neck is involved, it is preferable to use the four fingers.

In the cervicothoracic junction, a similar technique may be used if the patient is slim and the therapist has

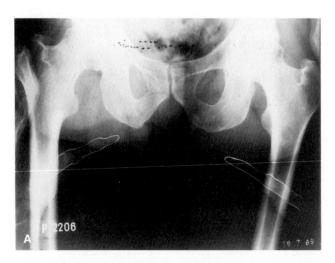
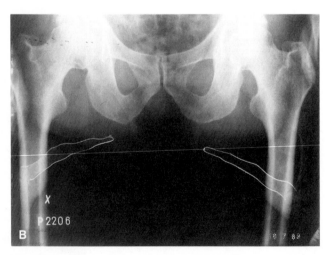

Figure 18.7 Palpatory illusion. **(A)** The tubera ischiadica are level, but not the palpating thumbs. **(B)** Improved position of the thumbs after treatment.

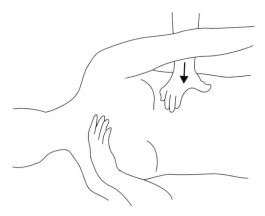

Figure 18.8 Moving the fascias around the chest.

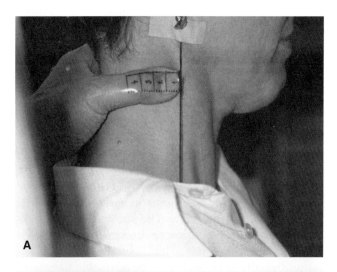

a large hand; if, however, this is not the case, we place both hands to the dorsal aspect with two thumbs over the spinous processes and the fingers on both sides above the patient's shoulders. We can now engage the barrier by a rotatory movement of both hands in one direction and spring it for diagnosis, and if there is a restrictive barrier we wait to obtain release. But we can also treat the soft tissues with a wringing movement with one hand and the thumb moving in a cranial direction. The other hand (with the thumb) moves in a caudal direction.

Dysfunctional deep fascias are most frequently found in elderly chronic patients with considerable restriction of movement. On examination of individual segments of the cervical spine in these cases, we find stiffness in all movement segments, but it is difficult to decide which segment is at fault. Here we have always had to treat soft tissue first; the result in such cases is an immediate, even dramatic, increase in the range of head rotation. If then there is still some movement restriction, we can easily diagnose the restricted segment.

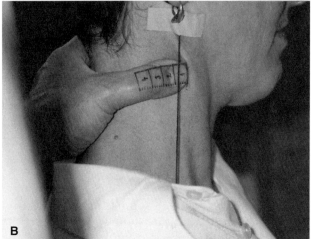

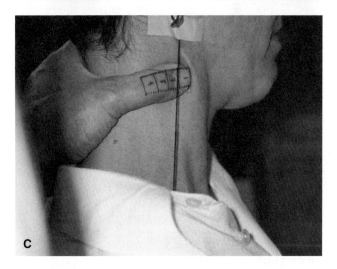

Figure 18.10 Moving the fascias on the neck. **(A)** Placing the thumb. **(B)** Engaging the barrier. **(C)** Springing the barrier.

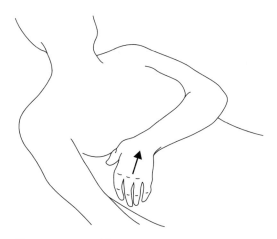

Figure 18.9 Self–treatment.

The Scalp

The scalp plays a similar role to that of the fascias: there are muscles that attach to it and movement restriction against the skull bears the same clinical characteristics as that of any other deep fascia. Clinically it can be considered as a continuation of the cervical fascia with which it seems to be closely connected. There is also often movement restriction there in similar conditions, i.e., in headache and vertigo.

For examination, we move or shift the scalp over the bone, preferably with the fingers of both hands, to compare mobility in several directions. Examination should include the forehead and the soft tissues covering the nose and jaw. The site of most frequent restriction is in the region of the mastoid processes. Care must be taken not to let the fingers slip over the patient's hair. At times it may be advisable to grasp a not too small area of hair to move the scalp, but this should never cause pain.

Wherever we engage the barrier, we spring it for diagnosis and when the barrier does not spring, we engage it and wait for release. The effect of such treatment shows the scalp to be a very important structure, with its close links to the cranio cervical junction and to the orificial system with the temporomandibular joint.

The Deep Fascias at the Extremities

As in the neck, mobility of soft tissue at the extremities is greatest around their long axis. Rotating the whole soft tissue pad, we examine mobility of the deep fascia against bone. We first engage the barrier and spring it for diagnosis and if a pathological barrier is found, it is engaged; after the usual latency, release follows. The alternative for therapy is a wringing movement between both hands placed around the extremity: one hand moves the soft tissue clockwise, the other (close to it) counter-clockwise. The moment tension between the hands is felt, the barrier is engaged, and after a short latency release follows.

This procedure can be applied to the arm, around the elbow, to the forearm, around the wrist; to the thigh, around the knee, to the leg, and around the ankle, wherever a pathological barrier is found.

Soft Tissue Lesions at the Heel

There are frequent painful conditions at the heel, where we may find a painful calcaneal spur, the attachment point of the plantar aponeurosis, and at the dorsal aspect of the heel, where the Achilles tendon is attached.

Tension in the plantar aponeurosis results most frequently from deep TrPs in the short muscles of the foot and from movement restriction in the joints between the tarsal bones and the tarso-metatarsal joints; these are treated by mobilization and/or relaxation. The soft tissue lesion related to a painful calcaneal spur affects the soft tissue pad on the plantar surface of the heel. This soft tissue pad has some mobility—it can be shifted with the thumbs of both hands in all directions against the underlying bone. In this direction we find a pathological barrier release is obtained by engaging the barrier and waiting (Fig. 18.11).

Tension at the attachment point of the Achilles tendon is caused by TrPs in the soleus; they are treated by PIR. Pain at the posterior aspect of the heel may, however, be caused by a painful lesion of the soft tissue between the Achilles tendon and the underlying bone. If this is the case, we produce a soft tissue fold between the thumb of one and the fingers of the other hand and reinforce this thumb with the thumb of the other hand. After engaging the barrier, we wait for release. Care must be taken that the thumb is so placed that it can penetrate into the narrow space between the tendon and bone (Fig. 18.12).

The Soft Tissue Between the Metacarpal and Metatarsal Bones

Mobility between the metacarpal and metatarsal bones depends on mobility of the soft tissue between these bones. Tension there, as in the skin fold between the fingers and/or toes, is most frequent in root syndromes with pain and/or numbness radiating into the toes.

Mobility or resistance to passive movement is examined by grasping two adjacent metacarpals (metatarsals) between the thumb and the forefinger of both hands and moving them in opposite directions, taking up the slack, and springing them first in one and then in the opposite (plantar or dorsal)

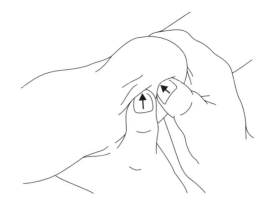

Figure 18.11 Shifting soft tissue at the heel pad.

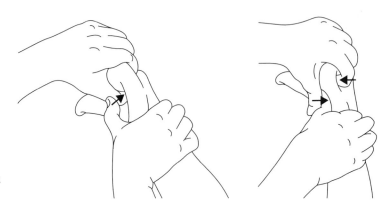

Figure 18.12 Stretching a soft tissue fold beneath the Achilles tendon in both directions.

direction. If increased resistance is found, we use a pincer movement (Fig. 18.13): the therapist places two thumbs on one metacarpal (metatarsal) on the dorsal aspect and two forefingers on the palmar (plantar) aspect of the adjacent bone. With gentle shearing pressure of his fingers he engages the barrier and waits for release.

As in the skin fold, increased resistance between the metacarpals or metatarsals is a true neurological sign of root involvement. Resistance between the second and third and the third and fourth metacarpal shows that the C7 root is involved and between the fourth and fifth metacarpal the C8 root; between the first and second and the second and third metatarsal the root L5 is

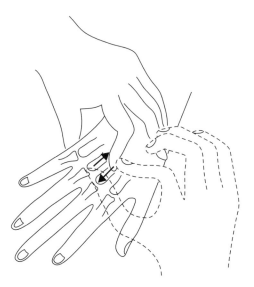

Figure 18.13 Pincer movement. With two thumbs on one metacarpal on the dorsal and two fingers on the neighboring metacarpal on the palmar aspect, the therapist moves one metacarpal in a dorsal and the neighboring in a palmar direction. He then reverses the position of the thumbs and fingers, moving the metacarpals in the opposite direction.

involved, and between the third and fourth and the fourth and fifth metatarsal the S1 root. These cases should first be treated at the interdigital fold, followed by mobilization of the metacarpals (metatarsals).

Periosteal Points

Tender or painful periosteal points most frequently result from overstrained muscles attached at these points. At examination we regularly find that mobility of the soft tissues covering these pain points is restricted in at least one direction, as compared to the the other side. On trying to shift these tissues in the restricted direction, we sense a pathological barrier that does not spring. A tangential movement across the pain point is painless. In the same direction we then engage the barrier and wait for release. Unlike friction or periosteal massage no pressure is exerted on the pain point and therefore this technique is much gentler and yet very effective. In fact, we encourage the patient to touch his pain point and ask him whether and to what extent he still feels pain.

Epicondylar Pain

Pain at the radial and the ulnar epicondyle of the elbow is one of the most frequent painful conditions we treat. Basically it is pain at the attachment points of strained muscles that need to be relaxed. As a rule, there is restricted joint play at the elbow and movement restriction in the cervical spine; in addition, we find that the soft tissues around and above the epicondyles cannot be shifted with the same ease in all directions, compared to the unaffected side, and that at least in one direction there is a pathological barrier. Examination is performed with the tip of a finger or the thumb. After finding the pathological barrier (Fig. 18.14) and taking up the slack, release is obtained. After treatment, the patient is asked to check his pain point.

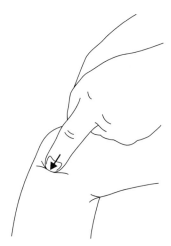

Figure 18.14 Examination (treatment) of soft tissue at the epicondyle.

Pain at the Spinous Processes, Particularly on the Low Lumbar Spine

Pain at the tip of the spinous processes is a frequent condition in low back pain and should be distinguished from other causes. The spinous processes are muscle attachment points and may be impinged if there is hypermobility on back bending. We rarely ever find a painful spinous process in elderly patients with Baastrup syndrome, i.e., hyperostosis at the edges of adjacent spinous processes, where they touch one another during back bending. However, young hypermobile patients, more frequently women, experience pain during back bending, i.e., when spinous processes touch each other.

At examination it is easy to provoke typical pain by very moderate pressure at the tip of the spinous process, most frequently that of L5, where lordosis is usually greatest on back bending. On closer examination, we can then find that the spinous process is very tender on one side but much less so on the other. On the painful side we can palpate increased tension (resistance to pressure) of the soft tissues adjacent to the bone. By pressure against the soft tissues in a ventral direction, parallel to the spinous process, we engage the barrier and wait to obtain release. During release our finger penetrates into the soft tissue without increasing pressure. Exerting pressure with the tip of the forefinger, we have to support the articulation between the second and third phalanx between the thumb and the index of the other hand. After this procedure we check tenderness.

Pain at the Spinous Process of the Axis

The most frequent pain point in the cervical area is probably the lateral edge of the spinous process of the axis. Very frequently the patient will demonstrate this pain point, with his finger, while bending his head to the opposite side, i.e., by rotating the axis and bringing the lateral surface of the spinous process toward the palpating finger. It is precisely in the position of side-bending to the opposite side that we have to examine this pain point.

Clinically, this pain point is usually found in movement restriction of C1/2 and C2/3, more frequently on the right side, if there is spasm in the levator scapulae, and in most conditions causing strain at the muscles of the shoulder girdle.

At examination, side-bending the patient's head to the opposite side, we shift the soft tissues overlying the lateral surface of the spinous process in a cranio-caudal and a latero-lateral direction, to find the pathological barrier, and compare with the non-painful side. After engaging the barrier, we wait for release. After this, the patient checks his pain point.

Pain at the Posterior Superior Iliaca Spina (PSIS)

This is a frequent, yet in our experience not specific, pain point in patients with low back pain and even pain from the hip joint. With the patient prone, the surface of the PSIS slopes roof-like from its medial prominence, in a lateral direction. It is in this direction that we have to examine mobility of the overlying soft tissue and also examine the barrier; if restriction is found, we compare the two sides. If we diagnose abnormality, we engage the barrier to obtain release, sliding in a lateral direction. The patient then checks for tenderness.

The Pes Anserinus of the Tibia

This is a frequent and important attachment point of the gracilis, sartorius, and semitendinosus. It is frequently tender in cox arthrosis and in referred pain from the segment L3/4. Lying on the medial surface of the tibia, the soft tissue covering it is easily shifted in all directions, and by taking up the slack and springing, pathological barriers are found and treated by engaging them and obtaining release. The patient then check the pain point.

The principles detailed here can be applied to any other periosteal pain point we may find.

Active Scars

The most dramatic effects of soft tissue treatment we obtain are when treating "active" scars.

It was in 1947 that Huneke (6) published his book dealing with scars treated by novocain (Impletol) infiltration. After injecting scars, symptoms frequently disappeared in painful lesions, which seemingly were in no way related to the scar. The effect was so prompt that it was termed "Sekunden effect." His successes were never accepted by the medical profession; however, they started an influential movement among German doctors who used the term "Neuraltherapie" (3,5). The effect was first attributed to the novocain. Later, however, similar effects were obtained by other substances, even gas, and in the end the needle alone proved effective. Many doctors who first became interested in "Neuraltherapie" later became involved in acupuncture.

By needling scars, very similar effects could be obtained as by injecting them with a local anaesthetic. The most unsatisfactory point of this development was lack of adequate diagnosis, i.e., how to determine when and what scar to treat, and also to find a reason why and in what way a scar can become pathogenic.

Pathomechanism and Diagnosis

The answer to the problem lies, in our opinion, in the role of soft tissues as we have shown so far. A scar penetrates all the layers of soft tissue from the skin to the bone or even into the abdominal cavity. If after injury (operation) everything heals normally, scar tissue fully adapts to the surrounding layers of soft tissue and functions normally. If, however, this is not the case, then soft tissue around such a scar cannot function normally, from the skin down to the deep fascia.

This is exactly what we find in "active" scars: there is increased skin drag at the site of the scar, the skin does not stretch normally, and the skin fold is thicker; scar tissue does not shift normally against underlying structures, particularly against bone, and if the scar penetrates into the abdominal cavity, we palpate the reresistance in some direction. In all these layers we can find pain points. These are most frequently found at one end of the scar. After burns, or osteomyelitis, we find flat scars covering mainly bone, which adhere to the bone and frequently are active. Active, dysfunctional scars therefore interfere with normal functioning of all soft tissues they penetrate and that surround them. These, fascia in particular, are chained up with TrPs, and joint dysfunction at a localization that can be at a great distance from the site of the scar. If, e.g., an active scar penetrating the abdomen is active, the abdominal wall cannot function normally, with repercussions throughout the entire motor system.

It is not, however, enough to make the diagnosis of an active scar. The patient does not come for treatment reporting scars; what he reports is back pain or headaches. It is therefore essential to determine the relevance of the scar in relation to the patient's problem. The case history can point in the direction of a scar: his back pain started not long after the injury (operation) that produced the active scar. The proof, however, lies in testing the effect of soft tissue treatment. For this we must strictly adhere to the rules of chain reactions as given in Chapter 33. The relevance of active scars is frequently such that if we fail to diagnose one it may cancel out the results of any other treatment.

Clinical Pearl

The Importance of Auditing the Patient's Response to Treatment as a Diagnostic Step

It is the first step in treatment that confirms or rejects our diagnosis. Therefore, we should never treat lesions immediately at examination, one after another; treatment must be postponed until the whole patient has been adequately examined. Only then can we decide which lesion to treat and determine its relevance. If there is an active scar, we must begin there and then re-examine (i.e., audit) wherever there was an abnormal finding. Only when most of the changes (TrPs, joint movement restrictions, etc.) have been relieved can we be sure that the active scar was relevant. This is, of course, of great importance for further treatment and/or rehabilitation, because if there is such a positive response, then rehabilitation also has to target the scar. When post-treatment audit proves that the treatment has improved the patient's relevant clinical signs, then this confirms that a "key link" has been found.

Clinical Picture

Because the concept of "active" scars has rarely been described in the literature, we have to rely on personal experience and particularly on 41 treated cases since 1998. During this period, we paid much greater attention to this problem and improved both diagnosis and therapy.

The most important advance has been made in the examination of scars and even in their detection. It is easy to find a scar on the surface of the body and to see whether it is smooth, drawn in, or even adherent to bone (at the extremities). It is, however, more difficult to detect active scar tissue in deeper layers or where there is no mark on the surface, as with a torn muscle. But even if the scar is obvious, the active deeper layers are not necessarily where we would expect them. This is the case after operation if the incision on the skin does not exactly correspond to where the operation actually took place, so that we find painful resistance in deep tissues at a distance from the site of the skin lesion. With increasing experience we now believe that all deeper layers of a scar are usually affected; however, good results can sometimes be obtained even after treatment of the superficial layers only. There the two ends of the scar are usually most active.

There may be no sign of activity at the surface but only, e.g., in the abdominal cavity. This has become an important factor now that operations are increasingly performed by laparoscopy, after which we find pathological barriers only in the deeper layers inside the abdomen. After purulent appendicitis with peritonitis, drainage of the abdominal cavity is necessary. The "culprit" may then be the scar after the drain, and not the appendectomy scar. We palpated a painful scar left by operation of a rectal carcinoma at the site where we examine the pelvic floor. At first we thought it was a TrP of the coccygeus muscle and treated it by relaxation, unsuccessfully. The patient improved dramatically after we applied (painful) local pressure, followed by release.

It can be seen from our material that the relevance of active scars is very high: 36 out of 51 cases. Patients may experience any type of pain in the motor system, from headache to neck, thoracic, and low back pain, including dizziness, but only rarely is it felt at the site of the scar. Most active scars were formed after appendectomy (almost half of our patients), but any type of scar may be involved.

Therapy

Because scars are situated mainly in the soft tissue and the scar itself consists of connective tissue, soft tissue techniques are the basic approach to treatment. Hot packs are a very useful auxiliary or preparatory method and exteroceptive stimulation (Appendix 18-A) is another important source of help, particularly for self-treatment.

To return to soft tissue manipulation, it should be applied to every tissue layer affected by the scar. At the surface we apply skin stretch, then we form a soft tissue fold of subcutaneous tissue wherever this is possible and stretch the fold. Folding may, however, be impossible in scars that are drawn in and buried deep in the tissues. In such cases only pressure must be applied, with the alternative being needling or injection. After abdominal operation, we have to look for resistance in the abdominal cavity. This must be examined very carefully. We exert pressure against

the pathological barrier to engage it and obtain release. This has to be sensed continually until the normal barrier is restored.

The last point has to be stressed because it has great importance not only for therapy but also for confirming or correcting diagnosis, because whenever we use our hands for treatment we are also in a diagnostic feedback relation with the patient. If the diagnosis of deep scar tissue is correct, release after engaging the barrier should take place. If, however, no release is obtained, this diagnosis has to be corrected and intra-abdominal pathology must be looked for!

In the case of flat active scars, such as those left after burns, scalding, osteomyelitis, or irradiation, we find adherence to the underlying bones, like that of fascias. In such cases, mobility of the scar has to be restored in all directions, just as with fascias, engaging the barrier and shifting. There may be no scar visible on the surface of the body, e.g., after a torn muscle, after deep injury, and now after operation under laparoscopy or by laser. In such cases, we have to look exclusively for resistance (pathological barriers) in the abdominal cavity and wait for release, both for therapy and for confirmation of our diagnosis. But even if there is a scar at skin level after operation, deeper structures may have been cut at a distance from the skin incision; in such cases, we have to palpate the site of scar tissue and treat the pathological barriers accordingly.

Some case histories illustrate this much underrated clinical problem.

Case 1 The patient P.H., born in 1951, male electrician manager of a firm, reported pain in his right lower abdomen since 1995. He was repeatedly examined but nothing pathological was found. After playing golf on April 4, 1999, he experienced excruciating pain the next day. Pain in the right lower abdomen and waist radiated into the right groin, testicle, and to the anterior aspect of the right thigh. He was completely immobilized.

As a child he had recurrent tonsillitis and in 1984 he underwent operation for chronic appendicitis. In 1997 he was treated for gastro-duodenal ulcer and received antibiotics to combat *Heliobacter pylori*.

He was first examined at the urological department, where renal colic was excluded. He was hospitalized on April 6 at the Neurological Clinic of the medical faculty in Prague Motol. There, in addition to neurological examination, the following laboratory tests were performed: complete blood and urine examination, examination of the cerebrospinal fluid, ophthalmological examination, examination of the lumbar spine (showing degenerative changes), MRI of the thoracic and lumbar spine, CT of the abdominal cavity, excretory urography, and more urological and surgical examinations, which all proved negative. Finally, psychological examination summed it up as follows: uncharacteristic acute stressful reactions to cumulative strain, triggered and accompanied by pain caused by a considerable extent to nociceptive neuro-psychological and conversion mechanisms.

After all these procedures the patient was sent to our rehabilitation clinic on September 9, 1999. There we found an antalgic posture with trunk anteflexion and pelvic shift to the left (right trunk deviation). On walking the patient took his weight off the right leg. Backbending caused immediate low back pain and pain in the groin. There was painful movement restriction at the L5/S1 segment.

Further examination revealed an unusually symptomatic appendectomy scar. It was surrounded by erythema and the patient reacted painfully even to gentle palpation. There was positive skin drag and restricted skin stretch; pathological barriers were found also in the subcutaneous tissues, particularly at both ends of the scar, and there was painful resistance in the abdominal cavity.

Treatment began by gentle skin stretch, although painful, and release was obtained after a few seconds, followed by relief of pain. This was followed by release also in the deeper layers of the scar. After some initial pain, relief was achieved after approximately 10 minutes of treatment. The patient straightened up and was able to walk normally. No restriction was then found between L5/S1. Further treatment was aimed at the scar until October 29. In addition to soft tissue techniques including fascia on the back, hot packs were applied to the scar. He was taught self-treatment by stroking and how to mobilize his lumbar spine.

Comment In this case, not only was pain localized in the right low abdomen but also was there a highly symptomatic scar, yet no one, particularly surgeons, would admit or suspect a scar to be of any importance, and because all lengthy and costly examinations were negative, the only diagnosis was psychiatric, and treatment by drugs was ineffective. Full recovery followed after scar treatment.

Case 2 The patient P.M., male, born 1974, sportsman, tore his left straight abdominal muscle, causing hematoma, while playing soccer in the spring of 1999. He experienced pain ever since. Pain was not related to any physical activity. He had never experienced pain before. He never was ill except for an appendectomy at the age of 2.

At examination on June 12, 2000, the only finding was tenderness at the lower end of the left straight abdominal muscle, which was treated by postisometric relaxation (PIR). He was sent for sonographic examination, which was negative.

There was no improvement on July 7, when painful TrPs were found at the iliacus muscle, the psoas, the short adductors, and the diaphragm on the left side. After PIR of the diaphragm, these findings immediately improved. He was shown self-treatment, but at control examination on July 27 he was not better. We found no TrPs at the diaphragm or at the psoas or iliacus. We found, however, that the patient was able to reproduce his pain by sit-ups, whenever he contracted his straight abdominal muscles. A very painful resistance was found there, which was needled (for diagnostic reasons). Needling reproduced his pain, and a hematoma was formed after needling.

On August 3, he was much improved and there was further relief after mere pressure, producing release. The patient fully recovered after soft tissue treatment combined with hot packs and stroking.

Comment Local tenderness with increased resistance in a muscle was mistaken for a TrP, supposedly related to other TrPs and was temporarily relieved by PIR. Only the correct interpretation of the pain point, as an active scar, helped to introduce effective treatment.

Case 3 V.B., born 1967, female, speech therapist reported pain in the cervico-thoracic region and at the shoulder blade, more on the left side, especially at night. She also has some headaches. Pain has gradually worsened since 1997.

After her second delivery of a baby of more than 4 kg, she experienced repeated high temperatures treated by antibiotics, but without diagnosis.

At examination on October 3, 2000, there were left-sided TrPs (chain reaction) beginning with the SCM, pectoralis, subscapularis, diaphragm, pelvic floor, a restricted fibula, and the left foot, with TrPs and restriction at the metatarso-phalangeal joints.

In addition, we found an intensely painful pressure point in the lower abdomen on the right side. After exactly locating the resistance in the abdomen, we obtained release. Immediately the entire pain chain from the feet up to the SCM disappeared.

On October 3, she called to say that she was still greatly improved. She was much improved also at control examination at the end of November.

Comment Although there was a typical left-sided chain reaction, which suggested treatment in the chain (see Chapter 33), possibly at the pelvic floor or even the feet (key regions), we also knew that before her symptoms began, she had a protracted delivery followed by high temperatures, suggesting some tear during child birth. Therefore, it seemed a good idea to look first for a possible active scar in her low abdomen. When this was found, also for diagnostic reasons, the indication was to treat this first.

■ CONCLUSION

This chapter is an attempt to show that the same judicious diagnostic and therapeutic methods can be systematically applied for soft tissues as in manipulation of joints and in treatment of trigger points, and that these methods should be distinguished from massage. An important part is devoted to diagnosis and treatment of scars, because in this field soft tissue techniques are particularly effective and because this very important problem has been widely neglected by health professionals, especially by surgeons whose role in producing scars is far from negligible. In addition, it seems that this type of treatment gives the most spectacular results.

Audit Process
Self-Check of the Chapter's Learning Objectives

- Can you identify the barrier phenomena in various tissues such as fascia, skin, muscle, and joint?

- Can you correlate the barrier phenomena with increased tension and pain in your patients?

- Can you release the barrier with various means such as stretch, post-isometric relaxation, ischemic compression, etc.?

■ REFERENCES

1. Chaitow L. Palpatory Literacy. Bath, UK: Torston, 1992.
2. Dejung B, Gröbli C, Colla F, Weissmann R. Triggerpunkt-Therapie. Die Behandlung akuter undchronischer Schmerzen im Bewegungsapparat mit manueller Triggerpunkt-Therapie und Dry Needling. Bern, Göttingen, Toronto, Seattle: Verlag H. Huber, 2003.
3. Dosch P. Lehrbuch der Neuraltherapie nach Huneke. Ulm: Haug, 1964.
4. Gatterman MI. Foundation of Chairopracric Subluxation. St. Louis: Mosby, 1995.
5. Gross D. Therapeutische Lokalanästhesie. Stuttgart: Hippokrates, 1972.
6. Huneke F. Krankheit und Heilung anders gesehen. Köln: Staufen, 1947.
7. Lewit K. Manipulative Therapy in Rehabilitation of the Locomotor System, 3rd ed. Oxford: Butterworth-Heinemann, 1999.
8. Lewit K, Liebenson C. Palpation—problems and implication. J Manip Physiol Ther 1993;16:586–590.
9. Lewit K, Janda V, Veverkova M. Respiratory synkinesis—polyelectromyographic investigation. J Orthop Med 1998;20:2–6.
10. Popolyanski YY, Popelyanski AY. Treatment of neurodystrophic changes in the locomotor system. Revmatologia 1984;84:66–70 (in Russian).
11. Travell JG, Simons DG. Myofascial Pain and Dysfunction—The Trigger point Manual, 2nd ed. Vol. 1. Baltimore, MD: Williams & Wilkins, 1999.
12. Ward RC. Foundations for Osteopathic Medicine, Glossary. Baltimore, MD: Williams & Wilkins, 1997.
13. Ward RC. Myofascial release concepts. In: Basmajian JV, Nyberg RP, eds. Rational Manual Therapeutics. Baltimore, MD: Williams & Wilkins, 1993: 223–242.

Exteroceptive Therapy

Helena Hermach

Tactile Perception and Its Influence on Muscle Tone

Although the child in the womb reacts to touch of the mother's hand by moving, one can only speak of tactile perception from the moment of birth. At the beginning of life, the whole body provides the point of contact with the support. At first the child raises up on the arms, reducing the area of contact with the body. Then later the child supports himself only by the four limbs, and when erect posture is achieved only the sole of the foot remains in contact with the support. Today, the chief point of contact is more often the caudal end of the body.

The child normally feels stroking and cradling as comforting, but if the reaction to stroking is repeated crying, this may be a warning signal for the future, and for normal motor development. It may signal increased tension, which could even develop toward spasticity. The area of support indicates whether muscular tension is increased, adequate, or lowered, with the child or even the adult in the recumbent position. The area of contact and the ability to use it for support determines the capacity for movement in space, for taking off, and regaining contact with the support.

The way the individual reacts to skin contact with the outer world tells us of his ability to accept, reject, interpret, and react to these contacts, whether adequately or not.

The skin is an essential conductor of the information from the outer world, which we need to form our idea of space: both the outer and the inner space. It is the skin and its tactile perception that tell us the difference between self and what is exterior to it. How much space do I occupy? Impaired or insufficiently developed tactile perception changes our orientation in space, and our understanding of our own position in space. Obviously this must affect how we move, i.e., the motor system.

Our perceptions are closely related to our psychological attitudes. What we perceive must be interpreted and our interpretation shows how we have perceived: as something pleasant, welcoming, or as disagreeable, hostile, traumatic.

If the skin contact is pleasant, we welcome the outer world, and vice-versa. On this depends certainty or uncertainty of our movement in space.

The better we perceive, the more readily we make finer distinctions; the ability to make fine distinctions is a sign of acute perception. In terms of tactile perception, this means distinguishing things by touch, what this tells us, and where we stand.

Our reactions are formed and our behavior develops according to the quality of our perceptions and the way we interpret them.

Behavior and movement are interrelated; thus skin tactile perception influences the motor system. This relationship, however, is even closer: it is the expression of tension in the skin, the subcutaneous tissue, and muscles, and it shows in changes in tension. In my experience, increased tension including muscles is a sign of increased skin sensitivity. Reduced tension indicates reduced sensitivity. Just as each individual has his own idea of the world, these reactions, too, are highly individual and we may find the reverse in some cases. The skin is not very sensitive and yet there is great tension. This may be the reaction of the whole organism to insufficient input of information, which has to be compensated for.

The important thing is that treatment can change tactile perception. The skin can be taught to perceive more, or less, to improve. Changes in perception induce changes in tension in the skin, the subcutaneous tissue, and muscles.

This phenomenon can be used for therapy. Subtly differentiated perception goes along with suitable tension in tissues and adequate muscle tension. The capacity of muscles to adapt to the required degree of tension is but the expression of good coordination. It can be said that adequate tactile perception accompanies properly coordinated motion. If I may exaggerate, should therapy result in perfectly balanced tactile perception, the patient would begin to move in a well coordinated manner, with the right orientation in space.

To fully use this knowledge, we must learn to examine skin sensitivity properly.

Assessment of Changes in Tactile Perception

Tactile perception is examined by the usual methods of neurological examination, preferably using a fingernail as an instrument. Scratching can be gentle or more forceful according to which part of the body is examined, making use of the dorsal surface of the fingernail. It slides over the skin. Scratching must be sudden to elicit a clear reaction. After a few repetitions, the reaction gradually changes, as the skin adapts to the stimulus. If there is no adaptation, it is a sign of hypersensitivity.

The reaction to this treatment is of two types: local and generalized; there may be neither. Roughly speaking, the more intense the distant reaction, the less it is adequate. There may be no local reaction, implying lowered perception, an adequate or normal reaction; or an exaggerated reaction, implying hypersensitivity. The latter presents itself as ticklishness or even pain.

There may be a paradoxical reaction; instead of jerking when the sole of his foot is stroked, for instance, the patient may hold his breath and stiffen the thoracic muscles. Any suggestion that the sole of his foot is sensitive may induce sweating and goose flesh. The most important generalized reactions are changes in respiration and perspiration. Both reveal lability of the whole organism, whereas changes in respiration also affect the motor function of the trunk. The patient's personality, cultural background, and momentary level of stress must be taken into account in assessing his reaction. We all have moments when we overreact.

How to Modify Tactile Perception

The sensitivity of the skin to tactile stimuli is not constant, but rather changes and adapts in the short-term. By stroking, however, sensitivity may change in the long-term, too, as the skin learns to feel and to distinguish, and the patient learns to interpret the changes.

Part of the effect of massage springs from its role of tactile stimulation, and certain massage techniques can be applied to this end, particularly those that are gentle and applied only to the surface of the body. Brushing is another well-known physiotherapeutic technique that can be used without risk on patients with lowered tactile perception. In cases of changed perception or hypersensitivity, the technique chosen must be either pleasant or at least bearable. A technique that causes discomfort will provoke a defense reaction and prevent normalization.

My own first method of choice in all cases of changed perception is stroking, over the largest possible area, slowly, and in smooth contact with the patient's skin. No tickling! The hand serves a feedback function, sensing changes in tension in the skin, subcutaneous tissue, and muscle. If these

are changes for the better, stroking can continue; if not, either the chief object of treatment has been missed or the stimulus was too weak. If the changes are not for the better, one must desist, reconsider the diagnosis, and decide whether the tactile stimulus was correctly chosen. Stroking has the advantage of excellent feedback, so that undesirable changes are felt at once by the experienced therapist. Stroking is most frequently directed along the axis of the body, on the buttocks, for instance, and across the body, whereas the abdomen can be stroked diagonally.

If the skin is excessively hypersensitive, the therapist has two alternatives: he can stroke the patient through a thin cloth or the patient may stroke himself for several minutes per day until he can bear the touch of the therapist's hand.

If an insensitive skin does not react sufficiently, the stimulus can be intensified by stroking faster, changing the pressure or direction, or by using rough material (e.g., Turkey toweling) or a soft brush. It must be borne in mind that good perception is the ability to react to delicate stimuli and that too rough means will not achieve this.

To achieve good coordination between the muscles, they must be capable of mutual interaction if the tonus in one muscle changes. There should be neither hypertonus nor hypotonus in either. The muscle should be able to relax and adapt to any situation. Success in changing muscle tone by whatever method implies a situation in which movement is ideally coordinated, without training or correction. In my experience, if muscular, subcutaneous, or skin tension has been improved by stroking, muscle coordination has also improved and thus has motor function in all its aspects.

Changes in Tissue Sensitivity After Operation (Scars)

Examining skin perception, it is essential to look at scars. To recognise a sensitive scar, one makes a thin fold of scar tissue; if the patient feels a pinching or burning sensation, the scar is sensitive. If after treatment by stretching and/or shifting the scar is still sensitive, one must seek a deep painful spot.

Sensitivity in the surrounding skin must be examined, not only the scar itself. Surgery may damage some nerves of the skin, making it either insensitive or (paradoxically) oversensitive. In both cases, skin perception must be restored, because as long as it is abnormal, tension in the subcutaneous muscles is also changed, causing them to react abnormally. Insensitive skin often signals slightly hypertonic muscles, and that the patient is not fully in control. Hypersensitive skin may present as paraesthesia or as pain, even referred pain.

Hypersensitivity may be so intense, where cloth touches the skin, that the patient cannot bear to be touched anywhere in that region. I call this the "taboo phenomenon": the patient also reacts very emotionally. Stroking must then be attempted through cloth or performed by the patient himself daily until he can accept the touch of another's hand. Once sensitivity is restored in the scar, the patient must check from time to time and stroke it again to see if the skin becomes less or overly sensitive.

The muscles below a painful scar are usually hypertonic and often painful. This may improve as skin sensitivity becomes normal.

The Foot, the Hand, the Mouth

Sensitivity of the skin to touch is highly individual, is not the same over the whole of the body, and changes with age.

The baby begins to recognize things by touch, first in the mouth and then using his hands. Soon he uses his feet to grasp things, until he needs them for standing, and later for walking.

For this, the feet provide support that is not passive: the body reacts to the ground on which it stands and from which it tries to rise.

We know that in the adult sensory brain cortex, the tongue and the mouth, the hand, (especially the thumb) and the foot occupy most space. These are thus the most important tactile entrance areas, and changes in their sensitivity will change the behavior of the individual as a whole.

Only in exceptional cases do I examine sensitivity of the tongue and mouth, but it is often necessary with babies. Abnormal behavior: a restless tongue, or one that moves too little, restlessness of the lower jaw or the lips, or a mouth that is always open, are indicative. To examine inside the mouth, I use a damp finger. It is a sign of hypersensitivity if the tongue reacts to my finger wildly and out of control, or if touching the tip of the tongue provokes the urge to vomit. If the tongue does not react to the finger moving over it, sensitivity is lowered. For treatment, the tongue, gums, and the inside of the mouth must be stroked with a damp finger. Adult patients continue this treatment themselves, whereas the mothers of babies and children can be trained to perform it. If the vomiting reflex is provoked very easily, treatment must be very gentle. In time the seat of irritation moves back to the root of the tongue.

It is difficult to determine the sensitivity of the hand, perhaps because our hands are constantly in use, handling objects or doing things. Only if there is good reason is it necessary. The patient sits in a relaxed position, with the hands palm upwards; in this position, the muscle tone of the hand flexors is usually slightly dominant. The fingers are curled a bit. I take the patient by surprise, lightly scratching his palm with two or three fingers. If there is no reaction, the hand is hyposensitive. Normally the hand withdraws for a very short moment, returning to a relaxed position. The hand is clearly hypersensitive if the reaction is to stretch the fingers; this can be confirmed by repeating the stimulus. The most effective therapy is either stroking or activities such as running the fingers through grains of rice, kneading dough, or modeling with plasticine. People with hypersensitive hands are often dexterous and creative, but they have to learn how to consciously relax their hands.

Examination of sensitivity of the feet should be routine; they are of crucial importance for upright posture and therefore for the position and functioning of the spine. The patient lies supine; without warning, the therapist draws the dorsal aspect of his thumbnail across the sole of the foot, from heel to toe. A normally sensitive foot will withdraw from the source of irritation with slight momentary flexion of the ankle, knee, and hip. If the foot does not react, it is hyposensitive; this means that it is unable to react adequately during walking or standing, lacking sufficient information from the terrain. An excessive reaction, or a general reaction of the body, shows that the foot does not adapt to the terrain, because of inadequate processing of that information. This must be treated by stroking the sole of the foot. The patient can then do this on his own, as well as practice walking barefoot at home, over grass, or pebbles outside.

In some cases the degree of sensitivity differs from one foot to the other. Here it is necessary to examine sensitivity elsewhere in the body: the shin, the thigh, the abdomen, the chest, the arms, and the face. We may find changed tactile perception on only one side of the body; this often occurs with marked right- or left-handedness. This asymmetry also affects motor function, leading to disturbance of the motor system as a whole. The patient must learn to be conscious of the "forgotten" side and learn to use it. Treatment begins with stroking the hyposensitive side of the body, with the patient continuing on his own.

The therapist must check to see whether symmetry has been restored. If the patient then stops self-treatment, the problem may recur, a danger he must be aware of.

Ticklishness, especially on the abdomen and chest, is another sign of hypersensitivity. It occurs most often where muscle tone in those areas is increased. This also disturbs muscle coordination there, respiration may be affected, and the motor function of the spine is inevitably disturbed as well. Ticklishness is an advance signal of pain, and it is very important to treat the sensitivity of the trunk in such cases.

The Individual Character Of Perception

The reaction of each patient must be considered in the context of the whole personality. What may seem an excessive reaction may be the norm for a temperamental person, whereas a reserved individual may show hypersensitivity by a "normal" reaction. It is essential to listen to the patient (his own words will show what he thinks of his pain,) and to observe his general behavior. There may be a strange reaction to our touching the skin, for instance, in patients whose emotional background is disturbed, as in unloved children, even after they have grown up.

A different degree of sensitivity on either side of the body suggests that the patient cannot locate the center of his body correctly and thus may not perceive his surroundings normally. On the less sensitive side, things are less "real" to him, and he is more likely to lurch into things on that side. This unequal distribution of sensibility is paralleled by emotional instability, but as such patients learn to feel their whole body and use the less sensitive side as well, when their sense of security improves.

Correct sensitivity of the feet is essential for balance and hence for a sense of security. If this is lacking, the patient tries to maintain stability in the erect position by overusing other muscles, e.g., in the pelvic and lumbar region, or the diaphragm and the thoracolumbar region, or by tension at the shoulders and the back of the neck, as well as in the masticator muscles. All these disturbances of muscular function show the chain reactions described by Lewit (1).

Subjects with oversensitive hands are sometimes prone to excessive cleanliness and to perfectionism.

Self-Treatment

The patient can treat skin sensitivity himself by:

1. Stroking the skin with his fingers
2. Stroking with soft towelling
3. Rolling a plastic rubber ball over the skin; rolling a tennis ball under the foot
4. Treading pebbles or wooden beads
5. Running rice, lentils, nuts, etc., through the fingers
6. Lying on a "mattress" of plastic balls or chestnuts; little children may play in a bath half-full of plastic balls or chestnuts
7. Stimulating with a soft brush (I rarely use this method)

One of the aims of therapy is to reintegrate the insensitive or hypersensitive region into the body image. There are right-handed patients who need to learn to use their left hand in certain circumstances; some patients need to learn to walk barefoot; others must become aware of their thorax, rolling over and over down hill.

■ REFERENCES

1. Lewit K. Manipulative Therapy in Rehabilitation of the Locomotor System. Oxford: Butterworth-Heinemann, 1999.

19

Manual Resistance Techniques

Craig Liebenson, Pamela Tunnell,
Donald R. Murphy,
and Natalie Gluck-Bergman

Learning Objectives
After reading this chapter, you should be able to understand:

- The different methods of muscle relaxation
- The physiology of muscle inhibition
- The key role of identifying the barrier to resistance and achieving a release phenomena
- How to lengthen the most clinically relevant muscles in the body
- Manual resistance techniques for joint mobilization and muscle facilitation

Introduction

The original manual resistance techniques (MRTs) have their origins in the proprioceptive neuromuscular facilitation (PNF) philosophy of physical therapy and the muscle energy procedures (MEP) of the osteopathic field. These techniques involve manual resistance of a patient's isometric or isotonic muscular effort. This resisted effort is typically followed by relaxation or stretch of a tense or tight muscle. MRTs are primarily used to relax overactive muscles or to stretch shortened muscles and their associated fascia. Many methods have been developed depending on the clinical goal. To achieve these positive clinical effects, MRTs take advantage of two physiological phenomena: post-contraction inhibition and reciprocal inhibition (RI). MRTs are invaluable workhorses in the rehabilitation of the motor system.

MRTs may also be used to facilitate or train an inhibited or weak muscle. Manual resistance allows the doctor or therapist to achieve precise patient positioning and control of movement not possible with machines or even free weights. Manual contacts also allow for varying proprioceptive stimulation to facilitate an inhibited muscle during active resistance. The value of clinician control over resisted exercise cannot be underestimated, especially when improved coordination and motor control are goals as important as strengthening. Moreover, whether MRTs are used to relax, stretch, or facilitate and train muscles, they fulfill an important role in patient education and activation by enabling the patient to gain guided kinesthetic awareness of how to perform home exercises in a safe and beneficial manner.

In the late 1940s, publications about the use of PNF to facilitate neurologically weak muscles appeared (13). Soon other publications followed, reporting that spasticity responded as well (18). This led to the development of various forms of PNF (i.e., hold–relax, contract–relax, etc.), which could be used for orthopedic as well as neurological problems. The osteopaths used MEPs primarily to mobilize joints; they also developed a variety of modifications that could be used to stretch shortened muscular and connective tissues and to strengthen weak muscles (27).

Manual medicine practitioners in Europe were not far behind in incorporating these new methods. Gaymans and Lewit wrote of success using these techniques for joint mobilization using specific eye movements and respiratory synkinesis to enhance the physiological effectiveness of the procedures (5,21). Later, Lewit (5) focused on a gentle muscle relaxation technique he termed post-isometric relaxation, similar to hold–relax, which was applied to the contractile portion of an overactive muscle (20).

Neurophysiology

There are two aspects to MRTs. The first is their ability to relax an overactive muscle (increased neuromuscular tension, "spasm" or trigger points). The second is their ability to increase extensibility of a shortened muscle or its associated fascia when connective tissue or viscoelastic changes have occurred. When using MRTs, it is essential to relax the neuromuscular (contractile) component of the muscle before attempting any forceful stretching manoeuvre. Often a "release phenomenon" occurs so that a length change occurs spontaneously while relaxing excessive neuromuscular tension (see Chapter 18). In such cases, treatment serves as a diagnostic test, confirming that the dysfunction is neuromuscular (contractile) in nature, rather than being caused by connective tissue shortening. Even if connective tissue/non-contractile pathophysiologic changes have occurred, it is still important to relax the neuromuscular apparatus before stretching. This inhibits the stretch reflex, allows more vigorous stretching to be tolerated well by the patient, and helps avoid damage to the muscle sarcomeres that may be associated with stretching of a non-relaxed muscle.

Clinical Pearl

Differentiating Neuromuscular Versus Connective Tissue Involvement in Decreased Muscle Length

- Length changes in muscles may be caused by neuromuscular or connective tissue factors.

- Often a muscle has a decreased length but only needs to be relaxed rather than stretched to achieve a normal resting length.

- The diagnostic test of weather the muscle's length deficit is caused primarily by neuromuscular factors is if it lengthens spontaneously after relaxation techniques such as PIR without requiring stretching methods.

- If the muscle does not lengthen after PIR, then it is likely that the muscle's reduced length is caused by connective tissue factors and stretching will be required.

Two fundamental neurophysiologic principles form the basis of these techniques' success. The first is post-contraction inhibition, which states that after a muscle is contracted it is automatically in a relaxed or inhibited state for a brief, latent period. The second is reciprocal inhibition (RI), which states that when one muscle is contracted, its antagonist is automatically inhibited. For instance, if the quadriceps is contracted this inhibits the hamstrings, thus allowing for easier relaxation or stretching of the hamstring. This is based on Sherrington's law of reciprocal inhibition. RI's purpose is to allow an agonist (i.e., biceps) to be able to achieve its action (flexion) unimpeded by its antagonist (i.e., triceps). In the past, various explanations have been proposed for how the effects of MRTs are achieved. Whereas only postcontraction inhibition and RI have been validated, other suggested mechanisms include autogenic inhibition, golgi tendon organ stimulation, reciprocal innervation, presynaptic inhibition of Ia afferents, resetting of the gamma system, and post-synaptic inhibition.

It has been demonstrated that the receptors responsible for this inhibition are intramuscular and not in the skin or joints (34). Measurements of Hoffman reflex activity, which represents the excitability of the motor neuron pool, show that it is inhibited for up to 25 to 30 seconds after an agonist or antagonist contraction, whereas during static stretching this inhibition only lasts approximately 10 seconds (7). This effect has been found to be neurologically mediated and is not a result of any mechanical effect (35).

Muscle fibers also have certain biomechanical characteristics that affect their stiffness. Skeletal muscle fibers are known to adapt to imposed demands. For instance, during growth, muscle length increases as new sarcomeres are added in series and individual fibers increase their girth (41). Prolonged immobilization of a limb joint in an extended or shortened position results in an increase or decrease in the number of sarcomeres, respectively (38,42). When immobilized in a shortened position, muscle stiffness increases (38). It has been observed that an increase in connective tissue occurs with immobilization in a shortened position (43).

Connective tissue proliferation is minimized if the immobilized muscles are placed in a lengthened position or their contractile activity is maintained with electrical stimulation (38,43). Therefore, either passive stretching or maintenance of contractile activity in immobilized muscle can prevent muscle shortening and connective tissue proliferation.

Shortened muscles that have been immobilized require approximately 4 weeks of treatment to return to their pre-immobilization length (38). Muscle stiffness in response to stretch varies on the basis of intrinsic molecular properties of muscle fibers. Muscles that are kept still increase their stiffness two-fold in just a few minutes (17). Conversely, oscillations and isometric and eccentric muscle contractions all reduce muscle stiffness (8,17).

This plasticity of muscle fibers in response to passive or active movement is described as thixotrophic behavior. Thixotrophy refers to changes in viscosity and resistance to deformation of the intrinsic molecular make-up of muscle fibers that result from shaking or stirring motions. Both intrafusal and extrafusal muscle fibers have thixotrophic properties (9).

Thixotrophic bonds are thought to occur between actin and myosin filaments (9,11). Such bonds or cross-bridges form easily in muscles. According to Hagbarth, "After stretching or passive shortening, it may take 15 minutes or more before muscle fibers spontaneously return to their initial resting length (9)." He also stated, "Strong isometric contractions and muscle stretching maneuvers are likely to dissolve preexisting actomyosin bonds and thereby reduce the inherent stiffness of the extrafusal muscle fibers (9)."

Evidence About Stretching

Although stretching implies a more forceful procedure than described in this chapter, the evidence regarding its effectiveness or lack thereof is important. A literature review evaluating stretching identified several key points for clinical application (37):

1. Whereas use of cryotherapy or heat can increase a stretch's effectiveness in increasing range of motion, "only warm-up is likely to prevent injury."
2. For healthy individuals, a single 30-second stretch per muscle group will increase range of motion; however, clinicians may need to increase the length of stretch or number of repetitions for certain individuals and for certain injuries or muscle groups.
3. PNF has been identified as the most effective technique to increase range of motion, but it is important to note that during PNF techniques, the targeted muscle often undergoes an eccentric contraction during the stretch which can increase risk of injury to the targeted tissues.
4. When the patient is an athlete who is concerned with injury prevention, evidence indicates that whereas warm-ups decrease the risk of injury, stretching does not, thus stretching may not be appropriate before commencing activity (32,33,36,37).

According to a literature review by Hebert and Gabriel, stretching before and after exercise does not reduce post-exercise muscle soreness. Stretching before does not reduce injury risk (10).

What evidence does exist is largely negative. The question is, can we generalize based on a few moderate quality studies—as Herbert and Gabriel have—that stretching is **proven to be ineffective** as preventive of injury (10)? At present, it seems the evidence of stretchings ineffectiveness is limited. Certainly, there is a dearth of evidence of stretching's effectiveness, but to say there is strong evidence of its ineffectiveness would be to overreach the literature.

A second issue is the fact that there may be subgroups of patients in whom stretching is effective, but when a study considers a heterogenous group to mistakenly be a single homogenous group this smaller subgroup can be missed (16). Future research involving stratification of subjects into reasonable subgroups is needed.

The literature suggests that such subgroups do exist (28). For instance, Biering-Sorenson found that increased trunk flexion mobility, not hypomobility, predicted future low back pain (LBP) in men (1). It has also been recently reported that patients with spondylolisthesis tended to be hypermobile, whereas those with spinal stenosis, disc prolapse, or degenerative disc disease tended to be hypomobile (26). Thus, if a large group of heterogenous individuals are clumped together into one single group, the effectiveness of specific interventions for each smaller subgroup would be missed (16).

Decreases in hip internal rotation have shown to correlate with LBP (2,3). Tight muscles (iliopsoas and gastrosoleus) are shown to be correlated with increased injury risk—especially of the knee—in male college athletes (14). McGill has recently found that decreased hip extension mobility is correlated with disabling LBP (25). Van Dillen reported that chronic LBP subjects had less passive hip extension mobility than asymptomatic subjects (40). Studies in adolescents have documented that future episodes of LBP are correlated with decreased hip extension mobility (15). Some controversy exists, however, because Nadler reported that hypermobility in the lower extremity was correlated with future LBP in college atheletes (30,31).

Finally, even if the question of the value of stretching was clear, it is quite possible that even more important as an injury preventive would be limbering or "warm-up" (6). At the present time, clinicians should consider carefully the individual needs of their patient. Some may require increases in mobility, whereas others certainly may not.

Different Methods

PNF is the most complex system of MRTs (41). In PNF, neuromuscular re-education is the goal. Manual contacts, patient pre-positioning, muscle contraction against resistance, irradiation, and verbal commands are all used in concert to begin the process of improving movement. Its most commonly used inhibitory techniques are hold–relax (HR), contract–relax (CR), and rhythmic stabilization. HR involves isometric resistance and is used mostly for pain relief. CR is used for relaxing and stretching tight muscles and related soft tissues. This method incorporates isotonic resistance and multiplanar, usually diagonal, movement.

Historically, it was thought that using both agonist and antagonist muscles created a neurophysiological summation of RI and post-contraction inhibition. More recent reviews of the literature indicate that during PNF techniques, muscle electrical activity increases with co-contraction of agonist and antagonist muscles taking place (37). PNF stretching activates an eccentric contraction of the targeted muscle group, which also appears to have an analgesic effect, permitting greater range of motion and relaxation to occur (24,29).

When osteopathic physicians used MRTs, they applied them to mobilize joints, as well as to strengthen and relax muscles. They called these methods muscle energy procedures (MEPs) (27). Using a language familiar to chiropractors, they described the area where movement was felt to be limited as a "pathological" barrier (see Chapters 18 and 21). If, while moving a joint or muscle through its physiological range of motion, premature or increased resistance is felt, this is considered a "pathological" barrier. MEPs were developed by the osteopaths as alternatives to thrust manipulation procedures for restricted joint mobility and required the use of gentle forces. They were also used on muscles in a way similar to PNF.

In Europe, manual medicine physicians soon began experimenting with these methods. Lewit and Gaymans (4) wrote of success using these techniques in an extremely gentle fashion. At first, they used the rhythmic stabilization approach borrowed from PNF. Later, Lewit (5) focused on the HR approach. He found that by positioning an overactive muscle at the pathological barrier (see chapter 18) and then resisting a very gentle isometric contraction, excellent relaxation and an improved resting length of the muscle could be achieved. Lewit termed this approach postisometric relaxation (PIR). Lewit and Gaymans (4) also incorporated specific eye movements, in which the patient is asked to look in the direction of contraction during the isometric phase of the procedure and in the direction of muscle lengthening/relaxation during the inhibitory phase. In addition, for most muscles, breathing in facilitates the contraction and exhaling aids relaxation in the overactive muscle. These enhancements were termed visual and respiratory synkinesis respectively. Lewit felt that only the gentlest force was required (5).

Janda, another European, used HR with significantly greater forces for treating true muscular and connective tissue shortening (22,23). This adaptation, termed post-facilitation stretch (PFS), is for chronically shortened muscles. The patient performs a maximal contraction with the tight muscle in a mid-range position. On relaxation, the doctor quickly stretches the muscle, taking out all the slack.

Evjenth and Hamberg's work stands as an authoritative approach to muscle stretching procedures (4). Their work shows for each joint and muscle the exact doctor and patient positions for performing HR. The various manual resistance techniques are summarized in Table 19.1.

Practice-Based Problem

Can Manipulation Be Applied to All Mobile Structures Possessing Movement Restrictions?

The goal of manipulation is to mobilize tissue. Generally, manipulation is considered only for joints with movement restriction. However, can it be applied to skin, soft tissue (fascia), muscle, or joint?

A tissue with a movement restriction has a "pathological barrier." In other words, it has a premature loss of mobility and/or its quality of end-feel is abnormal (e.g., poor joint play or resilence). Manipulation is designed to improve mobility (quantitatively or qualitatively). When a "pathological barrier" is perceived, the goal of manipulation is to achieve a "release phenomenon." Generally, release is achieved in joints with a thrust that creates cavitation.

Another Clinical Question Arises—Namely, Can a "Release Phenemona" Be Achieved Without Force?

Naturally, joints can be pulled (traction), rocked, or oscillated. Muscles can be lengthened to their barrier and then after post-isometric relaxation a "release phenomenon" can occur, thus mobilizing the barrier. Scars, fascia, and muscle can be lengthened and held. Merely holding and waiting during a latency can achieve the simplest of all "release phenomena."

Table 19.1 Manual Resistance Techniques

Proprioceptive Neuromuscular Facilitation
   a) Hold–relax
   b) Contract–relax
   c) Rhythmic stabilization
Muscle energy procedures
Post-isometric relaxation
Post-facilitation stretch

Practice-Based Problem (*continued*)

What Effect Can Repeatedly Cavitating a Joint Have on the Normal Protective Barrier? In Other Words, Can You Cavitate a Joint Over and Over Again?

Within a brief time-frame such as 15 minutes, you cannot achieve repeated audible releases in a joint capsule. There is a normal, non-pathological barrier that should be respected in tissues. If tissues are too frequently or too forcefully manipulated, the normal protective barrier can lose its function. Unfortunately, in the pursuit of the goal of improving tissue mobility, instability may be produced!

Classification of Tense and Tight Muscles

According to Janda, certain muscles tend toward hypertonus (including tightness/shortness) and others toward inhibition (and weakness) (see Chapter 10 and Table 10-1). He also has emphasized that it is possible to divide muscle hypertonicity into a variety of different treatment-specific categories (12). Muscle dysfunction is typically caused by either neuromuscular or connective tissue factors. Different types of dysfunction include reflex spasm, interneuron facilitation from joint dysfunction, trigger points, central nervous system influences (i.e., limbic system involvement), and gradual overuse (see Tables 10.2 and 19.2).

Types of Hypertonus According to Janda (12)

1. *Limbic system dysfunction*—Caused by psychological stress. You will see increased muscle tone diffusely over the shoulder–neck area, low back, and pelvic floor muscles. It can lead to headache, LBP, dysmenorrhea, dyspareunia, and urinary frequency. The effected muscles will be tender to touch and the whole area will be involved with a sharp line of transition between the dysfunctional area and the normal area. Trigger points (TrPs) may tend to develop in these muscles.

Table 19.2 Classification of Tight or Tense Muscles (12)

A) Neuromuscular
   1) Reflex spasm
   2) Interneuron
   3) Trigger point
   4) Limbic
B) Connective tissue
   5) Overuse muscle tightness

2. *Interneuron dysfunction*—The interneuron is the most delicate part of the reflex arc. It can become disrupted by aberrant afferent information being sent to it because of spinal or peripheral joint dysfunction. This then causes hypertonicity of the muscles that are segmentally related. These muscles will be predisposed to the development of TrPs and their "antagonists" will become reciprocally inhibited and hypotonic. This imbalance of activity can lead to faulty movement patterns because the CNS will tend to over-activate the hypertonic muscles in the patterns that they are involved in and under-activate the hypotonic ones. As movements are performed in this dysfunctional state, the faulty patterns become reinforced.

3. *Myofascial trigger points*—This is an area of local congestion within the muscle that comes about as a result of sustained shortening of a fascicle of muscle fibers. Trigger points are common pain generators and should be thought of not as disorders that *alter* function but as results *of* dysfunction.

Definition: a hyperirritable spot, usually within a taut band of skeletal muscle or in the muscle's fascia, that is painful on compression and that can give rise to characteristic referred pain, tenderness, and autonomic phenomena (39).

4. *Reflex spasm*—This is muscle spasm as a response to nociception. It frequently acts as a splinting mechanism, for example, antalgia caused by LBP or abdominal "rigidity" caused by appendicitis. Once the underlying pain process resolves, the muscle hypertonicity often remains and must be treated. This can lead to TrP or faulty movement pattern development. Continuous spontaneous EMG activity is seen.

5. *Muscle tightness*—This is a myopathological and neuropathological state in which the muscle becomes hyperactive and shortened most commonly because of overuse, especially in a postural function. The antagonist of the tight muscle can become reciprocally inhibited, thereby setting up an imbalance of activity. This imbalance of activity leads to the development of faulty movement patterns because the tight muscle becomes too readily activated by the CNS and tends to dominate the movement patterns that it is involved in and the inhibited muscle tends to be left out of the movement patterns in which it is involved. Every time these movement patterns are performed, the hyperactivity and hypoactivity are reinforced. This can also be a cause of joint dysfunction because of the altered distribution of pressures that is created on each side of the joint.

Making a precise assessment of soft tissue functional pathology helps to guide the treatment decision-making process. In the case of muscle tension or tightness, Table 19.3 shows what specific treatments are appropriate for each different type of dysfunction.

Clinical Application

Manually resisted exercises are the perfect bridge to active care because they take place in the treatment room with the doctor's guidance and instruction. The doctor provides appropriate resistance to specific movements that are being trained. When performing MRTs, it is helpful to realize that whereas historically there are many names (PNF, MEP, PIR, etc.) for different techniques, there are certain common elements to successful MRT application. MRTs involve isometric, concentric, or eccentric contractions. They are used to relax muscles, stretch muscles or fascia, mobilize joints, or facilitate muscles. The clinical indications for MRTs are summarized in Table 19.4.

MRTs have been presented as alternatives to thrust maneuvers, but in the context of this chapter they are primarily seen as complementary to traditional chiropractic and manual medicine methods. In as much as overactive or shortened muscles are related to a specific joint dysfunction, MRTs may indirectly mobilize a joint or at the very least make an adjustment more comfortable and long-lasting for the patient. Thus, their main application is in directly treating the muscular component so as to enhance the efficacy of joint adjustments. Both in acute situations in which muscular guarding (neuromuscular tension or "spasm") is present and chronic cases in which muscle and fascial shortening (connective tissue changes) is present MRTs serve as invaluable clinical tools.

MRTs may be used to relax tension in muscles before thrust manipulation. However, if we desire to stretch chronically shortened muscles or fascia, then chiropractic adjustments should precede any aggressive stretching. After an adjustment, MRTs can be

Table 19.3 Specific Treatment for Different Types Of Muscle Tension/Tightness (12)

Type	Treatment
1) Reflex	Cause (i.e., remove appendix)
2) Interneuron	Joint manipulation
3) Trigger point	PIR or ischemic compression
4) Limbic	Yoga, meditation, counseling
5) Muscle tightness	PFS or eccentric MEP

Table 19.4   MRT Goals (Indications)

1) Muscle inhibition/relaxation/decontraction
2) Muscle stretch
3) Fascial stretch
4) Muscle facilitation
5) Joint mobilization

used to reinforce neuromuscular reeducation and to instruct the patient for effective home exercise.

MRTs require active patient participation and are therefore less likely than passive modalities to encourage patient dependency. They are, however, more demanding of the patient. The use of reciprocal inhibition or gentle PIR methods is nearly always painless and, with a little patient education, simple to perform.

As compared to deep tissue massage (i.e., Graston technique), trigger point therapy (Nimmo, myotherapy, or receptor tonus), or active release technique (ART) MRTs can be a faster and less painful way of reducing increased muscle tension or normalizing trigger points or muscle tension. Exceptions to this would be if the patient is either very uncoordinated or simply unable to relax. Patients with difficulty relaxing often need moist heat, relaxation, and breathing exercises, and some type of gentle, non-painful massage (i.e., effleurage). The combination of MRTs and soft tissue procedures can be used with great effect. For instance, as the tissues are being massaged, if an area of tension is found the patient can be instructed to contract that tissue, then allow it to relax. This combination can often overcome even very stubborn "knots." The ART technique can easily be used in combination with MRTs to achieve a greater muscle inhibition.

Many times if a patient cannot tolerate deep soft tissue manipulation (i.e., Rolfing or transverse friction massage), MRTs may be used to reduce the sensitivity of the area. After MRT application, deep massage or ischemic compression techniques will usually be tolerable to the patient. Any massage or passive therapy runs the risk of encouraging patient dependency. To minimize this, and to re-educate the use and coordination of the treated muscle in the newly available range of motion, passive therapies should always be combined with some form of patient education, exercise, and self-treatment.

Positional release (i.e., strain/counterstrain) or osteopathic functional techniques are preferable to MRTs when it is difficult to find an active movement that does not provoke the patient's symptoms. In such cases, positional release methods (finding a painless muscle or joint position and holding there) are a painless and effective means to reducing irritability

and increasing motion in a patient with soft tissue pain.

MRTs and spray and stretch have quite similar goals and may be used interchangeably (39). Both are considered alternatives to dry needling and injection of anesthetic for relief of painful trigger points or periosteal attachment points (19). Spray and stretch is passive and thus may be better in the first stages of treatment when a patient has poor motor control (incoordination and difficulty relaxing) and pain levels are high. The strong inhibition of pain signals afforded by spray and stretch may be needed by some patients in the initial acute phase of care to quiet highly active trigger points. Those patients who are cold-intolerant may require even more passive methods such as heat, electrotherapy, osteopathic functional technique, joint mobilization, or massage. Spray and stretch can be used as an alternative to PFS for lengthening shortened connective tissue. Sometimes spray and stretch and various MRT techniques can be combined together. Trial and error often determines which approach has a greater inhibitory effect on the muscle for a specific patient. Because of Fluori-Methane's negative environmental profile, PIR and intermittent cold and stretch have been proposed as alternatives whenever possible (39).

An alternative to PFS for musculo-fascial shortening is the osteopathic myofascial release method. This typically involves lifting the involved soft tissue and stretching it perpendicular to its muscle fiber orientation (see Chapter 18). This method is often advantageous because it avoids engaging the stretch reflex. PFS, myofascial release, and deep tissue massage can often complement each other. Often, especially in recurrent and chronic conditions, neuromuscular and chronic muscle shortening dysfunctions co-exist and each component of the soft tissue dysfunction may need to be addressed in order to successfully resolve the patient's symptom.

The use of hot packs, ultrasound, electrical muscle stimulation, and other passive thermal or electrical modalities is common in musculoskeletal clinical care. These are sometimes appropriate in acute and subacute care but are inappropriate in rehabilitation beyond the phase of early soft tissue healing. Modalities can be useful for preparing the tissues for more active manual techniques but the treatment regimen should be transitioned to active care as early as possible.

MRTs have the advantage that while being easily tolerated like passive modalities, they also involve the patient in an active way, thus limiting patient dependency. The thrust of modern management of chronic pain is away from passive therapy (physical agents) toward active patient involvement in the rehabilitation process (see Chapters 1 and 14). This does not mean that passive therapies do not have a role to play, but that we must aim our patients toward functional restoration in activities of daily living. MRTs are ideal bridges between passive and active care.

To summarize, MRTs are invaluable for normalizing pathological barriers within joints and muscles. The pathological barrier is identified as the point within the normal range of motion of a joint or muscle where premature or increased resistance to motion is felt. The barrier may be caused by joint blockage, increased muscular tension, muscle shortening, or a combination of the three. MRTs are one method to eliminate this barrier and restore normal range of motion (ROM). They achieve this by relaxing the overactive muscle and/or mobilizing the hypomobile joint. When true joint blockage exists, a chiropractic adjustment is without peer as the treatment of choice. MRTs can stand on their own, but they are better as a complement to the adjustment and a bridge to exercise.

Rules for Application

When using MRTs, the more precisely we can facilitate contraction in the desired muscle fibers, the better our results will be. Table 19.5 summarizes some of the keys to achieving successful facilitation. When the clinical goal is to relax a muscle, a moment's attention to the patient's overall comfort and body positioning can greatly aid relaxation of the target muscle. Patient pre-positioning with respect to the specific target muscle will affect how easy or difficult it is to activate the muscle. Our verbal command is also important, not only for what we say but also for the inflection we use. Trial and error with each patient will reveal which commands activate the desired movement best. In general, telling a patient to push to the right or left is not as good as giving them an actual tactile target. When using facilitation techniques, it is helpful to place a contact on the muscle you wish to activate because manual contacts are facilitatory. Likewise, firm massage or goading while the patient attempts to contract the muscle may help to awaken a particularly inhibited muscle. Irradiation is sometimes used to facilitate a muscle which

---

Table 19.5 Facilitation Techniques

Pre-positioning
Hand contacts
Tissue stimulation
Verbal cues or commands
Irradiation

---

is especially "dormant." This involves using a synergistic muscle that is stronger to pull its inhibited neighbor into action.

Technique Principles

1. Patient positioning—the patient should always be placed in a position of maximum comfort. The muscle being treated should be placed in a position in which it is in a relaxed state and is not contracting against gravity. The muscle should also be placed in a position that is most advantageous for the recruitment of motor units to that muscle. During patient positioning the order in which you take up the slack may be altered to improve isolation of the target tissue (e.g., flexion, contralateral side bending, and ipsilateral rotation for the upper trapezius). This is called "winding-up" the muscle.

2. Engaging the barrier—the muscle should be elongated to the extent to which the full resting length is attained. The barrier is the point at which further lengthening would cause the muscle to go into a stretch reflex. It is important to carefully engage this barrier and not go beyond it.

3. Use of isometric contraction—the isometric contraction is either very gentle or hard, depending on whether the condition being treated is neuromuscular hypertonus (e.g., trigger points) or muscle tightness with connective tissue involvement. A good rule of thumb is "as little force as possible or as much as necessary." **The gentler contraction is always tried first because the trigger point being the most sensitive part of the muscle is isolated by a light contraction.** The position of the patient and the treated muscle should be such that the doctor or therapist can maintain stability and control at all times. The duration of the contraction is usually 4 to 10 seconds. This may be increased up to 30 seconds if little or no release is achieved with a 4- to 10-second effort.

4. Use of breathing and eye movements—most muscles become facilitated with inhalation and inhibited with exhalation. Also, certain muscles are facilitated when the eyes are moved in certain directions and are inhibited when the eyes move in the opposite direction. These physiological reflexes can be used to maximize the effectiveness of the manual resistance procedures.

5. Feeling the release—after the isometric contraction is let go, the patient breathes out and engages in inhibitory eye movements; it is important to wait to feel for the tension in the muscle to release. It is at this point that the muscle

Table 19.6 Safety Rules

1) Stretch over largest, most stable, least painful joint
2) Place joints in "loose-packed" position
3) Avoid uncoupled spinal movements
4) Do not stretch nerves if irritated

should be slowly guided to lengthen. This is **not a stretch!** Guide the muscle until a new barrier is engaged, at which time a second isometric contraction is begun and the process is repeated.

When using MRTs, there are various guidelines that help us to avoid irritating our patients. Care must be taken that related joints are not put in a position of strain (i.e., close packed position) during stretching. For example, when stretching the iliopsoas if the lumbar spine is allowed to extend too much, strain will occur in the low back. When stretching in the spinal column it is also important to avoid uncoupled movements. For instance, in the cervical spine proper coupling occurs when rotation and side-bending occur in the same direction (spinous process towards the convexity). In the lumbar spine it is the opposite, unless the spine is flexed. In the neutral or extended positions, normal lumbar coupling takes place when rotation and side-bending occur in opposite directions (the spinous process moves toward the concavity). This is important to incorporate when mobilizing joints with MRTs, and when stretching muscles that require slack be taken out in what would be an uncoupled manner for the underlying spinal joints.

An example of an uncoupled joint position is the cervical side bending away and rotation toward an upper trapezius muscle being stretched. Because this might strain the cervical spinal joints, we stretch almost completely over the upper back and shoulder area, avoiding any contraction or strong stretching in the neck area. The way that we "wind-up" the upper trapezius will reduce the potential for neck strain. Full flexion with slight ipsilateral rotation would be taken out first, then gently we would side-bend the neck away from the muscle, and then finally slack would be taken out of the upper back and shoulder regions to the barrier. The patient's contraction would be only from the shoulder in the direction of elevation. During relaxation and stretch, we would take out the slack over the larger, more stable shoulder and avoid taking out slack in the neck, except perhaps in flexion. This illustrates a general rule in MRTs that we should relax or stretch over the largest, most stable, and least painful joint (22,23).

Another principle is to avoid stretching related structures such as nerve roots if irritated (22,23). Hopefully every clinician knows not to stretch the hamstrings if the sciatic nerve is irritated. Similarly, femoral nerve irritation may contraindicate rectus femoris stretching and brachial plexus irritation may contraindicate scalene stretching. Any increase in radicular pain or symptoms, no matter how slight, strictly contraindicates these procedures.

Finally, pregnancy of either the patient or doctor contraindicates use of the PFS technique. Table 19.6 summarizes these important safety tips during stretching.

How we "wind-up" the muscle, in other words the order with which we take out the slack in the different planes of motion (rotation, flexion/extension, side-bending), can dramatically alter where the patient feels the stretch (22). Playing with this variable allows for better isolation of the specific muscle fibers requiring treatment. Most people use too much force when they first begin to use MRTs. The forces used during MRTs should be light. According to Lewit, the time of the contraction can be lengthened for up to 30 seconds if inhibition is not readily achieved using a 10-second contraction (20). Whether to adjust joints before or after MRTs is a common question. If there is a significant joint restriction in the pathway we are attempting to stretch through, then it is crucial to adjust first. Otherwise a manipulation can be achieved more easily and with less force if performed after the contractile elements have been relaxed. Table 19.7 lists different ways to improve MRT results.

Specific Procedures

One of the most useful MRTs is post-isometric relaxation (PIR). This is Lewit's modification of the gentle, indirect isometric MEP, which the osteopaths applied to joints (20). It is also similar to hold–relax. The main goal of PIR is relaxation (decontraction) of a hypertonic (contracted) or overactive muscle. This is the preferred method if the patient has difficulty relaxing or you simply want to use a "softer" approach until you gain the patient's trust. It is ideal for trigger points, joint mobilization, muscle spasm, and increased neuromuscular tension.

Table 19.7 Ways To Maximize MRT Results

1) "Wind-up" muscles to maximize isolation
2) Start gentle and add force only if necessary
3) Increase contraction time up to 30 seconds
4) Adjust restricted joints first

Post-Isometric Relaxation

Post-isometric relaxation (PIR) involves the following simple steps (20):

1. Position the patient appropriately for the muscle to be treated. Ensure that the patient is comfortable, fully supported, and at rest.

2. Passively lengthen the tense muscle to the point at which the first slight increase in resistance (pathological barrier) is felt. Avoid bouncing.

3. Have the patient contract the overactive muscle gently, with minimal effort, for approximately 10 seconds. This should be resisted with equal counterforce creating an isometric contraction. For most muscles, the patient should breathe in while contracting the muscle.

4. Have the patient breathe out, "let go," and relax the muscle fully. The doctor *pauses momentarily* and monitors for a decrease in resistance felt at the barrier. If resistance decreases, the muscle is gently, passively lengthened until a new barrier is felt, the next slight increase in resistance.

5. If no decrease in resistance is felt, the procedure is repeated at the same barrier and any of the modifications described may be used.

6. While remaining engaged at the barrier, three to five repetitions are performed per treatment session.

7. If relaxation is not achieved, try the following:
   - Be sure the patient breathes in during the contraction phase and exhales during the relaxation phase.
   - For most trunk and extremity muscles, the patient should look in the direction of contraction, then while relaxing look in the direction of stretch.
   - The duration of contraction may be lengthened for up to 30 seconds.
   - A harder contraction may be tried.
   - Starting from a mid-range position, isotonic resistance of movement by the antagonist muscle toward the restricted barrier may be used one to three times.

8. Once relaxation is achieved, have the patient contract the antagonist (RI) muscle isometrically in a rhythmic fashion by resisting the contraction in a pulsed manner.

9. After this has been accomplished, the patient should be instructed to perform active ROM exercise through the new range.

Clinical Pearl

Relaxation is a neurophysiological response that occurs in time; the time taken to relax varies from individual to individual, from muscle to muscle, from early to later stages of care, and even from repetition to repetition within a treatment session. Once relaxation has begun, it is key to allow it to continue for as long as it takes/continues, at times up to 30 seconds, so as not to cut-off the desired beneficial effect of treatment.

Success with this method depends on precise positioning of the body part so as to isolate the tense muscular bundles involved, accurate engaging of the barrier, and attention to overall patient comfort and response.

Visual and respiratory synkinesis, described in detail, are technique enhancements described by Lewit to improve the effectiveness of the PIR technique (21). Although part of the standard PIR technique, their use with any given patient is at the doctor's discretion. Remember that the goal of PIR is to elicit relaxation within a muscle. Because individuals vary in their response to factors such as strength of isometric contraction, duration of isometric contraction, practitioner tactile and verbal cues, and the use of eye movements and breathing, the skillful doctor or therapist remains alert to and continues to assess the patient's response to these variables. These factors then should be incorporated in the way that most effectively produces relaxation in the individual and muscle being treated.

Visual Synkinesis Visual synkinesis is based on the neurophysiological relationship between eye and body movements (21). This relationship exists to facilitate visual tracking of an object of interest and to assist body orientation during ADLs. For example, looking up causes cervical and trunk extension and thereby induces activation of the cervical and spinal extensors while inhibiting the flexors. Likewise, looking to the right causes right cervical and trunk rotation, activation of the muscles involved in right rotation, and inhibition of those involved in left rotation. Whereas these relationships are strongest in the trunk musculature, they can be used with good effect when treating extremity musculature as well. When there is no direct relationship between eye movement and the action of the muscle being treated, have the patient look in the direction the body part would move, if allowed, during the contraction. Assess the patient's response to your directions and modify accordingly. If the patient overactivates, ask for a gentler effort, use a quieter tone of voice, and/or have the patient simply think of looking in the desired direction.

1. Give the patient instructions to look in a specific direction, along with your instructions for isometric contraction of the target muscle. For example, for suboccipital PIR, instruct the patient to look up (toward their forehead) while gently isometrically activating the muscle.

2. As you instruct the patient to cease contraction and relax, have them also focus the eyes in the direction the body would move if the muscle being treated were to lengthen. For example, for the suboccipitals have the patient look down (toward their chin or toes) into flexion.

3. When working with patients, simplicity has its merits. When treating a muscle whose action is in three planes, use of eye movements in only one or two predominant planes of action is usually enough to achieve the desired facilitation and inhibition of the target muscle while avoiding confusion and anxiety about complex movements.

Respiratory Synkinesis Respiration also has a synkinetic relationship with muscle activation (21). In general, inhalation enhances muscle activation, whereas exhalation enhances muscle relaxation. The primary exception to this is when the body part treated is part of the respiratory apparatus and thus its motion is linked to facilitate the function of breathing. For example, the mandibular elevators (masseter and temporalis) are inhibited during inhalation and facilitated during exhalation.

Clinical Pearl

Breathing instructions are most effective when performed at the patient's own breath rhythm. Thus, before beginning, the practitioner should observe and coordinate with the patient's inhalation. Neither the natural inhalation nor the exhalation should be cut short if the best effect is to be achieved.

---

1. Have the patient breathe in during isometric contraction.

2. Have the patient breathe out during relaxation.

3. Have the patient return to their normal breath rhythm between repetitions and allow relaxation to take its full course as previously described.

Clinical Pearl

Watch the patient's response. Whereas some patients respond to breathing instructions well, others overactivate the treated muscle or even the whole body, thus increasing overall tension at the end of the procedure. Breathing instructions should be modified to elicit the desired level of response from the individual. A minimum repertoire of breathing related patient instructions would include "take a deep breath in," "take a little bit of a deeper breath in," and "take a nice deep breath in," accompanied by suitable tone of voice to either lessen/lighten/diminish or accentuate the response.

Post-Facilitation Stretch (PFS)

PFS is a second very valuable MRT (22,23). It involves the following steps:

1. Position the patient appropriately for the muscle to be treated. The patient must be comfortable, fully supported, and at rest.

2. Place the shortened muscle in a position approximately midway between the barrier and neutral resting position of the muscle; the barrier is not engaged.

3. Have the patient contract with maximum or near maximum effort for approximately 10 seconds. This should be resisted by the doctor to create a nearly isometric contraction.

4. Have the patient relax the muscle completely and fast. The doctor must feel that the patient has completely relaxed the muscle before performing the stretch.

5. When the patient has "let go" completely, perform a fast yet careful stretch to the new barrier, avoiding bouncing, and hold for up to 20 seconds.

6. Allow the patient to relax with the muscle in a mid-range position for 20 to 30 seconds.

7. Repeat three to five times per treatment session.

8. After this has been accomplished, the patient should be instructed to perform an active ROM exercise through the new range.

After stretching, advise the patient that it is normal to feel warmth, weakness, burning, or tingling in the stretched tissue. An appropriate series of such stretches would be six visits over a 2-week period.

Indications

- Myofascial shortening (viscoelastic stiffness)

In PNF, two of the most well-known MRTs are hold–relax (HR) and contract–elax (CR). HR involves positioning the patient at the barrier or "first stop" and pushing against resistance while asking the patient to hold. This creates an isometric contraction. In all other respects, HR is identical to PIR.

CR involves taking out the slack and then commanding the patient to "push against me" or "push toward. . . . (an object or target)." This encourages a concentric contraction because pushing implies movement, whereas holding implies staying stationary. Unlike PIR or HR, a greater force and accompanying movement are allowed. At the end of the contraction, RI may be used so that the patient actively takes out the slack themselves. This combination is often called contract–relax antagonist contraction (CRAC). This is preferred to HR if the patient is using a stronger muscle, which would be difficult for you to resist isometrically.

An alternative to PFS for stretching connective tissues is the osteopathic eccentric MEP. This involves starting at a mid-range position and having the patient push lightly against your resistance using approximately 20% effort. During the patient's contraction, the doctor lengthens the muscle. The patient must continue to contract lightly so that it is a lengthening or eccentric contraction. This is excellent for lengthening the non-contractile elements.

Table 19.8 summarizes the choice of MRT depending on the specific treatment goal.

Self-PIR and Self-Stretching

Self-treatment should be performed on a regular basis to prevent elevated neuromuscular tension or viscoelastic stiffness from recurring. Once or twice per day, key tense or stiff muscles may be gently stretched. Simple guidelines for self stretching are as follows:

1. If possible, perform simple warm-ups before stretching.
2. Gently take out the slack in the involved muscle until a gentle and comfortable pulling is felt.

3. Maintain good body posture so that no strain is felt anywhere else in the body.
4. Hold the stretch position for 10 to 20 seconds, taking out further slack as relaxation is achieved.
5. Breathe naturally, deeply, and slowly to encourage relaxation.
6. Repeat stretches at least twice per session and one to two times per day.
7. After stretching it is advisable to actively contract the muscle and move it through a full range of motion a few times.

Clinical Pearl

There should be no increased pain associated with the self-PIR or stretch procedure. Ideally, try to find the level of stretch at which you can feel the muscle easing into the stretch; this is part of the art of safe and effective stretching. If at any time you feel increasing tightness or discomfort, this is an indication of over-stretching and you should ease up accordingly into a level of stretch your muscle can relax into.

Selected MRT Procedures

MRT techniques can be used for a variety of purposes. They are alternatives to adjustments or soft tissue work. They are powerful facilitation and strengthening techniques. But they are most famous for their ability to relax muscles. Examples of each of these are described and pictured in detail.

PIR Procedures for Muscle Relaxation and Stretch

The format for this section is designed for easy clinical application. Readers are encouraged to refer to Chapters 10, 22, and 26 for more detail regarding specific tests, related strengthening exercises, or treatment

---

Table 19.8 Matching Therapeutic Goals to MRTs

	Inhibit Muscle	Stretch Muscle	Stretch Fascia	Mobilize Joint
PIR	+			+
HR	+	+		
CR	+	+		
PFS		+	+	
Eccentric MEP		+	+	

protocols. The following headings are used for most of the muscles described.

Referred Pain: Location of pain symptom

Clinical Result of Shortened Muscle: Related clinical findings

Activation or Perpetuation: What activates or perpetuates trigger point

Observation: Postural analysis

Trigger Point: Location

Periosteal Point: Location

Evaluation for Overactivity: How muscle over-activity would be identified

Evaluation for Muscle Shortening: Test for muscle tightness

Joint Dysfunction: Related joint dysfunction

Corrective Actions: Exercise and educational approach

PIR Technique:

   Patient Position

   Doctor Position

   Patient's Active Effort

   Direction of Muscle Lengthening:

Other PIR Stretches:

Self-PIR/Self-Stretches:

1. Hamstring

Referred Pain

- Lower buttock to upper medial calf

Clinical Result of Shortened Muscle

- Recurrent pulled hamstrings
- Anterior knee pain
- Fibular head dysfunction (long head of biceps femoris)

Activation or Perpetuation

- Compensation for weak gluteus maximus
- Compression of posterior thigh from a chair that is too high
- Being in a shortened position from prolonged sitting

Observation

- Increased muscle bulk in posterior thigh (two-thirds down)

Trigger Points

- Mid belly

Periosteal Points

- Ischial tuberosity
- Fibular head (biceps femoris)

Evaluation for Overactivity

- Knee flexion during prone hip extension test

Evaluation for Shortening

- Straight leg raising test of less than 90 degrees with the non-tested knee bent

Joint Dysfunction

- L5-S1
- T/L junction
- Fibular head

Corrective Action

- Relax/stretch the hip flexors if indicated
- Facilitate or strengthen the gluteus maximus
- Avoid prolonged sitting

PIR Technique (Fig. 19.1)
   Patient Position

- Supine
- Hip flexed and knee extended on involved limb
- Hip and knee flexed with foot on table on non-treated side

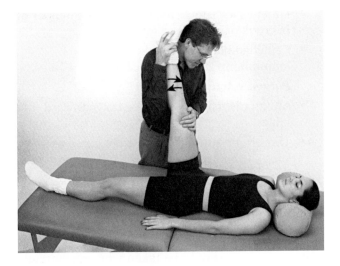

Figure 19.1 Hamstring PIR.

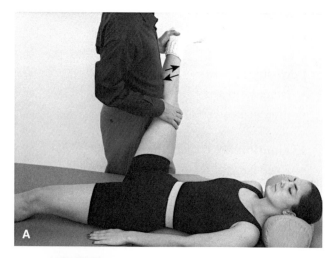

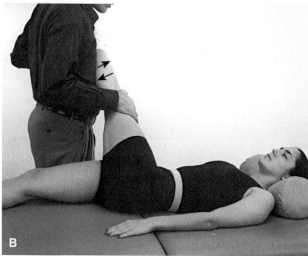

Figure 19.2 Medial and lateral hamstring PIR.

Doctor Position
- Standing on side of treated limb facing cephalad
- Patient's leg supported on doctor's shoulder or in crook of elbow
- Cephalad hand proximal to patella maintaining knee in extension

Patient's Active Effort
- Attempt is made to push leg down toward table
- This effort is resisted by the doctor so as to keep the contraction as close to isometric as possible

Direction of Muscle Lengthening
- Flexion of hi\p while maintaining knee in extension

Comment Care should be taken whenever stretching the hamstrings that the sciatic nerve tension tests

(Lesague's test, straight leg raise, or slump test) are negative (see Chapter 20 for neuromobilization methods). Also, in the case of lumbar joint irritability, the opposite hip and knee may be flexed to reduce strain on the lumbar spine.

Other PIR Stretches Additional hamstring PIR procedures are shown for the medial fibers (Fig. 19.2A), lateral fibers (Fig. 19.2B), and the one joint hamstring—the biceps femoris (Fig. 19.3).

Self-Stretches For hamstring self-stretches it is important that the back is stable. The patient should feel the stretch in the posterior thigh, but no strain in the lower back should be felt (Figs. 19.4, 19.5A, and 19.5B). The sacrum and hips should be kept resting on the floor and not permitted to lift or tilt posteriorly, which moves the stretch away from the hamstrings and moves it into the low back. If necessary, a small rolled towel or comparable support may be placed in the small of the low back to protect against lumbar flexion. During the supine or standing self-stretches once the final stretch position is achieved if the patient is instructed to perform an anterior pelvic tilt they will feel a greater stretch.

2. Hip Adductors

Referred Pain
- Groin, inner thigh, anterior or medial knee, medial shin

Clinical Result of Shorteneed Muscle
- Hip or SI disorders or medial knee pain
- Difficulty with squats

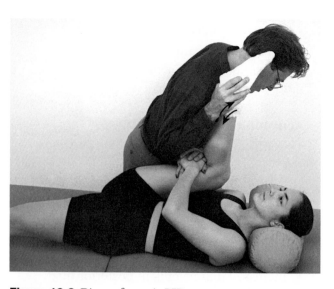

Figure 19.3 Biceps femoris PIR.

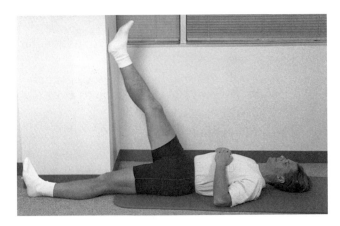

Figure 19.4 Hamstring self-stretch.

- Difficulty with activation of gluteus medius
- Lateral shift of pelvis to same side

Activation or Perpetuation
- hip arthritis, horseback riding, hill running, sudden overload (slipping)

Trigger Points
- Muscle belly

Periosteal Points
- Pubic symphysis
- Pes anserinus
- Medial femoral condyle

Evaluation for Shortening
- With patient supine, abduct thigh with knee extended; normal is 40 degrees
- If 40 degrees not reached, flex knee and observe if additional abduction possible
- If yes, long adductors (medial hamstrings) are tight
- If no, one-joint adductors are tight

Joint Dysfunction
- Hip joint

PIR Technique
  a) Supine Technique (Fig. 19.6)
    Patient Position
- Supine
- Leg abducted (knee flexed or extended to isolate one or two joint adductors, respectively) until resistance is felt

- Opposite leg is abducted slightly on the table to help stabilize the pelvis; knee is bent with the foot placed flat on the table
  Doctor Position
- Standing with one leg between patient's abducted thigh and the table. The weight of the patient's leg should be fully supported.
  Patient's Active Effort
- Patients attempts to push thigh into adduction
- This effort is resisted by the doctor's leg so as keep the contraction as close to isometric as possible
  Direction of Muscle Lengthening
- The doctor then takes out the slack into further abduction

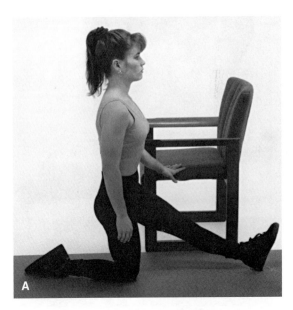

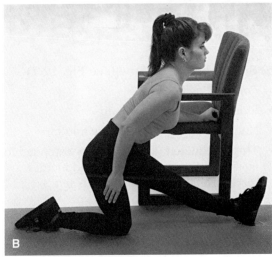

Figure 19.5 Hamstring self-stretch.

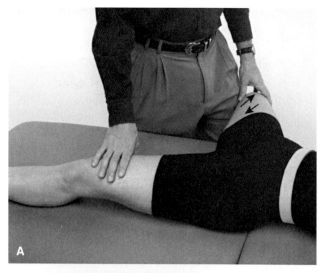

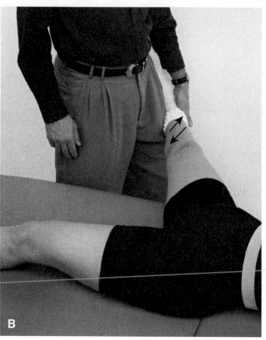

Figure 19.6 1- and 2-joint adductor PIR.

b) Side-Lying Technique (see Fig. 19.7)
Patient Position
- Side-lying involved side up
- Non-treated leg bent at knee and hip
- Thigh abducted (knee flexed or extended to isolate the one and two joint adductors, respectively) until resistance is felt

Doctor Position
- Standing behind patient
- Abducts patient's thigh, caudal hand hooking under patient's knee
- Cephalad hand stabilizes the pelvis

Patient's Active Effort
- Patient attempts to push thigh into adduction toward table
- This effort is resisted by the doctor's caudal arm so as to keep the contraction as close to isometric as possible

Direction of Muscle Lengthening
- The doctor then takes out the slack into further abduction

Self-Stretches Self-stretches are shown in Fig. 19.8.

3. Iliopsoas

Referred Pain
- Low back and SI joint, anterior thigh

Clinical Result of Muscle Shortening
- Poor hip extension

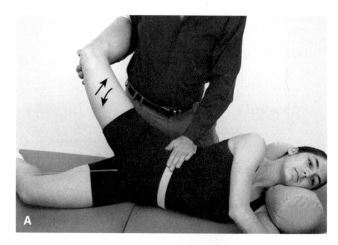

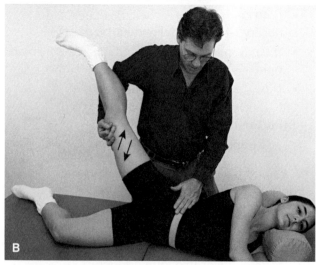

Figure 19.7 1- and 2-joint adductor PIR.

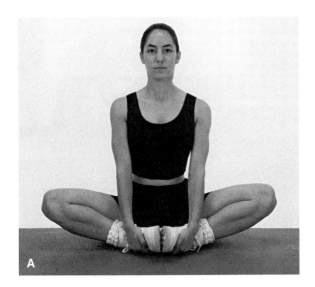

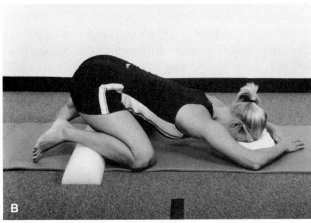

Figure 19.8 Adductor self-stretches.

- Forward-drawn posture
- Difficulty with the posterior pelvic tilt

Activation or Perpetuation
- Recent intervertebral disc syndrome
- Sway back (psoas must act as a checkrein)
- Prolonged sitting
- Compensation for weak abdominals

Observation
- Anterior pelvic tilt in standing
- Hip joints flexed in standing

Trigger Points
- Any where in muscle belly

Evaluation for Overactivity
- Inability to keep heels on the floor during knee bent sit-up

Evaluation for Shortening
- Modified Thomas test:
  - Supine patient's non-tested hip and knee are held maximally flexed by doctor
  - Tested leg is allowed to extend off table
  - Test is positive if:
    1. Thigh rests above horizontal (tight iliopsoas)
    2. Shin does not fall to vertical position (tight rectus femoris)
    3. Thigh is abducted, patella is deviated superolaterally, or a groove is visualized along the lateral thigh (tight TFL)

Joint Dysfunction
- T10-L1

Corrective Action
- Avoid prolonged sitting
- Facilitate and strengthen the abdominals and gluteals
- Relax/stretch the erector spinae

PIR Technique (Fig. 19.9)
Patient Position
- Supine
- Involved hip freely extending off end of table
- Contralateral hip and knee held in full flexion against chest
- Lumbar spine may be laterally flexed away from the psoas being treated
- Need sufficient table height to allow floor clearance of the treated leg, usually at least 40 inches

Doctor Position
- At same side of table as involved limb or at end of table
- One hand holds contralateral knee to chest, thereby stabilizing pelvis
- Other hand contacts treated thigh just proximal to knee

Patient's Active Effort
- Patient is instructed to raise involved knee up toward ceiling
- To enhance psoas isolation, patient may be instructed to supinate foot against resistance offered by therapist's leg
- This effort is resisted isometrically by the doctor

Direction of Muscle Lengthening
- Once the patient has fully relaxed, the doctor may take up the slack by extending the hip to

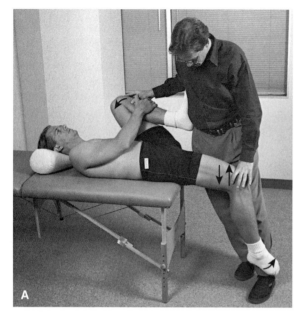

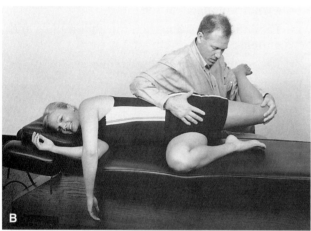

Figure 19.9 Iliopsoas PIR.

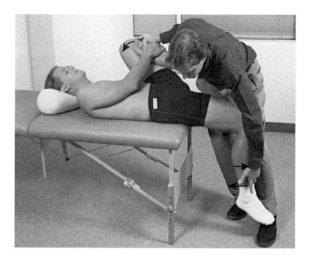

Figure 19.10 Rectus femoris PIR.

prone iliopsoas (Fig. 19.11). For the prone iliopsoas, the hip should be internally rotated and the spine laterally bent away. Care should be taken to avoid abducting the thigh. This is perhaps the most specific iliopsoas stretch, but it is a tremendous strain on the doctor unless an elevation table is used. If an elevation table is used, start in elevation and hold the thigh up while allowing the table to lower and simultaneously stretch the muscle while maintaining feel for the barrier.

Self-Stretches It is important when performing self-stretches for the hip flexors that the stretch is felt in the anterior hip or thigh and not in the low back. For its new end point while continuing to stabilize the opposite leg.

Comment At times the patient will report discomfort in the fully flexed hip (the one not being stretched). This may be provoked by the passive over-pressure required to flatten the low back. When this occurs it is often necessary to back off a little in the attempt to take all the lordosis out of the lumbar spine. A number of manual techniques may be helpful in relieving this discomfort. Hip joint traction, hip PIR mobilization, or PIR on the iliopsoas, TFL, gluteus medius, or adductors may help to ease the hip sufficiently to allow for comfortable full hip flexion.

Other PIR Methods Other related hip flexor PIR procedures include the rectus femoris (Fig. 19.10) and

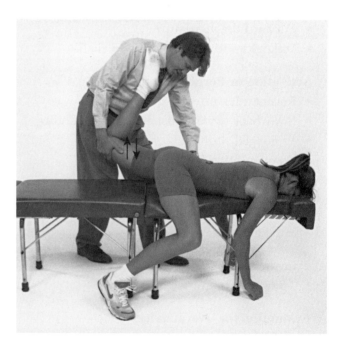

Figure 19.11 Iliopsoas PIR.

the iliopsoas, this is best accomplished if the patient holds a posterior pelvic tilt and internally rotates the hip while stretching (Figs. 19.12A and 19.12B). The rectus femoris stretch requires some knee flexion (Figs. 19.13A and 19.13B) and the ability of the patient to produce and maintain a braced lumbar spine.

4. Tensor Fascia Latae (TFL)

Referred Pain
* Lateral aspect of thigh to knee

Clinical Result of Shortened Muscle
* Knee extensor mechanism disorders
* Patellofemoral syndrome

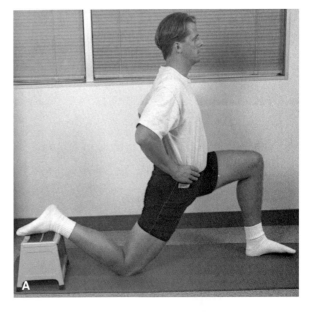

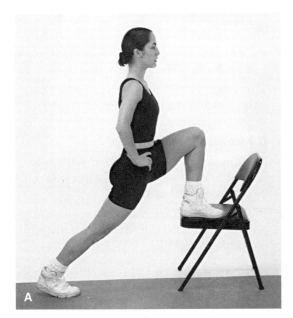

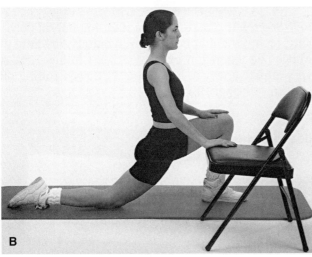

Figure 19.12 Iliopsoas self-stretches.

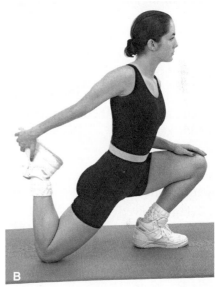

Figure 19.13 Rectus femoris self-stretches.

* SIJ problems
* QL myofascial disorders

Activation or Perpetuation
* Repetitive strain from running
* Lateral pelvic shift
* Forefoot instability (excessive pronation)
* Prolonged sitting, especially in bucket seats
* Bicycling
* Compensation for a weak gluteus medius

Trigger Points
* Superior portion of muscle

Observation
- Groove along iliotibial band
- Superolateral deviation of patella
- Tight of fibers seen or felt at superolateral patella

Evaluation for Overactivity
- Hip flexion during hip abduction (gluteus medius) test

Evaluation for Shortening
- Ober's test
- Resistance to adduction of thigh

Joint Dysfunction
- SI joint
- Patellofemoral joint

Corrective Action
- "Small/short foot" exercises
- Foot orthotics
- Facilitate and strengthen the gluteus medius
- Facilitate and strengthen the vastus medialis obliquus
- Foam roll

PIR Technique (Fig. 19.14)
Patient Position
- Side-lying involved side up
- Non-treated leg flexed at knee and hip
- Thigh adducted and extended until resistance is felt
Doctor Position
- Standing behind patient

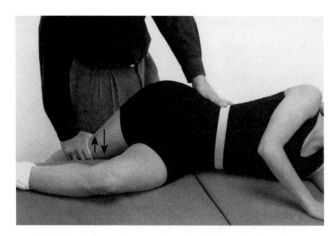

Figure 19.14 Tensor: fascia latae PIR.

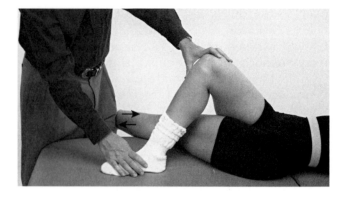

Figure 19.15 Tensor fascia latae PIR.

- Adducts patient's thigh with caudal hand above knee
- Cephalad hand stabilizes the pelvis
Patient's Active Effort
- Patient attempts to push thigh into flexion and abduction toward ceiling
- This effort is resisted by the doctor's caudal hand to keep the contraction as close to isometric as possible
Direction of Muscle Lengthening
- The doctor then takes out the slack into further adduction and extension without loss of pelvic neutral position
- In patients with patellofemoral syndrome, the patella should be stabilized medially while stretching the TFL.

Other PIR Methods The TFL can also be stretched with the patient supine (Fig. 19.15). This stretch will be felt in the quadratus lumborum (QL) if the TFL is not tight or if the low back is unstable.

Self-Stretches There is also a standing lateral pelvic shift technique that is often used before engaging in McKenzie extension exercises (see Chapter 15). A very effective way to loosen the TFL is by rolling on a foam roll (Fig. 19.16).

5. Piriformis
Referred Pain
- Posterior thigh, buttock and SI joint

Clinical Effects of Shortened Muscle
- SI disorders
- Entrapment neuropathy of sciatic nerve (pseudosciatica)

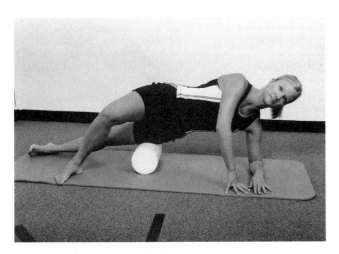

Figure 19.16 Tensor fascia latae foam roll mobilization.

Activation or Perpetuation

- Short leg
- Long drive with hip flexed and abducted
- Compensation for weak gluteus medius
- Balance or proprioceptive deficits, instability of ankle; turned out lower extremity position provides wider base of support

Observation

- Lower extremity/foot turned out in standing or supine position
- Pelvic rotation in standing

Trigger Point

- Muscle belly
- Muscular guarding elicited on light palpation over sciatic notch.

Evaluation for Overactivity

- Hip external rotation or pelvic rotation during hip abduction or gluteus medius test

Evaluation for Shortening

- Patient supine, flex hip less than 60 degrees, apply pressure through knee along the long axis of femur toward the hip, adduct the thigh fully then feel resistance to internal rotation of the hip

Joint Dysfunction

- L4/L5 and SI joint

Corrective Action

- Short foot exercises

- Improve seat or seated position
- Facilitate and strengthen gluteus medius
- Sensorimotor or balance training program as indicated
- Correct lower extremity instability

PIR Technique (Fig. 19.17)
Patient Position

- Supine
- Hip flexed approximately 45 degrees (maximum of 60 degrees)
- Knee flexed approximately 90 degrees

Doctor's Position

- Standing on involved side, facing patient
- Cephalad hand/forearm on patient's thigh supported by doctor's chest
- Cephalad hand pushes through knee along shaft of femur
- Doctor adducts patient's thigh
- Caudal hand grasps patient's calf or ankle/medial malleolus and produces internal rotation to barrier

Patient's Active Effort

- Patient pushes thigh outward into doctor's chest (abduction)
- Also pushes ankle inward in opposite direction, creating an external rotation force

Direction of Muscle Lengthening

- Once the patient has fully relaxed, the doctor adducts and internally rotates the patient's thigh to the new barrier

Other PIR Methods PIR can also be performed on the piriformis supine in adduction (Fig. 19.18A) in full flexion with the hip externally rotated (Fig. 19.18B)

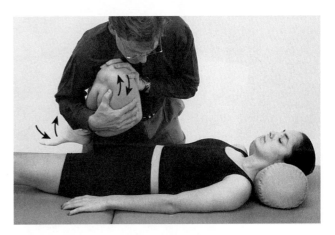

Figure 19.17 Piriformis PIR.

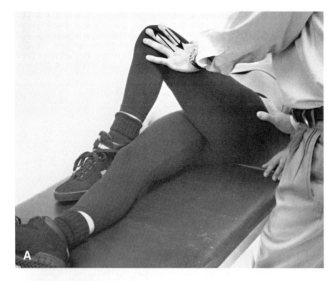

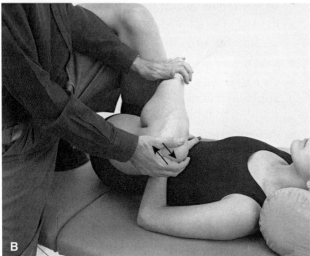

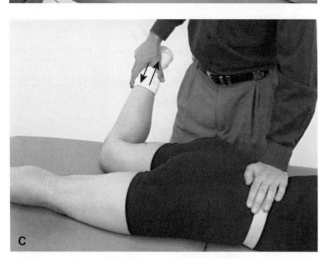

Figure 19.18 Piriformis.

or in the prone position (Fig. 19.18C) with the knee flexed 90 degrees.

Self-Stretches Self-stretches for the piriformis are possible in a variety of positions (Figs. 19.19A and 19.19B). Figure 19.20 shows a strong posterior hip capsule stretch that also addresses piriformis shortening (Figs. 19.20A to 19.20C).

6. Rectus Femoris/Quadriceps

The quadriceps as a group can be either weak or tight. The rectus femoris is prone to tightness and this is often mistaken for quadriceps tightness. Weak quadriceps typically lead to stoop rather than squat lifting technique and this creates lumbar overstress. Squats and lunges are the most functional exercises for training the quadriceps.

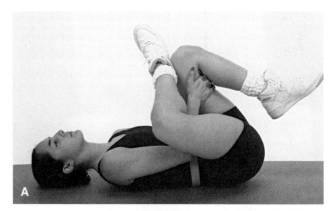

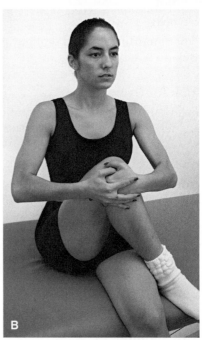

Figure 19.19 Piriformis self-stretches.

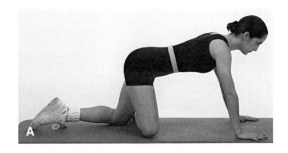

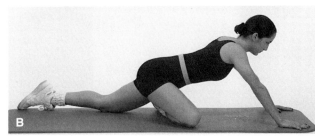

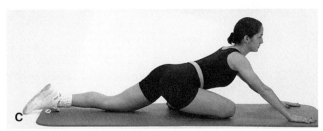

Figure 19.20 Posterior hip capsule and piriformis self-stretch.

PIR for the quadriceps can be easily performed in the prone position (Fig. 19.21).

Comment Care should be taken whenever stretching the quadriceps group that the femoral nerve tension tests are negative (see also Chapter 20).

7. Gluteus Maximus

Stretching this primary hip extensor is often not necessary. However, in very tight individuals it may be necessary. Susceptible individuals are those who perform repetitive forceful hip extension such as runners and swimmers. PIR for the gluteus maximus may be useful when the muscle houses trigger points; this is often the case in the patient with coccyx pain. The PIR technique is also a good way to facilitate this muscle for training with bridges and other strengthening exercises. Self-stretching is performed like the traditional Williams exercises or can be doctor assisted (Fig. 19.22).

8. Quadratus Lumborum (QL)

Referred Pain

- Lateral fibers refer to the iliac crest and lateral hip
- Medial fibers refer to the SI joint and deep in the buttock

Clinical Effects of Shortened Muscle

- Low back pain
- Posterior lower rib pain
- Perpetuation of SI disorders
- Abnormal hip hiking during gait
- Restriction of rib motion and respiratory dysfunction

Activation or Perpetuation

- Lifting with the trunk twisted
- Sustained side bending of trunk
- Sustained overload as in gardening or working in a stooped position
- Repeated trunk extension

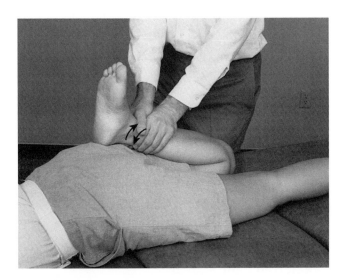

Figure 19.21 Quadriceps PIR.

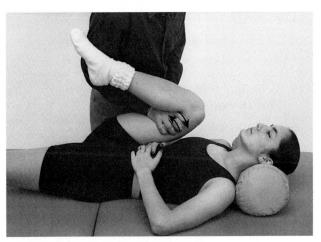

Figure 19.22 Gluteus maximus stretch.

Observation
- If unilateral, elevated ipsilateral ilium in standing
- If unilateral, ipsilateral lumbar side-bending in standing
- If unilateral, horizontal crease in flank
- If unilateral, appearance of floating ribs being pulled in
- If bilateral, increased lumbar lordosis

Trigger Points
- Beneath erector spinae muscle lateral to transverse processes
- Best palpated with patient side-lying

Periosteal Points
- Iliac crest and rib attachments

Evaluation for Overactivity
- During hip abduction testing in the side-lying position, monitor for early pelvic elevation

Evaluation for Shortening
- Screening test: Side-lying patient raises trunk up with hand or forearm under shoulder. Test is positive if the downside contour of the trunk does not form a smooth convexity from the sacrum to the lateral ribs (Fig. 11.15).

Joint Dysfunction
- T10-L1

Corrective Action
- Correct short leg
- Correct unlevel pelvis when sitting
- Facilitate or strengthen gluteus medius
- Teach proper lifting technique
- Avoid sustained or repetitive overuse

PIR Technique (Fig. 19.23)
Patient Position
- Side-lying, involved side down
- Pelvis tucked into posterior pelvic tilt with torso is slightly rotated backwards
- Hips and knees flexed 90 degrees with ankles crossed
Doctor Position
- At side of table facing patient
- Patient's knees resting on doctors caudal thigh

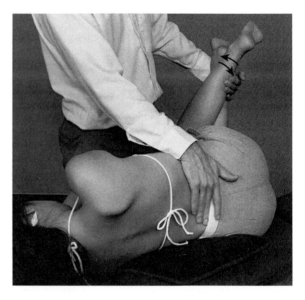

Figure 19.23 Quadratus lumborum PIR.

- Doctor grasps patient's ankles and raises them creating lumbar lateral flexion on the downside
- Cephalad hand free to palpate downside erector spinae muscles for contraction
Patient's Active Effort
- Patient pushes feet down towards floor
- After the patient has contracted for appropriate period he should be encouraged to "let go" or relax
Direction of Muscle Lengthening
- Ankles lifted, creating further lumbar lateral flexion as the muscle relaxes
- Degree of hip flexion and pelvic tucking may need to be modified to isolate the desired QL fibers during both contraction and stretch

Other PIR Methods A tight or tense QL can be relaxed or stretched in a variety of ways. Prone (Fig. 19.24A) and side-lying techniques are possible (Figs. 19.24B to 19.24D). Sometimes it is difficult to isolate the muscle with PIR, and active release techniques are thus a useful option.

Self-Stretches A standing self-stretch is shown in Figure 19.25.

9. Erector Spinae
Referred Pain
- SI joint, diffuse area in low back, buttock

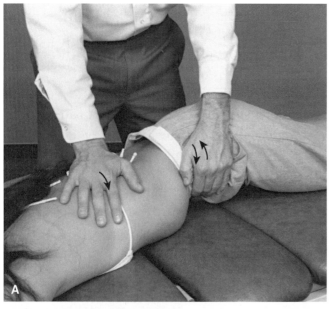

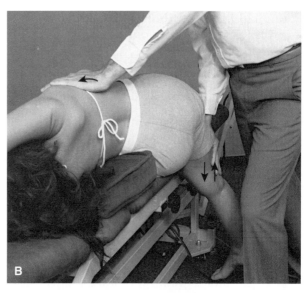

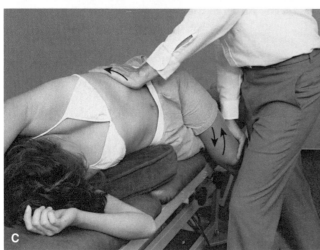

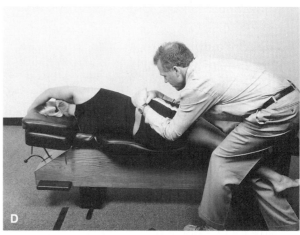

Figure 19.24 Quadratus lumborum PIR techniques.

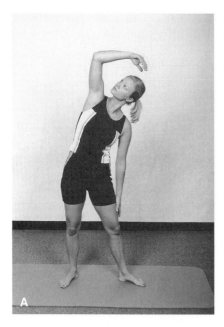

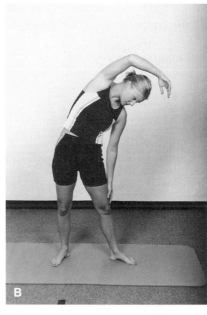

Figure 19.25 (A & B) Quadratus lumborum self-stretch.

Clinical Effect of Shortened Muscle

- Low back pain
- Inhibition of abdominals

Activation or Perpetuation

- Postural overstrain (sustained slumping or stooping)
- Sudden overload when lifting with back twisted or flexed
- Compensation for weak or inhibited gluteus maximus

Observation

- Increased lumbar lordosis
- Muscle hypertrophy at thoraco-lumbar junction

Trigger Point

- Any where in muscle belly

Periosteal Points

- Spinous processes of L4-S1

Evaluation for Overactivity

- During the hip hyperextension test, an early increase APT or lumbar lordosis signifies dynamic instability of the lumbar spine with overactivation of the erector spinae.

Evaluation for Shortening

- Failure of lumbar lordosis to reverse on fingertip to floor test or sit and reach test
- Fingertip to floor distance is not valid for lumbar flexibility because of effects of hip and pelvic motion, hamstring tension, and relative differences between arm, torso, and leg length

Joint Dysfunction

- Segment at corresponding level, especially L4/L5 and L5/S1

Corrective Action

- Strengthen abdominals
- Facilitate or strengthen gluteus maximus
- Teach neutral posture of lumbar spine and pelvis
- Teach proper lifting technique
- Strengthen quadriceps
- Lumbar support for chair

PIR Technique (Fig. 19.26)
Patient Position

- Side-lying, involved side up
- Down-side arm back and behind patient
- Upper torso is rotated forward with the up side arm hanging off table in front
- Down-side leg should be flexed at the hip and knee for stabilization
- Up-side hip is in slight extension so as to hang leg off back of table

Doctor Position

- Seated/standing in front of patient
- The doctor fixes pelvis at anterior superior iliac spine (ASIS) with one hand
- The other hand and forearm take a broad contact over upside lumbar muscles
- He then pushes the ASIS away and rotates the lumbar spine towards himself to take up the slack, engaging the barrier in the muscle.

Patient's Active Effort

- Patient is asked to turn his upper body back towards into the doctor's resistance while breathing in. The patient may also be instructed to look in direction they are turning.

Direction of Muscle Lengthening

- After contracting the patient is asked to relax and breath out naturally

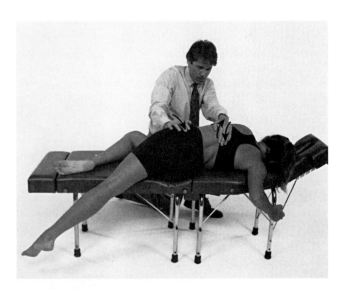

Figure 19.26 Erector spinae PIR.

• When the doctor feels the muscle has "let go," he then takes out the slack toward the new barrier

Other PIR Methods The erector spinae may also be stretched using a supine technique taught by Janda (Fig. 19.27) or a seated position (Fig. 19.28). In the latter case, care is taken to avoid uncoupled movements. If stretching in flexion, be sure to rotate and side bend to the same side. If stretching or mobilizing in a neutral or extended position, then place the patient in rotation and side bending to the opposite side.

Self-Stretches Self-stretches for the low back muscles are numerous (Figs. 19.29A–D). A simple self-PIR technique is also an excellent way for a patient to relax the low back (Fig. 19.30). It is pragmatic to have the patient explore which stretches are most comfortable and effective.

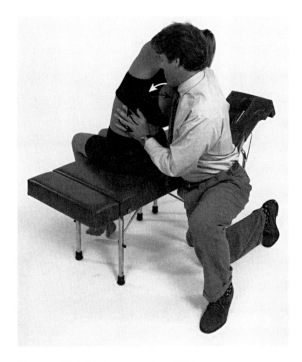

Figure 19.28 Erector spinae PIR.

Clinical Pearl

Stretching the lumbar spine into end-range flexion is contraindicated in patients with symptomatic disc problems. Such stretching should be reserved for healthy individuals after they are fully warmed-up. Also, such stretches should be avoided in the early morning of after prolonged sitting.

---

10. Lumbar Multifidi

PIR Technique (Fig. 19.31)
Patient Position
• Side-lying, involved side up
• Torso rotated backward
• Pelvis rotated forward
Doctor's Position
• At side of table in front of patient
• Cephalad forearm pushes shoulder backward
• Caudal hand and forearm rotate top side ilium forward
Patient's Active Effort
• Attempt is made to rotate torso forward while moving pelvis backwards
• This effort is resisted by the doctor to keep the contraction as close to isometric as possible.

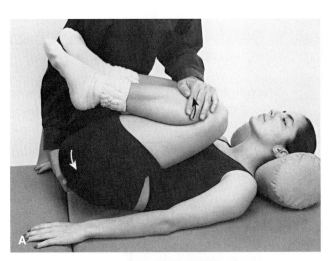

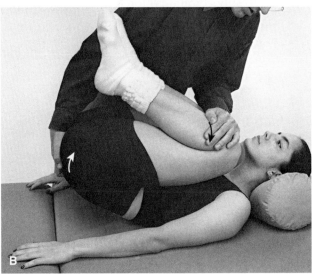

Figure 19.27 Erector spinae PIR after Janda.

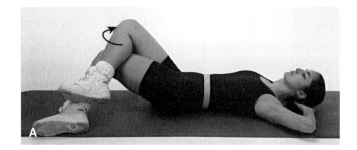

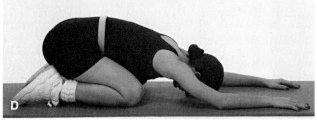

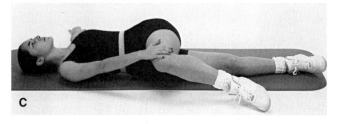

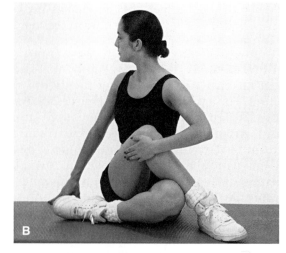

Figure 19.29 Erector spinae self-stretches.

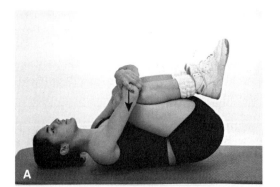

Direction of Muscle Lengthening

- Once the patient has relaxed fully the doctor may take the slack out toward the new barrier by pushing the shoulder backwards and pelvis forward

11. Posterior Cervical Muscles (Splenei, Semispinalis, Multifidi, Rotatores)

Referred Pain

- Up to suboccipital region
- Down to upper shoulder girdle
- Forehead

Figure 19.30 Erector spinae self-PIR.

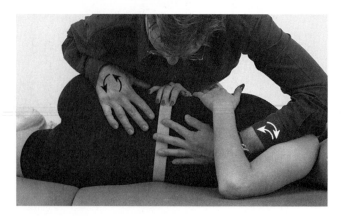

Figure 19.31 Multifidi PIR.

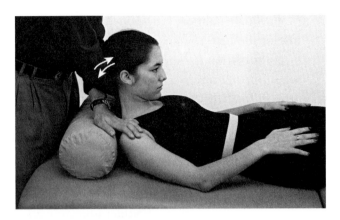

Figure 19.32 Semispinalis capitus PIR.

Clinical Result of Shortened Muscle

- "Short neck" or cervico-cranial hyperextension
- Cervical headaches
- Dizziness of cervical origin
- Cervical zygapophyseal joint disorders

Activation or Perpetuation

- Sustained neck flexion while reading and writing
- Forward-drawn or stooped posture
- Trauma (i.e., whiplash)

Trigger Points

- Occiput, suboccipital triangle to C4-C5
- Any where in muscle belly

Periosteal Points

- Transverse process of the atlas

Joint Dysfunction

- C0/C1 to mid-cervical

Corrective Action

- Train proper head on neck postural set (i.e., Alexander technique)
- Address forward weight-bearing posture (tight calves, hip flexors, and pectorals)
- Facilitate and strengthen gluteus maximus and deep neck flexors

PIR Technique
a) Semispinalis capitus (Fig. 19.32)
Patient Position

- Supine

Doctor's Position

- At the head of the table
- Patient's head may be supported by the doctor's crossed arms while the doctor's hands are placed on the patient's shoulders
- Bring head into forward flexion stopping as resistance is felt, or before if the patient perceives any stretching pain

Patient's Active Effort

- The patient will attempt to gently push the head back and breath in while the doctor offers a matching resistance
- After 5 to 10 seconds, the patient is instructed to "let go"

Stretch

- When the doctor perceives that the patient has fully relaxed, the patient is asked to take a deep breath in and out
- As the patient exhales and continues to relax, the doctor now takes up the slack in the muscle
- A new resting length should be achieved which is farther into forward flexion than before
- These steps can be repeated two or three additional times

b) Left Semispinalis Cervicis (Fig. 19.33)

Note this is an uncoupled movement for the cervical spine; therefore, if joint pain is provoked, lessen the side-bending component. Combine flexion with rotation and side-bending to the ipsilateral side. If there is provocation of joint pain, an adjustment should be performed first. Very gentle forces should be used in this technique (intermittent cold and stretch is an option).

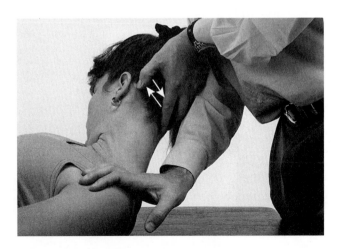

Figure 19.33 Semispinalis cervicus PIR (left).

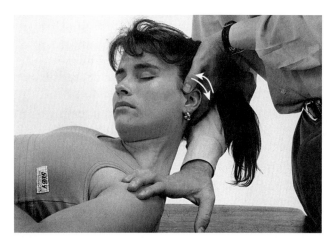

Figure 19.34 Splenius capitus/cervicus PIR (left).

c) Left Splenius Capitis/Cervicis (Fig. 19.34)

Combine flexion with rotation and side-bending to the contralateral side. Very gentle forces should be used in this technique.

d) Left Multifidi and Rotatores (Fig. 19.35)

First, full rotation then maximal flexion of the rotated head should be performed. Very gentle forces should be used in this technique.

12. Upper Trapezius

Referred Pain

- Along posterolateral neck to mastoid and temple

Clinical Effect of Shortened Muscle

- Headaches, especially temporal
- Neck pain
- Forward head posture and increased upper cervical extension
- Altered scapulo-humeral rhythm

Activation

- Occupational stress from sustained shoulder elevation
- Holding telephone between shoulder and ear
- Chair with armrests at wrong height or absent
- Desk, typewriter, or keyboard too high
- Compensation for weak lower fixators of the scapulae
- Habitual forward position of the shoulders
- Cervicothoracic kyphosis

- Inadequate support for heavy breasts
- Purse too heavy or shoulder strap too thin
- Compensation for short leg
- Shoulder elevation with respiration
- Emotional stress
- "Weight of the world on shoulders"
- Leg-length inequality

Observation

- Straightening/convexity of the neck–shoulder line contour ("Gothic" shoulder appearance).

Trigger Points

- Mid-belly, anterior edge, lateral

Evaluation for Overactivity

- Early elevation of shoulder girdle or excessive upper trapezius activity seen during shoulder abduction test

Evaluation for Shortening

- Laterally bend head away and rotate head toward side to be tested, with neck fully flexed
- Depress shoulder; positive finding is loss of resiliency

Joint Dysfunction

- Atlantooccipital
- Any other posterior cervical joint including the cervicothoracic junction

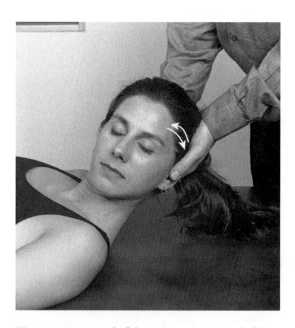

Figure 19.35 Multifidi and rotators PIR (left).

Corrective Actions

- Improve workstation ergonomics:
  - ○ Make sure elbows are properly supported by arm rests
  - ○ Correct desk, typewriter, and keyboard height
  - ○ Shoulders relaxed
  - ○ Elbows bent at 90 degrees
  - ○ Hands relaxed with wrist in "neutral position" on work surface
  - ○ Use of wrist rest at proper height
  - ○ Release tension using shoulder shrugs during "coffee breaks"
  - ○ Proper support bra with wider strap
  - ○ Smaller purse with wider strap over opposite shoulder
  - ○ Re-educate diaphragmatic breathing
  - ○ Facilitate and strengthen lower fixators of the scapulae

PIR Technique (Fig. 19.36)
  Patient Position

- Supine
- Head and neck are flexed, rotated toward and laterally flexed away from the side of stretch
- Arm on involved side is relaxed at the patient's side

  Doctor's Position

- Standing at head of table
- Crossed or uncrossed arm contact with one hand gently on the patient's shoulder and the other hand behind mastoid process
- "Wind-up" stretch by first taking out slack in full head and neck flexion, then gently in side bending away and rotation toward the involved side. Finally, take out the strongest slack in the direction of shoulder depression.

  Patient's Active Effort

- Attempt is made to bring shoulder into elevation toward the patient's ear ("shrug")
- This effort is resisted by the doctor so as to keep the contraction as close to isometric as possible
- A common error is for the patient to raise their shoulder up off the table rather than elevating it toward their ear

  Direction of Muscle Lengthening

- After the patient has contracted for appropriate period, he/she should be encouraged to "let go" or relax

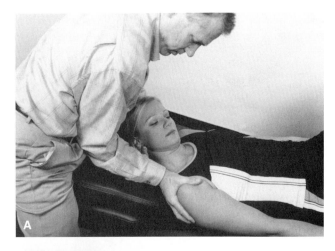

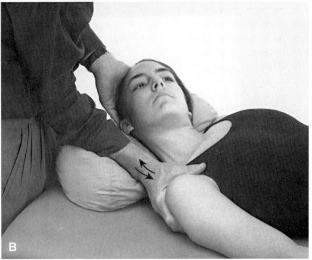

Figure 19.36 Upper trapezius PIR. **(A)** Correct. **(B)** Incorrect.

- After the muscle is felt to have relaxed, the doctor may take up the slack by depressing the shoulder as far as it will allow . . . or to the new barrier
- Some slack may also be taken out by increasing neck flexion, but no further slack should be taken out in the uncoupled side bending away and rotation toward the muscle

Self-Stretches An excellent self-stretch is shown in Fig. 19.37. Adding neck flexion to the barrier increases the specificity of this method. Self-PIR can easily be incorporated.

13. Levator Scapulae

Referred Pain

- Vertebral border of scapula
- Nape of the neck

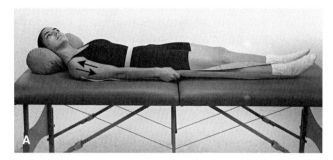

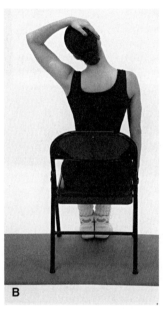

Figure 19.37 Upper trapezius self-stretches.

Clinical Effect of Shortened Muscle

- Pain on same side as patient turns head
- Torticollis
- Altered scapulo-humeral rhythm
- Limited upward rotation of the scapula

Activation

- Sustained neck rotation as in talking to someone sitting to the side
- Excessive telephone work
- Working over a desk with prolonged periods of neck flexion

Observation

- Slight bulge or double-wave appearance of neck–shoulder line appears above scapular insertion

Trigger Points

- Superior angle and medial border of scapula
- Push trapezius laterally to palpate full length of muscle

Periosteal Points

- Lateral surface of spinous process of C2

Evaluation for Shortening

- Laterally bend and rotate head away from tested side
- Apply gentle pressure to ipsilateral shoulder
- Positive test is lack of resiliency when pushing on shoulder

Joint Dysfunction

- C1/C2 and C2/C3
- Cervicothoracic junction

Corrective Actions

- Using a headset
- Rearranging computer monitor or reading material so that head does not need to be turned
- Facilitate and strengthen the lower fixators of the scapulae

PIR Technique (Fig. 19.38)
   Patient Position

- Same as for trapezius except that hand is turned palm up and anchored all the way under the back of the thigh and the neck is rotated away

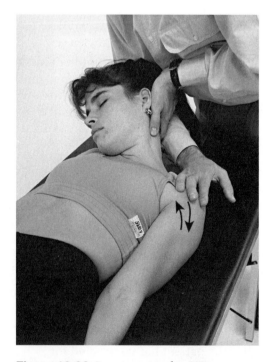

Figure 19.38 Levator scapulae PIR.

Doctor's Position

- At the head of the table on the side of involvement
- Arm closest to patient's head supports head while the hand contacts the patient's superior-medial border of the shoulder blade
- Outer arm crosses in front of the other arm so open hand can contact mastoid process
- Patient's neck is maximally flexed, then laterally flexed and rotated away from the involved side
- Take out all the slack in the direction of the shoulder depression and minimize forces on the head and neck

Patient's Active Effort

- Patient is instructed to gently try and elevate the shoulder blade
- This effort is resisted by the doctor so as to keep the contraction as close to isometric as possible

Direction of Muscle Lengthening

- Once the patient has fully relaxed, the doctor takes out the slack by increasing shoulder depression

Other PIR Methods PIR may also be used with resistance through the patient's elbow (Fig. 19.39).

Self-Stretches Self-stretches are shown without PIR (Fig. 19.40A) and with PIR (Figs. 19.40B and C).

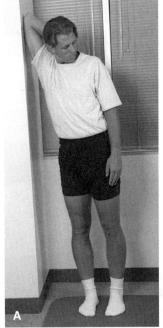
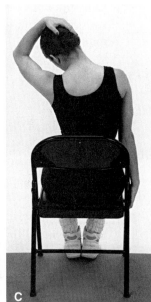
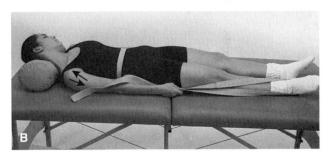

Figure 19.40 (A–C) Levator scapulae self-stretches.

14. Suboccipitals

Referred Pain

- Side of head, back of head, forehead, eyes

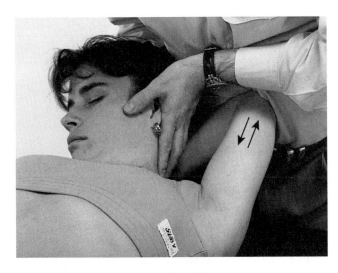

Figure 19.39 Levator scapulae PIR.

Clinical Effects of Shortened Muscle

- Occipital headache
- "Short neck"—cervico-cranial hyperextension

Activation

- Sustained flexion
- Maladjusted eyeglass frames
- Reading or writing
- Sustained extension
- Bicycle riding
- House painting
- Forward-drawn posture
- Weak deep neck flexors

Trigger Points

- Deep to trapezius and semispinalis capitus

Evaluation for Shortening

- Supine patient draws chin to chest
- Positive if gap of one or more finger's breadth remains

Joint Dysfunction

- C0/C1
- CT junction

Corrective Actions

- Improve forward-drawn posture
- Awareness training of "short neck" (i.e., Alexander technique)
- Book stand or writing wedge
- Computer monitor at correct height (center between mouth and nose)
- Strengthen weak deep neck flexors

PIR Technique

Patient Position

- Supine
- Chin slightly flexed to barrier

Doctor's Position

- At the head of the table
- One hand behind occiput, tractioning slightly
- Heel of other hand on forehead with fingers pointing toward chin

Patient's Active Effort

- Patient attempts to tilt head backwards patient is asked to look up toward forehead
- This effort is resisted by the doctor to keep the contraction as close to isometric as possible

Direction of Muscle Lengthening

- Once the patient has fully relaxed the doctor increases his traction force with his hand supporting the neck/occiput
- Then he takes out the slack into forward flexion using the heel of his hand on the forehead
- If the patients resist this forward flexion, you may ask the patients to actively tuck their chin in and then relax and they will have, in effect, inhibited the muscle in taking out the slack themselves and simultaneously use RI.

15. Sternocleidomastoid (SCM)

Referred Pain

- Over eye, frontal area, mastoid process, vertex, throat, temple

Clinical Effect of Shortened Muscle

- Headache (over eyes)
- Earache
- Decreased neck rotation

Activation

- Mechanical overload (excessive upper cervical extension)
  - Painting a ceiling
  - Watching a movie from the front row
  - Bicycle riding
- Sustained lower cervical flexion (overuse of checkrein/antigravity function)
- Sleeping on two pillows shortens SCM
- Postural stress (compensation to short leg)
- Uncorrected poor eyesight
- Forward head posture
- Weak deep neck flexors
- Shortened suboccipitals

Observation

- With shortening, the muscle belly is visibly prominent
- Head forward posture noted

Trigger Point

- Any where in muscle, particularly below mastoid process

Evaluation for Overactivity

1. Neck–head flexion should be tested in the supine position
2. The patient is asked to slowly raise the head into flexion in an arc-like fashion
3. Positive test would be if chin pokes during initiation of movement.

Joint Dysfunction

- C0-C1 and C2-C3

Corrective Actions

- Pillow should be tucked between shoulder and chin, NOT under shoulder
- Head-forward posture needs to be corrected (shortens SCM)
- Lumbar pillow may help to restore both lumbar and cervical curves
- Instruct patient in proper positioning of computer monitor

- Nearsightedness should be corrected
- Limit overhead work that overloads the check rein function of SCM
- Round-shouldered posture and increased thoracic kyphosis (tight pectoralis muscles) contributes to head-forward posture
- Strengthen weak deep neck flexors
- Stretch shortened suboccipitals

PIR Technique (Fig. 19.41)
Patient Position

- Supine
- Shoulders at head edge of table, so that the head is supported by the edge of the bench
- The head is rotated away from the involved side and the neck is allowed to extend slightly on the thorax, but the head is kept in slight flexion on the neck*.
- Hand is tucked under hip on treated side

Patient's Active Effort

- Patient attempts to raise head slightly, with minimal rotation (Fig. 19.41A)

Direction of Muscle Lengthening

- The doctor merely allows the neck to extend as far as it will on it's own while maintaining cervical rotation and upper cervical flexion. For the clavicular division, slack is also taken out into contralateral lateral flexion.
- Gravity is the only force that is required to take up the slack into extension (Fig. 19.41B)

Other PIR Methods and Self-Stretches If the cervical spine is irritable, the SCM may still be treated by pre-positioning in flexion and thus avoiding provocative extension positions (Fig. 19.42). These are ideal in office or self-treatment methods. This technique is often an excellent pre-thrust relaxation technique for a patient who "guards" excessively.

16. Scalenes

Referred Pain

- Pectoralis muscles, upper arm, radial forearm/hand, and rhomboids/medial scapula

Clinical Effects of Shortened Muscle

- Possible numbness or tingling in hands and/or fingers

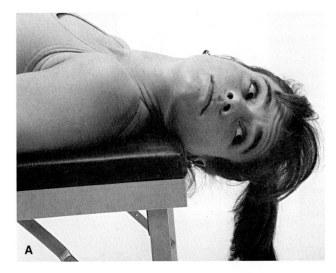

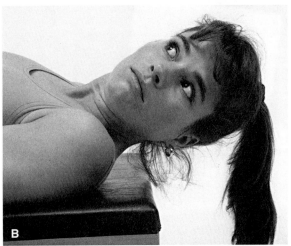

Figure 19.41 (A & B) Sternocleidomastoid PIR (self).

- DDx: ulnar distribution of dysthesia brachial plexus or subclavian vein radial distribution myofascial syndrome

Activation

- Forward-head posture
- Paradoxical breathing pattern and (excessive upper chest respiration) lifting of ribs/clavicle on inspiration
- Anxiety
- Tension in other elevators of shoulder girdle
- Holding the phone between shoulder and ear
- Excessive force used in repetion of lifting and pulling motions
- Leg-length inequality

---

*Contraindicated if any signs of vertebrobasilar insufficiency are noted.

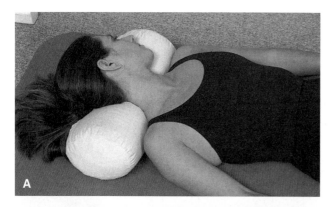

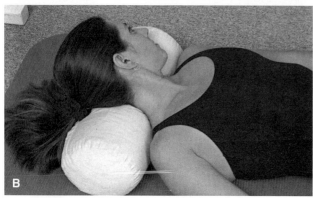

Figure 19.42 Sternocleidmastoid PIR.

Trigger Points

- Any where within anterior, medial, or posterior divisions of muscle
- Palpate and treat the scalenes with caution because of proximity of extremely sensitive neurovascular tissue

Joint Dysfunction

- Flexion fixations of cervical spine (anterior cervicals)
- First rib blockage

Corrective Actions

- Retrain diaphragmatic breathing pattern and lateral rib "bucket handle" motion
- Stress management

PIR Technique (Fig. 19.43)
Patient Position

- Supine, head and neck laterally bent to opposite side and slightly extended
- For anterior fibers, rotate head and neck to involved side

- Medial fibers no rotation
- Posterior fibers require the head to be rotated away

Doctor Position

- At the head of table
- Anterior fibers are isolated with heel of one hand on the upper ribs medially and the other hand just anterior to the mastoid process.
- Medial fibers require the heel of one hand on the upper ribs and the other hand on mastoid process.
- Posterior fibers require the heel of one hand on the upper ribs laterally and the other hand just posterior to the mastoid process (rib stabilizations not shown to assist in photographic clarity)

Patient Effort

- Patient attempts to side-bend back toward midline.

Direction of Muscle Lengthening

- Slack is taken out into greater contralateral lateral flexion and extension
- Rotation varies with targeted fibers as described

Concern If the neck is hypersensitive or any vertebrobasilar symptoms are present, this technique is contraindicated. Joint mobilization/manipulation may be necessary before using this method to ensure that the joints are not compressing, especially with respect to the scalene anticus stretch (Fig. 19.43A).

Other PIR Methods An alternative way to address scalene dysfunction is by pre-positioning the patient's neck in a stretch position and then stabilizing over the origin of the muscle over the anterior chest. Resistance to inspiration can be sufficient to achieve post-contraction inhibition. Slack can even be taken out with the hand over the anterior chest or clavicle to lengthen the shortened muscle. Rib stabilization may also be assisted by having the patient tuck the hand on the treated side under the ipsilateral hip.

Self-Stretches Self-treatment is easy and safe especially if extension is minimized (Fig. 19.44). Figure 19.45 shows a side-lying technique for performing self-PIR with gravity resistance.

17. Pectoralis Major

Referred Pain

- Anterior chest, breast, inner arm, and forearm

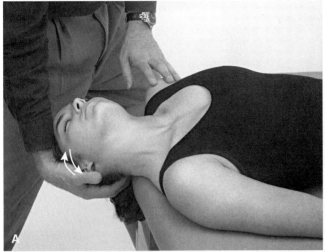

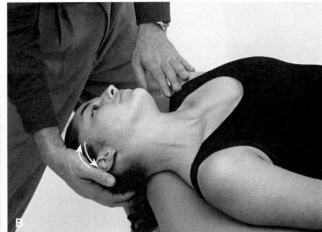

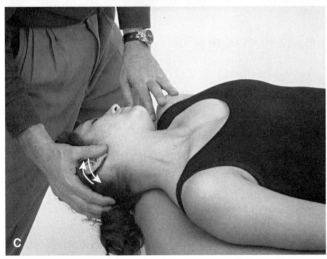

Figure 19.43 Scalene PIR. **(A)** Scalenus anterior. **(B)** Scalenus medius. **(C)** Scalenus posterior.

Clinical Effect of Shortened Muscle

- Cardiac ischemia-like pain
- Breast hypersensitivity
- Anterior humeral position can promote shoulder impingement syndrome

Activation

- Round-shouldered, kyphotic/slouched, head-forward posture

Observation

- Round shoulders
- Increased thoracic kyphosis
- Arms internally rotated
- Scapula abducted and protracted

Trigger Points

- Anywhere in muscle belly

Periosteal Points

- At rib attachments

Evaluation for Shortening

- Arm abducted 90 degrees and externally rotated
- Same with 100 to 120 degrees of abduction

Joint Dysfunction

- Upper ribs
- Glenohumeral joint

Corrective Actions

- Improve forward weight-bearing posture
- Facilitate and strengthen the lower scapular fixators, i.e., the middle and lower trapezeii and serratus anterior

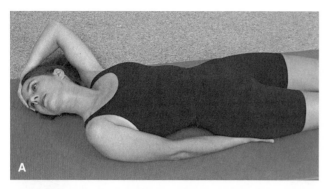

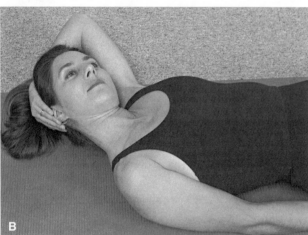

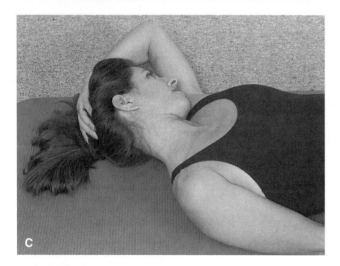

Figure 19.44 (A–C) Scalene self-stretch.

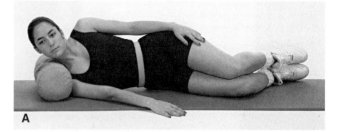

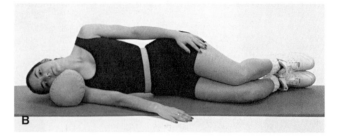

Figure 19.45 (A, B) Scalene self-PIR.

PIR Technique (Fig. 19.46)
Patient Position

- Supine
- Arm abducted 90 degrees and externally rotated

Doctor's Position

- At side of table on involved side
- One hand contacts the sternum or opposite clavicle
- Other hand grasps upper arm

Patient's Active Effort

- Attempt is made to raise arm
- This effort is resisted by the doctor to keep the contraction as close to isometric as possible

Direction of Muscle Lengthening

- Once patient has relaxed fully, the doctor may retract shoulder to new barrier
- It is important to stabilize the muscle insertion over the ribs firmly while taking up the slack to avoid torsion of the trunk and rib elevation

Concern If brachial plexus symptoms are encountered, PIR may be performed without stretch. The doctor should use good clinical judgement in application of these techniques; they may be contraindicated or warrant cautionary application in patients with a history of anterior shoulder instability.

Self-Stretches Self-stretching is very easy with the doorway or corner stretches. These stretches are most effective if the patient is instructed to maintain support of the body weight on the feet rather than hanging the body weight through the arms onto the door, which activates the pectoralis. Self-PIR or stretching may be performed as well with the patient lying supine on the mattress with the shoulder at the edge of the mattress and the arm hanging off the edge. For the more acute patient, or the patient requiring more stability, this same technique can be performed with the patient lying on the floor. The patient alternately lifts the arm slightly from the floor and relaxes it back to the floor. Where desired, this method allows for

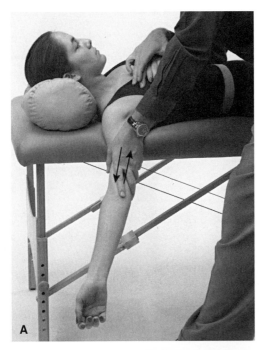

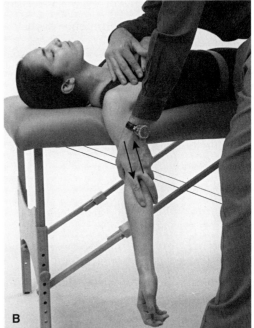

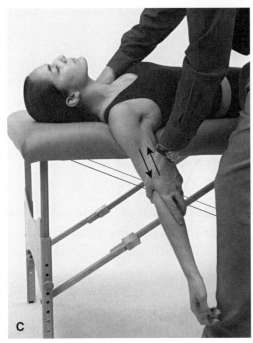

Figure 19.46 (A–C) Pectoralis major PIR.

decrease of tension and trigger points in the muscle without increase in length and mobility.

18. Pectoralis Minor

Clinical details are similar to those for pectoralis major. Application of PIR can cause nerve entrapment symptoms related to thoracic outlet syndrome.

Clinical Effects of Shortened Muscle

- Periosteal rib pain
- Thoracic outlet syndrome

Activation

- Sustained shoulder protraction
- Poor pattern of scapular depression.

Observation

- Scapular protraction with prominence of the inferior angle of the scapula.

PIR Technique (Fig. 19.47)

Patient Position

- Supine
- Arm abducted 80 degrees and externally rotated
- Hand hanging lower than shoulder

Doctor's Position

- Near head of table on involved side
- Cephalad hand contacts glenohumeral joint
- Caudal hand grasps arm

Patient's Active Effort

- Attempt is made to protract the shoulder by raising shoulder to ceiling while keeping hand lower than shoulder
- This effort is resisted by the doctor so as to keep the contraction as close to isometric as possible

Direction of Muscle Lengthening

- Once patient has relaxed fully, the doctor may take up the slack toward the new barrier by pushing the shoulder away from the clavicle and cephalad. The same cautions apply as to PIR for the pectoralis major. Ribs should be stabilized.

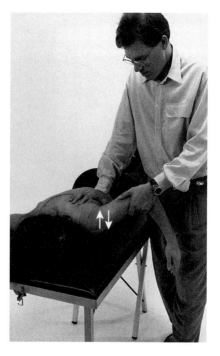

Figure 19.48 Pectoralis minor PIR.

Other PIR Methods A prone modification is shown in Figure 19.48.

19. Supraspinatus

Referred Pain

- Deltoid region, lateral upper arm, and elbow

Clinical Result of Shortened Muscle

- Painful abduction (painful arc)
- Difficulty reaching above shoulder
- Rotator cuff disorders (i.e., impingement syndrome) often result from tightness of the external rotators (infraspinatus, teres minor and supraspinatus)

Activating Factors

- Overhead work (i.e., weight lifting, throwing, swimming, etc.)
- Poor scapulo-humeral rhythm

Trigger Points

- In supraspinatus fossa deep to trapezius

Corrective Actions

- Avoidance of overhead work
- Cross-fiber massage
- Improve scapulo-humeral rhythm

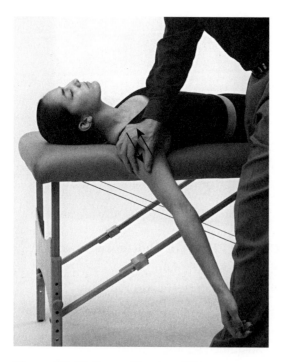

Figure 19.47 Pectoralis minor PIR.

PIR Technique

Patient Position

- Prone

Doctor Position

- Standing at the same side of the table as the involved shoulder
- The arm should be extended behind the patient
- With the elbow flexed 90 degrees, the upper arm should be adducted as far as it will comfortably go
- Place one hand against the upper arm and the other hand should grasp the patients wrist

Patient's Active Effort

- The patient is asked to gently push their upper arm out into abduction
- This is resisted isometrically
- The patient should follow the normal procedure for respiratory synkinesis to enhance the effects of treatment

Direction of Muscle Lengthening

- As the patient relaxes, the doctor should take up the slack into adduction

20. Infraspinatus

Referred Pain

- Anterior deltoid, shoulder, down the lateral forearm, and hand

Clinical Effects of Shortened Muscle

- Pain when sleeping on either side
- Difficulty reaching behind back to unhook bra
- Difficulty reaching back pocket for wallet
- Rotator cuff disorders (i.e., impingement syndrome) often result from tightness of the external rotators (infraspinatus, teres minor, and supraspinatus)

Activation

- Neglected shoulder overuse syndrome
- Altered scapulo-humeral rhythm
- Tight shoulder internal rotators

Trigger Points

- Infraspinatus fossa

Corrective Actions

- Sleep with involved side up and pillow under involved arm
- Improve scapulo-humeral rhythm

PIR Technique (Fig. 19.49)

Patient Position

- Supine
- The involved shoulder and upper arm should be supported by the table
- The arm is abducted and the elbow flexed 90 degrees

Doctor Position

- Abduct the arm and flex the elbow to 90 degrees
- Then allow the forearm to fall into as much internal rotation (forearm toward thigh) as gravity will take it
- Monitor that the shoulder does not begin to lift off the table; if necessary, stabilize the scapula into retraction with pressure on the anterior acromion

Patient's Active Effort

- With one hand on the arm above the elbow and the other hand on the dorsal aspect of the forearm, ask the patient to gently push the forearm up or backwards toward external rotation
- This should be isometrically resisted, again monitoring that the shoulder does not rise off the table

Direction of Muscle Lengthening

- When the patient has fully relaxed, take up the slack toward the new barrier into internal rotation while maintaining scapular stabilization

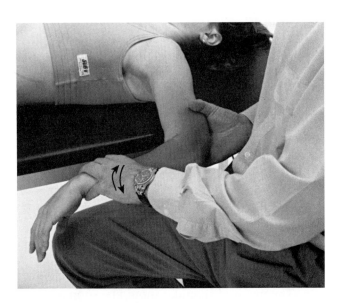

Figure 19.49 Infraspinatus PIR.

Concern Although this method is very simple to perform, care should be taken if the shoulder joint is hypersensitive.

Other PIR Methods An alternative method that reduces strain on the shoulder joint is accomplished with arm brought into full internal rotation and adduction across the front of the chest. To prevent subacromial impingement from occurring, strong traction is applied to the shoulder joint. This technique allows for the contraction and stretch to be felt at scapular attachment rather than the shoulder attachment of the infraspinatus.

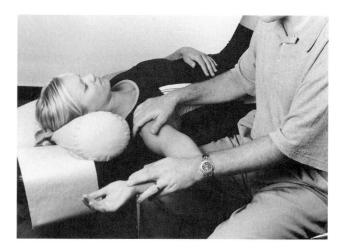

Figure 19.50 Subscapularis PIR.

21. Subscapularis

Referred Pain

- Posterior deltoid and posterior arm

Clinical Effects of Shortened Muscle

- Difficulty reaching back as in throwing
- Involved in "frozen shoulder"
- Promotes subacromial impingement and rotator cuff syndromes

Activation

- Shoulder overuse syndrome
- Lack of variety of motion in shoulder area
- Forward-drawn posture, especially tight pectorals

Trigger Points

- Ventral scapula
  #### Joint Dysfunction
- Glenohumeral joint
  #### Corrective Actions
- When lying on involved side, place pillow between arm and chest to maintain abduction
- When lying on uninvolved side, place pillow in front to prevent excessive abduction
- Improve scapulo-humeral rhythm
- Stretch pectoralis major, latissimus dorsi, teres major if tight

PIR Technique (Fig. 19.50)
Patient Position

- The patient should lie supine
- The involved shoulder should be supported by the table

Doctor Position

- On the same side of table as the patient's involved shoulder
- Abduct the arm and flex the elbow to 90 degrees
- Allow the forearm to fall into as much external rotation (forearm towards head) as gravity will take it
- Stabilize the humeral head posteriorly and monitor that the shoulder does not lift off the table

Patient's Active Effort

- With one hand on the arm above the elbow and the other hand on the ventral aspect of the forearm, ask the patient to gently push their forearm up or forward toward internal rotation
- This should be isometrically resisted, again monitoring that the shoulder does not significantly rise from the table

Direction of Muscle Lengthening

- When the patient has fully relaxed, take up the slack towards the new barrier into external rotation

Concern This technique is contraindicated if anterior instability is present. It also will be extremely pain provocative if a "frozen shoulder" is the problem. In either case the functional range for PIR may be limited to less than 90 degrees of shoulder abduction.

22. Gastrocnemius

Referred Pain

- Calf, posterior knee, and instep

Clinical Result of Shortened Muscle

- Forward weight-bearing posture
- Achilles tendinitis
- Plantar fasciitis

Activation

- Seat height too high
- High heels
- Too much driving (pushing on the accelerator)

Trigger Points

- Medial and lateral borders of muscle

Evaluation for Shortening

- With the patient supine dorsiflex the ankle without allowing the knee to bend. Should have 10 degrees of dorsiflexion. Check resting position of calcaneus as well as resistance to calcaneal inversion and eversion. Check palpatory tenderness of medial and lateral Achilles tendon.

PIR Technique (Fig. 19.51)
Patient Position

- The patient should lie supine with legs extended.

Doctor Position

- Standing at end of table and grasps heel of patient's foot with hand
- Passively dorsiflexes the patient's foot by leaning cephalad
- The patient's knee should not be allowed to flex

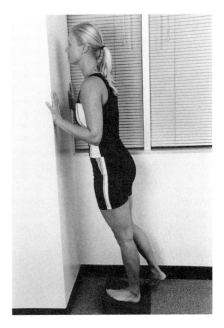

Figure 19.52 Gastrocnemius self-stretch.

Resisted Effort

- The patient attempts to plantarflex his/her foot (not toes)
- This should be isometrically resisted

Direction of Muscle Lengthening

- When the patient has fully relaxed, take up the slack toward the new barrier in ankle dorsiflexion.

Self-Stretches Self-stretching the gastrocnemius is best performed with the standing wall lean on a wedge (Fig. 19.52). It is essential that the knee is extended and the heel not rise up; weight should be felt on the heel throughout the stretch.

23. Soleus

Referred Pain

- Heel, posterior calf

Clinical Result of Shortened Muscle

- Forward weight-bearing posture
- Difficulty squatting

Observation

- Muscle hypertrophy in lower medial calf

Activation

- High heels

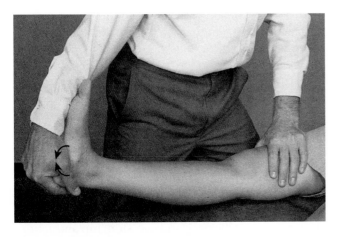

Figure 19.51 Gastrocnemius PIR.

- Excessive running
- Ankle instability; chronic ankle sprains

Trigger Points

- Superior and inferior muscle belly

Evaluation for Shortening

- Prone with knee bent 90 degrees; dorsiflex the ankle. Should have 20 degrees of dorsiflexion

PIR Technique (Fig. 19.53)
   Patient Position

- The patient should lie prone.
   Doctor Position

- Standing at the side of the table with the patient's knee in 90 degrees of flexion.
- Passively dorsiflex the patient's foot by pulling up on the heel while pushing down on the metatarsals.
   Resisted Effort

- The patient attempts to plantarflex his/her foot (not toes)
- This should be isometrically resisted
   Direction of Muscle Lengthening

- When the patient has fully relaxed, take up the slack towards the new barrier in ankle dorsiflexion.

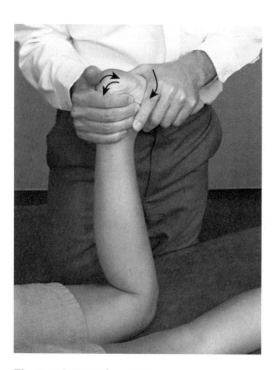

Figure 19.53 Soleus PIR.

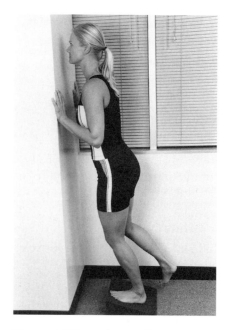

Figure 19.54 Soleus self-stretch.

Self-Stretch Self-stretch is accomplished as for the gastrocnemius except that the knee is flexed (Fig. 19.54).

Inhibition of Tonic Muscle Chains

Flexors, pronators, adductors, and internal rotator muscles of the upper and lower extremites are commonly found to be tense and/or shortened. Brügger proposed a sequenced treatment of key antagonist muscles as an inhibition of an entire chain of postural muscle hypertonia (see Chapter 16).

The treatment involves resistance of strong (40% to 80% of maximum effort) eccentric (lengthening) contractions of key inhibited antagonists. This is indicated when you want to release tension in multiple muscles simultaneously.

In the upper quarter, **eccentricly resist** finger and thumb abduction; wrist and finger extension and thumb abduction; forearm supination; shoulder external rotation; and shoulder abduction with external rotation. The resistance to shoulder abduction and external rotation is nearly identical to the final position of the PNF D2 upper extremity flexion, the "drawing a sword" position (Fig. 19.55).

In the lower quarter, **eccentricly resist** toe extension, ankle dorsiflexion, and eversion; hip abduction; and hip external rotation (Fig. 19.56).

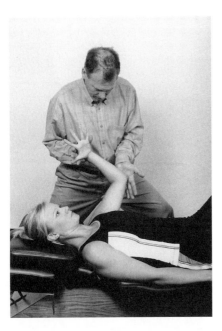

Figure 19.55 Brügger upper-quarter eccentric MRT.

PIR Joint Mobilization Procedures

1. Hip Joint Traction (Fig. 19.57)

Patient Position

- The patient should lie supine
- Involved leg is flexed at the knee and draped over the seated doctor's shoulder

Doctor Position

- Seated at the same side of the table as the involved hip, facing the patient
- Patient's leg is draped over the doctor's shoulder
- Contact is made over the patient's anterior hip with both hands and pulls arterior to

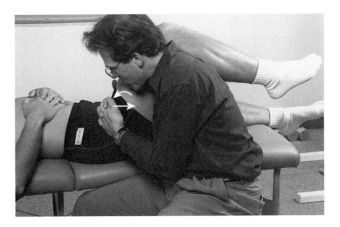

Figure 19.57 Hip joint traction PIR mobilization.

posterior to take out all available slack in posterior glide and hip traction

Resisted Effort

- The patient is instructed to pull his/her thigh towards their abdomen
- This should be isometrically resisted by the doctor
- The patient and doctor should be able to feel a contraction occurring in the anterior hip region

Direction of Mobilization

- Once the patient has fully relaxed, the doctor may take up the slack by increasing posterior glide to its new end point

2. Lumbar Spine Extension Mobilization (Fig. 19.58)

Patient Position

- The patient should be side-lying with their hips and knees flexed

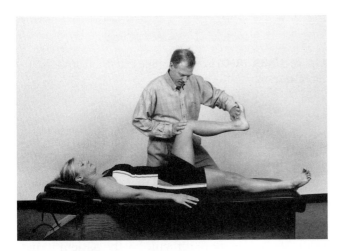

Figure 19.56 Brügger lower-quarter eccentric MRT.

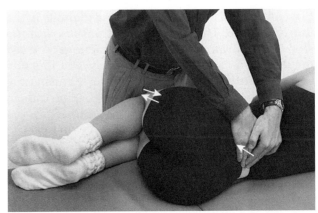

Figure 19.58 Lumbar spine extension PIR mobilization.

- Patient's knees protrude slightly over side of table
  Doctor Position
- Facing the patient
- Places fingers over adjacent lumbar spinous processes (one hand over the other)
- Patient's knees in contact with doctor's anterior thigh
- Doctor must take out all the slack in lumbar extension by pushing with his/her thigh into the patient's knees while stabilizing the vertebral segment above
  Resisted Effort
- The patient attempts to push knees into the doctor's thigh
- The patient's spine should be felt to kyphose or flex slightly
  Direction of Mobilization
- Once the patient has fully relaxed, the doctor feels an increase in segmental spinal extension via posterior movement of the inferior spinous process.
- The doctor maintains fixation of the superior segment while pushing with his/her thigh posteriorly against the patient's knees to the new barrier.

Self-Treatment Self-treatment of the lumbar spine into extension can be accomplished by performing the McKenzie prone on elbows, prone press-up, and standing extension exercises (Figs. 19.59A–C). Alternatively, if these are uncomfortable, the back extension stretch on the exercise ball is a very effective extension mobilization self-treatment (Fig. 19.60).

3. Thoracic Spine Extension Mobilization (Fig. 19.61)

PIR can be used to improve extension mobility in the thoracic spine. The seated patient pushes with the elbows downwards against the practioner's resistance. This is followed by mobilizing the thoracic spine into extension by simultaneously raising the patient's elbows while pressing into the spine with an opposing hand.

Self-Treatment The thoracic region can easily become kyphotic. Simple stretches to increase extension mobility should be prescribed. The sphinx on hands (Fig. 19.62) is performed like a cat–camel with the emphasis on the extension phase. Once the patient is feeling this in the mid-back, then the position should be held and fine-tuned. C0-C1 centration by

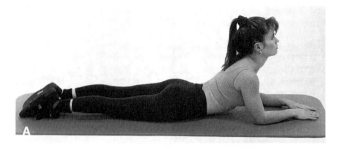
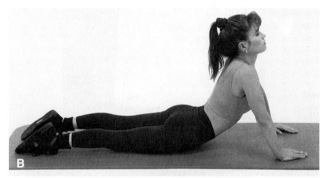
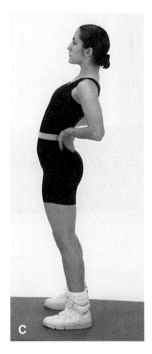

Figure 19.59 (A–C) Lumbar spine extension auto-mobilization.

nodding the head as if saying yes is a key. The scapulae should be cued to slide caudally. Active exhalation will facilitate the abdominal wall and prevent excessive lumbar lordosis so that the extension can be focused in the mid-dorsal region.

The sphinx on forearms is performed like the sphinx on hands (Fig. 19.63). Less range of motion is available so it is more difficult for the patient to perceive and isolate the motion.

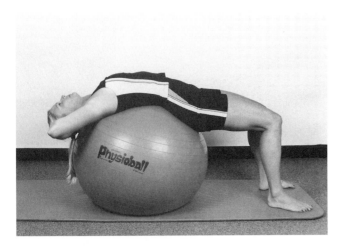

Figure 19.60 Back extension on the ball.

The upper back cat (Fig. 19.64) can be performed with a low chair or small gym ball. The key is to focus on the extension phase and find a comfortable/relaxed arm position where the stretch is felt in the mid-back, not in the shoulder joint.

The foam roll is an excellent tool for mobilizing the mid-back. It can be used in a variety of ways with the emphasis on increasing dorsal extension (Figs. 19.65 to 19.67).

4. Rib Mobilization

PIR can be used to help mobilize an upper costo-transverse joint. The technique requires the doctor to

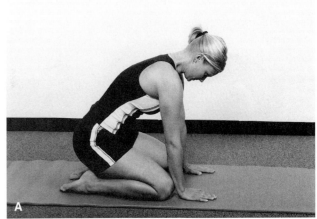
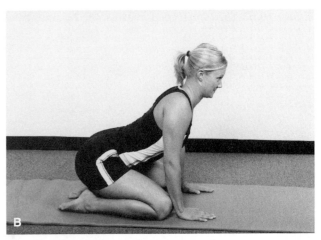

Figure 19.62 Yoga sphinx on hands. **(A)** Beginning position. **(B)** Final position.

contact the dysfunctional joint and reach the barrier in extension by raising the ipsilateral elbow. The patient is instructed to push the elbow downward, and after this is resisted and the patient relaxes, the joint may be mobilized (Fig. 19.68).

Facilitation Techniques

1. Lower Fixators of the Scapulae (Lower and Middle Trapezius)/Scapulo-Thoracic Facilitation (Fig. 19.69)

Patient Position
- The patient should be side-lying
- Involved side up

Doctor Position
- Seated or standing behind the patient
- Doctor places thumb or finger contact at inferior-medial border of the scapula

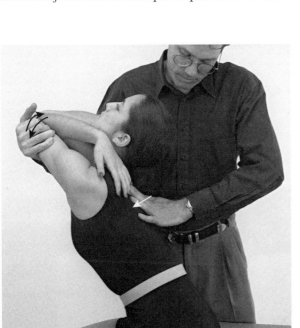

Figure 19.61 Thoracic spine extension PIR mobilization.

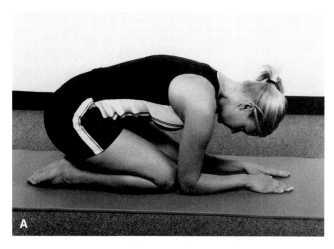
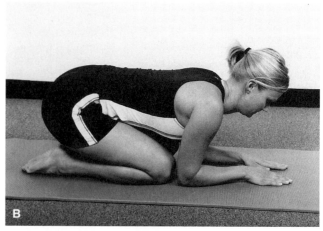

Figure 19.63 Yoga sphinx on forearms. **(A)** Beginning position. **(B)** Final position.

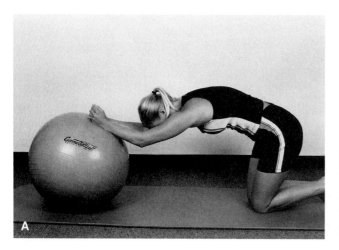
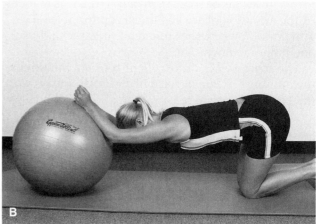

Figure 19.64 Upper back cat on the ball. **(A)** Beginning position. **(B)** Final position.

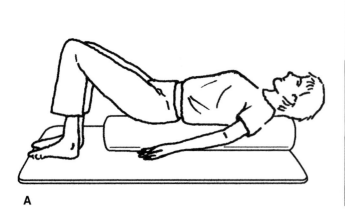
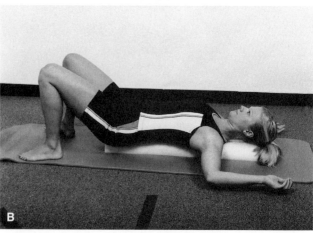

Figure 19.65 Foam roll—vertical. **(A)** Start position. **(B)** Progression.
(A) Reproduced with permission from gymballstore.com, "Improve your Posture" article.

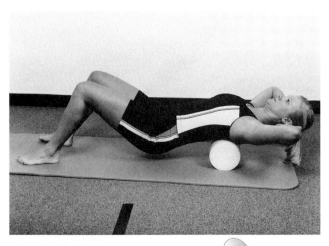

Figure 19.66 Foam roll—horizontal.

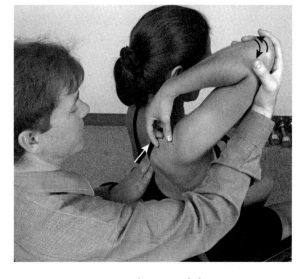

Figure 19.68 Upper rib PIR mobilization.

Patient's Active Effort

- The patient is instructed to pull the shoulder blade back toward the spine while avoiding any tendency to shrug or extend the shoulder
- This should be isometrically resisted at the inferior-medial border of the scapulae (or posterior shoulder)
- The patient may isometrically hold the adducted and depressed (back and down) position of the scapulae and perform the following:

- ○ Shoulder adduction/abduction
- ○ Shoulder flexion/extension

2. Middle Trapezius (Fig. 19.70)

Patient Position
- The patient should lie prone

Doctor Position
- Standing at side of table

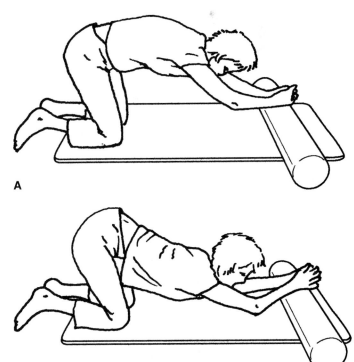

Figure 19.67 Foam roll—prayer. **(A)** Start position. **(B)** Final stretch position. Reproduced with permission from gymball-store.com, "Improve your Posture" article.

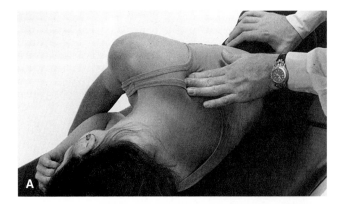

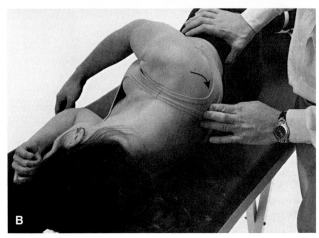

Figure 19.69 Scapulo-thoracic facilitation.

Patient's Active Effort
- Resistance may be applied to the inferior-medial border of the scapulae

3. Gluteus Medius Facilitation—Sister Kenny Method (Fig. 19.71)

Patient Position
- The patient should be side-lying with the lower hip and knee flexed

Doctor Position
- Standing behind the patient
- Contacts the gluteus medius insertion at the greater trochanter
- The doctor grasps the patient's leg under the flexed knee

Facilitation
- Rapid mobilization into abduction while applying "goading" stimulation to tendinous insertion
- Each mobilization should incrementally increase the range into hip abduction (may be

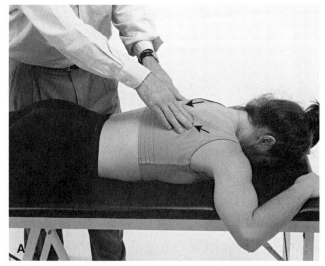

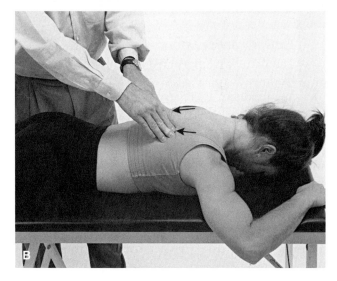

Figure 19.70 Middle trapezius facilitation exercise.

performed in a fast, ratchety manner four to eight times). Increased lumbar lordosis is to be avoided.
- After the mobilization is performed, the leg is placed into abduction, internal rotation, and slight extension, and the patient is requested to hold their leg up as the doctor suddenly lets the leg drop
- The muscle should be seen to quickly contract so that the leg does not drop

■ CONCLUSION

MRTs are invaluable tools when soft tissue lesions are considered primary or significant in the patient's functional pathology. In cases with marked guarding, MRTs will relax the patient and inhibit muscle tension,

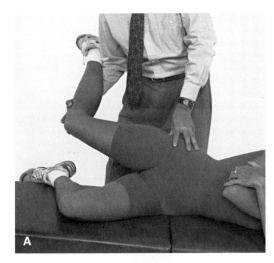

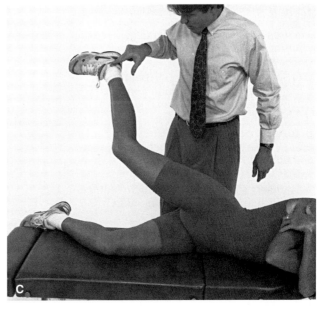

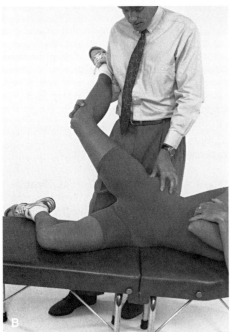

Figure 19.71 Gluteus medius facilitation.

thereby making joint mobilizations/manipulation easier to perform and longer lasting.

Generally, tense muscles should be relaxed and shortened myofascial tissue stretched as part of a rehabilitation program. Therefore, MRTs should be used alongside stabilization and functional training exercises.

MRTs are simple and allow patients to learn self-treatment. This enhances the doctor–patient relationship, encouraging the patients to become more actively involved in their own health care. Skilled and informed patients will be better able to manage minor aggravations of their symptoms on their own. This does not replace manual therapy, but in an era of diminishing third party reimbursement self-treatment becomes increasingly valuable.

Audit Process
Self-Check of the Chapter's Learning Objectives

- What are the different methods of muscle relaxation?

- What is the role of reciprocal inhibition and post-isometric inhibition in muscle relaxation?

- Is there a set duration for the length of isometric contraction in a muscle being relaxed?

- Is there a set duration for the length of time waiting for a release phenomena?

- Can you prescribe self-stretches for the most common muscles that tend to tightness?

■ REFERENCES

1. Biering-Sorensen F. Physical measurements as risk indicators for low-back trouble over a one-year period. Spine 1984;9:106–119.

2. Cibulka MT, Sinacore DR, Cromer GS, Delitto A. Unilateral hip rotation range of motion asymmetry in patients with sacroiliac joint regional pain. Spine 1998;23:1009–1015.

3. Ellison JB, Rose SJ, Sahrmann SA. Patterns of rotation range of motion: A comparison between healthy subjects and patients with low back pain. Phys Ther 1990;70:537–541.

4. Evjenth O, Hamberg J. Muscle Stretching in Manual Therapy: A Clinical Manual, Vol. 1. Alfta: Alfta Rehab, 1984.

5. Gaymans F, Lewit K. Mobilization techniques using pressure (pull) and muscular facilitation and inhibition. In Lewit K, Gutmann G, eds. Functional pathology of the motor system, Rehabilitacia supplementum, 10-11. Bratislava: Obzor, 1975:47–51.

6. Green J, Grenier S, McGill SM. Low back stiffness is altered with warmup and bench rest: Implications for athletes. Med Sci Sports Exerc 2002;34:1076–1081.

7. Guissard N, Duchateau J, Hainaut K. Muscle stretching and motoneuron excitability. Eur J Appl Physiol 1988;58:47–52.

8. Hagbarth KE, Hagglund JV, Nordin M, et al. Thixotrophic behavior of human finger flexor muscles with accompanying changes in spindel and reflex responses to stretch. J Physiol (Lond) 1985;368:323.

9. Hagbarth KE. Evaluation of and methods to change muscle tone. Scand J Rehabil Med Supple 1994;30:19.

10. Hutton RS. Neuromuscular basis of stretching exercises. In: Comi P, ed. Strength and Power in Sport: The Encyclopedia of Sports Medicine Series. London: Blackwell Scientific, 1992.

11. Herbert RD, Gabriel M. Effects of stretching before and after exercising on muscle soreness and risk of injury: Systematic review. BMJ 2002;325:468.

12. Janda V. Muscle spasm—a proposed procedure for differential diagnosis. J Man Med 1991;6:136–139.

13. Kabot H. Studies on neuromuscular dysfunction XIII: New concepts and techniques of neuromuscular reeducation for paralysis. Permanente Found Med Bull 1950;8:121–143.

14. Krivickas LS, Feinberg JH. Lower extremity injuries in college atheletes: Relation between ligamentous laxity and lower extremity muscle tightness. Arch Phys Med Rehabil 1996;77:1139–1143.

15. Kujala UM, Taimela S, Salminen JJ, Oksanen A. Baseline anthropometry, flexibility and strength characteristics and future low-back pain in adolescent athletes and nonathletes. A prospective, one-year, follow-up study. Scand J Med Sci Sports 1994;4:200–205.

16. Laboeuf-Yde C, Lauritsen JM, Lauritzen T. Why has the search for causes of low-back pain largely been nonconclusive? Spine 1997;22:877–881.

17. Lakai M, Robson LG. Thixotrophic changes in human muscle stiffness and the effects of fatigue. Q J Exp Physiol 1988;73:487.

18. Levine MG, Kabat H, Knott M, et al. Relaxation of spasticity by physiological techniques. Arch Phys Med 1954;35:214–223.

19. Lewit K, Simons DG. Myofascial pain: Relief by post-isometric relaxation. Arch Phys Med Rehab 1984;65:452–456.

20. Lewit K. Postisometric relaxation in combination with other methods of muscular facilitation and inhibition. Man Med 1986;2:101–104.

21. Lewit K, Berger M, Holzmuller G, Lechner-Sheinleitner S. Breathing movements: The synkinesis of respiration with looking up and down. J Musculoskel Pain 1997;5:57–69.

22. Liebenson CL. Active muscle relaxation techniques. Part I: Basic principles and methods. J Manip Physio Ther 1989;12:446–454.

23. Liebenson CL. Active muscle relaxation techniques. Part II: Clinical application. J Manip Physio Ther 1989;13:2–6.

24. Magnusson SP, Simonesen EB, Aagaard P, et al. Mechanical and physical responses to stretching with and without preisometric contraction of human skeletal muscle. Arch Phys Med Rehabil 1996;778:373–378.

25. McGill S, Grenier S, Bluhm M, Preuss R, Brown S, Russell C. Previous history of LBP with work loss is related to lingering deficits in biomechanical, physiological, personal, psychosocial and motor control characteristics. Ergonomics 2003;46:731–746.

26. McGregor AH, McCarthy ID, Dore CJ, et al. Quantitative assessment of the motion of the lumbar spine in the low back pain population and the effect of different spinal pathologies of this motion. Eur Spine J 1997;6:308–315.

27. Mitchell F Jr, Moran PS, Pruzzo NA. An evaluation of osteopathic muscle energy procedures. Valley Park: Pruzzo, 1979.

28. Moffroid MT. Distinguishable Groups of Musculoskeletal LBP Pts & Asymptomatic Control Subjects Based on Physical Measures of the NIOSH Low Back Atlas. Spine 1994;19:1350–1358.

29. Moore MA, Hutton RS. Electromyographic investigation of muscle stretching techniques. Med Sci Sports Exerc 1980;12:322–329.

30. Nadler SF, Malanga GA, Feinberg JH, Prybicien M, Stitik TP, DeFrince M. Relationship between hip muscle imbalance and occurrence of low back pain in collegiate atheletes: A prospective study. Am J Phys Med Rehabil 2001;80:572–577.

31. Nadler SF, Malanga GA, DePrince ML, Stitik TP, Feinberg JH. The relationship between lower extremity injury, low back pain, and hip muscle strength in male and female collegiate atheletes. Clin J Sports Med 2000;10:89–97.

32. Pope RP, Herbert RD, Kirwan JD. Effects of ankle dorsiflexion range and pre-exercise calf muscle stretching on injury risk in army recruits. Aust J Physiother 1998;44:165–177.

33. Pope RP, Herbert RD, Kirwan JD, Graham BJ. A randomized trial of pre-exercise stretching for prevention of lower-limb injury. Med Sci Sport Ex 2000;32:271–277.

34. Robinson KL, McComas AJ, Belanger AY. Control of soleus motoneuron excitability during muscle stretch in man. J Neur Neurosurg Psych 1982;45: 699–704.

35. Schieppati M, Crenna P. From activity to rest: Gating of excitatory autogenetic afferences from the relaxing muscle in man. Exp Brain Res 1984;56: 448–457.

36. Shrier I. Stretching before exercise does not reduce the risk of local muscle injury: A critical review of the clinical and basic science literature. Clin J Sports Med 1999;9:221–227.

37. Shrier I. Stretching before exercise: An evidence-based approach. Br J Sports Med 2000;32:271–277.

38. Tarbary JC, Tarbary C, Tardieu C, et al. Physiological and structural changes in cat's soleus muscle due to immobilization at different lengths by plaster casts. J Physiol Paris 1972;224:231.

39. Travell JG, Simons DG. Myofascial Pain and Dysfunction—The Trigger Point Manual, 2nd ed. Vol.1. Baltimore: Williams & Wilkins, 1999.

40. Van Dillen LR, McDonnell MK, Fleming DA, Sahrmann SA. The effect of hip and knee position on hip extension range of motion measures in individuals with and without low back pain. J Orthop Sports Phys Ther 2000;30:307–316.

41. Voss DE, Ionta MK, Myers BJ. Proprioceptive Neuromuscular Facilitation, Patterns and Techniques, 3rd ed. Philadelphia: Harper & Row, 1985.

42. Williams PE, Goldspink G. Longitudinal growth of striated muscle fibres. J Cell Sci 1971;56:448.

43. Williams PE, Catanese T, Lucey EG, et al. The importance of stretch and contractile activity in the prevention of connective tissue accumulation in muscle. J Anat 1988;158:109.

The Role of Active Release Technique in Rehabilitation

Clayton Skaggs and Charles Poliquin

Rehabilitative practice often involves conditions that are complicated by tightened muscles and/or their adjacent connective tissue structures. Soft tissue-related conditions and treatment are largely recognized (5,8,15,22,30), yet clinical research is lacking and has not produced conclusive results for standardizing diagnosis and treatment. However, the popularity for soft tissue treatment remains high among patients and practitioners. Active release technique (ART) has generated high interest in rehabilitative and sport medicine for its purported effectiveness with soft tissue problems. When applied to key soft tissues, ART can unload pain-generating structures and facilitate rehabilitation of functional deficits.

Indications

Soft tissue problems primarily involve connective tissue alterations as a result of trauma and/or sustained poor loading and movement. Connective tissue changes, commonly called adhesions, occur as a natural process of healing or in a protective role for loads caused by stress or tension (27). These areas of fibrosis represent the modified tissues that surround and link muscles, joints, and nerves. Leahy proposes that ART releases the adhesion and provides functional improvement sufficient to enhance healing and performance (20). Therefore, in most situations, the application of the ART procedure is to unload or improve the gliding of the pain provoking tissues. Importantly, applying ART to adhesions related in tissues related to the patient's activity intolerance and/or mechanical sensitivity is when this method is most valuable.

Myofascial Presentations

Janda's classification of muscle hypertonus includes functional components that are applicable for ART. Most indicated in this classification system would be the following: interneuronal dysfunction: myofascial trigger points and muscle tightness (see Chapter 19) (17). Interneuron dysfunction leading to altered tone is primarily caused by joint dysfunction. Murphy contends that interneuronal dysfunction can also be caused by muscle dysfunction as a result of dysafferentation of nociception, which will indirectly impact joint function (26). Accordingly, it has been suggested that increasing stretch on injured ligamentous structures improves their stress/strain properties and quantitative and qualitative cross-link formation (14). Therefore, ART protocols directed to problems with ligaments and joint capsules can assist in this process of injury restoration. Preliminary results suggest that ART used in combination with joint mobilization/manipulation is successful (4,10,19,20,28).

Studies have shown that controlled motion of injured soft tissues influences the healing process, giving improved functional outcomes (1,12,18). In the acute phase, the practitioner's task is to coordinate, through active and passive approaches, a balance between muscle regeneration and scar tissue formation. The protective splinting properties of scar tissue can inhibit muscle regeneration and decrease its qualitative formation for strength and stability (18). Early motion in the rehabilitation of repaired tendons of the hand improved gliding function and led to higher tensile stiffness and strength of the repair site (1,3,12). Thus, the proposed mechanism provided by ART would decrease scar tissue development and/or increase the early activation potential of the injured area for improved recovery.

ART has wide implications for the unresponsive chronic pain patient. Chronic patients typically have localized areas of hyperirritability and/or hypertonicity known as myofascial trigger points (22). Chapter 19 has discussed the importance of an active approach such as PIR for addressing trigger points. ART is complementary to PIR and can be used alongside it. When addressing connective tissue problems, ART is an alternative to eccentric muscle energy or post-facilitation stretch techniques (see Chapter 19).

Nerve Presentations

Nerve injury and/or entrapment represents a promising category of treatment for ART. Pain patterns caused by radicular pain or entrapment neuropathy can be identified by clinical testing (6,23,25,29). Butler and others have developed efficient protocols to identify mechanical sensitivities related to nerve irritation (see Chapter 20) (6,11,24). ART protocols have specific applications for common nerve syndromes and most importantly, the common sites of tension development or entrapment.

Minor nerve injury is likely within many of the vague musculoskeletal presentations that make up clinical practice. This category is sometimes classified as "neuropathic pain." This is pain that fails to match a classic pain pattern and shows limited abnormal findings electromyographically and/or radiographically (see Chapter 2) (7). In animal pain studies, it has been shown that fibrosis surrounding the nerve and its adherence to surrounding musculature is reported over the first few weeks following minor nerve injury (2). Although this fibrosis decreases, it is still present at 15 weeks. Importantly, these findings are manifestations of an acute, minor nerve compression and do not represent a gradual peripheral nerve irritation. Greening summarizes that "minor peripheral nerve injury can have effects at both ends of the spectrum; therefore, abnormal input from damaged or ischemic compression may cause pain and trigger central sensitization" (13). He suggests that mobilizing the surrounding neuronal tissue with techniques to optimize posture and function would improve nerve restoration and reduce chronic manifestations. Butler (6) has described neural processes with extreme detail and suggests that any method of easing stress at nerve injury sites or nerve irritation is going to improve restoration and healing. In presentations of "neuropathic pain" or unresolving limb pain, use of ART and its system of entrapment sites can be an efficient way to catalyze recovery before central sensitization occurs.

Performance and Strength Training

Clinical research suggests that nociceptive and non-nociceptive afferents modulate muscle activity locally and distal to the area of stimulation (9). Accordingly, ART applied to sites distal to the area of weakness can facilitate proximal strength and performance gains.

Contraindications

Contraindications for ART are common to most manipulative therapies. Treatment should not be applied that would compromise vascular or nerve

structures. Additionally, cases of organic pathology such as cancer or progressing nerve pathology such as cauda equina should be managed appropriately within common medical guidelines. Lastly, it is contraindicated, as with other manipulative therapies of this magnitude, to perform ART without appropriate training. Improper treatment can produce poor, inconsistent results and most importantly can cause harm.

Background and Principles of ART

ART was developed by Dr. Michael Leahy, a Colorado Springs chiropractic physician. His soft tissue management system contains more than 250 protocols for muscle lesions and nerve entrapments for the musculoskeletal system. Dr. Leahy proposes the concept identified as the "law of repetitive motion"(21). In this model, the extent of insult to the tissues is explained by four interrelated factors. These factors are related as the "number of repetitions" times the "force or tension of each repetition" (as a percent of the maximum muscle strength) divided by the "amplitude of each repetition" times the "relaxation time between repetitions." Out of this concept he justifies the mechanism of injury with apparently minor events. He describes that adhesions and fibrosis also develop along with local edema as a result of minor repetitive forces that lead to poor gliding mechanics and resultant pain as described.

Once tissue adhesion or tension is identified then treatment application can be applied. As is the case with most manual therapies, locating the most impor-

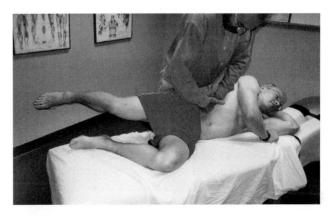

Figure 19A.1 ART of the psoas. The practitioner is applying manual tension superior and medial to the psoas. The patient begins with the hip and leg flexed and then proceeds to extend the leg and hip while the practitioner maintains his contact.

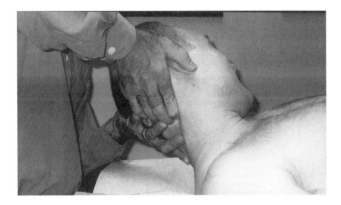

Figure 19A.2 ART of the rectus capitus major/minor (RCM). The practitioner applies superior and slightly lateral tension to the RCM. The practitioner then extends the upper cervical spine and rotates the head to the side of treatment. While tension is maintained on the RCM, the upper cervical spine is flexed and the head taken into the opposite rotation.

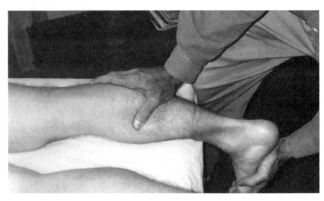

Figure 19A.3 ART to the gastrocnemius. The practitioner takes a contact with superior tension on the gastrocnemius. He then asks the patient to plantar-flex the ankle. While maintaining superior tension, the patient slowly dorsi-flexes the ankle.

tant lesion or "key link" structure is a critical factor in the success of the procedure. The common method of ART is to move the tissue from a shortened position to a lengthened positioned while maintaining tension on the local site of adhesion or tissue tension. A list of treatment principles, developed by Leahy, helps the practitioner in achieve the maximum result with minimum complication (9) (Table 19A.1).

It has often been said that "there is nothing new under the sun." The application of manual therapy or some form of massage to muscle with and without active motion has been proposed for many years, well before and since the development of ART (15,16,22). Like PIR or other manual therapy techniques ART is in fact an art and requires proper training and subsequent clinical experience to master.

Table 19A.1   A List of Treatment Principles and Guidelines When Applying Active Release Procedures

---

1. *Use soft contact:* Use the specific contact described in the protocol. Hands-on instruction is most beneficial in learning a proper touch.
2. *Begin active, work longitudinally:* For many reasons, this method effectively breaks the adhesions in and between tissues. Although restrictions may be found in any direction, it is most important to establish longitudinal freedom of motion within a muscle. Then, if necessary, treat in the other direction.
3. *Use active motion whenever possible:* This provides the patient with a sense of control and also inhibits pain. The methods of active motion are designed to maximize relative motion between tissues.
4. *Use slow motion:* If any motions are fast or quick, the tolerance of the patient is reduced and the muscle will tense.
5. *Evaluate patient tolerance:* The pressure and number of passes is always limited to patient tolerance. In general, three to five passes over a general area is the limit.
6. *Evaluate tissue tolerance:* It is sometimes necessary to delay a treatment because of tissue intolerance. This is indicated by physical as well as nonphysical indicators. When the tissue is sensitive from the previous treatment, it is better to delay the treatment and decrease the frequency of visits.
7. *Work along the direction of venous and lymphatic flow:* Bruising and lymphatic edema are almost completely avoided by accurate methods. When motions are made against venous or lymphatic flow they are very short.
8. *Frequency = alternate days:* Treatment frequency is never more often than alternate days. Daily treatment may lead to tissue intolerance and protracted treatment plans. In some cases, an even longer period between treatments is necessary.

Adapted from Leahy PM, seminar course notes 2000.

Clinical Correlation to Common Functional Patterns

Symptom complex: Low back pain

Pain generating structure: Lumbar facets

Overloading mechanism: Shorten hip flexors

Kinetic linkage: Altered hip extension

Symptom complex: Headache

Pain generating structure: Upper cervical facets

Overloading mechanism: Shortened suboccipital musculature

Kinetic linkage: Altered capital flexion

Symptom complex: Achilles tendonitis

Pain generating structure: Achilles tendon

Overloading mechanism: Shortened gastrocnemius

Kinetic linkage: Hyperpronation/weak foot intrinsics

■ REFERENCES

1. Akalin E, El O, Tamci S, et al. Treatment of carpal tunnel syndrome with nerve and tendon gliding exercises. Am J Phys Med Rehabil 2002;81:108.
2. Bennett G, Xie Y. A peripheral mononeuropathy in rat that produces disorders of pain sensation like those seen in man. Pain 1988;33:87.
3. Best T, Hunter K. Muscle injury and repair. Scientific principals of sports rehabilitation. Pain 2000;11:25.
4. Buchberger D. Posterior-superior glenoid impingement of the throwing shoulder: Evaluation and management. Sports Chiro Rehabil 2000;14:5.
5. Butler DS. Adverse mechanical tension in the nervous system: A model for assessment and treatment. Aust J Physiother 1989;35:227.
6. Butler DS. The Sensitive Nervous System. Adelaide, Australia: Noigroup Publications, 2000.
7. Campbell J, Raja S, Belzberg A, et al. Hyperalgesia and the sympathetic nervous system. Touch, temperature, and pain in health and disease: Mechanisms and assessments. Progress Pain Res Manage 1994;3:24.
8. Cyriax J. Textbook of Orthopedic Medicine. London: Bailliere Tindall, 1982.
9. Deriu F, et al. Non-nociceptive upper limb afferents modulate masseter muscle EMG activity in man. Exp Brain Res 2002;143:286–294.
10. Drover J, Herzog W. Influence of active release technique on quadriceps strength and inhibition. International Conference on Spinal Manipulation, 2002.
11. Elvey R. Treatment of arm pain associated with abnormal brachial plexus tension. Aust J Physiother 1989;32:224–229.
12. Gelberman R, Vande Berg BJ, Lundborg G, et al. Flexor tendon healing and restoration of the gliding surface. J Bone Joint Surg 1983;65:70.
13. Greening J, Lynn B. Minor peripheral nerve injuries: An underestimated source of pain? Manual Ther 1998;3:187.
14. Gomez M, Woo S, Amiel D, et al. The effects of increased tension on healing medial collateral ligaments. Am J Sports Med 1991;19:347.
15. Hammer W. Functional soft tissue examination and treatment by manual methods. New York: Aspen Publishing, 1999.
16. Hunter G. Specific soft tissue mobilization in the treatment of soft tissue lesions. Physiother 1994;80:15.
17. Janda V. Muscle spasm: A proposed procedure for differential diagnosis. J Man Med 1991;6:136.
18. Jarvinen M, Lehto M. The effects of early mobilization and immobilization on the healing process following muscle injuries. Sports Med 1993;15:78.
19. Leahy PM, Mock L. Myofascial release technique and mechanical compromise of peripheral nerves of the upper extremity. Chiro Sports Med 1992;6:139.
20. Leahy PM. Improved treatments for carpal tunnel and related syndromes. Chiro Sports Med 1995;9:6.
21. Leahy PM. Active Release Soft Tissue Management System. Course Manual. 1999.
22. Lewit K. Manipulative Therapy in Rehabilitation of the Motor System, 3rd ed. London: Butterworth-Heinemann, 2002.
23. McCombe PF, Fairband J, Cockersole BC, et al. Reproducibility of physical signs in low-back pain. Spine 1989;14:908–918.
24. McKenzie RA. Mechanical diagnosis and therapy for low back pain. In: Physical Therapy of Low Back Pain. New York: Churchill Livingstone, 1987.
25. McLellan DL, Swash M. Longitudinal sliding of the median nerve during movements of the upper limb. J Neurol Neurosurg Psych 1976;36:566.
26. Murphy D. Conservative Management of Cervical Spine Syndromes. New York: McGraw-Hill, 2002.
27. Pneumaticos S, Nobel P, McGarvey W, et al. The effects of early mobilization in the healing of Achilles tendon repair. Foot Ankle Int 2000; 21:551.
28. Schiottz-Christensen B, Mooney V, Azad S, et al. The role of active release manual therapy for upper extremity overuse syndromes—a preliminary report. J Occup Rehabil 1999;9:210.
29. Sunderland S. The nerve lesion in the carpal tunnel syndrome. J Neurol Neurosurg Psych 1976; 39:615.
30. Travell JG, Simmons DG. Myofascial Pain and Dysfunction: The Trigger Point Manual. Baltimore: Williams and Wilkins, 1993.

20

Neuromobilization Techniques—Evaluation and Treatment of Adverse Neurodynamic Tension

Michael C. Geraci,
Martin Lambert,
and Mark R. Bookhout

Introduction
General Concepts
Precautions and Contraindications
Evaluation of ANDT: The Lower Quarter
Evaluation of ANDT: The Upper Quarter
Treatment of the Container
Upper Quarter Protocol
Joint Dysfunctions
Cervical and Thoracic
Clavicular
Re-evaluation of ULNT and Neuromobilization

Learning Objectives
On completion of this chapter, you will be able to:

- Explain how the clinician can incorporate neuro-mobilization techniques as evaluation and treatment modalities.
- Identify the adverse neurodynamic tension (ANDT) test.
- Identify the indications for performing ANDT testing.
- Assess the difference between muscle and capsular tightness from ANDT in patients.

Introduction

The evaluation and treatment of adverse neurodynamic tension (ANDT) has been published by Elvey (15), Butler (5), Shacklock (33), as well as Slater (34). Their work has been presented in workshops and courses by Shacklock, Butler, Slater, and their co-workers (35) offered by the Neuro-Orthopedic Institute. All of these authors have helped in presenting this material and its clinical usefulness to physical therapists and physicians who treat musculoskeletal disorders. Greenman and the authors (1) of this chapter have combined the evaluation and treatment of ANDT and neuromobilization techniques with manual techniques and exercise. The scientific basis for the evaluation and treatment of ANDT has been presented by basic science experts and clinicians (2–6,8–14,16,18–26,28–33,37–42). In particular, Butler (7) in his new book, *The Sensitive Nervous System*, has dedicated a chapter on the subject of research and neurodynamics.

In this chapter, we discuss the general concepts, including the aim of treatment, consequence of mobilization of the nervous system, precautions, and contraindications. Even for the experienced clinician it is sometimes difficult to differentiate ANDT from muscle tightness, joint dysfunctions, and joint capsular patterns of tightness. By having a thorough understanding of the slump test and straight leg raise, as well as sensitizing and relieving maneuvers, one can differentiate hamstring tightness from ANDT in the sciatic nerve or one of its nerve roots. After testing for ANDT and before neuromobilization techniques are applied as a form of treatment, we explain why treating lumbar segmental dysfunction, sacroiliac/pelvic dysfunction, capsular tightness patterns, and muscular tightness patterns are performed first. These areas represent the so-called container and should be treated before the use of neuromobilization techniques. We also differentiate between rectus femoris tightness and ANDT in the femoral nerve and its associated nerve roots. Sensitizing and relieving maneuvers will help when applied to the prone femoral nerve stretch test, as well as the side-lying slump femoral nerve stretch test to differentiate muscle tightness from ANDT in the femoral nerve distribution. In this case, the container involves the upper lumbar segmental dysfunctions, along with sacroiliac/pelvic dysfunctions and capsular tightness, especially of the anterior hip capsule. Muscular tightness, especially of the psoas and rectus femoris muscles, often associated with anterior hip capsule tightness, is also discussed in detail.

In the upper quarter, rib dysfunctions and muscular tightness patterns will be differentiated from ANDT of the median nerve in particular. We describe in detail the use of the upper limb neurodynamic tests (ULNT), formerly the upper limb tension test (ULTT), as well as how they can be used as a barometer of improvement and a treatment modality after the container has been treated. In this case, the container relates to certain muscle tightness patterns of the scalenes and pectoralis minor and how they relate to the first through fifth rib dysfunctions. Also, cervical and especially thoracic segmental dysfunctions need to be treated when indicated. Stretching of muscular imbalances such as the scalenes, pectoralis minor, teres major, latissimus dorsi, and posterior shoulder capsule are also included. We then recommend re-checking the ULNT to determine whether a significant change in ANDT has occurred.

This chapter does not substitute or delve into the detail as described in Butler's (5,7) works, as well as the other authors mentioned. We encourage you to review the excellent work on the subject, which has been referenced. However, we include how the previous work on evaluation and treatment of ANDT is now incorporated into our practices using manual medicine techniques to correct joint dysfunctions, including manual stretching for tight muscles and joint capsules. Whenever possible, three-dimensional (3-D) self-stretches and functional exercises are shown to help maintain the correction and prevent recurrences by reinforcing the quality of movement during functional activities.

General Concepts

Several definitions as defined by Shacklock (35) help us in understanding of ANDT. Neurodynamics is described as the mechanisms and physiology of the nervous system as they relate to one another. The term "pathodynamics" applies to abnormal mechanical, physiologic, and responses produced from nervous system structures when their mechanics are tested. The nervous system is designed for movement. The spinal canal length is approximately 7 centimeters (cm) longer in flexion than in extension. Most of these length changes occur in the cervical and lumbar region. In the periphery, for example, from wrist and elbow flexion to wrist and elbow extension, the median nerve has to adapt to a nerve bed 20% longer. A length change, however, of 15% or more will interrupt blood supply to the nerve (36). We believe this argues against using sustained stretching and supports the use of on/off non-ballistic and proprioceptive neuromuscular facilitation (PNF)-type stretching.

To help in further understanding peripheral nervous system dynamics, as an example, the median nerve has the ability to slide up to 2 cm in relation to the nerve bed in the upper arm. Movement of the fingers and wrist can slide the nerve by 1 cm in the upper arm. These movement changes are accompanied by pressure changes (36). These pressure changes, for instance in the ulnar nerve at the elbow, can be doubled by neck and shoulder movement, and in the position used for the ulnar nerve tension test, pressure can be quadrupled.

Butler, Shacklock, and Slater (35,36) have stressed that the order of movement introduced when performing ANDT testing is important. They feel that the best way to assess ANDT is to first take up the component that "houses" the pathological changes and then to add tension through the other components. They also strongly advocate that the method of neurodynamic testing should include a starting position that is constant each time. Although the testing may be performed actively by the patient or passively by the examiner, we feel the best way to assess quality of movement throughout the range tested is passively. The operator needs to be able to feel for barriers to movement and note the onset of resistance, or if there is pain or other symptoms. Noting pain responses, including the area and nature of pain, are important but, most of all, we believe reproducing the patient's symptoms is the goal of adverse neurodynamic tension testing.

Testing for symmetry or asymmetry and comparing both sides usually is best performed by checking the asymptomatic side first and appreciating the importance of resistance throughout the asymptomatic side and then symptomatic side. One, at this point, may wonder, "what is the purpose of trying to mobilize the nervous system?" Butler and co-workers state that the aim of treatment is to restore normal movement and elasticity of the nervous system. The dispersion of intraneural edema, stretching of neural adhesions, increased blood flow and cerebral spinal fluid flow, as well as axonal transport, are all discussed in detail by Butler and his co-workers. Normalizing extraneural interfaces is also a consequence of mobilization of the nervous system, but this is probably best achieved by addressing dysfunctions of the container first.

One of the authors of this chapter has introduced the concept of using neuromobilization techniques after transforaminal epidural steroid injections that are performed under fluoroscopy (17).

Precautions and Contraindications

As with any technique, understanding the precautions and contraindications are essential, especially for the novice when it comes to understanding ANDT testing. Several precautions, although not absolute contraindications, include symptomatic cervical or lumbar disc herniations, irritable nerve root, presence of progressive neurologic deficits, as well as general health problems. These would include circulatory disturbances, either inflammatory or infective, and may be exemplified by the presence of Guillain-Barré or localized abscess. Other relative precautions are when central nervous system signs present, such as dizziness, or known spinal cord injury. A limiting factor may also be the patient who has severe unremitting pain that creates difficulty with a thorough examination and diagnosis. Caution is required when handling this type of patient.

Absolute contraindications include recent or worsening neurologic signs, as well as the presence of cauda equina lesions. A direct injury to the spinal cord, or the presence of a tethered cord, where the spinal cord is adhered to the meninges and canal, such that movements like neck flexion are transmitted to the cord and not the supporting structures, are examples in which neuromobilizations would be contraindicated. Spinal instability and cases of osteoporosis resulting in abnormal interfacing tissues are other examples of contraindications. A history of previous transient quadriplegia also is associated frequently with spinal instability.

Evaluation of ANDT: The Lower Quarter

The assessment of the patient with ANDT of the lower quarter starts by watching the patient's gait. Certain antalgic postures, especially the knee held in constant flexion, may indicate adverse tension in the sciatic distribution, in which the knee flexion allows for slackening of tension on the sciatic nerve. The forward-flexion test can be initiated from the head down with fingertips reaching down toward the floor, stopping the patient at the point where reproduction of the symptoms in the back or leg is felt. Then, the examiner may passively extend the patient's neck. If this either relieves or provokes the patient's symptoms, this is a sign that the symptoms are provoked by adverse neurodynamic tension rather than muscular tightness.

The Slump Test

The slump test (Figs. 20.1A to 20.1F) is gaining widespread use in the musculoskeletal clinician's practice. This test should not be thought of as a substitute for the straight leg raise, but as an additional and more sensitive test for ANDT that can be performed in the seated position. Once the patient has been placed in the slump seated position, we recommend active neck flexion, performed by the patient, to the point at which symptoms are reproduced. If symptoms

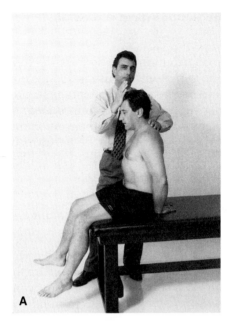

A

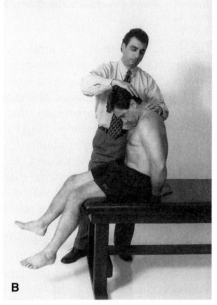

B

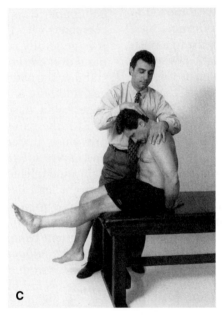

C

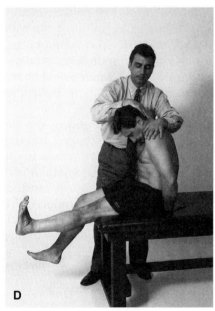

D

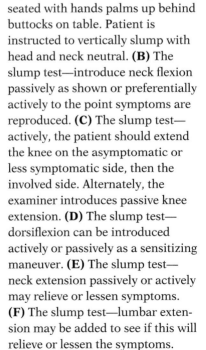

E

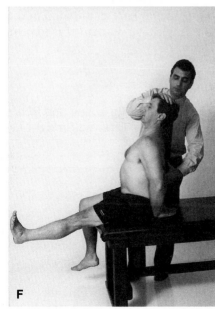

F

Figure 20.1 **(A)** The slump test—seated with hands palms up behind buttocks on table. Patient is instructed to vertically slump with head and neck neutral. **(B)** The slump test—introduce neck flexion passively as shown or preferentially actively to the point symptoms are reproduced. **(C)** The slump test—actively, the patient should extend the knee on the asymptomatic or less symptomatic side, then the involved side. Alternately, the examiner introduces passive knee extension. **(D)** The slump test—dorsiflexion can be introduced actively or passively as a sensitizing maneuver. **(E)** The slump test—neck extension passively or actively may relieve or lessen symptoms. **(F)** The slump test—lumbar extension may be added to see if this will relieve or lessen the symptoms.

are reproduced in the patient's classic distribution, the test may be stopped. However, if no symptoms are produced, we recommend adding knee extension passively by the examiner. The examiner can record the lack, in degrees, from full knee extension when adverse tension develops and note the patient's response. We also recommend using the terms "typical" to represent symptoms reproduced in the patient's distribution or partial distribution of symptoms, or "atypical" when ANDT develops, producing symptoms that are normally not felt by the patient but are still considered to be abnormal.

For example, if the patient assumes the slump position with neck flexion and then either active or passive knee extension is introduced on the left and this reproduces the patient's symptoms at 20 degrees from full knee extension, the test results should be recorded as follows: positive slump test on the left at 20 degrees from full knee extension, reproducing a typical response. This would be in contrast to a positive slump test on the asymptomatic right side at full knee extension, which would be recorded as follows: positive slump test on the right at full knee extension, with atypical response. When a typical response is found, one that reproduces the patient's symptoms, the test should be stopped and the limb held in the position at which symptoms first appeared. To differentiate in this case sciatic ANDT from hamstring or other muscle tightness, sensitizing and relieving maneuvers are then introduced (Table 20.1). Generally, the first relieving maneuver is to have the patient perform active cervical extension to see if symptoms are relieved or reduced. Please note that this may become a sensitizing maneuver if symptoms worsen or the site of the symptom changes. For example, the patient may feel that with neck extension, the symptoms in the posterior thigh and calf move to the lumbar spine and are eliminated in the lower extremity. If a sensitizing maneuver is to be introduced, gener-

ally passive or active dorsiflexion is most typically used. Dorsiflexion with eversion at the subtalar joint or plantar flexion with subtalar joint inversion can be introduced. Additional sensitizing and relieving maneuvers are listed in Table 20.1 and can most easily be performed actively by the patient, including left or right side-bending of the trunk.

The Straight Leg Raise (SLR)

With the patient supine, the straight leg raise (SLR) is performed (Figs. 20.2A to 20.2G). Again, active movement by the patient or passive movement by the examiner can be performed. However, one should keep in mind that as discussed under general concepts, by using passive movement the examiner is better able to appreciate resistance and note how that correlates with the onset of the patient's symptoms. It is generally recommended to stabilize with one hand over the anterior knee and patella, and even to stabilize the patella between the thumb and index finger, and note any attempt the patient has to flex the knee. Again, the examiner should note at what degree of SLR the patient reports symptoms. As discussed previously under slump testing, the terms "typical" and "atypical" can be applied the same way. Sensitizing and relieving maneuvers are also applied to the straight leg raise and are listed in Table 20.1. The most common one is adding ankle dorsiflexion and eversion or plantar flexion and inversion at the point the patient begins to feel symptoms during the base SLR test. Adduction and internal rotation of the hip may be introduced at the beginning or at the point symptoms are produced during the SLR. Neck flexion can also be added, either actively by the patient or passively by an assistant, if one is available.

If after adding the sensitizing and relieving maneuvers for the SLR and slump test there is no change in the patient's symptoms, one should think of muscular tightness especially of the hamstrings if symptoms are in the mid to upper thigh. When symptoms are located in the distal thigh or behind the knee, these often represent ANDT symptoms that will respond to sensitizing and relieving maneuvers that help to further clarify the situation.

In our clinical experience, treatment of the so-called container should be applied first, before neuromobilization techniques (Table 20.2). For the skilled manual practitioner familiar with various manual techniques, including high-velocity thrust (HVT), muscle energy techniques (METs), or joint play, they will have a system of evaluating for lumbar segmental dysfunctions. In particular, L_4 and L_5 segmental dysfunctions should be treated first. Sacroiliac and pelvic dysfunctions should be treated as well. After

Table 20.1 Sensitizing and Relieving Maneuvers for the Slump Test and Straight Leg Raise

Sensitizing	Relieving
Ankle dorsiflexion	Ipsilateral trunk
Ankle dorsiflexion/eversion	side-bending
Ankle plantar flexion	Neck extension
Ankle plantar flexion/inversion	Lumbar extension
Hip adduction/internal rotation	Trunk rotational
Contralateral trunk side-bending	movements
Neck flexion	
Trunk rotational movements	

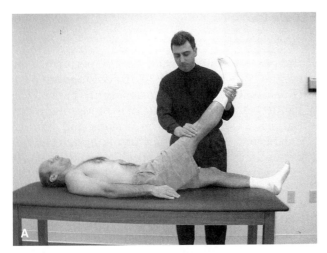
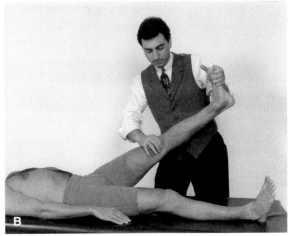
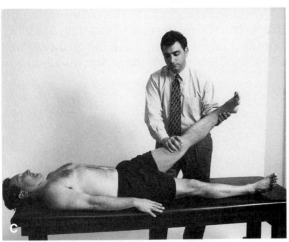
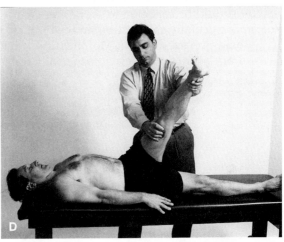
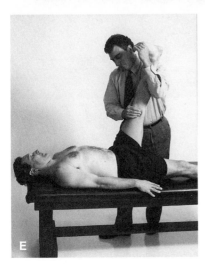
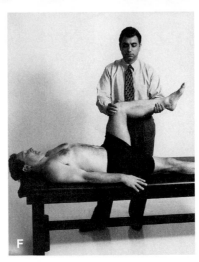
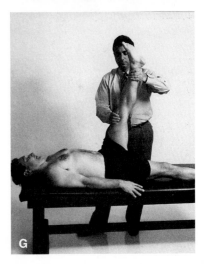

Figure 20.2 **(A)** The straight leg raise (SLR)—base test. Patient is supine, examiner introduces SLR with one hand, monitoring and stabilizing knee extension. **(B)** The SLR—sensitizing maneuver of dorsiflexion and eversion is added. **(C)** The SLR—sensitizing maneuver of hip internal rotation is added at point of symptom reproduction or at the beginning while the tested leg is still on the table. **(D)** The SLR—sensitizing adduction is added at the point of symptom reproduction or at the beginning. **(E)** The SLR—sensitizing maneuver of hip adduction, internal rotation, and dorsiflexion are all added at the point of symptom reproduction. **(F)** The SLR—starting position of the 90/90 SLR. (Alternate SLR position: note the hip is flexed first before the knee is extended.) **(G)** The SLR—knee is extended from the 90/90 position to point of symptom reproduction.

Table 20.2 Sequence of Treatment of the Container for Sciatic Adverse Neurodynamic Tension

1. Lumbar segmental dysfunction, especially L4 and L5
2. Sacroiliac/pelvic dysfunction
3. Capsular tightness, especially posterior hip capsule
4. Muscular tightness, especially piriformis/ hamstrings

any treatment to the lumbar, SI, or pelvic region, ANDT testing should be repeated to see if there is a difference, and especially a reduction, in the typical testing responses previously seen. Mobilization for any hip capsular tightness, if present, especially for the posterior hip capsule, can be performed in the supine (Figs. 20.3A and 20.3B) or standing position (Fig. 20.3C). After the posterior hip capsule mobilization, manual stretching of the muscular tightness patterns, especially the piriformis and hamstring, can be performed. The piriformis stretch can be performed supine or prone (Fig. 20.4A and 20.4B); however, we recommend standing, as seen in Fig. 20.4C. At this point it should be noted that the sequence of treating the container by treating the lumbar, SI, and pelvic dysfunctions first, primarily because they can be the source of tension and tightness patterns found in the capsule and muscles as mentioned.

Functional exercises for the piriformis and hamstrings should be performed to maintain flexibility and controlled mobility to improve the quality of motion. If ANDT still remains in the sciatic distribution after

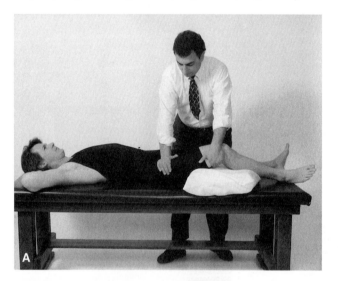

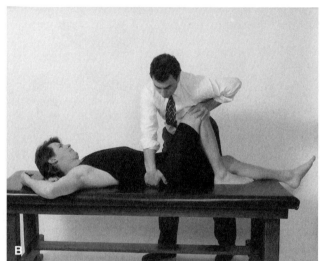

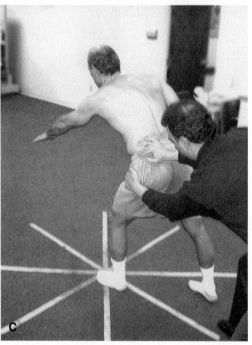

Figure 20.3 **(A)** Posterior hip capsular mobilization—patient supine as shown. With right lower extremity in the resting position of hip flexion/abduction to 30 degrees with slight external rotation. The examiner exerts a posterolateral force on the proximal femur with on/off technique until a normal glide is re-established. **(B)** Posterior hip capsular mobilization—patient supine as shown. Examiner places right hand under the posterior pelvis and the left hand on the anterior adducted knee. A posterolateral force is directed with on/off technique until a normal glide is re-established. **(C)** Posterior hip capsular mobilization— patient stands as shown. Examiner's right hand contacts the right proximal femur while the left hand contacts the right pelvis above the hip joint. The examiner pulls the femur posteriorly with the right hand while the patient reaches with both arms anteriorly at hip height.

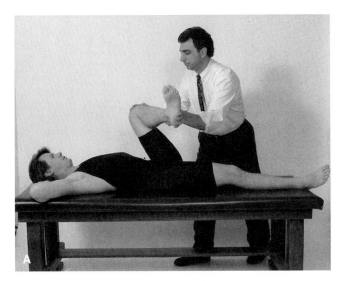

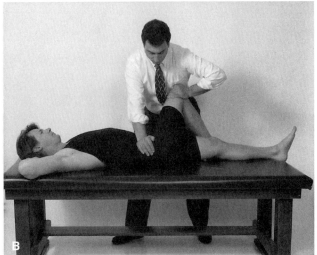

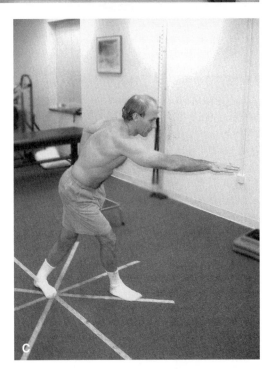

Figure 20.4 **(A)** Piriformis stretch—for tightness at more than 90 degrees. **(B)** Piriformis stretch—for tightness at less than 90 degrees. **(C)** Piriformis stretch—standing left side self-stretch.

treatment of the container has been performed, as described, the following neuromobilization techniques may be added.

Between the seated slump, supine SLR, and supine 90/90 straight leg raise, determine which of the three is the least pain-provocative and start with that position. Gradually progress to the most provocative position over time. This will vary from patient to patient. Neuromobilization techniques that should be added at this time include the slump slider (Fig. 20.5A), slump tensor (Fig. 20.5B), SLR (Figs. 20.2A to 20.2E), and supine 90/90 SLR (Figs. 20.2F and 20.2G). We recommend starting with the slump slider because it is often the least provocative of the different positions mentioned. The patient is ins-

tructed to add cervical extension with knee extension on the asymptomatic side first, performing 10 to 15 until tension reduces. This can be followed by the slump tensor position combining neck flexion with knee extension and adding varying degrees of adduction, internal rotation, dorsiflexion, and other sensitizing maneuvers. This can be followed typically by SLR from a 90/90 position and again adding dorsiflexion. The final sequence often used is SLR from the supine position, then adduction, internal rotation of the hip, and dorsiflexion of the ankle. It should be noted that all of these neuromobilization techniques should be performed with an on/off non-ballistic-type stretch and repeated 10 to 15 times or until tension is reduced.

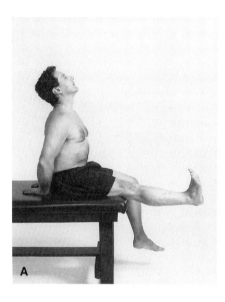

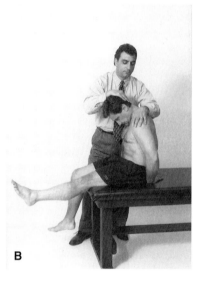

Figure 20.5 **(A)** The slump slider neuromobilization—patient extends the right knee as simultaneous neck extension is introduced to take tension off from above. **(B)** The slump tensor neuromobilization—patient extends the left knee while maintaining the slump position with neck flexion.

Femoral Nerve Stretch Test (FNST)

Also in the lower quarter, a common area that presents difficulty to a clinician in determining muscle tightness from adverse neurodynamic tension, is the rectus femoris and femoral nerve ANDT. The femoral nerve stretch test (FNST) can be performed prone (Figs. 20.6A and 20.6B) or in a side-lying slump position (Figs. 20.7A and 20.7B). Sensitizing maneuvers generally include the addition of active and/or passive neck flexion and relieving maneuver of active or passive neck extension. In the side-lying slump position, there is a distinct advantage to having an assistant perform the passive neck movements with the examiner controlling the thigh and leg movements. One should remember that sensitizing and relieving maneuvers are interchangeable in that a sensitizing maneuver may sometimes actually relieve symptoms and vice versa.

The concept of treating the container first also applies when addressing femoral nerve ANDT (Table 20.3). In this case, upper lumbar segmental dysfunctions, as well as SI/pelvic dysfunctions, should be treated first. Capsular tightness, especially of the anterior hip capsule, can be performed in the prone (Figs. 20.8A and 20.8B) or standing position (Fig. 20.8C). This should be followed by stretching of the corresponding tight musculature, in particular the psoas and the rectus femoris (Figs. 20.9A to 20.9C). Finally, functional exercises for the psoas in particular should be performed to maintain correction and be incorporated into a movement pattern to improve the quality of motion. At this point neuromobilizations, especially in the side-lying slump femoral nerve stretch test position, can be performed if an assistant is available to help the examiner. Sliders can be performed by having the assistant introduce neck extension while the examiner introduces knee flexion (Fig. 20.10A). Tensors can be performed with the neck in a flexed position and then introducing knee flexion (Fig. 20.10B). Also, if an examiner is with the patient without an assistant, neuromobilization for the femoral nerve can be performed in the prone position with the head off the table so that the patient can introduce active neck extension while the examiner introduces passive knee flexion in an on/off non-ballistic technique (Fig. 20.11A and 20.11B).

The actual neuromobilization techniques are advocated, as mentioned, using an on/off non-ballistic technique. The advantages to this technique are that it performs successive on/off mobilization of the muscle to reduce the gel phenomenon that occurs in muscles while mobilizing the connective tissue that surrounds the nerve. More importantly, perhaps using the on/off technique avoids reducing the blood supply to the nerve, which can occur when a stretch is held in a sustained manner. Different proprioceptive neuromuscular facilitation techniques can be added at this point for functional movement retraining.

Evaluation of ANDT: The Upper Quarter

Upper Limb Neurodynamic Tests (ULNT)

The purpose of this section is to introduce the concepts of upper limb neurodynamic testing and treatment. It is not intended to be a substitute for the extensive work pioneered by Elvy (15), Butler (5), and others (33–35). It will, therefore, take a more simplified approach to

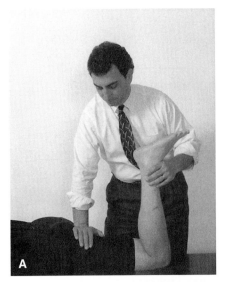

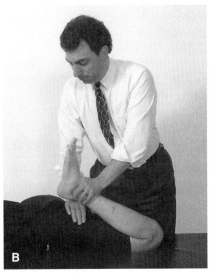

Figure 20.6 (A) Prone femoral nerve stretch test (FNST)—patient positioned as shown. Examiner flexes the left knee while stabilizing the pelvis at the ischium until symptoms are reproduced. **(B)** Prone FNST—normal flexibility of the rectus femoris and connective tissue around the femoral nerve should allow the heel to approximate the buttock. **(C, D)** Prone FNST—variations of head/neck flexion/extension movements to sensitize or relieve symptoms.

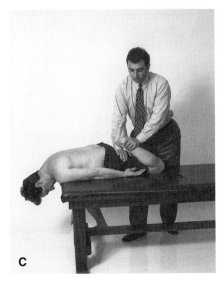

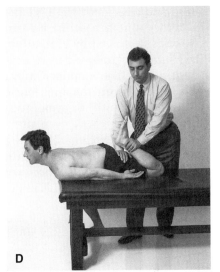

Figure 20.7 (A) Side-lying slump FNST—patient positioned as shown. One examiner controls flexion/extension of the head and neck while the other introduces hip extension then knee flexion or vice versa. Neck flexion shown here will usually increase symptoms. **(B)** Side-lying slump FNST—neck extension will usually decrease symptoms.

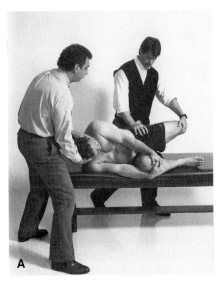

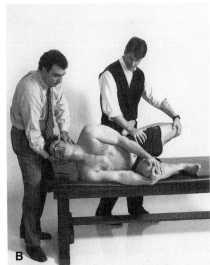

Table 20.3 Sequence of Treatment of the Container for Femoral Adverse Neurodynamic Tension

1. Upper lumbar segmental dysfunctions, especially L1 and L2
2. Sacroiliac/pelvic dysfunctions
3. Capsular tightness, especially anterior hip capsule
4. Muscular tightness, especially psoas/rectus femoris

evaluation of upper limb neural dynamic function so that we may introduce our approach to its treatment. The reader is strongly encouraged to read about these techniques in greater detail in the published works of Elvy and Butler. Our recommended protocol for evaluation and treatment of ULNT in the upper quarter is to determine a baseline measure for each of the base tests, followed by evaluation and treatment of "the container," followed by re-assessment of ULNTs. If treatment of "the container" fully resolves the underlying adverse neural dynamic tension (ANDT), no further neurodynamic treatment is necessary. If the ULNTs remain positive even after treating "the container," then neurodynamic mobilization may proceed as described later in the treatment section of this chapter. For simplification purposes, we only describe three of the four ULNTs described by Butler.

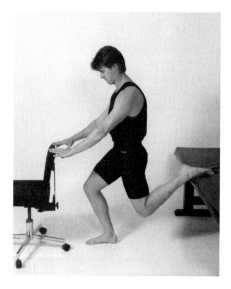

Figure 20.9 Rectus femoris standing self-stretch—left hip extension, posterior pelvic tilt, and increasing knee flexion provide the basis. Pelvic rotation and trunk side-bending when added make for a three-dimensional stretch.

Tests are considered positive when they reproduce the patient's symptoms.

ULNT 1 (Median Nerve Bias) The test position is described for your patient's right arm. Have your patient

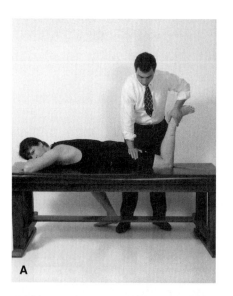
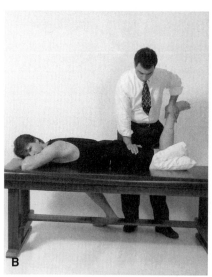
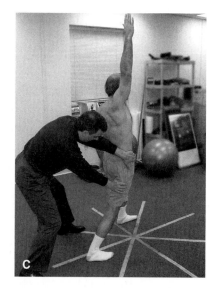

Figure 20.8 (A) Anterior hip capsular mobilization—position patient as shown. The examiner introduces an anterolateral force on the proximal femur with the right hand at the point the proximal femur comes off the table while introducing hip external rotation with the left hand. **(B)** Anterior hip capsular mobilization—alternate patient positioning with pillow under the distal thigh. **(C)** Anterior hip capsular mobilization standing—examiner applies an anterior force on the proximal right femur with the right hand while stabilizing the pelvis with the left hand.

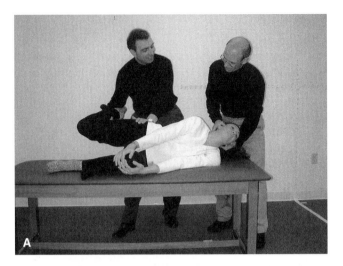
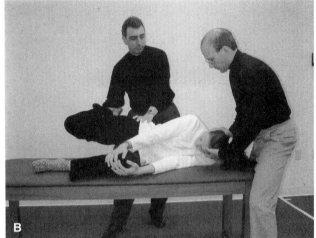

Figure 20.10 (A) FNST—slider neuromobilization. **(B)** FNST—tensor neuromobilization.

lie supine close to the edge of the table. The legs should be straight with the left arm by the side. A pillow is optional for comfort. Stand facing your patient.

1. Make a fist with your right hand and place it on top of your patient's right shoulder to prevent further shoulder elevation during the technique.
2. Rest the patient's right arm against your thigh as you grasp the patient's right hand with your left hand.
3. Slowly abduct the arm to approximately 110 degrees or to any increase in resistance, tissue tightening, or symptom provocation. The

patient's elbow remains flexed to approximately 90 degrees.

4. Rotate the forearm into supination.
5. Extend the wrist and fingers.
6. Externally rotate the shoulder (Fig. 20.12).
7. Carefully extend the elbow. This position is symptomatic in most patients so proceed cautiously (Fig. 20.13).

If symptoms are noted at any stage of ULNT 1, a goniometric measurement is taken to establish a baseline. Sensitizing maneuvers can include cervical side

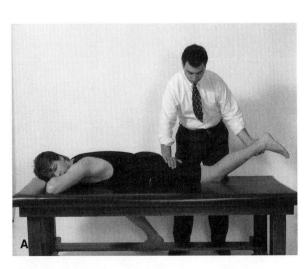
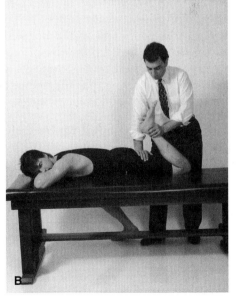

Figure 20.11 (A) FNST—neuromobilization, off technique. **(B)** FNST—neuromobilization, on technique.

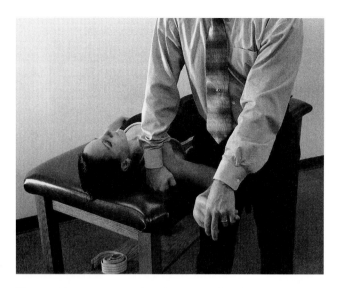

Figure 20.12 ULNT 1 (median nerve bias).

Table 20.4   Sensitizing and Relieving Maneuvers for ULNT 1 to 3

Sensitizing

1. Contralateral: Cervical side-bending to sensitize at ipsilateral cervical musculature
2. Ipsilateral: Cervical side-bending to sensitize at ipsilateral cervical intervertebral foramen
3. Cervical extension, contralateral side-bending with ipsilateral rotation to sensitize at ipsilateral anterior and medial scaleni

Relieving

1. Ipsilateral: Cervical side-bending to relieve at ipsilateral cervical musculature
2. Contralateral: Cervical side-bending to relieve at ipsilateral cervical intervertebral foramen
3. Cervical flexion, ipsilateral side-bending with contralateral rotation to sensitize at ipsilateral anterior and medial scaleni

bending away from the limb being tested to sensitize at the ipsilateral cervical musculature. Cervical side bending toward the tested limb will sensitize at the ipsilateral intervertebral foramen. Cervical extension, side-bending away, and rotation toward will sensitize at the ipsilateral anterior and medial scaleni. Relieving maneuvers can include cervical side-bending toward the tested limb to relieve at the ipsilateral cervical musculature. Cervical side-bending away from the tested limb will relieve at the ipsilateral intervertebral foramen. Cervical flexion, side-bending toward, and rotation away will relieve at the ipsilateral anterior and medial scaleni (Table 20.4).

ULNT 2 (Radial Nerve Bias) This is described for the patient's right arm. Have your patient lie supine with legs straight as you stand at the head of the table, facing the patient's feet. A pillow is optional for comfort. The patient should be positioned slightly diagonally across the table so that his or her right shoulder comes in contact with your leg and thigh.

1. Grasp the patient's right elbow with your left hand and hold the patient's right wrist with your right hand.
2. Depress the patient's shoulder girdle with your thigh.
3. Extend the patient's elbow.
4. Internally rotate the right shoulder and pronate the forearm.
5. Flex the wrist and fingers and deviate the wrist in an ulnar direction (Fig. 20.14).
6. Maintain this position as you abduct the patient's arm. (Fig. 20.15).

If symptoms are noted at any stage of ULNT 2, a goniometric measurement is taken to establish a baseline. Sensitizing and relieving maneuvers are the same as described for ULNT 1 and are listed in Table 20.4.

ULNT 3 (Ulnar Nerve Bias) The test is described for the patient's right arm. Position the patient in a supine position close to the edge of the table with the legs straight and the left arm at the side. A pillow is optional for patient comfort. Stand at the head of the table facing the patient's head.

1. Make a fist with your right hand and place it on top of your patient's right shoulder to prevent

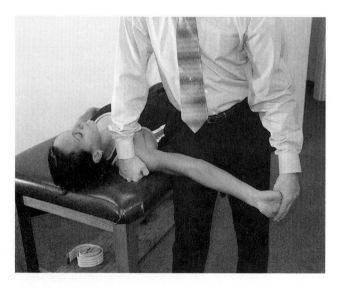

Figure 20.13 ULNT 1 (median nerve bias).

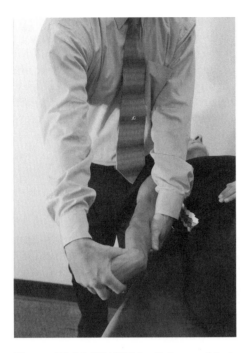

Figure 20.14 ULNT 2 (radial nerve bias).

further shoulder elevation during the technique.

2. Grasp the patient's right hand.

3. Rest your elbow on your thigh, minimizing shoulder abduction.

4. Extend the patient's wrist and fingers.

5. Pronate the forearm.

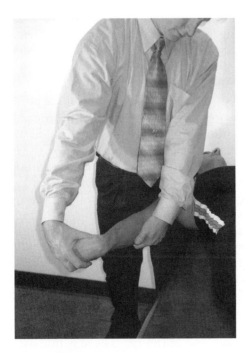

Figure 20.15 ULNT 2 (radial nerve bias).

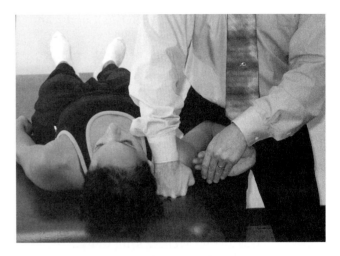

Figure 20.16 ULNT 3 (ulnar nerve bias).

6. Flex the elbow.

7. Externally rotate the shoulder.

8. Use your fisted right hand to depress the shoulder girdle (Fig. 20.16).

9. Abduct the shoulder (Fig. 20.17).

If symptoms are noted at any stage of ULNT 3, a goniometric measurement is taken to establish a baseline. Sensitizing and relieving maneuvers are the same as described for ULNT 1 and are listed in Table 20.4.

Treatment of the Container

The brachial plexus is formed from the ventral rami of C5-T1. Direct sites of potential mechanical irritation for the brachial plexus include:

1. Intervertebral foramen of the cervical spine

2. Scalene triangle

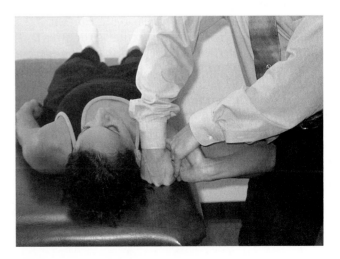

Figure 20.17 ULNT 3 (ulnar nerve bias).

3. Costoclavicular space between ribs 1 and 2 and clavicle

4. The posterior surface of the pectoralis minor

The median nerve and related vascular structures may be irritated by the following musculature: biceps brachii, pronator teres, flexor digitorum superficialis, flexor carpi radialis, and palmaris longus. All of these soft tissues are stretched during ULNT 1; however, in some cases, local myofascial techniques may be required to relieve neurovascular irritation. Dysfunction of the elbow, carpal, proximal, and distal radial ulnar joints, and interosseous membrane tightening may also cause neurovascular irritation and may require local treatment to relieve symptoms associated with a positive ULNT 1.

The radial nerve and its related vascular structures may be irritated by the following musculature: subscapularis, latissimus dorsi, teres major, all 3 heads of the triceps, brachialis, brachioradialis, and supinator. These muscles are stretched during ULNT 2; however, in some cases, local myofascial techniques may be required for relief of symptoms associated with positive ULNT 2. Dysfunction at the elbow, proximal radial ulnar joint, distal radial ulnar joint, and wrist may lead to compression and/or irritation of the radial nerve and related vascular structures. Evaluation and treatment of these joint dysfunctions may be necessary to relieve symptoms associated with a positive ULNT 2.

The ulnar nerve may be directly irritated by the following musculature: coracobrachialis, median head of the triceps, flexor carpi ulnaris, and flexor digitorum profundus. All of these soft tissues are mobilized during ULNT 3; however, in some cases, local myofascial techniques may be required to relieve neurovascular irritation. The ulnar nerve and related vascular structures may also be irritated by dysfunctions of the elbow and at the piso-hamate canal. These joints may require evaluation and treatment prior to relief of symptoms associated with a positive ULNT 3.

Other tissues may indirectly lead to irritation of the brachial plexus and related vascular structure. Dysfunction of ribs 3 to 5 and related thoracic vertebra may lead to spasm of the pectoralis minor muscle, which may cause irritation to the brachial plexus and related neurovascular structures. Disc herniation, stenotic changes, and/or dysfunction at C4-T2 may lead to irritation at C4-T1. Tightness and facilitation of the upper trapezius, levator scapula, and posterior shoulder capsule may lead to tightness and facilitation of those tissues that may result in irritation of the brachial plexus and neurovascular structures.

Upper Quarter Protocol

It is important for the examiner to ask the patient where he or she is feeling any applied manual intervention. If the patient is not feeling a stretch in the target tissue, then the examiner should not proceed with that particular technique and should move on to the next technique in the protocol described later. The following techniques are described with the patient lying on the left side or supine and can be simply reversed to evaluate and treat the corresponding tissues on the other side.

1. Posterior-to-anterior rib mobilization: With the patient positioned in left side-lying, the patient reaches forward with the right hand to expose the posterior aspect of the right rib cage. The primary ribs of concern are ribs 1 and 2, which may cause direct compression and irritation of the brachial plexus and related vascular structures, as well as ribs 3, 4, and 5, which may result in spasm of the pectoralis minor muscle, resulting in direct compression and/or irritation of the brachial plexus and related vascular structures. The anatomy of the ribs must be fully appreciated. Particular attention is paid to the fact that the ribs are not horizontal, but decline from posterior to anterior. The direction of the force must therefore be in line with this declination of each particular rib. The examiner places each thumb on the most posterior aspect of right rib 1. A springing maneuver is then applied from posterior to anterior, following the normal declination of the rib. An assessment is made as to whether the rib has mobility. It is not uncommon to find hypomobility of the entire mid to upper rib cage in our patient populations. If hypomobility is detected, the examiner then applies a gentle oscillating, posterior-to-anterior mobilization in the plane of the rib. These gentle oscillations continue until an improvement in mobility is detected. The same evaluative and treatment processes are conducted for ribs 2, 3, 4, and 5 (Fig. 20.18).

2. Anterior-to-posterior rib mobilization: The patient is lying on his or her left side. Have the patient place the right knee on the table, the right hand behind the head, and ask the patient to rotate the trunk backward as far as is comfortable while maintaining the right knee on the table. The examiner then uses each thumb along the costal aspect of the costochondral junction of rib 1, assessing the joint play in an anterior-to-posterior direction, appreciating the natural inclination of the ribs from this direction. If hypomobility is detected, the examiner then applies a gentle oscillating, anterior-to-posterior mobilization in the plane of the rib. These gentle oscillations continue until an improvement in mobility is detected. The same evaluative and

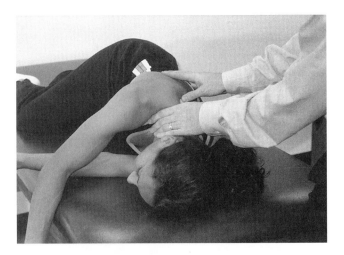

Figure 20.18 Rib mobilization—posterior-anterior.

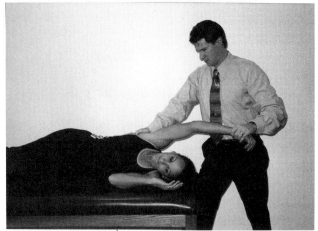

Figure 20.20 Teres major stretch.

treatment process is conducted for ribs 2, 3, 4, and 5 (Fig. 20.19).

3. Right teres major: The patient is lying on his or her left side. The patient's right scapula is retracted by the examiner's right hand. The examiner then grasps the patient's right upper extremity just proximal to the wrist, abducting the arm until a stretch is appreciated in the right scapulohumeral region. It is not uncommon for "pinching" to occur with this technique. The "pinching" may be alleviated by finding a position of comfort between the ranges of external and internal humeral rotation. This stretch is maintained until maximal lengthening has been accomplished (Fig. 20.20).

4. Left posterior shoulder capsule: The patient is lying on his or her left with the left arm abducted to 90 degrees. It is important that the left scapula is stabilized by the patient's positioning so that the left shoulder does not pro-

tract, because this will allow motion of the entire shoulder girdle and not localize it to the posterior shoulder capsule. Maintaining the elbow level with the shoulder, the patient's left arm is dynamically rotated internally to end range and back to the starting position. The dynamic on/off stretch is continued until maximal stretching has occurred. It is recommended that this stretch is performed in a dynamic on/off manner, because clinical experience has shown that static stretching of this structure evokes in patient's guarding and thus a less affect stretch (Fig. 20.21).

5. Right levator scapula/posterior scalene: The patient is lying on his or her left side. The patient is asked to tuck the left shoulder inferiorly toward the left hip as far as possible, while the head is gently rested on the table in a flexed and left side bent position. The patient's right scapula is then retracted, depressed, and

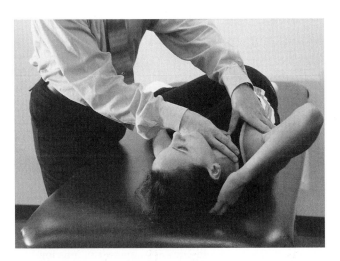

Figure 20.19 Rib mobilization—anterior-posterior.

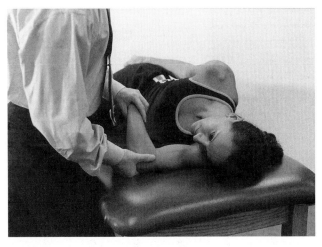

Figure 20.21 Posterior capsular stretch.

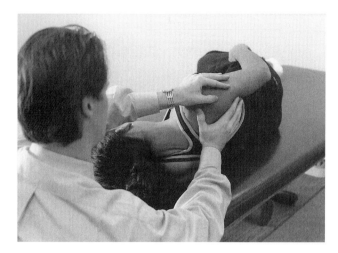

Figure 20.22 Levator scapula/posterior scalene stretch.

upwardly rotated (Fig. 20.22). A static stretch may be applied at this time. A contract/relax stretch is found to be most useful in this position, asking the patient to gently shrug the shoulder into your hands as you resist this motion. When the patient relaxes, the slack "is taken up in the tissue" and the scapula is then mobilized further into retraction, depression, and upward rotation. Once maximal gains have been met through scapular mobilization, the patient may be then asked to maintain his or her head on the table as he turns his head to the left, pausing for a second, and returning to the rest position (Fig. 20.23). When the patient resumes the initial starting position, it may then be possible to further mobilize the scapula into retraction, depression, and upward rotation. This process is continued until maximal stretching has occurred.

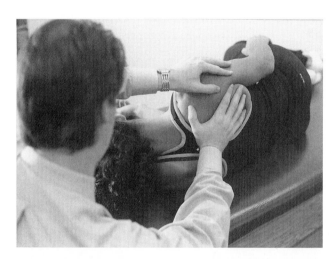

Figure 20.23 Levator scapula/posterior scalene stretch—rest position.

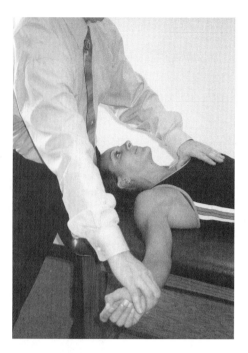

Figure 20.24 Rib mobilization—superior to inferior.

6. Superior-to-inferior right rib mobilization: The patient is placed in a supine position. The patient's right fifth rib is identified and then stabilized using the examiner's left thumb (Fig. 20.24). The examiner then grasps the patient's right upper extremity just proximal to the wrist joint and abducts the right arm in the frontal plane until tension in the tissues is appreciated (Fig. 20.25). The patient's right upper extremity is then returned to its normal rest position. This stretch is conducted in a dynamic manner to minimize any underlying adverse neural dynamic tension. This process

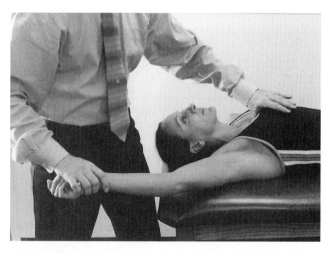

Figure 20.25 Rib mobilization—superior to inferior.

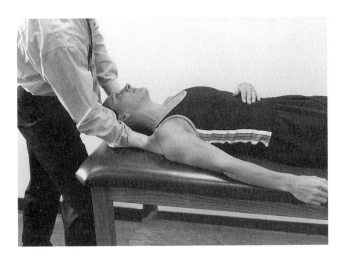

Figure 20.26 Pectoralis minor stretch.

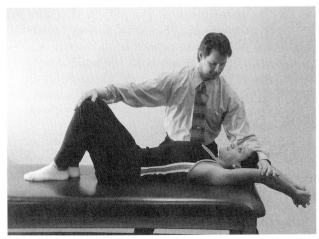

Figure 20.28 Latissimus dorsi—bilateral stretch.

is continued until maximal shoulder abduction is achieved. This process is then continued with ribs 4, 3, 2, and 1.

7. Right pectoralis minor: The patient is placed in a supine position. The patient's right scapula is passively depressed with the examiner's right hand (Fig. 20.26). The patient's right ribs 3 to 5 are identified and then depressed with the examiner's left palm. The patient's right upper extremity is then maximally elevated in the plane of the scapula (Fig. 20.27). The stretch may be provided either statically or dynamically and is continued until maximal lengthening has occurred.

8. Bilateral latissimus dorsi: The patient is placed in a supine position with the examiner at the right side of the table, facing the patient's head. The examiner's right hand is placed between the patient's right scapula and the table with the palm

facing upward as the patient's right scapula is passively depressed toward the foot of the table. The examiner then repeats this process with the patient's left scapula. This pre-positioning of the scapulae is performed to minimize the chance of shoulder impingement during this technique. The patient is then asked to clasp his hands together with elbows extended, flexing both shoulders maximally. The examiner's left arm then bridges both arms to maintain bilateral shoulder flexion (Fig. 20.28). The patient is then asked to bring his knees to his chest. The examiner then bridges the anterior surface of both legs, providing maximal hip and ultimately lumbar flexion from below (Fig. 20.29). The shoulder flexion is maintained statically, while the lower quarter is applied dynamically. This process is continued until maximal stretching has occurred.

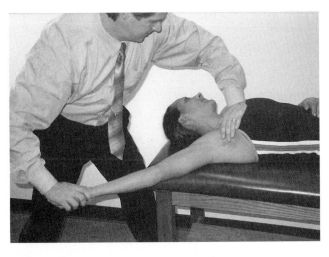

Figure 20.27 Pectoralis minor stretch.

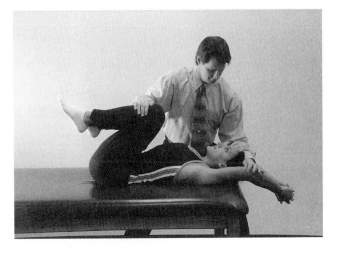

Figure 20.29 Latissimus dorsi—bilateral stretch.

9. Right upper trapezius: The patient is placed in a supine position. The patient is asked to slide to the end of the table so that the proximal portion of the scapula is off the table. The patient is then asked to abduct and externally rotate the right upper extremity with elbow flexed to 90 degrees. The examiner then uses his right hand to depress the patient's right scapula (Fig. 20.30). The patient's neck is then gently brought into flexion, left side-bending, and right rotation until a gentle stretch is appreciated (Fig. 20.31). This stretch is best performed as a contract relax technique with the patient asked to shrug his shoulder into your hand as you provide resistance, not allowing any motion to occur. On relaxation, the slack is taken up by further depressing the scapula and gently increasing cervical flexion, left side-bending, and right rotation. Another contract–relax technique that is considered useful is to ask the patient to tuck his chin in while maintaining the stretch position, followed by relaxation. On relaxation, the examiner is frequently able to further increase cervical flexion, left side-bending, and right rotation. The process is continued until maximal stretching has occurred.

10. Right sternocleidomastoid: The patient is placed in a supine position. It is important for the examiner to perform vertebral artery testing on the patient before sternocleidomastoid stretching to ensure its safe application. The patient is asked to slide to the end of the table until the proximal aspect of the scapula is just over the end. The patient's cervical spine is then passively rotated to the left. The patient's right clavicle is depressed and stabilized as the examiner slowly and gently lowers the patient's head over the edge of the table until a stretch is

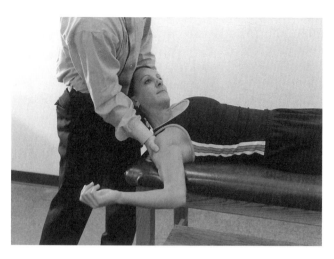

Figure 20.31 Upper trapezius stretch—finish position.

appreciated. This stretch may be maintained statically or may be performed dynamically. A contract–relax technique involves resisting clavicular elevation during deep inhalation, followed by further stretching with exhalation. The technique is continued until maximal stretching has occurred.

11. Right anterior and middle scalene: The patient is placed in a supine position. The patient is asked to slide to the edge of the table until the proximal scapula is just over the end. The examiner then uses the web space of his or her right hand to depress right ribs 1 and 2. The cervical spine is controlled anteriorly by the examiner's left shoulder placed on the patient's while the left hand firmly grasps the occiput (Fig. 20.32). The slack is taken up in the tissues in the following pattern: cervical retraction maintaining occipital flexion on C1; left cervical lateral translation, left cervical side-bending,

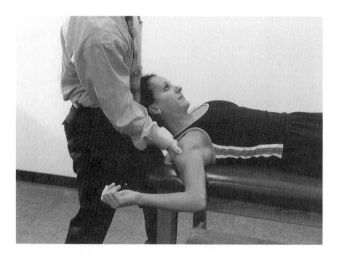

Figure 20.30 Upper trapezius stretch—start position.

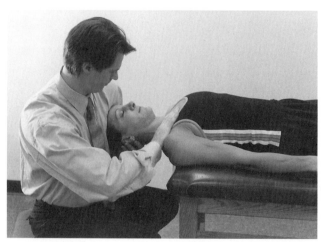

Figure 20.32 Anterior and middle scalene stretch.

and right cervical rotation (Fig. 20.33). The technique may be applied statically, dynamically, or using contract–relax by asking the patient to take a deep breath and pick the head up to look at his feet. The technique is continued until maximal stretching has occurred.

A summary of the upper quarter protocol is listed in Table 20.5.

Joint Dysfunctions

It is beyond the scope of this text to describe the specific evaluative and treatment techniques for a myriad of dysfunctions that may occur at the joints listed. They are included in this section to highlight their importance in the treatment of adverse neural dynamic tension.

Cervical and Thoracic

The C4-T1 vertebrae can cause neurovascular irritation of the ventral rami and spinal nerves of C4-T1 because of associated boney or disc pathology. Dysfunctions of the cervical spine may lead to tightness and facilitation of the scaleni, sternocleidomastoid, levator scapula, and upper trapezius musculature, which can cause neurovascular irritation. Dysfunctions of T1-T6 may result in dysfunction of ribs 1 to 5, which may also cause neurovascular irritation.

Clavicular

Dysfunction of the sternoclavicular and/or acromioclavicular joints may result in tightness and facilitation of the sternocleidomastoid, pectoralis minor,

Table 20.5 Upper Quarter Protocol for Treatment of Container for Adverse Neurodynamic Tension of Median, Radial, and Ulnar Nerves

1. Left side-lying
   a. Posterior to anterior right rib mobilization
   b. Anterior to posterior right rib mobilization
   c. Right teres major
   d. Left posterior shoulder capsule
   e. Right levator scapula/posterior scalene
2. Right side-lying
   a. Posterior to anterior left rib mobilization
   b. Anterior to posterior left rib mobilization
   c. Left teres major
   d. Right posterior shoulder capsule
   e. Left levator scapula/posterior scalene
3. Supine
   a. Superior to inferior right rib mobilization
   b. Superior to inferior left rib mobilization
   c. Right pectoralis minor
   d. Left pectoralis minor
   e. Bilateral latissimus dorsi
   f. Right upper trapezius
   g. Right upper trapezius
   h. Left sternocleidomastoid
   i. Right anterior and middle scalene
   j. Left anterior and middle scalene

*If the upper quarter protocol followed by neural mobilization fails to relieve ANDT, localized and direct treatment of precise cervical, thoracic, rib, sternoclavicular, acromioclavicular, and upper extremity joint dysfunction, as well as upper extremity myofascial dysfunctions, may be required. Based on this clinician's experience, this occurs only in a minority of cases.

trapezius, and coracobrachialis, all of which may cause neurovascular irritation.

Re-evaluation of ULNT and Neuromobilization

On evaluation and treatment of the tissues described, it is now appropriate to repeat the ULNTs. If the tests are now negative, there is no reason to apply neuromobilization techniques. If any tests remain positive, neural mobilization is indicated. This may be accomplished with either of two techniques: tensors or sliders.

A tensor is the positive base test taken to the point of the first barrier or pain provocation and then returned to the position of ease. It is described as a tensor because tension is being taken up at one end of the neural structure while the other end remains static. Conversely, a slider is the positive base test taken to the point of the first barrier or pain provocation to

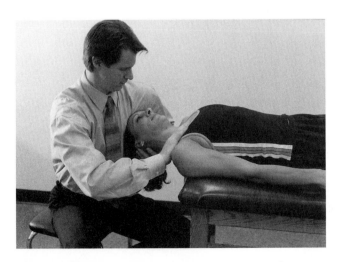

Figure 20.33 Anterior and middle scalene stretch.

increase the proximal neural tension while the cervical spine is side-bent toward the test limb to relieve the proximal neural tension. The upper extremity is then taken to the position of ease to relieve the distal neural tension while the cervical spine is side-bent away to increase the proximal neural tension. Cervical motion may be introduced either actively or passively, although passive motion is preferred to minimize cervical muscular tension. This procedure is described as a slider because the neural tissue is theorized to repeatedly slide distally then proximally as the process continues. Based on clinical experience, we recommend the use of sliders during repeated motion testing because we feel they are both safer and more effective than tensors.

If ANDT has been identified and measured, it is now appropriate to further test these structures using repeated motion testing similar to that advanced by McKenzie (see Chapter 15) (27). The process begins by identifying the positive ULNT(s) (Figs. 20.12 to 20.17). The positive ULNT is used as both the test and treatment using a slider (Figs. 20.34 to 20.39). This process is repeated for 10 repetitions. In the course of the 10 repetitions, the examiner attempts to assess the ease of the motion and whether the range is increasing or decreasing. If the range progressively decreases and/or the patient feels worse after 10 repetitions, the examiner can then infer that an inflammatory state exists and neuromobilizations are not indicated at this time. If the ROM remains the same or progressively increases and the patient reports no increase in symptoms after 10 repetitions, the examiner may infer that a restricted state exists. Neuromobilization is indicated in the presence of restricted states and treatment is performed in the same man-

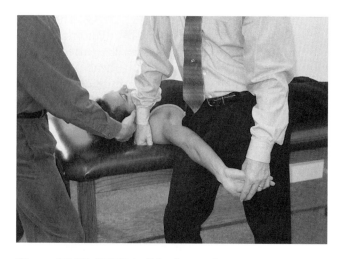

Figure 20.35 ULNT 1 slider for median nerve—on position.

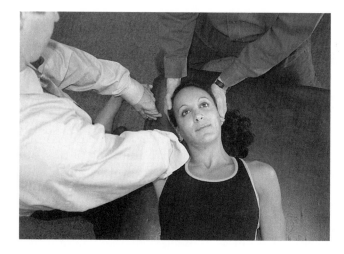

Figure 20.36 ULNT 2 slider for ulnar nerve—off position.

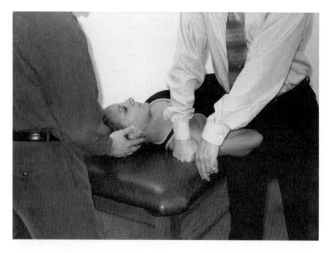

Figure 20.34 ULNT 1 slider for median nerve—off position.

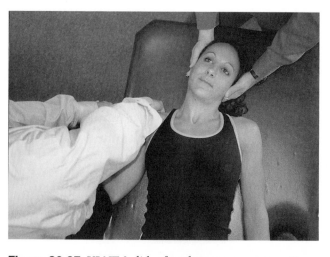

Figure 20.37 ULNT 2 slider for ulnar nerve—on position.

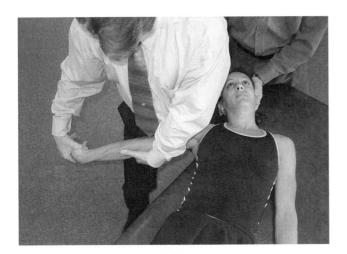

Figure 20.38 ULNT 3 slider for radial nerve—off position.

of ANDT is present after addressing the container, using on/off non-ballistic neuromobilizations can be very helpful in relieving the residual tightness or restriction in motion that is left. Incorporating functional exercises can help to maintain the correction and mobility while improving the quality of motion.

We owe a debt of gratitude to Butler and his coworkers for their groundbreaking clinical work in the assessment and treatment of ANDT, as well as their continued efforts to further refine these evaluation and treatment techniques. We hope by taking their concepts and combining the treatment techniques of joint mobilization, capsular, and muscular stretching, along with functional exercises, that we will have a more comprehensive treatment plan for patients with musculoskeletal disorders.

ner as the examination, continuing until the maximum ROM has been achieved.

■ CONCLUSION

The evaluation and treatment of ANDT is an important tool in the armamentarium of clinicians treating musculoskeletal disorders. The clinician must be able to differentiate capsular and muscular tightness patterns from ANDT. By adding sensitizing and relieving maneuvers, remembering that they are interchangeable, one can further confirm the presence or absence of ANDT. By using the concept of treating the container first, one will not be tempted to apply neuromobilization techniques before addressing and mobilizing associated joint, capsular, and muscular tightness patterns first. However, if some lesser degree

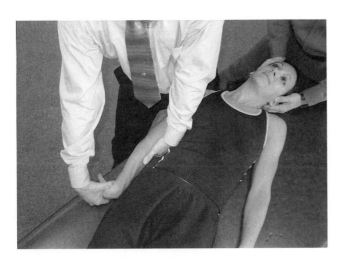

Figure 20.39 ULNT 3 slider for radial nerve—on position.

Audit Process
Self-Check of the Chapter's Learning Objectives

- Describe what a typical or atypical response is on adverse neurodynamic tension (ANDT) test.

- Define the precautions and contraindications to performing ANDT testing.

- Know how to treat the "container" before the treatment of ANDT.

- Know how to perform sliders to release ANDT.

■ REFERENCES

1. Bookhout MR, Geraci MC, Greenman PE. Exercise prescription as an adjunct to manual medicine. Course syllabus. 2001.
2. Breig A, Troup JDG. Biomechanical considerations in straight-leg-raising test: Cadaveric and clinical studies of the effects of medical hip rotation. Spine 1979;4:242–250.
3. Brody IA, Williams RH. The signs of Kernig and Brudzinski. Arch Neurol 1969;21:215.
4. Brudzinski J. A new sign of the lower extremities in meningitis of children (neck sign). Arch Neurol 1969;21:217.
5. Butler D. Mobilization of the Nervous System. Melbourne: Churchill Livingstone, 1991.
6. Butler D, Gifford L. The concept of adverse mechanical tension in the nervous systems. Physiother 1989;75:622–636.
7. Butler DS. The Sensitive Nervous System, 1st ed. Adelaide, Australia: Noigroup Publications, 2000.
8. Charnley J. Orthopedic signs in the diagnosis of disc protrusion with special reference to the straight-leg-raising test. Lancet 1951;1:186–192.
9. Cipriano JJ. Photographic Manual of Regional Orthopedic Tests. Baltimore: Williams & Wilkins, 1985.
10. Cram RH. A sign of sciatic nerve root pressure. J Bone Joint Surg Br 1953;35:192–195.

11. Deyerle WM, May VR. Sciatic tension test. South Med J 1956;49:999–1005.
12. Dommisse GF, Grobler L. Arteries and veins of the lumbar nerve roots and cauda equina. Clin Orthop 1976;115:22–29.
13. Dyck P. The femoral nerve traction test with lumbar disc protrusion. Surg Neurol 1976;6:163–166.
14. Edgar MA, Park WM. Induced pain patterns on passive straight-leg-raising in lower lumbar disc protrusion. J Bone Joint Surg Br 1974;56:658–667.
15. Elvey RL. Treatment of arm pain associated with abnormal brachial plexus tension. Aust J Physiother 1986;32:225–230.
16. Fahrni WH. Observations on straight-leg-raising with special reference to nerve root adhesions. Can J Surg 1966;9:44–48.
17. Geraci MC. Manipulations under anesthesia. In: Stanton DF, Mein EA, eds. Manual Medicine. Physical Medicine & Rehabilitation Clinics of North America. Philadelphia: W. B. Saunders & Co., 1996:910–911.
18. Goddard BS, Reid JD. Movements induced by straight-leg-raising in the lumbosacral roots, nerves, and plexus and in the intrapelvic section of the sciatic nerve. J Neurol Neurosurg Psychiatry 1965;28:12–18.
19. Hall T, Hepburn M, Elvey RL. The effect of lumbosacral posture on a modification of the straight leg raise test. Physiother 1993;79:566–570.
20. Herron LD, Pheasant HC. Prone knee-flexion provocative testing for lumbar disc protrusion. Spine 1980;5:65–67.
21. Hudgins WR. The crossed-straight-leg raising test. N Engl J Med 1977;297:1127.
22. Katznelson A, Nerubay J, Level A. Gluteal skyline (G.S.L.): A search for an objective sign in the diagnosis of disc lesions of the lower lumbar spine. Spine 1982;7:74–75.
23. Kernig W. Concerning a little noted sign of meningitis. Arch Neurol 1969;21:216.
24. Little H. The Neck and Back: The Rheumatological Physical Examination. Orlando, FL: Grune & Stratton, 1986.
25. Maitland GD. Negative disc exploration: Positive canal signs. Aust J Physiother 1979;25:129–134.
26. Maitland GD. The slump test: Examination and treatment. Aust J Physiother 1985;31:215–219.
27. McKenzie R: The Cervical and Thoracic Spine Mechanical Diagnosis and Therapy. Waikanae, New Zealand. Spinal Publications 1990.
28. Palmer ML, Epler M. Clinical Assessment Procedures in Physical Therapy. Philadelphia: J. B. Lippincott, 1990.
29. Philip K, Lew P, Matyas TA. The inter-therapist reliability of the slump test. Aust J Physiother 1989;35:89–94.
30. Postacchini F, Cinotti G, Gumina S. The knee flexion test: A new test for lumbosacral root torsion. J Bone Joint Surg Br 1993;75:834–835.
31. Rask M. Knee flexion test and sciatica. Clin Orthop 1978;134:221.
32. Scham SM, Taylor TKF. Tension signs in lumbar disc prolapse. Clin Orthop 1971;75:195–204.
33. Shacklock M. Neurodynamics. Physiother 1995;81:9–16.
34. Shacklock M, Butler D, Slater H. The dynamic central nervous system: Structure and clinical neurobiomechanics. In: Boyling JD, Palastanga N, eds. Grieve's Modern Manual Therapy: The Vertebral Column, 2nd ed. Edinburgh: Churchill Livingstone, 1994.
35. Slater H, Butler D, Shackloch M. Mobilization of the nervous system. Level-II: Clinical and pain sciences development: Part of a neuro-orthopedic approach. Course syllabus. 1996–1997.
36. Slater H, Butler D, Shackloch M. Mobilization of the nervous system. Initial course: Part of a neuro-orthopedic approach. Course syllabus. 1994–1995.
37. Slater H, Butler DS, Shacklock MD. The dynamic central nervous systems: Examination and assessment using tension tests. In: Boyling JD, Palastanga N, eds. Grieve's Modern Manual Therapy: The Vertebral Column, 2nd ed. Edinburgh: Churchill Livingstone, 1994.
38. Spengler DM. Low Back Pain: Assessment and Management. Orlando, FL: Grune & Stratton, 1982.
39. Urban LM. The straight-leg-raising test: A review. J Orthop Sports Phys Ther 1981;2:117–133.
40. Wartenberg R. The signs of Brudzinski and of Kernig. J Pediatr 1950;37:679–684.
41. Wilkins RH, Brody IA. Lasègue's sign. Arch Neurol 1969;21:219–220.
42. Woodhall R, Hayes GJ. The well-leg-raising test of Fajersztajn in the diagnosis of ruptured lumbar intervertebral disc. J Bone Joint Surg Am 1950;32:786–792.

21

Manipulation Techniques for Key Joints

George DeFranca

Learning Objectives

On completion of this chapter, you should be able to:

- Understand joint manipulation and its use in treating locomotor disturbances.
- Become aware of the barrier concept and the release phenomenon.
- Appreciate the reflex nature of the nervous system and its role in manipulative therapy.
- Become aware of clinically observed chain reactions and their key links.
- List contraindications to manipulative therapy.
- Be aware of the manipulative treatment of key joints commonly involved in disturbance of the locomotor system.

Introduction

Writing a chapter based solely on manipulation carries the risk of having the reader take the information out of context, thinking that treating functional disturbances of the locomotor system only involves manipulating joints. Conversely, observing firsthand the powerful effects of manipulation can seduce one into believing that it is all one needs to do. The manipulation and mobilization of joints has captured the interest of a variety of healers, doctors, and therapists for hundreds of years in their quest to treat a diversity of musculoskeletal pain syndromes. No doubt many of them have become seduced, if not enamored, by the allure of manipulative therapy's effectiveness. However, it is very short-sighted to think that using only one modality can treat an entity as diverse and complex as the locomotor system. This is especially so when dealing with the chronic patient population in which biomechanical compensations, muscular imbalances with their resultant altered movement patterns, global reaction of the locomotor system, and regional deconditioning dwarf the role of articular dysfunction. This chapter will hopefully be read with this in mind as the use of manipulation in dealing with a variety of key locomotor dysfunctions is discussed.

Manipulation

A distinction between "thrust versus non-thrust" techniques is often made; however, this terminology carries negative implications. Whereas thrust techniques refer specifically to joint manipulations, non-thrust techniques refer to mobilizations. Unfortunately, manipulation has been given a negative connotation by some, being described as too rough and even dangerous. Although its improper use can lead to such descriptions, it is inherently safe and its intended use is very effective at reducing pain and changing function throughout the locomotor system.

The term "thrust" should be used reservedly. It implies the use of force and gross movements, neither of which should characterize a therapeutic manipulation. Triano discusses in depth the mechanics of a manipulation and the reader is referred there for an excellent discussion on the topic.[37] Basically, joint manipulations are characterized by a sudden, impulse-like movement that takes a joint beyond its paraphysiological barrier and is usually associated with a click noise. The sudden movement is beyond the control of the patient, a situation that necessitates the utmost in patient relaxation and clinician control. Mobilizations entail oscillations or tractional movements that coax motion. They are slower and remain under the control of the patient.

Manipulation is a skillful art that demands much training and experience to become proficient in its use. A weekend course in manual technique does not qualify someone to perform expert manipulations anymore than singing in the shower prepares one for a concert tour. Manipulative therapy demands practice, experience, and ability.

Manipulation is performed to restore joint play at dysfunctional joints. It is thought to work by: 1) releasing entrapped synovial folds or plica; 2) relaxing hypertonic muscles; and 3) disrupting articular or periarticular adhesions.[35] Fibrosis of the periarticular tissues can be a result of trauma and inflammation, immobilization, and degenerative joint disease.

The Manipulable Lesion

Various terms describe the manipulable lesion. Gatterman discusses more than 100 terms related to spinal manipulable lesions.[12] Among these are subluxation, joint dysfunction, somatic dysfunction, fixation, joint blockage, and segmental dyskinesia. A variety of factors characterize a manipulable lesion, yet most of its underpinnings are unfortunately hypothetical.[7,37] Typically, static and dynamic mechanical dysfunctions create local inflammatory and biomechanical changes. In addition, remote functional and pathological changes in the locomotor system occur.

However, because manipulation is a force that imparts mobility, this characteristic of joint and soft tissue lesions should at least be taken into consideration. Yet lack of mobility alone is not a reliable criterion for technique selection. Subjective pain provocation was found to be a more accurate assessment.[19] In this regard, decreased regional and intersegmental motion should be looked for, especially in the presence of pain via provocative testing. Included with this is joint dysfunction, a painful loss of joint play, a central feature of the manipulable lesion according to Mennell.[30] A positive response to manipulative treatment is a logical but not too often thought of characteristic of the manipulable lesion.

Soft tissue changes such as thickening or atrophy of the periarticular tissues can be present and represent reflexogenic changes to segmental dysfunction. An interesting clinical observation is the disappearance of painful soft tissue changes after manipulation of the offending dysfunction. This can occur so quickly that a reflex etiology, versus an inflammatory cause, seems plausible. Pain and localized skin hypersensitivity also characterize the manipulable lesion, as does muscle spasm, especially if localized, and muscle imbalances. Myotendinoses, myosis, and attachment tendinosis represent painful reflex changes within the muscle, muscle belly, and attachment points of tendons or musculotendinous junctions, respectively.[8]

Joint Signs and Tension and Pain

What guides the practitioner in the use of manual techniques is the presence of "joint signs."[29] These are pain, restriction of motion, and spasm. Pain and tension form the vocabulary of the locomotor system, allowing it to convey its message of dysfunction. The locomotor system speaks to us softly, rarely shouting its message. It is the astute observer that will listen, look, and feel. Fortunately, the system usually communicates in a consistent and logical manner. Thus, to comprehend the locomotor system's language, we need to understand the relationship of tension and pain, the phenomenon of chain reaction patterns, and the reflex nature of the neuro-locomotor system.

Tension in the locomotor system is usually associated with pain—be it in a muscle, joint, or periosteal insertion points of muscles, ligaments ("pain" points), skin, or fascia. See Table 21.1 for a list of commonly found pain points. It represents the locomotor system's attempt to protect itself from a nociceptive stimulus. Tension is manifested in muscles as increased tone, spasm, or overactivity. Tension in joints pertains to joint dysfunction, that is, a lack of joint play with pain on testing motion. Skin, periosteal pain points, fascia, and even scars can palpate as tense, thickened, and painful structures. If you can identify and release tension in the locomotor system via the appropriate modality, function can be restored and pain can be reduced or eradicated. Mobilization or manipulation of joints and the stretching of tight, overactive muscles releases tension not only in the respective joints and muscles but also in their related periosteal insertion points. In addition, stretching and releasing tension in skin, scar tissue, fascia, and even viscera can have reflex effects on the rest of the locomotor system, resulting in changed function.

Pain can arise from tissue damage, inflammation, and pathoanatomy; however, with functional locomotor disturbances pain is perceived as a result of poor function. Tension anywhere in the system and improper function alone can trigger pain, the pain of dysfunction. This pain is not inflammatory but reflex in nature and can trigger various reflex responses in the entire locomotor system. Therefore, it is commonly observed that when tension and dysfunction are appropriately treated, pain diminishes or disappears immediately. Inflammatory pain does not.

Pre-Manipulative Provocative Testing

Before any manipulative thrust, a pre-manipulative provocative test should be conducted to assess for patient tolerance and pain and also to acquaint the patient with the technique to be used.[3] The manipulative technique is set-up with complete slack removal, yet a thrust is not delivered. During the technique's "dry run," an assessment is made as to patient comfort and their ability to relax as the joint in question is preloaded. The clinician also assesses his or her ability to properly set-up the technique and to gain a sense about the amount of slack that needs to be taken up. If no problems are encountered with this pre-manipulative maneuver, an actual manipulation set-up can then be made and a thrust safely attempted. Evidence of pain or the inability of the patient to relax mandates the alteration of technique administration. Submaximal manipulation or mobilization may then be used.

Post-Manipulation Side-Effects

Post-manipulative side-effects are common but relatively minor when compared to the more serious yet rare complications that can arise from manipulation.[16,34] The most common side effects encountered

---

Table 21.1 Common Pain Points: Areas of Painful Thickenings and Tension at Attachment Points Caused by Reflex Locomotor Disturbances or Related Local Joint and Muscle Dysfunctions

Nuchal line	Rib angles
Posterior arch of atlas	Xiphoid process
Tip of C1 transverse process	Pubic symphysis
Spinous processes	Iliac crest
Medial clavicle	Ischial tuberosity
Hyoid bone	Fibular head
Sternocostal joints	Calcaneus
Humeral epicondyles	Adductor tubercle
Styloid process	Pes anserine insertion

entailed local discomfort, radiating discomfort, headache, and fatigue, especially when the cervical and thoracic spine is manipulated. These can be predicted to some degree (Table 21.2). Senstad et al studied more than 1000 patients undergoing more than 4700 treatments and observed some predictors to the more common side effects of spinal manipulation mentioned.[34] Uncommon reactions such as dizziness and nausea were not associated with any specific predictors. Contraindications to manipulative therapy must always be kept in mind (Table 21.3).[15]

In their study, Senstad et al found that when only the thoracic spine was manipulated, more patients reported side effects than when the other spinal regions were solely treated.[34] Headaches were the most common side effect from cervical and thoracic spine manipulations. They also observed that the number of reactions increased as the number of spinal regions treated was increased from one to three. Younger subjects (27–46 years) were more likely to experience reactions when compared to older subjects (47–64 years). Women reacted adversely more commonly than men and more reactions were observed after the first two treatment sessions, but especially the first.

Because of these observations, one should be careful to limit treatment to one area on the first treatment session especially in younger women. Most importantly, force should not be substituted for skill, nor should there be a quest to satisfy the neurotic need to hear an audible click by either clinician or patient. One should keep in mind that 85% of these reactions are only mild to moderate in nature and that 74% are transient, disappearing within 24 hours.[34]

Axen et al[1] showed that low back pain patients who demonstrated the most favorable response to chiropractic manipulative treatment were those who reported immediate improvement after the first visit. Those patients that did not show early improvement did not respond favorably. Flynn et al[9] identified a clinical prediction rule whereby low back pain patients who responded favorably to manipulation had four out of five variables present (Table 21.4).

Table 21.2 Predictors of Adverse Reactions to Manipulative Therapy (Senstaad. LeBoeuf)

Female gender
Younger (27–46 years) vs. older (47–64 years)
First treatment
Thoracic spine treatment had greatest number of reported reactions
Cervical and thoracic spine when only one area treated (more than lumbar)

Table 21.3 Contraindications for Manipulative Therapy (12)

Relative contraindications

Acute disc herniation
Osteopenia
Spondyloarthopathy
Patient on anticoagulant medication
Bleeding disorders
Psychologic overlay
Hypermobility

Absolute contraindications

Progressive neurologic deficit
Destructive lesions, malignancies
Acute myelopathy
Unstable os odontoideum
Healing fracture/dislocation
Avascular necrosis
Bone infection
Segmental instability
Cauda equina syndrome
Large abdominal aortic aneurysm
Referred visceral pain
Long-term repeated manipulation with symptom relief lasting less than 1 day
Recognized secondary gain/malingering

The most important of these was the duration of symptoms being less than 16 days.

Reflex Nature of the Nervous System

It is also important to realize the reflex nature of the locomotor system by virtue of the nervous system. In this regard, the locomotor system should be considered as part of a "neuro-locomotor system" to accentuate the importance of the nervous system's input to its function. Aside from increasing mobility in restricted joints, manipulation affords a powerful means with which to reflexly stimulate the locomotor system globally. Afferent inputs from joints, muscles, skin, fascia, scars, and viscera can trigger local and/or remote reactions via direct or indirect nervous system connections. Therefore, the locomotor system can be affected by inputs from any one of these tissues by a variety of therapeutic modalities, some being more effective than others. The locomotor system, being totally interrelated and integrated neurologically, responds globally, not only locally, to any afferent input.[20,23] Joint manipulation of dysfunctional articulations affords a very powerful way to stimulate the neuro-locomotor system. The ner-

Table 21.4 Variables for Clinical Prediction Rule for Favorable Outcome of Manipulation

Duration of symptoms less than 16 days
Fear–Avoidance Belief Questionnaire work subscale
  score less than 19
At least one hip joint with less than 35 degrees of
  internal rotation
Lumbar spine segmental hypomobility
No symptoms distal to the knee

vous system relies on input from receptors, particularly those in the spine, pelvis, and periphery. These receptors yield direct information of the environment that we interface with. Key regions of proprioceptive input are the feet, pelvis, and upper cervical spine. It is no wonder why these areas are often the sites of treatment.

Reflex neuromuscular effects as a consequence to manipulation have been observed clinically and experimentally. Manipulation of the human spine and pelvis has been shown to cause electromyographic signals in the neck, back, and limb musculature.[17] Cervical manipulations caused responses in the neck and back muscles but not in the limbs. Thoracic manipulations caused responses throughout the entire back musculature and ipsilateral upper limb in the latissimus dorsi. Lumbar and sacroiliac manipulations caused responses in the entire back musculature and both upper and lower limb.

Chain Reactions

The locomotor system "thinks" in terms of function and its individual parts are integrated to work as a system. No part functions in isolation but rather is intimately linked to the entire locomotor system. Muscles and joints normally function together in groups, forming patterns of activation that create purposeful movements or stabilization. This occurs under the volitional direction of the nervous system or via involuntary reflex mechanisms. This is hardwired into the system. For instance, every muscle, joint, and related attachment point involved in the stance phase of gait is activated in a chain reaction fashion in a particular sequence.[22,24] These are the same joints and muscles that function in one-legged stance from heel strike to toe-off (Fig. 21.1). During the swing phase of gait, a different set of muscles and joints become activated as a functional myotatic unit (Fig. 21.2). Each link in the lower extremity kinetic chain functions within the confines of an integrated unit, one affecting the other.

The typical chain reactions found in the upper quarter, cervical spine, and upper thoracic spine can be organized into two main groups according to how they can be assessed clinically. The first group is named "C0-1: SCM: Scalene," whereas the second is named "C2-3: Levator: Trapezius."[3] Both chains can interrelate and make for a very confusing picture.

The C0-1: SCM: Scalene pattern involves the anterior aspect of the neck and trunk generally and is named after the major joint dysfunctions and muscle patterns of hypertonicity commonly observed (Fig. 21.3). The pectoral muscles are usually involved and together with the scalene muscles cause rib joint dysfunction and pain. The patient usually exhibits poor breathing patterns, headaches, neck pains, and a head-forward posture.

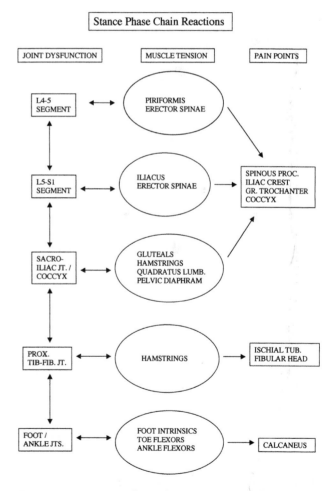

Figure 21.1 Stance phase chain reactions. Related joint dysfunctions, muscle tension, and associated pain points (attachment points) associated with the stance phase of gait. Note: chain reaction spans lower two lumbar levels/ sacroiliac joint to foot. Pain is posterior-lateral and posterior to ankle or heel.

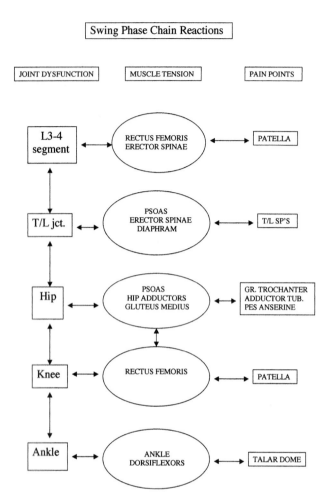

Figure 21.2 Swing phase chain reactions. Related joint dysfunctions, muscle tension, and associated pain points (attachment points) associated with the swing phase of gait. Note: chain reaction involves thoracolumbar, mid-lumbar, and even upper cervical segments together with hip and knee joints. Pain is anteriorly placed.

related dysfunctions. These chain reactions seem to follow the tenets of biomechanics, anatomy, and neurophysiology. In addition, certain articulations in the spine and extremities appear as key links in these chains that can trigger, support, or, with treatment, collapse their existence.

Key Links

Key links often occur at critical anatomical areas such as spinal transitional areas, areas of high innervation and control (craniocervical region, pelvis, and feet), are usually chronically dysfunctional (often clinically "silent"), or can commonly occur at the most distal link in kinematic chains. A key link maximally forces the locomotor system to compensate to its presence. Thickened and firm periarticular soft tissues are manifestations of chronic tissue changes. Substantially shortened and tight muscles or very

The C2-3: Levator: **Trapezius** pattern generally affects the posterior aspect of the body and is also associated with a head-forward posture, neck pain, and shoulder pain (Fig. 21.4). In addition, poor scapular control is usually a dominant issue. This pattern also can intermingle with this chain pattern.

Just as joints and muscles are programmed to function in groups, they can also become dysfunctional in groups in chain reaction-like fashion.[9,18–20, 20,23] When assessing and treating patients with disturbances of the locomotor system, it becomes readily apparent that these patterns of joint and muscle dysfunctions appear with an intriguing consistency (Table 21.5). This occurs so regularly that the finding of one dysfunction should lead the examiner to search for other

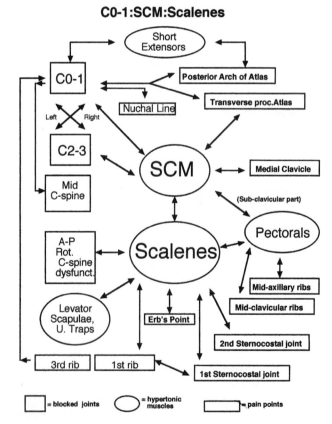

Figure 21.3 C0-1: SCM: Scalene chain reaction. Related joint and muscle dysfunctions with associated pain points (attachment points). Dysfunctions are anteriorly placed and blend with flexor–synergy muscles of upper extremity.

C2:Levator:Trapezius

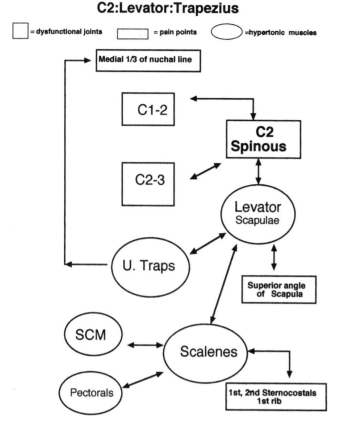

Figure 21.4 C2-3: Levator: Trapezius chain reaction. Related joint and muscle dysfunctions with associated pain points (attachment points). Dysfunctions are posteriorly places and blend with extensor-synergy muscles of upper extremity.

weak and inhibited muscles with atrophy are also important findings. For example, an asymptomatic yet dysfunctional cervicothoracic segment that is incredibly stiff with chronic soft tissue changes and a board-like lack of mobility can foster upper extremity pain syndromes. The upper extremity pain often draws the attention away from the underlying problem and a painful wrist or shoulder can be unsuccessfully treated for weeks or even months. Only when the cervicothoracic region is treated does the condition resolve. There can also be more than one key link activating the chain of dysfunctions.

Barrier Concept

When joints are moved beyond their neutral position, a slight resistance can be felt at some point. The barrier concept pertains to the normal or abnormal resistance to joint or soft tissue movement within their range of motion. It was originally described in the osteopathic literature as it pertained to articular motion. However, it is also observed in the gliding movements of soft tissues such as skin, subcutaneous tissue, fascia, muscle, and periosteal points near bone.

The barrier to motion can be physiologic or pathologic. Lewit defines the physiologic barrier as the first normal resistance to motion away from the neutral position of joints or soft tissues (Fig. 21.5).[24,25] This is common to the movement of all joints and soft tissues. It is very subtle, has a slight springy end feel, and its resistance is sensed gradually rather than

Table 21.5 Muscle–Joint Correlations: Tension in the Following Muscles Often Correlates With Joint Dysfunction in the Related Joint Listed

Muscle	Joint
SCM	C0-1, C2-3
Suboccipitals	C0-1
Scalenes	Mid and lower cervicals, upper two ribs
Levator scapulae	C1-2, C2-3
Pectorals	Upper ribs
Subscapularis	Glenohumeral joint
Psoas	T/L, hip joint
Quadratus lumborum	T/L
Rectus femoris	L3-4, hip, patellofemoral joint
Hip adductors	Hip, pubic symphysis
Piriformis	L4-5, coccyx
Iliacus	L5-1, coccyx
Biceps femoris	L5-1, sacroiliac joint, proximal tibiofibular joint

Adapted from Lewit (24) with permission from Butterworth-Heinemann.

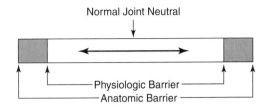

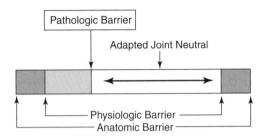

Figure 21.5 Barrier concept (19).

abruptly. Further movement into the range of motion will stretch and deform the soft tissue restraints until the anatomic limit of motion is reached, such as capsuloligamentous structures or bone-on-bone contact. The anatomic limit is not reached during normal active movements and is only engaged with passive over pressure. An elastic barrier is also present, being situated between the passive range and anatomic limit of a joint's motion. It is this barrier that is transgressed during manipulation, resulting in a click noise as the paraphysiologic space is entered.

A pathologic barrier occurs when resistance to movement is felt prematurely in the range. This is usually the case when dysfunction causes joint or soft tissue tension. In addition, a qualitative change in the barrier from a normal gradual springy nature to an abrupt end feel occurs. Little springing can be felt, whether in a joint or soft tissue structure. Being able to engage and release pathological barriers in joints and soft tissues is key in assessing and treating locomotor system dysfunctions.

Release Phenomenon

A characteristic of barriers is that they will release with mobilization, manipulation, or just a light sustained pressure being held against it for a few seconds. The barrier is then extended further into the joint's range of motion with a resultant increase in joint and muscle function. If the barrier concerns a soft tissue structure, it will yield on release. Abnormal resistance to passive movement of these tissues could be treated by simply engaging the barrier and waiting for tension to release in a matter of seconds.

This release in tension would result in not only decreased local pain but also remote reflex changes observed elsewhere in the locomotor system.

Manipulation Techniques

There are many fine techniques used to manipulate joints and only the more common ones are discussed in this chapter. The following section addresses techniques used to manipulate dysfunctions in the spinal transitional areas, pelvis, and foot/ankle joints. Unless otherwise stated, all joint manipulations explained in the following section describe manipulation of the right-sided articulation.

Post-Isometric Relaxation[24-26]

Post-isometric relaxation (PIR) is a gentle yet effective procedure used to mobilize restricted joints or release tension in soft tissue structures. It involves first taking a joint or soft tissue structure to its pathologic barrier. A light 10-second isometric contraction away from the barrier held by the patient is then resisted by the clinician. Respiratory and visual synkinesis can be used to enhance the inhibitory effect on the muscular system (see chapter 20). On relaxation, the key aspect of the procedure, an increase in joint or soft tissue mobility is observed, and the joint or soft tissue is taken to the next barrier. This affords a very safe, painless, and effective way to mobilize joints and soft tissues and can be used for any technique described in this chapter instead of a manipulative thrust.

Spinal Transitional Areas

The spinal transitional areas include the craniocervical, cervicodorsal, thoracolumbar, and lumbosacral regions. These are the areas where anatomy and function transition from one region of the spine into another. They are areas of biomechanical strain and are subsequently fertile soil in which key dysfunctions can develop.

Craniocervical Region

The craniocervical region is where the head is balanced on the neck and powerful mechanoreceptor influence resides. It includes the C0-1, C1-2, and C2-3 joints. Dysfunction here creates muscle tone changes commonly seen throughout the spine and locomotor system and is commonly associated with head and even face pain. One of the most important regions to assess and manipulate in the entire human spine when treating locomotor disturbances is the upper cervical area. It is rich in somatosensory input to the central nervous system and is associated with many reflexogenic affects on the entire locomotor system. Temporomandibular joint dysfunction is often associated with cervicocranial problems as are problems of equilibrium. Almost half of all cervical rotation takes place at one level, the atlantodental joint. The upper cervical spine's biomechanical importance is reflected by the fact that an entire branch of clinical chiropractic practice pays attention solely to it at the exclusion of other areas. Clinicians experienced in spinal joint manipulation frequently observe changes in subjective symptoms and objective signs occurring distant from the site of treatment. This is often profoundly observed when treating the upper cervical region.

Occipital-Atlantal Joint (Figs. 21.6 to 21.9)

Occipital-atlantal joint dysfunction is characterized by pain and stiffness over the joint found midway between the midline and the tip of the atlas transverse process. Soft tissue thickening is commonly palpated. Radiating pain can also be elicited. Subjective symptoms include upper neck pain and headaches. Pain referral to the eye or retro-orbitally is common, as is a sense of disequilibrium. A firm block to movement palpation in the suboccipital region is felt during a scan examination and joint restrictions can be found in both posterior-to-anterior and anterior-to-posterior rotations, lateral flexion, flexion, and anterior glide using specific passive segmental palpation techniques. Interestingly, rotation and lateral flexion are often restricted to the left, although bilateral restriction can occur. The left occipital-

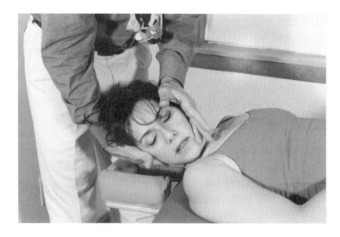

Figure 21.7 Occipital rotation manipulation. Occiput is rotated and laterally flexed on the upper cervical spine. Chin is pressed toward acromioclavicular joint. Pressure is on the zygomatic process and not mandible.

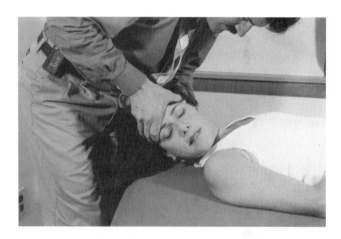

Figure 21.8 C0-1 Lateral flexion manipulation. Cervical rotation locks upper cervical joints and subtle lateral flexion movement is localized to occipital-atlantal joint with both hands.

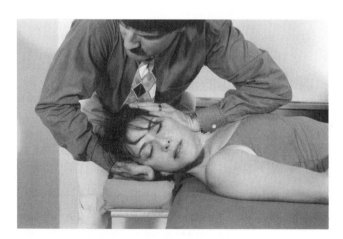

Figure 21.6 Occipital lift. Manipulation is a combination of rotation, lateral flexion, and axial traction. Rotation should not be maximal.

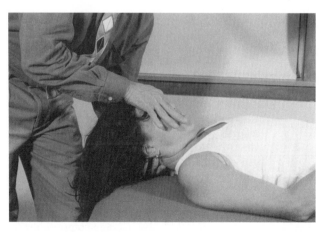

Figure 21.9 C0-1 Flexion mobilization. Atlas vertebra is stabilized by forefinger and thumb of inferior hand while superior hand mobilizes occiput with forehead contact.

atlantal joint is frequently involved, evidenced by tender thickened soft tissues overlying it. In addition, dysfunction of any of the upper three ribs, but especially the third, is commonly associated with occipital-atlantal joint dysfunction.

Muscle tension is typically found in the suboccipital and upper part of the sternocleidomastoid muscles. Pain on palpation can be elicited along the lateral one-half of the nuchal line and medial aspect of the clavicle, i.e., the origin and insertion of the sternocleidomastoid. The posterior arch of atlas may be tender because of suboccipital muscle tension and the tip of the atlas may also be painful.

Motion assessment of the occipital-atlantal joint entails observing the relationship between the transverse process of atlas, mastoid process, and angle of the jaw during test movements.[3] The small sulcus just anterior to the atlas transverse process is also used to assess changing relationships between the atlas and occiput. The test movements include end-range motion in rotation, lateral flexion, anterior glide, and flexion. It is critical to maintain the entire spine in a neutral position when assessing the cervical spine's mobility. Sitting with a slumped and kyphotic lumbar spine will create postural tension and falsely induce cervical joint restrictions.

Atlantoaxial and C2-3 Joints (Figs. 21.10 to 21.13)

Half of all cervical spine rotation takes place at one level—the atlantoaxial joint. Therefore, loss of rotational motion here forces the rest of the cervical spine to compensate for it. Headache is a common feature in joint blockage at this level, as is neck pain.

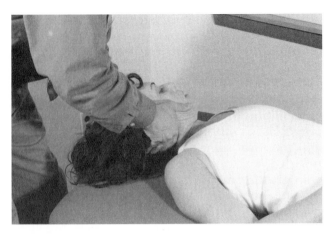

Figure 21.11 Manipulation C1-2, C2-3 in lateral flexion. The primary motion of lateral flexion is taken out with slight rotation added.

The C2-3 facet joint is one of the more common joint blockages in the cervical spine and is often the cause of an acute stiff and painful neck, the infamous wryneck. A common pain point seen with this dysfunction is also the lateral aspect of the C2 spinous. The facet joint palpates with restriction and painful thickening of the joint capsule. Muscle tension and trigger points can be found in the upper fibers of the sternocleidomastoid and trapezius muscles as well as the levator scapulae. Rotation and lateral flexion are usually blocked to the right with the right facet joint more frequently involved. Interestingly, Jirout has shown that when the chin is retracted into the neck while rotation is performed, any resultant restriction can be specifically localized to the C2-3 joint.[18] Interestingly, the contralateral occipital-atlantal joint is

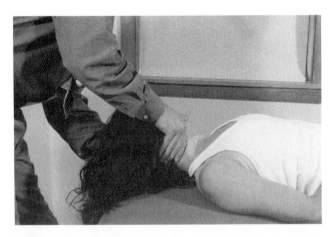

Figure 21.10 Manipulation C1-2, C2-3 in rotation. Primary motion of rotation is taken out at level of manipulation being sure not to rotate fully. Slight lateral flexion is added to bring joint to further tension.

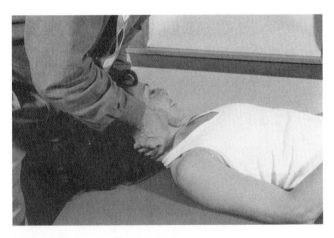

Figure 21.12 Flexion manipulation C2,3. Contact is made on the anterior aspect of the motion segment with index contact. Flexion is localized only to the level involved. Lower cervical segments entail more flexion than the upper segments.

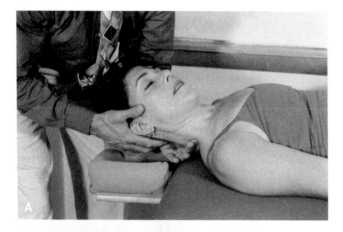

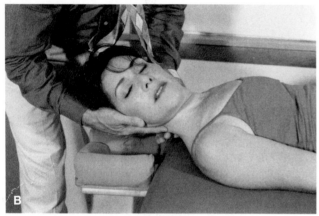

Figure 21.13 Anterior-to-posterior rotation manipulation C2-3. **(A)** Note the soft tissue pull of the lower anterior cervical skin and soft tissues by the clinician's left finger pulling from underneath and from the opposite side. **(B)** Soft tissue tension is maintained via the left index finger and a rotational pull move is performed to create an anterior-to-posterior manipulative force at the right C5,6 segment.

commonly associated with a painfully blocked C2-3 joint dysfunction.

Anterior-to-posterior rotation and lower cervical segmental flexion dysfunctions are commonly found with cervicobrachial conditions, ipsilateral upper extremity disorders, and side of handedness. A common clinical finding is a firm, painful end feel during flexion or rotation (anterior to posterior) over the C5 and C6 levels, especially with cervicobrachial conditions and ipsilateral upper extremity disorders. Movement restriction is commonly found on the side of handedness. Firm pressure applied to the anterolateral aspect of the lower cervical motion segments often elicits referred pain onto the upper anterior chest wall, upper arm, and/or upper back medial to the scapula- the so-called doorbell sign. Maigne[28] mentions that this upper back pain of cervical origin is quite consistent

and regularly found 2 cm lateral to the T5 and T6 spinous processes.[18] Scalene and pectoral muscle tension is commonly associated with anterior-to-posterior rotation and flexion dysfunctions.

Anterior-to-posterior rotational joint dysfunctions are commonly present, yet clinical awareness of their existence is often lacking. As a consequence, their presence is very often overlooked. These joint dysfunctions in the upper cervical segments are commonly associated with sore throats, especially in children. In the lower segments they are often found in conjunction with chronic upper cervical joint dysfunctions, upper extremity pain syndromes, scalene muscle trigger points, and thoracic outlet conditions. Pain from these lower cervical anterior-to-posterior rotation dysfunctions often causes pain in the medial scapular region, upper extremity, or anterior superior chest wall. Faye mentions a curious finding of the elicitation of a cough reflex when testing for this type of dysfunction at the atlas transverse process.[32]

Cervicodorsal Region (C6-T2) and Upper Ribs

The cervicodorsal region is where the mobile cervical spine transitions into the relatively immobile upper thoracic spine. In addition, powerful muscles link the cervical and upper thoracic spines, shoulder girdle, and upper ribs. The deep neck flexors originate on the cervical spine and insert as far down as the third thoracic segment. The cranial and cervical attachments of the deep extensors insert as far down as the sixth and even seventh thoracic segment. The iliocostalis cervicis links the ribs three through six to the mid and lower cervical spine. The scalene muscles link the cervical spine with the upper two and sometimes three ribs and the sternocleidomastoid muscle links the cervical spine with the sternum.

Movements of the upper extremity, by virtue of muscular attachments and function, influence this region heavily. This area is rich in chain reaction formations by virtue of its anatomical and biomechanical links. In addition, rib joint function of the upper three ribs must be considered.

Cervicodorsal joint dysfunction is often associated with upper extremity pain syndromes, especially those of the shoulder and wrist. Muscles commonly found to be in tension are the pectorals, subscapularis, sternocleidomastoid, scalenes, and upper and middle fibers of the trapezius, and levator scapulae.

This area is commonly stiff with soft tissue thickening present and in some cases being associated with a Dowager's hump appearance. A chronic forward-head posture, tight pectoral muscles and rounded shoulders, restricted upper rib articulations, and cervicodorsal spinal joint dysfunctions are commonly found together. In these cases, extension of only the upper cervical spine is often observed when backward bending of the neck and upper back is attempted.

Painful soft tissue thickenings are often observed segmentally and close observation will reveal that they occur unilateral to the side of facet joint dysfunction. The overlying skin will be painfully adherent to the spine, as is evidenced by restricted skin rolling.

Movement restriction is assessed in extension, rotation, and lateral flexion. This region is normally restricted in its range of motion due to the upper ribs. However, subtle joint play and shifting movements can and should be felt normally. Extension and lateral flexion joint dysfunctions are commonly found and respond well to manipulations. Both supine and prone manipulative techniques can be used (Figs. 21.14 to 21.18).[3]

Upper Rib Joints

The upper three or four costotransverse joints are commonly in dysfunction and found to be painful and stiff. Cervical and upper thoracic joint dysfunctions are often associated with coexisting costotransverse joint dysfunctions. A common example of this is the consistent finding of upper cervical joint fixations associated with joint dysfunction of the upper three costotransverse joints, most notably those of the first and third rib joints. The finding of one necessitates searching for the other. Trigger points

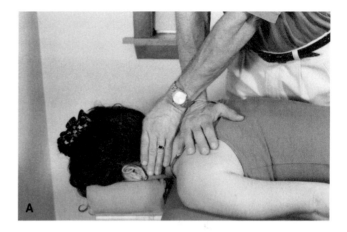

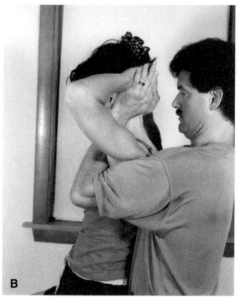

Figure 21.15 Upper thoracic spine. **(A)** The clinician is making an interspinous contact with the ulnar aspect of his right hand. The left hand is cupping the occiput and imparting axial traction. The thrust is directed into the table and slightly cephalad to impart extension. **(B)** Long axis distraction. Both hands traction occiput as the clinician's forearms resist the patient's attempt to bring elbows into adduction. Cervical spine is not flexed. Patient inhales, then exhales and for the manipulation, and the sternal contact impulse is anterior as occiput is lifted.

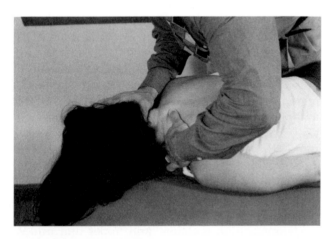

Figure 21.14 Lateral flexion manipulation upper thoracic spine. The cervicothoracic and upper thoracic segments are leveraged over the manipulating thumb contact. The head and neck are laterally flexed just until tension is generated at the correct segment. Rotation is imparted so that the face points away slightly. Thrust is performed with the contact hand only.

and muscle tension are often found in the pectoral and scalene muscles, as are painful restrictions of the related sternocostal joints.

The upper three rib joints are often involved with trauma to the neck, shoulder, or upper extremity and must be carefully assessed for pain and restriction in such cases. Additionally, the cause of neck ache and upper extremity heaviness that persists after cervical disc resolution can often be found in dysfunctional costotransverse joints of the upper three ribs.

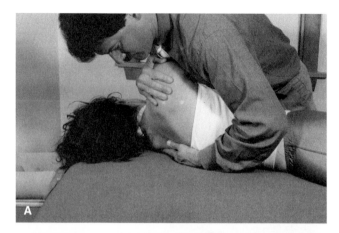

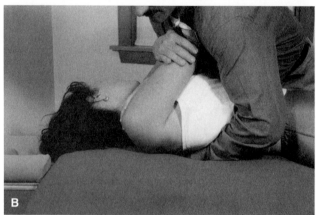

Figure 21.16 Supine manipulation of upper thoracic spine. **(A)** Contact is made with thenar aspect of hand. **(B)** A thrust is performed in the direction of the patient's humeri as the motion segment is leveraged over the contact hand. Simultaneously, the inferior hand quickly pulls the contact caudally.

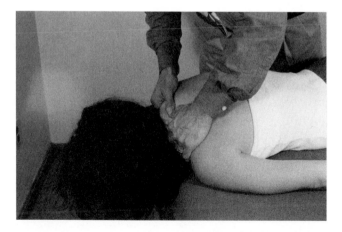

Figure 21.17 Circumduction mobilization of upper thoracic spine. Bilateral contact of the spino-laminar junction is performed with the thumb pads while the index fingers contact the anterior aspect of the cervicothoracic region. Circumductions or posterior-to-anterior pressures are applied.

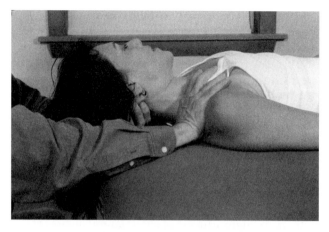

Figure 21.18 Cervicothoracic localized traction technique. The inferior hand contacts the T1 spinous process from above via the thumb pad and presses caudally. The superior hand cups the base of the occiput and upper cervical region and applies axial traction, thus gapping the C7-T1 segment. This localized traction can be performed as far down as one can reach.

Interesting anatomical relationships exist between the cervicothoracic spine and upper ribs. The powerful anterior and middle scalene muscles link the cervical segments to the first rib. The anterior scalene muscle originates from as high up as the third cervical vertebra, the larger middle scalene from the second vertebral segment, and sometimes the atlas. Both the anterior and middle scalene muscles insert on the first rib. The posterior scalene links the lower two or three cervical vertebrae to the second rib. It is tempting to ponder the importance of this relationship because a consistent finding on examination is joint dysfunction of the first and/or second rib joints associated with a painfully stiff ipsilateral C2-3 facet joint and scalene muscle tension.

Other muscles that attach to the first rib include the serratus anterior, subclavius, and intercostals. In addition, the costoclavicular ligament links the first rib to the shoulder girdle via the clavicle and the suprapleural membrane attaches to its undersurface along the inner border. The serratus anterior, levator costae, and intercostals also insert onto the second rib. As mentioned, the iliocotalis cervicis originates on the third through sixth rib angles and inserts on the cervical transverse processes of C4 through C6. A very important and overlooked muscle intrinsic to the cervicothoracic region is the serratus posterior superior, often causing myofascial pain in the upper back and upper extremity. The cervicothoracic junction epitomizes anatomical diversity and makes for a complex assessment of interrelated structures.

First Rib Painful dysfunction of the first costotransverse joint often presents as a deep ache in the root of the neck. Pulling and lifting movements using the arms are painful. Pain can sometimes be referred into the upper extremity and scalene muscle spasm and trigger points are commonly found. Lifting the head off the bed may irritate the pain caused by scalene contraction. Pain can also be elicited on deep inspiration. The upper fibers of the trapezius muscle are often in spasm and cervical rotation toward the painful side is restricted. Cervical extension is painful and flexion feels tight and restricted.

The angle of the first rib usually palpates more elevated when compared to the non-painful side. Grieve mentions that the patient with this condition presents with an antalgic attitude of slight lateral flexion of the neck towards the painful side while reaching across with the opposite arm to rest the fingers on the painful "yoke" region.[14] A subjective feeling of heaviness or "deadness" in the upper extremity is often reported.

The clinician can palpate the first ribs bilaterally behind the clavicles and ask the patient to inhale deeply, then relax, and exhale (Figs. 21.19 and 21.20). The dysfunctional first rib will palpate as elevated and stiff, seemingly remaining restricted in its inspiration phase. Interestingly, this is often noticed on the side of hand dominance. Its sternocostal attachment is exquisitely tender and can be palpated just under the medial end of the clavicle. The first rib can also be palpated using cervical spine movements.

Second and Third Ribs Second rib joint pain and dysfunction typically presents with painful prominences anteriorly at its sternal attachment and posteriorly at its angle. Springing a dysfunctional rib angle meets with resistance and pain. Pain can be referred to the shoulder and arm as a deep ache, numbness, or pins and needles. Patients are often only painfully aware of the rib's anterior attachment. A visible prominence of the anterior rib attachment just lateral to the sternal angle can be seen. Painful pectoralis fibers and trigger points are usually present. Cervical side bending, flexion, and extension provoke the upper pectoral pain.[14] As a differential point, careful palpation of the second rib angle is very painful, restricted, and elicits the patient's presenting pain while examination of the first and third rib angles do not.

The third rib, when painful and dysfunctional, creates anterior chest pain that leaves the patient with a sense that something is "stuck" there. Like the second rib dysfunction, a painful prominence can be palpated and even seen and deep chest pain is elicited on compression of the rib's anterior attachment. The posterior rib angle is also prominent and often exquisitely tender with palpably knotted and painful muscle tissue overlying it. An interesting consistent finding on examination is ipsilateral occipital-

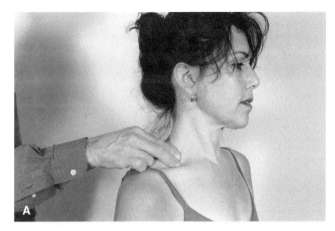

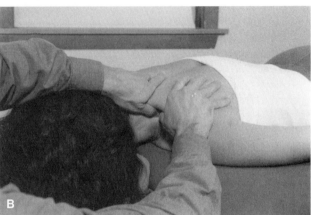

Figure 21.19 First rib palpation. **(A)** The first rib is found posterior to the clavicle and anterior and deep to the edge of the upper fibers of the trapezius muscle. **(B)** Both thumbs lift the upper edge of the trapezius muscle and contact the first rib from above. Similarly, a caudal glide mobilization can be performed.

atlantal joint dysfunction accompanying a third rib joint dysfunction.

With the patient prone, the rib angles of the second and third ribs can be palpated approximately 2.5 inches lateral to their respective thoracic spinous process. Care should be taken in not mistaking painful soft tissue thickenings for rib angles. The rib angle palpates as a hard bony structure, whereas firm and painful soft tissue changes can be moved aside to palpate the deeper rib angle. Both second and third ribs can be manipulated prone or supine (Fig. 21.21) similar to thoracic spine techniques with the exception that hand contacts are taken more laterally on the rib angles.

Thoracolumbar Region

The thoracolumbar region is where the thoracic spine and attached rib cage meet the lumbar spine. Power-

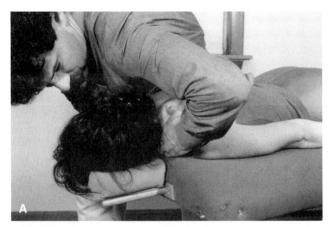

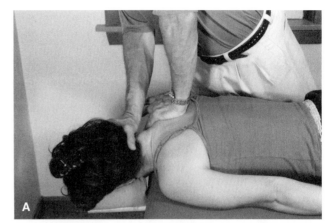

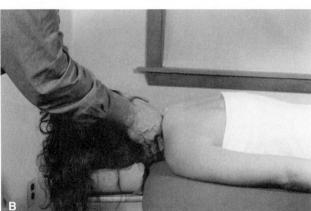

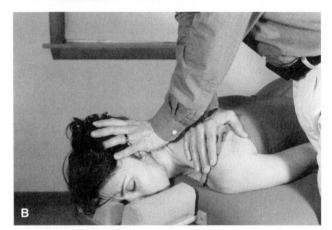

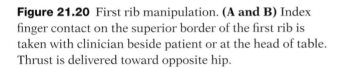

Figure 21.20 First rib manipulation. **(A and B)** Index finger contact on the superior border of the first rib is taken with clinician beside patient or at the head of table. Thrust is delivered toward opposite hip.

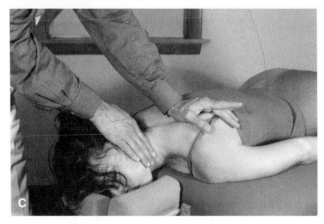

Figure 21.21 Manipulation of second and third ribs prone. **(A and B)** Pisiform contact is on rib angle while opposite hand takes up tissue slack with slight head and neck rotation and lateral bending. **(C)** From head end of table.

ful muscles span this junction including the quadratus lumborum, erector spinae, abdominal muscles, psoas, and diaphragm. This is a common area of dysfunction, often disrupting function at other spinal transitional regions. Problems with statics and posture commonly affect the thoracolumbar junction.

Anatomically this region sharply transitions between thoracic and lumbar characteristics, usually within one segment, because its upper aspect is thoracic in nature whereas its lower part is lumbar. This creates great strain focused into a small area, resulting in often vigorous reaction by the large muscles surrounding the region when dysfunction is present. Commonly the psoas major reflexly reacts to thoracolumbar joint dysfunction with tension and trigger points. In addition, the quadratus lumborum and erector spinae react likewise, with the quadratus lumborum being an important source of myofascial back pain.[5,36] Trunk rotation is often limited when this transitional region is dysfunctional. Thoracolumbar joint dysfunction commonly causes referred pain that is felt near the sacroiliac and lumbosacral regions and the iliac crest. Maigne found 40% of 350 patients with low back pain to have thoracolumbar joint dysfunction as the cause of their symptoms.[27] The thoracolumbar and lumbar regions are manipulated in like manner (Figs. 21.22 and 21.23).

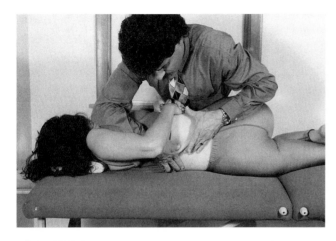

Figure 21.22 Thoracolumbar rotation manipulation. Counter-rotation tension is imparted to the spine, localizing manipulation to the desired level. Care must be taken not to strain costotransverse joints.

Lumbosacral Region

The lumbosacral region is the meeting place of the spine, pelvis, and lower extremities. Large powerful muscles in this region are often in imbalance and poor joint function, particularly in the sacroiliac joints, commonly cause symptoms. Being at the base of the spine, posture and spinal statics are influenced greatly here. Function of the lower extremities has a very large impact on the lumbosacral region, as well as the rest of the spine.

The sacroiliac joints are a common pain generator in lower back problems and have a major influence on the locomotor system.[6][11][2][31] Provocative stress tests can be applied to assess for pain and dysfunction. Palpation of sacroiliac joint motion is not very reliable; however, a constellation of signs and symptoms can aid in the diagnosis in conjunction with pain provocative testing.[21] Essentially, pain is localized to the joint, but can be referred into the buttock, thigh, groin, and even the leg and foot. Provocation tests are performed to localize a mechanical stress to the joint. The Patrick-Fabere, Gaenslen's, and Yeoman's tests are used to elicit pain. In addition, the posterior shear or thigh thrust test and compression and distraction tests are useful in eliciting sacroiliac joint pain.[21] Fortin mentions the Fortin finger test as a simple diagnostic measure for sacroiliac joint problems whereby the patient simply identifies the pain by pointing inferior and medial to the posterior superior iliac spine.[10]

Movements occurring at the sacroiliac joints are complex and controversial. The more accepted ones are nutation and counternutation.[6] Nutation is when the sacral base travels anterior and inferior while the apex moves posterior and superior. This occurs around a transverse axis through the S2 segment. Counternutation is the opposite motion. Manipula-

tion can be performed to either nutate or counternutate the sacrum at the sacroiliac joints and is more commonly manipulated in the side-posture position.[6][24] By placing the joint to be manipulated on the down side, the table stabilizes the ilium whereby a sacral contact can be taken to impart motion in the sacroiliac joint. Taking a sacral apex contact tends to counternutate the sacroiliac joint while taking a sacral base contact nutates it (Fig. 21.24A–D). The sacroiliac joint can also be nutated in the supine position (Fig. 21.25).

Extremity Joints

It is extremely common to find important joint dysfunctions in the extremity articulations that cause changes throughout the locomotor system, either locally or globally. This is epitomized by joint dysfunctions found in the foot/ankle complex and the proximal tibio-fibular joint, especially as it pertains to lower back problems. Other articulations of importance include the hip, acromioclavicular, sternoclavicular, and carpal joints. Glenohumeral joint dysfunctions are often dwarfed in importance by the more common myofascial dysfunction and muscular imbalances found in the shoulder region. A notable exception in this regard is a loss of joint play in caudal glide (Fig. 21.26).

The only articular connection between the upper quarter and trunk is via the strut-like clavicle with its two articulations, the sternoclavicular and acromioclavicular joints. Of these the acromioclavicular joint presents more commonly with joint dysfunction needing manipulation or mobilization compared to the sternoclavicular joint (Figs. 21.27 to 21.30).

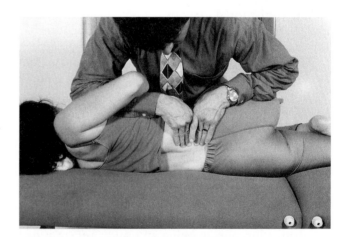

Figure 21.23 Lumbar lateral flexion manipulation. Fingers press from above to impart lateral flexion lack removal. A slight counter-rotation is applied to the spine and a thrust is made when the level is brought to tension.

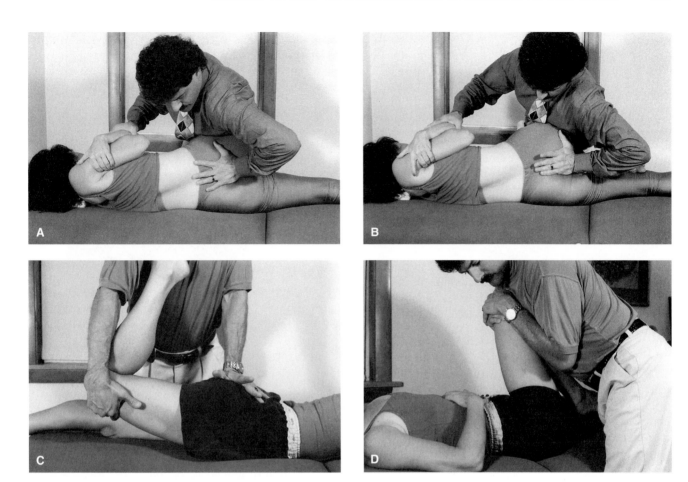

Figure 21.24 Sacroiliac joint manipulation. **(A)** Nutation in side-posture contacting sacral base on the down side. **(B)** To impart counter-nutation, a sacral apex contact on the down side would be made. **(C)** Sacral apex or base contact can be made with thigh extended to take joint to tension. **(D)** Posterior thigh thrust technique. More adduction can be used to affect the hip joint.

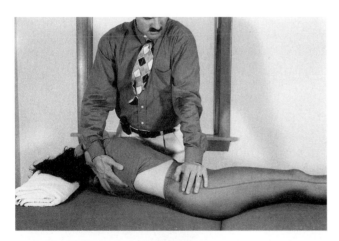

Figure 21.25 Sacroiliac joint manipulation, nutation in supine posture. Hips are positioned slightly closer to clinician and feet are place slightly away. The leg on the side of dysfunction is placed on top of the other leg. Trunk is rotated to tension while pelvis is stabilized against table with anterior superior iliac spine contact. Thrust is made toward table with contact hand on ASIS.

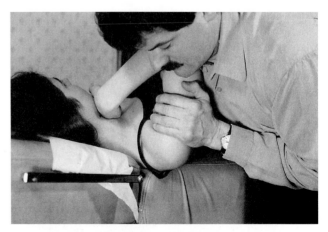

Figure 21.26 Caudal glide of glenohumeral joint. The most proximal aspect of the humerus is grasped and pulled posterior and caudally in an arcing motion.

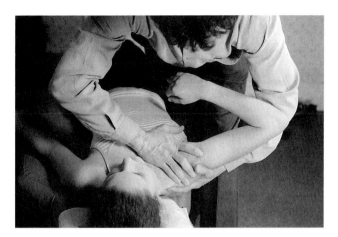

Figure 21.27 Sternoclavicular joint in long axis distraction. The scapula is cradled posteriorly while the clavicle is contacted anteriorly. The entire upper extremity is tractioned laterally at the sternoclavicular joint with the shoulder at 90 degrees of abduction.

The foot is the first part of our body to literally touch and assess our environment as we assume the upright posture and walk. Consequently, it is heavily endowed with receptors and intrinsic muscle control to constantly appraise the nervous system of terrain characteristics. The importance of this is reflected in foot anatomy. Of the 31 muscles that influence foot

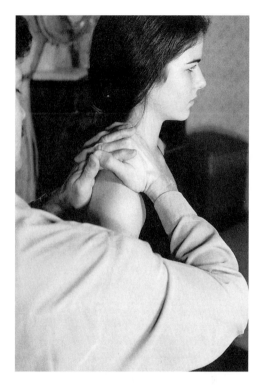

Figure 21.29 Acromioclavicular joint. Anterior-to-posterior compression is achieved with counter acting forces from the hand contacts on the distal clavicle anteriorly and the acromion posteriorly.

and ankle function, 20 are intrinsic to the foot alone, two on its dorsal aspect and 18 arranged in four layers underneath. Spindle activity from intrinsic muscle action, joint mechanoreceptors from foot articulations, and soft tissue receptors in the sole of the foot

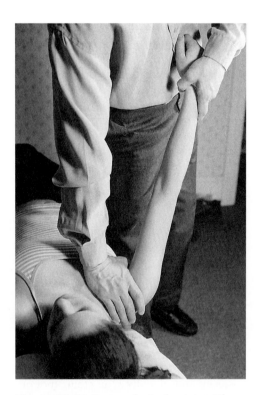

Figure 21.28 Sternoclavicular joint. The arm is tractioned while pressure is maintained at the medial aspect of the clavicle.

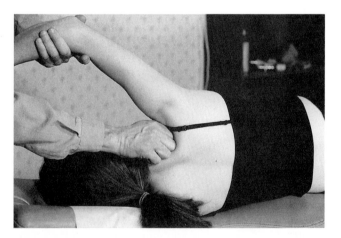

Figure 21.30 Acromioclavicular joint. Superior glide is achieved by blocking superior movement of the distal acromion with a thumb and bent index finger contact. The arm is elevated bringing the distal clavicle to tension at the joint.

comprise a complex sensory system that has local and global reflex effects on the locomotor system. Dys-afferentation from joint and soft tissue dysfunctions in the foot can be a powerful cause of reflex dysfunctions throughout the whole locomotor system.[33] Therefore, ankle and foot joint dysfunction must be assessed for and manipulated to achieve appropriate afferent input to the rest of the locomotor system (Figs. 21.31 to 21.37). This greatly aids in the rehabilitation of locomotor system disturbances.

The superior tibio-fibular joint seems to be another important articulation that, when in dysfunction, occupies the role of key link. It is interposed between the biceps femoris and peroneus longus tendons, structures theorized to aid in force transmission between the pelvis and foot, the so-called spine–leg mechanism.[38] Joint dysfunction can either occur locally or cause other more remote locomotor disturbances.[4,13,24] Manipulation is easy and effective (Fig. 21.38).

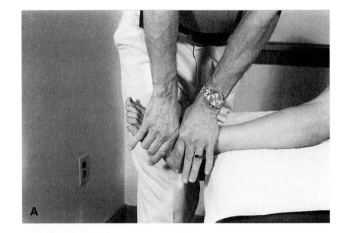

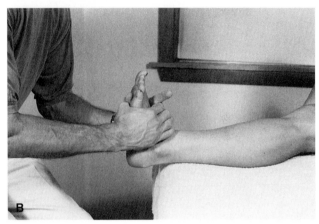

Figure 21.32 Tarsal joint manipulation: dorsal to plantar glide. **(A)** Palpation assessment with double web contact attempting to shift tarsals in dorsal to plantar glide. **(B)** Manipulation with left hand's middle finger placed over joint to be treated and reinforced by right hand. A pull move is used to impart dorsal to plantar movement.

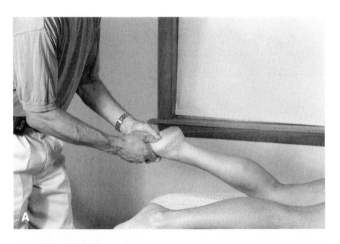

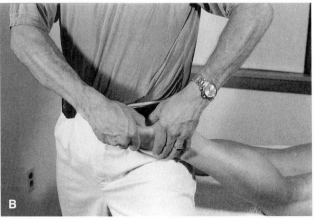

Figure 21.31 Tarsal joint manipulation: plantar to dorsal glide. **(A)** Double thumb contact is used to mobilize or manipulate from plantar to dorsal as traction along long axis of foot applied. **(B)** Tarsal joints are specifically plantar flexed using double thumb contract as fulcrum.

The hip joint can be thought of as being a part of the pelvis and, consequently, its normal function is critical in lower back and pelvic mechanics. Hip pain and joint dysfunction are common and readily force compensatory reactions by the spine, pelvis, and lower quarter. Appropriate hip joint mobility is necessary to spare the spine during bending and gait motions (Figs. 21.24D and 21.39).

■ CONCLUSION

While keeping in mind indications and contraindications, the use of joint manipulation, particularly of the spine, is both safe and effective. The locomotor system must be assessed and treated within the context of a "systems" approach rather than focusing on a particular joint, muscle, or related structure in

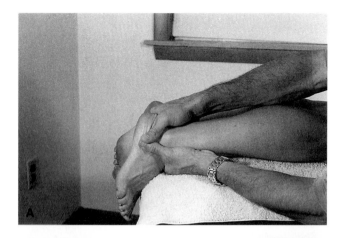

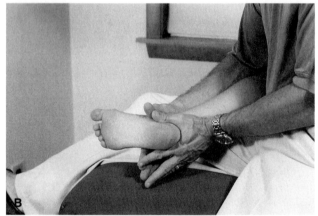

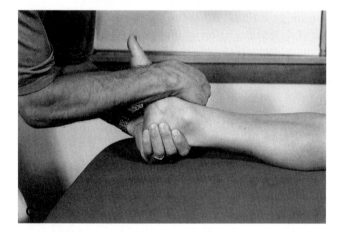

Figure 21.33 Subtalar joint manipulation. **(A and B)** The three joint play movements of long axis distraction, anterior and posterior rocking, and lateral and medial side tilt can be performed in either position. **(C)** Calcaneal contact from the medial aspect is made and a long axis pull move is used to manipulate subtalar joint. Other hand stabilizes tarsals.

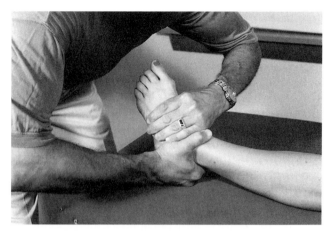

Figure 21.34 General foot joint mobilization: pronation–eversion. Calcaneal hand contact everts rearfoot as other hand inverts forefoot. The movement is reversed.

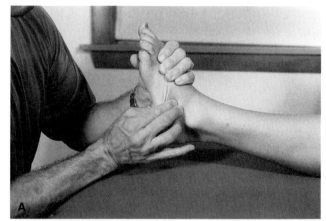

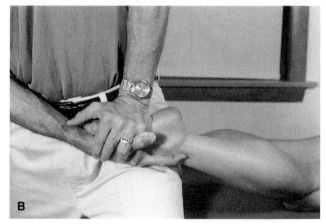

Figure 21.35 Calcaneocuboid joint manipulation. **(A)** Calcaneocuboid joint is mobilized specifically in either plantar to dorsal or dorsal to plantar glide. **(B)** Pisiform contact used to manipulate plantar to dorsal joint dysfunction at calcaneocuboid joint. Note that clinician's proximal thigh is used to stabilize foot.

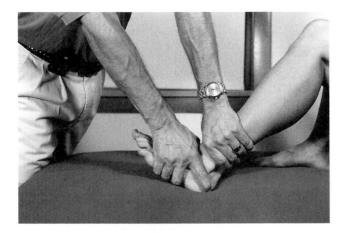

Figure 21.36 Ankle manipulation: anterior to posterior glide.

isolation. Spinal and extremity joint manipulations are performed not only to create mobility in areas that are restricted but also to stimulate the neuro-locomotor system globally via reflex nervous system activation.

In assessing the locomotor system, attention should be paid to the phenomena of chain reactions and their key links. In so doing, the clinician will gain more of an appreciation for the reflex function of the neuro-locomotor system. Key regions of dysfunction will be observed in spinal transitional areas and important extremity articulations as will consistent muscle–joint correlations. Tension and pain should be sought for in key muscles, joints, and attachment points to assess chain reactions. Release in their tension with treatment should serve to monitor treatment success.

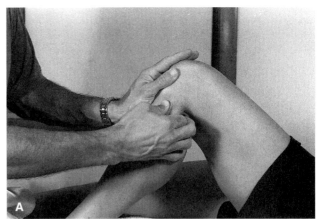

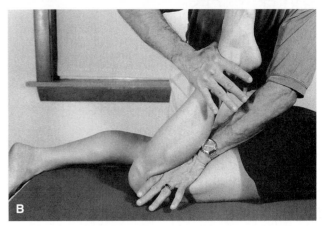

Figure 21.38 Proximal tibiofibular joint manipulations. **(A and B)** Two variations used to manipulate anterior to posterior and posterior to anterior glide movements. In **(B),** the ankle can also be dorsi and plantar flexed with one hand while the fingers on the other hand can monitor superior to inferior and inferior to superior glide motions at the fibular head.

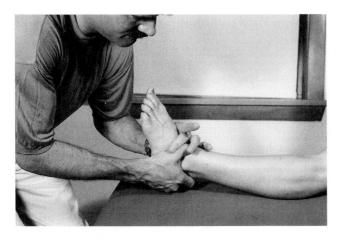

Figure 21.37 Ankle manipulation: long axis extension. The talus and the rest of the tarsals are grasped and pulled from underneath the distal tibiofibular mortise.

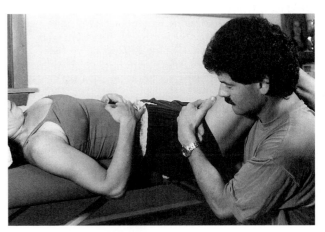

Figure 21.39 Hip joint long axis distraction. Hip is abducted as proximal-most femur is contacted and pulled laterally and toward the floor.

Audit Process
Self-Check of the Chapter's Learning Objectives

- Understand the functional chain reactions relating specific muscles and joints together.

- Understand how to mobilize or manipulate key joints.

- Discuss manipulative treatment of key joints commonly involved in disturbance of locomotor function.

■ REFERENCES

1. Axen I, Rosenbaum A, Robech R, et al. Can patient reactions to the first chiropractic treatment predict early favorable treatment outcome in persistent low back pain? J Man & Manipul Ther 2002;25:450–454.

2. Daly JM, Frame PS, Rapoza PA. Sacroiliac subluxation: A common, treatable cause of low-back pain in pregnancy. Fam Pract Res J 1991;11:149–159.

3. DeFranca GG. Evaluation of Joint Dysfunction of the Cervical Spine. In: Murphy DR, ed. Conservative Management of Cervical Spine Syndromes. New York: McGraw-Hill, 2000:265–305.

4. DeFranca GG. Proximal tibiofibular joint dysfunction and chronic knee and low back pain. J Manipulative Physiol Ther 1992;15:382–387.

5. DeFranca GG, Levine LJ. The quadratus lumborum and low back pain. J Manipulative Physiol Ther 1991;14:142–149.

6. DeFranca GG, Levine LJ. Pelvic Locomotor Dysfunction: A Clinical Approach. Gaithersburg: Aspen Publishers, 1996.

7. Dishman RW. Static and dynamic components of the chiropractic subluxation complex: A literature review [see comments]. J Manipulative Physiol Ther 1988; 11:98–107.

8. Dvorak J, Dvorak V. Manual Medicine. Diagnostics, 2nd ed. New York: Georg Thieme Verlag, 1990.

9. Flynn T, Fritz J, Whitman J, et al. A clinical prediction rule for classifying patients with low back pain who demonstrate short-term improvement with spinal manipulation. Spine 2002;27:2835–2843.

10. Fortin JD, Falco FJ. The Fortin finger test: An indicator of sacroiliac pain [see comments]. Am J Orthop 1997;26:477–480.

11. Galm R, Frohling M, Rittmeister M, et al. Sacroiliac joint dysfunction in patients with imaging-proven lumbar disc herniation. Eur Spine J 1998;7:450–453.

12. Gatterman MI. What's in a Word? In: Gatterman MI, ed. Foundations of Chiropractic Subluxation. St. Louis: Mosby, 1995.

13. Gillet H, Liekens M. Belgian Chiropractic Research Notes. Huntington Beach: Motion Palpation Institute, 1984.

14. Grieve GP. Common Vertebral Joint Problems, 2nd ed. New York: Churchill Livingstone, 1988.

15. Haldeman S, Chapman-Smith D, Petersen JDM. Contraindications and complications. In: Haldeman S,

Chapman-Smith D, Petersen JDM, eds. Guidelines for Chiropractic Quality Assurance and Practice Parameters. Gaithersburg, MD: Aspen Publishers, Inc, 1993:167–177.

16. Haldeman S, Rubinstein SM. The precipitation or aggravation of musculoskeletal pain in patients receiving spinal manipulative therapy. J Manipulative Physiol Ther 1993;16:47–50.

17. Herzog W, Scheele D, Conway PJ. Electromyographic responses of back and limb muscles associated with spinal manipulative therapy. Spine 1999;24:146–153.

18. Jirout J. The rotational component in the dynamics of the C2-3 spinal segment. neuroradiology 1979;17:177.

19. Keating JC, Jr, Bergmann TF, Jacobs GE, et al. Interexaminer reliability of eight evaluative dimensions of lumbar segmental abnormality. J Manipulative Physiol Ther 1990;13:463–470.

20. Kolar P. The sensomotor nature of postural function. Its fundamental role in rehabilitation of the motor system. J Orthop Med 1999;21:40–45.

21. Laslett M. Pain provocation sacroiliac joint tests: Reliability and prevalence. In: Vleeming A, Mooney V, Snijders CJ, et al, eds. Movement, Stability, and Low Back Pain. The Essential Role of the Pelvis. New York: Churchill Livingstone, 1997:287–295.

22. Lewit K. Chain reactions in disturbed function of the motor system. J Manual Med 1987;3:27.

23. Lewit K. Chain reactions in the locomotor system in light of co-activation patterns based on developmental neurology. J Orthop Med 1999;21:52–57.

24. Lewit K. Manipulative Therapy in Rehabilitation of the Locomotor System, 3rd ed. Boston: Butterworth-Heineman, 1999.

25. Lewit K. Soft Tissue and Relaxation Techniques in Myofascial Pain. In: Hammer WI, ed. Functional Soft Tissue Examination and Treatment by Manual Methods, 2nd ed. Gaithersburg: Aspen Publishers, 1999:479–532.

26. Liebenson C. Manual resistance techniques and self-stretches for improving flexibility/mobility. In: Liebenson C, ed. Rehabilitation of the Spine. Baltimore: Williams and Wilkins, 1996:253.

27. Maigne R. Low back pain of thoracolumbar origin. Arch Phys Med Rehabil 1980;61:389–395.

28. Maigne R, Le Corre F. New ideas on the mechanism of common adult dorsalgias. J Manual Med 1969;4:73.

29. Maitland GD. Peripheral Manipulation, 2nd ed. Boston: Butterworths, 1981.

30. Mennell JM. Joint Pain. Diagnosis and Treatment Using Manipulative Techniques. Boston: Little, Brown and Co, 1964.

31. Mierau DR, Cassidy JD, Hamin T, et al. Sacroiliac joint dysfunction and low back pain in school aged children. J Manipulative Physiol Ther 1984;7:81–84.

32. Schafer RC, Faye LJ. Motion Palpation and Chiropractic Technique: Principles of Dynamic Chiropractice. Huntington Beach: Motion Palpation Institute, 1989.

33. Seaman DR, Winterstein JF. Dysafferentation: A novel term to describe the neuropathophysiological

effects of joint complex dysfunction. A look at likely mechanisms of symptom generation. J Manipulative Physiol Ther 1998;21:267–280.

34. Senstad O, Leboeuf-Yde C, Borchgrevink C. Predictors of side effects to spinal manipulative therapy. J Manipulative Physiolog Ther 1996;19:441–445.

35. Shekelle PG. Spine update. Spinal manipulation. Spine 1994;19:858.

36. Travell JG, Simons DG. Myofascial Pain and Dysfunction. The Trigger Point Manual. Baltimore: Williams and Wilkins, 1983.

37. Triano JJ. The Mechanics of Spinal Manipulation. In: Herzog W, ed. Clinical Biomechanics of Spinal Manipulation. New York: Churchill Livingstone, 2000:92–190.

38. Vleeming A, Snijders CJ, Stoeckart R, et al. The role of the sacroiliac joints in coupling between spine, pelvis, legs, and arms. In: Vleeming A, Mooney V, Dorman TA, et al, eds. Movement, Stability, and Low Back Pain. The Essential Role of the Pelvis. New York: Churchill Livingstone, 1997:53–71.

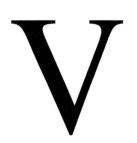

PART

V

Recovery Care Management (after 4 weeks)

Editor's Note

Those patients who are not recovering quickly in the first month of care have reached a crucial decision point. Since with each passing week those failing to recover become less likely to recover, it is essential to mobilize more pro-active methods in patient self-management. If reassurance, gradual reactivation, medication, and manipulation are the standard bearers in acute care, exercise and cognitive-behavioral therapy are the "gold standards" in subacute to chronic care.

This section covers modern approaches to active care, with an emphasis on improving motor control and muscular endurance. It is not sufficient to focus on "isolated" training of specific impairments. This must be combined with a focus on disabilities in activities of daily living, job demands, or sports and recreational activities and psycho-social issues affecting participation in these tasks. Self-care or management is guided by cognitive-behavioral principles such as supervised, graded exposures to specific feared stimuli and education in problem-solving abilities.

22

Sensory Motor Stimulation

Vladimír Janda, Marie Vávrová,
Alena Herbenová, and
Michaela Veverková

Introduction
Sensory Motor Stimulation Background
Therapeutic Approaches
Basic Concepts of Motor Learning
Sensory Motor Devices and Aids
Indications for the Sensory Motor Stimulation
Methodology
Overview of Sensory Motor Training
The Small (Short) Foot
Postural Correction
Corrected Stance on One Leg
Lunges
Jumps
Balance Boards (Rocker and Wobble)
Balance Sandals
The Sequence
Miscellaneous SMS Tools

Learning Objectives
After reading this chapter, you should be able to understand:

- The indications and purpose of sensory motor training
- The rationale and technique for training the small foot
- The rationale and technique for training postural correction
- The rationale and technique for training lunges
- The rationale and technique for training balance on balance boards and sandals

Introduction

Therapeutic approaches have been continuously changed with respect to our knowledge and progress of physiology. The original approach considered the motor system as an effector only and did not understand it's role with the afferent system as one functional unit. The result of this approach was the idea that motor performance is a result of isolated and separate, although coordinated, activation of individual muscles. The main concern of these techniques was activation of individual muscles or muscle groups in the hope that the new motor pattern will be developed automatically. Examples of such thinking are exercises prescribed according to muscle testing or the progressive resistance exercise program. The next evolution in thinking about exercise accepted that a movement cannot be accomplished without coordination of the afferent pathways and centers; thus, the realization that the motor system and the afferent system were closely linked.

Sensory Motor Stimulation Background

Therapeutic Approaches

Kabat developed and introduced into practice the concept of activation of afferent pathways as an approach to movement reeducation (20). In therapy, this concept is the basis of the proprioceptive neuromuscular facilitation (PNF) technique. This approach, and similarly others developed during the past few decades, such as that of Temple Fay, Bobaths, Vojta, Rood, to mention only some of the most important ones, systematically stress the muscle coordination and the importance of proprioceptive information. At present, it is understood that the afferent system does not have only an informative role, but that it participates substantially in motor programming and motor system regulation. Therefore, proprioceptive stimulation is stressed more and more.

The term proprioception was used for the first time by Sherrington to describe the sense of position, posture, and movement (30). Over time this term has been used in a much broader way, and today, although not quite correctly, it is used for nearly the entire afferent system.

It is understood today that splitting the function and/or dysfunction of the myo-osteo-articular system from the central regulatory nervous mechanisms is wrong. Both parts function as one inseparable functional unit and cannot be separated. Thus, any lesion or impaired function of any part of the peripheral motor system leads to adaptive mechanisms in the central nervous system and vice versa.

Probably the first one who, from the clinical point of view, noticed the relation between the lesion (injury) of the foot joints and incoordinated muscle function of the lower leg was Kurtz (22). However, apart from the fundamental experimental works of Wyke and Skoglund 1956, in clinics it was Freeman and co-workers who systematically considered some aspects of joint traumatology and the importance of impaired afference in the genesis of an unstable ankle joint (7–9,31,33). Freeman was also the first one who introduced in non-neurological cases a detailed evaluation of coordination and stressed the importance of muscle inhibition as an integral part of the clinical picture (8). Since the first paper of Freeman, the interest in this problem has increased (7). One of the most extensive works is the book of Hérveou and Messean, *Technique de Reeducation et d' Education Proprioceptive* (11).

In our clinic we started to work out our program, based to some extent on the papers mentioned, in 1970. To avoid problems in terminology and/or confusion, we have named our technique "sensory motor stimulation" (SMS) in the hope that this term will stress the unity between the afferent and efferent system without implicating any specific structure or function and will not lead to confusion with PNF.

Basic Concepts of Motor Learning

The principle of SMS is based in the concept of two stages of motor learning (10). The first stage can be characterized as an attempt to achieve a new movement performance and to work out the basic motor program. In this process, the brain cortex (predominantly the frontal and parietal) are strongly involved. This type of motor regulation has some advantages as well as disadvantages. On the one hand it enables the individual to achieve new skills; however, as it passes several synapses it is rather slow and because of the necessary conscious participation of the cortex it is tiring. Therefore, the brain tries to minimize the pathways and to simplify the regulatory circuits. This mechanism has been named as the second stage of motor learning. It enables a reduction of cortical participation and is thus, less tiring and much faster. However, if such a motor program has been fixed once, it is very difficult, if not impossible, to change it. Therefore, in motor reeducation the attempt has to be made to achieve a quality of movement patterns that are as close to the normal as possible.

To prevent the injury, and microinjury in particular, fast reflex muscle contraction is needed to protect the joints. The second stage of motor learning enables such a faster response, which in fact may play a decisive role in prevention. It has been shown

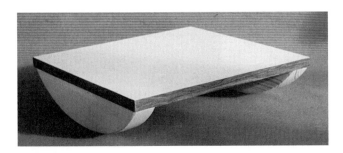

Figure 22.1 Rocker board.

that it is possible to accelerate by increased proprioceptive flow and balance exercises the muscle contraction approximately two-fold (4). In principle, in SMS an attempt is made to stimulate the proprioceptive system and those circuits and pathways that play an important role in regulation of equilibrium and posture.

From the afference point of view, excluding the skin exteroceptors, there are three areas that have the main proprioceptive influence. These are the receptors from the sole of the foot (Freeman), from the neck muscles (Abrahams), and the sacroiliac area (Hinoki) (1,7,12).

Afference from the sole receptors can be increased in different ways, e.g., by stimulation of the skin receptors or, more effectively, by active contraction of the foot muscles, with the emphasis on activity of the intrinsic muscles when forming the so-called small or short foot.

Clinical experience has revealed that activation in particular of the intrinsic muscles of the foot with only tonic activation of the toe muscles is most effective. Therefore, the "foot fist," as recommended for activation of proprioceptors by Ihara and Nakayama, is not used in this method (14).

The deep neck muscles contain, in comparison to the other striated muscles, many more proprioceptors (1). Abrahams has shown that these muscles should be considered as muscles for maintaining posture and equilibrium rather than muscles for producing dynamic movement. It should be mentioned that the deep tonic neck reflexes are the result of muscle activation and not of the neck joints, as it was mistakenly described originally.

The area of sacrum has been, in clinical practice, recognized as an important area to control posture and equilibrium only recently. The observation of Hinoki confirms this (12). However, at present it is not possible to differentiate whether it is the sacrum itself and its position or whether it is the sacroiliac joints that play the decisive role.

A special role has been recognized for the cerebellum and the whole spino-vestibulo-cerebellar regulatory circuit.

Sensory Motor Devices and Aids

In principle, various balance exercises are used. The equipment used is simple and inexpensive. The principles are not new and were introduced by Bobaths and others (3) for motor re-education of children with cerebral palsy. However, the application to chronic back pain patients is rather new and has been introduced only recently.

There are many exercise aids of various types, from wobble and rocker boards, balance shoes, various types of twisters and trampolines, and the Fitter. Wobble and rocker boards are made preferably from wood and not from plastic material, because wood stimulates the receptors more (Figs. 22.1 and 22.2). The average dimensions for the rocker board are: length, 35 cm; width, 25 cm; and height, 15 cm (6). The radius of the wobble board is, on average, 35 cm and the height is 15 cm. Exercises on the rocker board are easier; therefore, it is advisable to start with it.

The size of the balance shoes depends on the size of the foot. The sandals have to have a firm, not flexible, sole, with the modeled sole and the metatarsal support, because these help to configure the small foot. There should be just one strap over the forefoot and the heel should remain free, again to help to activate the muscles of the foot. The hemispheres are made from solid rubber, 5 to 7 cm in diameter, and placed in the center of the sole (Fig. 22.3).

The twister enables activation of the trunk and buttock muscles. When exercised in front of a mirror, one can visualize any asymmetry in muscle strength and/or asymmetrically performed exercise. We prefer to use of a flat twister 40 cm in diameter.

The Fitter (similarly as the twister), strictly speaking, is not a device for proprioceptive training; however, it substantially helps to improve coordination. There are several devices with similar function on the market. We use one that was developed by Fitter international from Canada (Fig. 22.4).

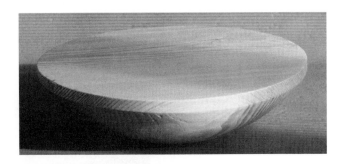

Figure 22.2 Wobble board.

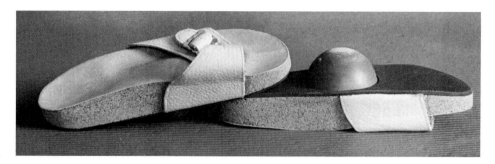

Figure 22.3 Balance shoes.

A minitrampoline is an excellent device to stimulate the proprioceptors of the whole body (Fig. 22.5). Unfortunately, the mostly used trampolines do not have sufficiently resilient material. The stimulatory effect is thus reduced. Springs of 15 to 18 cm in length provide a suitably unstable base, springs of less than 7 cm are of little proprioceptive value, although they decrease the compression of weight-bearing.

Exercise on gymnastic balls (mostly of 65 cm to 85 cm in diameter) are very efficient for kinesthetic stimulation and balance training.

Indications for the Sensory Motor Stimulation

SMS can be beneficially used as a part of any exercise program because it helps to improve muscle coordination and motor programming or regulation, and it increases the speed of activation of a muscle. It was used originally to improve the unstable ankle after an injury; however, it can be used for a variety of conditions (Table 22.1). Chronic back pain syndromes are one of the most important indications. Better control of the trunk, improved activation of the gluteal muscles, and thus better stability of the pelvis is achieved. There is a broad indication for sensory defects of neurological origin. Used carefully (to avoid injury), the method can help to compensate proprioceptive loss in aged subjects and thus to helps to prevent falls. Balance deficits have been correlated with an increased incidence of falls, and balance training has been shown to be an effective preventive intervention. However, this technique cannot be recommended for patients with acute pain syndromes.

Methodology

Overview of Sensory Motor Training

In this chapter the main principles of sensorimotor training are described. A more detailed description was published in Czech (17) and can be seen in Czech and English on videotape (15,16).

One of the most important advantages of this program is that it helps to improve not only the muscle imbalance but also, in particular, the most important motor activities such as standing, i.e., posture and gait. At the same time, the control of posture in daily activities, including those related to work and sport, is facilitated and improved automatically. Therefore, exercises performed in the upright position are the most important.

As a general rule—from a motor control perspective—a program to normalize relevant dysfunction in the periphery should be initiated before beginning the SMS exercises. This is because any pathological or unwanted proprioceptive information from the periphery results in functional, adaptative processes of the whole central nervous system. Therefore, attention should be paid first to the skin, fasciae, muscles, and joints, and their adjacent structures. Also, trigger points, whether active or latent, should be treated before beginning sensorimotor training.

Muscle imbalance, which is always present at least to some degree, should be improved first. This is particularly true in the case of severe muscle imbalance. The preparatory exercises include stretching of the tight muscles first, followed by strengthening the weak ones. The emphasis is placed on the specific patterns of coordination important for correct posture in standing.

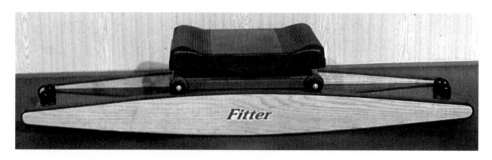

Figure 22.4 The Fitter.

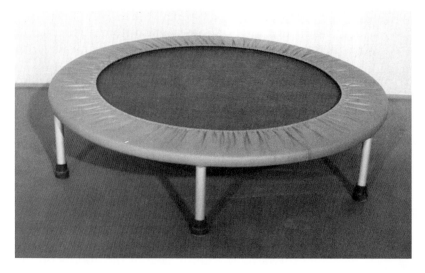

Figure 22.5 Minitrampoline.

To increase the proprioceptive flow, special attention is paid to forming the small (short) foot, the locking mechanism of the knee, stabilization of the pelvis, and, last but not least, the position of the head, neck, and shoulder girdle. Table 22.2 outlines the basic rules for administering SMS.

The exercises can be divided into those by means of which the transfer of weight or of the center of gravity is trained and those that train more the balance and muscle coordination in general. Both types of exercise aim to improve and stabilize posture.

The Small (Short) Foot

This term is understood as the shortening and narrowing of the foot. Stretched (neither relaxed nor flexed or extended) toes closely fitted (adhered) to the floor are pulled together with the metatarsal heads toward the heels (Fig. 22.6). Thus, both the longitudinal and transverse arches are increased.

Table 22.1 Indications for Sensory Motor Stimulation

- Post-traumatic, postoperative
- Chronic back and neck pain
- Faulty posture connected with respiratory dysfunction
- Hypermobility and instability in general (unstable ankle, knee, pelvis, spine)
- Less severe forms of idiopathic scoliosis
- Postpartum muscle imbalance
- Certain neurological conditions
- Prevention of falls in senior population
- Maintenance of general fitness

Table 22.2 Sensory Motor Stimulation Rules

The exercise program in the upright position follows several rules:

1. Correction is started from distal areas and gradually continued proximally. Therefore, modeling of the foot (feet) comes first, then correction of the position of the knees, then that of the pelvis, and finally that of the head, neck, and shoulders.
2. Exercises are performed barefoot because this increases both exteroceptive and proprioceptive input and enables the therapist to pay attention to better control. Last but not least, it helps to decrease the danger of injury.
3. Exercise should by no means provoke pain and should not lead to either physical (somatic) or mental (psychic) fatigue.
4. From the very beginning, special attention is paid to the awareness of posture (particularly feet, pelvis, and head).
5. All exercises should be first trained on a firm surface, then on balance devices.
6. The number of repetitions of each exercise should be between 10 and 20 in a typical treatment session. The more difficult exercises are repeated only 5 to 6 times.
7. Hold times for most of the exercises is 5 to 10 seconds.
8. The duration of a typical SMS training session varies. Balance shoe walking takes approximately 2 minutes in one treatment session, whereas other aspects of the routine can be longer (20 to 30 minutes in one treatment session).

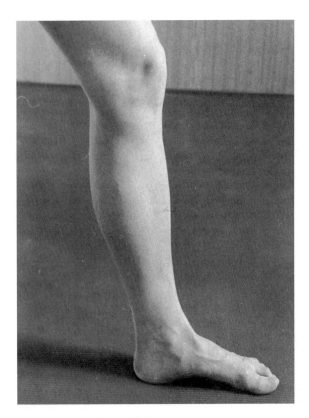

Figure 22.6 The small foot.

The small foot helps to increase afferent input, mainly from the sole. It improves the position of the body segments, improves the stability of the body in the upright position, and helps to improve the required springing moment of the foot during walking.

Before starting to train the small foot, attention has to be paid to foot mobility and awareness in most cases. To achieve this, we mobilize both the soft tissues and joints and stimulate both exteroceptors and mechanoreceptors, especially of the sole. Deep massage, brushing, tapping, and different stimulatory devices, e.g., small balls ("hedgehogs") or walking on pebbles are used.

Initially, formation of the small foot is difficult to perform in erect posture. Therefore, it is advisable to start the formation sitting, usually in three steps: sitting with passive modeling by the therapist, later semiactive (passively modeling by the therapist in combination with active patient effort), and finally active self-formation.

Passive Modelling of the Small Foot

The patient is seated at the edge of the chair with one foot forward. The entire sole of this foot is on the floor, toes and knee pointing forward, and the lower leg vertical to the ground. The therapist cups one hand behind the patient's heel and the other hand grasps the forefoot from above, gently squeezing the first and fifth metatarsals together (Fig. 22.7). Then, with vibratory movements, the therapist shortens and lengthens the sole of the foot.

This is repeated three to four times, followed by relaxation. By this procedure, the muscles responsible for the small foot formation are stimulated and longitudinal and transverse arch modeled. The therapist explains what he is doing while the patient watches and is asked to perceive and feel what happens during modeling of the small foot.

Active Assisted Modelling of the Small Foot

The position is the same. The therapist with one hand fixes the patient's heel from behind, and the other hand covers the forefoot (toes and metatarsals). The

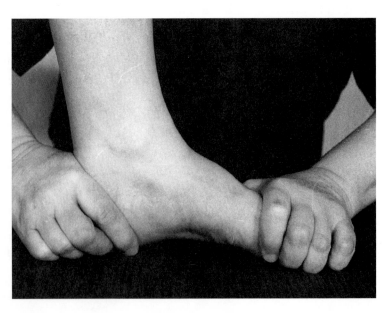

Figure 22.7 Passive modeling of the short foot.

Table 22.3 Clinician Options to Facilitate the Active Patient's Formation of the Small Foot

Option 1
The therapist facilitates the active modeling of the transverse arch by touching or slightly pushing with his finger at the top of the transverse arch (2nd metatarsal) from the dorsum of the foot. This pressure should aim to actively model the transverse arch. Similarly, the touch or slight pressure on os naviculare from the dorsum of the foot facilitates the active modeling of the longitudinal arch.

Option 2
Once the patient has learned to actively model the small foot, the therapist or the patient pushes on the knee from above in a downward direction, providing resistance and thus facilitating the small foot.

Option 3
The small foot can be more easily achieved when both feet work together with the inner edges of the feet firmly close together. The more advanced foot helps the less skilled one.

Table 22.4 Progressions to Challenge the Small Foot

Option 1
The patient holds the small foot and both externally and internally rotates the lower leg. The substitution by moving the knee from side to side (the movement in the hip) must be avoided.

Option 2
The small foot is modeled with the knee in various angles of knee flexion: 70° (easier) to 100° (harder).

The most common mistakes:
Flexion of the toes and lifting of the head of the 1st metatarsal and of the inner edge of the foot (inversion).

patient pushes slightly with the plantar surface of the stretched toes against the floor and tries to narrow the forefoot and pull it toward the heel. Thus, both the longitudinal and transverse arch of the foot are increased. The therapist helps to correct the movement with slight pressure on the toes from above to prevent flexion of the toes.

Another facilitation can be achieved when the therapist brings the first and the fifth metatarsal together. Table 22.3 describes a few additional options for the therapist to facilitate active modeling of the small foot by the patient.

Active Modelling of the Small Foot

The position of the patient is the same. The patient voluntarily models the small foot by narrowing the forefoot and pulling it toward the heel. Each trial is followed by relaxation of the foot muscles. Table 22.4 describes progressions to enhance the training of the small foot.

The next step is voluntary forming of the small foot on the leg positioned in front of the other while standing (Fig. 22.8). The aim is to teach the patient to form the small foot on the non-weight-bearing/front leg, which is less difficult than forming the small foot with the load of the weight of the body.

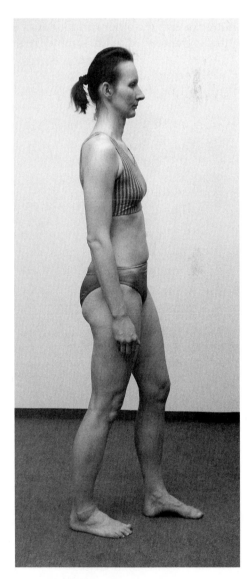

Figure 22.8 Active formation of the small foot on the front leg (in stance).

Postural Correction

The basic position for most exercises in the standing position, both on the floor and with labile devices, is the so-called corrected stance. The corrected stance is achieved by the following stages:

First Stage (First Stage of Obtaining Information)

The feet are parallel, hip-width apart, and toes pointed forward. The patient slowly leans his body forward from the ankle joints so the weight is transferred/shifted to the forefoot region (Fig. 22.9). The movement has to be stopped before the patient falls over. The heels remain fixed on the floor and the lower extremities, together with the pelvis, the trunk and head are in alignment. The therapist guides the movement by touching the patient's chest with one hand and his buttocks with the other and monitors whether the weight was transferred to the forefoot region.

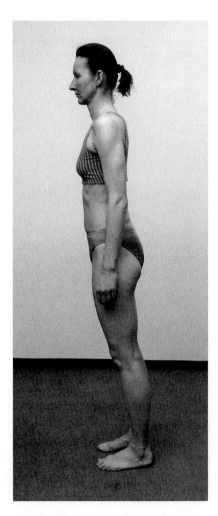

Figure 22.9 Postural correction with forward lean from the ankles (first stage).

The aim is to achieve the conscious feeling of foot contact with the floor, to increase activity of the foot muscles, and to improve awareness of the whole body posture.

Second Stage (Second Stage of Obtaining the Information)

The position of the feet is the same as in the first stage. Slight flexion in the knees (approximately 20°) is added with external rotation in the hip joints. Thus, the axis of the knee joints moves toward the outer edge of the feet. The body leans forward and the weight is transferred/shifted to the forefoot. The heels remain firmly on the floor.

Through activation of the hip external rotators, and forward shifting of the body weight, activity of the foot and lower extremity muscles is increased. Forming of the arches of the feet and correction of the pelvis and upper parts of the body are begun automatically. Awareness of the feet, the posture, and body position in the space is achieved.

Corrected Stance

The feet are positioned the same as in the second stage. First, the small foot is voluntarily formed, then slight flexion in the knees (unlocked position) follows with external rotation in the hip joints. The body leans slightly forward from the ankle joints to achieve equal distribution of weight to the three main support areas of the foot (namely the heel and the heads of the first and the fifth metatarsals) and the toes. The patient is asked to push the soles of the feet (including toes) into the floor and stretch his body upward along the vertical axis, all the way from the heels of the feet to the top of the head (vertex) (Fig. 22.10).

This achieves further correction of the posture. The abdominal wall flattens, the head is held elevated, and the shoulders are broadened and pulled down along the sides of the body.

Activation of the muscles participating in upright posture is increased with the curves of the spine maintained in physiological alignment. The posture becomes more stable from the feet, through the pelvis and trunk, and up to the head.

Corrected Stance on One Leg

The programme continues with corrected stance on one leg (Fig. 22.11). Then half-step forward is performed with weight evenly distributed between legs. The weight shifts forward until the trunk and head forms one line with the back leg. Half-step backward is performed by gradually shifting the weight backwards while moving the buttock of the back leg towards the heel with trunk in vertical position (Fig. 22.12).

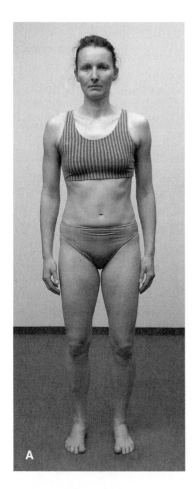
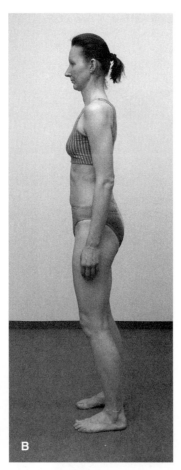

Figure 22.10 Corrected stance.

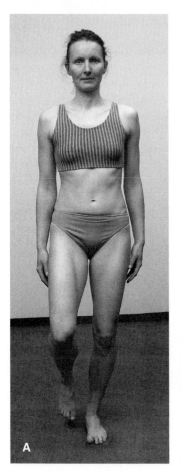
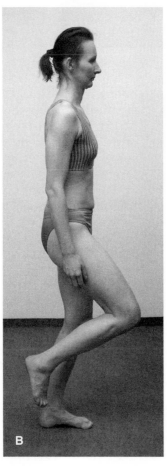

Figure 22.11 Corrected stance on single leg: **(A)** front view; **(B)** side view.

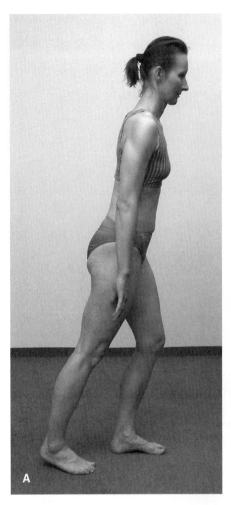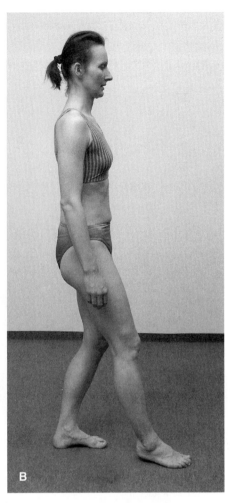

Figure 22.12 Half steps:
(A) forward; **(B)** backward.

To increase demands and proprioceptive flow, first pressure and then pushes in different directions toward the pelvis, shoulders, or both are added by the therapist. The patient must maintain appropriate muscle activation throughout.

Lunges

The next steps are lunges. In this exercise we evoke situations in which the patient is losing balance and then gaining it again. The speed of muscle contraction and control of the posture are trained. The goal is to perform fast lunges that accelerate reaction and improve control and are thus effective for preventing injuries of the lower extremity joints, the spine, and falls resulting from poor coordination.

Procedure

From corrected stance, the trunk leans forward in the ankle joints. The center of gravity/weight shifts forward above the forefoot until the heels start to lift up. At the moment of the loss of balance (the body is

falling forward), the equilibrium/balance has to be regained by stepping with one leg forward (Fig. 22.13). This has to be performed quickly and landing of the foot has to be soft and springy. If performed correctly, at the end range there is a small foot formed, the knee is stabilized or "locked" in flexion (at 90° maximum) on the front/stance leg, and the back leg is supported on the tip toe. The whole body is elongated (along the long axis of the body) and from the heel up to the head makes one line. The small foot reinforces the stability of the knee.

At the beginning it is advisable to use a shorter lunge. The therapist gives the security to the patient standing in front of him and touching his shoulders or sternum from front. Different variations of lunges are possible, e.g., stepping forward in different directions and/or with different movements of the arms (e.g., as in walking pattern) (Fig. 22.14).

Mistakes

The wrong timing of the movement or the lunge is not performed automatically (as a protective reaction)

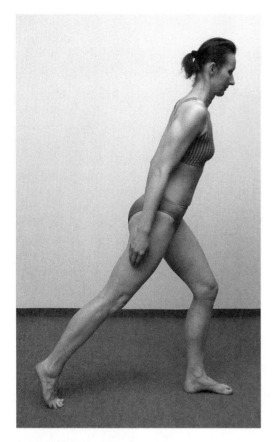

Figure 22.13 Lunge.

in the moment of danger of falling (as a result of the loss of balance/equilibrium). It is done voluntarily before the balance is actually threatened. Hard landing of the foot shows uncorrected foot. The trunk is not in the same line with the back leg and the patient bends forward or backward, sometimes even with the hyperlordosis. The knee moves medially (internal rotation in the hip), the ankle joint tends to valgosity with overload of the medial longitudinal arch of the foot.

Jumps

Lunges are followed by jumps on both legs and then on one leg (Fig. 22.15).

Balance Boards (Rocker and Wobble)

Each exercise (corrected stance, single leg stance, step forward and backward, lunges, jumps) is performed first on the floor and then on the rocker board, and later on the wobble board (Fig. 22.16). Only when the patient achieves sufficient skill in less demanding exercises is he allowed to move to the next, more difficult ones. Jumping on the labile boards is recommended only for advanced and well-trained patients.

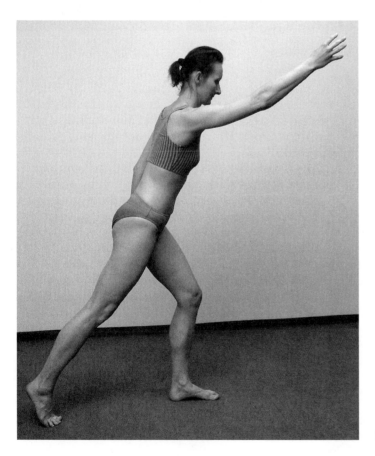

Figure 22.14 Lunge (walking pattern).

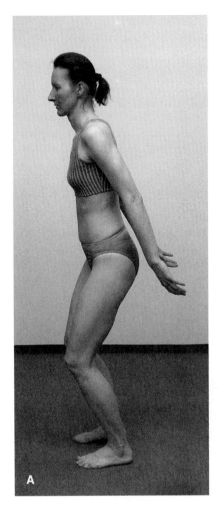
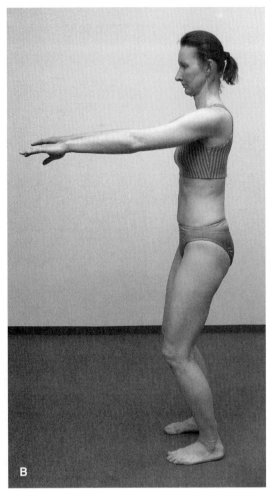
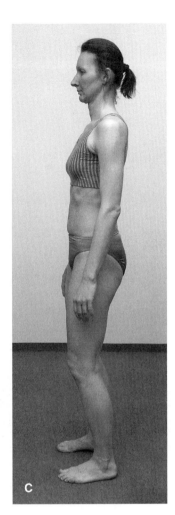

Figure 22.15 Jumps: **(A)** starting position; **(B)** landing; **(C)** final position.

The level of difficulty can be further increased by the addition of different variations, such as movements of the upper extremities, squatting, rocking, catching a ball, etc, and gait training on the labile boards.

Pushes toward the pelvis, trunk, and shoulder girdles in different directions, combined with perpendicular pushes of the labile board, significantly increase the proprioceptive flow to the central nervous system (Fig. 22.17). This facilitates the spino-vestibulo-cerebellar pathways. This activation brings sometimes quite surprising and fast therapeutic effects. This technique has been introduced into therapeutic practice only recently, although for diagnostic purposes it was described by the French neurologist Foix in 1903 and has since been used in clinical neurology for diagnosis of cerebellar lesions (3).

Balance Sandals

Gait training on balance shoes is exceptionally useful for long-term therapy, and patients usually like them more than other exercises (Fig. 22.18). Balance shoes, when used correctly, increase demands on the entire postural mechanism and automatically, without conscious effort, help to correct and stabilize posture.

As with other exercises, a certain amount of voluntary control is needed at the beginning of balance shoe training. Several important aspects must be considered:

The sole of the foot must be held closely to the molded surface of the shoes. This is achieved by the activity of the muscles which form the small foot. The foot works together with the shoe as a functional unit. This should be maintained during the whole training session.

The subject controls his posture voluntarily at first, particularly the position of the pelvis, shoulder girdles, and head.

The feet should be held parallel and the steps should be short and quick.

The knees should be flexible, not rigid.

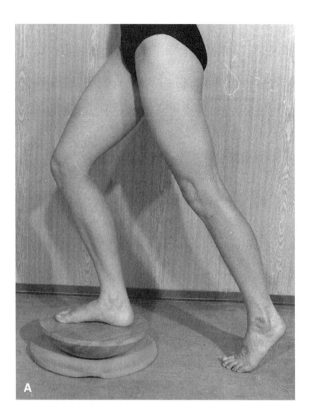
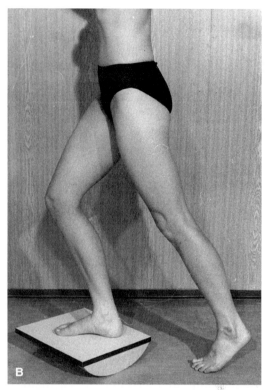

Figure 22.16 Lunge on balance boards: **(A)** wobble board; **(B)** rocker board.

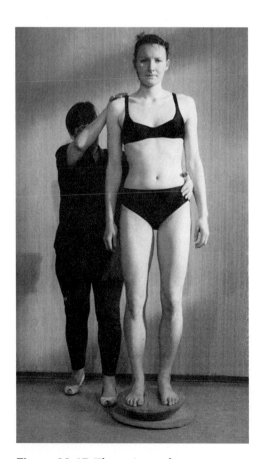

The landing of the shoes should be soft and quiet. Vertical and lateral shift of the pelvis should be avoided.

The Sequence

First Stage—Preparatory Stage

We start with teaching the stance. The patient uses firm support and learns to stand maintaining the bal-

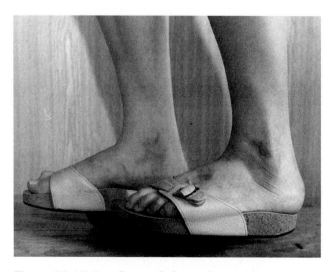

Figure 22.17 Therapist pushes.

Figure 22.18 Standing on balance shoes with support.

ance sandals in horizontal position, parallel with the floor, with the feet held parallel and the soles and toes adhered to the surface of the sandals. The therapist corrects the posture of the patient as he shifts from one leg to another in place. Usually it is very helpful to correct the pattern in front of the mirror.

Second Stage—Walking on the Shoes With the Help of the Therapist

The patient stands facing the therapist using support of his shoulders. First, the patient walks in place, and then walks with the support of the therapist. The therapist can facilitate the activity of gluteus maximus by touching or slightly pushing against anterior side of patient's hips; at the same time, the correction of the pelvis is achieved.

The Third Stage—Independent Walking

Walking forward, backward, and sideways are trained (Fig. 22.19). In many unpublished poly-EMG studies performed at Clinic of Rehabilitation Medicine at Vinohrady Faculty Hospital in Prague, a pronounced

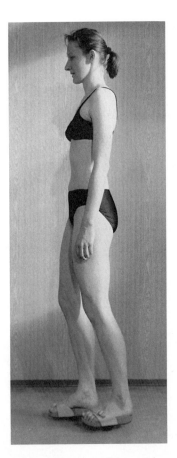

Figure 22.19 Walking with balance shoes.

increase of the activity in the muscles of the pelvis and trunk (particularly gluteus medius, gluteus maximus, errector spinae in lumbar region, rectus abdominis) has been found when exercising on the balance sandals. This was shown to persist with barefoot walking.

Balance sandals training achieves and sustains an improvement in muscle function during upright posture. Another advantage is the possibility to train advanced patients in small groups. Patients can also train with balance shoes at home or at the workplace.

According to our clinical experience, it is more effective to walk on balance shoes for a short time (1 to 2 minutes) several times per day. At the beginning, usually a few meters or steps are sufficient. With the first signs of fatigue, the patient should take a short rest and then walk several meters or steps again. The daily dose should not exceed 10 to 15 minutes.

In general, the improved posture becomes evident within a few weeks of training. One study has demonstrated more effective activation of glutei muscles within 1 week of training (4). The rate of motor unit recruitment increased, as well as gluteal activity and the difference between activation of the gluteals barefoot and in balance shoes walking decreased.

In another unpublished study, we were able to demonstrate that the abdominal recti, if hypotonic or inhibited, were better-activated during the curl-up after using the shoes for 1 week (5). This could be related to both the speed of motor units recruitment and total amount of EMG activity.

Miscellaneous SMS Tools

When training on the Fitter, gliding movements from side to side and from anterior to posterior direction are performed (Fig. 22.20). The demands on maintaining erect posture, coordination, and balance are increased. It improves the postural stability in general and specifically lateral stability of the pelvis achieved by increased activation of the gluteus medius. Estimation of body asymmetries is less recognizable when compared to the twister.

The twister is a device that allows possible improvement of the activation of the trunk and buttock muscles. In addition, the twisting movements specifically activate the deep intrinsic spinal muscles. It is easy to control the symmetry of the exercise while training on the twister. This is favorable because it helps correct asymmetries that develop as a rule in back pain patients and are sometimes difficult to recognize. The twister does not specifically increase proprioception, but it improves coordination and automatizes trunk and pelvic control.

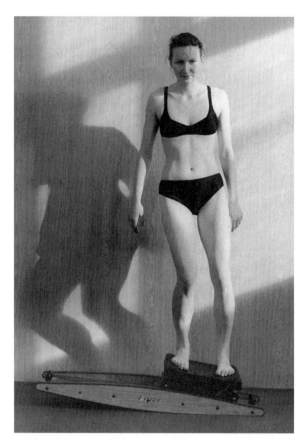

Figure 22.20 Training the gluteus medius on the Fitter.

Rollers and gymnastic or exercise balls have recently gained popularity in treatment of back pain patients, although they were used for decades in the treatment of children with cerebral palsy. One of the advantages of using balls in the treatment of back pain is that the trunk or spine stability can be trained in unloaded positions with the weight of the body fully or partly supported by the ball. From this point of view they are safe because they minimize the danger of the spine injury. They can be used in pain-free positions to prevent muscle inhibition. The activity of the muscles is achieved automatically as a reaction to the ball movement, which is important for gaining the normal movement patterns or normal motor behavior. The incredible variety of exercises, especially with regard to the potential positions that can be used, improve kinesthetic awareness, balance control, and spinal stability. Thus, they are very useful for postural training in general (see Chapter 26).

The minitrampoline is a device that is particularly useful. Jogging or jumping activates proprioception much more effectively than a similar exercise performed on a firm floor (Fig. 22.21). In addition, it

protects the joints because it functions as a shock absorber. Exercises on a trampoline do not need to be performed in an upright position only, but may also be performed while sitting, which is particularly effective in strengthening the abdominal muscles. Also, minitrampoline exercise in four-point kneeling is recommended for elderly women with kyphosis caused by osteoporosis (Fig. 22.22).

■ CONCLUSION

The SMS program deals, above all, with the upright posture of the body. Its aim is to improve function of the postural system or more precisely the motor program that controls the posture in a vertical position, particularly in stance and gait.

In fact, all functions of this system are trained—that is assuming and maintaining the upright posture balance during stance and dynamic stability (postural behavior during the movement). The emphasis is placed on the optimal posture that includes the straightening and stabilization of the axial organ/spine (21).

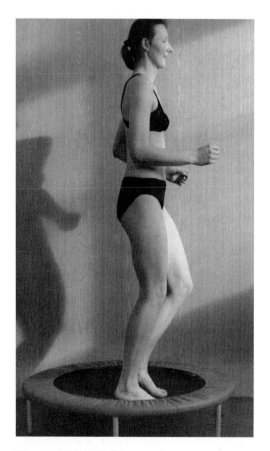

Figure 22.21 Walking on the minitrampoline.

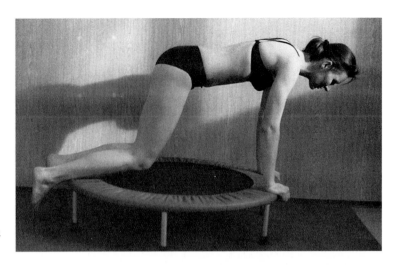

Figure 22.22 Four-point kneeling on the minitrampoline.

Thus, one of the main goals of SMS is to activate the stabilizing muscles. The activity of both stabilizing systems, described in literature as local and global stabilizing system, are trained (2,27). The role of the local stabilization system in spinal intersegmental control is highlighted in relation to the motor control changes described in low back pain patients and their treatment. The literature deals mostly with the dysfunction of the local stabilizing system in the lumbar region (26,32), but similar dysfunctions have been found also in the cervical spine (19).

In stability of the trunk (spine), a significant role is played by regulation of intra-abdominal and intra-thoracic pressures, which depend on appropriate activity of the diaphragm, abdominal wall (particularly transversus abdominis), pelvic floor and the deep spinal intrinsic muscles (13,27–29). One clinical study has demonstrated the immediate release of trigger points in the diaphragm and thoracic erector spinae after the active contraction and relaxation of pelvic diaphragm (23).

In SMS, the corrected stance position through the activity of the feet muscles (the "small" foot) and external hip rotators helps to stabilize the pelvis. The lumbar spine tends to adopt so-called neutral position (24,25) in which the lumbar part of multifidus plays an important role (24,25,27). At the same time, the activity of transversus abdominis is also achieved by flattening the abdominal wall, whereas the inspiratory position of the chest must be avoided.

Through elongation of the body, other parts of the spine are further straightened. The vizualization of the long axis of the body contributes to further increase of the activity of deep muscles of the spine, with deep muscles of the neck included. It is generally known that mere vizualization of the movement is able to increase the muscle tone. It can be presumed that in this case the muscle tone is increased especially in muscles with exclusively tonic function—deep mus-

cles of the spine. The activity of the intersegmental muscles of the neck elicited through vizualization is mentioned in literature (18).

The activity of pelvic floor (and thus also transversus abdominis) can be increased in corrected stance when leaning the body forward with the simultaneous pressure of the soles against the floor (clinical experience).

Thus, in true corrected stance, the coordinated activity of pelvic floor and transversus abdominis, with the neutral position in lumbar spine maintained, facilitates the postural role of diaphragm, which participates on stabilization of the spine. The stability of the spine (particularly lumbar spine) is achieved.

The maintenance of the upright posture, particularly long-lasting maintenance (as trained in corrected stance), is not possible without tonic activity of the local stabilizing system of the whole spine.

The training on labile surfaces and dynamic exercises increases the demands not only on the local stabilizing system but also on the global one, or more precisely on their coordination. Signs or symptoms of hyperactivity of the global stabilizing system, e.g., pathological distribution of muscle tone, the loss of optimal curves of the spine, tendency to inspiratory position of the chest, or faulty breathing pattern is possible to observe and, if necessary, correct voluntarily. Tests for the spine (trunk) stability and balance are included in the examination of the patient before the program is started. In case of severe insufficiency, particularly of the local stabilizing system, special attention is paid in preparatory exercises.

Repeated disturbance of balance with the element of speed increases (by means of automatic protective reactions) the alertness and accelerates the ability of muscles to achieve "maximum" contraction (increased rate of motor unit recruitment). At the same time, the ability of postural system to predict threatening the stability and balance from outer and inner environment (patient's own body) is gained. Thus, the postural system is able to start its stabilizing process in time and sufficiently before it is "threatened" from outside or before the fast volitional movement is started. The aim is to avoid the risk that arises from the movement elicited on the faulty posture—that is, the damage or injury particularly of joints (both of the the spine and extremities) and its passive stabilizing system.

Clinical experience shows that even after short training periods of SMS, the stability of posture and balance are improved; also, the fixed motor stereotypes or programs are more easily broken and the new ones automatically achieved. At the same time, the performance of everyday movements is facilitated and accelerated.

The movement variety and thus the deftness that is important for coping with the accidental situations in which the fast and coordinated reaction of the motor system is needed are increased. This is very important in prevention of microinjuries (and injuries) of the spine, which are one of the causes of back pain syndromes and their recurrences.

The SMS method has a wide spectrum of indication. It can be used successfully in postural defects of different origin: posttraumatic, postoperative, chronic back pain, faulty posture in children and adolescents, postural defects connected with childbirth (pelvic floor, abdominals), and with respiratory dysfunction, various forms of hypermobility, or instability (both spine and extremity joints). Children, adults, and seniors can use the exercise, as can athletes and people with sedentary lifestyles. It could also be included in back school programs. Thus, it may become a part of many therapeutical programmes that aim to improve or gain the upright posture and its stability. It also can be used in neurological cases and, in fact, in all situations in which the defect of afference can be presumed. In principle, there are no contraindications of the method. It is not suitable for acute pain condition (of posttraumatic and postoperative) or for the complete sensory loss and for patients who are unable to cooperate.

The SMS program is not a fixed or rigid one; rather, it must be adapted to the individual problems and needs of the patient.

SMS is a process of sensorimotor learning and its name points out the importance of sensory afference for movement control. Increased flow of afference from all resources necessary for facilitation of the function of the postural system are used, particularly somatosensory and vestibular afference, with the emphasis on the role of proprioceptive afference.

The need to stimulate proprioceptors is even greater today than a few decades ago. Our lifestyles have changed substantially and are associated with a general decrease in sensory (proprioceptive) stimulation.

Thus, the elements of SMS should take part in every movement education, including the general and special and, naturally, the therapeutic one.

Audit Process
Self-Check of the Chapter's Learning Objectives

- What are a few indications for sensory motor training?

- What is the difference between passive modeling, active assistance, and active performance of the small foot?

- In postural correction, where should pressure be felt in the feet?

- What is the procedure for performing the lunge?

- What exercises can be performed on the rocker and wobble boards?

- How does the clinician initiate balance sandal training?

■ ACKNOWLEDGMENT

The authors would like to express their thanks for cooperation on the chapter to Craig Liebenson. We especially appreciate his effort, which led to the new edition of this chapter. We believe this method still continues as an important part of physiotherapy treatment, not only in our country but also abroad. Our great thanks belong also to Pamela Tunnell for her sensitive and precise correction of the English text.

■ REFERENCES

1. Abrahams VC. The physiology of neck muscles. Their role in head movement and maintenance of posture. Can J Physiol Pharmacol 1977;55:332–338.

2. Bergmark A. Stability of the lumbar spine. A study in mechanical engineering. Acta Orthop Scand 1989;230(suppl):20–24.

3. Bobath K, Bobath B. The facilitation of normal postural reactions and movement in treatment of cerebral palsy. Physiother 1964;50:246.

4. Bullock-Saxton JE, Janda V, Bullock MI. Reflex activation of gluteal muscles in walking. Spine 1993;18:704–708.

5. Bullock-Saxton JE, Janda V, Bullock MI. Reflex activation of abdominal muscles during a curl up. Unpublished 1994.

6. Burton AK. Trunk muscle activity induced by three sizes of wobble (balance) boards. J Orthop Sp Phys Ther 1986;8:70–76.

7. Freeman MAR, Wyke BD. Articular contributions to limb muscle reflexes. J Physiol (Lond) 1964;171:20P–21P.

8. Freeman MAR, Dean MRE, Hanham IWF. The etiology and prevention of functional instability of the foot. J Bone Joint Surg (Br) 1965;47B:678–685.

9. Freeman MAR, Wyke BD. Articular reflexes at the ankle joint. An electromyographic study of normal and abnormal influences of ankle joint mechanoreceptors upon reflex activity in leg muscles. Br J Surg 1967;54:990–1001.

10. Guyton AC. Basic Neuroscience. Philadelphia: WB Saunders, 1987.

11. Herveou C, Messean L. Technique de reeducation et d education proprioceptive. Paris: Maloin ed., 1976.

12. Hinoki M, Ushio N. Lumbosacral proprioceptive reflexes in body equilibrium. Acta Otolaryngol 1975;330(Suppl):197–210.

13. Hodges PW, Butler JE, McKenzie D, Gandevia SC. Contraction of the human diaphragm during postural adjustments. J Physiol 1997;505:239–548.

14. Ihara H, Nakayama A. Dynamic joint control training for knee ligament injuries. Am J Sports Med 1986;14:309–315.

15. Janda V, Vavrova M. Sensory Motor Stimulation: A Video. Presented by JE Bullock-Saxton, produced by Body Control Systems, Brisbane, Australia, 1990.

16. Janda V, Vávrová M. Sensory motor stimulation (video), 1990, in Czech.

17. Janda V, Vávrová M. Sensory motor stimulation. Rehabilitacia 1992;3:14–35, in Czech.

18. Jirout J. Reaction of the cervical vertebrae on assumed changes in the shape of the cervical spine. Československá neurologie a neurochirurgie 1989;2:75–77, in Czech.

19. Jull G. Deep cervical flexor muscle dysfunction in whiplash. J Muskuloskel Pain 2000;8:143–154.

20. Kabat H. Central mechanisms for recovery of neuromuscular function. Science 1950;112:23–24.

21. Kolář P. The sensomotor nature of postural functions. Its fundamental role in rehabilitation on the motor system. J Orthop Med 1999;1:40–45.

22. Kurtz AD. Chronic sprained ankle. Am J Surg 1939;44:158–160.

23. Lewit K. The stabilizing system of the lumbar spine and the pelvic diaphragm. Rehabilitace a fyzikální lékařství 1999;2:46–48.

24. Liebenson C. Rehabilitation of the Spine: A Practitioner's Manual. Baltimore: Williams & Wilkins, 1996.

25. Norris C. Back Stability. Champaign: Human Kinetics, 2000.

26. Panjabi MM. The stabilizing system of the spine. Part 1. Function, dysfunction, adaptation and enhancement. J Spinal Dis 1992;5:383–389.

27. Richardson C, Jull G, Hodges P, Hides J. Therapeutic Exercise for Spinal Segmental Stabilization in Low Back Pain. London: Churchill Livingstone, 1999.

28. Sapsford RR, Hodges PW, Richardson CA. Activation of the abdominal muscles is a normal response to contraction of the pelvic floor muscles. Japan: International Continence Society Conference, abstract, 1997.

29. Sapsford RR, Hodges PW, Richardson CA, Cooper DA, Jull GA, Markwel SJ. Activation of pubococcygeus during a variety of isometric abdominal exercises. Japan: International Continence Society Conference, abstract, 1997.

30. Sherrington CS. On reciprocal innervation of antagonistic muscles. Proc R Soc 1907;79B:337.

31. Skogland S. Anatomical and physiological studies of knee joint innervation in the cat. Acta Physiol Scand 1956;36 (Suppl 124):1–101.

32. Stanford M. Effectiveness of specific lumbar stabilization exercises: A single case study. J Manual Manip Ther 2002;10:40.

33. Wyke BD. The neurology of joints. Ann R Coll Surg Engl 1967;41:25–50.

23

Facilitation of Agonist-Antagonist Co-activation by Reflex Stimulation Methods

Pavel Kolář

Learning Objectives

After reading this chapter, you should be able to understand:

- The role of agonist–antagonist muscle co-activation and functional joint centration
- The relationship between developmental kinesiology and muscle balance/imbalance
- The stages of neurodevelopment of upright posture
- The use of reflex locomotion methods techniques involving creeping and rolling movements to facilitate muscle balance and joint centration
- The relationship of coordination between the abdominal wall and diaphragm for promoting spinal stability

Introduction

Two types of motor behavior result from the structure and function of the nervous system. One manifests itself by motor function as a result of motor learning. This consists of conditioned reflexes, which are formed by constantly repeated stimuli. The second is automatic learned motor functions, which are termed motor stereotypes.

The nervous system produces motor functions that appear in the same way from one generation to the next. These genetically determined factors of motor behavior are called motor patterns. Muscle function is encoded in motor patterns, which develop as the central nervous system (CNS) matures. Motor patterns, i.e., the reactions of the motor system to afferent stimulation, represent the programs of the CNS. The response to a given stimulus depends on the level of integration in the CNS. The reactions of specific stimuli described so far are at the spinal and brain stem level. This level of organization corresponds to phenomena such as the supporting reaction, the crossed extension reflex, gait automatism, segmental cutaneous motor reflexes, deep tonic neck reflexes, vestibular reflexes, etc. In addition to these reactions (programs), it is now possible to demonstrate motor patterns integrated above the brain stem level. These programs mature only in the course of postural ontogenesis.

If a 1-year-old is lifted by one arm and the leg of the same side from the supine position and held horizontal (Collis horizontal reaction), a characteristic motor response is obtained (Fig. 23.1). This response, if repeated, is constant, with the child reacting in the same way each time. This response does not result from motor learning but will be the same in all children of the same age with a normal CNS. The type of

response depends on postural function resulting from muscular co-activation, corresponding to the stage of maturity reached by the CNS.

Motor patterns at this level of integration are neglected by clinicians and by neurophysiologists, despite their fundamental clinical significance. In this chapter we demonstrate that these motor functions, which though genetically determined, are controlled and integrated on a higher than brain stem level and can be explained by mechanisms of the ontogenesis of posture.

Central and Reflex Changes of Muscle Function

To fully appreciate muscular function it is necessary to describe, study, and understand not only its anatomy but also its function under the control of the CNS. It has been pointed out that muscle activity is the result of very complex reflex processes, which are better termed programs, because their nature is processing information by very complex and in many ways unknown physiological mechanisms. The relationship between receptors and effectors cannot be explained by a simple reflex pathway, but only by a program worked out by the CNS.

If there is disturbed activity of the CNS or of any other part of the human organism, including visceral organs, there will be repercussions in the somatic, i.e., muscular system. There are, however, only two types of response.

1. Inhibition, with signs of hypotonus, decreased activity and weakness.
2. Hypertonus, spasm, rigidity, and even spasticity.

In most cases, these changes affect only the contractile elements. However, they may affect connective tissue, resulting in shortening, or even contracture. In this case, the muscle cannot reach its full length. At a certain point contracture can change the alignment of joints the muscle is related to, even in the neutral position. Even when slowly stretched, the full range of movement cannot be reached (8).

Changes in muscular function, whether caused by hyperactivity or hypoactivity, can affect the whole muscle or group of muscles, or only a small part of it. If it is only a small localized lesion, it is called a trigger point (TrP). It consists of only a few muscle fibers with a decreased threshold to stimulation. In voluntary movement they contract first, but uneconomically. In the center of the TrP, the fibers are in a state of contraction, whereas at the periphery the fibers are distended and inhibited. This can be called intramuscular incoordination.

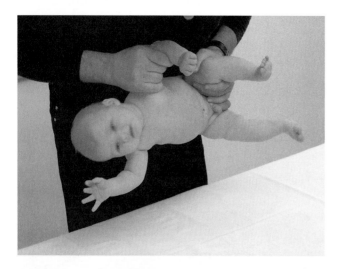

Figure 23.1 The Collis horizontal reaction.

The muscle may not be weak in itself, but it may not function well because its attachment point is insufficiently fixed. A muscle must have a punctum fixum. Thus in resisted flexion of the wrist, the attachment point of the wrist flexors must be stabilized by the muscles that stabilize the elbow, and the elbow in turn by the shoulder girdle. In this way, stabilization of attachment points depends on a chain of muscles. Disturbed function of a muscle can therefore be caused by dysfunction of a far-distant muscle.

groups and in other groups inhibition, ending up in atrophy. This is true, e.g., in organic lesions of the CNS. Those muscles that tend to develop spasm in acute poliomyelitis are the same as those that in the chronic stage of the disease produce contracture, and in patients with cerebral palsy (with signs of spasticity) cause spastic contracture. Their antagonists, however, are inhibited.

The same muscles that are likely to produce contracture and those that incline to inhibition in lesions of the CNS can be found to be hypertonic or weak respectively in disturbed posture.

As the shoulder girdle is stabilized by the abdominal muscles in the upright position, wrist flexion can be impaired by dysfunctional abdominal muscles. In this way, the condition of the abdominal muscles may change the quality of wrist flexion. This principle holds for specific muscular activity. It follows therefore that the functioning of any muscle is determined not only by its specific function but also by its stabilization. Insufficient stabilization is a very frequent cause of muscular dysfunction. Unfortunately, muscle function is usually examined without adequate regard to stabilization. This takes place automatically and unconsciously, programmed by the CNS. It is very important in treatment of disturbance of motor function to analyze the chain of muscles determining the stabilizing function.

The following characteristic features of these changes in function are:

1. They are interrelated, i.e., they are never isolated, but form chain reactions.
2. The dysfunctional chains are not at random, but follow definite rules.
3. Muscular dysfunction goes hand in hand with functional changes of joints, skin, fascia, periosteum, and even visceral organs.

Muscular Imbalance

There is clinical and experimental evidence that some muscles are inclined to inhibition (hypotonus, weakness, inactivity), and other muscle groups are likely to be hyperactive with a tendency to become short (2–4,6,7,9). This fact was already known. Janda, however, was the first who showed that the ensuing imbalance followed certain rules, which are sufficiently constant and characteristic to be called syndromes (the upper and lower crossed syndrome, the stratification syndrome) (see chapter 10).

A number of pathological conditions produce hypertonus and even contracture in some muscle

Muscular Imbalance and Its Nature

The muscular system reacts according to certain rules. What, then, are the common features of muscles with a tendency to hypertonus, hyperactivity, and tightness, to spasticity, and even to spastic contracture in cerebral lesions? The same question can be asked about muscles tending to inhibition. In what function do these muscles differ?

The contemporary theory suggests that the two muscular systems have opposite characters. One basic feature stems from their function against gravity. Janda distinguishes tonic muscles with a tendency to shortness, and even contracture with a mainly postural function (3,4), hence the term postural muscles. It is, however, questionable which position (posture) is formative in the first place. Which position is decisive in opposing gravity? Janda considers gait to be the basic typical human motor activity (see chapter 10). He further explains that we stand on one leg during 85% of the time spent walking. He considers the muscles responsible for erect posture during a given stage of walking to be postural muscles in the true sense of the word (5,7).

Physiologists have shown that the two types of muscles differ in both function and structure. The same difference is also found in the nervous structures in control of these muscles, for it is the type of motor neurons that determine the type of muscle fiber. It is therefore better to speak of tonic and phasic motor units. Tonic motoneurons, i.e., small alpha motor cells, innervate red muscle fibers, whereas phasic motoneurons (large alpha cells) innervate white muscle fibers. In humans, both types of motor units are present in every muscle, in different proportions. Such muscles are "mixed." According to the preponderance of one or the other type of motor units, tonic (postural) and phasic (kinetic) muscles can be distinguished. Contraction and decontraction is slower in tonic than in phasic motor units.

Having understood the functional and morphological difference between the two antagonistic muscular systems, this difference is particularly striking from the point of view of phylogenesis and ontogenesis. This also provides a more specific and effective approach for treatment of disturbances resulting from the functional antagonism of the two systems.

The Development of Muscle Function in Light of Postural Ontogenesis

It is common knowledge that unlike most animals, humans are immature at birth, both in function and even morphologically. The CNS matures in the course of postnatal development, as does useful muscular function. The position of the joints, and posture, are the essential items of ontogenesis. This is to a great extent because of the stabilizing function of muscles acting interdependently. The specific bipedal erect posture matures during ontogenesis with trunk rotation and abduction and outward rotation of the arms. Thus, also, the development of joint position is determined by muscles responsible for coordinated stabilization of their attachment points.

The morphological development of the skeleton takes place at the same time (the shape of the hip joint, the plantar arch, spinal curvature, etc.) depending on the postural and stabilizing function of the "phasic" muscles, which are phylogenetically younger. Thus, intrauterine evolution continues in function and in morphology and is accomplished at the age of 4 years, when gross motor function has reached full maturity. This development can be illustrated at the shoulder blade. It does not stop at birth; during pregnancy, the shoulder blade begins to descend in a caudal direction, and if this does not take place, Sprengel deformity results.

Under normal conditions, CNS maturation continues at the shoulder blade after birth as the maturation of muscle function causes it to descend further. After the fourth week, the caudal part of the trapezius and the serratus anterior come into play. The stabilizing function of other muscles, in particular, of the abdominal muscles and even the diaphragm, is essential to facilitate outward rotation of the caudal angle of the shoulder blade, resulting in abduction of the arm to more than 90 degrees. This represents the most recent stage in the evolution of the scapulae's position.

In infantile lesions of the CNS, the muscles responsible for posture and stabilization do not function, and neither the descent nor outward rotation of the shoulder blade takes place. The shoulder blade remains in the neonatal position, i.e., elevated as a result of pull by the upper trapezius and the levator scapulae (Fig. 23.2). This is also the case in bad posture because of incomplete maturation. Only humans can fix the shoulder blade to the thorax in a

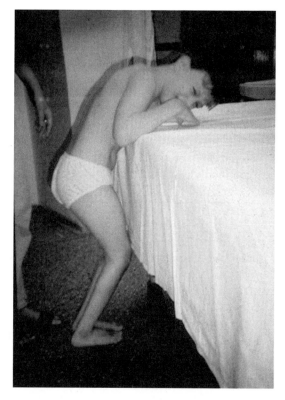

Figure 23.2 Child with spastic diparesis. The posture corresponds to the neonatal stage of development and morphological immaturity.

caudal and outward rotated position. This function matures only during postural ontogenesis after birth. The muscles responsible for this position are very prone to inhibition, and similar disturbances can be observed in other parts of the human skeleton.

Not unlike posture, the position and stabilization of joints results from coordinated muscular activity under the control of the CNS. This follows logically from the development of some characteristic positions of the body (prone, supported on elbows, "oblique" sitting, standing erect), and also from the positions the joints take up in the course of primitive locomotion. Studying the separate phases of locomotion "frozen phases" Janda helps us to understand posture better and to infer joint position at each stage of motion (5,7). In the case of locomotion, on all fours we obtain the sum of momentary positions beginning with the starting position and reaching the opposite end position of side-bending, rotation, and anteflexion and retroflexion.

Postural Ontogenesis— Motor Programs

Muscular synergy develops during evolution, following patterns stored in the brain. The infant does not need to be taught how to lift his head, to grasp a toy, to turn around, or to move on all fours. All this occurs automatically in the course of maturation of the CNS by muscular coordination. These functions are genetically determined. Postural activity of the muscles comes into play automatically depending on optic orientation and the emotional needs of the child. This activity ensures active posture, i.e., all possible positions in the joints determined by their anatomical shape. Morphological development of the skeleton depends on postural function of the muscles. Understanding the kinesiology of postural development is essential for both the diagnosis and treatment of the locomotor system (10).

The Development of Functional Joint Centration

The position of joints is controlled from infancy (even during movement) by coordinated co-contraction of antagonists. It is also linked up with muscles providing joint stabilization. The co-activation pattern of antagonists develops between the fourth and sixth week of infancy. Well-balanced activity of antagonists guarantees well-centered joints. This depends only on a normally developed CNS. Any abnormality of the CNS causes abnormal joint position. This is very important for diagnosis, particularly in the early stage of development.

The concept of functional centration is essential to understand the relationship between joints and muscles. The terms "centration," "decentration," "subluxation," and "luxation" used mainly in orthopedics describe the morphological and/or pathological condition of joints. Functional centration, however, implies maximum load bearing, i.e., the best possible distribution of the load at the articular surfaces. In other words, it implies maximum contact of articular surfaces during each position in the course of movement.

A good example is the hip joint. If functional centration is to be maintained during flexion, there must be abduction and outward rotation at the same time. Thus, only maximal contact of the articular surfaces can be achieved. Under the same conditions the axis of rotation, too, is at the center of the joint cavity and of the femoral head. As flexion decreases, outward rotation and abduction decreases as well, and there is none in extension.

If hip movement is separated into individual stages, with each stage being correctly centered from one extreme to the opposite end position, a sum of "frozen" articular positions is obtained, i.e., of coupled flexion, rotation, and abduction. Maximum contact of the articular surfaces also produces maximum facilita-

tion of muscle activity. Kabat's diagonal movements make excellent use of this principle.

The weight lifter can serve for illustration. He puts himself into a position in which the spinal column, the hip joints, the knees, etc. are loaded most favorably. His joints are centered during all the stages of weight lifting to bear the maximum load. In any other position the articular surfaces would be incongruent, risking tissue damage. This is an example of the balanced function of antagonists and goes hand-in-hand with well-balanced loading of the spinal column, its discs, and articulations.

The same principle of joint centration is adhered to during all the stages of postural ontogenesis because of balanced muscular activity. This principle holds for the spinal column because of the activity of the deep intrinsic back muscles, the deep neck flexors, and the abdominal muscles. Under their control, the optimum position of the individual segments is achieved in the sagittal plane. In this way, the most favorable loading of the intervertebral discs and the centration of intervertebral joints is achieved. It constitutes a motor program forming spinal curvatures in the sagittal plane. This postural program is completed during the fourth month. It is the posture we have seen in the weight lifter.

Further differentiation of muscle function from the fifth to the seventh month enables the child to achieve a well-centered posture, even during trunk rotation, having learned how to turn from prone to supine and back. A well-centered posture both in the sagittal plane and during rotation can be maintained only if the CNS develops normally. According to Vojta, this degree of maturity is never attained in 30% of children (1,11,13). In such children, faulty posture and muscular imbalance begin at an early stage of their development.

It must be particularly stressed that muscular synergy related to this model of evolution always depends on body posture as a whole and not that of a particular segment. Decentration of a single joint has its effect on the centration of all the other joints. The interrelation of all body segments is best demonstrated by Vojta's method of reflex locomotion. If stimulation is performed in a position of decentration, e.g., of the head, not a single joint will be correctly centered. In conclusion, correct centration of joints can be considered an important sign of normal function of the CNS.

Motor Programs During Individual Developmental Stages

During each stage, partial motor patterns mature representing the basic elements of adult motor behavior

The Neonatal Stage

During this stage of development, the posture of the infant is unbalanced (Fig. 23.3). The point of gravity is in the sternal and umbilical region. In this unbalanced posture there is neither a differentiated function nor any point of support. The whole body rests on the surface. If prone, the child lays on one half of the body from the cheek to the chest as far as the umbilicus. The upper and the lower extremities are in flexion, unable to give any support. The same unbalanced posture can be seen with the baby supine (Fig. 23.4).

This neonatal posture is given here in detail:

- The hand—the fingers are flexed and in ulnar flexion, there is also flexion at the wrist
- The elbow is in flexion and pronation
- The shoulder is protracted and in internal rotation
- The shoulder blade is elevated
- The spine is in flexion
- The pelvis is in anteversion
- The hip joint is in flexion and internal rotation
- The knees are flexed, the legs rotated outward
- The foot in plantar flexion

In the neonatal period, the tonic muscular system is in complete control. As we have pointed out, all the anatomical structures of the skeleton at this stage are immature, too. This holds for the angle of anteversion and the colodiaphyseal angle of the femur, the plantar arch, the plateau of the tibia, leg rotation, and the horizontal position of the collar bones, etc. These are related to the formative influence of the postural function of the phasic muscular system: the abductors and outward rotators at the hip, the

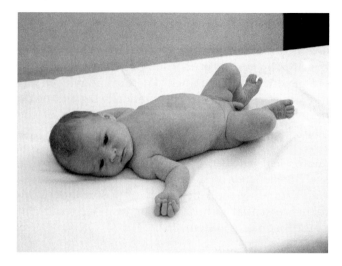

Figure 23.4 Posture at birth: supine.

spinal extensors, the short extensors at the knee, the tibialis anterior, the peroneal muscles etc. Because no higher centers of nervous control are as yet functioning and the tonic system is in complete control, there is no postural balance and it is yet possible to elicit certain motor responses (programs), which are integrated at the spinal level of control.

The Suprapubic Reflex

On slight (not nociceptive) pressure at the upper edge of the symphysis extension and inward rotation at the hip, extension at the knee, plantar flexion of the feet, and fanning out of the toes takes place (Fig. 23.5). This response is symmetrical on both lower extremities.

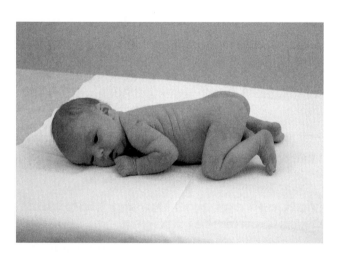

Figure 23.3 Posture at birth: prone.

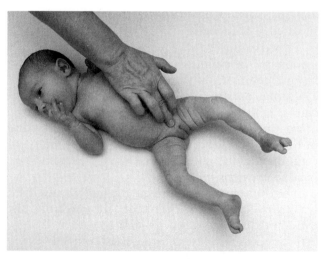

Figure 23.5 Suprapubic reflex.

Support Reaction

The baby is held under the armpits and the soles of his feet are stimulated (Fig. 23.6). The response is extension (support) of both lower extremities. If this reflex continues for some time, it can be mistaken for the infant attempting to stand.

Automatic Gait

This reflex is elicited similarly to the previous one; however, in this case, only one sole is stimulated (Fig. 23.7). Triple flexion of the opposite extremity takes place. In this reflex, the infant demonstrate a walking pattern on an involuntary basis.

The Crossed Extension Reflex

With the baby supine and the lower extremity flexed at the hip and knee, slight pressure is exerted against the knee in the direction of the hip joint (Fig. 23.8). Extension and inward rotation at the hip, extension of the knee, plantar flexion of the foot, extension at the metatarsophalangeal, and flexion at the interphalangeal joints take place in the other lower extremity.

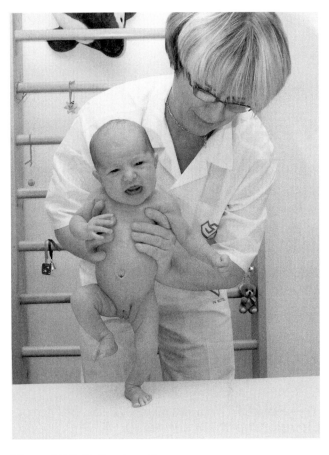

Figure 23.7 Gait automatism.

Calcaneal (Heel) Reflex

The heel is tapped and the hip and knee are in a semiflexed position (Fig. 23.9). Extension of the knee and hip takes place.

In all the motor programs given, we find a reciprocal response of antagonists on stimulation, i.e., for

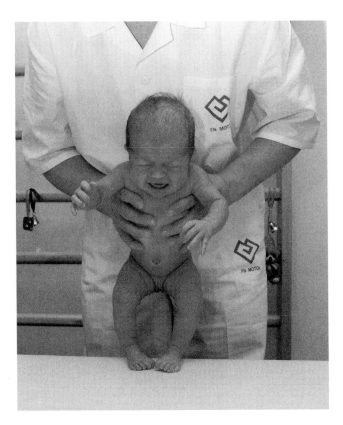

Figure 23.6 Support reaction.

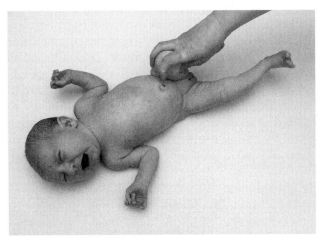

Figure 23.8 Crossed extension reflex.

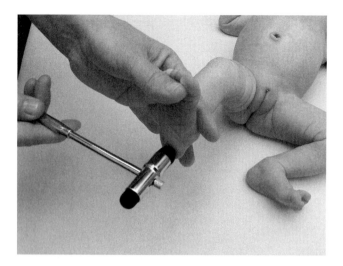

Figure 23.9 Heel reflex.

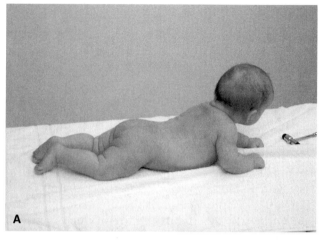

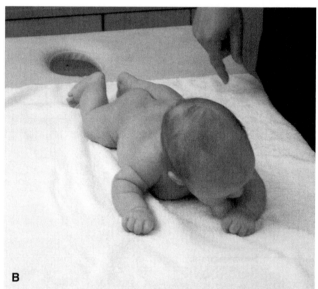

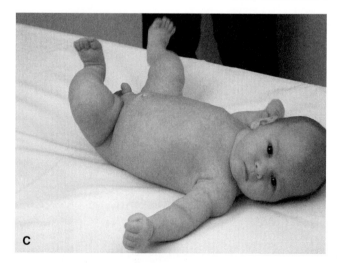

Figure 23.10 First stage of erect posture after optic orientation between 4 and 6 weeks **(A–C)**.

every reflex response of one muscle, its antagonist is inhibited.

The Fourth Through Sixth Week of Motor Development

Optic fixation appears between the fourth and sixth week and with it the infant's orientation in space. It begins to lift the head against gravity (Fig. 23.10). In this way, the head is lifted beyond its base of support and supports itself on the forearms. The upper arms are no longer in a frontal plane, they move toward the sagittal plane by adduction and flexion at the shoulder. At the same time, the point of gravity moves in a caudal direction toward the symphysis, and anteflexion of the pelvis decreases. It must be stressed that lifting the head first is in no way an isolated movement but that this goes hand in hand with the upper extremity providing support to lift the thorax, changing in this way the entire body posture. This depends on precisely coordinated muscular function providing stabilization. This all-around change of posture is automatic; however, it depends on the child's mental development and is encoded in locomotor ontogenesis.

Higher levels of CNS control come into play when optic fixation is established. The characteristic features of this stage are:

1. The spinal motor patterns disappear or are hidden, i.e., the supporting reaction, the gait automatism, etc.
2. Muscular co-activation appears, resulting in a balanced activity by simultaneous action of

antagonists and their mutual reciprocal facilitation and inhibition.

3. "Phasic muscles" begin to take part in the stabilization of posture. As a consequence, muscles with a tendency to weakness take part in the maintenance of posture as links of a chain. These muscles, as pointed out, are not true phasic muscles and, in view of their postural function, should be better-considered as phylogenetically and ontogenetically younger postural muscles. The most important phasic and tonic muscles are listed in Table 23.1.

The End of the First and the Beginning of the Second Trimenon

At 3.5 months, the first support base is defined and the points of support can be shown to be the elbows and the symphysis with the infant prone (Fig. 23.11). If supine, the area of support is formed by the upper part of the gluteal muscles, the scapular region, and the linea nuchae (Fig. 23.12). Posture is fully determined at this stage, controlled by the CNS. Spinal straightening, ensured by well-balanced activity of the deep extensors and flexors, can be observed starting at the occipital level and ending at sacrum.

Table 23.1   Muscles With Predominately Phasic and Tonic Function

Tonic Muscles	Phasic Muscles
adductor policis	abductor pollicis brevis
flexor digiti minimi	opponens pollicis
interossei palmares	interossei dorsales
palmaris longus	extensor digiti minimi
flexor digitorum superficialis	
flexor digitorum profundus	extensor carpi radialis
flexor carpi ulnaris	extensor carpi ulnaris
flexor carpi radialis	extensor digitorum
	abductor pollicis longus
pronator teres	abductor pollis brevis
pronator quadratus	
biceps brachii brevis	anconeus
brachioradialis	triceps brachii lateral and medial heads
triceps brachii long head	teres minor
	infraspinatus
subscapularis	supraspinatus
pectoralis major	serratus anterior
pectoralis minor	deltoideus
teres major	biceps brachii longus
latissimus dorsi	trapezius—lower part
coracobrachialis	rhomboidei
trapezius (middle and upper)	abdominal muscles
levator scapulae	extensors and outward rotators of the hip joint
	vastus medialis and lateralis
neck extensors	hip joint abductores
sternocleidomastoideus	gastrocnemius
scaleni	peroneal muscles
quadratus lumborum	longus colli
	longus capitis
iliopsoas	rectus capitis ant.
rectus femoris	
hip joint adductors	
tensor fascie latae	
ischiocrural muscles	
soleus	
foot adductors	

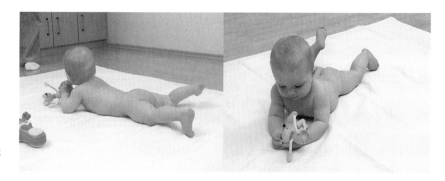

Figure 23.11 Posture when prone at 3.5 months.

Equilibrium between the lower and upper fixators of the shoulder blade is established: in the course of the fourth month, stabilization of the spinal column in the sagittal plane matures. This forms the basis of the stepping forward (grasping) and support function of the extremities, which involves rotation of the spinal column. Maturity of the spine in the sagittal plane is also necessary for the grasping function of the upper extremity. Further development depends on this basic synergy. Turning over, sitting, standing, getting on all fours, and so on can be achieved only if there is stability in the sagittal plane. The spinal column thus provides the basis for stabilizing the muscles of the extremities, playing the role of a punctum fixum. If there is any abnormality, there will also be dysfunction at the extremities. This relationship is, however, reciprocal. Development in the sagittal plane that is not ideal can always be observed even later (during adulthood).

The muscular interplay described, very well-defined from the kinesiological point of view, is essential for erect posture. It represents a genetically fixed model, specific exclusively for the human species, and deter-mines the formation of the characteristic spinal curvatures (kyphosis and lordosis) in the sagittal plane. It is very important that this model can be evoked by Vojta's method of reflex locomotion in the neonatal stage of development, at a time when the anatomical structures are not yet fully developed. This proves the genetically determined formative role of postural function.

Motor Development From the Second Half of Trimenon

At age 4.5 months, the child is able to grasp an object when lying prone. The head, the upper extremity, and the shoulder are lifted against gravity. If the CNS functions normally, the spine and the extremity joints are in a centered position, and the support is of a triangular shape, formed by the elbow, the anterior superior iliac spine of one side, and the medial epicondyle of the femur of the opposite side (Fig. 23.13). Thus, the support pattern of the lower extremity is partially formed. In this model of development, the fist is formed with radial flexion. At the same time, there is thumb flexion with abduction of the fingers. Lifting of the upper extremity prone is possible only if muscle pull of the opposite weight-bearing extremity is directed distally to the point of support.

At age 4.5 months, the child lying supine is able to lift his pelvis, supporting himself on the thoracolumbar junction, which is stabilized by muscular coactivation. This point of support enables the child to grasp an object situated above mid-line while supine. At this stage, the chest can also be asymmetrically stretched with the child supine. In this way, the lower shoulder becomes the point of support, which, too, is possible only if there is distal muscle pull. From this position, trunk rotation can follow with the spine straight, a function completed by the end of the sixth month. Two oblique muscle chains appear at this time. The first produces pelvic rotation in the direction of the supporting upper extremity. Muscle contraction starts at the obliquus abdominis internus on the side to which the chin is turned, pass-

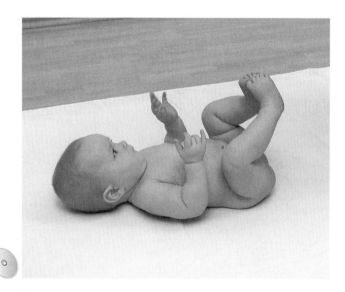

Figure 23.12 Posture when supine at 3.5 months.

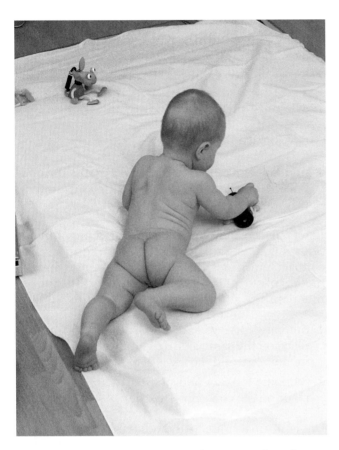

Figure 23.13 Posture at 4.5 months: support based on the elbow, the anterior superior iliac spine of one side, and the medial epicondyle of the opposite knee.

ing by the transversus abdominis to the obliquus externus of the opposite side (Fig. 23.14). The dorsal muscles take part in the co-activation synergy. The second oblique chain taking part synergistically in rotation is formed by the abdominal muscles with the pectoralis major and minor of both sides, producing rotation of the upper part of the trunk and straightening at the shoulder (Fig. 23.15).

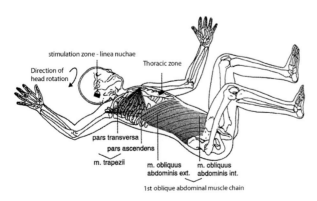

Figure 23.14 The first oblique muscle chain according to Vojta.

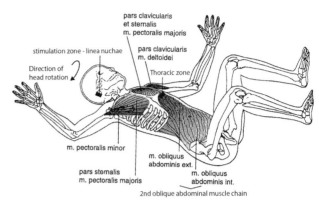

Figure 23.15 The second oblique muscle chain according to Vojta.

When turning over from supine to prone, one leg is supporting and the other is "swinging" (stepping forward). The arms behave in an analogous way. The reciprocal movement pattern has been finished, i.e.:

1. The supporting leg (which takes off) moves into inward rotation, adduction, and extension, and the other leg moves in external rotation, abduction, and flexion at the hip. The other articulations function analogically, i.e., their movement has a reciprocal pattern.

2. The muscles of the supporting leg exert a pull in a distal direction, i.e., "the punctum fixum" is distal and "the punctum mobile" is proximal. The muscles of the swinging (stepping forward) leg, however, have their punctum fixum proximal while the punctum mobile is distal.

3. Thus, muscle pull is differentiated at this stage of development, i.e., in the supporting leg (arm) the joint cavity moves against the head of the joint, whereas in the swinging leg (arm) the head moves against the joint cavity.

It is characteristic for locomotion during the fifth and sixth month that the supporting and swinging extremities are ipsilateral. Differentiated muscle function is established, by which is meant an opposite direction of muscle pull in swinging and supporting extremities. In stepping forward or grasping, the extremity muscles pull against a fixed point (punctum fixum) located proximally. The femoral and humeral heads move against the joint cavities. However, in the supporting extremities the situation is the opposite. In support function, the extremity muscles pull against a fixed point located distally. Now, the joint cavities move against the femoral or humeral heads.

We mean the direction of muscle pull, i.e., the location (proximal or distal) of the fixed point ("punctum fixum") against which the muscles pull and the movement of the joint head and cavity. The swinging (grasping) and the support extremity behave in the same way. The only difference is that the movement is reciprocal.

The oblique sitting position develops from both the prone and the supine position. The points of support are the gluteus medius and the hand. The grasping upper extremity is flexed at the shoulder at an angle above 120 degrees. Crawling on all fours develops from this position. The next step is for the child to stand up and walk toward the side. This is followed by true bipedal locomotion. After the age of 6 months, the supporting and swinging function of the arms and legs takes on a contralateral pattern. Thus, the "swinging" or grasping arm is on the side of the supporting leg and vice versa. The course of the movement of the stepping forward and the supporting extremity is the same. The difference is in the punctum fixum, which in the former is proximal and in the latter distal. There are two basic models of the phasic movements. The stepping forward (grasping) and support function may be either contralateral or ipsilateral. This coordinated muscular activity is genetically programmed. It stabilizes the spinal column in the sagittal plane (fourth month) and later develops the function of swinging (stepping forward, grasping) and support. It forms the basis of our "motor subconsciousness." All joint positions result from muscular synergies maturing during early development. The range of movement depends not only on the anatomical structures but also on the muscles and muscular synergies performing the movement. Muscular synergies resulting in this model always depend on body posture, never that of a single segment. This functional goal explains the relationship between the anatomical structure of muscles and joints and their function.

Summary

Motor development in infancy is automatic, depending on optical orientation and the emotional needs of the child. It is genetically determined, developing the motor functions that form the basis of our automatic subconscious motor behavior. Two basic functions play a decisive role in this context:

1. The development of stabilization in the sagittal plane at the end of the fourth month. At this period, the muscular stabilizing function matures, enabling the spinal column to adopt ideal weight-bearing posture. If the CNS functions normally, the principles of neurophysiology

and biomechanics must be in harmony. Stabilization in the sagittal plane forms the basis for every phasic movement.

2. The development of specific phasic movements. These are the swinging (stepping forward or grasping) function and the take off. They are closely related to the stabilizing function and develop at a precise date. Grasping takes place first from the side (third month), later from the mid-line (4.5 months), and finally across the mid-line (fifth to sixth months). The other extremity provides the function of support or take off.

Later in the development, the stepping forward (grasping) and support (take off) functions occur on contralateral sides. In other words, there are two models of stepping forward and support (taking off) functions:

1. Stepping forward and support (taking off) take place on the same side. (e.g., the left arm is moving forward and the leg is also stepping forward)
2. Stepping forward and support (taking off) take place on the contralateral side

Under normal conditions, both the stepping forward and support function take place according to a biomechanically ideal pattern when all the joints are functionally centered. This can be true only if there is normal maturation of the CNS.

Reflex Locomotion

Partial motor functions maturing in the course of postural development, such as postural stabilization in the sagittal plane, the swinging, and the support function (ipsilateral and later on opposite sides) can be evoked by reflex stimulation. This constitutes a new and fundamental principle that has changed our understanding of the motor system, i.e., its functional pathology controlled by the CNS.

It is possible to evoke partial movement patterns by innocuous pressure (pressure must be in the correct direction and vary in intensity) at stimulation points (Fig. 23.16), which are points of support. Two types of complex responses result: reflex turning over (Fig. 23.17) and reflex creeping (Figs. 23.18 to 23.20) are both described by Vojta (12). They are general patterns in which the entire muscular system is involved in a well-defined coordinated way, and all levels of the CNS are involved. The movement evoked by stimulation involves the partial patterns described. Thus, in reflex turning over, we may observe partial movements according to the stage of development: lifting the legs over the table and keeping them in

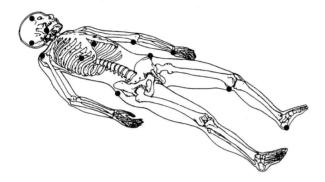

Figure 23.16 Stimulation zones.

triple flexion and abduction (fourth month), grasping over the midline (4.5 months), combined with turning to the side (fifth month), turning to prone position (sixth month), lying on the side using the elbow as a support (seventh month), oblique sitting position (eighth month), crawling on all fours (tenth month), walking sideways (twelfth month). These general patterns controlled by the CNS are constant and can be reproduced.

By stimulation of reflex zones in a given position, involuntary muscle activity is evoked, including the orofacial system. This response is constant and purposeful. The genetically programmed locomotor pattern is as follows:

1. By evoked muscle activity, the point of gravity is transferred and the body is supported automatically at given points. These points are genetically determined and represent structures that play an important role in upright posture. At these sites we find a great number of muscular and/or ligamentous attachment points rich in receptors. If stimulated, muscle activity is directed toward these points of support. The initial position in which stimulation takes place determines the zone of support. The automatic choice of the support point is made by stereognosis, i.e. by awareness of the point of contact and its position in space (making no use of vision), related to the body scheme. Therefore, no matter whether the body is lying on the side, supine, or prone, there will be the same response to the same stimulation, but the point of support will change.

2. The stabilizing system in the sagittal plane will be activated (fourth month). The spinal column, the thorax, and the shoulder blade automatically adopt the ideal position of maximum load bearing as the principles of neurophysiology and biomechanics are in harmony. The pattern of stabilization in the sagittal plane is the constant response to stimulation whether stimulation takes place when lying on the side, prone, or supine. Only the points of support are changed.

3. Stabilization of the spinal column is followed by the swinging (grasping) and support function of the extremities which is coupled with spinal rotation. The oblique abdominal muscles come into play. The choice of the ipsilateral or contralateral pattern of swinging (grasping) and the supporting extremity depends on the initial position. This, too, is automatic depending on head position and visual orientation. The mechanism of swinging (grasping) and mechanism of taking off is always identical, but in the opposite sense. On the swinging leg, we find:

- The hip in flexion, external rotation, and abduction
- The knee in flexion and external rotation
- The foot in dorsal flexion and supination
- On the grasping, upper extremity:
- The shoulder in flexion, external rotation, abduction
- The elbow in supination and slight flexion
- The hand in extension, supination, and radial flexion

The supporting extremity moves in the opposite way. During the movement, all the joints are perfectly centered. The direction of muscular pull differs in the two patterns: in the swinging (grasping) extremity the punctum fixum is proximal and the punctum mobile distal; in the supporting limb, it is the reverse. In the former the head of the joint moves against the joint cavity, in the latter the joint cavity moves against the head. This model can be evoked throughout life, at every age. It differs, however, in the adult, because the response to stimulation is under the control of the cortex. In everybody, however, there will be changes in respiratory function that enhance the stabilization of the spinal column and the thorax, and also changes in muscle tonus, including those muscles that are not completely under the control of our will. To increase facilitation in addition to zone stimulation, we can also resist the locomotion movement (stepping forward) isometrically.

Postural Function of Phasic Muscles

The phasic muscles start their postural activity after the age of 6 weeks, as pointed out. As the CNS matures, these muscles play an increasingly important part in posture and its stabilization, and greatly influence the formation and shape of anatomical

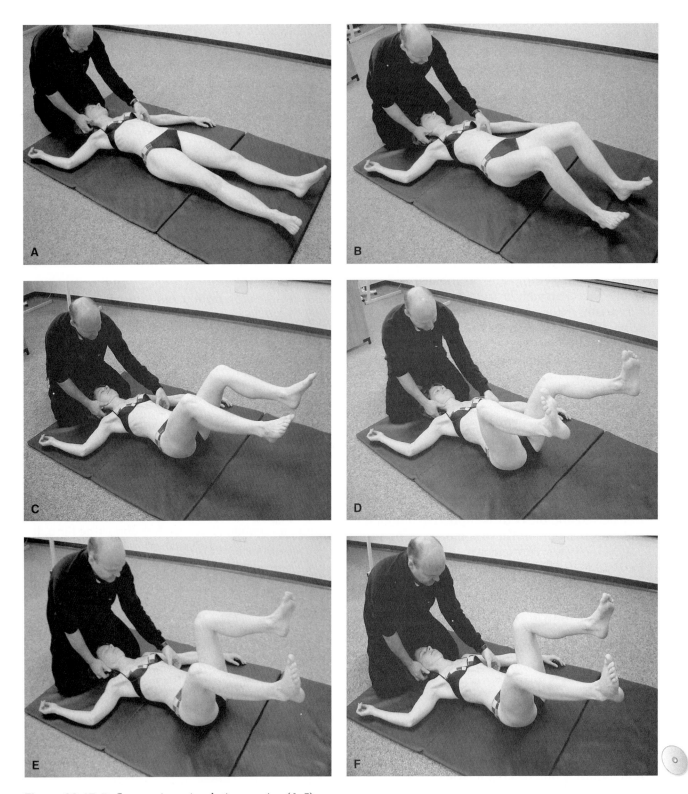

Figure 23.17 Reflex turning stimulation: supine (**A–I**).

structures. The development of postural function of the phasic muscles is completed by the age of 4 years, when the central motor control of gross mobility has matured. At this stage of development, the child can attain at each joint the opposite position to that of the infant at birth (Fig. 23.21). This was earlier described for the shoulder blade and is further demonstrated on the entire upper extremity.

At birth, the position of the upper extremity is characterized by fingers in flexion and adduction, the

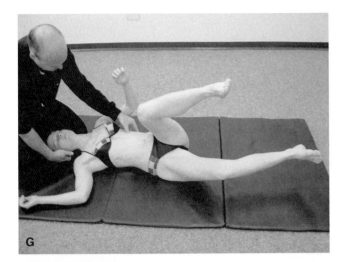

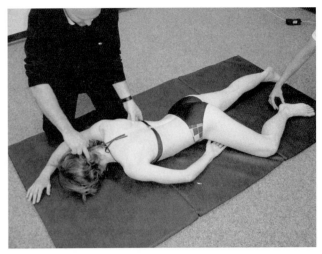

Figure 23.18 Reflex creeping—basic position for stimulation.

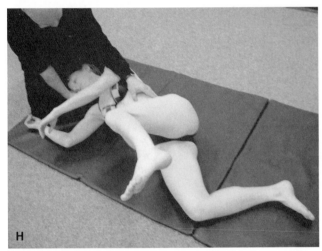

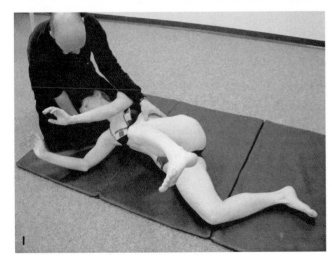

Figure 23.17 (*Continued*)

wrist in ulnar and palmar flexion, the elbow in pronation and flexion, and the shoulder in protraction, adduction, and internal rotation. Posture is under the predominant influence of the phylogenetically older tonic system. At full postural maturity,

the child can acquire a posture in which the fingers are extended and in abduction, the wrist in extension and radial flexion, the elbow in supination and extension, and the shoulder in depression, abduction, and external rotation (Figs. 23.22 A–D and 23.23 A and B). A similar development takes place in other body segments.

This posture is the youngest from the phylogenetic and ontogenetic point of view, and this also goes for its structure (no animal can attain a similar position with respect to the anatomical shape of the joints and even the muscles, responsible for posture). The muscles or their parts involved in posture are phylogenetically young in their postural function (active only in humans) and tend to become weak. It is often expressed that tonic muscles are mainly concerned in posture ("postural muscles") and phasic muscles in movement ("kinetic muscles"). But both types have dual functions participating in both posture and movement.

Ontogenesis clearly shows that the decisive difference between the two systems consists in the timing of their development, i.e., at which period they are integrated into the postural function. Muscles with a tendency to weakness, i.e., the phasic muscles, come into play later; hence, they are younger with regard to their postural function. This postural function is also related to the developmentally youngest morphological structures. This system is not only young but also very fragile. The postural activity of phasic muscles goes hand in hand with central nervous control at a higher level of integration, compared to the neonatal period. It is of great clinical importance that at this higher level of integration a different interplay between different muscle systems are achieved than on the spinal or brain stem level. Motor programs at the spinal and

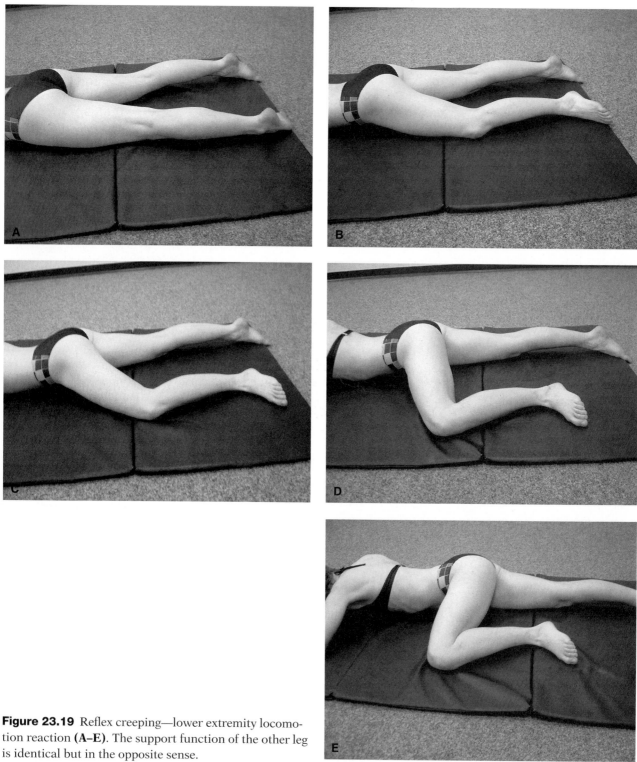

Figure 23.19 Reflex creeping—lower extremity locomotion reaction **(A–E)**. The support function of the other leg is identical but in the opposite sense.

brain stem level function mainly by reciprocal inhibition of the antagonist (activation of the muscle causes inhibition of its antagonist), as can be seen from neonatal reflex activity. Co-activation patterns develop only as higher levels of integration mature. At the same time neonatal reflexes are inhibited.

Phasic muscles are involved in postural activity as a whole, as a system, and its activity automatically changes posture. The moment the deep neck flexors become activated (when between the fourth and sixth week the child lifts its head), all the other phasic muscles take part in postural function by

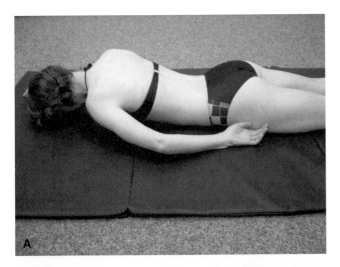

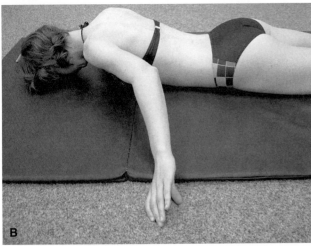

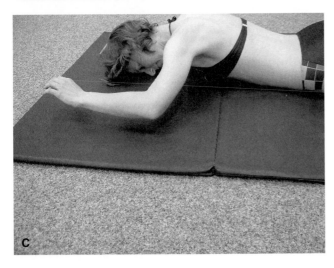

Figure 23.20 Reflex creeping—upper extremity locomotion reaction **(A–C)**. The support function of the other arm is identical but in the opposite sense.

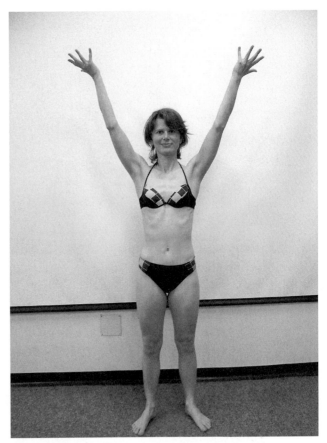

Figure 23.21 Posture reached at the age of 4 years.

means of their interacting attachments, including the external rotators and abductors of the hip joint, the external rotators and abductors of the shoulder, and the deep spinal extensors, the lower fixators of the shoulder blade, and other muscles of the same system. This represents a highly integrated global reflex stabilization function.

It can be shown that this program involves both the tonic and the phasic system as a whole and that the two cooperate in stabilizing posture by reflex action. If only a single phasic muscle is weak, not only is joint position automatically changed but also will inhibition irradiate into the entire system. Equilibrium between the two systems will change in favor of the tonic system. The tonic system predominates in stabilizing posture. By restoring the function of a single phasic muscle, however, inhibition of the entire tonic system will occur. If, e.g., we enhance the postural activity of the lower fixators of the shoulder blade, we lower the tension not only of their antagonists, i.e., the upper fixators of the shoulder blade, but also of tonic muscles at a distance, e.g., of the hamstrings (increasing the range of hip flexion). Resisting external rotation at the shoulders, extension at the elbow, supination, or

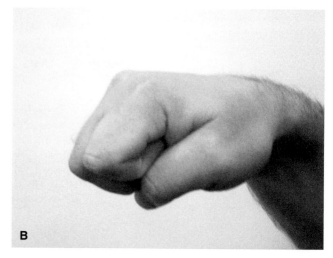

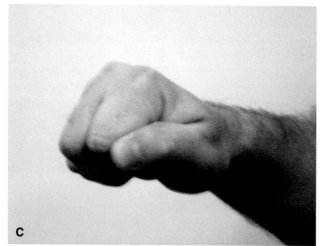

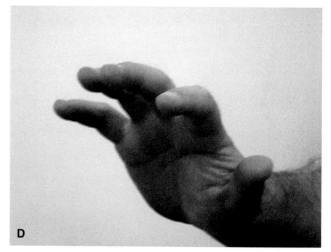

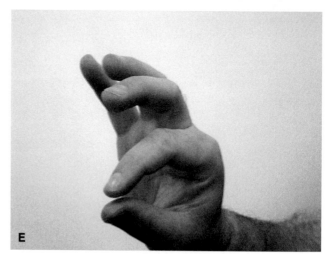

Figure 23.22 Development of hand position from birth to 9 months **(A–E)**.

finger extension, not only will the antagonists of each muscle be inhibited but also will the tonic muscles be affected at a distance, e.g., the hamstrings may cause a change in the straight leg raising test. This higher level of integration results in new types of reflex relations, which can be estab-

lished between muscles situated far apart. In this connection, the upper part of the trapezius (a tonic muscle) is an antagonist not only of the lower part of trapezius but also of the vastus medialis in the system of phasic muscles. Such reflex relations are established on a higher than brain stem level.

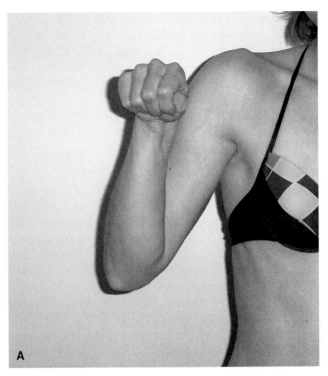

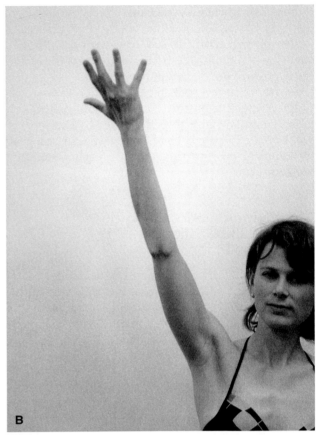

Figure 23.23 Development of posture at the shoulder girdle up to 4 years **(A, B)**.

The Influence of Gravity on Function and Structure

The development of the postural function of phasic muscles is closely related to maturity or immaturity of the skeleton.

At birth, for example, the extremity abductors and outward rotators have no postural function. This can first be traced at the age of approximately 6 weeks. It not only changes posture but also influences anteversion and the colodiaphyseal angle of the femur. Insufficiency of the postural function of the abductors and external rotators results in anteversion and valgosity of the hip joint. The muscles necessary to attain the highest stage of morphological development are the middle and posterior part of the abductors and the outward rotators of the hip joint. These muscles belong to the phasic system with a tendency to inhibition.

Another example is the foot. The longitudinal axis of the calcaneus lies laterally because of the position of the talus at birth, and the heel is high because the calcaneus has not yet slipped under the talus. The calcaneus reaches this position underneath the talus thanks to the postural activity of the short muscles of the foot and the tibialis anterior, tibialis posterior,

and the peroneal muscles. The shape of the longitudinal arch is not complete until the age of 4 years, i.e., when the postural function of all the pertinent muscles has been fully developed. In cerebral palsy the foot remains at the neonatal or even at an earlier stage, because the function of the muscles has failed to mature. The same is true in children with a central disturbance of coordination.

Thus, the phasic muscles determine the shape of most anatomical structures, including also the colodiaphyseal angle and the angle of anteversion at the hip joint, the plateau of the tibia, the transverse arch of the foot, the horizontal position and the torsion of the collar bones, the spinal curvatures, etc. Thus, a mature phasic muscle system ensures morphological maturity at the age of 4 years. Absent or faulty stabilizing postural function of phasic muscles not only causes faulty posture similar to that of patients affected by neonatal cerebral palsy but also causes typical changes in the skeleton: coxa valga antetorta, a kyphotic spinal column, an oblique tibial plateau, an insufficiently developed foot with valgosity, genua valga, and pelvic anteversion.

In almost 30% of the child population, there is some degree of faulty posture caused by dysfunction of the phasic muscles, which also affects the skeleton (1,11,13). Systematic weakness of the phasic muscles is also characteristic in old age, with insufficient extension of the spine, restricted elevation of the arms, faulty posture during trunk rotation, etc. The entire system tends to revert to an earlier neonatal postural model. Protective posture caused by joint pathology shows a similar pattern, as described by Cyriax, but was never explained. Here again we can see that pathological posture reverts to an earlier stage of development.

Developmental Kinesiology of Spinal Stabilization in the Sagittal Plane

The CNS program controlling the development of stabilized erect posture starts at the beginning of the second month. It is not restricted to the head and neck, but results in a change in the entire body posture. Spinal straightening, i.e., balanced co-activation of the muscles on the dorsal and ventral body aspect, is complete by the end of the fourth month. It is related to the first basis of support, i.e., for the prone position the triangle formed by the elbows and the symphysis, and for the supine by the glutei, the scapular region, and the linea nuchae (Figures 23.11 and 23.12).

At this stage of development, the foundations of stabilization of the spine in the sagittal plane are laid. Only on this basis can phasic movement be achieved. Any disturbance of stabilization will be evident in phasic movement. Stabilization in the sagittal plane, the prerequisite of physiological centered spinal posture, therefore requires:

1. The co-activation of the dorsal and ventral musculature. This is of crucial importance for physiological ("centered") posture, i.e., optimum static function. This applies in particular to the deep neck flexors and the abdominal muscles, and to the extensors of the spinal column on the dorsal aspect. Only this co-activation can achieve a centered position and provide optimum static function.

2. The cooperation of antagonistic muscles that are attached to the thorax and the shoulder blades. Both these anatomical structures transfer muscle pull to the spinal column. This applies particularly to the cooperation of the inferior serratus anterior and abdominal muscles, and, also, the scapular adductors and the pectoralis major.

3. The integration of the diaphragm into stabilization by respiration.

The muscles of the stabilization system function as a unit; they are interdependent. If one muscle is weak or overactive, this never remains isolated, affecting the static and dynamic function of the entire spine—the individual segments will be no longer in a centered position.

The Cervical and Upper Thoracic Region

Erect posture (centration) of the cervical spine develops after the age of 6 weeks. In an anatomic sense, the cervical spine ends at C7, but from a functional perspective it ends at T4, because the upper thoracic spine participates in flexion, extension, as well as in side bending and rotation of the head. This is borne out by the anatomy of the most important muscles that extend the cervical spine and originate in the mid thoracic region.

The extensors of the cervical spine are the semispinalis cervicis, semispinalis capitis, splenius capitis, splenius cervicis, and longissimus cervis muscles. These muscles originate at T4, T5, and T6. At this stage of development, extension is further enhanced by the rhomboids and the middle and lower trapezius in cooperation with the serratus anterior, which serves as a punctum fixum for the spinal extensors. The serratus anterior, however, can fulfill its stabilizing function only if its attachment points are stabilized by the abdominal muscles.

Erect posture, i.e., correct centration of the cervical spine, is possible only if there is activity of the muscles on the ventral aspect, i.e., the longus colli and primarily the longus capitis, in addition to those on the dorsal aspect. These muscles also originate at the level of the upper thoracic spine and prevent reclination (i.e., back-bending) of the head and cervical hyperlordosis. The balanced co-activation of these muscles ensures correct centration and prevents overstrain of the sternocleidomastoids and the scaleni. In pathological cases, there is reclination of the head and flexion/extension takes place only at the cranio-cervical junction. When this occurs, normal development of the entire spinal column is impaired. Centration of the cervical spine also depends on the stabilizing function of the deep extensors of the mid thoracic spine. They provide the punctum fixum for the deep extensors of the cervical spine. Their weakness is accompanied by hyperlordosis, inhibition of the deep neck flexors. Activity of the deep neck flexors and extensors depends on stabilization of their attachment points, which in turn depend on a muscular chain. For instance, if the lumbar section of the diaphragm and the lateral section of the abdominal muscles do not function, forward-bending of the head occurs with substitution of the sternocleido-mastoids for the deep neck flexors, with the result being a chin poke.

The Lower Thoracic and the Lumbar Spine

There is a similar close relationship between the function of the lumbar and lower thoracic spine as there is between the cervical and upper thoracic spine down to the mid thoracic region (T5). This results, too, from the anatomy of the relevant muscles. Erect posture of the thoracic and lumbar spine develops in close relation to the cervical spine. This is related to the anatomy the muscles. Straightening of the thoracic and lumbar spine is closely related to that of the cervical spine. Activity of the spinal extensors must be kept in balance by simultaneous activity of the abdominal muscles and the diaphragm, resulting in the correct centration of individual segments. The abdominal muscles with the diaphragm become involved in posture at the same stage of development as the deep extensors. Both the oblique abdominal muscles and the rectus originate from the lower ribs, beginning at T5. This anatomical and functional relationship enhances erect posture under the control of the CNS. If this stabilizing function is disturbed either by hyperfunction or hypofunction, the static function of the spine is compromised.

The interplay of the abdominal and back muscles with the diaphragm and the pelvic floor must be understood. At birth the diaphragm is still in an oblique position while the pelvic floor has no postural function, nor is there any postural synergy between the intrinsic back and the abdominal muscles. As the intrinsic back musculature comes into play, the spinal column straightens. The thorax with the ribs is stabilized by the caudal pull of the abdominal muscles. The ribs are steeper than in the newborn stage. Straightening up of the spine in concert with stabilizing activity in the abdominal muscles alters the punctum fixum for the attachments of the diaphragm, thus bringing the diaphragm into a horizontal position.

This is as specific for humans as is erect posture. Increased intra-abdominal pressure and decreased pelvic anteversion through the pull of the abdominal and gluteal muscles enable the pelvic floor to perform its postural function. The coordinated function of the diaphragm with the abdominal muscles is crucial for the anterior stabilization of the lumbar spine. Stability of these structures is decisive also for the thoracic and cervical spine because they form their punctum fixum. The postural function of the pelvic floor is brought about by increased intra-abdominal pressure and a change in pelvic anteversion by the activity of the abdominal muscles.

Postural Ontogenesis and the Function of the Diaphragm

If the CNS develops normally, the diaphragm will be the chief respiratory muscle. At the same time, it forms part of the co-activation pattern resulting in erect posture. These functions mean that posture exerts a great influence on respiration, and respiration on posture. As erect posture develops, the diaphragm finds its horizontal position at the end of the fourth month. If the diaphragm contracts, it flattens and is resisted by the abdominal wall. In co-activation with the abdominal muscles, it produces intra-abdominal pressure. This plays an important role in stabilizing the lumbar spine. Thus, the diaphragm not only is the main respiratory muscle but also stabilizes posture. Its activity depends also on the position of the spine and the thorax, which act as a punctum fixum. The inspiratory position of the chest together with thoracolumbar hyperlordosis impairs the activity of the diaphragm in all of its three sections. Activity of the lumbar section of the diaphragm is particularly impaired and the stabilizing co-activation of the abdominal muscles is lacking. Respiratory activity is transferred mainly to the thorax and via the auxiliary respiratory muscles to the cervical region. Under normal conditions, however, the diaphragm with the abdominal muscles and the spinal extensors stabilize the punctum fixum for the psoas at the thoracolumbar junction.

Muscular Imbalance in Disturbed Co-activation and Impaired Spinal Stabilization in the Sagittal Plane

The spinal column forms a fulcrum stabilizing muscles, which relate to the extremities, i.e., a punctum fixum. Faulty position of the spinal column is accompanied by functional imbalance of the muscles of the pelvic and shoulder girdle and the extremities. The reverse is also true.

Erect posture (sagittal plane function) is completed at an earlier stage than vertical stance. As pointed out, the postural model, i.e., well-balanced muscular co-activation resulting in optimum loading of the spine, is completed during the fourth month. At this early stage of development, the final basic posture is established. It remains unchanged even when the child stands up and during further postural development, but it adapts to the varying areas of support. A child with even a slight lesion of the CNS (approximately

30%) never reaches this ideal level of co-activation between the two functional systems (1,11,13). The posture of such children when standing is never truly erect. Generalized muscular imbalance caused by faulty development is the cause of future faulty posture. Hence, it requires treatment at this initial stage. Similar muscular imbalance need not, however, be caused by abnormal development, but by affections at a later stage, which result in reflex changes of a stereotypical character.

The muscles responsible for well-centered posture (the deep stabilizers) act as a functional unit. Hypofunction or hyperfunction of a single muscle never remains isolated but involves the entire complex by affecting the points of attachment. We therefore find that weakness of the pelvic floor is usually accompanied by weakness of the deep neck flexors and vice versa. This interrelation is very important for treatment. This functional unit is young from the phylogenetical standpoint.

Insufficiency of the deep flexors is characteristic for the cervical region. This results in head reclination with hyperextension of the lower cervical spine. The upper thoracic spine is in a forward-drawn position. Neck rotation is not proportional throughout the cervical spine and is therefore restricted. Fixation by the serratus is insufficient and therefore the rhomboids and the lower and middle trapezius cannot achieve erect posture in the cervical spine. The upper trapezius, the levator scapulae, sternocleidomastoids, and the scaleni predominate and function also as auxiliary inspiratory muscles.

Normally, co-activation of the abdominal wall, spinal extensors, and the diaphragm controls intra-abdominal pressure and centrates the low thoracic and lumbar spine. Weakness of the abdominal wall and insufficient intra-abdominal pressure result in permanent pelvic anteversion and increased lumbar lordosis. This is frequently accompanied by diastases of the abdominal muscles. Weakness of the abdominal wall not only induces hyperlordosis and pelvic anteversion but also prevents extension of the thoracic spine below T5. Lumbar lordosis thus ends in the low thoracic region, most frequently at the thoraco-lumbar junction, and kyphosis starts from this level. In the kyphotic segments there is no extension. The thorax is in an inspiratory position and there is obliquity of the diaphragm. The intercostal spaces do not widen at inhalation and the thorax is lifted as a whole. Thus, inhalation takes place by contraction of the auxiliary respiratory muscles. This condition goes hand-in-hand with weakness of the pelvic floor. At the same time there is disturbed co-activation of the serratus anterior and the lower trapezius, which normally straightens the thoracic spine and facilitates the transversus abdominis.

The mid thoracic spine, i.e., the transitional vertebra T5, plays a very important role both in ontogenesis and in pathogenesis. It represents the punctum fixum, from where the cervical spine straightens and where the most important postural muscles originate: the splenius cervicis and capitis, the longissimus capitis and the longus colli, and where the longigissimus thoracis is attached. The abdominal muscles also originate from the fifth rib. This is the level where the lumbar lordosis ends because of muscular co-activation.

In normal posture, T5 forms the apex of the thoracic kyphosis or the end of lumbar lordosis. Thus, the area from T4 to T6 is the region that functionally divides the upper and lower half of the human body.

Clinical examination of this section of the spine is particularly important. Only if there is well-balanced muscular activity in the entire motor system is it possible to straighten up below T5. It appears that almost every disturbance of muscle activity related to the spinal column as well as to the extremities will affect this region, keeping it in flexion, with kyphosis and movement restriction into extension below T5. The extent of this fixed kyphosis varies but can reach as far as to the thoraco-lumbar junction in some cases. Abnormality of the spine in the sagittal plane results from faulty activity of the oblique abdominal muscles. Thus, rotation of the spine, too, depends on stabilization of the spine in the sagittal plane.

Normal and Abnormal Kinesiology of Respiration: Its Relationship to Spinal Stabilization

Movement of the thorax plays an essential role in respiration. It is formed to comply with the movements of breathing. The muscles involved can be described as inspiratory and expiratory, and as main and auxiliary respiratory muscles. Auxiliary muscles come into play only when great effort is required or under pathological conditions.

During respiration the ribs are raised and lowered, moving around an axis starting at the head of the rib and ending at the transverso-costal joint, in a dorso-lateral direction. Torsion of the rib is most important for movement. There are three types of torsion:

1. Around the thorax
2. Along the lower edge of the rib (if placed on its edge on a table the rib touches it only at two points)
3. Twisting—at its dorsal end it is almost vertical, and in front oblique, pointing in a ventro-cranial direction.

Curvature of the ribs is important for the enlargement of the thoracic cavity. The joints between the ribs and the sternum have very tight capsules, allowing only slight movement. The ventral ends of the ribs are raised together with the sternum. In this way, the thoracic cavity widens in the sagittal plane. It should be noted that during inhalation the sternum should also move forward.

This is accompanied by rotation in the sternoclavicular joints. The clavicle does not move and the sternum rotates at the sternoclavicular joint. (The cavity at manubrium sterni moves against the articular head of the clavicula). The axis of the neck of the lower longest ribs (Ribs 6–8) runs in a dorso-lateral direction, which makes the thoracic cavity widen in the frontal plane. This movement may be disturbed in pathological cases. The upper ribs move much less under normal conditions. If the development of the CNS is normal, the diaphragm is the main respiratory muscle, but it also stabilizes posture.

The diaphragm flattens and acts against the resistance of the abdominal wall. It controls intra-abdominal pressure in cooperation with the abdominal muscles and the pelvic floor, which are also important for stabilization. Its activity depends on the position of the spine and the thorax, which form a punctum fixum. If the thorax is in inhalation position with the sternum and the ribs raised, and the thoracolumbar junction in extension, then activity of the diaphragm is impaired in all its three sections. This particularly affects its lumbar section. Respiration is then limited to the thorax, which is pulled upward by the auxiliary muscles. The diaphragm and the abdominal muscles stabilize the thoracolumbar junction, providing a punctum fixum for the iliopsoas. In this way, physiological respiration stabilizes the lumbar spine. Examination of respiratory and stabilization function is therefore an essential part of examination and treatment of the locomotor system.

Examination of the Deep Stabilization System of the Spine in the Sagittal Plane

Disturbance of spinal stabilization is an important factor in back pain and other conditions. We have to bear in mind that any purposeful movement first requires spinal stabilization. Stabilization also plays an important role in compensation and normalization of dysfunction. Control of spinal stabilization is therefore a prerequisite for successful therapy.

Diagnostic Tests

1. **Diaphragm test—lateral abdominal wall activation:** Examination sitting erect or supine. We palpate below the last ribs at the lateral aspect of

the abdominal wall. The patient is told to press against our hands, which press gently against the side of his abdominal muscles during exhalation, when his thorax is lowered. The spinal column must remain straight during examination; no spinal flexion should be observed.

Muscular activity at the waist is also palpated during inhalation. This test serves to examine to what extent the diaphragm is able to perform its stabilizing function (Fig. 23.24A with the patient seated; Fig. 23.24B with the patient supine).

Signs of Impairment The patient exerts minimal counterpressure or none at all. He may show some activity during exhalation, but none during inhalation. Quite often he is not aware that he could acti-

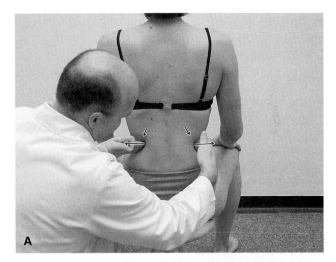

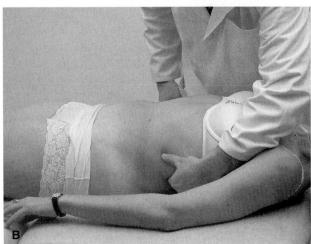

Figure 23.24 We ask the patient to press against our fingers: assessment of the patient's ability to activate the diaphragm (especially its lumbar part) together with the lateral parts of the abdominal muscles, with the ribs remaining in the caudal position. **(A)** Examination with the patient sitting **(B)** Examination with the patient lying supine.

vate those muscles. This shows lack of cooperation between the diaphragm and the lateral part of the abdominal muscles, creating an eccentric and finally isometric contraction. The pelvic floor also takes part in this muscular co-contraction, essential for the control of intra-abdominal pressure that stabilizes the lumbar spine from in front. The patient substitutes for this dysfunction by exaggerated activity of the rectus abdominis, particularly of its upper part, which is connected with the anterior paramedial part of the diaphragm, and by increased activity of the paravertebral muscles, especially at the T/L junction level. A patient unable to control the activity of the diaphragm in co-contraction with the lateral portion of his abdominal muscles is most likely to have low back pain. If this activity is asymmetrical at examination, disc herniation between L4/5 or L5/S1 is probable. Such a herniation can be asymptomatic; the patient does not have to have symptoms of spinal root irritation.

2. Diaphragm test—stabilization of expiratory thorax position: Examination supine with the legs extended or in slight flexion, followed by examination in the erect seated position. Supine, the patient exhales. With our palpating hands, we encourage the patient to move his thorax as far as possible with the sternum in a caudal direction (Fig. 23.25). We hold the patient's chest in this expiratory (caudal) position and ask him to relax the abdominal wall completely. He is then asked to inhale while maintaining the caudal position of the thorax. With our hands we follow the movement of the sternum (we palpate the lower part of it) and the low false ribs (later-

ally from the medioclavicular line) (Fig. 23.26). Inability to maintain the caudal position of the chest during inspiration indicates poor spinal stabilization; there is insufficient functional cooperation between the diaphragm and the abdominal wall. The patient cannot properly control intra-abdominal pressure. During the test we also check if the lateral aspect of the patient's abdominal wall protrudes below the last ribs. If this area bulges, it is a sign of good cooperation between the posterior part of the diaphragm (where eccentric contraction takes place) and the lateral group of abdominal muscles that also work eccentrically. This muscular cooperation is crucial for spinal stabilization.

With the patient seated, we palpate at the costal angle of the lower ribs (Fig. 23.27) and follow rib movement during inhalation and exhalation. Under normal conditions, these ribs move in a lateral but not in a cranial direction; the caudal position is possible even during the inhalation. If the patient is in good control of his stabilizing functions, he should be able to perform this lateral rib movement even without breathing. He thus demonstrates his ability to control the lumbar section of his diaphragm. This is very important for the stabilization of the lumbar spine.

Signs of Impairment If the deep stabilizers are insufficient, the patient cannot control chest position during breathing. The initial position is cranial, i.e., the inspiratory position of the chest. The axis connecting sternal and lumbar attachments of the diaphragm is oblique (normally it is horizontal). The

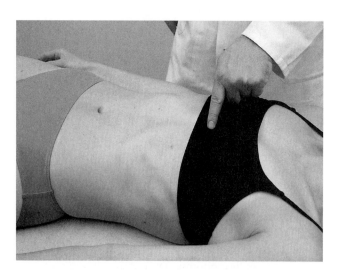

Figure 23.25 Assessment of the patient's ability to stabilize the chest during respiration. The sternal bone should reach the caudal position.

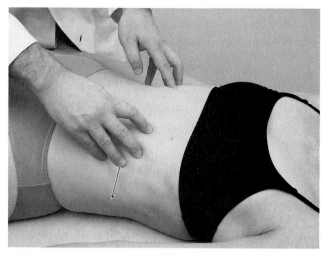

Figure 23.26 Palpatory assessment of false rib movement: the therapist notes whether the movement takes place in the cranial or lateral direction. The arrow indicates the direction of rib movement under physiological conditions.

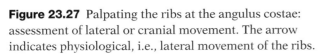

Figure 23.27 Palpating the ribs at the angulus costae: assessment of lateral or cranial movement. The arrow indicates physiological, i.e., lateral movement of the ribs.

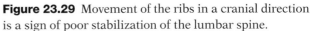

Figure 23.29 Movement of the ribs in a cranial direction is a sign of poor stabilization of the lumbar spine.

lumbar attachment points are lower than the sternal. During inhalation the chest reaches an even more cranial position (Fig. 23.28); its lower part does not widen and the axis becomes steeper. The patient cannot inhale while keeping his chest in a caudal position (Fig. 23.29). By examination at the angelus costae during inhalation and exhalation, we observe cranio-caudal, but not lateral, movement. The intercostal spaces do not widen. By transmitting muscular activity, the thorax enhances stabilization. If, however, the thorax moves in a cranio-caudal direction during respiration, mainly by the activity of the auxiliary respiratory muscles, without stabilization in

the transverse plane, there is no control of intra-abdominal pressure by the abdominal walls. Intra-abdominal pressure normally increases when we make any purposeful movement with our extremities.

3. **Hip flexion test:** Examination of the patient sitting erect with legs apart and hanging down freely. The patient flexes one hip against gravity or slight resistance and we assess to what extent he stabilizes the thoracolumbar spine. During hip flexion, the iliopsoas is activated and its point of origin must be stabilized. Under normal conditions, we assess the contraction of the muscles of the abdominal wall as abdominal pressure increases. It is important to observe the tension of the abdominal and the function of the paravertebral muscles (Fig. 23.30).

Signs of Impairment Insufficient stabilization is evident in increased activity of the paravertebral muscles and of the rectus abdominis, mainly of its upper section. There is minimum activity of the lateral part of the abdominal wall palpated at the waist. Under such conditions, every contraction of the iliopsoas is performed with an insufficiently stabilized lumbar spine. There is increased tension in the paravertebral muscles and we may even find discrete lateral shift of the thoracolumbar junction toward the flexing leg during hip flexion (Fig. 23.31).

4. **Intra-abdominal pressure test:** The patient is supine with legs bent at the hips and knees at right angles in abduction and slight external rotation (with clinician's support); the distance between the knees should be approximately the breadth of the shoulders. This is the correctly centered position from the functional point of

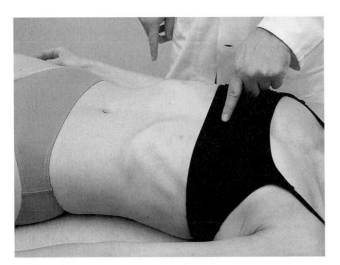

Figure 23.28 Movement of the sternum in a cranial direction. The patient is unable to maintain the caudal position of the chest and so cannot stabilize the lumbar spine from the front.

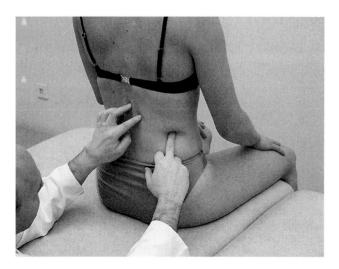

Figure 23.30 During examination, we palpate the T/L junction and lateral abdominal muscles below the lower ribs.

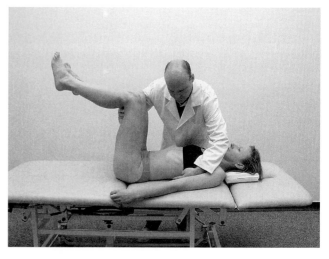

Figure 23.32 The patient's posture corresponds to the developmental stage at which stabilization of the spine in the sagittal plane has been fully accomplished.

view (Fig. 23.32). The patient is told to support himself at the thoracolumbar region by the activity of the abdominal wall. The clinician slowly remove support. This tests the quality of stabilization of the T/L junction by muscular activity and intra-abdominal pressure.

Signs of Impairment The first signs are revealed at the starting position. The rectus abdominis has a convex shape. Below the lower ribs, however, a concavity at the level of the costal angle can be noticed (Fig. 23.33). At the caudal part of the lateral abdominal muscles on the side of the quadratus lumborum, the abdominal wall bulges because of muscular hypo-

activity. Trying to straighten the thoracolumbar junction (for support) increases tension in the rectus abdominis and in the paravertebral muscles, with no activation of the lateral abdominal muscles (Fig. 23.34). This is a sign of insufficient co-activation of the lumbar section of the diaphragm and the abdominal muscles, which is essential for stabilization of the lumbar spine. We also note whether there is diastases of the abdominal wall, which is another sign of insufficient stabilization. Diastases frequently increases if the patient tries to support himself at the thoracolumbar junction.

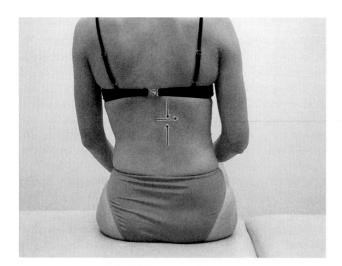

Figure 23.31 If there is abnormality, we find lateral shift of the T/L junction, increased tension of the paravertebral muscles, and of the m. rectus abdominis, and poor stabilization of the lateral abdominal muscles.

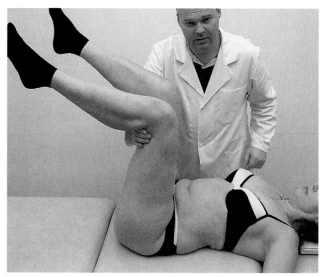

Figure 23.33 Insufficiency of the stabilization system results in hyperextension of the T/L junction; m. rectus abdominis predominates, and the chest is in a cranial position.

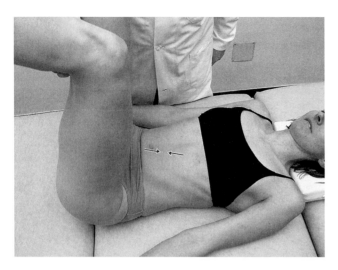

Figure 23.34 Any attempt to straighten the T/L junction results in hypertonus of the m. rectus abdominis and paravertebral muscles, whereas the lateral abdominal muscles remain hypoactive.

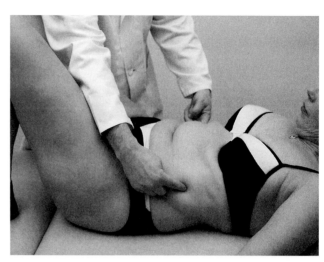

Figure 23.35 Evaluation of rib movement during trunk flexion. Movement in the lateral direction is pathological. Diastases of the rectus abdominis can frequently be observed.

5. **Trunk flexion test:** The patient is supine with the arms along the body. The patient slowly bends his trunk. For examination, we palpate the rib movements. The lowest false ribs are palpated in the medioclavicular line and their movement is assessed.

Signs of Impairment When there is insufficient stabilization, the ribs deviate to the side and there is lateral bulging of the abdominal wall (Fig. 23.35). Cranial movement of the navel is a sign of upper rectus abdominis overactivity.

6. **Arm lifting test:** The patient is supine or standing erect. With the thorax in a caudal position, the patient lifts his arms. Activity at the thorax is assessed. If stabilization by the abdominal muscles is normal, the thorax should not be lifted during shoulder movement at full range (Fig. 23.36).

Signs of Impairment When the patient lifts his arm, the thorax moves up as stabilization by the abdominal muscles is insufficient (Fig. 23.37).

7. **Neck flexion test:** Examination with the patient supine with the legs extended. The patient slowly bends his head and neck. We assess the muscles performing the movement and those which stabilize their attachment points (Fig. 23.38 A and B).

Signs of Impairment The patient moves with the head in a forward-drawn position because of exaggerated activity of the sternocleidomastoids and the scaleni. There is hyperactivity in suboccipital mus-

cles and in spinal extensors. The lower ribs move in a lateral direction during the test and sometimes even cranially. The activity of the deep flexors is inhibited not only by their weakness (which may not be apparent) but also by the lack of attachment point stabilization. During neck flexion the clavicle should not move cephalad.

8. **Seated neck straightening test:** Sitting erect. The patient is asked to straighten the cervical spine. The point of gravity of the head should move in a dorso-cranial direction (Brügger's erect seated position).

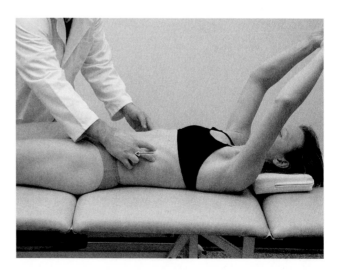

Figure 23.36 We assess chest position during shoulder flexion. Normally, the patient should maintain the caudal position of the chest throughout the whole movement.

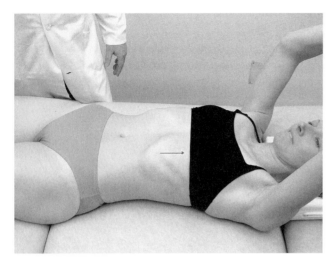

Figure 23.37 If there is poor muscular stabilization, the chest moves in a cranial direction during shoulder flexion.

Signs of Impairment In dysfunction, we frequently see that straightening up begins at the thoracolumbar region (as though the axis of rotation was there) (Fig. 23.39A) or at the cervicothoracic junction, but not at T4/5, where it should start (Fig. 23.39B). Extension of the mid thoracic spine is impaired. There is increased tension of the paravertebral muscles and of the adductors of the shoulder blade. Because extension of the mid and low thoracic spine is insufficient, the patient activates the sternocleidomastoid, the suprahyoid muscles, and the scalene when trying to straighten up segment T4/5. Stabilization of the thorax is insufficient. This insufficiency prevents the patient from being able to compensate adequately for stability challenges. Under such conditions all exercises will be useless.

9. **Extension test:** The patient is prone and supports himself on his hands. The patient straightens his cervical and upper thoracic spine. Below T5, extension takes place from one vertebra to the next in succession. The shoulder blades remain abducted and in a caudal position. Straightening his arms, the patient pushes himself up and exhales. The patient moves to make the symphysis the main point of support.

Signs of Impairment Insufficient extension of the mid thoracic spine and exaggerated extension of the thoraco-lumbar region. Tension in the paravertebral muscles greatly increases. The shoulder blades move together and upwards (Fig. 23.40).

Treatment of Insufficient Stabilization of the Spine

There is controversy about whether we should strengthen the abdominal, back, or other muscles and whether to train proprioception by wobble boards, gymnastic balls, or other methods. However, it is too little realized that in the majority of cases we are unable to ensure the correct initial position essential for any type of exercise. There is then a lack of stabilization and the effectiveness of the exercise program is questionable. We should be aware that the chain of muscles required for any specific movement must be secured by stabilization of muscular attachment points.

Muscular coordination will greatly differ according to differences in stabilization. It is, for example,

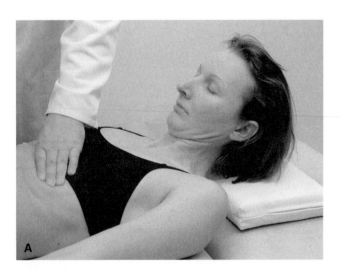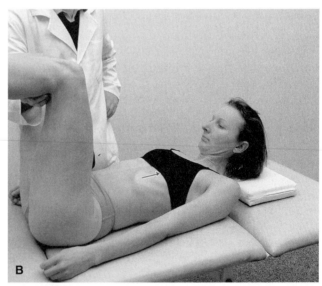

Figure 23.38 Flexion of the cervical spine is examined while the chest is fixed in a caudal position **(A)** Cranial movement of the chest prevents activation of the deep neck flexors **(B)**.

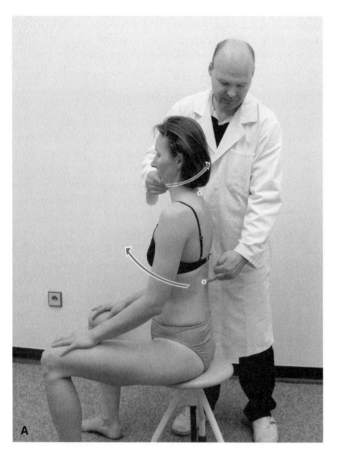
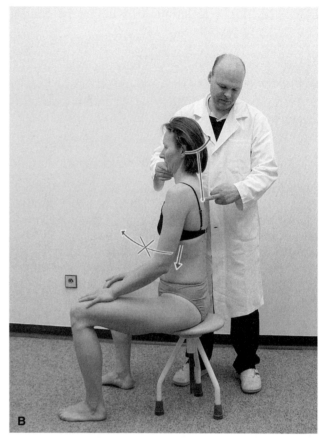

Figure 23.39 Straightening up of the spine starts at the level of the T/L junction and either the chest moves cranially or the movement starts from the lower segments of the cervical spine **(A)**. The patient cannot straighten the mid-thoracic spine **(B)**.

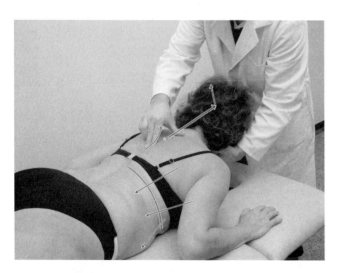

Figure 23.40 During spinal extension, the thoracic spine does not straighten. Tonus in the paravertebral muscles increases and is maximal around the T/L junction. The patient cannot fix his shoulder blades in abduction and caudal position.

a great difference whether external rotation of the shoulder occurs with the shoulder blade stabilized by the trapezius or by the serratus anterior with the lateral abdominal muscles, or whether neck flexion takes place with the thorax in inhalation or exhalation. Stabilization results from the activity of a muscular chain that is not under the control of our will, nor do we know how to activate it deliberately. To make these muscles work, neither instruction nor explanation is effective. Reflex mechanisms or manual fixation are required to start with.

To be able to compensate for dysfunction, the patient must control spinal stabilization or else he will overburden the system. Every type of exercise, including sensory motor training or gym balls, depends on correct stabilization as a prerequisite of effective therapy.

There are three basic approaches to improving stability, depending on whether the case is acute or chronic, or whether our aim is prevention. It also depends on whether the patient is able to react adequately to our instructions or whether he cannot control his movements.

1. Reflex locomotion
2. Control of respiration
3. Treatment based on instruction and manual control of stabilization.

Making Use of Reflex Stimulation

Stimulating reflex zones activates muscles for a definite purpose. The spinal column, the shoulder blades, and the thorax are brought into an ideal position of maximum load bearing by the activated muscles. In this position, muscle pull is most favorable. The response to stimulation is constant: the thorax settles in a caudal position, respiration is without any cranial displacement of the sternum or ribs, the ribs move in a lateral direction, and the intervertebral spaces widen. The diaphragm contracts regularly in all its sections and arrives at the horizontal position. The abdominal muscles together with the serratus anterior provide fixation of the thorax and there is balanced activity of the rectus abdominis and the lateral abdominal muscles. The thoracic spine extends by the activity of the deep intrinsic muscles. The thoracolumbar junction is centered and stabilized by the activity of the diaphragm, the abdominal muscles, and the spinal extensors, so that the psoas can flex the hip joint. The accessory respiratory muscles relax by reflex action and the deep neck flexors are brought into postural activity. The shoulder blades move in a caudal direction and are fixed by the balanced activity of the serratus anterior and the adductors. In this way, the spinal column is stabilized in the sagittal plane as a prerequisite for the stepping forward and support functions. The response will be the same in any position in which we choose to stimulate. The intensity of the reflex response can be enhanced by resisting against the stimulated movement.

Reflex stimulation of the stabilizing function is indicated mainly in the chronic stage of locomotor disturbance in patients with little ability to form new motor stereotypes. It is an attempt to achieve better voluntary control of stabilization by reflex stimulation. Reflex stimulation is particularly useful in an adult who is not fully conscious (e.g., after trauma or after a stroke). We may thus influence postural tonus, provoke muscle activity, preventing spasticity and contracture. Reflex locomotion is helpful in patients in intensive care units unable to cooperate. It also helps in patients with lesions of the spinal cord, in particular in the early stages. Making use of inborn mechanisms, we are able to activate specifically the muscle chains responsible for respiration. This is important in patients with respiratory disturbances, because they are unable to control the respiratory muscles.

Treating Pathological Respiration

This has the greatest impact on intra-abdominal pressure regulation and spinal stabilization. The prerequisite for normal stabilization is that the thorax is in a position like during ontogenesis, or as a result of stimulation, i.e., with the sternum and the ribs in a caudal position. The sternum moves only in a ventro-dorsal (dorso-ventral) direction (not cranio-caudal), with the axis of movement being in the sternocostal and not in the acromioclavicular joints. The caudal position of the sternum and the ribs is essential for the eccentric contraction of the abdominal wall during inhalation. The diaphragm flattens and contracts in all its parts. Thus, the patient widens his abdomen not only anteriorly but also the lateral and lumbar part of the abdominal wall must also distend proportionally. The constant height of the sternum with the ribs in the sagittal plane is essential for a balanced activity of the abdominal, serratus anterior, and pectoral muscles. Respiratory movements are taught first with the patient supine (Fig. 23.41), and only gradually in more demanding positions. The basic task is to teach the patient to breathe with the sternum in a caudal position, moving it only antero-posteriorly. The thorax must widen in the transversal plane. Only under such conditions can the diaphragm and the abdominal muscles fulfill their stabilizing function.

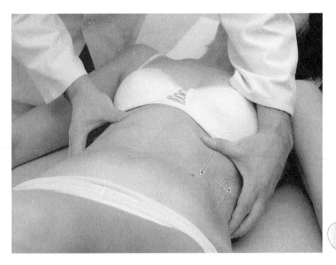

Figure 23.41 We have to teach the patient how to breathe and maintain the caudal position of the chest. The chest must not be lifted. During inspiration the anterior and also the lateral and lumbar sections of the abdominal wall must distend.

Patient's Voluntary Activity

The patient's voluntary activity is used in carefully chosen positions, fixed by the therapist, to control stability of transmission systems (e.g., the shoulder blade, the thorax). The aim is to teach the patient how to change the stabilization function. Some techniques and their modification are demonstrated.

- The patient is supine, the legs are lifted with the hip and the knees flexed at right angles and abducted, the knees are approximately as far apart as the shoulders breadth and in slight external rotation. This is the position of functional joint centration and muscular facilitation. The sternum and the thorax are moved down first during exhalation under the therapist's manual control. The lower section of the thorax must widen. In this position, the patient is asked to support himself at the thoraco-lumbar junction, which forms a punctum fixum. Then he slightly lifts his buttocks, activating the abdominal muscles. He should not, however, draw in the pelvis. We fix the lower ribs from above with our hands at the level of the attachments of the lateral abdominal muscles to enhance their caudal position. In this way, the diaphragm and the lateral abdominal muscles are automatically brought into action. This can be felt at the waist (Fig. 23.42).

Mistakes to be Avoided When slightly lifting the buttocks, the ribs must not be moved up by the activity of the rectus abdominis and the ventral section of the diaphragm. This is seen when the abdomen bulges in front, without contraction of the lateral abdominal muscles. It is also a mistake if retroversion of the pelvis occurs, as is adduction of the shoulder blades accompanied by increased activity of the paravertebral muscles.

- The patient is prone with hands clasped behind his head. In this position, care must be taken that the upper trapezius is relaxed. Support is given to the arms and shoulders to help the patient into extension. The patient is helped to fix the shoulder blades in a caudal position and abduction. Extension is most important in the mid-thoracic spine. In this position it is essential that the patient supports himself at the symphysis while his shoulder blades remain fixed. In this way, centration of the thoracolumbar region is achieved, and the lateral abdominal muscles and the lumbar part of the diaphragm are activated.

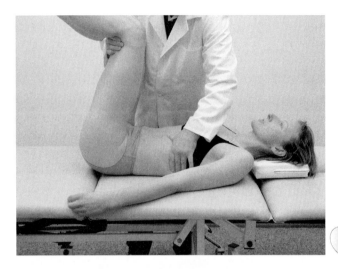

Figure 23.42 Activation of the abdominal press with the diaphragm in the caudal position. We fix the patient's ribs and chest in a caudal position and ask him to support himself at the area of the T/L junction and slightly lift the buttocks up from the table.

Mistakes to be Avoided The patient flexes the thoracic spine while seeking support at the symphysis. He adducts his shoulder blades.

- The patient is prone, supporting himself on his hands. He straightens the cervical and the upper thoracic spine. Below T5, the vertebrae move into extension one after the other, only into mid position, i.e., to achieve centration. The patient pushes himself up by pressing on his palms. The movement is to make the symphysis the point of support. In this position, maximum caudal movement of the thorax is attempted during exhalation. At this moment, the patient is told to exert pressure against our resistance underneath the costal angle of the lower ribs, i.e., at the laterodorsal aspect of the abdominal wall. Extension should not be greater than 45 degrees above horizontal (Fig. 23.43).

Mistakes to be Avoided The patient adducts the shoulder blades. When contracting his abdominal muscles and the diaphragm, he increases flexion of the thoracic spine. The patient is unable to keep his thorax in a caudal position during the pushup.

Motor Patterns and Trigger Points

In addition to muscular imbalance between ontogenetically older and younger muscles, it is important to show the principles of chain reaction between muscles

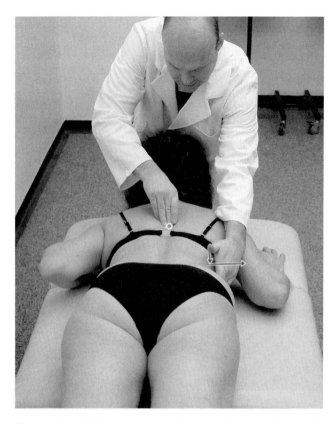

Figure 23.43 The patient straightens the area of the mid thoracic spine while keeping his chest in a caudal position and activating the diaphragm and the deep abdominal muscles.

with local differences in tension, in particular muscles harboring trigger points (TrPs). We may assume that their origin is nociception. Their interconnection is by no means haphazard but follows rather strict rules. If we release one TrP, we obtain release in TrPs much further away. Localized changes in muscle tension will also affect joint function by changing the articular pattern. A TrP is never an isolated change in function. A number of authors have pointed out that TrPs are to some degree interconnected. The description of individual chains has so far been empirical, without neurophysiological explanation.

Here, too, developmental kinesiology has brought about a change. The existence of inborn motor patterns points the way for a new functional understanding. The development of posture shows that the highest level of control of inborn motor patterns is not at spinal or brain stem level, but above the latter. This, too, forms the basis of our motor behavior. Two patterns play an essential role in succession:

1. Spinal posture in the sagittal plane (which matures at the age of 3.5 months [Figs. 23.11 and 23.12]).

2. The stepping forward and support function of the extremities in connection with trunk rotation.

These functions mature in succession during the motor development. Motor patterns can be seen in the course of the individual phases of the postural development. It is important that they are parts of the global locomotor pattern. This pattern is inhibited by the cerebral cortex but can be evoked by reflex mechanisms not only in children but also in adults.

The locomotor pattern is made up of purposeful joint movements from one extreme position to its opposite. If, for instance, we stimulate the reflex pattern of the hip joint, it starts in one leg in extension, adduction, and internal rotation, and it ends in flexion, abduction, and external rotation. In the other leg, the opposite reciprocal movement takes place at the same time, i.e., starts in flexion abduction and outward rotation and ends in extension, adduction, and internal rotation. At the forearm, the movement starts in maximum pronation and ends in supination (at the other arm it will be the reverse, i.e., from maximum supination into maximum pronation).

The wrist moves on the stepping forward side from flexion and ulnar deviation into extension and radial flexion (and it will be the reverse on the opposite side). The principle is the same for all joints. For each joint there is a well-determined movement as part of a motor pattern. The anatomical structure determines the biomechanically ideal joint movement. The neurophysiological and biomechanical principles make up the normal motor pattern. Each position the joint adopts in the course of the motor pattern may be called "frozen." This is controlled by muscles that stabilize it (fixation by muscular attachments). The angle at which a joint is placed determines the activation of specific parts of the muscles that stabilize the joint in a given position at a given moment (Fig. 23.44).

The role of the TrP is to immobilize the joint in certain positions or locomotor stages ("frozen positions"). The articular pattern is changed automatically as the joint is immobilized in that position or stage of movement. The TrP is found in the part of a muscle that stabilizes that particular locomotor stage or position. The angle at which we examine a joint activates different portions of the stabilizing muscle. In other words, when the joint is at a different angle it affects different sections of the stabilizing muscles. For example, in a given position of the arm only a specific section of the pectoralis muscle will respond. In addition there will be a chain of TrPs in muscles that stabilize the attachment points of this part of the pectoralis. They will

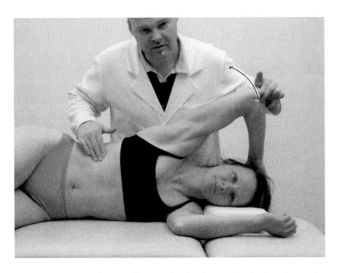

Figure 23.44 The angle at which the articulation is positioned determines which parts of the muscles will be activated and which parts of the muscles providing stabilization will be activated.

be found in those fibers that are functionally connected with the fibers of the pectoralis harboring the TrP. Thus, if the pectoralis muscle is active, its attachment point must be stabilized by other functionally related muscles. Other parts of the abdominal muscles, of the adductors (retractors), of the shoulder blade, and also of the adductors and abductors of the hip, etc., must be activated if the angle of arm abduction is changed. Attachment point stabilization automatically occurs under the control of the CNS. Every joint position is stabilized during movement by muscle function.

Chains of TrPs can therefore be explained by the synergy of stabilizing muscles or their parts that correspond to a specific position or stage of movement ("frozen position") of the locomotor pattern. Reflex changes like TrPs are never isolated. They require immobilization of a certain position by a chain of stabilizing muscles. Thus, if we find a TrP in the pectineus, another will be found in the corresponding part of its antagonist, i.e., in the posterior part of the gluteus medius, and also in the corresponding part of the pectoralis, with an attachment point at the fifth rib, in the upper part of the subscapularis, and in the adductors of the shoulder blade, with attachment points at the T5/6 level, etc.

Principles of Examination and Correction of Pathological Articular Patterns

The basis for examination and treatment of disturbed function is the function of muscles and joints

determined by a program under central control. The principles are as follows:

1. First, we try to make the joint move according to its pre-programmed pattern. For this, it is important to know the pattern of locomotion which is most favorable with regard to its mechanism. Therefore, the joint is examined under dynamic, not static, conditions. Because examination is passive, no resistance should be felt close to the neutral point of the joint. If there is abnormality, this pattern is changed. We feel some resistance and normal movement is substituted in a characteristic way, like a detour, with the movement not being smooth, as though a certain phase has had to be left out. This "derailment" is very characteristic.

   If we examine the segment L5-S1, passive flexion is produced at the hip joint, with the patient lying on the side, rotating at the same time the pelvis and trunk, which corresponds to the stepping-forward pattern (Fig. 23.45). At the stage when the segment L5-S1 comes into play, i.e., at the end of the stepping-forward stage, we sense resistance and a change (substitution) of the movement pattern. This is felt like resistance, producing a lateral deviation of the pelvis. This deviation is a very sensitive sign of a movement restriction in segment L5-S1.

2. Correct positioning plays a key role in therapy. For this, we have to find the phase of the motor

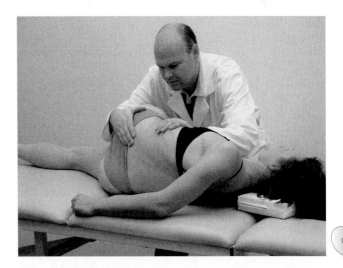

Figure 23.45 Mobilization of the lumbar spine making use of the stepping-forward function of the leg. During mobilization, our fixation must prevent incorrect substitution patterns.

pattern in which resistance has been found at examination. This position has to be fixed; then, we have to overcome the resistance, the pathological substitution, by manual contact and complete the full range of the locomotor pattern. By mobilization, we prevent the joint moving in an abnormal way by using our hands. Thus, we obtain the effect of mobilization, i.e., normal joint pattern including joint play. If, for example, we mobilize the segment L5-S1, we position this segment to make it move in the pattern of stepping forward (Fig. 23.46). By manual fixation, we prevent lateral movement of the pelvis (i.e., substitution) and move on into flexion. We do not mobilize by a movement of joint facet translation, but only by correcting the movement that is part of the normal pattern. This principle can be applied to joints in general.

Another possible way to correct articular patterns is by specific activation of muscles. We first take up the slack in a joint and the patient makes a "stepping-forward movement" with his leg, against resistance. The patient is required to exert only minimum resistance. In this way, muscular stabilization is obtained, securing the segment to be mobilized. By resisting the stepping-forward pattern, we change the muscle tension at the segment we intend to mobilize, including the deep stabilizers, which are not under the control of the patient's will (Fig. 23.47). This effect can also be produced by stimulation of specific zones. Stimulation has to be performed in the position in which the slack of the joint

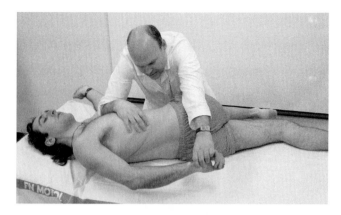

Figure 23.47 After taking up slack in the segment to be mobilized, resist the stepping-forward function of the arm (supination, extension, and radial duction). The force developed by the patient should only be minimal.

to be treated has been taken up (Fig. 23.48). Muscle facilitation takes place automatically. In this way, muscle tension is normalized and mobilization takes place.

■ CONCLUSION

An attempt has been made to integrate the principles of developmental kinesiology with those of both neurophysiology and biomechanics. They comprise basic motor functions that form the basis of a diagnostic and therapeutic system. This principle is universal. Most techniques apply the principles of the developmental program, in particular of precise joint

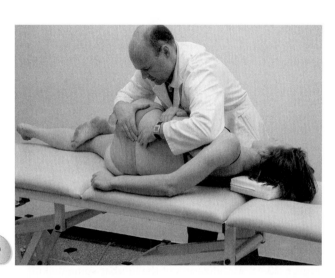

Figure 23.46 Mobilization of the segment without making use of movement patterns.

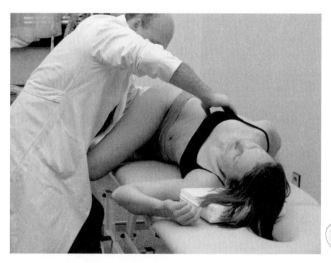

Figure 23.48 After taking up the slack in the segment to be mobilized, we stimulate the appropriate zones.

centration, of balanced muscular stabilization, and even of restoring proprioception.

The development of human erect posture helps us to understand chain reactions of functional lesions of the motor system. Without understanding the anatomical and functional, co-contraction of muscles would be meaningless.

Developmental kinesiology of course plays a key role in the assessment of early development in infancy and in the detection of even the slightest motor lesion in the earliest stages when therapy is most effective.

Developmental kinesiology enables us also to assess the prognosis of children with cerebral palsy. It is even possible to assess the relation between what has been achieved by treatment and what could have been achieved under optimum conditions. It is therefore possible to assess the effectiveness of rehabilitation.

Audit Process
Self-Check of the Chapter's Learning Objectives

• What are the chief landmarks in neurodevelopment of the upright posture that an infant/child achieves from ages 1 month to 4 years?

• How would you position a patient in the supine position to perform reflex locomotion in rolling?

• How would you position a patient prone to perform reflex locomotion in creeping?

• How can you test and train coordination of the abdominal wall and diaphragm?

■ ACKNOWLEDGMENT

This chapter would not have been possible without Alena Kobesova's editing suggestions and translation.

■ REFERENCES

1. Costi GC, Radice C, Raggi A, et al. Vojta's seven postural reactions for screening of neuromotorial diseases in infant. Research of 2308 cases. Ped Med Chir 1983;5:59.

2. Janda V. Movement Patterns in Pelvic and Thigh Region with Special Reference to Pathogenesis of Vertebrogenic Disturbances. (Czech.) Thesis. Prague: Charles University, 1964.

3. Janda V, Stara V. The role of thigh adductors in movement patterns of the hip and knee joint. Courier. 1965;September:563–565.

4. Janda V. Postural and phasic muscles in the pathogenesis of low back pain. XIth Congress ISRD. Dublin Proceedings. 1969:553–554.

5. Janda V. What is the typical posture of man? (Czech). Cas lek ces. 1972;111:32:748–750.

6. Janda V. Muscle and joint correlations. Proceedings IV Congress FIMM. Praha 1974. Rehabilitacia Suppl. 1976;Suppl:10–11, 154–158.

7. Janda V. On the concept of postural muscles and posture. Austr J Physiother 1983;29:S83–S84.

8. Janda V. Muscle spasm—a proposed procedure for differential diagnosis. J Man Med 1991;6:136–139.

9. Janda V. Muscle strength in relation to muscle length, pain and muscle imbalance. In: Harms-Rindahl K, ed. Muscle Strength. New York: Churchill Livingstone, 1993.

10. Kolár P. The sensomotor nature of postural functions: Its fundamental role in rehabilitation. J Orthop Med 1999;2:40–45.

11. Lajosi F, Bauer H, Avalle C. Early diagnosis of central motor disturbances by postural reflexes after Vojta. Barcelona: XIV International Congress of Pediatrics, 1980 (abstracts).

12. Vojta V. Die cerebralen Bewegungstoerungen im Kindesalter, 4te Auflage. Stuttgart: Ferdinand Enke Verlag, 1988.

13. Vojta V. Mozkove hybne poruchy v kojeneckem veku. Vcasna diagnosa a terapie. Crerebral motor disturbances in babies. Early diagnosis and treatment. Prague: Grada-Avicenum [book translated from German original: "Die zerebralen Bewegungsstorungen im Sauglinsalter]. 1993:29,30,71,89,94,103,108, 112,114,115.

24

Yoga-Based Training for Spinal Stability

Jirí Čumpelík and František Véle

Learning Objectives

After reading this chapter, you should be able to understand:

- The contributions of the diaphragm, transverse abdominus, and inter-costal and deep spinal intrinsic muscles to normal respiration
- The relationship between thoracic spine mobility and function of the cervical and lumbar spines
- The physiological differences between lower abdominal, lower chest, upper chest, and whole-body breathing exercises
- How recumbent spinal exercises for the deep "intrinsic" muscles can improve mid-thoracic joint mobility and lumbar spine stability

Introduction

The greatest problem with back pain is its chronic and recurrent nature. Even though manual techniques have been proven effective in removing pain and restoring restricted movement, if the real cause of the problem is not addressed, relapse regularly occurs. Even closely followed home exercise programs are not able to suppress the chronic nature of back pain.

Understanding the postural program provides a key in correction of recurrent back pain. A special program stored in the central nervous system (CNS) controls postural muscles. Its function is to control and stabilize posture, protect spinal joints, and prevent the effects of micro-trauma (18). The postural program gradually adapts to "civilized" environmental conditions, like prolonged periods of sitting, and loses efficiency as its pattern is continuously altered. This altered CNS program needs repair to prevent the repeated damage of micro-trauma on the joint structures (15).

Local manual treatment, even when effective, may address the acute symptoms but often cannot correct the underlying "cause," which is altered control of the postural motor program.

Postural muscles have different functions in stabilizing posture. Short inter-segmental muscles, close to the joint, stabilize individual segments. Long superficial muscles stabilize larger sections of the spine (3). Postural stability can be flexible or rigid. Flexible stability results from individual activation of the short deep muscles, whereas rigid flexibility comes from the activation of the long superficial muscles. Though each type of stability has independent control, the two are interdependent (3). Examination methods rarely differentiate between flexible and rigid stability. Our clinical experience shows that this differentiation is vital in the diagnosis and treatment of spinal dysfunction.

We can demonstrate the difference between rigid and flexible stability with a simple experiment: Instruct a patient to bear down and tighten his abdomen to stabilize posture. Then, pertubate his shoulder with two fingers in several directions while observing his reaction. Next, instruct the patient to relax and concentrate on abdominal breathing. Again, try to move his shoulder in several directions while observing his reaction. Compare these two reactions.

In the first part of this experiment, the body is held firm, like a rod, and there is a lot of compensatory activity in the leg muscles. Stability is rigid and the shoulder can easily be moved. In second part of the experiment, the compensated reaction to the perturbation is distributed between different segments of the body and the shoulder cannot be easily moved. Although the body is flexible, it is clearly more stable (7).

We have made a pilot study to make this experiment objective. Using a posturograph, we measured the time required to return to a state of stability after an external impact destabilized the trunk. A correlation has been found between breathing patterns and time. In the habitual chest breather, it took 2.5 seconds to return to a normal state of stability after an impact. Consistently, in abdominal breathers, it took an average of 1.5 seconds to return to stability. It appears from this experiment that the body requires less time to stabilize when the flexible stabilization system is dominant than when a more rigid stability predominates (7).

The short, deep muscles of the spine are affected in many back pain syndromes. Panjabi's work (14) has proven that these muscles help to maintain the spinal joints in proper position and to protect them against damage especially in the "neutral zone." The short inter-segmental muscles have greater abundance of muscle spindles than the long, more superficial muscles. More kinesthetic information coming from the muscle spindles of these short muscles allows greater CNS control of them (4).

The principle control of posture is associated with minute position changes of individual spinal segments. This observation was reinforced during our ongoing studies of breathing mechanics. We have established through clinical experience that the stabilizing postural muscles are also active in breathing mechanics (17). The dynamics of movement during respiration depend on postural stability. The same muscles that create flexible stability also support normal breathing mechanics. If an external load demands, the CNS will protect the spine first, at the expense of modifying breathing mechanics (see Chapters 5 and 17). A good example of this is the way we automatically hold our breath when we have to make a sudden stop while driving a car. This disturbance of the normal motor program, which initially occurred to meet an emergency demand, can get "fixed" in the CNS and become a habitual pattern long after the "emergency" is over.

If we know how to interpret breathing movements, valuable indirect knowledge about the function of the deep intrinsic muscles can be gathered. Dysfunction in the diaphragm, inter-costals, abdominals, pelvic floor, and deep spinal intrinsic muscles can be easily seen during examination of breathing mechanics, as discussed in section III: yoga-based respiratory exercises.

This chapter describes exercises based on yoga principles. We thank Swami Dewa Murti (8) and Dr. Swami Gitananda (9) for sharing their knowledge. The goal of our yoga-based exercises is to repair the altered CNS postural and respiratory programs and to restore spinal stability. Throughout the chapter we emphasize the quality of movement and attempt to enhance the quality of the motor program controlling the movement.

The Clinical Role of Respiratory Mechanics

Breathing Mechanics

The diaphragm, inter-costal muscles, transversus Abdominis (TrA), muscles of pelvic floor, and the deep intrinsic muscles of the spine are all muscles with either a horizontal or an oblique orientation that can be segmentally activated. They participate as core stabilizers in respiratory mechanics as well as in postural function (7).

The diaphragm is the prime mover and initiator in respiratory mechanics. It is a horizontally oriented membranous dome that separates the thoracic and abdominal cavities. Most anatomists divide it into three sections: lumbar, costal, and sternal (11). Others claim eight separate sections on each side (6). All sections insert into the central tendon of the diaphragm, forming a rounded aponeurosis with no bony attachment in the middle of this flat muscle.

Basmajian (1,2) using EMG has substantiated that voluntary control of individual motor units is possible. His findings support our clinical experience that individual sections of the diaphragm are able to be activated separately as well as together as a unit. This ability to learn to activate each part of the diaphragm allows the success of localized segmental breathing, which is currently used in respiratory therapy.

Diaphragmatic movement is divided into two phases:

1. Vertical movement.

   In this first phase, the central tendon moves up and down during expiration and inspiration and the rib cage does not change in diameter. The abdomen is vaulted outward during inhalation and pulled "in" toward the spine during exhalation. There is a partnership between the diaphragm and TrA throughout this phase of movement.

2. Horizontal movement.

   In this second phase, the vertical shift of the central tendon of the diaphragm stops, caused by increasing abdominal pressure, and the TrA does not allow the abdomen to vault "out" further. The central tendon is now fixed and the diaphragm supports rib movement by enhancing activity of the inter-costal muscles. The movement of the ribs is like a fan opening and closing laterally and dorsally.

Effect of Yoga-Based Respiratory Exercises on Spinal Function

Breathing is an involuntary action. So, it seems unreasonable to think that one needs to be taught how to breathe. Yet breathing can be modified in various ways, not just momentarily, but habitually. Unhealthy breathing "habits" often develop without our awareness. With the help of breathing exercises, it is possible to restore normal abdominal and chest movements associated with efficient breathing and postural function. The ultimate purpose of the following exercises is to change the respiratory program until it is efficient and habitual. At this point, the postural program also has the opportunity of optimal function.

The reader will note that throughout these exercises, co-activation between the diaphragm, TrA inter-costal muscles, and the deep spinal intrinsic muscles is being established. Also, throughout the exercises, the intrinsic muscles must stabilize the spinal segments and correct the extension and flexion tendencies made by movements of the ribs and abdominal muscles during breathing.

In a functional and mobile spine, the physiological movement of the cervical spine starts from T4 and progresses upward, and the movements of the lumbar spine from T6 and go downward. Extension and flexion of the thoracic spine continues through a lengthened spine into the cervical and lumbar regions. This is in keeping with Kolar's theory of neurodevelopment (Chapter 23).

When restriction of extension is present in the area of T1-T4, there is overstrain of the neck caused by hyperextension of the upper cervical spine. Keeping the sternum down and increasing abdominal pressure is the remedy for removing the restriction of upper thoracic movements (see Chapters 23 and 26). As practice continues, the deep muscles of the thorax relax and more differentiated movement of the ribs become possible. As this occurs, many patients feel improvement of functional problems in their neck, shoulders, and arms.

A similar pattern exists in the thoraco-lumbar spine. If movement restriction is found in the area of T6-T12, there is a tendency toward lumbar hyperextension, which must be corrected during the exercise. As practice continues, greater mobility of whole thoracic spine occurs by the enhanced coordination between the mobility of spinal segments and movements of the ribs.

Regular practice of these exercises will enhance mobility as well as coordinated movement of the spine. It is suggested that joint fixation in the spine or in the ribs should be treated first by manipulation or mobilization. In chronic cases, local mobilization can relieve local problems temporarily, but resolution of the condition is only possible by repairing the faulty respiratory program controlled by the CNS.

The primary goal of these yoga-based exercises is the prevention of motor faults. These exercises can also be very effective therapeutically. Breathing and spinal exercises are considered an integral part of daily hygiene, much like brushing one's teeth. When practiced regularly, these exercises keep the body and mind not only in good condition but also in good communication. The greatest benefit aside from an increased sense of vitality and well-being may lie in an enhanced ability to detect dysfunction in one's own body at early stages, when correction is most appropriate.

Yoga-Based Respiratory Exercises

Exercises Enhancing and Controlling Normal Respiratory Motion

The trunk is functionally divided into three respiratory sections: lower, middle, and upper. Breathing exercises are divided into four primary groups that are categorized by the anatomical and functional regions being influenced:

1. Lower abdominal breathing exercises enhance the core relationship between the diaphragm and abdominal and pelvic floor muscles.
2. Lower chest breathing exercises enhance the normal lateral excursion of the lower rib cage and relationship between inter-costal muscles, diaphragm, and deep spinal intrinsic muscles.
3. Upper chest breathing exercises enhance the fan-like movement of the upper rib cage and the relationship between the muscle activity of inter-costal muscles and deep spinal intrinsic muscles.
4. Whole-breathing exercises integrate the functional relationship and enhance the coordinated movement of all three sections.

As described, when respiration is normal, all three sections are functioning optimally and in mutual coordination (16). A complete program of breathing exercises must address all three sections: lower, middle, and upper in all three directions of movement and anterior, lateral, and posterior.

Before beginning these exercises, it is essential to assess the initial pattern of breathing. This is easily done in the lower abdomen by putting the palms sequentially on the lower part of the abdomen, first just under the navel, then on the sides, and finally on the back at the same level. Then, the same scan can be repeated in the middle and upper chest. Nine areas are evaluated. Finally, integration between all three parts can be compared by moving the hands during respiration. Start by putting the left palm on the middle chest and right palm on the abdomen. At full inhalation, shift the right hand from the abdomen to the upper part of the chest. Move the hands in both exhalation and inhalation. Evaluate the range of movement below the palms. The facilitating exercises that follow are used to improve movement in areas where movement is restricted, asymmetric, or even absent.

The best posture for this group of exercises is the kneeling position, while sitting on the heels. In this position the spine is straight, the ribcage and the abdomen are able to move freely, and breathing is optimized. If it is difficult to assume this position, other postures, such as sitting on the edge of a chair, can be used. The choice of position is dependent on individual comfort. Any posture that allows the spine to be maintained in the same position is acceptable (Fig. 24.1).

The scanning exercise allows the patient to assess his control of respiratory movement. The exercise provides valuable feedback so that progress can be monitored as practice continues. If difficulty in control of movement in a specific area (lower abdominal or middle or upper chest) was found in this scanning exercise, we suggest that you go to the exercises that facilitate greater control of movement in that specific area that are described here.

Exercises Facilitating Breath Control

Exercises Facilitating Lower Abdominal Breath Control

Exercise A. (Fig. 24.2) Facilitates the diaphragm's first phase of movement with maximum activity of the sternal part of the diaphragm. When performed correctly, there will be improvement of co-activation between the deep spinal intrinsic, diaphragm, TrA, and the inter-costal muscles.

Basic Position

- Sit on the heels, with spine straight and with the arms relaxed at the side.

Movement
Inhalation

1. As the abdomen starts to vault "out," rise up with slight flexion in the hips to a kneeling position with the spine straight.

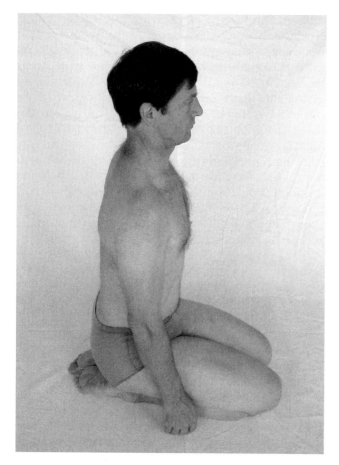

Figure 24.1 Beginning position respiratory training, kneeling.

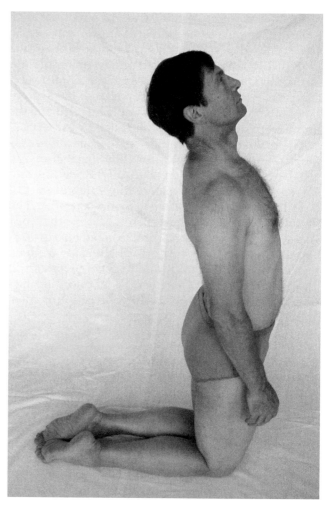

Figure 24.2 Facilitating sternal part of diaphragm.

2. Continue inhalation by increasing extension of the spine starting at T12/L1 (NOT the L/S junction). This extension enables greater lowering of the central tendon.

3. Keep the arms and sternum relaxed and the eyes open.

4. Be careful to avoid cervico-cranial hyperextension.

   Exhalation

1. Begin exhalation by drawing the navel toward the spine.

2. Return the neck and the entire spine to a neutral position.

3. Lower to the starting position of sitting on the heels and exhale completely.

Repeat this exercise three to six times.

Exercise B. (Fig. 24.3) Facilitates the diaphragm's first phase of movement with maximum activity of the costal part of the diaphragm.

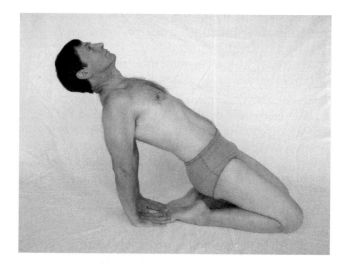

Figure 24.3 Facilitating costal part of diaphragm.

Basic Position

- Sit on the heels, bend back putting the palms of the hands on the mat behind, point the fingers forward, and touch the toes. Rest the weight of the upper body on the hands and relax in this position. The back is arched and the neck is elongated.

Movement

Inhalation

1. As the abdomen starts to vault "out," raise the buttocks off the heels and arch the back from T12/L1 (NOT the L/S junction) to the highest comfortable level.

2. Complete the inhalation by continuing to extend the spine to end-range while the ribs remain relaxed and the sternum remains lowered.

3. Allow the neck to lengthen and follow the extension of the spine.

   (Be sure to avoid cervico-cranial hyperextension. As the spine becomes more flexible, extension of the mid to lower cervical spine often becomes more natural.)

Exhalation

1. Begin exhalation by drawing the navel toward the spine.

2. Stabilize the spine and lower to the starting position with a neutral spine and exhale completely.

   Repeat this exercise three to six times.

You may point the fingers away or bend at the knuckles if this position is uncomfortable to the wrists. In time, work toward the proper hand position.

Exercise C. (Fig. 24.4) Facilitates the diaphragm's first phase of movement with maximum activity of the lumbar part of the diaphragm.

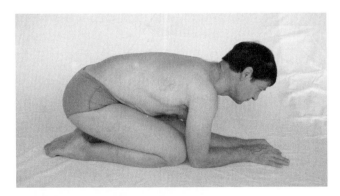

Figure 24.4 Facilitating lumbar part of diaphragm—kneeling sphinx on forearms.

Basic Position

- Sit on the heels, kneel with forearms on the floor, elbows touching knees, palms down and open, fingers pointed away and the entire spine lengthened (avoid cervico-cranial hyperextension).

Movement

Inhalation

1. Vault the lower abdominal area "out," expanding more in a latero-posterior direction as the spine remains lengthened.

Exhalation

1. Concentrate on the contraction of the latero-posterior abdomen and try to make the waist small.

2. This time, the navel is not drawing in toward the spine, but supporting the side movement of the waist.

3. With each breath out, focus on bringing the lumbar spine closer to the mat and continuing the thoracic spine extension. The oblique abdominals and the large superficial back muscles are relaxed and not active during this exercise.

Note: In many cases, the lumbar spine begins this exercise in a kyphotic position. It often takes time for the large muscles of the spine to relax and for extension to be possible. Co-activation between the diaphragm, TrA, and the multifidi muscles must be monitored. Instruct the patient to bring the spinous processes closer together during exhalation and hold the spine still during the next inhalation, maintaining the extension.

Stay and breathe in this position for a few minutes, and then relax.

Exercise Facilitating Middle Breath Control

Exercise A. (Fig. 24.5) Facilitates the diaphragm's second phase of movement and rotational movement of the ribs, especially in the side and back.

Basic Position

- Sit on the heels with the hands "palm down" and directly in front of the knees. Keep the arms straight and slightly pressed to the floor. Extend and elongate the spine. Neck discomfort in this position is often caused by immobility of the upper thoracic vertebra. Be careful to avoid cervico-cranial hyperextension. This will become easier once upper thoracic extension coupled with keeping the sternum down can be maintained.

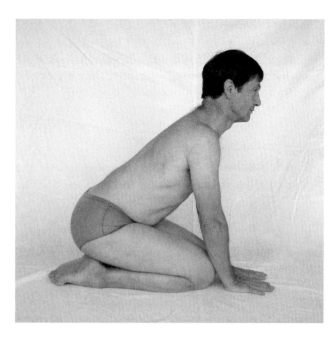

Figure 24.5 Middle breath control, kneeling sphinx—kneeling sphinx on hands.

Movement

Inhalation

1. Expand the rib cage allowing the ribs to rotate and "fan-open," especially in the back.
2. Maintain the extended position of the spine.
3. This position facilitates movement in the middle chest area and makes it difficult to breathe into the lower and upper areas.

Exhalation

1. Relax the chest and allow the ribs to rotate and "fan-closed."
2. Continue to lengthen the entire spine and further increase the thoracic lordosis.
3. With each breath out, focus on bringing the spinous processes of T6-7 closer to the mat while relaxing and closing the ribs.
4. Stay in this position for several minutes and keep focused on breathing.

Note: There is a co-contraction between the diaphragm, intercostals and multifidi muscles during this exercise. The spine remains extended during both inspiration and expiration. The multifidi are actively correcting the tendency toward flexion and extension, whereas the ribs are moving during breathing. The chest is relaxed and allows rib movement while the sternum remains still. The large superficial muscles of the back are relaxed. Co-activation of the diaphragm, TrA, and multifidi occurs naturally in this position,

facilitates the second phase of diaphragmatic movement, and enhances the movements of the ribs and spine.

Exercise B. (Fig. 24.6) Facilitates the diaphragm's second phase of movement and rotational movement of the ribs, especially in the front and side.

Basic Position

- Sit with the legs extended, lower the trunk using the elbows for support, rest the forearms and hands on the mat, and arch the spine.

Movement

Inhalation

1. Allow the ribcage to expand and the ribs to rotate "open" like a fan.
2. Relax into full thoracic lordosis with the peak at T6.
3. Allow the neck to be lengthened and extended. Be careful to avoid cervico-cranial hyperextension.
4. Actively maintain the spine in this arched position.

Exhalation

1. Stabilize and maintain extension while focusing directly on the motion of the ribs.
2. Rotate the ribs "closed" with a relaxed chest and lowered sternum.
3. Stabilizing the thoracic spine in extension is a key to this exercise.

Exercise C. (Fig. 24.7) Facilitates the diaphragm's second phase of movement and rotational movement of the ribs in the middle chest.

Basic Position

- Supine with legs extended, heels together, back arched, neck extended, and top of the head and elbows touching the mat (and weight-bearing).

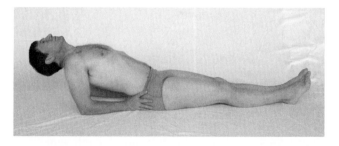

Figure 24.6 Middle chest breathing leaning back.

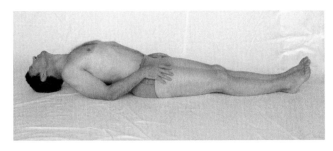

Figure 24.7 Middle chest breathing supine.

The forearms may be used to gain this position, and then relax the hands on the thighs.

Movement

Inhalation

1. Relax into full thoracic lordosis with the peak at T6. Allow the entire spine to be lengthened.
2. Expand the rib cage laterally and rotate the ribs "open" like a fan while keeping the sternum relaxed and lowered.
3. Actively maintain the spine in extension.

Exhalation

1. Maintain extension and focus on the ribcage.
2. Rotate the ribs "closed" while relaxing the chest and keeping the sternum lowered.
3. Completely exhale and move into even greater T6 extension.
4. Stabilizing the thoracic spine in extension is essential to allow relaxed movement of the ribs.

Exercises Facilitating Upper Breath Control

Exercise A. (Fig. 24.8) Exhalation is usually more difficult than inhalation in the upper chest; therefore, the exercise below emphasizes facilitation of exhalation.

Basic Position

- Sit on the heels with the head and spine in an erect position, arms along the body, and fingers interlaced behind.

Movement

Inhalation

1. Maintain an erect spine and take a deep breath in.

Exhalation

1. Slowly exhale and bend forward until the head touches the floor in front of the knees.

2. At this point, all of the breath should be expelled.
3. Raise the arms over the shoulders and head as far as comfortably possible with either the fingers interlaced or the hands open and palms up.
4. Relax in this position for a few seconds without breathing in.
5. Rapidly pulse the arms further away and expel the remaining air from the lungs with three short thrusts of the arms. (Do not inhale.)

Inhalation

1. Lower the arms and use the breath to lift the body; with a neutral spine, return to the starting position.

Repeat this exercise six to 12 times, until the upper chest is relaxed with greater freedom of movement in the ribs and shoulders.

Exercise B. (Fig. 24.9) Facilitates the movement of the upper ribs opposite head rotation. Exhalation is usually more difficult than inhalation in the upper chest; therefore, the exercise below emphasizes facilitation of exhalation.

Basic Position

- Begin in a kneeling position and move forward until the upper chest is resting on the ground with the head turned to the right, resting on the left cheek. Outstretch the arms at a 120-degree angle, arch the spine with the buttocks raised as far as comfortably possible toward the ceiling, flex the hips, and rest the weight of the body on the upper chest (not on the cheek) and on the knees.

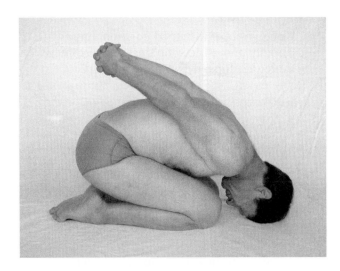

Figure 24.8 Upper breath control, exhalation.

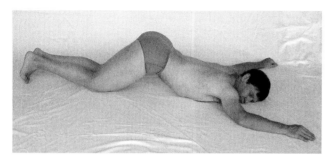

Figure 24.9 Upper breath control, with rotation.

Movement

Inhalation

1. Allow the ribs to move on the right, the opposite side of head rotation. The rotation of the ribs on the right raises the ribcage slightly "up."

Exhalation

1. Lower the ribcage and allow the ribs to rotate "closed" while relaxing the chest and shoulders and using the weight of the body to deepen the exhalation and reach the end range of movement.
2. Slowly breathe six to 12 times in this position. Then, repeat with the face turned to the right for an additional six to 12 breaths to facilitate the left side of the upper chest.
3. To come out of this position, place the hands under the shoulders and perform a gentle push up, relax, and slowly return to an erect sitting position.

Exercise Facilitating Whole-Breath Control

Exercise A (Figs. 24.10 and 24.11)

Basic Position

- Kneel in the quadruped position, hands directly under the shoulders, knees directly under the hips, legs hip width apart.

Movement

Inhalation

1. The abdomen vaults and progressively expands the lower, middle, and upper chest to the side while the spine progressively arches the lower, middle, and upper back and, lastly, raises the head up.

Exhalation

1. The abdomen starts drawing the navel to the spine and slowly closes the ribs in lower, middle,

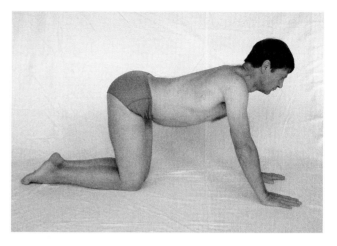

Figure 24.10 Whole breath control, inhalation position.

and upper chest, while the spine progressively rounds the lower, middle, and upper back and, lastly, relaxes the neck and lowers the head toward to the floor. Breathe and move slowly and simultaneously, segment by segment, with intention.

Repeat three to six times, relax, and return to the kneeling position.

Note: During inhalation, fill the lungs first in the lower abdomen, then the middle and upper chest, and during exhalation empty the lungs in the same sequence, again, the lower abdomen, then middle, and, lastly, upper chest.

Clinical Pearl

The oblique muscles should not contract during either relaxed inhalation or exhalation.

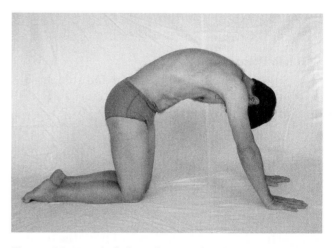

Figure 24.11 Whole breath control, exhalation position.

The Effect of Yoga-Based Spinal Exercises on Spinal Function

The spinal exercises were derived from human loco-motion, respectively, from the torsional movements of the spine while walking. Human gait is fully automatized as fixed movement programs in the CNS. Unfortunately, faulty habits of movement modify this program, such as after prolonged period of pain. Correction is a difficult task if the modified program continues longer than necessary.

Spinal exercises are aimed at the prevention of functional disorders of the "axial organ," a Czech term from the work of Vojta (19) (referring to the head and spine including the thoracic cage and pelvis). These exercises can also be used therapeutically to correct specific dysfunction. They are performed in a horizontal position to avoid axial pressure and lessen the influence of the postural program, which runs continuously in the vertical position. This also allows better concentration and helps build a new correct program that is less influenced by acquired incorrect posture and movement. By changing the position of the legs, we change the torsional movement in different levels of the spine. Outstretched legs target segments in the lumbar spine, whereas bent legs tend to target thoracic spinal segments.

The close linkage between control of "axial" movement and control of breathing is of special importance throughout these exercises. In the first phase of practice, the concentration is aimed at smooth, controlled rotation of the head and the pelvis. Once this is achieved, synchronization of head and pelvic rotation can be coordinated. Simply put, when the head is fully rotated to one side, the pelvis should be fully rotated to the opposite side. As movement continues in the opposite direction, the coordination and pace between head and pelvis remain constant. Neither the head nor the pelvis should reach center or the point of full rotation before the other. Movement should be continuous; jerky movements and stopping should be avoided. After controlled and synchronized movement is obtained, one can begin to introduce control of the breath with the exercise.

Breathing and posture are used to enhance stability. Each exercise begins with activation of the diaphragm in inhalation to move the central tendon inferiorly. This will be experienced as horizontal motion in the abdominal and lower rib cage regions. A common substitution pattern that should be avoided is vertical lifting of the rib cage upwards during inhalation. The rib cage should be completely relaxed so it hangs down on a lengthened spinal column. Next, voluntary co-activation of the oblique abdominals, transverse abdominus, and serratus posterior inferior is encouraged to stabilize the thoraco-lumbar (T/L) spine in a "centrated" posture (avoiding hyperlordosis). Finally, spine rotation exercises are performed while holding this stable T/L posture.

By achieving a relaxed rib cage on a lengthened spine with horizontal respiration and centration of the T/L spine, all the deep stabilizers of the spine—abdominal wall (not merely rectus abdominus), diaphragm, multifidi, and pelvic floor muscles—will be activated. The result will be increased abdominal pressure, which, according to Kapandji, increases stability and reduces axial pressure on the discs (11).

Practicing spinal exercises is also a method to learn voluntary control and "correction" of spinal movement. The biomechanics of this motion is quite complex, so much so that it is still not totally defined in the literature. True total voluntary control of this complex movement would be an insurmountable task! In reality, the performance of the movement remains subcortical. The mind is focused not on the specific action of the muscles but rather on control of the movement itself. While performing the exercise, one can feel whether the movement is "jerky" or uncoordinated. Through practice the perceived "fault" can be corrected. Direct control of intrinsic movement is not inherent, but improved coordination can be "learned." Deep, motivated concentration and patience is the prerequisite for learning this skill.

Clinical Pearl

- Many symptoms of functional and postural imbalances are corrected when function of the deep spinal intrinsic muscles is normalized and coordination of movement is restored. For instance, if gait takes place with a rigid thoracic spine and reduction in the normal contralateral pelvic-torso rotation, then this training can easily restore a more normal gait function.

The aim of these yoga-based spinal exercises is to maintain (or restore) normal function of the motor program. This is accomplished by accessing volitional control of movement through facilitating the powerful afferent mechanisms that link the intrinsic muscles, core stabilizers, and respiratory program with improved motor coordination. The exercises enhance both CNS regulation and expression of the motor program.

As with all exercise, individual ability and level of comfort must be monitored when prescribing thera-

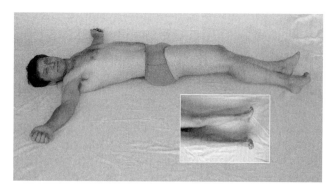

Figure 24.12 Spinal twist—feet apart.

peutic or home care programs. The spine is less stable when the respiratory portion of the exercise is not included. Because of the torsional motion of the exercises, patients with active disc problems should proceed with caution. Always stay within a pain-free range of motion. Moving slowly will enhance control. Even after dysfunction is corrected, these exercises can be an integral part of a daily program of spinal wellness.

Spinal Exercises

Supine Exercises

Exercise 1 (Fig. 24.12)
   Basic position

- Lie supine, legs straight, feet hip width apart, arms outstretched in a T position at shoulder level, shoulders lowered and relaxed, palms open and facing the ceiling.

   Breathing

- Take a deep breath in and hold it. Monitor that the abdominal cavity expands transversely in all 360 degrees without lifting of the rib cage in a cephalad direction. Voluntary muscular effort of the deep spinal stabilizers will be necessary to avoid cephalad movement of the lower anterior rib cage (see chapter 23). Imagine a lengthened spinal column throughout this exercise. Intra-abdominal pressure is high in this position, the rib cage is lowered, and the diaphragm is fully activated and held in position. The glottis does not need to be closed to hold the breath in. Once this pattern is established, breathe lightly throughout the training, but avoid the tendency to lift the rib cage in a cranial direction.

Note: This new motor skill initially may be challenging, but with practice this position can be held for longer periods of time. Encourage the patient to do as much as comfortably possible. Ability will increase with consistent practice. For those who are unable to activate the diaphragm and deep stabilizers in this manner, the exercise can initially be performed while breathing normally until the motor skill is developed to do the exercise as described.

Movement

- Rotate the pelvis to the left, lifting the right hip off the mat, while coordinating the rotation of the head to the right. Shoulders stay on the mat. The trunk rotation should take place around its long axis while deviation of the pelvis and neck is kept to a minimum. The movements should be slow and controlled.

- Go to the end range of motion possible with ease and comfort (if possible), with the chin touching the left shoulder and the big toe of the left foot touching the heel of the right foot. Continue with a slow and coordinated motion back to the other side. As you move from one side to the other, do NOT stop in the middle, but continue with coordinated motion to the opposite side. Attempt to reach the "middle line" simultaneously with the chin and the feet! Stopping at the end range of motion for additional stretch is permitted.

- Repeat the movements alternately four to five times or as long as the breath can be comfortably held.

- After each exercise, relaxation should follow.

Relaxation for Supine Exercises: (Fig. 24.13)

- *Inhale* and slowly raise the hands, shoulders and knees while arching the low back and extending the neck. Heels, buttocks, elbows, and head remain touching the mat.

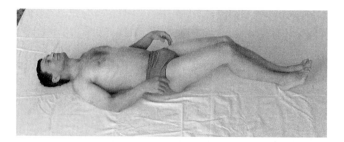

Figure 24.13 Relaxation exercise.

- Hold this position a few seconds.
- *Exhale,* relax, and drop to the original supine position turning the head to either side.
- Repeat two to three times

Supine Exercise Variations

All of these exercises are performed supine using the same breathing and counter-rotation of the pelvis and head staying within the individual's range of comfort and ability. Relaxation follows each exercise.

Exercise 2 (Fig. 24.14)
Variation of Basic Position

- Legs straight with the right foot crossed over the left ankle.

Movement

- As the pelvis rotates to the left, movement pivots on the left heel. The big toe of the right foot touches the mat as the chin approaches the right shoulder at full rotation. Pivot on the left heel as the pelvis rotates to the left. The big toe of the left foot touches the mat as the chin approaches the left shoulder at full rotation.
- Repeat the movements four to five times or as long as the breath can be comfortably held.

Exercise 3 Perform the same exercise with the left foot crossing the right at the ankles.

Exercise 4 (Fig. 24.15)
Variation of Basic Position

- Heel of the right foot is placed between the first and second toe of the left foot.

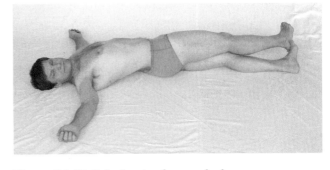

Figure 24.15 Spinal twist, feet stacked.

Movement

- Pivot on the left heel. When the pelvis is rotated fully to the left, the big toe of the right foot touches the mat and the chin moves toward the right shoulder. When the pelvis is rotated fully to the right, the small toe of the right foot touches the mat as the chin approaches the left shoulder.
- Repeat the movements four to five times or as long as the breath can be comfortably held.

Exercise 5 Perform the same exercise with the left heel placed between the first and second toe of the right foot.

Exercise 6 (Fig. 24.16)
Variation of Basic Position

- Right side of the right ankle is placed just above the left kneecap.

Movement

- The right knee touches the ground (if possible) at full rotation in both directions as the chin rotates to the opposite shoulder.

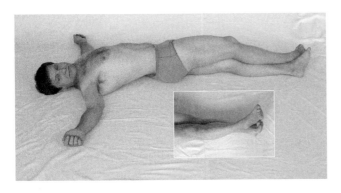

Figure 24.14 Spinal twist, ankles crossed.

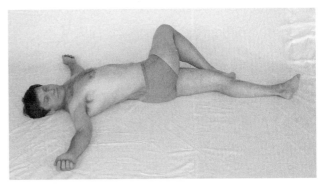

Figure 24.16 Spinal twist, Figure 4 option.

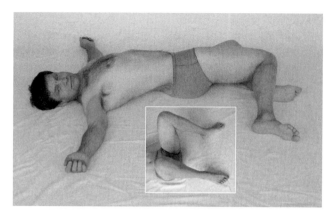

Figure 24.17 Spinal twist, knees bent, feet wide.

- Repeat the movements four to five times or as long as the breath can be comfortably held.

Exercise 7 Perform the same exercise with the left ankle placed just above the right kneecap.

Exercise 8 (Fig. 24.17)
Variation of Basic Position

- Feet on the mat, knees bent and hip width apart.

Movement

- As the pelvis rotates to the right, the right knee touches the mat, the left knee touches the right heel, and the chin moves toward the left shoulder. The opposite occurs in left rotation.
- Repeat the movements four to five times or as long as the breath can be comfortably held.

Exercise 9 (Fig. 24.18)
Variation of Basic Position

- Feet on the mat, knees bent and together.

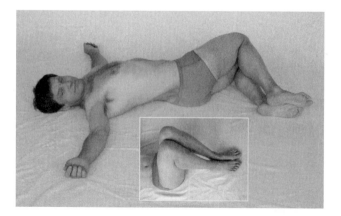

Figure 24.18 Spinal twist, knees bent and together.

Movement

- The right knee touches the mat and the knees stay together during right pelvic rotation. The left knee touches during left rotation.
- Repeat the movements four to five times or as long as the breath can be comfortably held.

Exercise 10 (Fig. 24.19)
Variation of Basic Position

- Knees bent, together and lifted toward the chest (touching the chest if possible).

Movement

- The right knee touches the mat during right pelvic rotation, the left knee touches during left rotation.
- Repeat the movements four to five times or as long as the breath can be comfortably held.

Exercises 11 and 12 These spinal exercises can also be performed in the side-lying and prone positions (Figs. 24.20 and 24.21).

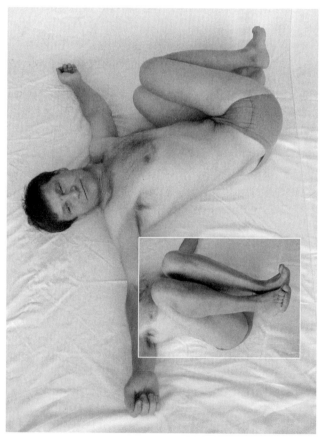

Figure 24.19 Spinal twist, knees to chest.

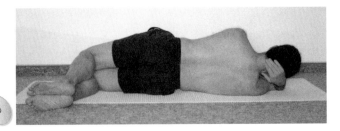

Figure 24.20 Side-lying spinal twist, knees bent.

Additional Yoga-Based Exercises

Abdominals

Effect of Yoga-Based Abdominal Exercises on Spinal Function

The yoga-based exercises that follow help to coordinate muscle function and improve stability of the spine. In addition, these exercises also indirectly improve the function of the visceral organs by influencing intra-abdominal pressure. Function of the abdominals cannot be measured by the strength of a dynamometer test, but by their ability to activate during activities of daily living, in particular during lifting and respiration.

Functional strength depends on the synergism of abdominal activation and co-activation of all the core stabilizers. The strength of each separate muscle is not as important as the coordination between them. Learning to control contraction of individual muscles in coordination with other core stability muscles helps to facilitate the postural program. As our studies have shown, posture is more easily corrected when the diaphragm takes an active role in the process.

The rectus abdominis has three tendonous insertions that separate the muscle into four parts. These four parts are capable of functioning independently. Learning to isolate the activation of the recti enables it to support the function of other muscles, most notably the transverse abdominis (TrA) and the diaphragm. To control and separately activate the abdomen as a horizontal wave over and under the navel, the TrA abdominis and the diaphragm must have coordinated function in all their parts.

The first abdominal exercise increases awareness of TrA and diaphragmatic control. The activation and relaxation of the abdomen occurs in the form of a horizontal wave made possible by the support of intrinsic co-activation on each level. These exercises challenge all the muscles involved in maintaining intra-abdominal pressure (5).

The second abdominal exercise causes relaxation of the abdominal muscles by manipulating pressure in the thoracic cavity. By expanding the thorax without breathing "in," a negative pressure is created in the chest, the diaphragm is passively pulled "up" into the thorax cavity, and the abdominal muscles are able to relax. This exercise also influences the muscles of the pelvic floor.

The third, fourth, and fifth abdominal exercises are extensions of the second exercise. In these exercises, pressing the thighs with the hands provokes the postural reaction. This results in an isolated contraction of the rectus abdominis. Through this manipulation of periodic activation and relaxation of the rectus abdominis, pressure in the abdominal cavity is altered and also the muscles of the pelvic floor are being influenced. Pressure changes indirectly control the function of the visceral organs through mechanical and CNS influence.

Common abdominal exercises accentuate the more superficial layer of abdominal muscles (recti and obliqui) rather than the deep transversus muscle and their separate control; they target strength and esthetics. Our goal is core spinal stability and optimal function of the abdominal organs. Strengthening the abdominal muscles is not only achieved by increasing their force but by obtaining awareness and control over all participating components and harmonizing their function (10). If we accept this principle of abdominal training, there is no limit to the many exercises that can be created to support and integrate our body/mind function.

Author's note: The next series of exercises requires a great deal of control and coordination. We encourage the reader to keep practicing and not to dismiss the exercises as "too difficult" if they cannot be performed on the first attempt.

The need to practice with total concentration and a relaxed body cannot be overstated. Over time, the benefit to the postural program and of course to the patient will be well worth the effort.

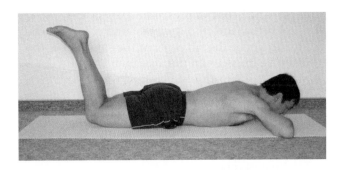

Figure 24.21 Prone spinal twist, knees bent.

Abdominal Exercises

Exercise 1

Basic Position

- Begin in a standing position with the legs hip width apart. Bend the knees and rest the hands on the thighs.

Movement

Inhale

1. Hold the breath and without breathing out push the chest and diaphragm "down," allowing the abdomen to vault "outward" as in the spinal exercises.

2. Without breathing out or changing the diameter of the chest, draw the lower abdominal wall "in" toward the spine and relax. The chest and diaphragm actively maintain abdominal pressure as it is altered by co-activation of the abdominals, intrinsics, and pelvic floor muscles.

3. Continue to alternate a coordinated wave of "out" and "in" abdominal motion.

4. Repeat this movement 10 to 15 times or as long as the breath can be comfortably held.

Exhale

1. Exhale and relax.

Repeat this exercise three to five times.

Note: Holding a constant chest position allows abdominal pressure to be maintained. Regular practice of this exercise increases awareness of the deep muscles of the lumbar spine, TrA, diaphragm, and pelvic floor.

Exercise 2 (Fig. 24.22)

Basic Position

- As described, standing with bent knees, hands leaning on thighs

Movement

Exhale

1. Exhale fully, without breathing in, expand the chest. The negative pressure will pull the diaphragm "up" into the chest and create a hollowing under the rib cage. At the same time, the negative pressure in the abdomen will pull the abdominal muscles "in" toward the spine.

2. Hold this position with the rest of the body as relaxed as possible for a few seconds.

Inhale

1. Inhale and relax

Repeat this cycle of movement 10 to 15 times.

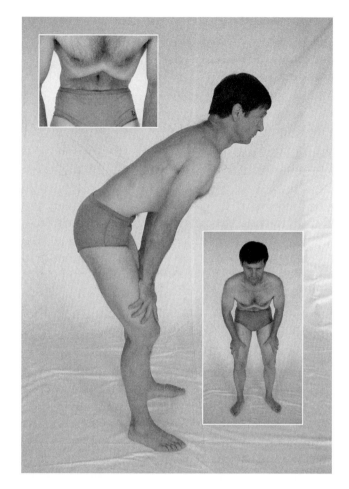

Figure 24.22 Lower abdomen drawing in.

Note: The rhythm of this exercise as well as the amount of time that the breath is held is determined by individual comfort and ability. Coordination and control are achieved through regular practice and repetition, not by overstraining. Patients are encouraged to proceed to exercise 3 only after control is achieved in exercise 2.

Exercises 3, 4, and 5 allow control over the rectus abdominal muscle.

Exercise 3 (Fig. 24.23)

Basic Position

- As described, standing with bent knees, hands leaning on thighs

Movement

Exhale

1. Exhale fully, expand the chest, and pull the diaphragm "up" as in exercise 2.

2. While maintaining this position with the breath held out, apply a downward pressure alternately with the right and then left hand on the thighs.

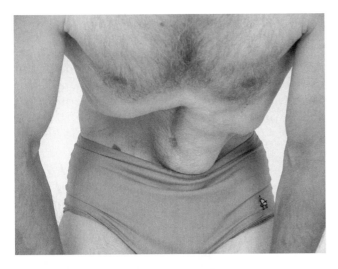

Figure 24.23 Unilateral rectus abdominus activation.

The rectus abdominus on the same side as the pressing hand will be activated. By alternating the pressure of the right and left hands, the right and left rectus are facilitated individually, which induces the separate function of each side.

3. Repeat this movement three to six times or as long as the breath can be comfortably held.

Inhale

Inhale and relax.

After the breath has returned to normal, the exercise can be repeated.

Exercise 4 (Fig. 24.24)
Basic Position

- As described, standing with bent knees, hands leaning on thighs

Movement
Exhale

1. Exhale fully, expand the chest and pull the diaphragm "up" as in exercises 2 and 3.

2. While maintaining this position with the breath held out, apply a downward pressure simultaneously with both hands on the thighs.

3. Applying pressure with both hands causes synchronous activation of both recti as well as separate facilitation of the recti from all other abdominal muscles.

4. Repeat this movement three to six times or as long as the breath can be comfortably held.

Inhale

1. Inhale and relax.

After the breath has returned to normal, the exercise can be repeated.

Exercise 5
Basic Position

- As described, standing with bent knees, hands leaning on thighs

Movement

This exercise is a combination of exercises 4 and 5.
Exhale

1. Exhale, expand the chest, and pull the diaphragm "up," as in the previous exercises.

2. Apply a downward pressure with the right hand facilitating the right rectus and briefly hold it.

3. Slowly, start to release the pressure on the right as the pressure is increased on the left hand, facilitating the left rectus.

4. Continue this sequence of alternating pressure on the right and left, right and left, etc. As the recti are alternately activated, a circular wave-like movement appears across the abdomen.

5. Repeat this movement three to six times or as long as the breath can be comfortably held.

Inhale

1. Inhale and relax.

After the breath has returned to normal, the exercise can be repeated beginning on the left and moving the wave to the right.

Note: Do not overstrain. The best results in gaining control over this movement will occur from repeating the exercise frequently rather than prolonging the holding of the breath in one exercise.

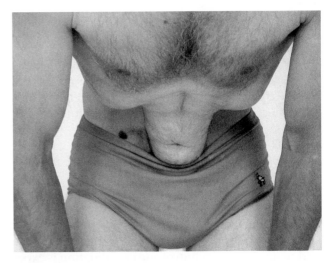

Figure 24.24 Synchronous, bilateral rectus abdominus activation.

Mastering the ability to create negative pressure in the abdomen (exercise 2) and relaxing the abdominal muscles will result in enhanced ability to gain control over the rectus abdominis (exercises 3, 4, and 5).

Pelvic Floor Muscles

Contraction of the pelvic floor can be used to facilitate activation of either the transverse abdominis or the multifidi. This is particularly useful as a coaching tool with patients who are having difficulty coordinating contraction of the core stabilizers with the global muscles.

The pelvic floor muscles have an integral role in breathing mechanics, postural and movement programs, as well as an influence on the internal organs. The relationship between core stabilization and respiratory mechanics must be normal for the pelvic floor to function optimally (the reverse is also true!). Any dysfunction of the spinal stabilizing system or respiration will ultimately result in dysfunction of the pelvic floor. Treatment of this area is as significant as restoring normal co-contraction of the diaphragm, intercostals, TrA, and multifidi muscles.

Effect of Yoga-Based Pelvic Floor Exercises on Spinal Function

The important function of the pelvic diaphragm must not be overlooked in the treatment of back pain (12,13). Pelvic floor exercises are traditionally used in yoga to gain control over the pelvic diaphragm to improve function of the spine and visceral organs. The exercises are combined with breathing. The aim is controlled muscle contraction, which, in time, leads to fine control and voluntary access to the CNS motor and respiratory programs.

Pelvic floor exercises play an integral part in normalizing the postural and respiratory programs. It is important to practice these exercises slowly and gently so to achieve isolated contraction of the deep muscles and avoid activation of the larger, global muscles. Concentration and a relaxed body are prerequisites. The best posture is sitting on the heels, but any posture that allows an erect spine may be used. The exercises can be performed in the side-lying position if it is difficult to activate the muscles while seated. More advanced exercises, not presented in this chapter, include variations in manipulating intra-abdominal pressure with the help of breathing mechanics.

As with the abdominal exercises, it may take time and practice before control and coordination is experienced. In the beginning, all the muscles in the area may contract together. Isolated contraction and control can be gained in each region with practice. These exercises are useful for everyone throughout their lifetime to maintain elasticity and good muscle control. They are also of significant therapeutic benefit to those with weak or dysfunctional sphincters, seen often with urinary incontinence, uterine prolapse, and in women with postpartum.

Pelvic Floor Exercises

In yoga, the exercises are divided into three areas: levator ani, urogenital, and perineum. Anatomically, the pubococcygeus division of the levator ani muscle is responsible for parts A and B. For ease of reference, we are calling the posterior exercise "levator ani," the anterior exercise "urogenital system," and the middle exercise "perineal muscles."

Exercise for Levator Ani
Basic Position
- Sit on the heels or on the edge of a chair with a straight spine.

Movement
1. Relax and begin to focus on the rhythm of the breath.
2. Bring the attention to the anus, Inhale, draw the anus "upwards" for a few seconds, and then release it.
3. Perform this drawing "up" movement slowly, with control, and repeat it rhythmically 10 to 15 times.
4. Exhale and relax.

Exercise for Urogenital System
Basic Position
- Sit on the heels or on the edge of a chair with a straight spine.

Movement
1. Relax and begin to focus on the rhythm of the breath.
2. Bring the attention to the urethra. Inhale and draw the urethra upward. (The muscles active in this exercise are the same as those that stop the flow of urine when contracted. Performing this drawing "up" movement will cause the testes in men and the vagina in women to move upward.)
3. Hold this contraction as long as the breath can comfortably be held.
4. Exhale and relax.
5. Repeat this exercise three to six times frequently throughout the day.

Isolating and contracting the correct muscles occurs through practice. It is recommended that you first gain control over exercises A and B before you begin exercise C.

Exercise for Perineal Muscles

Basic Position

- Sit on the heels or on the edge of a chair with a straight spine.

Movement

1. Relax and begin to focus on the rhythm of the breath.

2. Bring the attention to the perineum. Inhale and draw the perineum upward. For better understanding, you can imagine that you are pulling up and releasing a small cone placed in the middle of this area. The other muscles of the pelvic floor are relatively relaxed.

3. Contract and lift the perineum and then release it slowly.

4. Repeat this movement rhythmically three to six times.

This motion is often difficult to isolate. Results will be achieved with consistent practice.

Audit Process
Self-Check of the Chapter's Learning Objectives

- Describe the specific role of different muscles in each phase of respiration.

- What is the role of flexion fixations of T6-T12 in disturbing the normal function of the cervical and lumbar spines?

- How do you perform lower abdominal breathing exercises that enhance the core relationship between the diaphragm, abdominal, and pelvic floor muscles?

- How do you perform lower-chest breathing exercises to improve lateral excursion of the lower rib cage?

- How do you perform upper-chest breathing exercises to mobilize the fan-like movement of the upper rib cage?

- How do you perform whole-breathing exercises to enhance the coordinated movement of all three sections?

- How can recumbent spinal exercises for the deep "intrinsic" muscles improve mid-thoracic joint mobility and lumbar spine stability?

■ ACKNOWLEDGMENT

The authors thank Maria Perri for substantial contributions to this chapter as well as her trusted correction of the English text.

■ REFERENCES

1. Basmajian JV, Samson J. Standardization of methods in single motor unit training. Am J Phys Med 1973;52:250–256.

2. Basmajian JV, Baeza M, Fabrigar C. Conscious control and training of individual spinal motor neurons in normal human subject. J New Drugs 1965;5:78–85.

3. Bergmark A. Stability of the lumbar spine: A study in mechanical engineering. Acta Orthop Scand 1989;230:20–24.

4. Bogduk N. Clinical Anatomy of the Lumbar Spine and Sacrum, 3rd ed. London: Churchill Livingston, 1999:104–105.

5. Cresswell AG, et al. The effect of an abdominal muscle training program on the intra-abdominal pressure. Scandinavian Journal of Rehabilitation Medicine 1993;26:79–86.

6. Crisco JJ, Panjabi MM. The intersegmental and multisegmental muscles of the spine: A biomechanical model comparing lateral stabilizing potential. Spine 1991;7:793–799.

7. Cumpelík J, Véle F, Strnad P. Respiratory movement and stability of the spine in memorial volume In: Jelinek K, Chalupova M, eds. Diagnosis, Therapy and Prevention Through Movement. UK: FTVS, 2001.

8. Deva Murti S. Yoga praxis. New Delhi: International Yoga center, 1971.

9. Gitananda S. The correction of breathing difficulties by yoga pranayama. The all India yoga chikitsa seminar. Quilon, Kerala: Satya Press, 1971.

10. Hemborgg B, et al. Intra-abdominal pressure and trunk muscle activity during lifting. IV. The causal factors of the intra-abdominal pressure rise. Scand J Rehab Med 1985;17:25–28.

11. Kapandji LA. The Physiology of the Joints, vol. 3. The Trunk. Edinburgh: E & S Livingston, 1974.

12. Lewit K. Manipulative Therapy in Rehabilitation of the Locomotor's System, 3rd ed. Oxford: Butterworth, 1999:27–29.

13. Lewit K. Relation of faulty respiration to posture, with clinical implications. Journal of the American Osteopathic Association 1980;8:525.

14. Panjabi MM. The stabilizing system of the spine. Part 1. Function, adaptation and enhancement. J Spinal Dis 1992;5:383–389.

15. Richardson C, Jull G, et al. Therapeutic Exercise for Spinal Segmental Stabilization in Low Back Pain. Scientific Basis and Clinical Approach. London: Churchill Livingston, 1999:50–52.

16. Sára R, Smutný J, Čumpelík J, Veverková J. Evaluation of breathing dynamic. Scientific paper. CMP FEL ČVUT è. CTU-CMP-2001-23, 2001.

17. Véle F, Čumpelík J, Pavlů D. Reflections on the Problem of "Stability" in Physiotherapy. Rehabilitace a Fyzikálnílékařství 2001;8:103–105.

18. Véle F. Kineziologie pro klinickou praxi. Praha: Grada Publishing, 1997.

19. Vojta V, Peters A. Vojta's Principe. Praha: Grada Publishing, 1995.

■ ADDITIONAL BIBLIOGRAPHY

1. Acland RD. The Video Atlas of Human Anatomy. Tape 3: The Trunk. Baltimore: Williams & Wilkins, 1998.

2. Chaitow L. Clinical Application of Neuromuscular Techniques, vol 1. The Upper Body. London: Churchill Livingstone, 2000:50–52.

3. Donisch EW, Basmajian JV. Electromyography of deep back muscles in man. Am J Anat 1972;133:18.

4. Jirout J. Radiographic signs of the function of the intrinsic muscles of the spine. In: Paterson JK, Burn, eds. Back Pain, an International Review. London: Kluwer Academic Pub. Dordrecht, 1990:391.

5. McGill SM. Kinetic potential of the lumbar trunk musculature about three orthogonal orthopaedic axes in extreme postures. Spine 1991;16:809–815.

25

Spinal Segmental Stabilization Training

Paul W. Hodges and
Gwendolen A. Jull

Learning Objectives
After reading this chapter, you should be able to understand:

- How the central nervous system controls spine motion
- The relationship between motor control and spinal biomechanics
- The typical changes in motor control with spinal pain
- How to assess and rehabilitate abnormal motor control of the spine

Introduction

Recent studies suggest that spinal pain is associated with changes in motor control that are, to some extent, similar to deficits identified in nervous system pathology. Because control of spinal motion and stability are dependent on the contribution of trunk muscles, it is suggested that these changes in control may compromise the integrity of the spine and predispose the spine to injury or re-injury. Although individual muscles respond in a variety of ways to spinal pain, a consistent finding has been impairment in the control of the deep trunk muscles. The changes in the control of these muscles appear to be a non-specific response to the presence of pain, irrespective of pathology. These findings are consistent with hypotheses based on clinical observations of trunk muscle function in low back pain (LBP) (74,77,111,113,115). The purpose of this chapter is to present evidence of the strategies used by the central nervous system (CNS) to control and move the spine, relate this to the biomechanics of the spine, discuss changes in motor control with spinal pain, and present a clinical strategy to assess and rehabilitate this system.

Basis for Motor Relearning in Spinal Pain

Biomechanics of Spinal Control

The spine is inherently unstable and is dependent on the contribution of muscles in addition to the passive elements of the spine (101). Although trunk muscles must have sufficient strength and endurance to satisfy the demands of spinal control, the efficacy of the muscle system is dependent on its controller, the CNS (101). The challenge is immense for the CNS to move and control the spine despite constant changes in internal and external forces. The CNS must continually interpret the status of stability, plan mechanisms to overcome predictable challenges, and rapidly initiate activity in response to unexpected challenges. It must interpret the afferent input from the peripheral mechanoreceptors, vestibular apparatus, and visual system, compare these requirements against the "internal model of body dynamics," and then generate a coordinated response of the trunk muscles so that the muscle activity occurs at the right time, at the right amount, and so on. To further complicate this issue, it is critical to investigate two separate but related components of spinal control: control of spinal orientation and control of intervertebral translation and rotation.

Control of Spinal Orientation and Intervertebral Motion

Many models of the spine consider stability in terms of the ability of the spine to withstand compressive forces and resist buckling (16,25,32). Although this is an essential component of stability, it is important to also consider the control of intersegmental translation and rotation during movement (102) (Fig. 25.1). It has been shown that if the spine is modeled with one segment with no muscle attachment, the spine is as stable as having no muscle (25). Thus, segmental control is an essential component for spinal stability. It is important to consider that the CNS may use different muscles and strategies to control the individual aspects of spinal control.

The principles of control of orientation and intersegmental motion also apply to the pelvis. The orientation of the pelvis must be controlled around the three orthogonal axes; however, there is also the requirement to control the relationship between segments of the pelvis. In upright positions, the sacroiliac joint is subjected to considerable shear force as the mass of the upper body must be transferred to the lower limbs (123,125). This segmental control of the pelvis is controlled not only by the shape and structure of the sacroiliac joint (form closure) but also by compressive forces across the SIJ via muscle contraction (force closure) (124,125). Different muscles are likely to control each aspect of stability of the pelvis.

Muscle Control of Orientation and Intervertebral Motion

Consistent with the division of the spinal control into two elements, there is likely to be a division in mus-

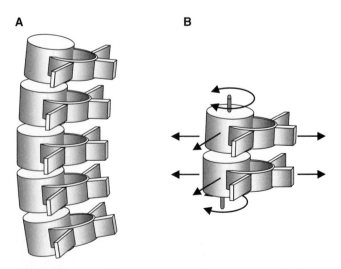

Figure 25.1 Stability of the spine involves control of **(A)** orientation of the spine and **(B)** intersegmental motion.

cles that contribute to each element from an anatomical and biomechanical perspective. Several authors have made distinction between muscle groups based on their specific contribution to control of motion and stability (9,33,69,118). Notably, Bergmark defined muscles as either "local" or "global" based on anatomical characteristics (Fig. 25.2). Whereas simple division of muscles into groups is likely to oversimplify the complex control of spinal motion and stability, it provides a useful definition to consider clinically. Global muscles attach from the pelvis to the thorax, have a large moment arm to move the spine, and are involved in the control of external forces. Examples of the global muscles include rectus abdominis, obliquus externus abdominis, obliquus internus abdominis, and the thoracic erector spinae. Muscles such as the lateral fibers of quadratus lumborum and anterior parts of psoas also meet these criteria. In contrast, local muscles attach directly to the vertebrae and are involved in the control of intervertebral motion. Bergmark included muscles such as the lumbar multifidus in this group; however, other muscles that satisfy these criteria are transversus abdominis (TrA), intertransversarii, interspinales and posterior fibers of psoas. The lumbar portions of longissimus and iliocostalis have one attachment to the lumbar vertebrae and share some features of the local system. The local system has only a limited ability to influence the control of orientation and similarly the global system has only a limited ability to control intervertebral motion. In fact, any contribution made by the global system to the control of intervertebral motion occurs as a result of compressive forces exerted by co-activation of antagonist global muscles. While compression can assist in the control of shear and rotation forces, this is associated with a "cost." First, global co-activation increases the compressive load on all of the lumbar vertebrae, resulting in increased intra-discal pressure and loading through the posterior elements; second,

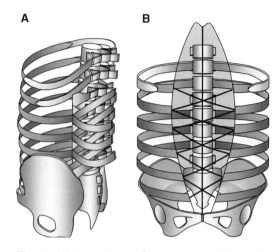

Figure 25.3 Anatomy of transversus abdominis. Posterolateral view (**A**) showing the attachment of TrA to the spine via the thoracolumbar fascia. Anterior view (**B**) showing the anterior fascias.

antagonist global muscle co-activation results in a restriction of spinal motion or "rigidity" of the spine. In contrast, local muscles allow controlled spinal motion and have the ability to control individual segments rather than providing a general compressive force across the spine.

Contribution of Transversus Abdominis to Spinal Control

TrA is a sheet-like muscle that attaches from the inguinal ligament, iliac crest, thoracolumbar fascia, and the lower six ribs (Fig. 25.3). The attachment to the spine is via the three layers of the thoracolumbar fascia. The posterior layer of the fascia attaches to the spinous processes, the middle layer to the transverse processes, and the anterior layer runs over quadratus lumborum (142). The contribution of TrA to spinal control is complex. Its muscle fibers have a relatively horizontal orientation and, therefore, it has minimal ability to move the spine. However, it may contribute to rotation (22,41,132). Its contribution to spinal control is likely to involve its role in modulation of intra-abdominal pressure (IAP) and tensioning the thoracolumbar fascia. TrA has been shown to be the abdominal muscle most closely associated with the control of IAP, (22,24) and recent data confirm that spinal stiffness in increased by IAP (54,56). Fascial tension may directly restrict intervertebral motion or provide gentle segmental compression via the posterior layer of the thoracolumbar fascia (35). For sacroiliac support, TrA acts on the lever formed by the ilia to increase anterior compression of the SIJ (125); this has been confirmed in vivo (116).

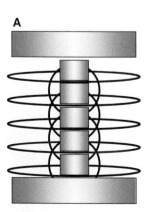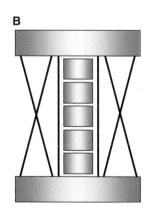

Figure 25.2 Local (**A**) and global (**B**) classification of muscles based on anatomical characteristics.

Contribution of Lumbar Multifidus to Spinal Control

Multifidus has five fascicles that arise from the spinous process and lamina of each lumbar vertebrae and descend in a caudo-lateral direction (90). The most superficial fibers of each fascicle cross up to five segments and attach caudally to the ilia and sacrum. In contrast, the deep fibers attach from the inferior border of a lamina and cross a minimum of two segments to attach on the mamillary process and facet joint capsule (87) (Fig. 25.4). The superficial fibers are distant from the centers of rotation of the lumbar vertebrae, have an extension moment arm, and can control the lumbar lordosis (90). In contrast, the deep fibers have a limited moment arm and have only a minor ability to extend the spine (102). Whereas many trunk muscles are suited architecturally to the control of spinal orientation, most have a limited ability to control intervertebral shear and torsion (11,102). The deep fibers of multifidus are ideally placed to control these motions. Multifidus can control intervertebral motion by generation of intervertebral compression localized to a few segments (141). The proximity of deep multifidus to the center of rotation results in compression with minimal extension moment to be overcome by antagonistic muscle activity. In addition, multifidus may be able to contribute to the control of intervertebral motion by direct opposition of anterior rotation and translation of the vertebrae (90), or via tensioning the thoracolumbar fascia as it expands on contraction (36). Several studies have provided in vitro and in vivo evidence of the ability of multifidus to control intervertebral motion (79,141).

Mechanisms of Motor Control of the Spine

The CNS must determine the requirements for spinal stability and generate appropriate muscle responses to meet the demands placed on it by internal and external forces. While all muscles contribute to spinal stability, the evidence presented suggests that the activity of specific muscles may be coordinated to contribute to different elements of control. To further complicate the task of spinal control, many of the trunk muscles also contribute to other functions such as respiration and continence. These functions must be coordinated with the contribution of these muscles to spinal control. This section addresses the normal strategies for motor control of stability and how this changes in LBP.

Strategies for Spinal Control

The CNS has two primary strategies for the control of the spine: feed-forward or "open" loop strategies for situations in which the outcome of a perturbation is predictable and the CNS can plan strategies in advance, and feedback or "closed" loop strategies in which responses are generated in reaction to afferent input (visual, vestibular, proprioception, etc.) from unpredictable perturbations (Fig. 25.5) (120). In addition, because of time taken to initiate a response, the CNS may also generate an underlying level of tonic activity to increase the muscle stiffness and act as the first line of defense against an unexpected perturbation (72). In general, normal function involves a complex combination of these strategies.

Feed-forward control of the spine is possible if the CNS can predict the outcome of a perturbation. In general, the CNS initiates a sequence of muscle activity in advance of the perturbation to prepare the body. Feedback-mediated control involves activation of the trunk muscles in response to an external perturbation that is unpredictable. In this situation, afferent input from mechanoreceptors in the muscles, ligaments, joint capsule, and skin or visual and vestibular input triggers a response to overcome the perturbation. The third type of control strategy is related to both feedback and feed-forward control and involves

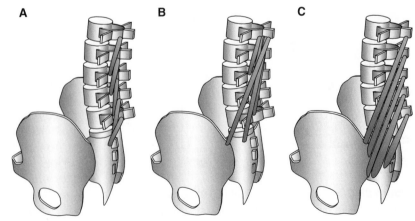

Figure 25.4 Anatomy of multifidus. **(A)** Deep fascicles of multifidus attach from lamina to lamina and lie close to the center of rotation of the lumbar vertebrae. **(B)** Deep and superficial fascicles arising from the spinous process of L1. **(C)** Superficial fascicles arising from the spinous processes of lumbar vertebrae.

Feedback mediated control   Feedforward mediated control

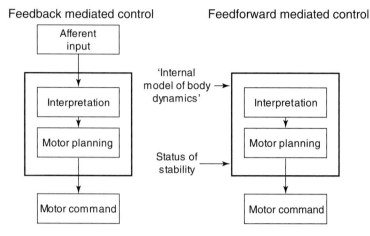

Figure 25.5 Feed-forward and feedback mechanisms for control of the spine.

modulation of the "tone" in specific muscles to provide an underlying degree of stability to the joints. This activity increases the stiffness (i.e. the property of muscles to act as springs) of muscles that surround the joints (9,32). Muscle stiffness provides control of forces applied to a joint and is available before even the shortest reflex response could be initiated (72). The absolute level of tone or stiffness can be modulated by afferent input from mechanoreceptors. Responses of the multifidus muscle have been identified with stimulation of the mechanoreceptors in the lumbar intervertebral discs and sacroiliac joints in pigs (66–68) and supraspinous ligament in humans (126). Each of these control strategies has been considered for the spine.

Separate Control of Intervertebral Motion and Orientation

Studies of feed-forward and feedback control of the trunk suggest that the CNS uses separate strategies for the control of intervertebral motion and orientation of the spine. Initial studies of the deep muscles investigated locomotion and trunk movements (22,104). In these tasks, the superficial abdominal and extensor muscles were active in a manner that was specific to direction (i.e., erector spinae activity during trunk extension when a flexion moment was imposed on the spine, or rectus abdominis and obliquus externus abdominis activity during trunk flexion when an extension moment was imposed on the spine). However, TrA and deep multifidus were tonically active and not influenced by the direction of movement (22, 104). This tonic and phasic activation has been confirmed in limb movements (49,50) and for the quadriceps muscle (112).

More precise evidence of this differential control has come from investigation of predictable challenges to spinal stability caused by rapid limb movements.

Early studies of arm movements showed activity of leg muscles and erector spinae prior to flexion of the arm (4,8,145). More recently, studies have confirmed that TrA and deep multifidus are activated as a component of this anticipatory response (60,61,96). Furthermore, while the response of the superficial muscles is linked to the direction of force (4,55,61), activity of TrA and deep multifidus is independent of the direction of force (Fig. 25.6) (55,61,96). That is, the superficial muscles are active to control the orientation of the spine while the deep muscles provide non-direction–specific control of intersegmental motion. An important additional finding of these studies is that the CNS does not make the spine rigid by co-activation of the superficial muscles, but instead uses controlled movement to help counteract the applied forces (53,55). The differential control of the deep and superficial muscles has been confirmed in neurophysiological experiments that have manipulated task parameters (63).

Thus, feed-forward studies indicate that the CNS uses specialized strategies for each element of spinal control (i.e., non-direction–specific, early, tonic co-activation of the deep muscles and direction-specific, phasic activation of the superficial muscles). This is supported by studies of feedback-mediated control. Many studies have investigated activity of the superficial muscles in response to external perturbations such as catching a load in box held in front of the body (86,140), translation of the support surface (42,82), or addition of a load to the trunk (23). These studies report direction specific activity of the superficial muscles to maintain spinal orientation. In contrast, studies of TrA report activity irrespective of the direction of force (23).

In summary, these studies identify four principles of control of the deep muscle system: (1) early recruitment; (2) tonic activity; (3) co-activation of deep muscles; and (4) activity that is controlled independently of the superficial muscles. These factors are important to consider in development of rehabilitation strategies.

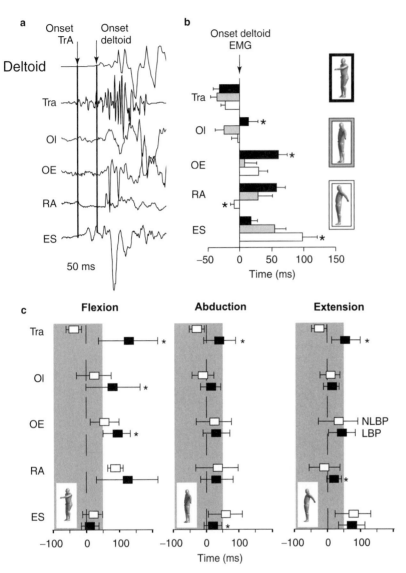

Figure 25.6 Normal and abnormal activation of the trunk muscles in association with rapid movements of the upper limb. **(A)** Raw EMG activity from a control subject in association with rapid arm movement. The onset of activity of TrA precedes that of deltoid indicating feed-forward activation to prepare the spine for the perturbation from arm movement. **(B)** Group data showing the onset of EMG activity of the trunk muscles relative to that of deltoid with movement of the arm in three directions. Whereas the onset of activity of the superficial abdominal muscles and erector spinae is dependent on the direction of limb movement (i.e., matched to the requirement to control spinal orientation), the onset of TrA is independent of movement direction. (Adapted from Hodges PW, Richardson CA. Experimental Brain Research 1997;114: 362–370.) **(C)** Data for subjects with recurrent LBP and matched control subjects. Zero indicates the onset of deltoid EMG. The onset of TrA activity was delayed with movement in each direction, thus failing to prepare the spine for the perturbation from limb movement. (Hodges PW, Richardson CA. Spine 1996;21:2640–2650.)

Factors That Complicate the Motor Control of the Spine

Regardless of whether TrA acts via IAP or fascial tensioning, its contribution is dependent the diaphragm and pelvic floor muscles, which control displacement of the abdominal contents. Studies have confirmed that activity of these muscles occurs in conjunction with TrA during arm movements (49,50,52,65). However, their involvement in spinal control presents a challenge to the CNS because these muscles also have respiratory and continence functions. Recent studies of repetitive limb movements confirm that tonic activity of these muscles (and TrA) can be sustained with superimposed modulation of activity to meet respiratory demands (49,50). In a mechanical sense, the diaphragm and TrA co-contract tonically, yet during inspiration diaphragm activity is increased and the muscle shortens, and TrA decreases

its activity and lengthens. The converse pattern occurs during expiration. However, this may be compromised by respiratory disease or when respiratory demand is increased (57).

This has important clinical implications. First, it is important to ensure that a back pain patient can coordinate the postural, respiratory, and continence functions of the trunk muscles. Second, patients with respiratory or genitourinary dysfunction may have difficulty during retraining. Third, it has been suggested that in some cases people with LBP may have excessive recruitment of the superficial abdominal muscles for expiration.

Changes in Motor Control With Pain

Many studies have investigated changes in the trunk muscles in LBP. Most have evaluated the strength and endurance of the trunk muscles with variable results. For instance, some show reduced strength and endurance (127), whereas others do not (129). It has been suggested that these changes may be more related to inactivity than pain (129). The importance of changes in strength and endurance is unclear as maximum strength and endurance are infrequently required in function and these parameters indicate little of how the muscles are used. Alternatively, studies have evaluated the activation of the trunk muscles, including the deep muscles, during a range of tasks. A consistent finding of these studies is that the activation of the deep muscles is impaired and that of the superficial muscles may be augmented.

Activity of abdominal muscles has been investigated in association with rapid limb movements (59, 62). These studies investigated people with chronic recurrent LBP when their pain was in remission. The most consistent finding was delayed activity of TrA with limb movement in all directions. Thus, activity of TrA was absent in the period before movement (Fig. 25.6C). This may indicate a compromise in the control of intervertebral motion. Activity of the superficial abdominal muscles was delayed only with specific movements. A major finding was that the change in TrA activity could not be explained by inhibition of the response or delayed transmission in the CNS, as the delay was different for each movement direction (i.e., there was a change in strategy, not a greater delay for the message to be transmitted to the motoneuron). This has been confirmed in neurophysiological studies that show that unlike the normal situation, the strategy used to control TrA is similar to the other superficial abdominal muscles in LBP (48). Possible mechanisms for pain to affect motor control are presented in Figure 25.7.

Few studies have investigated the motor control of multifidus in LBP. Preliminary studies report reduced activity of the deep multifidus during functional tasks (88,122). In contrast, changes in multifidus have been reported that may be indirectly associated with changes in control. For example, studies report changes in muscle fiber composition (108) and increased fatigability (10,117). In addition, reduced cross-sectional area of multifidus has been identified as little as 24 hours after the onset of acute, unilateral LBP (47).

In contrast to the impairment identified in the deep muscles, several studies have indicated an augmented activity of the superficial muscles. For example, when a load is removed from the trunk there is an increased time to turn off the obliquus externus abdominus (OE) and thoracic erecto spinae (ES) in people with LBP (107). In addition, when people are given LBP in an experimental setting by injection of hypertonic saline into the back extensor muscles, the

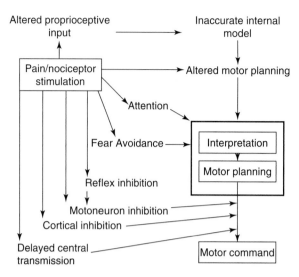

Figure 25.7 Possible mechanisms for the effect of nociceptor stimulation and pain on the motor control of the spine.

erector spinae no longer have periods of reduced activity between heel strikes in gait (3) and the superficial ES do not turn off at the end of lumbar flexion (144,146). Thus, data appear to indicate that the deep local muscles and the superficial global muscles are commonly affected in an opposite manner by the presence of pain. Hypothetically, this may result in reduced efficiency of intervertebral control. As mentioned, the superficial muscles are inefficient for providing control at the intervertebral level and can only do so at the cost of increased spinal loading and coactivation. As a result, a degree of the output of these muscles must be diverted to intervertebral control. This is likely to compromise the ability of these muscles to deal with the control of orientation. One possible mechanism for this effect is that the CNS may augment the global muscle activity to splint and restrict motion of a region of the spine to protect it from injury or re-injury. As a result, the deep muscle activity may be redundant and reduced. This follows the hypothesis of Cholewicki et al (17), who suggested that excessive activity in the superficial muscles might be a measurable compensation for poor passive or active segmental support (e.g. by the deep muscles).

The mechanism for pain and nociceptor stimulation to affect motor control is poorly understood. Pain could affect motor output at any level of the motor system including the cortex, the motoneurons, reflex pathways, and areas "upstream" of the motor cortex involved in motor planning. Studies have identified changes in motoneuron excitability (92), decreased cortical excitability (133), and changes in sensitivity of muscle spindles (105) in association with pain. However, the available data suggest that the change in motor control identified in LBP may be caused by a change in motor planning. Consistent with this hypothesis, pain changes activity of areas of the brain involved in motor planning (26). Although the exact mechanism is unknown, pain may have a direct affect on motor planning or may affect planning as a result of the attention demanding nature of pain or stress associated with pain. Further studies are required to investigate these possibilities. Alternatively, pain may not directly affect motor control, but indirectly via the influence of pain on proprioception. In chronic pain, non-nociceptor mechanoreceptors may contribute to excitation of second order nociceptor neurons (121) and pain may alter of proprioceptive feedback (14). Thus, pain may affect motor planning indirectly via inaccurate feedback.

An important consideration is whether changes in motor control occur as a result of the pain or whether incompetent motor control strategies lead to inefficient spinal control, and thus microtrauma, nociceptor stimulation, and pain. While neither possibility can be ruled out, injection of hypertonic saline into the lumbar longissimus muscle to produce transient pain changes the activation of the trunk muscles in a manner similar to that identified clinical pain (51). Changes in global muscle activity were different for individual subjects. This variability of the superficial muscles response to pain is consistent with clinical observations. However, it is likely that the motor control changes may also precede LBP. For example, Janda (69) identified that many people with chronic back pain also had minor neurological signs and slow reaction times have been shown to increase the risk of injury (128). Regardless of which came first, pain or motor control dysfunction, a patient presents with pain and the task is to break the cycle.

Summary

The CNS uses different strategies to control different muscles to control different elements of stability. Though much of this discussion has involved two important muscles, TrA and multifidus, it is likely that other muscles may contribute and some muscles may share features of both groups. Whereas several factors complicate the motor control of stability, such as respiration and continence, the most potent influence to this system is pain. Pain has several main effects on the deep muscles: (1) delayed activation; (2) phasic activation; and (3) loss of independent activation. Rather than training general strength and endurance, a major focus of rehabilitation is to restore

these aspects of motor control using contemporary motor relearning principles.

Application to the Cervical Spine

The cervical spine is a multi-segmental flexible column. In normal function, it must allow appropriate head movements in three dimensions in space, yet maintain mechanical stability of the head–neck system at any given orientation. The cervical spine must also distribute load from the weight of the head as well as the loads of the upper limb in posture and function (139). It is estimated that the osseoligamentous system contributes approximately 20% to the mechanical stability cervical spine, whereas 80% is provided by the surrounding neck musculature (103).

Muscle Control in the Cervical Spine

Twenty-three pairs of muscles act on the head–neck complex. In line with functional requirements, muscle interactions in the cervical region are complex and often a single muscle may perform multiple tasks (80). In addition to kinetic and dynamic supporting functions, the muscles of the neck are intimately related with reflex systems concerned with stabilization of the head and the eyes, vestibular function, and proprioceptive systems. The latter serve not only local needs in the neck but also needs for postural orientation and stability of the whole body (27,81,143). Therefore the cervical spine presents a multi-segmental, multi-muscle complex that is required to switch its control operations between intrinsic kinetic and mechanical demands, proprioceptive reflexes, and vestibulocollic reflexes, and still achieve an appropriate co-ordinated response (81).

Much of the research concerned with the patterns of neck muscle behavior during orientating and stabilizing activities has been performed on quadruped animal models. With very few exceptions, EMG experiments in humans have been limited to superficial muscles or selected deep muscles. Movement is produced and controlled by complex patterns of muscle action involving various muscle synergies (27,83–85,89).

Analogous to muscle control of the lumbar spine, Bergmark's (9) simple functional division between the superficial, more multi-segmental muscles and the deeper muscles layers can be applied to the cervical region. Cervical muscle architecture is complex. Of the dorsal muscles, the superficial splenius capitus and cervicus have long parallel muscle fascicles suited to torque production and orientation of the whole spinal and head. The deeper semispinalis capitus and cervicus are quilted by internal tendons and tendinous inscriptions and the longissimus capitus is fleshy and closely adhered to bone at multiple sites. The deepest suboccipital muscles are some of the smallest muscles in mass and length, although they have simple structure in their connections between the atlas, axis, and occiput. The deep cervical multifidus is intimately blended with the capsule of the zygapophyseal joints (39), indicating its local function. Ventrally, the superficial sternocleidomastoid comprises a contiguous sheet of muscle arising from the mastoid process to the sternum and clavicle. Though it will move and control the head, it has no attachment to the cervical vertebrae themselves. The three divisions of the scalene muscles, which span the rib cage to the cervical vertebrae, have tendinous origins and insertions. The deep longus capitus is characterized by an aponeurosis, which covers much of the muscle and serves as an attachment for many muscle fascicles. Rectus minor and lateralis are small and deeply placed muscles that were unable to be dissected cleanly from the bone (80). The longus colli is composed of complex, braided fascicles of fibers adherent to the ventral surface of all cervical vertebrae. The fascicles, which have their origins and insertions on the vertebrae themselves, are intrinsic to the cervical spine.

Thus, the morphology of the muscles supports the basic model of a deep muscle envelope consisting of muscles from the dorsal and ventral sides, which surrounds and controls the cervical segments, whereas the more superficial muscles are better configured to control spinal orientation and produce and guide neck and head movement. This functional division into deep and superficial muscles may oversimplify some complex interactions between various muscles for control during both voluntary and reflex postural adjustments and movements of the cervical region. Nevertheless, there is some evidence to support the basic hypothesis in relation to cervical segmental stability.

Direction specificity of activity has been identified in the superficial neck muscles in response to direct head displacing forces or postural perturbations (38,83–85,93). Patterns appear to be consistent for an individual but can vary between individuals (83). Activity of the deep and superficial neck muscles has been quantified non-invasively from shifts in signal relaxation times of T2-weighted magnetic resonance images (19). These authors demonstrated synergistic activity of deep and superficial muscle layers in the various planes of motion. However, in contrast to the superficial semispinalis capitus and splenius capitus, the deep multifidus, semispinalis cervicus group had a high T2 index before exercise, suggesting an important postural function for these muscles. Furthermore, when the relative activity of all muscles was calculated across the movements of flexion, extension, and lateral flexion, the results revealed co-contraction of the deep flexor muscles, the longus capitus, and colli, and dorsally the multifidus, semispinalis cervicus, and splenius capitus. This supports Mayoux-Benhamou et al's (93) concept that the longus colli and dorsal neck muscles form a muscle sleeve to support the cervical spinal segments in functional movements. Winters and Peles (143), in studying the interaction of several neck muscles by computer modeling, noted that if only the large muscles of the neck were simulated to produce movement, regions of local segmental instability resulted particularly in near upright or neutral postures. Deep muscle activity was required in synergy with the larger muscle activity to stiffen or stabilize the segments, especially in functional mid ranges.

There is a particular role for the deep neck flexors in support of the cervical curve. In the upright posture, the neck extensors counter the gravitational pull on the head. Contraction of the larger posterior muscles, which span the normal lordotic cervical curve, also creates a tendency toward buckling of the spine (143). Furthermore, the compressive weight of the head bends the spine in the sagittal plane producing a greater lordosis (103). Longus colli is the only muscle with attachments confined to the cervical vertebrae and thus the potential to counteract these forces and support the curve. Though little to no activity of longus colli has been recorded in resting posture, activity in longus colli increases when load is applied to the head (29,135). This is consistent with the increased need to support the cervical curve. The relationship between the cervical curve and the longus colli has been investigated with computerized tomography confirming that a greater lordosis is associated with a smaller cross sectional area of longus colli (94). Furthermore, when the subjects perform a neck-lengthening maneuver, there is electrical silence in the extensors, even when a load is placed on top of the head, affirming the supportive role of longus colli (93). The deep longus capitus has not been studied directly, but its morphometry and intimate relationship and synergy with the longus colli in its action, particularly on the skull and upper cervical joints, indicate that it has some functional features in common with longus colli.

Changes in Neck Pain

Changes in muscle structure with neck pain were observed in the biopsy studies of cervical muscles conducted by Uhlig et al (131) and Weber et al (138) in persons undergoing surgery for chronic neck pain of a variety of origins and varying duration. In total, 205 biopsy samples were taken variously from the sternocleidomastiod, omohyoid, and longus colli muscles in 37 patients who had an anterior surgical approach, and from the rectus capitus posterior major, obliquus capitus inferior, splenius capitus, and trapezius in 29 patients who had a posterior surgical approach. They documented the percentage composition of type 1 (slow-twitch oxidative), type IIA (fast-twitch oxidative glycolytic), type IIB (fast-twitch glycolytic), and type IIC (transitional) muscle fibers (indicating muscle transformation).

Signs of muscle transformation were evident in all muscles, but the flexor muscles had higher, above-normal counts of transitional fibers (55%) when compared to the extensor muscles examined (40%). The direction of the transition in neck muscle fiber type was always from type 1 slow twitch fibers to type 11B fast-twitch fibers which, from a functional perspective, could compromise the muscles' supportive holding or endurance capacity. A notable finding was that muscle transformation was independent of the underlying cause of neck pain. In respect of pathological change, atrophy and fatty infiltration, similar to that identified in the lumbar multifius, have been identified in the deep suboccipital muscles by using magnetic resonance imaging in small samples of subjects with chronic upper cervical dysfunction (2,40,95).

Concomitant with these studies, general changes in neck flexor and extensor strength and endurance or fatigability have been identified in patients with chronic neck pain (7,34,106,134). Janda (71) pointed to functional deficiencies in the neck flexors and particularly the deep neck flexors in neck pain patients and the adverse effects this impairment would have on the cervical joints. This sparked clinical interest in this muscle group, and several studies then emphasized cranio-cervical flexion in tests of neck flexor strength and endurance and identified problems in neck pain patients (6,31,37, 130,137). However, the basic functional differentiation between the deep and superficial muscles, as well as the findings of specific deficits between muscles in the low back, revealed the need to have a clinical test that might better separate the synergists. The more maximal tests previously used make differentiation between performance of deep and superficial neck flexors quite difficult. Also, a high load maximal test may not reflect the deep muscles' functional requirement of sustaining a low-level contraction to support the cervical joints in functional postures and movements (19,115). A different clinical test was required to better target the deep neck flexors, the longus colli, and longus capitus in

relative isolation from superficial flexors. The initial focus on these muscles in clinical testing does not dismiss the presence of, or consequence of, impairment in the neck extensors. Rather, the kinematics of the cranio-cervical and cervical regions and resultant differing actions of the superficial and deep neck flexors presented an opportunity for some differential testing of the flexor muscle layers in a clinical setting, which is not readily available for the neck extensor muscles.

The clinical test that our group developed was based on an analysis of the cranio-cervical flexion action, the anatomical action of the deep longus capitus, and longus colli muscles. It was presumed that if the discreet movement was performed under low load conditions, in supported supine lying, it could be expected that the longus capitus and longus colli muscles would principally perform the action and little work would be required from the sternocleidomastoid (SCM) and anterior scalene muscles. The SCM attaches to the mastoid process and effectively in this position is a cranio-cervical extensor, and the scalenes have no attachments to the cranium. Indirect quantification of the deep flexor muscle contraction was gained by inserting an air filled pressure sensor (Stabilizer, Chattanooga Pacific) between the testing surface and the back of the neck. A contraction of the longus colli causes a subtle flattening of the cervical lordosis (93), which could be registered as discrete increases in pressure in a progressively staged cranio-cervical action. Our initial study revealed that patients with cervicogenic headache had poorer performance in the test and were unable to achieve, control, and hold the pressure levels that could be achieved by asymptomatic subjects (73), suggesting impairment in the deep neck flexors. Surface EMG has been used to investigate the associated activity in the superficial flexors (SCM) during the staged cranio-cervical test. Results in subjects with persistent whiplash-associated disorders indicated that patients with neck pain were unable to achieve the controlled pressure levels with the staged cranio-cervical test (suggesting a poorer capacity in the deep neck flexors) as achieved by the asymptomatic subjects and this was associated with higher measured activity in the superficial neck flexors, a probable compensatory change in motor planning to assist the neck pain subjects to perform the nominated task (76).

Changes in motor strategies have also been found in superficial muscles spanning the neck, such as the upper trapezius, in neck pain patients (5,30,98). Although the primary function of these muscles relates to the shoulder girdle (83), alterations in function of the girdle muscles are considered clinically to negatively impact on cervical pain syndromes (97).

Strategies for Motor Re-education

The evidence thus far suggests that there are specific changes in the strategies used by the CNS to control the spine and this consistently involves impaired activity of the deep muscle system. On this basis, our primary goal of rehabilitation is to retrain control rather than increase the strength and endurance of the trunk muscles. Whereas there are several possible strategies that could be proposed to retrain this control, it is unlikely that general exercise for the trunk such as sit-ups and back extension exercises would achieve the goal of restoring the coordination between the trunk muscles. A strategy that our group has developed since the early 1990s is to use the principles of motor relearning and skill acquisition similar to those commonly implemented in the management of neurological disorders such as stroke. This approach aims to train cognitive control of the deep muscles and then through a series of steps to integrate this into automatic function (115).

Motor Relearning Approach

The nervous system has considerable potential for plasticity and learning. The motor relearning approach to the rehabilitation of movement disorders is characterized by several goals including improvement of motor performance (increased precision, decreased error), improved performance consistency (decreased variability), persistence of improvements (continued improvement over time leading to permanent improvement), and the adaptability of the skill to a variety of environments (novel contexts, decreased feedback, changes in physical or personal characteristics). Numerous motor learning strategies have been presented in the literature to achieve these goals. A key strategy described in the literature involves practice of "parts" of movement rather than the "whole" movement (91). When a skill is trained in parts, the attention demand is reduced to allow attention to be focused on a single element. Several techniques have been described for part-task training. These include *segmentation* and *simplification* (91). In the *segmentation* approach, the task is broken up into smaller parts to be practiced as an independent unit and then the practiced elements are integrated together progressively to practice the complete skill. A key feature of this strategy is selection of the specific features of a movement that are impaired or dysfunctional (i.e., "essential components") and then implementation of strategies that optimize the performance of that component (e.g., using cognitive strategies). At a later stage, it is important to perform the interdependent parts of a task together,

and to integrate the trained components in a functional context (15). From the evidence presented, the component of movement that is impaired in normal function is the activity of the deep muscle system (the activity of this system is delayed, more phasic, and no longer independent of the superficial muscles). Thus, the focus of rehabilitation is to train this component, independently from the superficial muscles, and then incorporate it back into function. In the *simplification* approach, the movement or its parts are simplified to increase the ease of movement performance. *Simplification* may be achieved by changing parameters such as reduction of the postural load (e.g., commencement of training in supported positions), reduction of attention demands, reduction of speed of the task, or using additional strategies to augment the performance (e.g., reduction of swelling to reduce reflex inhibition, positioning to decrease load, improved accuracy of feedback (e.g., ultrasound imaging).

Although the motor learning approach has a strong foundation in physiology, it may be argued that activation of the deep muscles in a voluntary and independent manner is artificial. This is, first, because these muscles are rarely, if ever, recruited in function without activity of the superficial muscles (although their activity is independent of the superficial muscles); and second, the activity of these muscles occurs automatically and not normally dependent on volition. On this basis, it may appear that this approach to reeducation may not be optimal. However, the goal is to re-establish the specific skilled control of the deep trunk muscles. By cognitive training of the deep muscles independently from the superficial global system we have the opportunity to train these muscles to perform their specific task (i.e., early activation, tonic activation, independent activation). Although the deep muscles may be active in a variety of exercise maneuvers (for instance, it is likely that TrA is active even during a simple sit-up), it is unlikely that simple activation of a muscle is sufficient to lead to change in the strategy used by the CNS to control these muscles. Furthermore, return to normal function, without training, is not sufficient to restore normal control. For instance, activity of TrA is delayed in people in remission from recurrent LBP despite the activity of this muscle in functional tasks (59). Furthermore, when people return to normal function after an episode of LBP, the size of multifidus does not return to normal without specific exercise intervention (45).

Motor learning occurs in three main stages: cognitive, associative, and autonomous phases (28). In the *cognitive phase,* the focus is on cognitively oriented problems. All elements of the movement performance are organized consciously with attention to feedback, movement sequence, performance, and instruction during repetition and practice. This phase is characterized by frequent, large errors and variability. Animal studies have identified an increased size of the hand area of the sensory cortex during the cognitive phase of motor learning of a task involving interpretation of sensory information from the hand (109). In addition, the area of the cortex over which transcranial magnetic stimulation produces an evoked response in muscles of the upper limb is increased with training (18). In motor relearning for LBP, the goal of the initial phase of motor relearning is to cognitively contract (although this may not be how the deep muscles are controlled in normal function) to increase the precision and skill of the contraction of the local muscles. The second stage is the *associative phase*, in which the fundamentals of the movement have been acquired and the cognitive demands are reduced. The focus moves from simple elements of performance of the task to consistency of performance, success and refinement. Correspondingly, the frequency and size of errors are reduced. In this stage, many repetitions are required in a variety of contexts to reduce the cognitive demand of the task. The final stage of motor learning, the *autonomous phase*, is achieved after considerable practice and experience. The task becomes habitual or automatic and the requirement for conscious intervention is reduced. Ideally, for the patient with LBP this is the goal of training. Whereas there is evidence of efficacy of the training approach for the management of symptoms of LBP (see later), there is also preliminary evidence that training can result in a change in the automatic activation of the local system. In two case studies, cognitive training of TrA was associated with a change in the timing of activity of this muscle in a limb movement task (78). Importantly, this task was not specifically trained, which suggests that there is transfer of automatic activation between tasks after training. Additional evidence suggests that this approach to training produces a change in automatic control comes from a study of people with patellofemoral pain. In this study, specific cognitive activation of the oblique fibers of vastus medialis resulted in a change in recruitment of this muscles during locomotion and tasks that challenged the stability of the knee (20).

Implementation of Motor Relearning Strategies in LBP

Several key concepts are important to consider in the implementation of motor relearning in musculoskeletal pathology. An important element of motor learning is the provision of augmented feedback.

Feedback can be generally divided into two main types: knowledge of performance and knowledge of results (120). Put simply, feedback that provides knowledge of performance relates to ongoing sensory/perceptual information provided during the movement, whereas knowledge of results provides feedback of the outcome of the movement. In the early cognitive phase, it is critical to provide accurate feedback of the quality of contraction and whether the goal is achieved. Because training attempts to improve the quality more than the quantity of contraction, it is the knowledge of performance that is paramount to the success of training. Each of the sensory systems, including visual, auditory, proprioceptive, and vestibular information, may be used to provide each form of feedback. This feedback may be intrinsic (naturally occurring) or augmented/enhanced in some way. Augmented feedback may include palpation, observation, EMG, and ultrasound imaging. However, there are several factors to consider. First, it is important that the patient is able to interpret the feedback appropriately. Second, patients should be encouraged develop the perception of contraction in addition to using feedback during training so that they do not become dependent on the feedback. Third, delayed removal of feedback may prolong rather than facilitate improvement and it should be withdrawn as appropriate.

Another concept to consider is that skill acquisition is often described as a reduction of the unnecessary muscle activity (120). Relearning control of the local system is no different, and the first improvement that may be noted is a reduction in the activity of the global muscles. As the skill is perfected, the amount of unwanted global activity during the performance of the task is decreased.

A critical component of skill learning is that the performance of the skill can be transferred to different conditions in which the environment, personal characteristics, or predictability are changed. To optimize transfer, it is considered essential to sequentially progress the task from easy to more complex situations. If the aim is to transfer a skilled movement to functional tasks, then it is necessary to progress to function. More specifically, it may be necessary to replicate sensory characteristics (e.g., limitation of visual feedback), environmental contexts (e.g., unstable surfaces, distractions), and personal contexts (e.g., anxiety, fatigue (96)) to ensure that the elements of the skill can be transferred to specific contexts (91).

To progress a patient with LBP through the normal phases of motor learning, the basic sequence that needs to be undertaken is: (1) skill learning; (2) precision training; (3) activation in a variety of contexts; (4) integration of the skill into tasks that include activation of the superficial trunk muscles; and (5) specific functional retraining to ensure the appropriate coordination of deep and superficial trunk muscles is maintained in a functional context.

Evidence of Efficacy of Motor Relearning in Musculoskeletal Conditions

Four randomized controlled clinical trials provide evidence of efficacy of motor relearning in the management of musculoskeletal pain. Two deal with LBP, one with cervicogenic headache, and another with patellofemoral pain. The first study investigated people with chronic LBP associated with spondylolisthesis (100). Subjects were allocated to participate in either a motor relearning program or a control group. The training period lasted for 10 weeks. At the end of training and at 30 months after training, there was a significant reduction in pain and disability in the subjects in the motor relearning group. There was no significant change in the control group.

The second study involved training in people with acute first episode of unilateral LBP (45). This group was selected because they have a reduced cross-sectional area of multifidus, ipsilateral to their symptoms (47). The intervention for this study involved a 4-week program of motor relearning focused on multifidus in conjunction with TrA. Subjects in the control group were encouraged to return to normal activity. After 4 weeks, all pain and disability measures had recovered in all but one subject. This is consistent with epidemiological data for this patient group. However, the size of multifidus had only recovered in motor control training group (45). The follow-up data provide potent evidence for the efficacy of the approach. After 3 years, people in the control group were 12.4-times more likely to have further episodes of pain that those in the exercise group (44).

In a recent trial of people with cervicogenic headache associated with cervical joint dysfunction, specific motor relearning for the deep neck flexors was found to be effective in the reduction of symptoms (i.e., frequency and intensity of headache and neck pain). Furthermore, this improvement was associated with improved performance of the clinical test of craniocervical flexion (75).

Evidence has also come from the implementation of motor relearning strategies for the management of pain at peripheral joints. In a recent study, specific motor relearning was used to re-establish the normal coordination of the medial and lateral muscles of the vastii group in patellofemoral pain (20). This training followed similar principles to those described here for the trunk muscles and resulted in a change in the automatic recruitment of the vastii in a variety of tasks. In addition, this was associated with a significant improvement in pain and disability.

These studies provide evidence for the efficacy of motor relearning strategies in the management of musculoskeletal pain. However, further studies are required to test these strategies in other patient groups and to compare them to other exercise interventions. An important concept to consider for the future is the identification of the patient groups for which this strategy is most effective.

Additional Factors

The discussion presented is based on a biomechanical model of back pain, that is, that the perpetuation of pain is caused by repeated microtrauma/trauma and repeated irritation of peripheral nociceptors, potentially with peripheral sensitization. However, it is accepted that once LBP becomes chronic, pain may be perpetuated by changes in the CNS. In this case it is important to consider that a multifaceted approach to management may be required and several factors require consideration. First, for transfer of training to be effective, patients may need to practice trunk muscle control in contexts that challenge factors such as fear of pain. Second, the clinical efficacy of motor relearning strategies may be influenced by factors independent of the improvement in biomechanical control of the spine, for instance, an improved control of the deep muscles of the trunk may provide the critical step required to reduce the threatening nature of pain. Finally, the specific proprioceptive input from contraction of the intrinsic spinal muscles may influence sensory perception. Many of these factors are the topic of further investigation (96a).

Clinical Assessment of Motor Control

Introduction

Assessment of motor control of the deep muscles has two inherent problems. First, the muscles are deep, which makes it difficult to assess their activation using non-invasive methods. Second, the aim is to assess motor control, not strength or endurance. Ideally, this could be assessed with intramuscular EMG recordings of the deep muscles in simple tasks such as rapid arm movement (59). However, this is not practical clinically and other techniques must be developed. This will involve compromises. Over the past approximately 10 years, our group has developed a series of tests that can provide an indirect indication of motor control of the deep muscles

(114,115). It is important to acknowledge that there are several weaknesses of these tests and it is important to consider that they provide a clinical judgment of the quality of control of the muscles but are not ideal objective tests for research purposes. Efforts are being made to identify improved methods of assessment, but at present these tests appear to be the most clinically appropriate. Despite these concerns the validity of the tests has been confirmed, that is, the tests provide information of motor control of the deep muscles. One study has compared the outcome of the clinical test with the latency of TrA during an arm movement task. There was agreement between tests. People who performed the clinical test well also had early activation of TrA and those who performed the test poorly had delayed activation of TrA (64). In a further study, performance of the test could be used to distinguish between people with and without LBP (13). While this section deals primarily with assessment of deep muscle activity, it is also important to assess the superficial global muscles. Techniques are described in other chapters for comprehensive assessment of this system. The aim of this section is to provide an overview of the strategies for assessment and rehabilitation of the deep muscle system with guidelines for progression of training. A detailed description of the assessment and rehabilitation strategies can be found in Richardson et al (115).

Assessment of Deep Muscle Function

Assessment of Motor Control of TrA

The assessment of motor control of TrA involves evaluation of the ability of a person to cognitively perform the skill of contraction of TrA independently from the global muscles (Fig. 25.8). The parameter that is measured is the precision of the task. As TrA lies deep to the oblique abdominal muscles, a combination of techniques is required to determine how well a patient is able to activate this muscle. These include observation, palpation, pressure biofeedback, and EMG biofeedback. It is possible to also use ultrasound imaging to observe the contraction of TrA (Fig. 25.8) (46); however, this is currently not commonly available in clinical practice. Contraction of TrA involves narrowing the waist and inward movement of the lower abdomen, thus any attempt to activate the muscle must involve this maneuver. As mentioned above, independent activation of TrA is a skill and requires practice, even in people without a history of LBP. Before the activation can be assessed it is necessary to teach the skill. This can be performed in any body position, but it is often useful to have the patient in a position with the abdomen dependent to

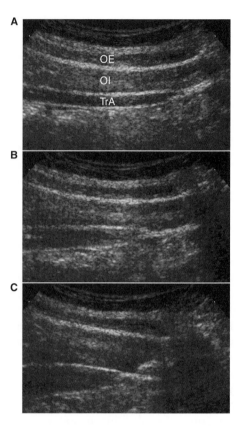

Figure 25.8 Ultrasound images of the abdominal wall at rest **(A)**, during independent contraction of TrA **(B)**, and general contraction of all abdominal muscles **(C)**. Image is a transverse image of the abdominal wall with the transducer placed between the rib cage and iliac crest on the left side. The right side of the image is medial. During muscle contraction the thickness of the muscles increases.

increase the awareness of the movement of the abdominal wall. Positions such as side-lying or four-point kneeling may be useful. However, this latter position is often not ideal for training because it is difficult for the patient to relax the superficial abdominal muscles. It is important to describe to the patient the anatomy of the muscle (for example, the description of the muscle as a corset can be useful) and the contraction that is required (i.e., **slow and gentle** inward movement of the lower abdomen). It may be helpful, but not essential, for the patient to separate breathing from the contraction, because it is often difficult to coordinate the two functions initially. An instruction such as "breath in and out, and then without breathing in, slowly and gently draw the lower abdomen in toward the spine, without moving the spine or pelvis." Some patients will be unable to cease respiration and accurate timing of instruction is required. Once the patient has practiced several repetitions, the contraction can then be tested more formally.

As mentioned, the basis of the test of TrA activity is to assess how precisely the person has performed the contraction of TrA. Thus, the performance of the task is assessed in two ways: (1) identification of signs that TrA is active and (2) identification of evidence that there is activity of the other muscles. The test can be performed in any body position (Fig. 25.9), although performance of the test in prone allows additional tools to be used to judge the performance of the task (e.g., pressure cuff; see later). Key factors that can provide evidence of TrA contraction include observation of slow inward movement of the lower abdomen and palpation of tightening with the fingers placed approximately 2 cm medial and inferior to the anterior superior iliac spine (43). In this region there is a large superficial bulk of obliquus internus abdominis (OI) and a deep, largely fascial area of TrA. If OI is active, this will be felt as a bulge; however, if TrA is active, without OI, this will be felt as a deep tensioning. Surface EMG recordings are not suitable for evaluation of the activity of TrA because there is no region of the abdomen in which TrA lies superficially.

If the test is performed in prone position, a pressure cuff can be placed under the abdomen to provide additional information of TrA contraction (Stabilizer, Chattanooga, TN). With the patient lying prone, the cuff is placed under the abdomen so that the navel lies in the center of the cuff and the distal edge is at the level of the anterior superior iliac spines. The cuff is inflated to approximately 70 mm Hg and the subject is instructed to slowly and gently draw the abdomen in. The ideal response is to be able to reduce the pressure by contraction of TrA by 4 to 6 mm Hg, to hold it reduced for 10 seconds, and to repeat this 10 times while breathing normally (115). It is generally ideal to watch the patient rather than the pressure dial for the first contraction to ensure that the patient has not simply flexed the lumbar spine by posteriorly tilting the pelvis or thoracolumbar flexion. If this occurs, the pressure will reduce, but not because of TrA contraction. TrA contraction draws the abdominal wall toward the spine and lifts it off the cuff, thus reducing the pressure. In contrast, contraction of the superficial abdominal muscles flattens the abdominal wall and either produces no change in the pressure or may cause it to increase. It is important to consider that this indirect measure of TrA activity is only one of a range of factors that must be assessed to confirm the precision of the task.

Several techniques are available to assess inappropriate activity of the superficial muscles during the performance of the TrA contraction. Again, observation and palpation are the primary skills, but EMG biofeedback can provide additional information. These signs and their possible interpretation are presented in Table 25.1.

At the completion of the assessment, the clinical outcome is judged from the precision of the independent activation of TrA. This can be reported as the signs that indicate TrA is active and signs that the superficial muscles were active (e.g., palpation, observation, EMG, pressure change, and ultrasound imaging). No single factor, such as pressure, is sufficient and a composite of measures is required to make accurate clinical judgment. It is important to identify the specific strategy used by the patient (e.g., which muscles, what sequence and what quality) because

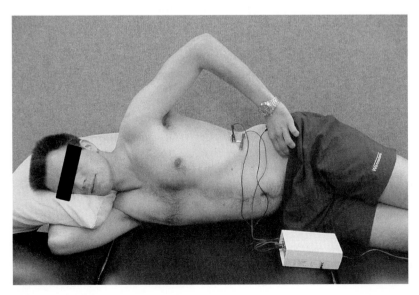

Figure 25.9 Activation of transversus abdominis. To ensure that the skilled contraction of TrA is being performed optimally, this patient is using feedback of contraction of TrA by palpation medial to the anterior superior iliac spines and is using EMG biofeedback with electrodes placed over the lateral fibers of obliquus externus abdominis to gain feedback of excessive activity of this muscle.

Table 25.1 Signs of Overactivity of the Superficial Abdominal Muscles During Independent TrA Contraction

Sign	Interpretation
Inward movement of upper abdomen	OE or RA activity
No movement of lower abdominal wall	OE or RA activity
Depression of rib cage	OE or RA activity
Thoracolumbar flexion	OE or RA activity
Rapid or "jerky" contraction	OE or RA activity
Posterior pelvic tilt	OE or RA activity
Inability to relax the abdomen	OE or RA activity
Expiratory activity of OE or RA with expiration in supported position	OE activity
Lateral expansion of waist	OE activity
Palpable/observable muscle activity over lower ribs	OE activity
Tight vertical band in anterolateral abdominal wall	OE activity
Increased EMG activity with electrodes placed over the OE over the angle of the 8th or 9th rib or on the lateral abdominal wall	OE activity
Increased EMG activity with electrodes placed over RA	RA activity
Palpable contraction over the muscle belly of RA	RA activity
Palpable bulge medial and inferior to the ASIS	OI activity
Contraction of the thoracolumbar erector spinae	Present to counteract the flexion moment of the superficial abdominal muscles
Quick deep inspiration	Inward movement of the abdominal wall produced by generation of negative pressure in the thorax

this information will be used to guide the initial stages of retraining. It may be necessary to evaluate the contraction in multiple positions to confirm all aspects of the assessment. Ultrasound has potential to provide an additional measure of activation of TrA and the other abdominal muscles (46). Recent studies have confirmed that it is possible to measure contraction of TrA and OI from changes in muscle thickness and shape with ultrasound imaging; however, it is not possible to assess OE in this manner (58). This technique is currently being investigated further and in future this may provide an important component of the assessment (46,115). One advantage of this technique is that it may allow identification of *independent* activity of TrA without the need to isolate the contraction.

Assessment of Motor Control of the Lumbar Multifidus

Assessment of contraction of the lumbar multifidus involves similar principles to those described for TrA. The test evaluates the ability to cognitively perform the skill of contraction of multifidus, particularly the deep fibers, independently of the superficial fibers. For multifidus, it is also useful to palpate the relaxed muscle, because changes in muscle consis-

tency may be present. If a person has acute LBP, there is likely to be a reduction in cross-sectional area of the muscle of approximately 30% (47). In the chronic situation when there is fatty infiltration into the muscle (1), the consistency of the muscle may be changed. Information gained from palpation of the relaxed muscle is important to compare with the results of the test of activation. For palpation, the patient lies prone. A pillow may be placed under the pelvis or abdomen to assist relaxation. Palpation is best performed by moving across the muscle fibers, starting at L1 and testing each level down to S1. The muscle size should increase in the caudad direction. The muscle consistency between sides can be compared by sinking the thumbs into the muscle belly.

The test of multifidus activation involves an isometric "swelling" contraction of the muscle (115). Because the aim of the test is to activate predominantly the deep muscle fibers (i.e., the fibers that have been suggested to be most important for intervertebral control (96), it is not sufficient to perform an anterior pelvic tilt by contraction of the long superficial fibers of the muscle. To teach the contraction, it is important to provide an explanation of the anatomy of the muscle and the type of contraction that is required. It may be necessary for the therapist to demonstrate the contraction or for the patient to palpate an isometric contraction of a limb muscle. The therapist then sinks the thumbs or an index finger and thumb into the multifidus for the patient to push against by swelling the muscle (Fig. 25.10). A useful instruction may be "breath in and out, without breathing in, slowly and gently swell the muscle out into my fingers, without moving your spine and pelvis, and start breathing normally." The ideal response is to palpate a slow gentle increase in deep tension under the fingers, which is symmetrical, can be held for approximately 10 seconds and can be repeated 10 times. Because of the deep placement of the segmental fibers of multifidus, it is difficult to be certain that these fibers are active. Several features can provide indirect evidence. One is that the increase in tension is slow, gentle, and deep, and another is whether the contraction of multifidus is accompanied by contraction of TrA but not the other abdominal muscles. This has been considered clinically to suggest predominant activity of the deep fascicles. If the superficial abdominal muscles are active,

this generally occurs to overcome the extensor moment generated by the superficial extensor muscles. Signs that suggest that the contraction of multifidus is not independent are listed in Table 25.2. Similar to the test of TrA, the outcome of the assessment is judged by interpretation of the observation, palpation, and EMG findings. Ultrasound may also provide a more accurate indication of activity of the deep muscle fascicles (46).

Assessment of Motor Control of the Deep Neck Flexors

Assessment of the motor control of the deep neck flexors follows similar principals to that described for the deep lumbar muscles and based on an analysis of the cranio-cervical flexion action. The patient lies supine with a pressure sensor (Stablizer, Chattanooga, TN) placed under the cervical spine (Fig. 25.11). The sensor is pre-inflated to 20 mm Hg, which is sufficient to fill the space between the bed and the back of the neck without pushing the neck into a lordosis. The test requires the person to perform progressive repetitions of the cranio-cervical action to discretely increase the pressure by 2 mm Hg incremental targets from 22 mm Hg to a maximum of 30 mm Hg. Assessment is in two phases. The first is to analyze the pattern of the cranio-cervical flexion movement. Movement should be of an increasing range of cranio-cervical flexion with each progressive stage of the test (27a). A common poor movement strategy is substitution with head and neck retraction, which is accompanied by overuse of the superficial neck flexors. This over-activity of the superficial muscles can be either palpated or recorded with surface EMG electrodes placed over the muscle belly. The second phase of the test is conducted once the patient can perform the cranio-cervical flexion action. This phase tests the patient's ability to hold (approximately 10 seconds) the cranio-cervical flexion position in each stage of the test on repeated occasions. The average level of the test that can be achieved by pain-free subjects with ranges between 26 and 28 mm Hg (73,76). Patients with neck disorders can usually only achieve 22 to 24 mm Hg, (75).

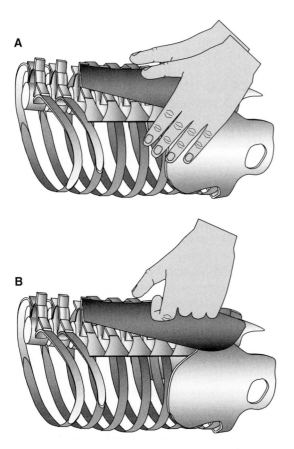

Figure 25.10 Technique for palpation of contraction of multifidus. Fingers are placed on either side of the spinous process. Pressure is applied to the muscle to give feedback of contraction and quality of contraction is palpated.

Assessment of Superficial Muscle Function

As mentioned, it is important to comprehensively assess the specific nature of the changes in control of the superficial global muscles. The activity of these muscles may be impaired or augmented and may present as more generalized dysfunction of movement

Table 25.2 Signs of Overactivity of the Superficial Abdominal Muscles During Independent Multifidus Contraction

Sign	Interpretation
Anterior pelvic tilt	Activity of long ES or superficial multifidus
Palpable contraction of long ES	Long ES activity
Contraction of superficial abdominal muscles	OE or RA activity to overcome the extension moment of the long ES or superficial multifidus
Posterior pelvic tilt	Inappropriate movement to push into the therapists fingers
Gluteal muscle contraction	Excessive effort

control. Many methods are available to assess the function of this system using tests that evaluate the relative timing of muscle activation in limb movement tasks (12,70), control of the trunk and pelvis during limb movement tasks (74,118), and functional tasks such as locomotion. These tests are described in detail

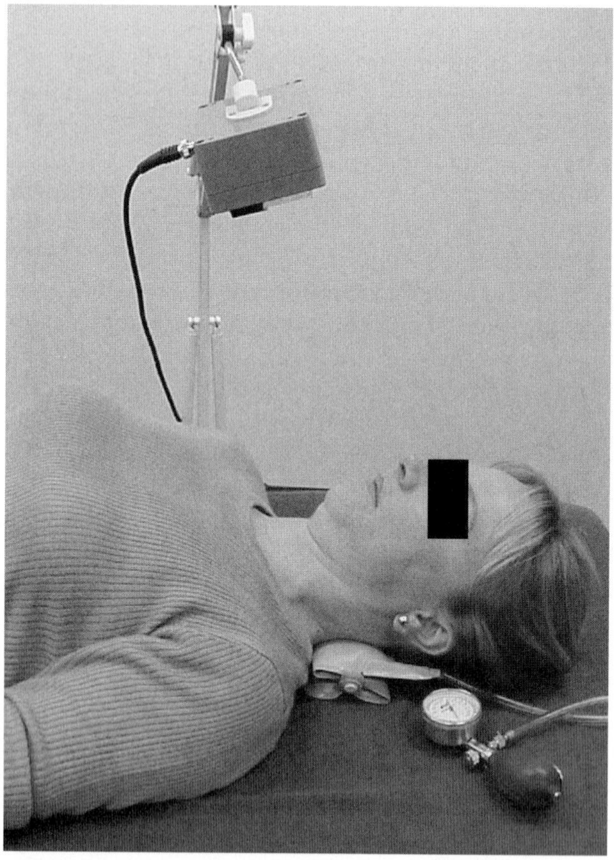

Figure 25.11 Clinical test of deep neck flexors. The pressure cuff is placed under the cervical spine and the patient gently drops the chin to increase the pressure in incremental steps. EMG electrodes could be placed over the sternocleidomastoid to record excessive activity of this muscle.

elsewhere and are important to consider in the overall management of the motor control deficits.

Summary

At the completion of the assessment, the therapist should have a detailed understanding of patient's ability to activate the deep muscle system and the strategies that used during the performance of the test maneuvers. Precise identification of these faults is critical because it directs the strategies implemented in the early stages of motor relearning.

Clinical Options for Re-education Motor Control

In the motor relearning approach, for the management of patients with low back or neck pain, the task is to re-educate the component missing in normal function, (i.e., early, tonic recruitment of the deep muscles independent from the superficial muscles), followed by reeduction of normal integration of activity of all trunk muscles into function. The treatment approach is detailed for the low back, but similar principles apply to management of the cervical region. The goal of treatment can be achieved by moving through four rehabilitation phases.

Phase 1: Activation

The first phase in the management of patients with back pain is the formal motor skill training. In this phase, patients are taught to cognitively perform the skilled activation of TrA and/or multifidus, independently of the superficial muscles. Techniques can be divided into two categories: techniques to decrease the activity of the superficial muscles and techniques to increase the activity of the deep muscles. The specific techniques that are used will depend on the findings of the assessment. For instance, if a patient has excessive recruitment of OE, then techniques to decrease this activity will be used first. However, if a patient has no over-activity but is unable to initiate a contraction of the deep muscles, the strategy will be very different and directed at using a facilitation strategy to increase the activity of the deep muscle. The aim of this phase is to teach the patient to perform a gentle isometric contraction of TrA and/or multifidus independently from the superficial muscles. Low-level contraction of these muscles is sufficient to control intervertebral motion (17) and studies indicate that activation of less than approximately 20% of maximum is common in function (55). Thus, the focus of training is low-level tonic activity. The following sections provide several options to reduce over-activity of the superficial muscles and increase activity of the deep muscles.

Techniques to Decrease the Activity of the Superficial Muscles

(i) Positioning—often it is necessary to use a supported position such as side-lying, supine, or supported standing to simplify the task by aiding relaxation of superficial muscles. To relax the long erector spinae, it may be useful to allow the patient to rest over a pillow.

(ii) Decreased effort of contraction—often patients will perform the contraction too hard and fast and reduction of effort can reduce this over-activity.

(iii) Feedback of contraction—EMG biofeedback, visual feedback with a mirror, tactile feedback with palpation.

(iv) Quiet breathing techniques—teaching a patient to perform normal diaphragmatic breathing with abdominal movement and bi-basal rib cage movement (i.e., increased lateral diameter of the rib cage), or statically holding the breath on inspiration.

(v) Active relaxation techniques—techniques such as contract–relax, connective tissue massage, and imagery.

(vi) Neutral position of the spine—placing in the patient in a neutral spine position with natural lumbar, thoracic, and cervical curves may aid in decreasing over-activity or "hanging" on the superficial muscles.

Techniques Available to Increase the Activity of the Deep Muscles

(i) Positioning—for TrA positions in which there is a gravity stretch on the muscle can make it

easier to contract; however, position is often guided by the requirement to reduce the over-activity of the global muscles.

(ii) Neutral spine position—placing the patient either actively or passively in a neutral spine position with natural lumbar, thoracic, and cervical curves may aid in activation of the deep muscles.

(iii) Co-activation of the pelvic floor—studies have shown that submaximal contraction of the pelvic floor muscles is associated with facilitation of activity of TrA (119). Patients should be instructed in the anatomy of the pelvic floor muscles (e.g., a sling of muscle that runs from the pubic bone to the coccyx) and provided with strategies to learn the contraction. For instance, using instructions such as "gently contract the pelvic floor muscles as if you are trying to stop the flow of urine." This instruction works well with men and women. The emphasis should be on performance of a slow gentle contraction and may be performed in isolation or with the instruction to extend the contraction up into the lower abdomen.

(iv) Co-activation of the other deep trunk muscles—for example, contraction of TrA may increase the activity of multifidus.

(v) Feedback—palpation of TrA contraction medial and inferior to the ASIS; mirrors for observation. Palpation of multifidus requires care with arm placement.

(vi) Adequate explanation of the type of exercise (low load control exercise) and muscle anatomy.

(vii) Imagery.

(viii) Demonstration.

Implementation

It is generally necessary to use a combination of strategies to achieve the most optimal independent contraction of the deep muscles. Improved activity may present as either an improvement in the pattern or an increase in the pressure change in the cuff, although the latter is not critical. At the end of this process, it should be possible to identify the strategy that worked best for the patient, the number of contractions that can be performed in a session (up to 10 10-second contractions), and to identify a strategy to ensure that the patient will perform the correct contraction at home. This latter task is often best achieved by feedback strategies such as palpation or observation in a mirror. It is generally best to train one muscle to start with. In the early stage of skill acquisition, fatigue occurs rapidly and it is advisable to cease practice when this occurs to prevent repetition of the incorrect task. Because of the complex nature of the exercise, patients will often find it difficult to practice frequently. In this early phase, patients are encouraged to perform their individual number of contractions (e.g., three times, 5-second contraction) for three to four sessions for the day.

Phase 2: Skill Precision

Once a patient can perform the independent contraction of one muscle, the next phase is to improve the precision of the task. Several goals are important to achieve: improved precision of the local muscle activation (increased number of repetitions and increased holding time), co-activation of local muscles including TrA and multifidus, coordination with breathing, progression to static functional positions, and progression to light dynamic tasks (Fig. 25.12). The ultimate goal of this phase of rehabilitation is to improve the patient's confidence and skill with the contraction so that they can cognitively perform the contraction accurately, with minimal feedback, without having to rely on specific facilitation strategies and to be able to perform the contraction in a variety of contexts (positions, support surfaces, etc).

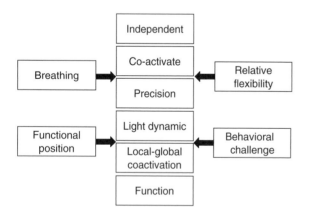

Figure 25.12 Steps for progression of motor relearning program for management of spinal pain. The middle column indicates the critical steps for progression of exercise. The additional elements to the sides are important components that need to be addressed as early as possible but at a point where they can be achieved successfully.

Co-Activation of Deep Muscles

In many cases, activation of one local muscle is associated with co-activation of the other muscles in the group. For instance, when TrA is active there is often concurrent recruitment of multifidus. For optimal control of intervertebral motion, it is ideal for the deep muscles to be co-activated. If this does not occur spontaneously, effort must be placed on achieving co-activation. In some patients this may require repetition of the initial process of identification of the ideal strategy for activation for the second muscle. In others it may simply require a change of position or increased feedback of the opposing muscle or the addition of a new strategy such as pelvic floor contraction to initiate activity of the other muscles. Once co-activation has been achieved then it is important to improve the precision of the co-activation.

Improved Precision of Deep Muscle Activation

A step in the process of improving the confidence of the contraction is to improve the precision of the skill by repetition. The patient is encouraged to increase the number of repetitions that can be performed and increase the duration of the contraction, up to approximately ten 10-second contractions. It is an advantage if the patients can determine when they have performed the contraction precisely because this will allow them to independently progress the number and duration of contractions. Patients should be encouraged to reduce the dependence on feedback of contraction and aim to perform the contraction cognitively without relying on facilitation strategies.

Coordination With Breathing

It is critical for the patient to be able perform normal diaphragmatic breathing (i.e., bi-basal rib cage expansion and abdominal movement) while maintaining the contraction of the local muscles. Many people have difficulties with this task, because the local muscles must be able to coordinate the respiratory modulation of activity as well as low-level tonic activity. In all patients it is important to assess the efficacy of the coordination of the respiratory and tonic activity of the deep muscles. For assessment it is necessary to evaluate all three major motions that occur with breathing, i.e., abdominal displacement (anterior displacement), bi-basal rib cage expansion (increased lateral and antero-posterior rib cage expansion), and upper chest motion (elevation and anterior displacement). In general, it is expected that the proportion of the total rib cage to abdominal motion will be approximately 60:40. When patients begin to breath while holding a contraction of TrA and multifidus, three main groups can be identified: (1) patients who can hold the tonic contraction of the deep muscles as respiration is continued at normal depth with respiratory movement in all three areas of the trunk (i.e., the ideal response); (2) patients who can hold the tonic contraction but use shallow upper chest breathing with minimal motion of the rib cage or abdomen; and (3) patients who loose the contraction of the local muscles with initiation of respiration. Training will be different for each group. It may be necessary to use relaxed positions and feedback of basal rib cage expansion to train this coordination. In general, the patient is encouraged to contract the local muscles and then add breathing to the tonic local muscle activity. At first it may be necessary to use shallow inspiratory movement and then progress through a gradual increase in lung volume with emphasis on maintenance of tension in the abdominal wall and multifidus. It is normal for the abdomen to move with respiration; the key is to sustain tension in the muscles, despite the change in muscle length.

Progression to Static Functional Positions

As soon as possible, but not too early, it is important to progress to functional upright positions such as sitting and standing. This may be difficult because of excessive recruitment of the superficial muscles. However, it is important to consider that once a person adopts a weight-bearing position there may be activity of the superficial muscles to keep the body upright and overcome the effects of gravity. The goal is for the person to be able to maintain the contraction of local muscles relatively independent of the global muscles. It may be necessary to make intermediate steps toward upright positions such as supported standing against a wall or supported sitting. The progression would be to reduce the amount of support. In this phase it may be necessary to introduce postural correction. Commonly, patients are encouraged to adopt a neutral spinal position. This position is the mid-position of the joints and generally involves a thoracic kyphosis and lumbar lordosis (not a thoracolumbar extension, which is commonly identified). This position is particularly important, because it is in this position that the passive system has its smallest contribution to spinal control and the system is dependent on the contribution of muscle. However, it is important to remember that the spine was designed to move, and movement of the spine is used to aid in the absorption of force. Thus, it is not ideal to encourage a patient to maintain a static neutral spinal position without variation, but rather to encourage activation of the deep muscles in a variety of positions and movements. As an intermediate step to normal movement, the neutral spinal position may be appropriate as a goal. However, to optimize loading of the spine and minimize effects such as creep, in sustained tasks it may be optimal to encourage patients to sustain the neutral spinal position for specific functions. Once the patient can perform the contraction in functional positions, it is then possible to dramatically increase the frequency of training. Ideally, by this stage the patient should be training the deep muscles for several repetitions every hour. It is through repetition that the system is being trained to automatically activate the local muscle system in function.

Progression to Light Dynamic Tasks

Once the local muscle contractions can be performed "confidently" in upright postures, it is appropriate to begin the more complex task of adding spinal movement. In this phase, the goal is to maintain tonic contraction of the deep muscles while the spine is moved. A useful task to initiate this phase of training is walking. In walking it is essential to allow the pelvis and spine to move and not be held statically to minimize the energy expenditure of locomotion. Thus, it is important that the patient be aware that the goal is to maintain the contraction of the local muscles in conjunction with small amplitude movement with phasic contraction of the global muscles superimposed over the local muscles. In this phase, it is critical that the patient is aware of the perception of contraction of the deep muscles, because the superimposed global muscle activity will mask the underlying local muscles. For a patient to progress to walking, it may be necessary to attempt intermediated steps such as forward/backward and side-to-side weight shift, then stepping with support, and finally unaided stepping. Because the goal is for the activation of the local muscles to become automatic without conscious contraction, it is important to gradually reduce the cognitive input. This can be achieved by repetition of the contraction at intervals during walking training rather than consciously sustaining the contraction throughout the task.

Phase 3: Superficial and Deep Muscle Co-activation

An important phase in progression is to teach a patient to coordinate the activity of the deep and superficial muscles without the global muscles taking over. There are many options to train a patient in this phase. The basic premise is to co-activate the local muscle system and then use load to activate the global muscles in a phasic direction specific manner. For example, if a subject lying prone is asked to co-activate the deep muscles and, then, without moving the spine or pelvis, lifts a leg, the mass of the leg introduces a rotary force on the pelvis and spine and the global muscles must contract to overcome this force and maintain the lumbo-pelvic position (74,110,113,118). Thus, the patient has co-activated the deep and superficial muscles appropriately. It is important to ensure that the contraction of the local system is maintained during the task. This is largely dependent on the perception of the patient as the activation of the global muscles precludes the palpation of the deep muscles. In this case, ultrasound imaging may be useful to observe changes in deep muscle activity (115).

There are many options available for this phase of training. In general, any technique that encourages controlled addition of load to the trunk with an emphasis on low load, isometric contractions, control of joint position, and co-activation may be appropriate. Examples include rhythmic stabilization techniques from proprioceptive neuromuscular facilitation (136), leg-loading tasks (74,110,113,118), Pilates exercises, Swiss ball exercises (21), unstable surfaces, and sensory motor integration techniques (70). Using these methods, progression can be achieved by increasing the load or speed or decreasing the stability of the environment. It is important to match the difficulty of the tasks to the demands of the lifestyle of the patient, and it is beneficial if the exercises are functionally relevant to the patient. The outcome of an assessment of the global muscles may direct the specific features of the exercise intervention. For example, if the patient has a flexion, extension, or rotation problem, then the exercise intervention for the global muscles will be more ideal if it specifically addresses these issues (118).

Phase 4: Functional Re-education

The final phase of training is functional re-education. There are several important points to consider. First, the specific functions that are trained must be based on the demands of the patient and the outcome of the subjective assessment. Second, the normal principles of skill learning are applied, that is, the task is broken down into individual elements and then put together as the elements are perfected. Third, the patient is encouraged to perform low-level tonic contraction of the local muscles during the performance of the task. For instance, if a patient has difficulties associated

with a tennis serve, the first step is to break the task into its components; each component is practiced with tonic co-activation of the deep muscles. As the tasks are perfected, the patient is encouraged to walk through the task, gradually increasing the speed and force. Ideally, the cognitive intervention for local muscle contraction should be reduced as the training progresses.

Treatment Considerations

Several factors are important to consider regarding the implementation of treatment strategies. First, it is ideal to use motor relearning strategies in conjunction with other treatment strategies. In the biomechanical model, training the control of the deep muscles can improve the control of the intervertebral joints. Thus, any technique that can directly affect tissue healing or manage other aspects of the pain experience can only be beneficial. Furthermore, in this light it is possible to see that these techniques may be beneficial in many different patient groups, but the extent to which it may have an effect on symptoms will be dependent on the specific pathology. There are several patient groups in which it has been argued that these techniques are optimal including patients with clinical signs of instability (99), spondylolisthesis (100), and acute LBP (45).

Second, in terms of application of the exercise intervention, the time taken to achieve results, the frequency of treatment, and whether the patient will need to continue the exercises for an extended period or can cease on resolution of symptoms is dependent on the individual and is guided by rate of progress and follow-up. Third, we believe that the precision of training is critical and the treatment outcomes may be faster and more successful when a patient is not progressed too soon. Further research is required to validate this issue.

Audit Process
Self-Check of the Chapter's Learning Objectives

- How does the central nervous system control spine motion?

- How is spinal biomechanics altered with typical manifestations of poor motor control in the neck and low back?

- What are some basic assessments for abnormal motor control in the neck and low back?

- What are some basic exercises to isolate key "weak links" in the neck and lumbo-pelvic regions?

Editor's Note:

Recent Developments in Research on the Deep Spinal Stabilizers

A study of a variety of abdominal exercises found that abdominal hollowing supine without lumbo-pelvic motion was ideal for isolating the Tr A.

Urquhart DM, Hodges P, Allen TJ, Story IH: Abdominal muscles recruitment during a range of voluntary exercises. Manual Therapy 2005, 10:144–153.

Recent data confirms that coordination of the abdominal muscles involving feedforward activity in the TrA can be restored with training of specific coordinated activation of the trunk muscles.

Tsao H, Hodges P: Specific abdominal retraining alters motor coordination in people with persistent log back pain: submitted for publication; 2005.

A subgroup of subacute neck pain patients without LBP have been found to be at heightened risk of future LBP. The inability to perform abdominal hollowing identifies individuals who are 3–6 times more likely to develop future LBP than asymptomatic people who are able to perform the same task.

Moseley GL: Impaired trunk muscle function in subacute neck pain: etiologic in the subsequent development of low back pain? Manual Therapy 2004, 9:157–163.

When the asymptomatic controls completed the active straight leg raise (ASLR) task, the transversus abdominus contracted in a feed-forward manner. However, when individuals with long-standing groin pain completed the ASLR task, the onset of transversus abdominus was delayed ($P < 0.005$) compared with a control group. There were no differences between groups for the onset of activity of internal oblique, external oblique, and rectus abdominus (all $P > 0.05$).

Cowan SM, Schache AG, Brukner P, Bennell KL, Hodges PW, Coburn P, Crossley KM. Delayed onset of transversus abdominus in long-standing groin pain. Med Sci Sports Exerc. 2004; 36:2040–5.

Study participants with LBP had a significantly smaller increase in TrA thickness with isometric leg tasks compared with controls. No difference was found between groups for OI or OE. Similar results were found for EMG. People with LBP had less TrA EMG activity with leg tasks, and there was no difference between groups for EMG activity for OI or OE.

Ferreira PH, Ferreira ML, Hodges PW. Changes in recruitment of the abdominal muscles in people with low back pain: ultrasound measurement of muscle activity. Spine. 2004:15;29:2560–6

Both insidious onset neck pain and whiplash groups had measurable dyfunctions during each stage of the cervico-cranial flexion test compared to the control subjects. Specifically, it was reported that EMG signal amplitude in the sternocleidomastoid is elevated (all $P < 0.05$), and there was a significant shortfall from the pressure targets ($P < 0.05$).

Jull G, Kristjansson E, Dall'Alba P. Impairment in the cervical flexors: a comparison of whiplash and insidious onset neck pain patients. Man Ther. 2004;9:89–94.

■ REFERENCES

1. Alaranta H, Tallroth K, Soukka A, Heliaara M. Fat content of lumbar extensor muscles in low back disability: a radiographic and clinical comparison. J Spinal Disord 1993;6:137–140.
2. Andrey MT, Hallgren RC, Greenman PE, Rechtien JJ. Neurogenic atrophy of suboccipital muscles after a cervical injury. Am J Phys Med Rehabil 1998;77:545–549.
3. Arendt-Nielsen L, Graven-Nielsen T, Svarrer H, Svensson P. The influence of low back pain on muscle activity and coordination during gait: a clinical and experimental study. Pain 1996;64: 231–240.
4. Aruin AS, Latash ML. Directional specificity of postural muscles in feed-forward postural reactions during fast voluntary arm movements. Exp Brain Res 1995;103:323–332.
5. Bansevicius D, Sjaastad O. Cervicogenic headache: The influence of mental load on pain level and EMG of shoulder-neck and facial muscles. Headache 1996;36:372–378.
6. Barber A. Upper cervical spine flexor muscles: age related performance in asymptomatic women. Aus J Physiother 1994;40:167–171.
7. Barton PM, Hayes KC. Neck flexor muscle strength, efficiency, and relaxation times in normal subjects and subjects with unilateral neck pain and headache. Arch Phys Med Rehabil 1996;77:680–687.
8. Belenkii V, Gurfinkel VS, Paltsev Y. Elements of control of voluntary movements. Biofizika 1967;12:135–141.
9. Bergmark A. Stability of the lumbar spine. A study in mechanical engineering. Acta Orthop Scand 1989;60:1–54.
10. Biederman HJ, Shanks GL, Forrest WJ, Inglis J. Power spectrum analysis of electromyographic activity: discriminators in the differential assessment of patients with chronic low back pain. Spine 1991;16:1179–1184.
11. Bogduk N, Twomey LT. Clinical Anatomy of the lumbar spine. New York: Churchill Livingstone, 1991.
12. Bullock-Saxton JE, Janda V, Bullock MI. Reflex activation of gluteal muscles in walking with

balance shoes: an approach to restoration of function for chronic low back pain patients. Spine 1993;18:704–708.

13. Cairns MC, Harrison K, Wright C. Pressure biofeedback: a useful tool in the quantification of abdominal muscular dysfunction? Physiother 2000;86:127–138.

14. Capra NF, Ro JY. Experimental muscle pain produces central modulation of proprioceptive signals arising from jaw muscle spindles. Pain 2000;86:151–162.

15. Carr JH, Shepherd RB. A motor relearning program for stroke. London: Heinemann, 1987.

16. Cholewicki J, McGill SM. Mechanical stability of the *in vivo* lumbar spine: Implications for injury and chronic low back pain. Clin Biomech 1996;11:1–15.

17. Cholewicki J, Panjabi MM, Khachatryan A. Stabilizing function of trunk flexor-extensor muscles around a neutral spine posture. Spine 1997;22: 2207–2212.

18. Classen J, Liepert J, Wise SP, Hallett M, Cohen LG. Rapid plasticity of human cortical movement representation induced by practice. J Neurophysiol 1998;79:1117–1123.

19. Conley MS, Meyer RA, Bloomberg JJ, Feeback DC, Dudley GA. Noninvasive analysis of human neck muscle function. Spine 1995;20:2505–2512.

20. Cowan S, Bennel K, Crossley K, Hodges P, McConnell J. Physiotherapy treatment alters recruitment of the vastii in patellofemoral pain syndrome. Med Sci Sports Exer 2002;34:1879–1885.

21. Creager CC. Therapeutic Exercises Using the Swiss Ball. Executive Phys Ther 1994.

22. Cresswell AG, Grundstrom H, Thorstensson A. Observations on intra-abdominal pressure and patterns of abdominal intra-muscular activity in man. Acta Physiol Scand 1992;144:409–418.

23. Cresswell AG, Oddsson L, Thorstensson A. The influence of sudden perturbations on trunk muscle activity and intra-abdominal pressure while standing. Exp Brain Res 1994;98:336–341.

24. Cresswell AG, Thorstensson A. Changes in intra-abdominal pressure, trunk muscle activation and force during isokinetic lifting and lowering. Eur J Appl Physiol Occup Physiol 1994;68:315–321.

25. Crisco JJ, Panjabi MM. The intersegmental and multisegmental muscles of the lumbar spine: A biomechanical model comparing lateral stabilizing potential. Spine 1991;7:793–799.

26. Derbyshire SW, Jones AK, Gyulai F, Clark S, Townsend D, Firestone LL. Pain processing during three levels of noxious stimulation produces differential patterns of central activity. Pain 1997;73:431–445.

27. Dutia MB. The muscles and joints of the neck: their specialization and role in head movement. Prog Neurobiol 1991;37:165–178.

28. Fitts PM, Posner MI. Human performance. Belmont, CA: Brooks/Cole, 1967.

29. Fountain FP, Minear WL, Allison PD, Function of longus colli and longissimus cervicis muscles in man. Arch Phys Med Rehabil 1966;47:665–669.

30. Fredin Y, Elert J, Britschgi N, Nyber, V, Vaher A, Gerdle B. A decreased ability to relax between repetitive contractions in patients with chronic symptoms after trauma of the neck. J Musculoskel Pain 1997;5:55–70.

31. Fulton I. The upper spine flexor muscles-do they get the nod? An investigation of muscle performance in normal asymptomatic male subjects. Proceedings of Manipulative Physiotherapists Association of Australia. Adelaide, 1989.

32. Gardner-Morse M, Stokes IAF, Laible JP. Role of muscles in lumbar spine stability in maximum extension efforts. J Orthop Res 1995;13:802–808.

33. Goff B. The application of recent advances in neurophysiology to Miss M. Rood's concept of neuromuscular facilitation. Physiother 1972;58:409–415.

34. Gogia PP, Sabbahi MA. Electromyographic analysis of neck muscle fatigue in patients with osteoarthritis of the cervical spine. Spine 1994;19:502–506.

35. Gracovetsky S, Farfan H, Helleur C. The Abdominal Mechanism. Spine 1985;10:317–324.

36. Gracovetsky S, Farfan HF, Lamy C. A mathematical model of the lumbar spine using an optimized system to control muscles and ligaments. Orthop Clin North Am 1977;8:135–153.

37. Grimmer K. Measuring the endurance capacity of the cervical short flexor muscle group. Aus J Physiother 1994;40:251–254.

38. Gurfinkel VS, Lipshits MI, Lestienne FG. Anticipatory neck muscle activity associated with rapid arm movement. Neurosci Lett 1988;94:104–108.

39. Gurumoorthy D, Twomey LT. A morphological study of the deep muscles of the cervical region. Proceedings Manipulative Physiotherapists Association of Australia, Blue Mountains, Australia, 1991.

40. Hallgren RC, Greenman PE, Rechtien JJ. Atrophy of suboccipital muscles in patients with chronic pain: a pilot study. J Am Osteopath Assoc 1994;94: 1032–1038.

41. Hemborg B. Intraabdominal pressure and trunk muscle activity during lifting. Doctoral dissertation, Department of Physical Therapy, University of Lund, 1983.

42. Henry SM, Fung J, Horak FB. EMG responses to maintain stance during multidirectional surface translations. J Neurophysiol 1998;80:1939–1950.

43. Hides J, Scott Q, Jull G, Richardson C. A clinical palpation test to check the activation of the deep stabilizing muscles of the spine. Intern Sports Med J submitted for publication.

44. Hides JA, Jull GA, Richardson CA. Long term effects of specific stabilizing exercises for first episode low back pain. Spine 2001;26:243–248.

45. Hides JA, Richardson CA, Jull GA. Multifidus muscle recovery is not automatic after resolution of acute, first-episode low back pain. Spine 1996;21:2763–2769.

46. Hides JA, Richardson CA, Jull GA, Davies SE. Ultrasound imaging in rehabilitation. Aus J Physiother 1996;41:187–193.

47. Hides JA, Stokes MJ, Saide M, Jull GA, Cooper DH. Evidence of lumbar multifidus muscle wasting ipsi-

lateral to symptoms in patients with acute/subacute low back pain. Spine 1994;19:165–177.

48. Hodges P. Changes in motor planning of feedforward Postural responses of the trunk muscles in low back pain. Exp Brain Res 2001;141:261–266.

49. Hodges P, Gandevia S. Activation of the human diaphragm during a repetitive postural task. J Physiol (Lond) 2000;522:165–175.

50. Hodges P, Gandevia S. Changes in intra-abdominal pressure during postural and respiratory activation of the human diaphragm. J Appl Physiol 2000;89:967–976.

51. Hodges P, Moseley G, Gabrielsson A, Gandevia S. Acute experimental pain changes postural recruitment of the trunk muscles in pain-free humans. Soc Neurosci Abstr 2001;27:304.11.

52. Hodges PW, Butler JE, McKenzie D, Gandevia SC. Contraction of the human diaphragm during postural adjustments. J Physiol (Lond) 1997; 505:239–248.

53. Hodges PW, Cresswell AG, Daggfeldt K, Thorstensson A, Three dimensional preparatory trunk motion precedes asymmetrical upper limb movement. Gait Posture 2000;11:92–101.

54. Hodges PW, Cresswell AG, Daggfeldt K, Thorstensson A, In vivo measurement of the effect of intra-abdominal pressure on the human spine. J Biomech 2001;34:347–353.

55. Hodges PW, Cresswell AG, Thorstensson A. Preparatory trunk motion accompanies rapid upper limb movement. Exp Brain Res 1999;124:69–79.

56. Hodges PW, Eriksson AEM, Shirley D, Gandevia SC. Lumbar spine stiffness is increased by elevation of intra-abdominal pressure. Proceedings of the International Society for Biomechanics, Zurich, Switzerland, 2001.

57. Hodges PW, McKenzie DK, Heijnen I, Gandevia SC. Reduced contribution of the diaphragm to postural control in patients with severe chronic airflow limitation. Proceedings of the Thoracic Society of Australia and New Zealand, Melbourne, Australia, 2000.

58. Hodges PW, Pengel L, Herbert R, Gandevia SC. Ultrasound measurement of changes in muscle geometry over a range of isometric contraction intensities. Muscle Nerve 2003;27:682-692.

59. Hodges PW, Richardson CA. Inefficient muscular stabilization of the lumbar spine associated with low back pain: A motor control evaluation of transversus abdominis. Spine 1996;21:2640–2650.

60. Hodges PW, Richardson CA. Contraction of the abdominal muscles associated with movement of the lower limb. Phys Ther 1997;77:132–144.

61. Hodges PW, Richardson CA, Feedforward contraction of transversus abdominis in not influenced by the direction of arm movement. Exp Brain Res 1997;114:362–370.

62. Hodges PW, Richardson CA, Delayed postural contraction of transversus abdominis associated with movement of the lower limb in people with low back pain. J Spinal Disord 1998;11:46–56.

63. Hodges PW, Richardson CA. Transversus abdominis and the superficial abdominal muscles are controlled independently in a postural task. Neurosci Lett 1999;265:91–94.

64. Hodges PW, Richardson CA, Jull GA. Evaluation of the relationship between the findings of a laboratory and clinical test of transversus abdominis function. Physiother Res Int 1996;1:30–40.

65. Hodges PW, Sapsford RR, Pengel HM. Feedforward activity of the pelvic floor muscles precedes rapid upper limb movements. Proceedings of the V International Physiotherapy Congress, Sydney, Australia, 2002.

66. Indahl A, Kaigle A, Reikeras O, Holm S. Electromyographic response of the porcine multifidus musculature after nerve stimulation. Spine 1995;20:2652–2658.

67. Indahl A, Kaigle A, Reikeras O, Holm S. Sacroiliac joint involvement in activation of the porcine spinal and gluteal musculature. J Spinal Disord 1999;12:325–330.

68. Indahl A, Kaigle AM, Reikeras O, Holm SH. Interaction between the porcine lumbar intervertebral disc, zygapophysial joints, and paraspinal muscles. Spine 1997;22:2834–2840.

69. Janda V. Muscles, central nervous motor regulation and back problems. New York: Plenium Press, 1978.

70. Janda V. Pain in the locomotor system—a broad approach. Melbourne: Churchill Livingstone, 1984.

71. Janda V. Muscles and motor control in cervicogenic disorders: Assessment and management. New York: Churchill Livingstone, 1994.

72. Johansson H, Sjolander P, Sojka P. A sensory role for the cruciate ligaments. Clin Orthop Rel Res 1991;268:161–178.

73. Jull G, Barrett C, Magee R, Ho P. Further characterization of muscle dysfunction in cervical headache. Cephalalgia 1999;19:179–185.

74. Jull G, Richardson C, Toppenberg R, Comerford M, Bui B. Towards a measurement of active muscle control for lumbar stabilization. Aus J Physiother 1993;39:187–193.

75. Jull G, Trott P, Potter H, Zito G, Niere K, et al. A randomized controlled trial of physiotherapy management for cervicogenic headache. Spine 2002;27:1835–1843.

76. Jull GA. Deep cervical neck flexor dysfunction in whiplash. J Musculoskel Pain 2000;8(1/2):143–154.

77. Jull GA, Richardson CA. Rehabilitation of active stabilization of the lumbar spine. New York: Churchill Livingstone, 1994.

78. Jull GA, Scott Q, Ricardson C, Henry S, Hides J, Hodges P. New concepts for the control of pain in the lumbopelvic region. In: Proceedings of the World Congress of Low Back and Pelvic Pain. Vienna, Austria: 1998.

79. Kaigle AM, Holm SH, Hansson TH. Experimental instability in the lumbar spine. Spine 1995;20: 421–430.

80. Kamibayashi LK, Richmond FJR. Morphometry of human neck muscles. Spine 1998;23:1314–1323.

81. Keshner EA. Controlling stability of a complex movement system. Phys Ther 1990;70:844–854.

82. Keshner EA, Allum JHJ. Muscle activation patterns coordinating postural stability from head to foot. New York: Spinger-Verlag, 1990.

83. Keshner EA, Campbell D, Katz RT, Peterson BW, Neck muscle activation patterns in humans during isometric head stabilization. Exp Brain Res 1989;75:335–344.

84. Keshner EA, Cromwell RL, Peterson BW. Mechanisms controlling human head stabilization. II. Head-neck characteristics during random rotations in the vertical plane. J Neurophysiol 1995;73:2302–2312.

85. Keshner EA, Peterson BW. Mechanisms controlling human head stabilization. I. Head-neck dynamics during random rotations in the horizontal plane. J Neurophysiol 1995;73:2293–2301.

86. Lavender SA, Mirka GA, Schoenmarklin RW, Sommerich CM, Sudhakar LR, Marras WS. The effects of preview and task symmetry on trunk muscle response to sudden loading. Human Factors 1989;31:101–115.

87. Lewin T, Moffett B, Viidik A. The morphology of the lumbar synovial joints. Acta Morphologica Neerlanco Scand 1962;4:299–319.

88. Lindgren K-A, Sihvonen T, Leino E, Pitkänen M, Manninen H. Exercise therapy effects on functional radiographic findings and segmental electromyographic activity in lumbar spine instability. Arch Phys Med Rehabil 1993;74:933–939.

89. Lu WW, Bishop PJ. Electromyographic activity of the cervical musculature during dynamic lateral bending. Spine 1996;21:2443–2449.

90. Macintosh JE, Bogduk N. The detailed biomechanics of the lumbar multifidus. Clin Biomech 1986;1:205–231.

91. Magill RA. Motor learning: Concepts and applications. New York: McGraw-Hill, 2001.

92. Matre DA, Sinkjaer T, Svensson P, Arendt-Nielsen L. Experimental muscle pain increases the human stretch reflex. Pain 1998;75:331–339.

93. Mayoux-Benhamou MA, Revel M, Vallee C. Selective electromyography of dorsal neck muscles in humans. Exp Brain Res 1997;113:353–360.

94. Mayoux-Benhamou, MA, Revel M, Vallee C, Roudier R, Barbet JP, Bargy F. Longus colli has a postural function on cervical curvature. Surg Radiol Anat 1994;16:367–371.

95. McPartland JM, Brodeur RR, Hallgren RC. Chronic neck pain, standing balance, and suboccipital muscle atrophy—a pilot study. J Manip Physiol Ther 1997;20:24–29.

96. Moseley GL, Hodges PW, Gandevia SC. Deep and superficial fibers of lumbar multifidus are differentially active during voluntary arm movements. Spine 2002;27:E29–E36.

97. Mottram S. Dynamic stability of the scapula. Man Ther 1997;2:123–131.

98. Nederhand MJ, Ijerman MJ, Hermens HJ, Baten CT, Zilvold G. Cervical muscle dysfunction in chronic whiplash associated disorder Grade 11 (WAD-11). Spine 2000;25:1939–1943.

99. O'Sullivan PB. Lumbar segmental "instability": clinical presentation and specific stabilizing exercise management. Man Ther 2000;5:2–12.

100. O'Sullivan PB, Twomey LT, Allison GT. Evaluation of specific stabilizing exercise in the treatment of chronic low back pain with radiologic diagnosis of spondylolysis or spondylolisthesis. Spine 1997;22:2959–2967.

101. Panjabi MM. The stabilizing system of the spine. Part I. Function, dysfunction, adaptation, and enhancement. J Spin Disord 1992;5:383–389.

102. Panjabi MM, Abumi K, Duranceau J, Oxland T. Spinal stability and intersegmental muscle forces. A biomechanical model. Spine 1989;14:194–200.

103. Panjabi MM, Cholewicki J, Nibu K, Grauer J, Babat LB, Dvorak J. Critical load of the human cervical spine: an in vitro experimental study. Clin Biomech 1998;13:11–17.

104. Pauly J. An electromyographic analysis of certain movements and exercises: I. Some deep muscles of the back. Anat Rec 1966;155:223–234.

105. Pedersen J, Sjolander P, Wenngren BI, Johansson H. Increased intramuscular concentration of bradykinin increases the static fusimotor drive to muscle spindles in neck muscles of the cat. Pain 1997;70:83–91.

106. Placzek JD, Pagett BT, Roubal PJ, Jones BA, McMichael HG, Rozanski EA, Gianotto KL. The influence of the cervical spine on chronic headache in women: A pilot study. J Man Manip Ther 1999;7:33–39.

107. Radebold A, Cholewicki J, Panjabi MM, Patel TC. Muscle response pattern to sudden trunk loading in healthy individuals and in patients with chronic low back pain. Spine 2000;25:947–954.

108. Rantanen J, Hurme M, Falck B, Alaranta H, Nykvist F, Lehto M, Einola S, Kalimo H. The lumbar multifidus muscle five years after surgery for a lumbar intervertebral disc herniation. Spine 1993;18:568–574.

109. Recanzone GH, Merzenich MM, Jenkins WM, Grajski KA, Dinse HR. Topographic reorganization of the hand representation in cortical area 3b owl monkeys trained in a frequency-discrimination task. J Neurophysiol 1992;67:1031–1056.

110. Richardson C, Jull G, Toppenberg R, Comerford M. Techniques for active lumbar stabilization for spinal protection: A pilot study. Aus J Physiother 1992;38:105–112.

111. Richardson C, Toppenberg R, Jull G. An initial evaluation of eight abdominal exercises for their ability to provide stabilization for the lumbar spine. Aus J Physiother 1990;36:6–11.

112. Richardson CA. Investigations into the optimal approach to exercise for the knee musculature. PhD Thesis. The University of Queensland, 1987.

113. Richardson CA, Jull GA. Concepts of assessment and rehabilitation for active spinal stability. Edinburgh: Churchill Livingstone, 1994.

114. Richardson CA, Jull GA. Muscle control—pain control. What exercises would you prescribe? Man Ther 1995;1:2–10.

115. Richardson CA, Jull GA, Hodges PW, Hides JA. Therapeutic exercise for spinal segmental stabilization in low back pain: Scientific basis and clinical approach. Edinburgh: Churchill Livingstone, 1999.

116. Richardson CA, Snijders CJ, Hides JA, Damen L, Pas MS, Storm J. The relation between the trans-

versus abdominis muscles, sacroiliac joint mechanics, and low back pain. Spine 2002;27:399–405.

117. Roy SH, DeLuca CJ, Casavant DA. Lumbar muscle fatigue and chronic low back pain. Spine 1989;14:992–1001.

118. Sahrman S. Diagnosis and Treatment of Movement Impairment Syndromes. St Louis: Mosby, Inc, 2002.

119. Sapsford RR, Hodges PW, Richardson CA, Cooper DH, Markwell SJ, Jull GA. Co-activation of the abdominal and pelvic floor muscles during voluntary exercises. Neurourol Urodyn 2001;20:31–42.

120. Schmidt RA, Lee TD. Motor Control and Learning: A behavioral emphasis. Champaign, Illinois: Human Kinetics Publishers, 1999.

121. Siddall PJ, Cousins MJ. Pain mechanisms and management: an update. Clin Exp Pharmacol Physiol 1995;22:679–688.

122. Sihvonen T, Lindgren KA, Airaksinen O, Manninen H. Movement disturbances of the lumbar spine and abnormal back muscle electromyographic findings in recurrent low back pain. Spine 1997;22:289–295.

123. Snijders CJ, Vleeming A, Stoeckart R. Transfer of lumbosacral load to iliac bones and legs. Part 1: Biomechanics of sale bracing of the sacroiliac joints and its significance for treatment and exercise. Clin Biomech 1993;8:285–294.

124. Snijders CJ, Vleeming A, Stoeckart R. Transfer of lumbosacral load to iliac bones and legs. Part 2: Loading of the sacroiliac joints when lifting n a stooped posture. Clin Biomech 1993;8:295–301.

125. Snijders CJ, Vleeming A, Stoekart R, Mens JMA, Kleinrensink GJ. Biomechanical modeling of sacroiliac stability in different postures. Spine: State of the Art Reviews 1995;9:419–432.

126. Solomonow M, Zhou BH, Harris M, Lu Y, Baratta RV. The ligamento-muscular stabilizing system of the spine. Spine 1998;23:2552–2562.

127. Suzuki N, Ohe K, Inoue H. The strength of abdominal and back muscles in patients with low back pain. Central Japan J Orthop Traumatol 1977;20:332–334.

128. Taimela S, Kujala UM. Reaction times with reference to musculoskeletal complaints in adolescence. Percep Motor Skills 1992;75:1075–1082.

129. Thorstensson A, Arvidson Å. Trunk muscle strength and low back pain. Scand J Rehabil Med 1982;14:69–75.

130. Treleaven J, Jull G, Atkinson L. Cervical musculoskeletal dysfunction in post-concussional headache. Cephalalgia 1994;14:273–279.

131. Uhlig Y, Weber BR, Grob D, Muntener M. Fiber composition and fiber transformations in neck muscles of patients with dysfunction of the cervical spine. J Orthop Res 1995;13:240–249.

132. Urquhart D, Story I, Hodges P. Rotation transversus abdominis. Proceedings of the VIth International Physiotherapy Congress, Sydney, Australia, 2002.

133. Valeriani M, Restuccia D, Di Lazzaro V, Oliviero A, Profice P, Le Pera D, Saturno E, Tonali P. Inhibition of the human primary motor area by painful heat stimulation of the skin. Clin Neurophysiol 1999;110:1475–1480.

134. Vernon H, Steiman I, Hagino C. Cervicogenic dysfunction in muscle contraction headache and migraine: a descriptive study. J Manipulative Physiol Ther 1992;15:418–429.

135. Vitti M, Fujiwara M, Basmajian JV, Iida M. The integrated roles of longus colli and sternocleidomastoid muscles: an electromyographic study. Anat Rec 1973;177:471–484.

136. Voss DE, Ionta MK, Myers BJ. Proprioceptive Neuromuscular Facilitation : Patterns and Techniques. New York: Lippincott Williams & Wilkins, 1985.

137. Watson DH, Trott PH. Cervical headache: an investigation of natural head posture and upper cervical flexor muscle performance. Cephalalgia 1993;13:272–284.

138. Weber BR, Uhlig Y, Grob D, Dvorak J, Muntener M. Duration of pain and muscular adaptations in patients with dysfunction of the cervical spine. J Orthop Res 1993;11:805–810.

139. White AA, Panjabi M. Clinical Biomechanics of the Spine. Philadelphia: J. B. Lippincott, 1990.

140. Wilder DG, Aleksiev AR, Magnusson ML, Pope MH, Spratt KF, Goel VK, Muscular response to sudden load. A tool to evaluate fatigue and rehabilitation. Spine 1996;21:2628–2639.

141. Wilke HJ, Wolf S, Claes LE, Arand M, Wiesend A. Stability increase of the lumbar spine with different muscle groups: A biomechanical in vitro study. Spine 1995;20:192–198.

142. Williams PL, Warwick R, Dyson M, Bannister LH. Grays Anatomy. London: Churchill Livingstone, 1989.

143. Winters JM, Peles JD. Neck muscle activity and 3-D head kinematics during quasi-static and dynamic tracking movements. New York: Springer-Verlag, 1990.

144. Yoshimoto K, Itami Y, Yumamoto M. Electromyographic study of low back pain. Jpn J Rehabil Med 1978;15:252.

145. Zattara M, Bouisset S. Posturo-kinetic organization during the early phase of voluntary upper limb movement. I. Normal subjects. J Neurol, Neurosurg Psychiatry 1988;51:956–965.

146. Zedka M, Prochazka A, Knight B, Gillard D, Gauthier M. Voluntary and reflex control of human back muscles during induced pain. J Physiol (Lond) 1999;520:591–604.

26

Functional Stability Training

Craig Liebenson

Learning Objectives
After reading this chapter, you should be able to understand:

- The indications for each major exercise group
- How to find the patient's functional range
- How bracing and breathing are used during training
- How to train muscular endurance
- How to audit correct exercise performance
- How to progress patients with functional–stability training
- How to troubleshoot if the patient is having trouble with an exercise

Introduction

Exercise is considered a "gold standard" in the management of patients with spine-related pain and disability. It has been shown to be safe and effective for patients. Before rehabilitation occurs, the patients' functional goals (activity intolerances) and functional deficits (relevant impairments) should be identified. This provides a starting point and an end point for the exercise prescription.

Modern therapeutic exercise emphasizes a behavioral and neurophysiologic approach. From a behavioral perspective, gradual reactivation, pacing, and graded exposures to feared stimuli frame the management of the self-care program. Neurophysiologically, the emphasis is on spine instability or poor motor control, which is now understood to be a key feature of spinal dysfunction responsible for activity limiting back problems.

Scientific Underpinnings

How Muscles Stabilize the Spine

Muscles stabilize joints by stiffening like rigging on a ship (Fig. 26.1). According to Cholewicki and McGill, spine stability is greatly enhanced by co-contraction of antagonistic trunk muscles (5). Co-contractions increase spinal compressive load, as much as 12% to 18% or 440 N, but they increase spinal stability even more, by 36% to 64% or 2925 N (14). They have been shown to occur during most daily activities (32). This mechanism is present to such an extent that without co-contractions, the spinal column is unstable even in upright postures! (12).

Co-contractions are most obvious during reactions to unexpected or sudden loading (26,33). Stokes has described how there are basically two mechanisms by which this co-activation occurs (45). One is a voluntary pre-contraction to stiffen and thus dampen the spinal column when faced with unexpected perturbations. The second is an involuntary reflex contraction of the muscles quick enough to prevent excessive motion

that would lead to buckling after either expected or unexpected perturbations (4,9,26,33,45,51).

Tissue injury is a result of repetitive end-range loading (see chapter 5). A stable spine is able to avoid injurious, repetitive end-range loading via the buttressing effect of agonist–antagonist co-activation in maintaining the integrity of the "neutral zone." The neutral zone is the inner region of a joint's range of motion (ROM) where minimal resistance to motion is encountered (40). This inner region's mobility is restricted by passive ligamentous factors alone, and when it is expanded joint instability is said to exist, which places greater demands on the muscles to stabilize a joint. Thus, the most observable and measurable sign of instability is not joint hypermobility, but rather excessive agonist–antagonist muscular co-activation (2).

Various studies have pointed out how important the motor control system is for preventing spinal injury. Ironically, when under load, the spine is best stabilized, but when "surprised" by trivial load at a vulnerable time such as in the morning or after prolonged sitting, the spine stability system is most dysfunctional (1,38). Inappropriate muscle activation during seemingly trivial tasks (only 60 Newtons of force) such as bending over to pick up a pencil can compromise spine stability and potentiate buckling of the passive ligamentous restraints (2). This motor control skill has also been shown to be more compromised under challenging aerobic circumstances (36). The basic science aspects of the spine stability system are presented in greater detail in chapters 2 and 6.

Motor Control Problems and Low Back Pain

Radebold et al have shown that there is a predictable muscle response pattern to sudden trunk loading in individuals with low back pain (LBP) (41). This includes delayed initial activation, over-activation, and delayed subsequent relaxation of muscles. Researchers in Queensland, Australia have found that delayed activation of the transverse abdominus during arm or leg movements distinguishes LBP patients from asymptomatics (21,22). However, according to Canadian scientists, focusing on a single muscle is like focusing on a single guy wire (25). Research from the University of Waterloo in Canada has found that while certain muscles such as multifidus and transverse abdominus may have special relevance in distinguishing LBP subjects from asymptomatic individuals, these muscles are part of a much bigger orchestra responsible for spinal stability (25).

Sufficient stability, according to McGill, is defined as the amount of muscle stiffness necessary for stability along with a safety margin (see chapter 5 the section on stability: The Foundation). Cholewicki and

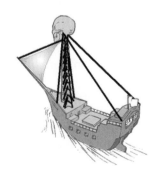

Figure 26.1 Rigging on a ship.

colleagues showed that modest levels of co-activation are necessary, but if a joint has lost its stiffness greater amounts of co-activation are needed (6,7).

Marras et al have reported that there is a different pattern of antagonist muscle co-activation (kinematic ability) in LBP individuals than in asymptomatics (31). Patients were found to have greater spine load and greater kinematic compromise during lifting tasks. Altered kinematics were strongly related to spine load, being able to predict 87% of the variability in compression, 61% in anteroposterior shear, and 65% in lateral shear. The kinematic picture for the LBP individual showed excessive levels of antagonistic muscle co-activation, which reduced trunk motion but also increased spine loading.

Efficacy: Evidence of Effectiveness for Spine Stability Training

Australian researchers have reported that multifidus atrophy occurs with acute LBP (18). The atrophy does not spontaneously go away when the pain does (19). However, motor control training does restore the multifidus and reduces long-term recurrence rates (20).

O'Sullivan et al showed that specific spine stabilization exercises achieved superior outcomes to isotonic exercises in chronic patients with spondylolysthesis (39). In a large, randomized, controlled clinical trial, Timm showed that exercise was superior to passive care in treating failed back surgery in patients (47). In this study, a further comparison of exercise types showed that low-technology exercise (McKenzie and stabilization) was superior to high-technology exercise (isotonics & Cybex).

Stuge et al found that stabilizing exercises were superior to traditional physical therapy for pelvic girdle pain after pregnancy (46). The stabilization group had lower pain intensity, disability, higher quality of life, and less impairments. The results persisted at 1 year check postpartum.

Yilmaz et al (2003) administered an 8-week stabilization program to postoperative lumbar microdiscectomy patients (52). It was compared to home exercise and to no exercise. At week 12, superior results were achieved in pain, function, mobility, and lifting ability for the stabilization group. Supervised stabilization training was superior to home exercises, which was superior to no exercise.

Safety: Is Spine Stability Training Safe?

Safe exercises for acute and subacute low back patients should have favorable biomechanical load profiles. It is known that without muscles, the spine buckles at 90 N. Yet during routine ADLs, loads 20-times that (2000 N) are routinely encountered

Table 26.1 Exercise Profiles (12,37,38,40,45)

Safe Exercises

1. Quad single leg raise—2000 to 2300 N
   • Opposite arm/leg raise—approximately 3000 N
2. Side bridge on knees—less than 2000 N
   • Side bridge on ankles—2600 N
3. Curl-up—2000 N

Unsafe Exercises

   • Sit-ups, bent knee—3350 N
   • Sit-ups, straight knee—3500 N
   • Curl-up on ball—4000 N
   • Prone superman—4300 N

(40). Thus, proper functioning muscles controlled by the central nervous system enable stability to be maintained. In fact, demanding ADLs involve loads of approximately 6000 N, and the NIOSH work demand limit is 6400 N (12,37,45). Elite weight lifters manage, through highly skilled motor control strategies, to safely lift loads of nearly 20,000 N (McGill personal correspondence). McGill recommends that for subacute exercise training, a safe limit is approximately 3000 N (38). Table 26.1 lists a number of exercises with safe and unsafe load profiles.

Clinical Application

Training Basics

Specificity of Training

The specificity principle is often referred to as the SAID Principle, which stands for specific adaptation to imposed demands. This means that the locomotor system will specifically adapt to the type of demand placed on it. Evidence shows that training leads to length, task, and speed specific changes (28,42,43). For example, long-distance running will improve cardiovascular endurance, but not speed. Also, if a person regularly weight-trains with maximal resistance and few repetitions, this will produce greater strength or power gains, but little endurance gains.

During the first 1 to 2 months of training, rapid improvement, as much as 100%, in weight-lifting ability occurs. However, if unrelated tasks are attempted, gains will be less than 20%.

The more similar the exercise is to the actual activity (position, whole body coordination, speed, resistance, etc.), the greater the likelihood that improvements in function at home, sports, or work will occur. This is known as the transfer-of-training effect. Therefore, if training programs do not address the specific functional needs of the individual, the goal cannot be achieved.

Endurance Training

Practice-Based Problem

Most traditional exercise programs focus on muscle strengthening. Why will this not help the LBP patients and what type of program is needed?

Cholewicki's work has demonstrated that sufficient stability of the lumbar spine is achieved with modest levels of co-activation of the paraspinal and abdominal muscles (7). According to McGill (see chapter 5), patients and athletes must be able to maintain sufficient stability throughout the duration of an activity, especially when unexpected perturbations are accidentally encountered. Thus, to maintain a stability margin of safety when performing tasks, endurance, not strength or power, is required.

Endurance training of agonist and antagonist co-contraction ability about a joint has been shown to improve joint stability by enhancing muscle stiffness (2). This does not require a very strong muscular effort. Hoffer and Andreasson showed that efforts of just 25% of maximum voluntary contraction (MVC) provided maximal joint stiffness (23). A prolonged tonic holding contraction at a low MVC is ideally suited to selectively train type 1 tonic muscle fiber function. According to McArdle et al, tonic fibers only operate at levels less than 30% to 40% MVC (34).

Isometric holds should be no more than 7 or 8 seconds based on recent infrared spectroscopy indicating rapid loss of available oxygen in muscles contracting at mild to moderate levels of intensity (<50% of MVC) (35).

Practice-Based Problem

Patients in pain are often fearful that exercise will make them worse. Is it possible to educate them that there is an unforeseen risk of not exercising?

Muscle strength is lost faster with rest than it is gained with exercise

- Muscle strength is lost at the rate of 3% to 7% per day of rest.

- Muscle strength improves 0.5% to 1% per day with training.

Cooper D, Fair J. Reconditioning following athletic injuries. Phys Sports Med 1976;4:125.

Table 26.2 Stability Training Variables

- Intensity: submaximal, less than 50% of single repetition maximum (1 RM)
- Sets and repetitions: start with 1 set of approximately 6 repetitions
  - Progress to 1 set of 12 repetitions
    - Further progress after the reverse pyramid approach of adding a second set of 8 repetitions, and then a third set of 4 reps
- Hold times: emphasize endurance by holding for 1 to 2 breaths (6 to 10 seconds)
- Form: movements should be performed slowly with appropriate form for motor control training and injury prevention
- Frequency: daily or twice daily to improve motor control
- Duration: up to 3 months required to re-educate movement patterns in a patient with chronic pain

---

The variables in stability training include intensity, sets, repetitions, hold times, form, frequency, and duration (Table 26.2).

Psychology of Training

Patient reactivation is a gradual process. Behavioral medicine or sports psychology tenets of "paced activity" and the relationship between hurt and harm should be discussed with the patient. Many LBP patients have excessive fear–avoidance beliefs or catastrophizing behaviors that promote a passive, symptom-driven approach, excessive pathoanatomic diagnostic testing, and a poor prognosis (30). At the other end of the spectrum are individuals who are overly aggressive, which can lead to a "boom or bust" mentality.

The middle path is best exhibited by the modern emphasis on quota-based graded exposures (30). This operant conditioning model successively demonstrates to patients that hurt does not necessarily equal harm, and that activity—contrary to the patient's pain expectancy or fear–avoidance beliefs—is actually beneficial. In graded exposures training (GET), the patient's activity levels are gradually increased in a step-wise manner limited by quota, not pain (11,29). For individuals at the other end of the spectrum who ignore pain and continue with or complete activities that may be harmful, GET is equally important (49). GET or pacing is important and ensures that either too little or too much activity is avoided (3,16,17).

It is important that the clinician prescribes only those exercises that have a large safety/stability margin. Such exercises should be mutually agreed on with the patient. They should be performed to a quota even if mildly uncomfortable. In chronic pain patients, the expectancy of re-injury is typically based on an activity avoidance belief or catastrophizing tendency and not an actual experience (10,48). Ciccione and Just showed that in susceptible individuals, there is discordance between pain expectancies and actual pain intensity with activities (8). Vlaeyen et al have demonstrated that GET can change the individual's fears and beliefs (48).

GET starts with baseline testing to identify feared activities (activity intolerances). Initial quotas should be set to sub-threshold levels to assure success. Then, patients are gradually exposed to their feared stimuli so they can experience that it is safe to do so (13,50). Post-treatment auditing of previously provocative maneuvers is crucial to "prove" the effectiveness of the program.

Practice-Based Problem

Chronic pain patients frequently expect to find a cure. Is this realistic? Even if manipulation (soft tissue or articular) achieves temporary relief, is it beneficial for the patient to attribute to the health care providers intervention rather than self-care? Also, because recurrences are the rule rather than the exception, should we tell chronic patients to expect them?

Patients should be given self-care advice before passive interventions so that they attribute to the self-care (see chapter 15). Such positive attribution to self-management is motivational (16,17). The McKenzie system is designed to facilitate this self-attribution via its rigorous audit process (post-treatment re-evaluation).

Chronic patients should be educated to expect relapses. Flare-ups are not failures to manage the pain. The challenge is to learn how to better self-manage such "flare-ups" (16,17). It is important for patients to learn that there are both first-aid and preventive, conditioning self-care programs. Chronic patients must master both.

How to Determine an Appropriate Starting Point for a Patient's Exercise Program

Individualizing the exercise prescription necessitates that the clinician have a strategic plan. What follows is a step-by-step guide to customize the right exercise for each patient.

First, identify the patient's activity intolerances (AI). This is derived from a history of things in his daily life he is having trouble performing. Restoring these functional abilities should be mutually agreed on as the goal of care.

Second, identify the patient's capabilities or functional deficits. This is derived from an examination of capabilities, and is termed the patient's functional range (FR). Dennis Morgan defines this as "the range of movement which is both painless and appropriate for the task at hand." The FR emerges from a rigorous functional assessment of both a patient's mechanical sensitivities (MS)—what the patient feels—and abnormal motor control (AMC)—what the clinician observes. Whenever possible, the patient's functional capacity or deficits should be quantified with reliable tests that have normative databases. This is a key to establishing the patients initial baselines that will be used later to monitor progress.

Third, identify exercises and supportive treatments that can close the gap between the patient's functional goals (activity intolerances) and capabilities. The exercises prescribed should ideally be performed without MS or AMC and be relevant for the patient's goals and deficits.

Fourth, regularly audit (re-check) the patient's AIs and FR (AMC and MS) to determine if the exercises are achieving the twin goals of reducing AIs and enhancing capabilities. McGill calls this finding the positive slope with the exercise(s). The goal is to find this as quickly as possible. However, in severe, acute pain when inflammation is predominant, or in disabling, chronic pain cases in which central sensitization is present, it can take a few sessions of empirical trial to establish the unique exercise prescription that yields a positive slope. Follow this audit frequency:

- AIs—
  ◦ Beginning of each session: verbally audit
  ◦ Weekly: Patient-Specific Functional Scale (PSFS)
  ◦ Monthly: region-specific outcome tool such as the Oswestry or Neck Disability Index
- MS—
  ◦ Re-examine at the beginning of each visit

- ○ Re-examine immediately after the exercise(s) are performed and at the end of the treatment session
- AMC—Re-examine at least once per week

Table 26.3 summarizes this prescriptive approach.

Motivating patients to stay in their painless range is easy. When the patients are in acute pain, they should avoid what hurts them. In this phase, hurt and harm may go hand-in-hand. The art of the McKenzie approach is successfully examining the patient to find the painful (or pain peripheralizing) movement and the pain centralizing or reducing movements. Once this is done it is easy to teach the patient what positions and movements to avoid and which to repetitively perform by recommending those that reduce or centralize symptoms.

Clinical Pearl

McKenzie says, "If you adopt certain positions or perform certain movements that cause your back to 'go out,' then if we understand the problem fully we can identify other movements and other positions that, if practiced and adopted, can reverse the process. You put it out—you put it back in."

McKenzie R. The McKenzie Institute International pamphlet 1998.

Motivating patients to perform exercises appropriately (biomechanically correctly) is not so easy. Pain is not a sufficient guide. In fact, patients often use "trick" movement patterns, with excessive global muscle substitution, to increase repetitions, thereby reinforcing dysfunction, for instance, stooping excessively during squat exercises. Unfortunately, many dysfunctional movements don't hurt in patients with chronic pain. Also, certain movements such as stretches for tissues that have adaptively shortened do hurt but are not harmful.

Table 26.3 Identification of the Rehabilitation Prescription

1. Identify AIs
2. Identify the FR (MS and AMC)
3. Prescribe exercise in the patient's FR
4. Perform ongoing re-evaluation/audit

Clinical Pearl

In approaching treatment, the clinician must answer two basic questions:

1. Does the patient present with unwanted global muscle activity?
2. If so, which muscles are problematic?

These questions must be answered to institute best-practice therapeutic exercise.

Richardson C, Jull G, Hides J, Hodges P. *Therapeutic Exercise for Spinal Stabilization in Lower Back Pain*. Edinburgh: Churchill Livingstone, 1999:126.

How to Progress a Patient's Exercise Program

The manner by which patients acquire the skill of "core" stability during functional activities generally follows certain established stages of motor learning (Table 26.4) (44). These may be unnoticed by the patient, but the astute clinician guides the patient effortlessly through these stages with the help of encouraging and facilitory cues, contacts, resistance, commands, etc.

The first stage of motor learning is the cognitive–kinesthetic stage. Most patients have poor kinesthetic awareness of how to produce and/or control motion of their problem area. In this first stage the patient learns to "discover" how to move an important region such as the lumbo-pelvic, scapulo-thoracic, or cervico-cranial. They acquire the skill to perform the movement and then to limit it to a "painless" or pain centralizing range. Examples include the following:

Lumbo-pelvic control—cat–camel

Scapulo-thoracic—shoulder rolls or Brügger position

Cervico-cranial—nodding of the head as if saying "yes"

Movement control then progresses to the second stage of motor learning called the associative stage. This is entered when the patient has sufficiently developed the kinesthetic awareness to move within his FR so that he can safely and appropriately perform more complex exercises using a "key" region.

Table 26.4 Stages of Motor Learning

- Conscious awareness
- Associative
- Autonomous control

For instance, a progression in level of motor control difficulty occurs when a movement progresses from simple, unresisted concentric motions (i.e., cat-camel) to one requiring isometric "core" stabilization during peripheral mobilization (i.e., quadruped single leg reach)

The third stage of motor learning is the autonomous stage. This is accomplished when the patient does not have to think about the exercise to perform it properly. This is demonstrated when the patient can control lumbo-pelvic posture during an exercise despite unexpected perturbations from a labile surfaces (i.e., stability pad, mini-trampoline) or from the clinician (quick, gentle pushes). In this way, the unexpected nature of "real life" situations involving sudden movements and jostles are trained.

Because many patients lack the motivation to concentrate during exercise training, it is crucial to reach the autonomous stage of an exercise as quickly as possibly. Additionally, the most functional exercise that the patient can perform with good stability is always a wise choice because compliance will be better. Gary Gray terms this "attacking success" (15). Vladimir Janda also emphasized this point by suggesting that exercises such as sensory–motor training on a rocker board were preferred to cortically demanding training such as complex floor exercises because it automatically trained the stability system without requiring much voluntary control (24).

Part of the art of prescribing exercises is determining how long to stay with exercises that require the patient to hypervigilently (voluntarily) control posture versus having the patient practice simple, functional movements that they automatically (involuntarily) perform with good "core" control. This is an important clinical issue because modern stabilization training may require 4 to 6 weeks of practice before abdominal hollowing can be learned (39). Karel Lewit (27) sums it up thusly, "remedial exercise is always time consuming, and time should not be wasted . . . We should not attempt to teach patients ideal locomotor patterns, but only correct the fault that is causing the trouble."

Table 26.5 Variables by Which to Progress Patients

- Unloaded to loaded (gravity)
- Simple to complex (uniplanar to triplanar or isometric to concentric to eccentric)
- Slow to fast
- Endurance to strength to power
- Increasing resistance
- Stable to labile (decreased points of support or use of unstable surfaces like ball or board)

There are innumerable different ways to progress patients. Table 26.5 outlines a few of the most important ones.

During training, what the clinician does is often more important than what the patient does (Table 26.6). For instance, there are ways to facilitate improved motor control by changing the patient's position. If a patient has trouble coordinating the side bridge, then they can be placed kneeling on heels and perform a more reactive, simpler pattern by raising their trunk upright. Hand contacts can be changed to train bracing by moving from the lumbar spine to the ilium when challenging the patient's resistance to twisting. Tissue stimulation can be facilitory, for example, when the gluteus medius is goaded at its tendinous insertion. Most importantly, verbal cues or commands should be neurolinguistically experimented with to see if varying tones or verbal targets are best. For instance, if a person is asked to perform a bird dog with neutral spine, one person might respond to the cue to keep their back horizontal while another might require the cue to keep their hips square. Even props can be used such as balancing a water bottle on the spine during the bird dog, which the patient is encouraged not to let drop.

It is essential to establish baselines from which a patient's progress can be monitored objectively (Table 26.7). One should identify the patient's movements or positions that reproduce their characteristic pain (MS) (e.g., trunk flexion). Also, iden-

---

Clinical Pearl

The goal of supervised training is to find the self-care methods that the patient feels confident will help him achieve his functional goals. This is the practical application of helping the patient achieve self-efficacy (see chapter 14).

Table 26.6 Facilitation Techniques

- Pre-positioning
- Hand contacts
- Tissue stimulation
- Verbal cues or commands
- Props

Table 26.7 Setting Baselines

- Identify the patient's MS
- Identify the patient's AMC
- Identify the patient's quantifiable functional deficits

---

tify their key abnormal motor control patterns (AMC) (e.g., hip extension). Finally, identify their relevant quantifiable functional deficits (e.g., side bridge endurance). Such baselines should be regularly reassessed to provide an independent, functional barometer of a patient's progress besides their report of pain.

The Exercises

Increasing physical performance ability, in particular spinal fitness, requires that exercises with acceptable load profiles are used. Muscle challenge should be high, but joint compressive penalty should be minimized (37). This requires that a motor control approach is taken to muscle fitness training. Additionally, the exercises should be progressed toward functional goals that incorporate how the individual actually uses their body in their daily life.

A step-wise approach to reducing AIs and restoring function has been developed. Once advice has been given about how to spare the spine during activities of daily living (ADL) (see chapter 14), and the safety of exercise discussed, then a progressive approach beginning with exercises with a wide stability/safety margin are prescribed to quota. The goal is to improve motor control by emphasizing coordination during simple movements designed to stabilize the back (i.e., hip hinging). Such introductory exercises are then progressed by adding low-load endurance challenges. Finally, exercises are progressed to include functional or performance components that mimic as closely as possible the actual ADL, work, or sports demands the individual faces (Table 26.8).

Table 26.8 Main Types of Spinal Rehabilitative Training

1. Stability training (coordination, endurance)
2. Functional integrated training (FIT)

Stability Training

Practice-Based Problem

Can you prescribe treatment for pain patients which will expand their "functional range"?

In stability training postural control, muscle balance and pain reduction or centralization is the focus. The goal is to train coordination and endurance with safe, low-load activities. This requires an emphasis on the cognitive–kinesthetic awareness stage of motor control (44).

Clinical Pearl

Training Hints

1. Remind patients that limbering movements should be performed slowly and at different times throughout the day, especially in the morning.

2. Stabilization exercises should be performed slowly (up to 10 seconds per repetition) up to 10 repetitions at least once per day.

3. Approximately 6 weeks to 3 months are necessary to have a training effect.

4. Always have the patient demonstrate the exercise on the next office visit to correct any errors that they may have adopted.

5. Whenever possible, have the patients work toward mimicking activities that they do in real life as part of their exercise.

When a patient has a lot of MS with normal ranges of motion, especially if there is referred or radicular pain, the McKenzie approach of prescribing movements, which centralizes referred pain and avoids movements that peripheralize the symptoms, is strongly recommended. In disc patients, these movements often involve end-range positions such as extension. The key is to regularly re-check the patient's MS to confirm that the patient's overall FR is expanding.

Once the patient learns to move and position the spine in fundamental ways, then a progression to more complex exercises and functional activities can occur. There are always two aspects to the decision of whether a patient is ready to progress. The first is concerned with MS, and the second with AMC. The sooner in the program actual functional activities are trained the better, but it is necessary at each step that (a) MS is not increased, and (b) that motor control is re-educated. Stability training involves functional centration or "neutral posture" of key joints, normal respiration (i.e., no breath-holding), and avoidance of abnormal patterns of muscle substitution. If, for instance, an exercise increases MS by either peripheralizing symptoms or increasing painful ROMs on post-exercise auditing, then the correct introductory training has not been achieved. Similarly, even if MS is decreasing but the patient is not learning how to perform simple movement patterns with good form, he is not ready to progress.

Clinical Pearl

All patients require reactivation, but the specific exercises needed vary from individual to individual. Thus, the exercise prescription is not given to the patient on day 1, rather it is found over the course of care!

What follows is an atlas of the functional stability training exercises. Table 26.9 shows the exercise blueprint followed in the atlas. Table 26.10 lists the exercises which have a primarily tissue (spine) stabilizing function.

Table 26.9 Exercise Blueprint

- Indications
- Procedure
- Progressions
- Evaluation
  - Errors: Common errors observed by the clinician—AMC
  - Patient Audit: What the patient should feel—no MS
- Troubleshooting

Table 26.10 Tissue-Stabilizing Exercises

1. Cat camel
2. Bracing
3. Quadruped—bird dog
4. Side bridge
5. Dead bug
6. Curl-up
7. Bridge
8. Hamstring curls
9. Back extensions
10. Sphinx with chin tuck
11. Wall angel
12. Push-up

1. Cat-Camel

Indications

- LBP
- Lower back stiffness
- Warm-up

Procedure

- Kneel on all fours
- Explore "functional range" (FR) and find trunk flexion or extension bias
- Stay in FR. Bias the movement to the comfortable range.
- Gently mobilize in both directions (Fig. 26.2A and B). This should be slow and smooth. Breathe normally throughout.

Evaluation

Errors

- Moving outside of FR
- Stretching rather than gently mobilizing
- Bending elbows
- Hips not over knees

Patient Audit (What The Patient Should Feel)

- Reduction in low back stiffness

Troubleshooting

- Stay in patient's functional range (i.e., if flexion is painful limit exercise to pain-free ROM)

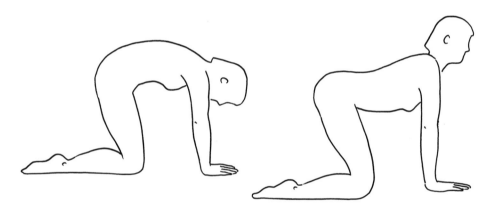

Figure 26.2 Cat-camel.

2. Bracing

Indications

- LBP
- Create a "safety margin" with all trunk exercises/activities

Procedure

- Explore "functional range" (FR) and find "neutral spine" posture—slight lordosis
- Tense muscles in 360° around the lower lumbar spine while continuing to breathe naturally
- Practice bracing in a variety of positions (supine, prone, quadruped, sitting, and standing)

Evaluation

Errors

- Moving outside of "neutral spine" posture by:
  ○ Posterior pelvic tilting
  ○ Kyphosing lumbar spine
  ○ Extending from thoraco-lumbar junction
- Holding the breathe

Patient Audit (What The Patient Should Feel)

- Tightening of the "core"

Progressions

- Once the patient has KA of bracing, challenge it by offering resistance to external perturbations (expected/unexpected, slow/fast) in different planes, especially the transverse plane
  ○ This works best in the Vleeming, Janda hip extension, quadruped, dead bug, and standing positions
- Add a more intense brace and heavy breathing challenge to exercises such as the abdominal curl and side bridge

Troubleshooting

- Have the patient relax the "core" and then gently press a few fingers lateral to medial into the side oblique muscles.
  ○ The patient should push with their muscles out into the clinician's fingers
- This can be tried with the anterior abdominal wall in all four quadrants
- It can be tried with the extensor muscles
- A more advanced version is to have the patient try to press out with the "core" muscles anteriorly and posteriorly simultaneously

3. Quadruped Leg Reach or Opposite Arm/Leg Reach (Bird Dog)

Indications

- LBP
- Faulty hip extension
- Poor trunk extensor endurance (Sorensen's test)
- Neck pain, whiplash, or headache associated with Co-C1 dysfunction

Procedure

- Quadruped leg reach: Pre-position spine in slight lordosis
- Perform abdominal brace
- Reach back or sweep the floor with the leg until the leg is in line the with back without arching or rotating the spine (Fig. 26.3A)
  - Start by keeping the foot along the ground until adequate lumbo-pelvic stability is mastered

Progression

- Quadruped opposite arm/leg reach: Perform with opposite arm and leg reaches (or sweeps) (Fig. 26.3B)
- Another progression is to approximate the knee and hand in the midline during the exercise
- Frontal or transverse plane arm raises (Fig. 26.4)

Evaluation

Errors

- Rounding the back
- Hyperextending the spine and poking the chin (Fig. 26.3C)
- Rotating the torso (Fig. 26.5A and B)
- Shrugging the shoulder
- Insufficient abdominal brace
- Breath-holding

Patient Audit (What The Patient Should Feel)

- Abdominal effort and balance challenge without low back strain

Troubleshooting

- Peel back to performing only a quadruped arm reach
- Put a water bottle or larger diameter object on the lower lumbar spine and have the subject try to balance it during the exercise
- Relax/lengthen the psoas
- Facilitate the abdominal brace with manual contact on the abdomen, or by offering perturbations to the trunk which the patient volitionally resists

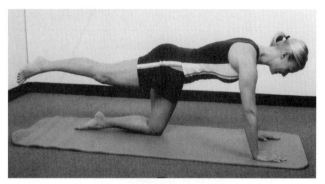

A

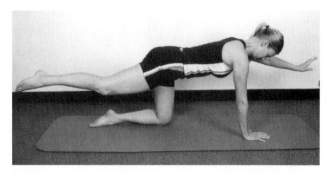

B

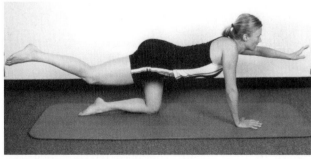

C

Figure 26.3 **(A)** Quad leg reach. **(B)** Quad opposite arm and leg reach. **(C)** Poor form, lumbar hyperextension and chin poking.

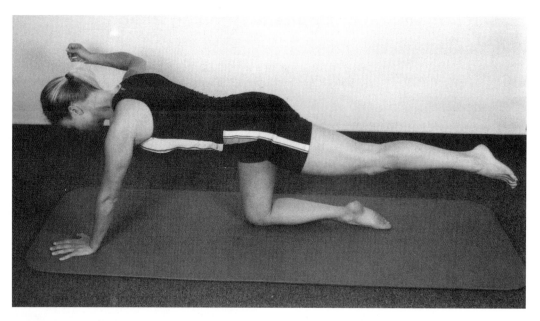

Figure 26.4 Transverse plane arm raises.

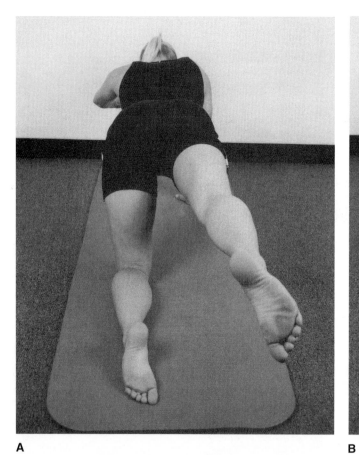

A

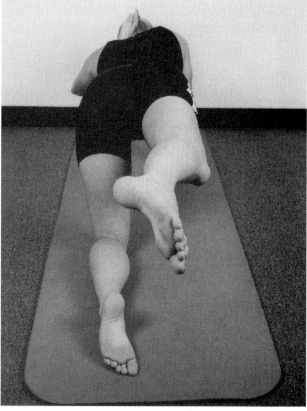

B

Figure 26.5 **(A)** Rotation controlled. **(B)** Over-rotated.

4. Side Bridge

Indications

- LBP
- Poor side bridge or abdominal endurance

Procedure (Fig. 26.6A and B)

- Side bridge on knees: begin side-lying, propped up on forearm
- Hips and knees should be bent slightly
- "Square" pelvis so that the spine is not sagging towards the floor
- Perform abdominal brace
- Then raise your hips up and forward until your knees, hips, and shoulders are aligned

Progression

- Perform side bridge on knees with a twist by slightly rolling body without torsioning at the lumbar spine
- Perform side bridge on ankles with body in a plank position (Fig. 26.7A and B)
- Perform rollover (Fig. 26.7C and D)
- During isometric hold, take a few deep breathes while maintaining abdominal brace
- Another alternative is to remain in the front plank position and perform a transverse plane arm reach (Fig. 26.8A and B)

Evaluation

Errors

- Rounding the back
- Raising the pelvis straight up without aligning the shoulder, hip, and knee
- On the ankle roll, excessive torsioning of the shoulders versus the pelvis (Fig. 26.7E)

Patient Audit (What The Patient Should Feel)

- Oblique abdominal effort without much shoulder discomfort

Troubleshooting

- Perform abdominal bracing
- Perform hip hinge from a kneeling position (Fig. 26.9A and B)
- Use both arms for support (Fig. 26.6C)
- If there is significant shoulder pain, buttress shoulder with opposite hand or perform plank roll standing and leaning against a wall

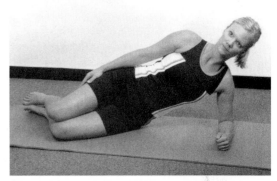

A

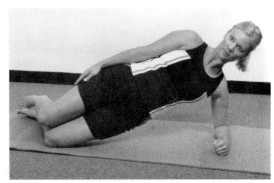

B

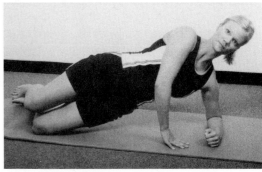

C

Figure 26.6 **(A)** Side bridge from knees, start position. **(B)** Side bridge from knees. **(C)** Side bridge, using hand for support.

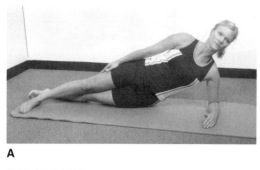

A

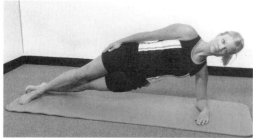

B

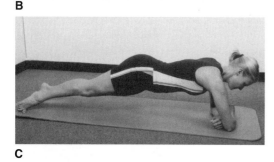

C

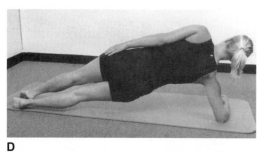

D

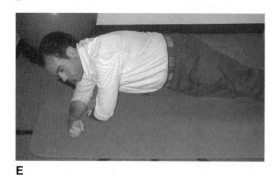

E

Figure 26.7 **(A)** side bridge from ankles, start position. **(B)** Side bridge from ankles. **(C)** Side bridge from ankles, with roll. **(D)** Side bridge from ankles, roll completed. **(E)** Side bridge from ankles, poor rolling with shoulder leading.

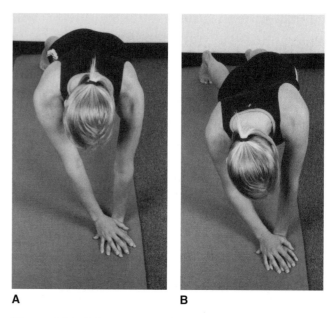

A   **B**

Figure 26.8 **(A)** Transverse plane arm reach with control. **(B)** Transverse plane arm reach, poor control.

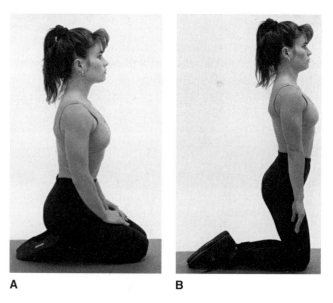

A   **B**

Figure 26.9 **(A)** Hip hinge from kneeling position, start position. **(B)** Hip hinge from kneeling position.

5. Dead Bug

Indications

- Subacute or chronic LBP problems
- Dysfunctional Vleeming's, abdominal, or side bridge function

Procedure

- Beginner dead bug: Lay on your back with right leg straight and left leg bent at the knee with foot on the floor
- Place the palm of right hand under the small of lower back
- Raise the left arm overhead supported on the floor
- Perform abdominal brace, without holding your breath
- Slowly draw the opposite arm and leg, which are straight, together over your abdomen (Fig. 26.10A and B)
- Bring them back to the start position

Progression

- Advanced dead bug: Perform with both feet off the floor (left bent 90° at the hip and knee) (Fig. 26.11A and B)
- Beginner and advanced dead bugs on half or full foam rolls (Figs. 26.12A and B, and 26.13)
- Dead bug with twist: perform dead bug with arms and legs slowly turning in opposite directions while maintaining firm abdominal brace while holding a medicine ball (Fig. 26.14)
- Dead bug on half or full foam: Perform with arms overhead holding a medicine ball (Figs. 26.15A and B, and 26.16)
  ◦ Be sure to "crunch" the lower ribs down without performing a posterior pelvic tilt
  ◦ Vary this by holding arm position and perform marching movement with legs
  ◦ Try to maintain "crunch" and move arms either further overhead or side to side

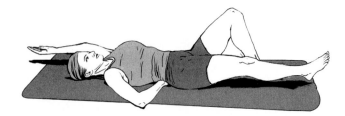

A

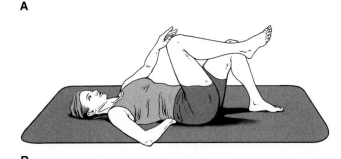

B

Figure 26.10 (A) Dead bug beginner, start position. Reproduced with permission from Liebenson CS. Spinal stabilization—an update. Part 3—training. J Bodywork Movement Ther 2004;8;2:286. **(B)** Dead bug beginner. Reproduced with permission from Liebenson CS. Spinal stabilization—an update. Part 3—training. J Bodywork Movement Ther 2004;8;2:286.

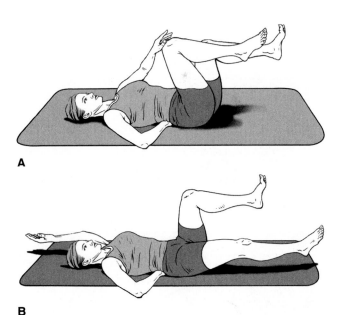

A

B

Figure 26.11 (A) dead bug advanced, start position. Reproduced with permission from Liebenson CS. Spinal stabilization–an update. Part 3—training. Journal of Bodywork and Movement Therapies, 8;2:287, 2004. **(B)** dead bug advanced. Reproduced with permission from Liebenson CS. Spinal stabilization—an update. Part 3—training. J Bodywork Movement Ther 2004;8;2:287.

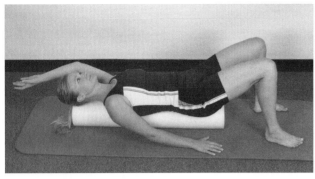

A

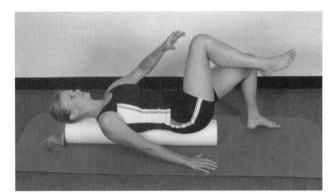

B

Figure 26.12 **(A)** Beginner dead bug on foam, start position. **(B)** Beginner dead bug on foam.

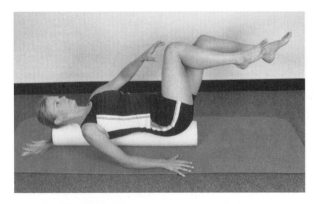

Figure 26.13 Advanced dead bug on foam.

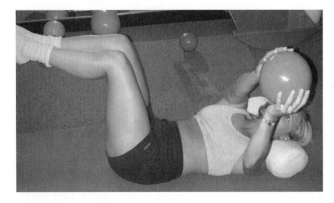

Figure 26.14 Dead bug with twist.

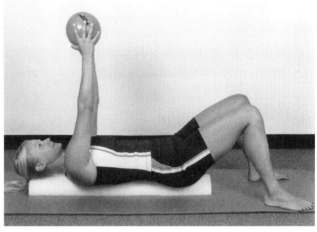

A

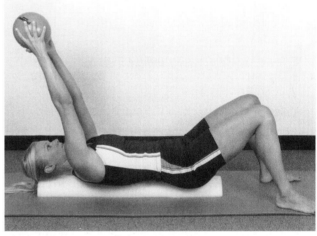

B

Figure 26.15 **(A)** Dead bug on foam with medicine ball, start position. **(B)** Dead bug on foam with medicine ball overhead.

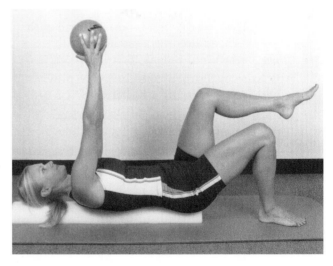

Figure 26.16 Dead bug on foam with medicine ball overhead, advanced.

Evaluation/Audit

Common Errors

- Letting go of abdominal brace or "crunch"
- Allowing back to extend too much

Patient Audit (What The Patient Should Feel)

- Abdominal effort, without lower back compression, ache, or strain

Troubleshooting (Complementary Treatments)

- Perform bracing of abdominal muscles by crunching lower ribs inferiorly (exhalation position) (Fig. 26.17A and B)
  - Avoid posterior pelvic tilting
  - Hold while breathing in and out
  - Avoid rounding shoulders or poking chin forward
- Perform isometric dead-bug with twist against manual resistance (Fig. 26.17C)
- Mobilize T4-8
- Inhibit/lengthen psoas
- Angle lunge with reach or pulley core twists

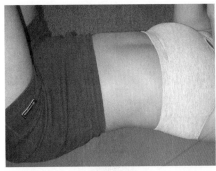

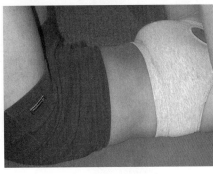

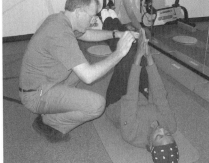

Figure 26.17 (**A**) Crunch start position with ribs elevation in inhalation position. (**B**) Crunch final position with ribs depressed in exhalation position. (**C**) Isometric dead bug with manual resistance.

6. Curl-up

Indications

- Subacute or chronic LBP (contraindicated in acute disc patients)
- Nerve root compression caused by spinal stenosis
- Poor abdominal or side bridge function

Procedure

- Basic: Place hands behind the small of back with elbows resting on mat
- One knee bent and one straight
- Perform abdominal brace
- Raise trunk up from point just below the shoulder blades, without flexing lower spine, hinging at the xiphoid (Fig. 26.18A)
- Reverse leg position half way through the set

Progression

- Advanced: Perform with elbows off mat (Fig. 26.18B)
  - Brace with abdominal muscles vigorously and perform a few deep exertional breaths
- Perform oblique curl up by lying on greater trochanter while performing crunch from the contralateral inferior-lateral rib cage (Fig. 26.19)

Evaluation/Audit

Common Errors

- Curling trunk or losing lumbar lordosis
- Sternocleidomastoid overactivity, chin jutting, or poking (Fig. 26.18C)

Patient Audit (What The Patient Should Feel)

- Abdominal effort without back strain

Troubleshooting (Complementary Treatments)

- Psoas inhibition/lengthening

Transverse plane facilitation (e.g., angle lunges with reaches or pulley twists)

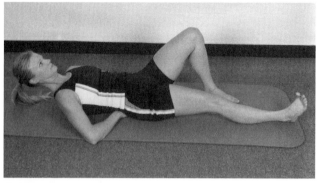

A

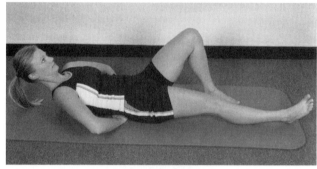

B

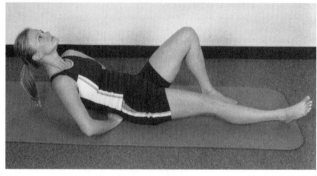

C

Figure 26.18 (**A**) Basic curl-up. (**B**) Advanced curl-up. (**C**) Curl-up, poor form—chin poke.

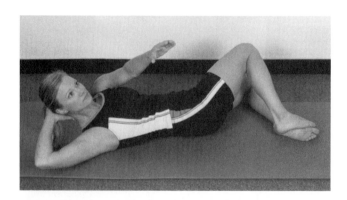

Figure 26.19 Oblique curl-up.

7. Bridge

Indications

- Subacute or chronic LBP
- Hip/knee or ankle pain
- Gluteus maximus insufficiency (also gluteus medius)
- Positive modified Thomas test

Procedure

- Bridge with band: Supine, hook lying position (feet under knees)
- Slightly externally rotate thighs
- Squeeze the gluts and slowly raise pelvis up
- This can be performed without a band, but to facilitate the gluteus maximus and medius, add resistance to thigh abduction and external rotation either manually or with a band (Fig. 26.20)

Progression

- Perform single leg bridge in an isometric manner by maintaining bridge while alternating lower leg raise (Fig. 26.21)
- Perform single leg bridge in an isotonic manner by bridging up and down on one leg

Evaluation/Audit

Common Errors

- Not squeezing gluts enough
- Hyperextending the low back
- Letting go of abdominal brace

Patient Audit (What The Patient Should Feel)

- Gluteal effort, without low back strain or hamstring cramping

Troubleshooting (Complementary Treatments)

- Increase resistance (manually or with band) to external rotation
- Brings heels closer to buttocks, particularly if hamstrings are overactive
- Inhibit or lengthen psoas
- Squats

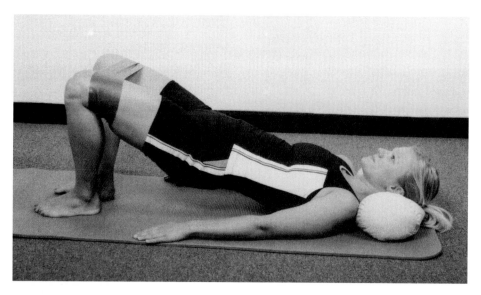

Figure 26.20 Bridge with band.

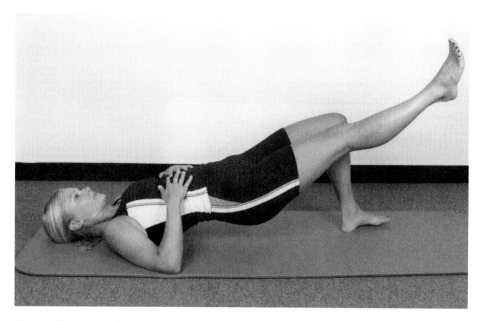

Figure 26.21 Single-leg bridge.

8. Hamstring Curls

Indications

- Knee pain
- Tight hamstrings

Procedure

- Hamstring curl start position: Straighten legs and place heels on apex of ball
- Co-contract gluteals and abdominals while maintaining "neutral" spine (slight lordosis) and bridge the pelvis up (Fig. 26.22A and B)
- Hamstring curl basic exercise: Once this elevated position can be held stable for a few repetitions, pull the ball toward buttocks with the heels by flexing the knees (Fig. 26.23A and B)

Progression

- Advanced hamstring curl: Start with knees flexed almost 90°
- Bridge up and pull heels closer to buttocks (Fig. 26.24A and B)
- Lower and return to start position
- Progress further by performing single leg hamstring curl in each of these positions (Fig. 26.25A and B)

Evaluation/Audit

Common Errors

- Not controlling the ball
- Hyperextending or kyphosing the lumbar spine

Patient Audit (What The Patient Should Feel)

- Effort should be felt primarily in the hamstrings along with the calf muscles

Troubleshooting (Complementary Treatments)

- Adjust the SIJ or fibular head
- Peel exercise back to simply bridging up and down instead of rolling the ball in

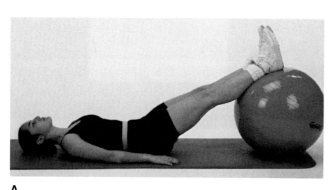
A

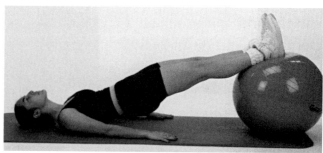
B

Figure 26.22 (A and B) Hamstring curl start position—bridging.

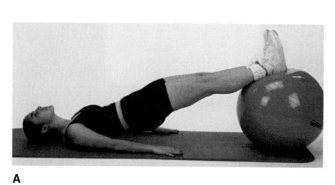
A

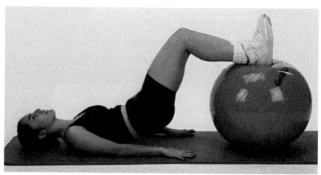
B

Figure 26.23 (A and B) Basic hamstring curl.

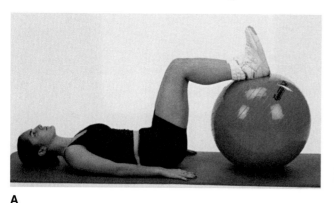
A

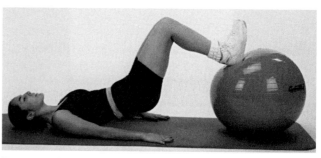
B

Figure 26.24 (A and B) Advanced hamstring curl.

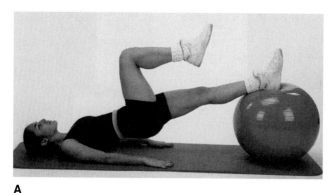
A

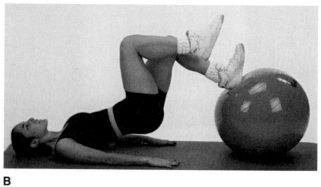
B

Figure 26.25 (A and B) Single-leg hamstring curl.

9. Back Extensions

Indications

- Subacute or chronic LBP
- Fail trunk extensor endurance test (Sorensen)
- Prevention of LBP

Procedure

- Beginner back extension: Begin nearly vertical with anterior superior iliac spine supported at edge of bench or support (Fig. 26.26A)
- Perform hip hinges while maintaining slight lumbar lordosis

Progression

- Gradually increase angle until horizontal position is tolerated (Figs. 26.26B and C)
- Alternative position:
  - Superman on ball: Perform over a gym ball with hip hinge used rather than spine extension to achieve horizontal position (Figs. 26.27A and B)
    - Arm position can be modified to simulate the Brügger exercise with forearm supination and finger abduction

Evaluation/Audit

Common Errors

- Hyperextending lumbar spine
- Kyphosing the lumbar spine

Patient Audit (What The Patient Should Feel)

- Hamstring and gluteal muscles working along with the back muscles

Troubleshooting (Complementary Treatments)

- Peel back to quadruped opposite arm and leg reach

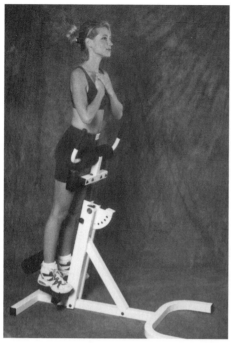

A

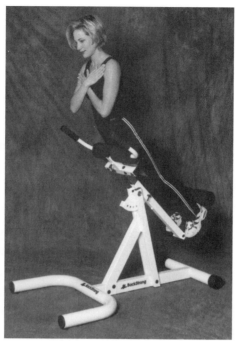

B

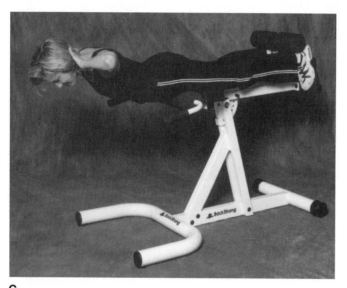

C

Figure 26.26 **(A)** Beginner back extension exercise. **(B)** Intermediate back extension exercise. **(C)** Advanced back extension exercise.

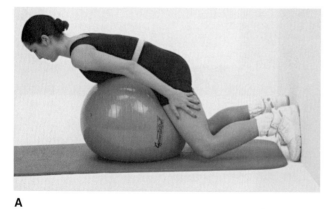

A

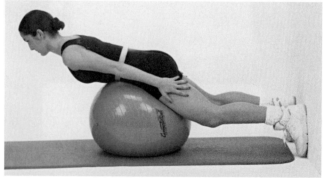

B

Figure 26.27 **(A and B)** Superman on ball.

10. Sphinx with Chin Tuck

Indications

- Neck pain
- Headache
- Whiplash

Procedure

- Prone sphinx with chin tuck: Lay prone propped up on forearms
- Allow upper back to sag down with shoulder blades retracting and shrugged, and chin jutting out (Fig. 26.28A)
- Glide head and neck back while nodding chin in, depressing and protracting scapulae (Fig. 26.28B)
- Hold this position while breathing normally and lengthening spine through the top of the head
- Nodding neck exercise: Throughout the day, perform the postural correction in upright positions by raising sternum, lengthening neck, and nodding chin (Figs. 26.29A and B).

Evaluation/Audit

Common Errors

- Not retracting scapulae to start with
- Substituting cervical retraction instead of gentle C0-C1 flexion (nodding)
- Not protracting or depressing scapulae

Patient Audit (What The Patient Should Feel)

- The ability to nod the head while gliding the head upward
- Shoulder blades coming together (retracting) to start exercise and then separating (protracting) in exercise's final position

Troubleshooting (Complementary Treatments)

- Mobilize T4-8
- Passively model nodding in a supine position
- Actively model nodding sitting or standing
- Mid-thoracic extension while maintaining the thorax in a caudal position (see Fig. 23.43).

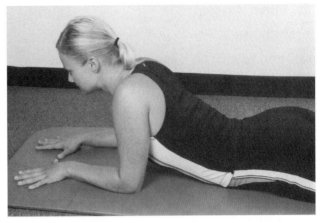

A

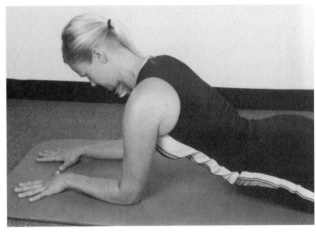

B

Figure 26.28 Prone sphinx with chin tuck: **(A)** beginning position and **(B)** final position.

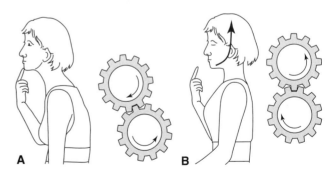

A   B

Figure 26.29 (A and B) Nodding neck exercise. Reproduced with permission from Liebenson CS. Functional reactivation for neck pain patients. J Bodywork Movement Ther 2002;6;1:68.

11. Wall Angel

Indications

- Shoulder or neck pain
- Failure during wall angel test
- Poor posture

Procedure (Fig. 26.30)

- Standing wall angel: Stand with feet approximately 4 inches from wall, shoulders back, and the arms, head, and buttocks flush against the wall
- Arms out to sides and bent at the elbows (cactus or "under arrest" position)
- Place radial side of wrist/hand on wall
- Flatten back against the wall with a sternal crunch

Progression

- Move flexed arms along wall up and down without shrugging shoulders or poking chin
- Perform with the wall slide (see Fig. 26.46).

Evaluation/Audit

Common Errors

- Ulnar contact instead of radial
- T/L not flat versus wall
- Shoulder shrugging

Patient Audit (What The Patient Should Feel)

- Mid back effort, without neck strain

Troubleshooting (Complementary Treatments)

- Mobilize T4-8
- Perform wall angel sitting on low stool or supine on floor to reduce effects of gravity

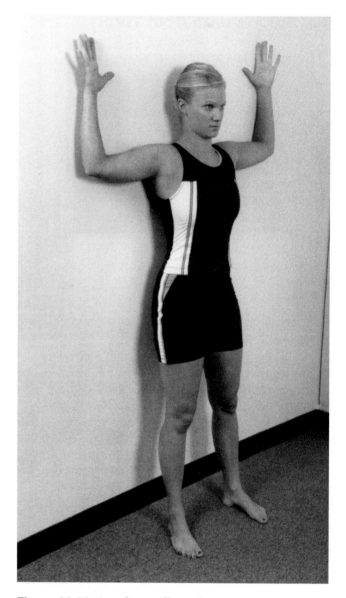

Figure 26.30 Standing wall angel.

12. Push-up

Indications

- Shoulder or upper quarter pain
- Failure in push-up test

Procedure

- All fours rock: In quadruped position perform a push-up
- When finishing the push-up, perform a full protraction (push up with plus) (Fig. 26.31A–C)
- Rock side to side, hand to heel, and diagonally

Progression

- Perform push-up with a plus in tripod position on one hand
- Perform push-up with a plus with legs on ball (Figs. 26.32A and B)

Evaluation/Audit

Common Errors

- Kyphosing
- Not protracting fully
- Poking chin

Patient Audit (What The Patient Should Feel)

- Upper back effort

Troubleshooting (Complementary Treatments)

- Perform push-up with a plus versus wall (Fig. 26.33A–C)

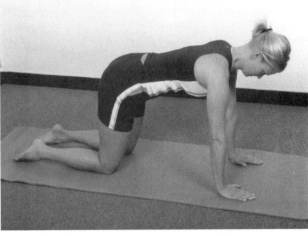

A

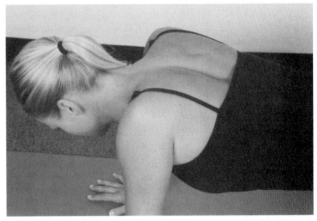

B

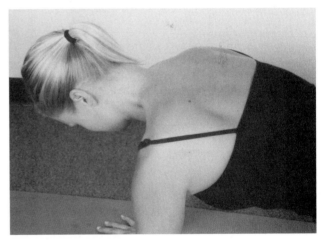

C

Figure 26.31 **(A)** Isometric push-up: all fours rock, beginning position. **(B)** Scapular motion only: retraction. **(C)** Scapular motion only: protraction.

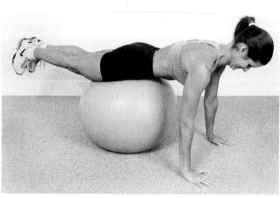
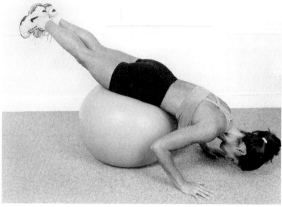

A

B

Figure 26.32 (A) Push-up with a plus on ball—start. Reproduced with permission from DeFranca C, Liebenson CS. The Upper Body Book. San Diego, CA: The Gym Ball Store, 2001. **(B)** Push-up with a plus on ball—end. Reproduced with permission from DeFranca C, Liebenson CS. The Upper Body Book. San Diego, CA: The Gym Ball Store, 2001.

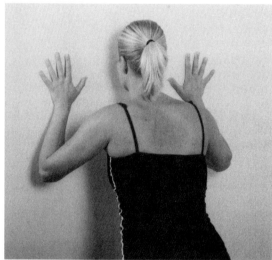

B

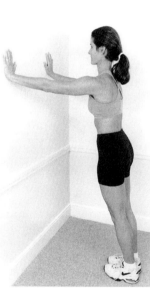

A

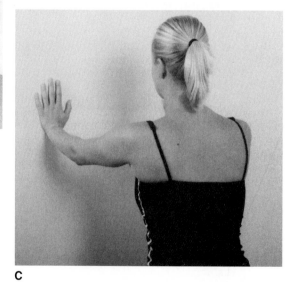

C

Figure 26.33 (A) Push-up with a plus vs. wall. Reproduced with permission from DeFranca C, Liebenson CS. The Upper Body Book. San Diego, CA: The Gym Ball Store, 2001. **(B)**–Push-up on wall, retraction. **(C)**–Push-up on wall, protraction.

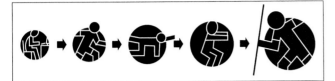

Figure 26.34 Reactivation–reconditioning continuum.

Functional Integrated Training (FIT)

Practice-Based Problem

How can we make training as functional as possible so it will stabilize the patient in the home and during sport and occupational activities?

Functional stability training is goal-oriented. Nonfunctional positions such as recumbent may be used as stepping stones to isolate and "groove" stability patterns. However, as soon as possible, "core" stability must be trained in exercises mimicking the demands the patient faces in during home, occupational, and recreational activities.

The sooner in the program actual functional activities are trained, the better. But it is necessary at each step that the movement is in the patient's functional range—reducing MS and AMC—while being as functional as possible.

Unless functional training occurs, there is no guarantee that the individual will be stable during "real world" challenges. Examples of functional training include squats, lunges, pushing, pulling, catching, carrying, etc. For more fit individuals, and to enhance performance or prevent injury in demanding sports or occupations, stability patterns may be further challenged by the addition of unstable surfaces such as balance boards and gymnastic balls. This provides enhanced proprioceptive stimulation that facilitates motor learning.

Clinical Pearl

Morgan emphasizes the motor control aspects of identifying the patient's functional range.

"After the patient has learned the limits of his or her functional range, conditioning and training for activities of daily living can safely begin . . . The patient must develop the coordination to control and feel the back position. Such coordination must become second nature so that the habit is maintained during all activities . . ."

Morgan D. Concepts in functional training and postural stabilization for the low-back-injured. Top Acute Care Trauma Rehabil 1988;2:8–17.

Reactivation progressions should continue until the patient's FR includes home, sports, and occupational demands (Fig. 26.34). Athletes will require high-level performance training, which will also include strength/power, agility, and speed challenges. These would be superimposed on the three levels of training already described. A frequent training error in programs designed for highly fit individuals is the performance of trunk or spine exercises with high-level strength or agility demands, without proper motor control. A step-wise approach built on a foundation of conscious–kinesthetic awareness of appropriate motor control is the best guarantee of injury prevention when performing high-level activities with a narrow safety/stability margin. Table 26.11 lists exercises that are functionally oriented.

Table 26.11 Functional Training Exercises

1. Sensory motor training
2. Squat
3. Lunge
4. Functional (balance) reach
5. Pulley
6. Core resistance

1. Sensory Motor Training

Indications

- Poor posture (e.g., wall angel)
- Poor balance (one-leg standing test)
- Lower quarter pain

Procedure

- The small foot: For all balance exercises, if hyperpronation is present, pre-position in subtalar neutral by having the patient grip with their toes, slightly externally rotate hips, or perform a "small foot" (approximation of medial calcaneus and great toe to raise the longitudinal arch) (Fig. 26.35A)
  - The clinician may assist the formation of the small foot by passively modeling or actively assisting it (Fig. 26.35B)
- Janda/Vele forward lean: maintain corrected upright posture and then sway forward without lifting heels (Fig. 26.36A and B)
  - Practice side-to-side sways as well

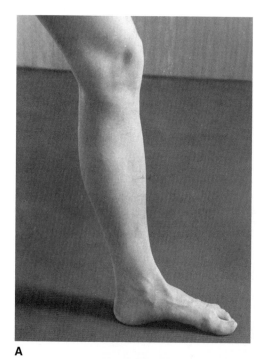

A

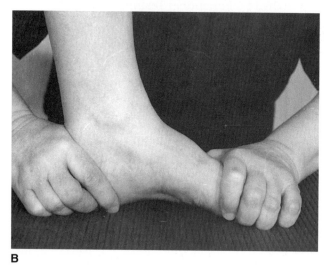

B

Figure 26.35 **(A)** Active small foot formation. **(B)** Passive modeling of small foot.

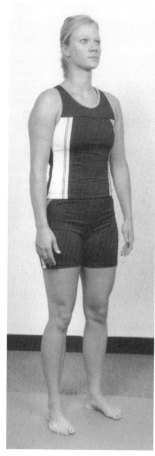 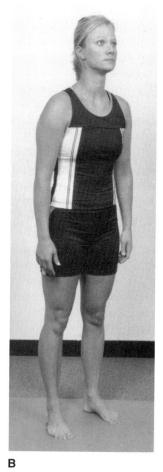

A **B**

Figure 26.36 **(A)** Vele/Janda forward lean, start position. **(B)** Vele/Janda forward lean.

- Perform tandem stance exercises (heel to toe) with eyes open (EO) and eyes closed (EC) (Fig. 26.37)
- Single leg stance (Fig. 26.38A and B)
  - Start in doorway EO
  - Progress to EC

Progression

- Progress floor balance exercises to foam pads of varying stiffness (Fig. 26.39A and B)
- Progress to balance board training (Fig. 26.40)
  - Start in sagittal plane
    - Rock board back and forth from ankle joint
    - Progress to holding board still and finally to standing on one leg with board static
  - Progress to oblique and frontal planes and then finally to wobble board
  - Step-ups on rocker (sagittal) or wobble board
  - Static hold with single arm raise over head with light weight in hand
- Balance sandals (Fig. 26.41A and B)
  - Tiny steps, raising knees
  - March in place
  - Progress to forward/backwards/sideways

Evaluation/Audit

Common Errors

- Rocker board sagittal hinging from waist, not ankle
- Subtalar hyperpronation
- Sandals—toes lift; sandal not horizontal

Patient Audit (What The Patient Should Feel):

- On forward lean: toes gripping
- Rocker board: calves
- Balance sandals: gluteal muscles

Troubleshooting (Complementary Treatments)

- Passive modeling and active assistance of "small" foot (subtalar neutral)
  - If necessary, add facilitation by lightly stroking the skin with a brush or fingernails
- Single-leg stance can be "peeled back" to tandem stance or double stance if AMC is present

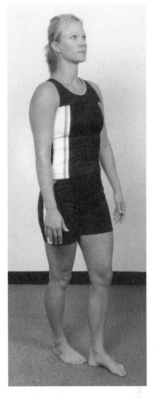

Figure 26.37 Tandem stance.

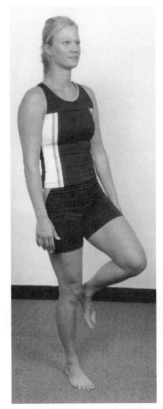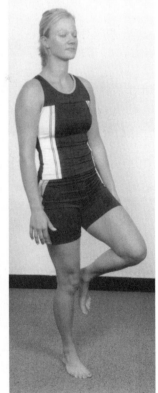

A   B

Figure 26.38 (A and B) Single-leg stance.

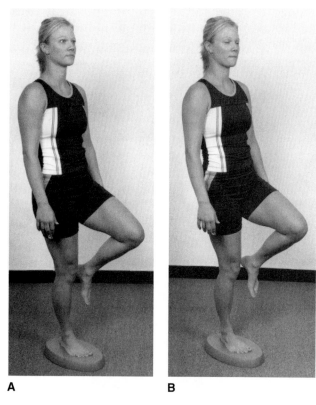

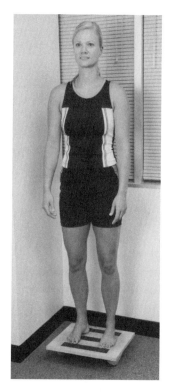

A   **B**

Figure 26.39 (A and B) Single-leg stance, labile surface.

Figure 26.40 Rocker board training.

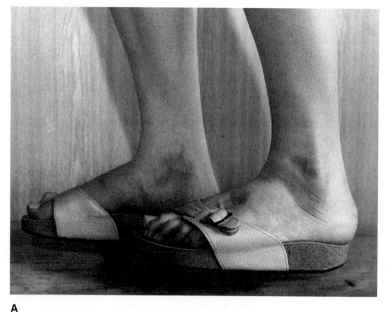

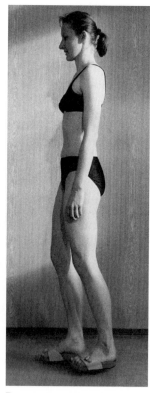

A

Figure 26.41 (A) Standing on balance sandals. **(B)** Walking with balance sandals.

B

2. Squat

Indications

- Poor posture (e.g., positive wall angel)
- Dysfunctional hip extension, abduction, squats/lunges, or balance
- LBP, especially disc problems
- Lower quarter pain
- Preventive functional training and performance enhancement

Procedure

- Perform hip hinge while rising from a chair
  - Correct and incorrect (Fig. 26.42A and B)
- Perform various squats with feet shoulder-width apart
  - Squat with gym ball (easiest)
    - maintain lumbar lordosis by keeping sacrum in contact with the gym ball (Fig. 26.43A and B)
  - Squat facing wall (Fig. 26.44A and B)
    - arms overhead to maintain lumbar lordosis
  - Squat with back to wall
    - reach for wall with gluteals
    - find furthest position from the wall where balance can be maintained and the wall can still be reached
    - Correct and incorrect (Fig. 26.45A and B)

Progressions

- Wall slide (Fig. 26.46A and B)
  - start in wall angel position; maintain hand position
  - perform abdominal crunch from lower ribs and slide down wall to simultaneously stretch the latissimus dorsi
- Perform squat on labile surface (Fig. 26.44C)
- Perform single leg squat facing the wall (Fig. 26.47A and B)
  - maintain lordosis
  - keep pelvis level
  - keep knee from passing anterior to toes

Evaluation/Audit

Common Errors

- Losing lordosis
- Poor balance on heels
- Valgosity of knees and hyperpronation of the feet (Fig. 26.48A)
- Patello-femoral shear (Fig. 26.48B)
- Single-leg squat
  - Valgosity (Fig. 26.49A)
  - Trendelenberg (Fig. 26.49B)
  - Trunk flexion
  - Hyperpronation (Fig. 26.49C)

Patient Audit (What The Patient Should Feel)

- Gluteal effort without back strain

Troubleshooting (Complementary Treatments)

- Mobilize T4-8
- Inhibit/lengthen adductors
- Add resistance band to thighs to facilitate external rotation of hips (Fig. 26.45C)
- Actively brace with abdominals to reduce lower back strain and hyperextension
- Peel back to bridges
- Clam shells
- Sensory motor training
- Wall ball

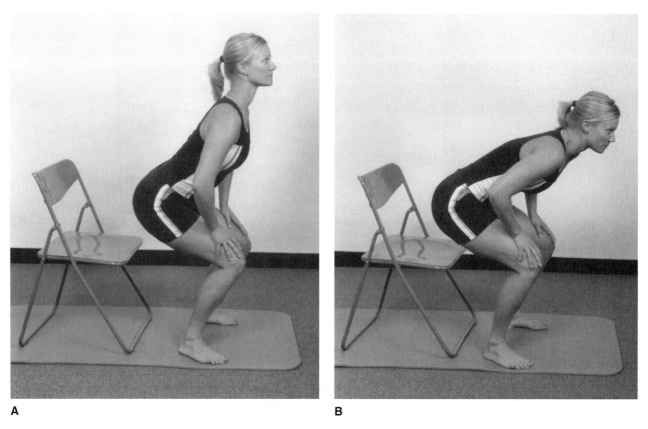

A   B

Figure 26.42 **(A)** Hip hinge, correct. **(B)** Hip hinge, incorrect.

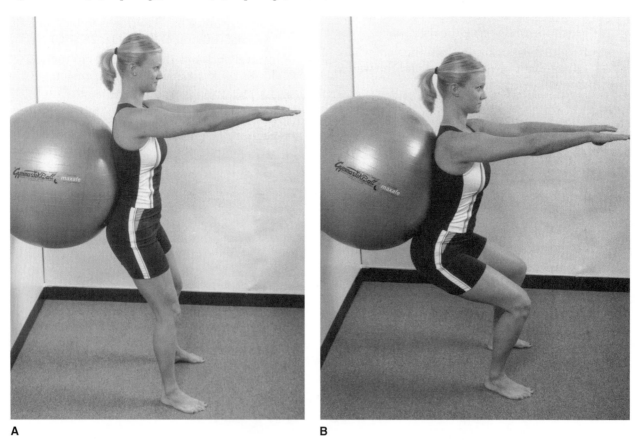

A   B

Figure 26.43 **(A)** Ball squat, start position, **(B)** Ball squat.

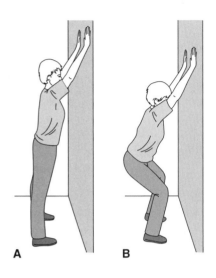

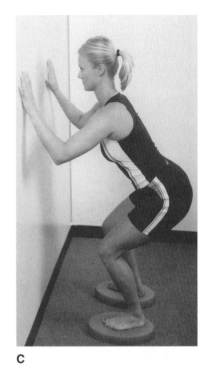

Figure 26.44 **(A)** Squat facing wall, start position. Reproduced with permission from Liebenson CS. Activity modification advice: Part II—squats. Journal of Bodywork and Movement Therapies, 7;4:229, 2003. **(B)** Squat facing wall. Reproduced with permission from Liebenson CS. Activity modification advice: Part II—squats. Journal of Bodywork and Movement Therapies, 7;4:229, 2003. **(C)** Squat facing wall, on foam pads.

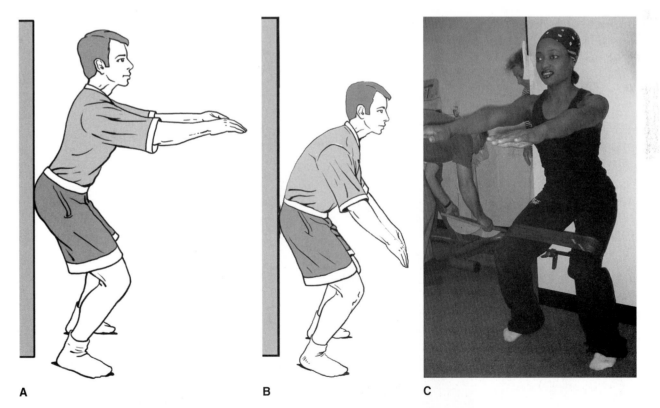

Figure 26.45 **(A)** Squat with back to wall. **(B)** Squat with back to wall—incorrect form. **(C)** Squat with band resistance.

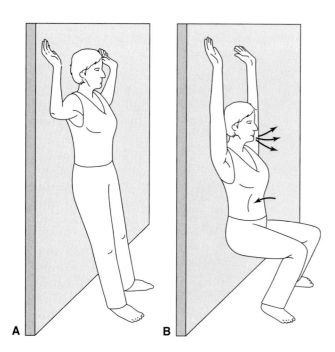

Figure 26.46 (A) Wall slide, start position. Reproduced with permission from Liebenson CS. Mid-thoracic dysfunction (Part Three): Clinical Issues. J Bodywork Movement Ther 2001;5;269. **(B)** Wall slide. Reproduced with permission from Liebenson CS. Mid-thoracic dysfunction (Part Three): Clinical Issues. J Bodywork Movement Ther 2001;5;269.

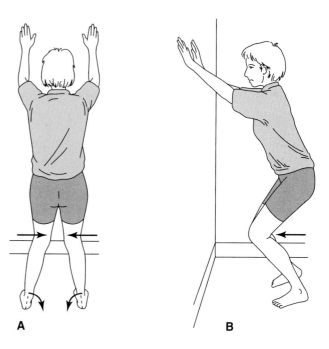

Figure 26.48 (A) Squat, valgus and hyperpronation. Reproduced with permission from Liebenson CS. Activity modification advice: Part II—squats. J Bodywork Movement Ther 2003;7;4:228–232. **(B)** Squat, patello-femoral shear. Reproduced with permission from Liebenson CS. Activity modification advice: Part II—squats. J Bodywork Movement Ther 2003;7;4:228–232.

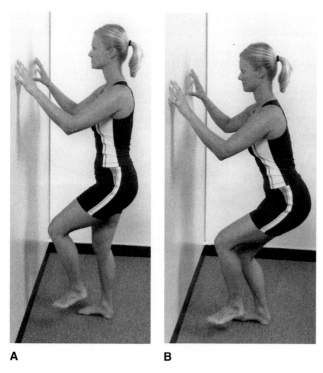

Figure 26.47 (A) Single-leg squat, start position. **(B)** Single-leg squat.

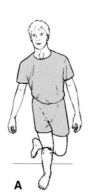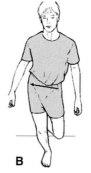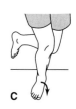

Figure 26.49 (A) Single-leg squat with valgosity. Reproduced with permission from Liebenson CS. Functional exercises. J Bodywork Movement Ther 2002;6:111. **(B)**–Single-leg squat with Trendelenberg sign. Reproduced with permission from Liebenson CS. Functional exercises. J Bodywork Movement Ther 2002;6:111. **(C)** Single-leg squat with hyperpronation. Reproduced with permission from Liebenson CS. Functional exercises. J Bodywork Movement Ther 2002;6:110.

3. Lunge

Indications

- Subacute or chronic LBP
- Hip/knee or ankle pain
- Gluteus maximus insufficiency or dysfunctional squats/lunges or balance
- Positive modified Thomas test
- Preventive functional training
- Performance enhancement

Procedure

- Forward lean and step (Janda lunge)
  - See forward lean and sway under Sensory–Motor section
  - Lean forward slowly (Fig. 26.50A)
  - When heels begin to lift, step forward
  - Land softly without knee passing forward of toes (Fig. 26.50B)
  - Keep body in straight line from back heel to hip to shoulder
  - Rear leg should bent at knee and forefoot
- Use star diagram to guide lunges at different angles—forward lunge (Fig. 26.51A)
- Add arm motions to "groove" normal movement patterns
  - Arms overhead to facilitate lordosis on forward lunge with arms overhead (Fig. 26.51B)
  - Angle lunge with reach: arm reach (push) across body to facilitate supination of contralateral subtalar joint and external rotation of lower limb (Fig. 26.52)
  - Backhand or frisbee toss: arm reach (pull) away from body to facilitate supination of ipsilateral subtalar joint and external rotation of lower limb (Fig. 26.53A and B). Also facilitates ipsilateral scapular retraction and extension of the thoracic spine

Evaluation/Audit

Common Errors

- Lumbar kyphosis (Fig. 26.51C)
- Subtalar hyperpronation
- Poor balance or weight shifting ability

Patient Audit (What The Patient Should Feel)

- Hip stretch, without knee pain

Troubleshooting (Complementary Treatments)

- Mobilize T4-8
- Inhibit/lengthen psoas
- Squats
- Peel back to forward lean with step

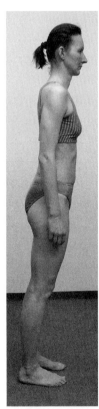
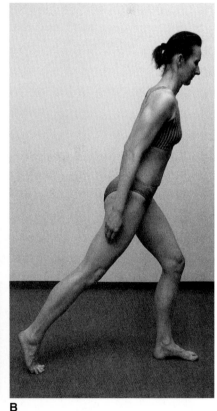

A   B

Figure 26.50 (A) Forward lean. (B) Forward lean with step (Janda lunge).

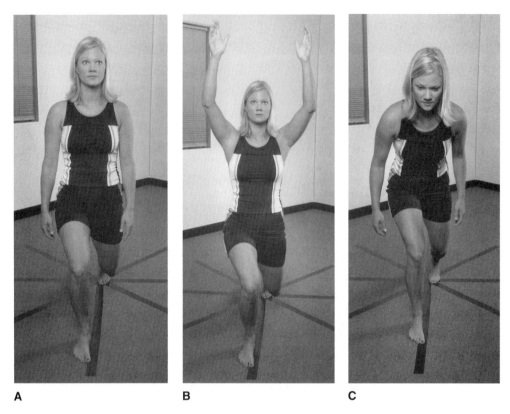

A   B   C

Figure 26.51 **(A)** Forward lunge. **(B)** Forward lunge with arms overhead. **(C)** Forward lunge with kyphosis.

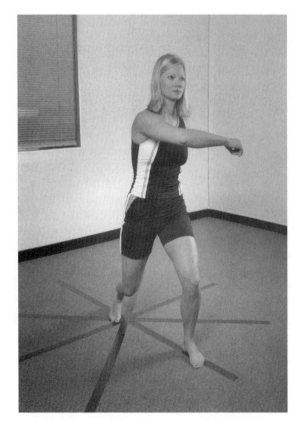

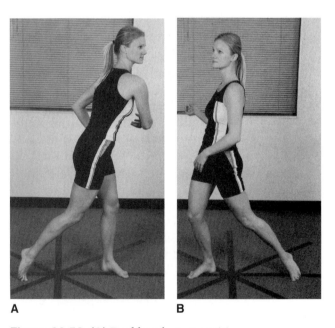

A   B

Figure 26.53 **(A)** Backhand, start position. **(B)** Backhand.

Figure 26.52 Angle lunge with reach (push).

4. Functional (Balance) Reach

Indications

- Subacute or chronic LBP, hip/knee, or ankle pain
- Gluteus maximus or medius insufficiency
- + modified Thomas test
- Preventive functional training and performance enhancement

Procedure

- Stand on star diagram and reach at different angles with leg (Fig. 26.54A–D)

Progressions

- Perform combined arm and leg motions (running man) (Fig. 26.55A and B)
- Add resistance from pulley (Fig. 26.56A and B)

Evaluation/Audit

Common Errors

- Trendelenberg position
- Loss of balance

Patient Audit (What The Patient Should Feel)

- Gluteal effort, without knee or back strain

Troubleshooting (Complementary Treatments)

- Perform functional reach with support (see Fig. 34.22L)
- Mobilize T4-8
- Inhibit/lengthen psoas
- Two- or one-leg squats
- Lunges
- Sister Kenny facilitation of gluteus medius (Fig. 19.71)
- Clam shell exercise (Fig. 26.57A and B)
- Wall ball (Fig. 26.58A and B)
- One-leg bridges

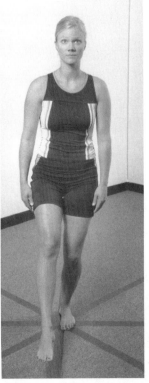
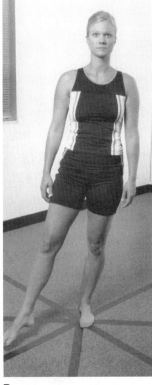

A   B

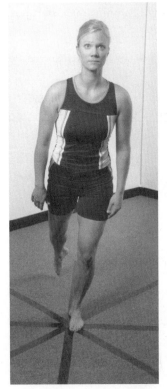
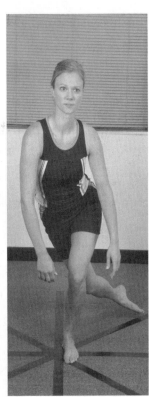

C   D

Figure 26.54 (**A**) Balance reach, forward. (**B**) Balance reach, antero-lateral. (**C**) Balance reach, posterior. (**D**) Balance reach, postero-lateral (bowler position).

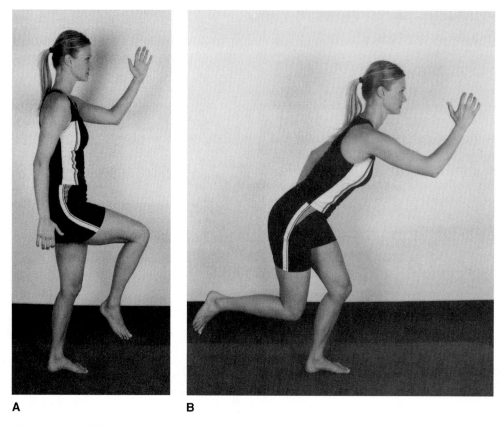

Figure 26.55 **(A)** Running man, start position. **(B)** Running man.

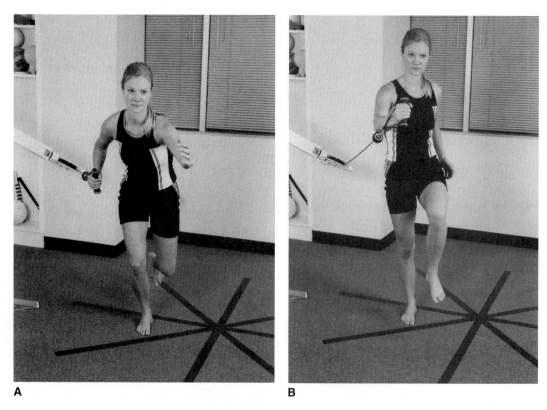

Figure 26.56 **(A)** Running man with cable, start position. **(B)** Running man with cable.

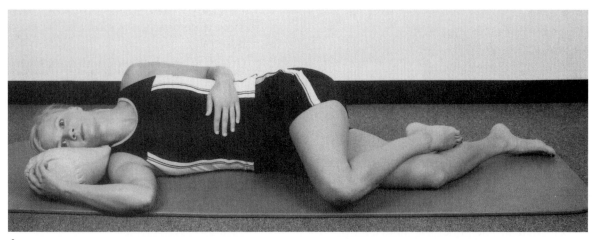

A

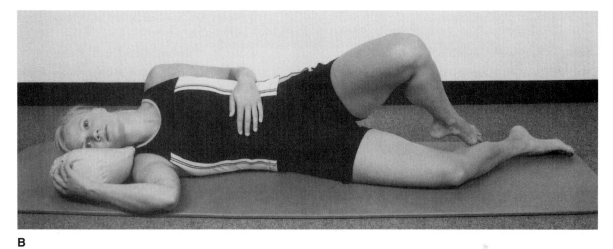

B

Figure 26.57 **(A)** Clam shell, start position. **(B)** Clam shell.

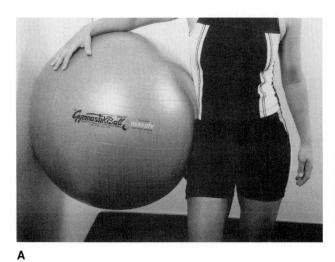

A

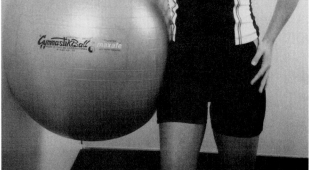

B

Figure 26.58 **(A)** Wall ball, start position. **(B)** Wall ball.

5. Pulley

Indications

- Back or upper quarter pain
- Preventative functional training or performance enhancement

Procedure

- Punch with step (pushes) (Fig. 26.59A and B)
  - Stand in a semi-squat position
  - Ensure that the pulley is not above shoulder level and that the patient is not shrugging shoulders
  - Perform a simple punching maneuver
  - Emphasize motion in the back hip
- Sword (pulls) proprioceptive neuromuscular facilitation (PNF) motion (Fig. 26.60A and B)
  - Rotate forearm externally during motion
  - As arm moves away from body, be sure that the hand leads the elbow to avoid deltoid over-activation and resultant shoulder impingement
- Seatbelt PNF motion (Fig. 26.61A and B)
- "Lawn mower" pulls (Fig. 26.62A and B)

Progressions

- Single-leg weight shifts
  - Standing on one leg, hold pulley handle and perform weight shift as if pushing or pulling (Fig. 26.63A and B)
  - Perform with little or no arm motion
  - Should feel this in the hip, especially the gluteus medius
- "Wood chop" down (Fig. 26.64A and B)
- "Wood chop" up (Fig. 26.65A and B)
- Core "pull"(Fig. 26.66A and B)
  - Keep arm at side and use trunk muscles and hip motion
  - Progress by adding shoulder external rotation (Fig. 26-66C)
- Core "punch" (Fig. 26.67A and B)
  - Keep arm at side and use trunk muscles and hip motion
  - Progress by adding shoulder internal rotation

- Push/pull core twist
  - Start in semi-squat position with elbows flexed 90°
  - Grasp pulley handle in both hands
  - Perform turning motion from hips and shoulders back and forth
  - Avoid twisting pelvis against the shoulders (e.g., twisting the spine)
- Pull downs (Fig. 26.68A–E)
  - Two legs and one leg
  - Kneeling
  - Maintain lordosis and perform as hip hinge with lower rib crunch
- Sport specific activities
  - Pushes (tennis forehand, overhand throw, volleyball spike)
  - Pulls (tennis backhand, golf swing)

Evaluation/Audit

Common Errors

- Starting in a slump posture
- Shoulder shrugging
- Poor balance at the end of the motion
- Pelvic or shoulder unleveling during the exercise
- Failure to supinate the lower quarter kinetic chain of the front leg

Patient Audit (What The Patient Should Feel)

- Shoulders, trunk, and hip/pelvis are turning as a unit
- With higher weights abdominal effort

Troubleshooting (Complementary Treatments)

- Mobilize T4-8
- Inhibit/lengthen psoas of back leg
- Angle lunge

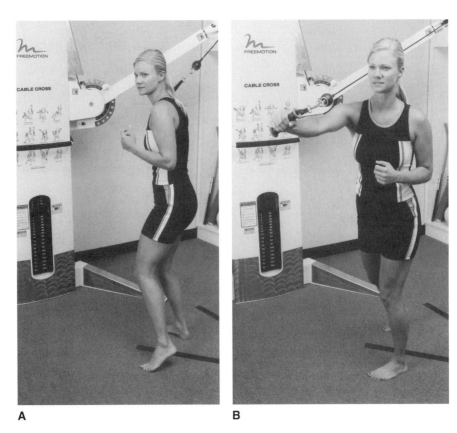

A   B

Figure 26.59 **(A)** Punch with step, start position. **(B)** Punch.

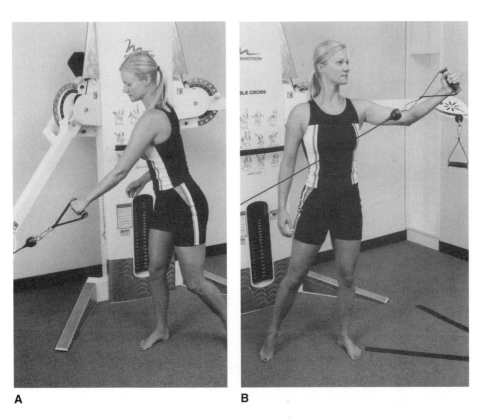

A   B

Figure 26.60 **(A)** Sword, start position. **(B)** Sword.

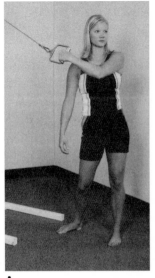
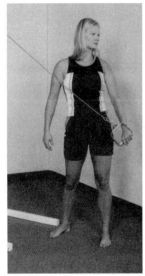

A B

Figure 26.61 **(A)** Seatbelt, start position. **(B)** Seatbelt.

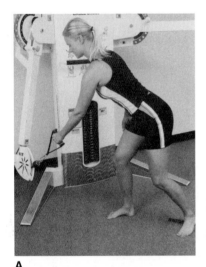
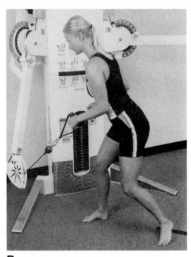

A B

Figure 26.62 **(A)** Lawnmower, start position. **(B)** Lawnmower.

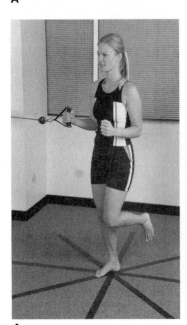
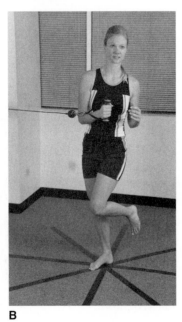

A B

Figure 26.63 **(A)** Single-leg weight shift during punch, start. **(B)** Single-leg weight shift during punch.

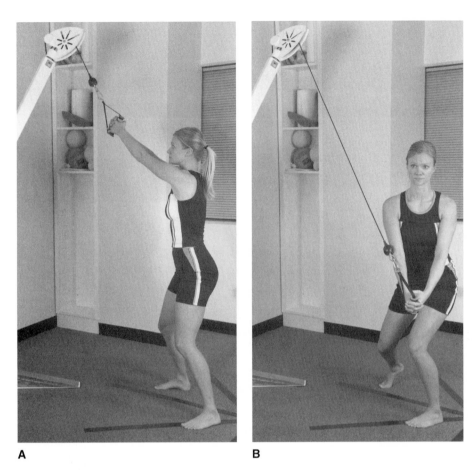

Figure 26.64 **(A)** Woodchop down, start position. **(B)** Woodchop down, end position.

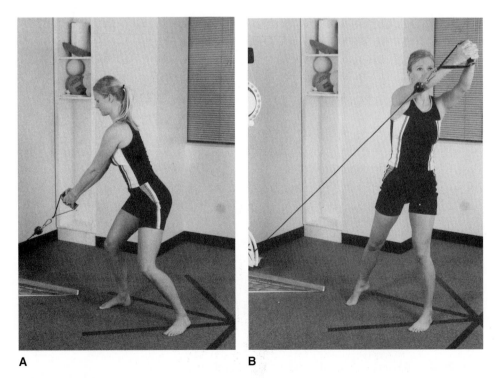

Figure 26.65 **(A)** Woodchop up, start position. **(B)** Woodchop up, end position.

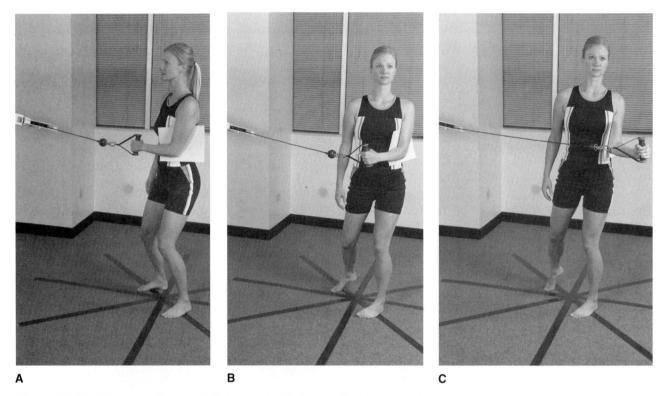

A   B   C

Figure 26.66 **(A)** Core pull, start. **(B)** Core pull. **(C)** Core pull with external rotation.

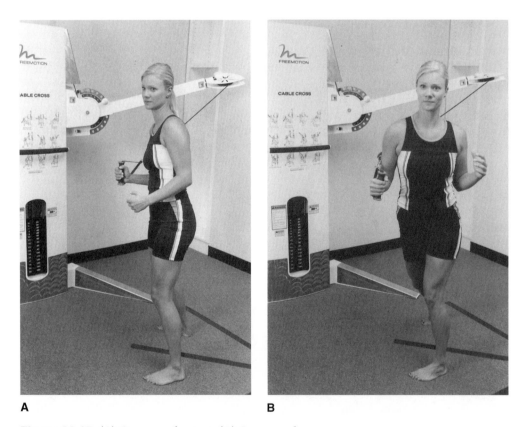

A   B

Figure 26.67 **(A)** Core punch, start. **(B)** Core punch.

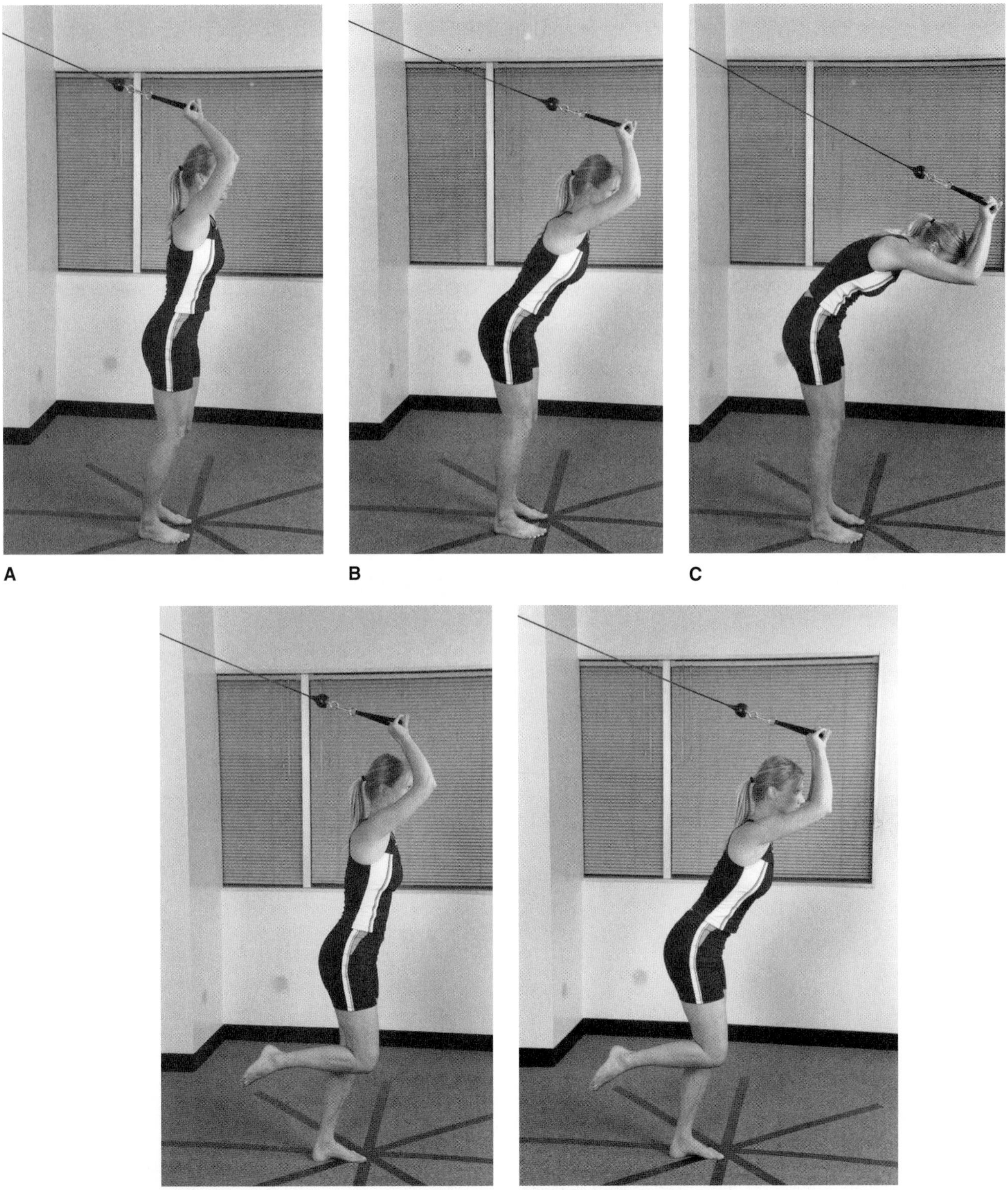

A B C D E

Figure 26.68 **(A)** Pull down, start. **(B)** Pull down, correct position. **(C)** Pull down, incorrect position. **(D)** Single leg pull down, start. **(E)** Single leg pull down.

6. Core Resistance

Indications

- Vleeming's test positive
- One-leg standing balance test positive
- Side-bridge or abdominal endurance tests positive
- Advanced exercise for preventive functional training or performance enhancement

Procedure

- Stand on Bosu and balance
  - Perform mini-squats
  - Cue firm abdominal bracing and then offer manual resistance through hands or stick (vertical or horizontal) (Fig. 26.69A)

Evaluation/Audit

Common Errors

- Poor balance
- Shoulder shrugging on resistance
- Insufficient bracing

Patient Audit (What The Patient Should Feel)

- Abdominal effort with resistance

Troubleshooting (Complementary Treatments)

- Train on rocker boards
- Squats/bridges
- Peel-back to dead bugs with resistance (manually or with stick) and stick resistance in squat position without Bosu (Fig. 26.69B)

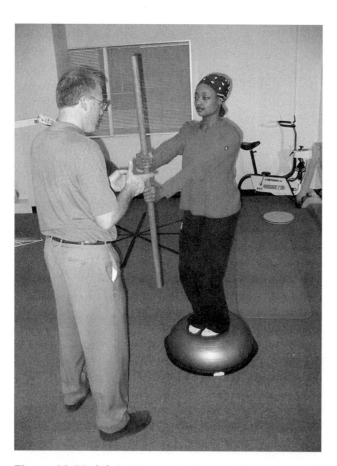
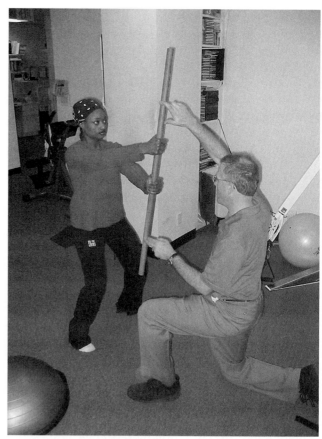

Figure 26.69 **(A)** Semi-squat on Bosu with resistance challenge. **(B)** Squat with resistance challenge via stick.

■ CONCLUSION

Therapeutic exercise should be safe and effective. Motor control exercise places the emphasis on wide margins of stability, endurance training, and functional activities. Such a program is easy to incorporate into the clinical setting, requiring little in the way of costly equipment. Supervision is required to weed out AMC and determine the specific routine that reduces the patient's AIs and MS. The ultimate goal of such training is that the patient learns a self-care program that they are motivated to continue with long after their supervised regimen ends.

Audit Process
Self-Check of the Chapter's Learning Objectives

- What are the indications for squat and lunge training?
- What is the breathing advice during functional–stability training?
- How is muscular endurance training different from strength training?
- What should a patient feel during the dead bug exercises?
- Besides increasing sets, repetitions, and resistance, how can functional–stability exercises be progressed?
- If the side bridge is difficult for a patient to perform, what troubleshooting options exist?

■ REFERENCES

1. Adams MA, Dolan P. Recent advances in lumbar spine mechanics and their clinical significance. Clin Biomech 1995;10:3–19.
2. Andersson GBJ, Winters JM. Role of muscle in postural tasks: spinal loading and postural stability. In: Winters JM, Woo SL-Y, eds. Multiple Muscle Systems. New York: Springer-Verlag, 1990:375–395.
3. Butler D, Moseley L. Explain Pain. Adelaide, Australia: Noigroup Publications, 2003.
4. Carlson H, Nilsson J, Thorstensson A, Zomlefer MR. Motor responses in the human trunk due to load perturbations. Acta Physiol Scand 1981;111:221–223.
5. Cholewicki J, McGill SM. Mechanical stability of the in vivo lumbar spine: Implications for injury and chronic low back pain, Clin Biomech 1996;11:1–15.
6. Cholewicki J, Panjabi MM, Khachatryan A. Stabilizing function of the trunk flexor-extensor muscles around a neutral spine posture. Spine 1997;22:2207–2212.
7. Cholewicki J, Simons APD, Radebold A. Effects of external loads on lumbar spine stability. J Biomechan 2000;33:1377–1385.
8. Ciccione DS, Just N. Pain expectancy and work disability in patients with acute and chronic pain: A test of the fear avoidance hypothesis. J Pain 2001;2:181–194.
9. Cresswell AG, Oddsson L, Thorstensson A. The influence of sudden perturbations on trunk muscle activity and intraabdominal pressure while standing. Exp Brain Res 1994;98:336–341.
10. Crombez G, Vlaeyen JW, Heuts PH, et al. Pain-related fear is more disabling than pain itself: evidence on the role of pain-related fear in chronic back pain disability. Pain 1999;80:329–339.
11. Fordyce WE, Brockway JA, Bergman JA, Spengler D. Acute back pain: a control-group comparison of behavioral vs traditional management methods. J Behav Med 1986;9:127–140.
12. Gardner-Morse MG, Stokes IAF. The effects of abdominal muscle coactivation on lumbar spine stability. Spine 1998;23:86–92.
13. Goubert L, Francken G, Crombez G, Vansteenwegen D, Lysens R. Exposure to physical movement in chronic back pain patients: no evidence for generalization across different movements. Behav Res Ther 2002;40:415–429.
14. Granata KP, Marras WS. Cost-benefit of muscle cocontraction in protecting against spinal instability. Spine 2000;25:1398–1404.
15. Gray G. Total Body Functional Profile. Wynn Marketing, Adrian MI, 2001.
16. Harding V, Williams AC de C. Extending physiotherapy skills using a psychological approach: Cognitive-behavioral management of chronic pain. Physiotherapy 1995;81:681–687.
17. Harding VR, Simmonds MJ, Watson PJ. Physical therapy for chronic pain. Pain—Clinical Updates, International Association for the Study of Pain 1998;6:1–4.
18. Hides JA, Stokes MJ, Saide M, Jull Ga, Cooper DH. Evidence of lumbar multifidus muscle wasting ipsilateral to symptoms in patients with acute/subacute low back pain. Spine 1994;19:165–172.
19. Hides JA, Richardson CA, Jull GA. Multifidus muscle recovery is not automatic after resolution of acute, first-episode of low back pain. Spine 1996;21:2763–2769.
20. Hides JA, Jull GA, Richardson CA. Long-term effects of specific stabilizing exercises for first-episode low back pain. Spine 2001;26:e243–e248.
21. Hodges PW, Richardson CA. Delayed postural contraction of the transverse abdominus associated with movement of the lower limb in people with low back pain. J Spinal Disord 1998;11:46–56.
22. Hodges PW, Richardson CA. Altered trunk muscle recruitment in people with low back pain with upper limb movements at different speeds. Arch Phys Med Rehabili 1999;80:1005–1012.
23. Hoffer J, Andreassen S. Regulation of soleus muscle stiffness in premamillary cats. J Neurophysiol 1981;45:267–285.
24. Janda V. On the concept of postural muscles and posture in man. Aus J Physioth 1983;29:83–84.
25. Kavcic N. Grenier S, McGill SM. Determining the stabilizing role of individual torso muscles during rehabilitation exercises. Spine 2004;29:1254–1265.

26. Lavender SA, Mirka GA, Schoenmarklin RW, Sommerich CM, Sudhakar LR, Marras WS. The effects of preview and task symmetry on trunk muscle response to sudden loading. Human Factors 1989;31:101–115.

27. Lewit K. Manipulative therapy in rehabilitation of the motor system, 3rd ed. London: Butterworths, 1999.

28. Lindh M. Increase in muscle strength from isometric quadriceps exercise at different knee angles. Scand J Rehabil Med 1979;11:33–36.

29. Lindstrom A, Ohlund C, Eek C, et al. Activation of subacute low back patients. Physical Ther 1992;4: 279–293.

30. Linton SJ Cognitive behavioral therapy in the prevention of musculoskeletal pain: description of a program. In: Linton SL, ed. New avenues for the prevention of chronic musculoskeletal pain and disability. Amsterdam: Elsevier, 2002.

31. Marras WS, Ferguson SA, Burr D, Davis KG, Gupta P. Functional Impairment as a Predictor of Spine Loading. Spine. 2005;30:729–737.

32. Marras WS, Mirka GA. Muscle activities during asymmetric trunk angular accelerations. J Orthop Res 1990;8:824–832.

33. Marras WS, Rangarajulu SL, Lavender SA. Trunk loading and expectation. Ergonomics 1987; 30:551–562.

34. McArdle WD, Katch FI, Katch VL. Exercise physiology, energy, nutrition and human performance, 3rd ed. Philadelphia: Lea Febiger, 1991:384–417.

35. McGill SM, Hughson R, Parks K. Lumbar erector spinae oxygenation during prolonged contraction: Implications for prolonged work. Ergonomics 2000;43:486–493.

36. McGill SM, Sharratt MT, Seguin JP. Loads on the spinal tissues during simultaneous lifting and ventilatory challenge. Ergonomics 1995;38: 1772–1792.

37. McGill SM. Low back exercises: prescription for the healthy back and when recovering from injury. Resources Manual for Guidelines for Exercise Testing and Prescription, 3rd ed. Indianapolis: American College of Sports Medicine, Baltimore: Williams and Wilkins, 1998.

38. McGill SM. The Biomechanics of Low Back Injury: Implications on Current Practice in Industry and the Clinic. J Biomechanics 1997;30:465–447.

39. O'Sullivan P, Twomey L, Allison G. Evaluation of specific stabilizing exercise in the treatment of chronic low back pain with radiologic diagnosis of spondylolysis or spondylolysthesis. Spine 1997;24: 2959–2967.

40. Panjabi MM. The stabilizing system of the spine. Part 1. Function, dysfunction, adaptation, and enhancement. J Spinal Disorders 1992;5:383–389.

41. Radebold A, Cholewicki J, Panjabi MM, Patel TC. Muscle response pattern to sudden trunk loading in healthy individuals and in patients with chronic low back pain. Spine 2000;25:947–954.

42. Rutherford OM. Muscular coordination and strength training, implications for injury rehabilitation. Sports Med 1988;5:196.

43. Sale D, MacDougall D: Specificity in strength training: A review for the coach and athlete. Can J Sport Sci 1981;6:87.

44. Shumway-Cook A, Woollacott M. Motor control-Theory and practical applications. Baltimore: Lippincott Williams & Wilkins, 1995.

45. Stokes IAF, Gardner-Morse M, Henry SM, Badger GJ. Decrease in Trunk Muscular Response to Perturbation With Preactivation of Lumbar Spinal Musculature. Spine 2000;25:1957–1964.

46. Stuge B, Laerum E, Kirkesola G, Vollestad N. The effect of a treatment program focusing on specific stabilizing exercises for pelvic girdle pain after pregnancy. A randomized controlled trial. Spine 2004;29:351–359.

47. Timm KE. A randomized-control study of active and passive treatments for chronic low back pain following L5 laminectomy. J Orthop Sports Phys Ther 1994;20:276–286.

48. Vlaeyen JWS, De Jong J, Geilen M, Heuts PHTG, Van Breukelen G. Graded exposure in the treatment of pain-related fear: a replicated single case experimental design in four patients with chronic low back pain. Behav Res Ther 2001;39:151–166.

49. Vlaeyen JWS, Morley S. Active despite pain: the putative role of stop-rules and current mood. Pain 2004; 110:512–516.

50. Vowles KE, Gross RT. Work-related beliefs about injury and physical capability for work in individuals with chronic pain. Pain 2003;101:291–298.

51. Wilder DG, Aleksiev AR, Magnusson ML, Pope MH, Spratt KF, Goel VK. Muscular response to sudden load. A tool to evaluate fatigue and rehabilitation. Spine 1996;21:2628–2639.

52. Yilmaz F, Yilmaz A, Merdol F, Parlar D, Sahin F, Kuran B. Efficacy of dynamic lumbar stabilization exercise in lumbar microdiscectomy. J Rehabil Med. 2003;35:163–167.

Proprioceptive Taping—An Adjunct to Treating Muscle Imbalances

Clare Frank, Wendy Burke, Cindy Bailey

Introduction

Proper proprioceptive information is integral to motor regulation (2,3,6,8,11). Proprioception involves the integration of information from mechanoreceptors in the skin, muscle, fascia, tendons, and articular structures with visual and vestibular input at all central nervous system levels to allow perception of static and dynamic position sense and force detection. The afferent input from these mechanoreceptors provide the basis for the central nervous system to regulate movement by altering the muscle balance and motor recruitment patterns for the task at hand. The muscular system has been described by Janda as "lying at a functional crossroad" (7) because it is influenced by stimuli from the central nervous system and the musculoskeletal system. The production and control of motion in normal and pathologic states involves the interdependence of all the structures of these systems. Dysfunction in any component of these systems is ultimately reflected in the muscular system in the form of altered muscle balance, coordination, and motor performance. Muscle imbalance is a systemic change in the quality of muscle function that results in altered joint biomechanics leading to pain, dysfunction, and eventually degeneration, as well as altered proprioceptive information, leading to adaptive changes in central nervous system regulation. Proprioceptive deficits are considered important factors that perpetuate muscle imbalances, impaired movement patterns, and, ultimately, the recurrences of chronic pain syndromes (6–8).

The success of any rehabilitation program involves improvement of all peripheral structures involved, treating the key impairments, muscle imbalances, and improvement of central motor control and programming. Numerous ways to facilitate the proprioceptive system have been introduced through the use of balls, wobble boards, and shoes, foam rolls, and, more recently, the use of tape (1,5,11). Taping of muscles is a useful adjunct to provide proprioceptive feedback to the central nervous system through direct or indirect reduction of pain associated with movement, reduction of edema, inhibition of overactive muscles, facilitation of underactive muscles, and promotion of joint alignment. The exact mechanisms by which proprioceptive taping is effective are not yet clear, but the articular, Myofascial, and cutaneous structures are regarded to have important roles in influencing proprioception (11). This appendix attempts to briefly discuss the different types of tapes that are available with particular attention to Kinesiotex tape and, secondly, how kinesiotaping techniques may be used to provide proper proprioceptive input to imbalanced muscle groups and, thus, improve movement patterns.

Types of Tape

There are currently three basic types of tape and taping techniques used in the rehabilitation setting, each of which has its specific uses and shortcomings. Athletic tape is fairly rigid and is widely used to stabilize joints by restricting movement of respective joints and soft tissue. Application requires an underwrap on the skin before taping to prevent blistering as a result of friction between the skin and the tape. Because of the compressive nature of athletic taping, the tape must be removed immediately after the activity to prevent skin irritation and circulatory complications.

The second type of taping technique involves the usage of two different kinds of tape, typically, cover roll and leukotape. This technique was initially developed by Jenny McConnell, an Australian physiotherapist, for the treatment of patello-femoral syndromes. There is some evidence that taping of the patella in conjunction with retraining of the quadriceps muscle through the use of electromyographic feedback alters the relative activity of the vastus lateralis and medialis obliquus during quadriceps activation (4,5). The McConnell taping approach has since expanded to other joints to include the shoulder, foot, and ankle.

The third kind of tape, Kinesiotex, was developed and manufactured by Kenzo Kase, a Japanese chiropractor, in an effort to decrease pain, decrease edema, assist muscle function, and, ultimately, improve joint function (9,10). Kinesiotex is designed to simulate human skin in thickness and weight. In addition, it has an elastic component that allows it to stretch 30% to 40% beyond its original length. Unlike other tapes that restrict movement, Kinestiotex allows for full range of movement while providing support to the muscle. Another unique feature of Kinesiotex is the type of adhesive used. Because it is heat-activated, it allows the tape to be worn for several days, including in the shower or in the pool without peeling off. The inherent wavy design of the adhesive in the tape also helps to channel away sweat, salts, and toxins from the skin, allowing for fewer skin reactions. Finally, the tape is hypoallergenic and latex-free, which makes it "skin-friendly" for patients with sensitive or fragile skin, such as patients with diabetes, fibromyalgia, or rheumatoid arthritis.

Kinesiotaping Techniques

Kinesiotaping has been widely used in the treatment of post-surgical edema to promote lymphatic drainage (9,10) (Fig. 26A.1) Unlike traditional taping techniques that use tape for compression, multiple thin strips of Kinesiotex are applied lightly to the surface of the skin over and beyond the edematous area. A rippling effect of the superficial skin occurs when this elastic tape is applied over the stretched fascia, opening up channels through which the lymph may flow freely secondary to the reduced interstitial pressure in the epidermis.

Another unique feature of kinesiotaping is in the treatment of muscle spasms and muscle weakness. Traditional athletic taping often places a joint in a neutral position through the compressive layers of tape over the area to restrict the extremes of motion to prevent injury. However, kinesiotaping is applied directly to the injured muscle itself from its proximal and distal attachments. Application of this technique

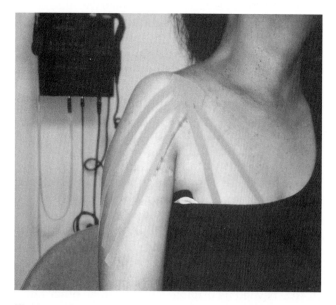

Figure 26A.1 Taping for lower extremity lymphadema.

therefore requires a thorough understanding of muscle anatomy and muscle fiber orientation. Because of its elastic property, the tape will attempt to achieve zero tension by recoiling toward the anchor, much like holding a rubber band with one hand and pulling it with the other. With that in mind, application of the tape from the muscle's origin to its insertion will tend to facilitate the muscle, whereas application of the tape from insertion to its origin will tend to inhibit the muscle activity. Determination of the type of kinesiotaping technique used depends on the acuity of the dysfunction and treatment goals. For example, treatment is directed at supporting the extensor muscles of the elbow and wrist in the painful stage of lateral epicondylitis. Taping from the muscle's insertion to its origin for muscle inhibition is thereby indicated. However, when the muscle is no longer in spasms and a controlled exercise program is indicated, taping from origin to its insertion to facilitate the muscle would then be appropriate. Joint position and associated range of motion are also achieved as a result of improving the balance of muscle activity around the joint.

Kinesiotaping and Muscle Reeducation

Clinically, two muscle systems have been differentiated by Janda (6–8), that is, muscles that are prone to develop shortness or tightness and muscles that are prone to develop inhibition and weakness. The changed relationship between these muscle systems results in muscle imbalances with subsequent clinical consequences. For example, hip hyperextension is a critical event during the terminal phase of the gait cycle. Inadequate hip extension caused by an imbalance between shortened hip flexors and weakened glutei muscles over time will result in a dysfunctional movement pattern in which hip extension is compensated by an increase in lumbar lordosis. In a patient with low back pain with this muscle imbalance, restoring adequate hip extension is imperative to reduce further stress on the lumbar segments. Kinesiotaping directed at inhibiting the shortened hip flexors and facilitating the gluteal muscles may be used in conjunction with manual techniques and exercises to restore hip extension. Altering muscle function through kinesiotaping provides the proper feedback to the body part and, consequently, the stimulus to the patient to consciously correct the movement pattern. Taping is continued until the patient has learned to actively control the movement in the desired fashion or the effects on symptoms are maintained when it is not worn. The proper movement hip extension pattern can be reprogrammed over time and with enough repetitious feedback.

Kinesiotaping in the Treatment of Pelvic Crossed Syndrome

Based on the elastic properties of kinesiotex tape, taping can be directed to facilitate underactive muscles and inhibit overactive shortened muscles. In the pelvic crossed syndrome, as described by Janda (8) the muscles that are often inhibited or weakened are the gluteus maximus, gluteus medius, and abdominals, whereas the muscles that are often shortened and tight are the hip flexors and lumbar extensors. Kinesiotaping can be used very effectively to facilitate these inhibited muscles in conjunction with stretching of the shortened tight muscles (Fig. 26A.2). As shown in the Fig. 26A.2, the tape is applied in from proximal to distal attachments to facilitate the gluteus maximus and medius muscles. For example, to facilitate the gluteus maximus, the base of the tape is first applied on its proximal attachment on the posterior ilium and then anchored on the greater trochanter after the hip is taken through the maximum pain-free flexion range of motion.

Kinesiotaping in the Treatment of Upper Crossed Syndrome

The posture in the upper crossed syndrome (7) is often exhibited in a push-forward position of the head and rounded shoulders, causing mechanical strain on the cervical segments and associated musculature necessary to support the head. The muscles that are often shortened are the pectoralis major, upper trapezius, and levator scapulae, whereas the muscles that are often inhibited or weakened are the deep cervical flexors and mid and lower trapezius. In addition to posture retraining and stretching of the shortened muscles, kinesiotaping may be used to facilitate the postural awareness of the patient (Fig. 26A.3) and inhibiting the overactive muscles. For postural taping, the scapula is first positioned in neutral as much as possible. The base of the tape is first applied anterior to the acromioclavicular joint and then placed over the scapula in the direction of the inferior angle and thoracic spine. To inhibit the upper trapezius (Fig. 26A.4), the base of the tape is first applied at the lateral border of the acromium and then placed along the muscle belly to the base of the occiput, whereas the cervical spine is side-bent and rotated away.

■ CONCLUSION

Although the exact mechanisms by which proprioceptive taping is effective are unclear, its clinical effects are significant and immediate, especially in relieving pain, promoting altered movement patterns, and allowing earlier progression of rehabilitation. Taping, in conjunction with manual therapy, therapeutic exercises, and patient education, is a useful adjunct in treating muscle imbalances and impaired movement patterns.

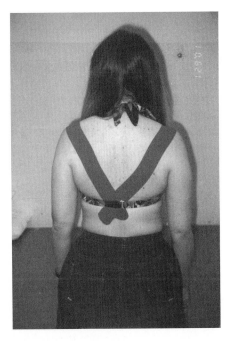

Figure 26A.3 Taping for postural support.

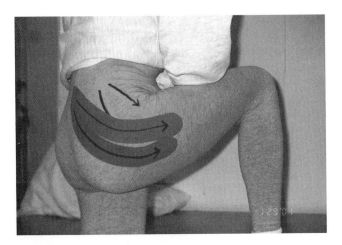

Figure 26A.2 Taping for facilitating gluteus maximus and gluteus medius.

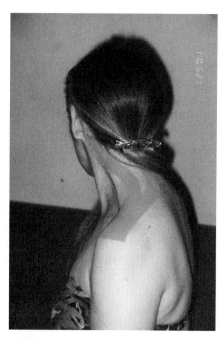

Figure 26A.4 Taping for upper trapezius inhibition.

■ REFERENCES

1. Bullock-Saxton JE, Janda V, Bullock MI. Reflex activation of gluteal muscles in walking with balance shoes: an approach to restoration of function for chronic low back pain patients. Spine 1993;18 :704–708.

2. Bullock-Saxton JE. Local sensation changes and altered hip muscle function following repetitive ankle sprain. Phys Ther 1994;74(1):17–31.

3. Bullock-Saxton JE. The influence of ankle sprain on muscle recruitment during hip extension. Int J Sports Med 1994;15:330–334.

4. Cerny K. Vastus medialis obliques/vastus lateralis muscle activity ratios for selected exercises in persons with or without patellofemoral pain syndrome. Phys Ther 1995;6:672–683.

5. Gilleard W, McConnell J, Parsons S. The effects of patellar taping on the onset of vastus medialis obliquus and vastus lateralis muscle activity in persons with patellofemoral pain. Phys Ther 1988;78: 25–32.

6. Janda V. Muscles, central nervous motor regulation and back problems. In: Korr M, ed. Neurobiologic mechanisms in manipulative therapy. New York: Plenum Press, 1986:27–41.

7. Janda V. Muscles and cervicogenic pain syndromes. In: Grant R, ed. Physical Therapy of the Cervical and Thoracic Spine: Clinics in Physical Therapy. New York: Churchill-Livingstone, 1988: 153–166.

8. Jull G, Janda V. Muscles and motor control in low back pain. In: Twomey LT, ed. Physical Therapy for the low back: Clinics in Physical Therapy. New York: Churchill-Livingstone, 1987.

9. Kase, K. Illustrated Kinestio Taping, 3rd ed. Tokyo: Ken'I Kai, 1994.

10. Kase K, Taksuyuki H, Tomoki O. Kinesio Perfect Taping Manual. Albuquerque, NM: Universal Printing & Publishing, Inc, 1996.

11. Lephart SM, et al. The role of proprioception in the management and rehabilitation of athletic injuries. Am J Sports Med 1997;25:130–137.

27

Global Muscle Stabilization Training—Isotonic Protocols

Neil Osborne and Jonathan Cook

Learning Objectives
After reading this chapter, you should be able to:

- Understand the principles underpinning isotonic training in rehabilitation
- Be conversant with the literature pertaining to isotonic training protocols
- Outline key elements in the design of successful isotonic training
- Understand how and when isotonic training may be incorporated into the motor control (stabilization) model of spinal rehabilitation
- Define normal parameters in strength, endurance, and ratios of the spinal musculature.
- Devise an assessment strategy for the rehabilitation candidate requiring isotonic training
- Select appropriate exercises for an individual's particular requirements

Introduction

Origins

The aim of this chapter is to describe the development, rationale, and detail of a global spinal stabilization rehabilitation model currently in use at the Anglo-European College of Chiropractic (AECC).

This particular brand of rehabilitation is consistent with the contemporary trend toward patient-centred active care (17,43,51,54) and derived from a number of influences, many of which are described in detail throughout this book. However, the catalyst for the development of such a program came from the AECC's MSc Program, developed in response to a demand from the profession for a formalized, post-graduate, university-validated Master's degree, the rationale for which has been previously described (8).

A large component of the MSc Clinical Chiropractic was spinal rehabilitation. Students were exposed to a number of models, many of which were described by contributors to this book and its predecessor, including Vladamir Janda, Karel Lewit, Craig Liebenson, Howard Vernon, and Alan Jordan.

The authors of AECC's approach, and of this chapter, have reviewed the literature underpinning the described models and have integrated the emerging issues. The model is heavily based in the literature, objectively monitored with validated outcome tools (see chapters 8 and 11), and is continually undergoing critical review.

Major Influences

Perhaps the most significant underpinning concept of the program is the promotion of "correct form." In this there must be an appreciation of the "deconditioning syndrome" (see Chapters 1, 2, 5, 25, and 26) and promotion of local and global stabilization procedures.

Local Stabilization

Local stabilization is the promotion of key muscle group activity at a local segmental level (within the low back or neck). The goal is to ensure good local stability before addressing the deconditioned global musculature.

The most convincing spinal work to develop in this area has been performed by a team of Australian researchers who began by noting a marked local segmental atrophy of multifidus in the lumbar spine secondary to acute low back pain. They went on to observe continued de-stabilization of the lumbar spine resulting from the transverse abdominus inhibition and then began developing a protocol to restore the functional cocontraction of these muscles as seen in healthy individuals (19–21,23–25). Adequate co-contraction is described as a prerequisite to lumbar spine stability (21,24,25) and has been shown to stabilize the sacroiliac joint (48). The training involves isometric cocontraction of the multifidus and transverses abdominus and then the superimposed training of global muscles, through which the individual learns to resist destabilizing load to the spine. A parallel exercise has also been developed for the cervical spine. In themselves such stabilization exercises do not seem to increase the size of the paravertebral muscles, when measured with computerized tomography, and other strengthening exercises need to be added to the program. Simple dynamic (isotonic) and static-dynamic (stabilization) exercises have been shown to be equally effective in this respect (11).

This apparently simple co-contraction exercise and its cervical spine equivalent, cervico-cranial flexion:, are described in chapter 25.

McGill, however, describes, in his excellent book on the subject (42), the limitations of purely prescribing transverse abdominus activity as a prerequisite to exercise. He argues that the work that has come out of Australia (19,20,23,24,25) has lead to some confusion in the literature, as it is being interpreted as an adequate prerequisite to isotonic or stabilizing exercises. Whereas he agrees that the work is very useful because it has identified aberrant motor control patterns in patients with low back pain and can be used to re-educate this motor control pattern, McGill argues that, as a core stabilizing exercise, it is inadequate. In electromyography studies, McGill and coworkers (31) have compared muscle activity of the low back and presented a sensible and convincing argument that bracing is superior to simply promoting transverse abdominus activity (31,41,42). He argues that the "stability index" for the low back, because of the bracing exercise, is vastly superior to abdominal hollowing and affords greater low back protection. The argument is, perhaps, flawed in one respect; in that he equates the "gross" abdominal hollowing to the specific isolation of the transverse abdominus, which has been promoted by the Australian workers (19,20,23, 24,25). Not withstanding, the message that bracing, rather than transverse abdominus activity alone, needs to be a prerequisite is clear.

The model that has been adopted by the authors of this chapter is that the transverse abdominus is isolated as described by Richardson and coworkers (19,20,23–25) to ensure activation of multifidus, and is then followed by a bracing procedure, before any subsequent exercise.

At AECC, all patients are educated to exercise with well-controlled posture, local stability (through co-contraction or cervicocranial flexion), and controlled breathing. The mastery of this is a prerequisite to other exercises and the promotion of "good form" is a strictly observed principle.

Interestingly, Joseph Pilates, a boxer and German national interned in England during World War I, developed the "Pilates technique." He devised a set of exercises that "made sense" to him and the promotion of a "navel-to-spine" policy before exercise has been practiced by interested individuals ever since. Pilates is has a much less refined, albeit remarkably similar, principle and has significant overlap with the establishment of what is now understood to promote "local" or "core" segmental stability.

Global Stabilization

Global stabilization involves the promotion of muscular stabilization through the training of multi-segmental muscles. The literature is replete with articles detailing the effectiveness of regional strength and endurance training, with perhaps the most relevant reviews of this work conducted in 1995 and again in 1996 by Jordan and Maniche (26,36), who concluded that such aspects as dose, intermediate and long-term goal setting, and supervision of patients are among the factors most likely to yield benefit. The vigorous approach taken with the patient with low back pain aims to redress the balance of deconditioning and fits well with the observation that the strongest physical predictor for chronicity seems to be lumbar extensor stamina (7,26,32,36).

To combine the two principles, i.e., to perform the isometric local stabilization exercises before and during all further vigorous isotonic exercise is central to AECC's approach to rehabilitation. The ultimate goal (albeit perhaps on occasion impossible to achieve) is not to allow the patients to move onto global stability/isotonic training until they can satisfactorily activate the local stabilizers.

Furthermore, it is hoped that this local stability promotion will become "automatic" through repetition, the promotion of "form," and the use of sensory motor training procedures (see chapters 22, 25, and 26).

Considerations in Successful Isotonic Training

Exercises have been advocated for spinal pain for more than 100 years. Various multidisciplinary programs have been designed and studied, but the majority of clinical trials investigating the effects of exercise intervention for low back and neck conditions have involved isotonic training. There is more evidence and literature regarding this form of spinal rehabilitation than any other (2,3,7,15,22,26,28,36,37,45).

The literature cited within this section is not intended to be exhaustive, but rather is intended to present the main arguments underpinning the model described.

Key Factors for Successful Isotonic Training

As with other forms of rehabilitation, the main aims are the restoration of functional capacity by facilitating healing processes (treatment) and the strengthening of weakened tissues (prophylaxis). Isotonic strength and endurance training has several physiological and psychological benefits (26,36).

- Muscle strength gains
- Strengthened connective tissues
- Neurophysiological improvements
- Improved capillary blood perfusion to muscle
- Improved discal nutrition
- Increased bone mineral content
- Improved physical condition
- Increased production of endogenous opioids
- Positive psychological elements

Reviewing the trials using isotonic training, there are conflicting conclusions in terms of pain, disability, and function regarding the outcomes of such programs. Consequently, in an attempt to make sense of these apparently contradictory conclusions, Jordan and Manniche began analyzing the published trials to identify what the successful trials had that the less successful lacked (26,36).

Despite considerable investigation in the area, the ideal training program has not yet been (and may never be) identified, because studies comparing one type of exercise to another are sparse and inconclusive. However, the conclusions of Jordan and Manniche's provide essential, evidence-based guidelines for the design of a successful isotonic program, such that the conditions for effective training may be specified.

These conditions include dosage, duration, relative disregard for pain, and supervision and compliance.

Dosage

Effective training requires sufficient dosage. Research in low back and neck training suggests that most benefit occurs with a greater amount of exercise and an increasing number of repetitions (2,15,22,30,45).

Endurance training is primarily targeted in an isotonic program, at least in the initial stages. Endurance loading maximizes blood flow, thereby maximizing healing. Furthermore, emphasizing improvements in the tonic holding capacity (endurance) of the spinal stabilizers is in keeping with most schools of thought in spinal rehabilitation.

Endurance is typically trained in the deconditioned patient with loading at 30% to 40% maximum voluntary contraction (MVC) and performing three sets of 12 to 14 repetitions. It is suggested that spinal musculature endurance levels will increase by 100 to 150% within 8 weeks in typical deconditioned individuals (3,28,37).

For those patients whose occupations or activities involve abnormally high levels of spinal loading (e.g., athletes, heavy labourers), additional protection to the spine may be provided through increased strength. Strength training requires loads of 70% to 80% MVC, performing one to two sets of 8 to 12 repetitions. Maximal strength gains after 8 weeks will be approximately 25% to 40% (3,28,37). However, the development of strength is usually a secondary consideration. Clearly, in such cases careful consideration needs to be given to muscle imbalances and the promotion of core stability.

Duration

Meaningful results have been obtained for the spine in terms of duration of exercise programs, suggesting that reasonable strength gains and subjective improvement occur with supervised training for a minimum of 8 weeks, with two to three sessions per week (2,3,6,29,30,37). The duration of the session should not exceed 1 hour.

The period of training may be increased for postoperative patients (e.g., disc surgery), with the length of training for such patients reaching as much as 3 to 4 months (38).

The training sessions should be high intensity. Trials looking specifically at the differences in outcome between high- and low-intensity programs demonstrate superior benefits from high-intensity exercise (3,6,15,16,22,29,30,37).

Relative Disregard of Pain

To maximise psychological benefits, it is important that pain is not the main indicator in setting dosages and performing the exercises. Focus should be placed on restoring functional capacity and understanding that pain improvements will tend to occur gradually and as a secondary effect. If the approach becomes "let pain be your guide," the program is less likely to be less successful (1), and therefore positive reinforcement that "hurt" does not necessarily equal "harm" is recommended. Caution is recommended and each case needs to be judged on the individual's pain tolerance and fear–avoidance behavior.

There may be several clinical exceptions to the "disregard of pain" concept, which are beyond the scope of this chapter; however, a notable example would be peripheralization of pain (McKenzie concept) (see Chapter 15).

Supervision and Compliance

Compliance is perhaps the single most important and predictive issue in the program. Some early attempts at rehabilitation programs reported drop-out rates as high as 50% to 70% (14), largely because of factors other than a worsening of symptoms. More recently, it has been suggested that comorbidity and an expectation of barriers to completing a program leads to less likelihood of compliance (4).

Ideally, training should be performed in a supervised setting. Although there will be inevitable therapeutics gains, unsupervised exercise programs lack accountability of form and compliance, and progression cannot be as effectively monitored; consequently, drop-out rates are high. In 1989, Reilly and Lovejoy (46) observed 91% compliance to a supervised program compared to 31% in an identical program in which the patients were not supervised. As a result, at 6 months the supervised group showed significantly greater improvements in aerobic fitness, strength, and pain. Such a finding has been echoed by other studies (40).

There is also a case for prescribing additional unsupervised daily home exercises on the days when formal training does not take place. This may assist in reducing dependency and encouraging self-help. However, the balance of evidence clearly emphasizes the importance of supervised training.

The comprehensive literature analysis of Jordan and Manniche's (26,36) suggests that small cohorts of ideally four to five patients are most beneficial, because patients in such settings tend to become mutually supportive. Instructors should be "inspiring, creative, and always striving to lead patients away from stereotypic patient roles."

Advantages of an Isotonic Program

With studies advocating various forms of spinal rehabilitative training, the clinician is left to choose which components to include in a program. The choice includes local stabilization training, flexibility exercises, sensorimotor stimulation, aerobic fitness training, isotonic training, and isometric (global muscle) spinal stabilization tracks. Clinical opinion and research evidence purports benefits of each approach.

However, isotonic training programs have several obvious benefits:

a) They use a standardised framework within which specific dosages and exercise modifications may be set for the individual. This approach may be less tissue specific but it is *easier* to apply in non-specific musculoskeletal pain.

b) Goal setting is simple and functional progress is self-evident. Regularly achieving dosage goals has obvious physical benefits for the individual as well as being a potent psychological motivator.

c) Isotonic exercises require a relatively low supervisor to patient ratio. Once the patients master the relatively simple exercise procedures, they can become largely independent. Other rehabilitative procedures such as co-contraction or isometric spinal stabilization tracks (e.g., the Bridge exercises; see Chapters 25 and 26) require high levels of precision, tuition, and monitoring; therefore, they require ongoing intensive levels of one-to-one supervision.

d) Outcome measures are easier to apply because each patient undergoes the same training program. A more tissue specific approach requires more variation in exercise procedures, making it more difficult to compare like with like.

What and How to Train

Many studies have identified the link between spinal pain and reduced strength, specifically endurance of the spinal stabilizers. This evidence primarily concerns patients with chronic low back or neck pain.

In a study of 912 adults, Biering-Soerensen (7) identified the strong correlation between lumbar extensor weakness (reduced endurance) and the likelihood of first-time low back pain developing. Patients with chronic low back pain were also shown to have poor lumbar endurance compared to those without, a finding strongly supported by the work of Luoto in 1995 (35). Furthermore, good isotonic endurance seems to protect against occupationally related back pain (50).

However, such a static back endurance test, arguably, becomes a test of pain, rather than an endurance test, in those with low back pain.

Further, Rissanen (49) demonstrated a comparative weakness of the low back flexors and extensors in chronic low back pain patients. The same finding was derived from a large-scale trial by Schifferdecker-Hock et al (52), who also noted flexor/extensor weakness in chronic neck pain patients. Jordan (28) showed a strong correlation between chronic neck pain and neck weakness compared to age-matched asymptomatic subjects. Restoring, or at least improving, strength and endurance in the neck or low back has a significant impact on chronic pain, function, and disability (6,7,28,35,43,45,49).

In a study of 594 people between ages 35 and 54, Alaranta et al (2) attempted to establish normative static back endurance values and, although their results were further broken down into age ranges, occupation (white collar/blue collar), and sex, the mean normative values for females ranged between 62 and 122 seconds, and for males between 73 and 131 seconds.

Ratio Promotion

One key aspect in the implementation of isotonic training exercises is attention to the restoration of normal strength ratios. The relationship in terms of maximum voluntary contraction between the flexors, extensors, and lateral flexors is invariably disrupted by injury and/or chronic pain in the low back and neck (5,28).

Considering the neck in asymptomatic individuals, the ratio between extensor and flexor strength should be in the region of 1.7:1 (28); and the relationship of the lateral flexors should be equal. The ratio in chronic neck pain patients tends to be approximately 1:1 (27,28), suggesting that whereas both flexors and extensors weaken with chronic pain, the greatest degree of weakening is in the extensors.

The main exception to this rule is in hyperextension injuries, in which the neck flexors undergo the greatest degree of weakening. Consequently, during isotonic training, dosage and goal setting should be modified to restore the "normal ratio" while strengthening each individual muscle group.

The situation is rather less predictable in the low back, but attempts at a calculation consider the normal strength ratio between extensors and flexors to be approximately 1.3:1 (5,27,28). Once again, in the chronic low back pain patient, the ratio tends to be approximately 1:1. Therefore, dosage and goal setting should once again reflect restoration of the normal ratio.

Task-Specific

Although the advantages of isotonic, gym-based programs are clear for the practitioner because they are easy to implement and generic exercises for several people can be prescribed, this can also be their downfall. There has been a long-accepted principle in sports rehabilitation (specific adaptation to increased demand [SAID]) that when returning to a particular sport after a period of recuperation, aspects of that sport should be carefully implemented into the program. For example, a javelin thrower should have slow, controlled, javelin throw–like exercises, with weight and pulley resistance while adopting a correct stance and using the torso to generate force in the same way that they would in their sport. The program will progress in terms of speed and force and gradually culminate in a "mimicking" of the throw.

The same principles should apply to all rehabilitation programs. So, for the low back, part of the assessment for the patient should involve an individual assessment of their activities of daily living (ADL), especially those movements that produce pain, and their program should promote strengthening to address these ADLs. This approach is referred to by some as work-hardening.

The Model

The program developed at AECC combines isotonic training for the global stabilizers with local stabilization training, muscle relaxation work, and sensorimotor stimulation. It is implemented in three stages.

Three-Stage Approach

Stage 1

Stage 1 is the transition from passive to active care with techniques, exercises, and advice to enhance the patient's response to treatment, and to prepare the patient adequately for isotonic training as necessary. It therefore involves the progression along the continuum between passive and active and is implemented by the practitioner as part of the regular treatment sessions. Largely, it involves the promotion of home stretching exercises (chapters 19 and 24) and the introduction of local stability exercises.

The emerging evidence supports the concept that local stabilization should precede global stabilization (3,6,23,29,30,42). Consequently, a formal assessment of local stabilizer function (co-contraction) in the low back and cervico-cranial flexion in the neck (chapter 25) is also performed at this early stage. Deficits in local stabilization are addressed through the initiation of co-contraction or cervico-cranial flexion training on a daily basis.

In the case of transversus abdominus and multifidus co-contraction, it is intended that before training isotonically, the patient will be capable of passing the level 1 test (10 10-second multifidus contractions and the same transversus contractions with pressure biofeedback reduction of approximately 6 to 10 mmHg). For cervical rehabilitation, the ideal standard on cervico-cranial flexion testing is 10 10-second contrac-

tions with a pressure increase of approximately 8 to 10 mmHg. For those patients who are unable to achieve these ideal standards, their "best effort" is recorded and then observed throughout the program to ensure continued improvement, or at least no worsening.

On occasion we have witnessed patients who achieve little or no competency in local muscle contraction, yet whose results on completion of the isotonic program are excellent. Notwithstanding, the interpretation of "best evidence" would suggest that as long as compliance remains unaffected, core stability should be promoted before global exercises.

Once the patient is identified as a good candidate for the intensive 10-week program, referral to the program is made.

Stage 2—Isotonic Training

After assessment, the patient will then undergo a 10-week, twice weekly, supervised program, in which most of the emphasis is on isotonic training. The basic procedure for endurance training is described in Exercise 27-1. The exercises are described in Exercises 27-2 to 27-12. All isotonic exercise are preceded with co-contraction and bracing.

Exercise 27-1 The Endurance Range

A simple and effective approach to setting dosage in isotonic resistance training, with weights, is to determine the level of resistance at which an individual can perform 3 sets of 12 repetitions (if they cannot perform this, then this will become the first goal). At subsequent training sessions, the individual attempts to increase the number of repetitions until they attain 3 sets of 20 repetitions.

At this point the resistance is increased (perhaps by only 5%) and the dosage reverts back to 3 sets of 12 repetitions, and the process is repeated.

The application of this principle in the isotonic rehabilitation setting is worthy of merit, even when the resistance is body weight and cannot be changed, such as in dorsal raises. In this example, 3 sets of 12 is the initial goal, even though an individual only may be able to perform 3 sets of 6 initially. With time they should be able to build to 3 sets of 12 and then to 3 sets of 20, adding small weights to their hands (as an advancement) if necessary.

All of the exercises described in the following Tables use this principle, described by Mooney et al., (2001) when setting doses.

Mooney V, Pozos R, Vleeming A, Gulick J, Swenski D. Exercise treatment for sacroiliac pain. Orthopedics 2001;24:29–32.

Exercise 27-2 Angle Bench Dorsal Raises (Back Lifts)

The Procedure

The prone patient is placed with L4 over the center of the roller—"Navel over center of roller."

They are then instructed to perform the co-contraction and to maintain a regular breathing rate while elevating themselves into 5° of lumbar extension. If they are to be assisted, then the supervisor assists by lifting the patient's arms. Repetitions are performed at breathing rate with hands beside head in double-sided salute position.

Between each set they are advised to rest, crouching back on their haunches, with the shoulders dropped low, until their heart rate recovers.

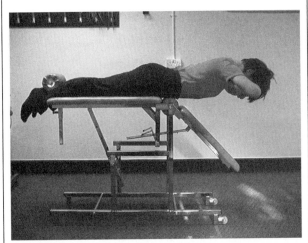

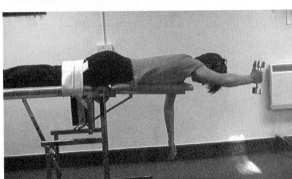

Advancement

Holding free-weight by forehead

Dynamic/Static Option

Between each repetition, they hold for 5 seconds. Increasing 10 to 20 repetitions for a maximum of 3 sets. This seems to increase the cross-sectional area of multifidus more effectively.

Exercise 27-3 Abdominals (Curl Downs Plus Alternative) (Figs. 27.2 and 27.3)

The Procedure

Seated, knees flexed to 90°, shoulders flexed to 90°.

Perform co-contraction and hold.

Lower trunk over count of "3," trying to resist most difficult part (just before shoulders touch down).

Heels must NOT leave floor. If unable to maintain heel contact, start with feet further out and draw in during maneuver.

Return to upright in a straight line using arms by sides—pressing, symmetrically off the floor.

DO NOT hold patient's feet down.

Digging heels into the floor accompanied by a posterior pelvic tilt and co-contraction will further de-facilitate iliopsoas.

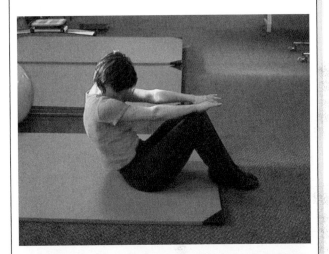

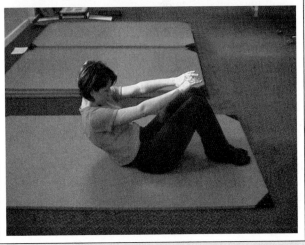

(continued)

Exercise 27-3 Abdominals (Curl Downs Plus Alternative) (Figs. 27.2 and 27.3) *(continued)*

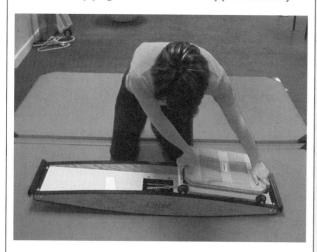

Advancement

Holding free-weight across the chest (albeit unusual for anyone to achieve this)

Alternatives (to be used if peel back required from curl-downs)

1) Fitter. Kneeling in co-contraction, shoulders centered above trolley. Push down firmly and slide trolley from side to side maintaining shoulders centered above fitter (NO TRUNK ROTATION). This must be slow and controlled.

2) Gym ball sit-ups. Co-contraction maintained throughout. Pelvis sits on front of ball (not on top). Hands across chest. Limit depth of curl-down to 45° off horizontal. Some patients can only do this with feet secured. This is not ideal because it activates the ilipsoas but is on occasion unavoidable.

3) See chapters (5 and 26) for the low force approaches of Stuart McGill.

However, a recent study investigating the effects of lumbar extensor training on changes in the cross-sectional area of the lumbar multifidus in chronic low back pain patients suggests a slight modification of dorsal raises and leg raises to achieve optimum results (12). The authors showed that in 10 weeks of training, significant hypertrophy of the multifidus was achievable using 5-second static holds between the concentric and eccentric phases of dorsal raises and leg raises (the quadruped exercise was also used). Interestingly, the same exercises without static holds and co-contraction–based exercises alone were

Exercise 27-4 Leg Extensions

Correct Procedure

Patient in reverse position, prone, on angle bench with greater trochanters at level of roller, and the bench angled down. Set bench two levels down from horizontal.

Canvas belt secures patient to bench (diagonally across sacrum) to help avoid use of arms (lats) in action.

Knees remain completely extended throughout action.

Try to maintain co-contraction throughout.

Extend from straight leg from hips until legs in straight line with torso. May help to tell patient to dorsiflex ankles.

DO NOT HYPEREXTEND. Action performed slowly to avoid hyperextension.

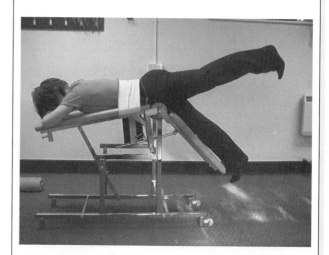

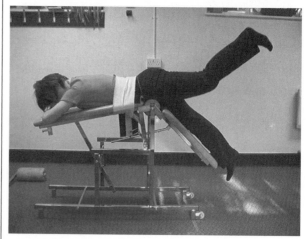

Alternatives

1. Single-leg raise. Action must come from gluteals and hip, NOT from rotation of the torso.

2. Knees start in flexion and extend with hips

3. Double leg raises

(continued)

Exercise 27-4 Leg Extensions *(continued)*

4. IF lumbar extension is the primary movement, ask the patient to pre-contract them, before leg extension.

Advancement

Add ankle weight.

Exercise 27-5 Lateral Raises (Side Lifts)

Correct Procedure

Side-lying on angle bench, iliac crest to upper edge of board.

Lower board angled downward to first setting.

Upside leg extended at knee, hip at 0°.

Downside leg flexed bringing ankle against upside calf to secure legs under leg restraint.

Start with upper board at just below 0° horizontal.

Raise torso without twist until just above neutral and lower.

Ensure the pelvis remain perpendicular to the bench.

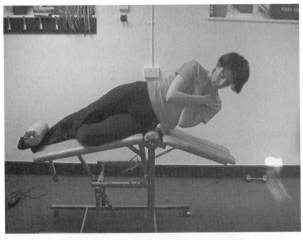

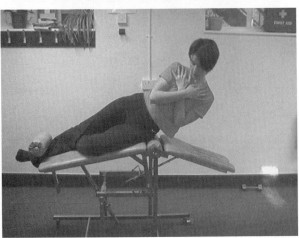

Exercise 27-5 Lateral Raises (Side Lifts)

Progression

Not initiated until patient capable of 4 to 5 sets of dorsal raises (12 repetitions).

Start on 2 sets 5 each side (may provide assistance/spot).

Advance to 2 sets of 10

Maximum 2 sets of 10 with upper board lowered as far as 45°.

Advancement

Add free-weight across the chest

Alternatives

See chapters 5 and 26 for the side-bridge approach of Stuart McGill

Exercise 27-6 Gym Ball Squats

The Procedure

The patient performs and holds co-contraction. The patient stands with a gym ball between the small of the back and a wall. Then perform squats with the weight against the ball, ensuring that the patient does not flex/extend the back. Maintain co-contraction.

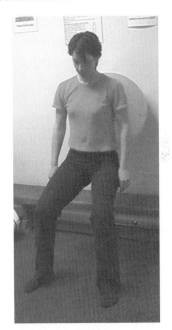

Advancement

Further advancement with hand weights.

Also, free-standing squat, with hand weights or barbell.

Notes

Wide-based squats are better for gluteal activity, narrow squats (with a medicine ball held between the knees) are better for activation of the VMO.

Exercise 27-7 Abduction

The Procedure

Maintain neutral sideways standing posture and knee extension throughout. Maintain gentle co-contraction

Ask the patient to abduct leg to approximately 30° and ensure it is "pure," without hip hike, rotation, or flexion.

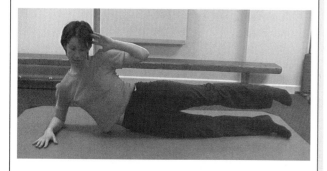

Alternative

Side-lying. Down-side leg flexed at the knee for stability. Abduct the straight top leg.

Advancement

Add ankle weight.

Exercise 27-8 Adduction

The Procedure

Maintain neutral sideways standing posture and knee extension throughout. Maintain gentle co-contraction

Adduct leg to approximately 20° in front of stance leg.

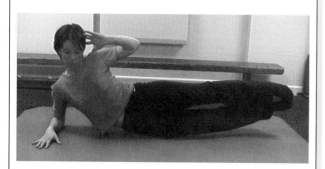

Alternative

Side-lying. Top side leg flexed at the hip in front of the body. Adduct the straight down-side leg advancing with ankle weights as necessary.

Advancement

Add ankle weight.

Exercise 27-9 Pull-Downs

The Procedure

Wide grip on the bar with correct, erect posture and co-contraction

May be performed sitting or standing. Pre-contract lower scapulae stabilizers and depress the shoulder—look for (the incorrect) hike of trapezius.

Pull down to sternum in front of head.

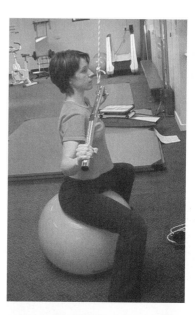

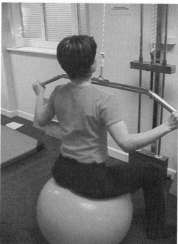

Exercise 27-10 Neck Machine

Correct procedure

Cervico-thoracic junction level with lever arm axis of rotation.

Shoulders level and relaxed, hands on grips sit erect with thighs >90° (to decrease the use of the feet).

Then activate lower scapula stabilizers and perform co-contraction and deep neck flexion.

Perform all movements within the pain-free ROM

Rest between sets 30 seconds to 1 minute.

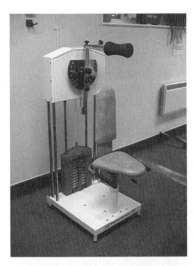

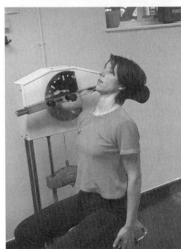

Extension

Arm level with external occipital protuberance. Extend without recruitment of trunk or limb muscles. DO NOT push through feet. Add deep neck flexion/cervical cranial flexion (as described in chapters 25 and 26)

Exercise 27-10 Neck Machine *(continued)*

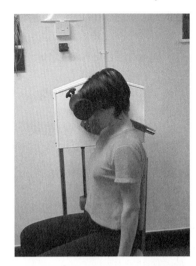

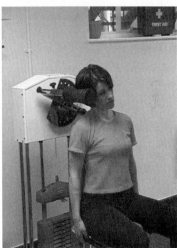

Flexion

Pad level with lower forehead, above the bridge of the nose.

Lateral Flexion

Shoulders remain level throughout. Pad positioned just above ear.

Progression

Progressed by incremental increases in resistance. Aiming gradually toward extensors 1.7: 1 flexors ratio.

Maximal/comfortable levels should be achieved during assessment.

Note

At the start of each ROM, a "warm-up" set of repetitions with 0.5 kg of resistance should be performed.

(continued)

Exercise 27-11 Reverse Fly

The Procedure

Patient prone on bench with suitable weight in hand and extend arms with slight elbow flexion, shoulders at 90° abduction. Co-contraction.

Shoulders must be depressed throughout and ensure scapular retraction is attained (main aim of exercise) and watch for over active trapezius (shoulder elevation).

Alternatives

Wall angel or floor angel (often preferred by patients)

Advancement

Perform over a gym ball in superman position.

Exercise 27-12 Supine Fly

Correct Procedure

Supine on bench with suitable weight dumb bells. Arms abducted to 90° with slight elbow flexion. Bring weights up until they touch, and then lower.

Maintain shoulder depression throughout.

Alternatives

Push-ups, but watch for winging and superior migration of the shoulder (overactive upper trapezius).

Bench press.

Exercise 27-13 Gym Ball Phasic— Dorsal Raises

The Procedure

Feet against wall or secured, shoulder-width apart. Lying prone in straight line over ball so navel is just clear of ball. Co-contraction. Hands beside forehead. Lowering until hands as far as possible and extending to just above neutral.

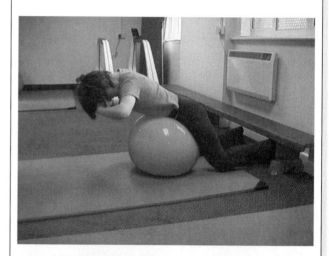

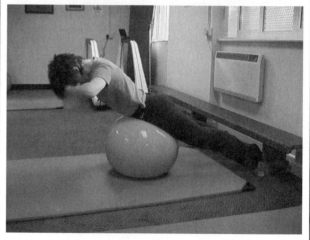

Notes

Similar to aspects of the superman track and promotes good stability because of labile surface.

shown to have no significant effect on the cross-sectional area of the multifidus in chronic low back pain sufferers.

It is intended that a significant degree of competence will develop in all aspects of the patient's exercises and independence will gradually develop. Although not individually supervised at every visit, the rehabilitation supervisor will ensure that adequate progression is demonstrated through self-report, objective outcome questionnaires, functional tests, and demonstration of increasing independence.

Stage 3—Discharge and Independent Exercise

The core exercises in this section are described in Exercises 27-13, 27-14, and 27-15.

Successful outcome of stage 2 must clearly involve functional and symptomatic improvement but, perhaps more importantly, must have promoted self-reliance and an absence of fear–avoidance behavior. Consequently, and somewhat paradoxically, success-ful candidates will remove themselves from stage 2 into their own environment, to continue at home, with gym ball phasic exercises or conventional gym exercise sessions.

Patient Selection and Assessment

In developing and incorporating rehabilitation in to chiropractic care, it is essential to decide on a system

Exercise 27-14 Gym Ball Phasic—Leg Raises

The Procedure

Prone over gym ball resting forearms on floor. Trochanters to apex of ball. Co-contraction.

Raise legs as describes for angle bench hip extension, and maintain a posterior pelvic tilt.

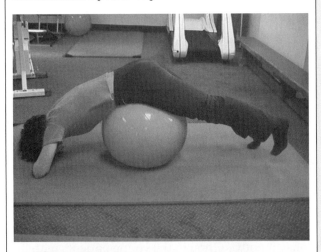

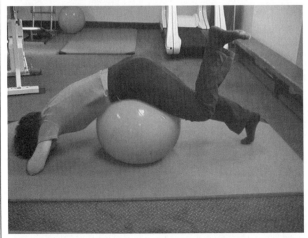

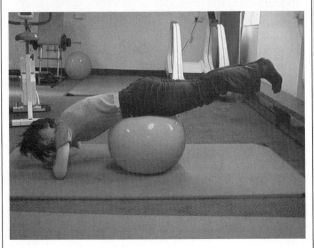

Notes

Promotes good stability because of labile surface.

Exercise 27-15 Gym Ball Phasic— Lateral Raises

The Procedure

A difficult exercise and the patient should take care.

Side-lying on gym ball with upside leg forward, and feet secured at base of wall. Main point of contact on gym ball = greater trochanter.

Cross arms across chest. Raise and lower laterally.

Notes

Promotes good stability because of labile surface, but difficult to master. Requires supervision in early stages because of trunk flexion recruitment.

of identification for suitable candidates. Most importantly, a screen of "red flags" is necessary to rule out sinister pathology and ensure the condition considered for isotonic training is of a mechanical origin likely to respond to rehabilitation (see Chapter 7). It is chiefly the chronicity predictors that provide indicators as to who is most likely to benefit from a course of training (Chapter 9).

Basic Premises for Referral

There are six basic premises dictating referral to stage 2:

1. The chief predictor for chronic ongoing pain and disability appears to be chronicity itself (54), and this is the most common reason for referral to the rehabilitation unit. The majority of clinical trials of intensive isotonic training select patient populations with long-standing pain diagnosed as being of spinal origin (2,3,7,15,26,27,36, 37,45).

2. If chronicity describes ongoing rather than episodic spinal pain, recurrence of symptoms forms a second key referral indicator. This is supported by previous work showing high recurrence rates at 1 year (84%) of low back pain in patients with confirmed segmental multifidus atrophy (21).

3. The diagnosis of discogenic pain forms another key referral criterion. This is considered especially important for various reasons. Discal injuries have a relatively poor prognosis and surgical intervention is more common. Furthermore, because of the highly segmental nature of the injury, the potential segmental inhibition of the local stabilizing system and consequent destabi-

lization are considered to strongly predispose to future recurrent pain and disability. Intervention through isotonic training is considered appropriate in the post-surgical patient or after successful passive care (7,26,36,52).

4. The fourth standard criterion for referral is failure to respond. This encompasses a failure to improve at all with passive treatment and/or a plateau of progress. At such a point, a further rehabilitation assessment may well be appropriate.

5. Traumatic onset of spinal pain necessarily constitutes an important reason for isotonic training, because muscle tissue injury and pain-related inhibition inevitably occur. Typical within this category are the whiplash-associated disorders.

6. Finally, given the potential for any acute pain to become chronic (10), should a patient wish to begin a course of rehabilitation, it is inevitably encouraged.

Achieving Compliance

Compliance is a major issue in the successful outcome of an intensive rehabilitation program. Failure to perform the program with to the standard required or a failure to attend inevitably adversely affects the outcome (14,18,46).

To reduce non-compliance, several issues need to be considered:

1. The cost and time commitment are discussed with the patient before referral to the program. A start date is agreed when the patient will be able to attend consistently over a (minimum) 10-week period. Failure to identify this will lead to (i) non-acceptance into the program, (ii) a program with reduced supervision, or (iii) a home-based program but only undertaken if the supervision–compliance relationship is discussed.

2. The nature of the training program is also discussed in detail. The patient should know what to expect once training begins.

3. Also at this stage, the likely benefits to the patient are discussed. Because the literature and our own experiences support improvement in pain intensity, frequency of episodes, and duration of episodes in the average patient undergoing such programs, these are identified as the likely changes. However, because no patient is truly "average," it is necessary to explain that the specific benefits to the individual are unpredictable. They are also counselled that improvement may not be seen until the sixth week (38).

4. Also, the "relative neglect of pain" MUST be discussed with the patient.

5. Appropriate patient selection is paramount because despite the insistence of many insurance companies, rehabilitation is not for everyone! Compliance is only maintained IF the individual is motivated or open to such motivation. The staff may encourage this, but largely this is up to the individual.

6. Finally, selection of the appropriate rehabilitation supervisor is essential and should not be underestimated. Positive reinforcement, encouragement, and an understanding nature are probably the most important attributes that the supervisor can have when dealing with the de-conditioned pain sufferer. Good initial intentions and motivations are easily eroded if early attempts at exercise exacerbate the problem. The skill of the supervisor is to encourage, enthuse, and motivate the patient beyond initial early discomfort toward individual goals.

Consequently, although the young patients with first time, post-acute low back pain are excellent candidates in whom to promote rehabilitation and prevent chronicity, they are unlikely to commit to an extended supervised program. Conversely, the individual who has suffered recurrent bouts of pain and has "been everywhere" with limited success and "wants to do something for himself" may be ideal and, moreover, motivated.

Exclusion Criteria

Most of the exclusion criteria for isotonic training are those that are exclusion from rehabilitation in itself. These range from undetected or uncontrolled hypertension, the presence of pathology, etc., and are largely beyond the scope of this chapter. However, there are clinical considerations that may lead to the patient being excluded from rehabilitation. It may be desirable for the rehabilitation supervisor to conduct cardiovascular assessment to ensure heart rate and blood pressure responses to exercise are within normal limits and to use a suitable questionnaire.

Although it is rare to exclude an individual who is motivated to attend rehabilitation from isotonic training protocols, the authors have modified the original "disregard of pain" concept, because a number of people did not cope well with this approach. Most of these individuals demonstrated significant fear–avoidance behavior (demonstrated through such measures as the Bournemouth Questionnaire; chapter 8) and required a less vigorous approach. Consequently, although patients are encouraged to set their own goals and are "pushed" to achieve these, a number are removed from isotonic training and transferred to an alternative program initially, progressing to isotonics at a later stage.

Furthermore, in the case of neck pain, the authors have noted that patients need to have a relatively full and painless range of motion and need to be in a period of remission to progress well. Largely, the more acute neck pain sufferer will be put on active range of movement exercises, cervical spine sensorimotor training, and eye–neck coordination protocols, rather than isotonic training machines.

Assessment

Individual assessment and prescription that are tailored to individual's needs, rather than general low back or neck programs, have been shown to be more effective than programs (13). Assessment procedures integrating various aspects of muscle function for spinal disorders have been devised. Tests of strength and endurance, which assist the prescription of, and emphasis on, isotonic exercise, are supported by tests of local muscle function, muscle tone, and length imbalance and sensorimotor function.

In completing these examination routines, the examiner identifies deficits in the various parameters of muscle function as it pertains to spinal stabilization, so that rather than merely "blanket" prescription of isotonic training an integrated package of exercise procedures tailored to the individual's requirements may be devised.

Assessment Criteria

As with clinical assessment, there are few pathognomonic tests in rehabilitation assessment, so the clinician must use judgement in the interpretation of the information that can be gleaned from the gamut of tests at their disposal. The initial tests aim to identify general muscle imbalance:

- Posture: Postural analysis through the methods described by Janda and by Liebenson is applied as a general screen. Postural syndromes (e.g., upper crossed syndrome, lower crossed, etc.) are identified along with more local abnormalities (e.g., lumbar lordosis length, sacral angle etc.) (chapter 10).
- Movement Patterns: These allow the examiner to more specifically assess the combined function of global musculature as it pertains to joint stabilization during movement. Evidence of muscle over activity or shortening can be correlated with findings on specific muscle

length analysis and posture. The key patterns assessed are the trunk flexion, hip extension and hip abduction movement patterns for the low back and trunk lowering, neck flexion, and arm abduction for the upper body (chapter 10). Further associated motion assessment, e.g., the squat or lunge test may also be appropriate. (Chapter 34)

- Muscle Length: Assess muscle lengths of the postural groups, which are prone to hypertonicity and may have a role in perpetuating or predisposing to recurrence of spinal–related conditions. (Table 27.1)
- Local Stabilization Tests: Muscle control of the local stabilizers is tested through pressure biofeedback of transversus abdominus contraction and palpation tests of multifidus for the low back and through the measurement of cervico-cranial flexion endurance/coordination in the neck. These procedures are described in chapter 25.
- Sensorimotor Function: Sensorimotor function as it pertains to low back stabilization is assessed through the one-leg stand test, Hautant's test, Unterberger's test, and Fukada-Unterberger's test. Additionally, head repositioning accuracy may be sought and retrained to promote the cervico-occular reflexes (47). These tests may be selected based on historical indicators.

All the information provided through these examination procedures provides prescriptive indicators for the exercises, which may be used to complement the isotonic training.

More specific information pertaining to isotonic training may be provided through the following quantifiable local stabilization, isometric, and isotonic tests:

1. Quantifiable abdominal muscle tests: such as the prone abdominal drawing in test and various trunk flexor tests as described in chapter 11 are useful for establishing baselines from which to judge progress with abdominal exercise routines.

2. Isometric endurance of the erector spinae: identified by Bierring-Soerenson as having a strong correlation with the development of first time low back pain and with recurrence (7), this test is valuable prescriptively and as an outcome measure. Subsequent trials have further sought to clarify the reliability and specificity of this test (33,34,44), and it has been criticized as being too dependent on motivational factors, but it remains one of the best-known methods

Table 27.1 Postural Muscles of the Low Back and Neck

Low-Back Groups	Neck Groups
Lumbar extensors	Neck flexors
Gluteals	Neck extensors
Abdominals	Neck lateral flexors
Abductors	Sub-occipital muscles
Adductors	Lower trapezius
Quadriceps	Pectorals
Hamstrings	Serratus anterior
Latissimus dorsi	
Multifidus & transverse abdominus	Deep neck flexors

for assessing lumbar extensor endurance. One possible limitation of this test is that it measures static isometric endurance. Because the training is isotonic, the authors feel a more dynamic test may be more appropriate as an outcome measure (9).

3. Dorsal raises: The lumbar extensors can be tested isotonically, a test which is preferred by the authors. Isotonic testing of the erector spinae involves the use of an angle bench and requires the patient to perform their maximum number of dorsal raises. When to stop is the decision of the patient, but the patient is guided to continue until unable to perform another repetition without fatigue or pain to 5° extension (see art in Exercise 27-2). The test is performed through angles of flexion rather than from neutral to extension because of length/tension relationship issues and because this is more representative of typical acts of daily living (ADLs) and directly comparable to the program being undertaken. This test has previously been described in the literature (34,43). To further assess reliability and help establish normative data, a further study of normal subjects is currently in press (9). Currently, our observations are that in the chronic low back pain population, a typical range of values is 10 to 25 repetitions.

4. Isometric testing of maximum voluntary contraction (M.V.C.) in the cervical spine: This may be assessed by a digital strain gauge attached to the "neck machine." The reliability of this device and normative data have been published (28). An alternative method is through the use of a sphygmomanometer, in which forces of the neck are measured when a patient pushes into the blood pressure cuff, which is pre-inflated to 20 mmHg (53).

5. Jull's cervico-cranial flexion test: Jull has described a simple screening test for deep neck flexor weakness (53). This is a progressive test of cervico-cranial flexion motion, coordination, and endurance using a pressure biofeedback device (see Chapter 25).

Prescription

Detailed assessments allow the identification of deficits in the musculoskeletal stabilizing systems, allowing a fairly "lesion-specific" approach to prescribing corrective interventions/exercises.

When prescribing an exercise regime, the primary intervention is the relaxation and if necessary stretching of overactive or shortened muscle groups, followed by the promotion of local stabilization (stage 1). This advances through the exercise program (stage 2) to self-reliance (stage 3).

The prescribed program needs to be flexible enough to allow all deficits to be trained within a single rehabilitation session (usually 45 to 60 minutes) if necessary, or alternatively to focus on a particular weakness. Within a largely standardized framework, there is room to de-emphasise or even omit exercise tracks in which the patient has demonstrated competence to focus on areas of weakness. For example, the patient may demonstrate little or no sensorimotor or muscle length problems but may have obviously inadequate global and local muscle activity. Alternatively, some patients (such as athletes) may demonstrate excellent flexibility, strength, endurance, and balance but fail a test of co-contraction and demonstrate segmental multifidus atrophy, indicating a need to concentrate almost entirely on local stabilization training.

Local muscle deficit is trained with continued local stability training, and the global deficit is targeted through the prescription of isotonic exercises, as identified in exercises 27-2 to 27-12. Most patients will perform all the exercises, but the muscle groups trained hardest will be identified and corrected according to Table 27.2.

The emphasis placed on each depends on the performance during the assessment, with specific regard for the lumbar flexors and extensors. The emphasis must depend on the correction of normal strength ratios.

The co-contraction track for spinal stabilization involves a high degree of specificity, and methods such as pressure biofeedback and real-time ultrasonography have been used by their developers (19,20,23–25) to ensure the correct action at every stage of advancement. Once the patient is on the isotonic resistance equipment, there is no guarantee that co-contraction is maintained; we must rely on the patient's kinaesthetic awareness of the correct contraction. As Richardson states:

"At the present time there are no methods for checking if appropriate control of segmental motion is occurring during functional tasks."

There is also a case for incorporating the equivalent cervical method of local stabilizer recruitment, i.e., lower scapular stabilizer contraction and cervicocranial flexion, to isotonic neck exercises. But this is complex and requires a high level of competency to ensure the correct procedure.

Considering the integration of sensorimotor training with isotonic exercise, the literature does not appear to offer any specific guidelines. Therefore, it is logical to address these issues in parallel. The patient may initiate sensorimotor training (such as balance board tracks and one-leg stand exercises) at the same time as isotonic exercise.

In the later stages of the low back program, the aspects of sensorimotor, co-contraction, and endurance training become integrated when exercises such as dorsal raises, leg raises, and lateral raises are transferred from the angle bench to the gym ball, i.e., from a stable to a labile surface. This leads to stage 3, independence and discharge.

Holding co-contraction while performing dorsal raises on a labile surface such as the ball is clearly an advanced exercise, but it could be argued this pro-

Table 27.2 Correlation of Functional Test, Isotonic Exercise, and Muscle Groups Trained

Test	Example of an Isotonic Procedure	Muscle Groups
Isometric endurance test Dorsal raise test Hip extension movement pattern	Dorsal raises	Lumbar extensors Hamstrings Gluteals
Hip extension movement pattern	Wide-stance bench squats Hip extensions	Gluteals
Trunk flexion movement pattern Quantifiable abdominal muscle test	Curl-downs, sit-ups, crunches, gym ball curl-ups, fitter	Abdominal muscles
Hip abduction movement pattern	Side raises or side-lying abductions/adductions	QL, hip abductors/adductors
Neck flexion movement pattern of Janda Jull's cervico-cranial flexion test Neck flexors M.V.C.	Resisted flexion on neck machine (note ratio)	Cervical flexors
Neck extensors M.V.C.	Resisted extension on neck machine (note ratio)	Cervical extensors
Neck lateral flexors M.V.C.	Resisted flexion on neck machine (equal ratios)	Cervical lateral flexors

vides multiple therapeutic benefits. For that reason alone, it could be argued that the spinal stabilization exercises (chapter 26) are superior to the gym-based isotonic approach.

Concurrent Passive Care

Given that the benefits of the program will not typically become apparent until several weeks after commencement, it is inevitable that most patients will experience some ongoing, or even increased, discomfort in the early stages of training.

Manniche (38,39) noted that in a low back pain population, improvements were not felt until 5 to 7 weeks of rehabilitation. Clearly, concurrent passive care is appropriate for most patients until their symptoms improve and they achieve greater independence.

Although a "relative disregard" of pain is advocated, we have become more pragmatic as the program has developed and have not instructed people to continue to work until our goals are met, rather until their goals are met. Additionally, the Bierring Sorensen test has now been, largely, removed from the program because we found that a number of people had a retrograde step before rehabilitation caused by their sustained holding of this position. Also, this test, in the symptomatic patient, is no longer one of endurance but rather a test of pain tolerance.

Post-Isotonic Program

Reassessment

Reassessment may be formal (as in the initial referral to the program) or informal (taking place in the gym during an exercise session) and, largely, toward the end of the program the patients are in three categories:

1. Discharge and move to independence. Many people gradually go through an informal reassessment and leave the rehabilitation center having made significant gains and move on to a gym or independent home-based program.

2. Failure to respond. The literature suggests that the average time for a rehabilitation program is between 8 and 12 weeks, with response expected within 5 to 7 weeks (5). Clearly, not everyone is "average" and a failure to respond by 6 to 8 weeks is likely to require a formal reassessment. The patients' goals and expectations are revisited and a re-evaluation of their performance undertaken. In our experience, and if they are willing to continue beyond such a point, most people respond

IF they can master co-contraction and exhibit good "form" in their exercises.

3. A significant proportion of people are not "exercise-types" and recognize their own shortcomings. They realize that they will not continue alone at home (with phase 3) and prefer to continue at the rehabilitation center. Their own program will be negotiated individually such that it will give them weekly (or every 2 weeks) contact with the rehabilitation staff, allowing periodic supervision and advancement. They will also continue at home.

Cases

Case 1—Mrs. R. (Ratio Correction)

Mrs. R., a 63-year-old woman, had been suffering from periodic, recurrent bouts of low back pain since her first acute episode at the age of 28. In recent years the bouts had become more frequent and more persistent and, although she had previously enjoyed long periods of relief from passive treatment, she was now having continuous trouble. Mrs. R. had been a competitive swimmer since her younger years and continued to swim (breast stroke) some significant distance "at least three times per week."

Mrs. R. stood with a lower-crossed posture. Her hip extension movement pattern demonstrated early activity of the bilateral erector spinae. The leg abduction pattern showed tightness of the iliopsoas and her trunk flexion pattern was normal, although she was not capable of performing sit-ups without lifting her feet. Mrs. R.'s Biering-Sorenson test (erector spinae endurance) exceeded 240 seconds.

Her history of swimming is typical of an individual who does not cross-train sufficiently. Her erector spinae endurance is exceptional for her age (and typical of a dedicated swimmer) but it is significantly out of balance with the strength of the abdominal muscles. Clearly, training her low back musculature was not important.

Her program involved the redressing of this balance and, after 8 weeks, she was significantly better. Abdominal work is now incorporated into her training regime.

Case 2—Mr. J. (The 10-Week Program Is Only "Average")

Mr. J., a 43-year-old man, was referred to the rehabilitation center by his medical practitioner. He had been off work for the past 30 months after a fall from his horse, which caused "intractable weakness" in his low back. The pain was constant at 5 on a scale of 10, and "any exercise" aggravated the pain to 8 to 9 on a scale of 10. He had been signed off work as permanently disabled but was keen to attempt anything that may help. He had not ridden a horse since the accident.

Mr. J. took 4 weeks to master the co-contraction exercise. At that stage he still could not be assessed for erector spinae endurance because it was felt that this would aggravate his pain. His movement patterns were normal in terms of movement sequences and patterning, although generally "weak."

Mr. J. was an extreme example of the deconditioned patient. After 20 weeks in the rehabilitation gym, after beginning with co-contraction and building up through gym ball phasic exercises and the use of the "fitter" for abdominal work, he became fully independent. He was reduced to weekly and then two weekly visits and discharged approximately 6 months after his first exercise assessment. He converted part of his house into a dedicated low-technical gym and continues his exercises.

Mr. J. has begun horse riding again and works as a counsellor in drug and alcohol abuse.

Case 3—Mr. B. (the Importance of Local Stabilization)

Mr. B. is a 32-year-old tri-athlete who is, needless to say, very fit. He trains daily and conducts a sensible cross-training regime, involving cycling, running, swimming, and gym work. However, despite this activity he experiences back pain with running. He has experienced little relief from various practitioners of passive care, despite allowing them a "reasonable" window of time to treat him.

Mr. B.'s strength tests were normal, with the major deficit identified in his assessment being the inability to hold and maintain co-contraction, and it was this that was trained, largely outside of the rehabilitation gym environment—something that can be achieved by the dedicated sportsman. Mastering this simple exercise afforded him a significant decrease in the severity of the pain, which now only comes mildly and towards the end of an event.

■ CONCLUSION

Training the spinal stabilization system requires a combination of fine motor control and isotonic exercises. One of the most important reasons to include isotonic programs is that many patients are highly motivated to work out in gyms, thus making greater compliance with such a program feasible. Naturally, by combining the principles of local stabilization motor control into global stabilization exercises, greater safety and effectiveness can be anticipated.

Audit Process
Self-Check of the Chapter's Learning Objectives

- What are the principles underpinning isotonic training in rehabilitation?

- Outline the key elements in the design of an isotonic training which are likely to improve the program's effectiveness.

- What is core stability and why is it important?

- Define normal strength and endurance measurements and the ratios of agonist–antagonist relationships?

- Devise an assessment procedure.

- For any given spinal muscle group insufficiency, which isotonic exercises might be used in its correction?

■ ACKNOWLEDGEMENTS

The authors thank Zoe Scott for her contribution to this chapter and, moreover, for her invaluable contribution to the Rehabilitation Centre at AECC.

■ REFERENCES

1. Alaranta H, Hurrri, Heliovaara M, Soukka A, Harju R. Intensive physical and psychosocial training program for patients with chronic low back pain. Spine 1994;19:1339–1349.

2. Alaranta H, Hurrri, Heliovaara M, Soukka A, Harju R. Non-dynamometric trunk performance tests: Reliability and normative data. Scan J of Rehab Med 1994;26:211–215.

3. Alaranta, H, Hurri H. Non-dynamometric performance tests; reliability and normative data. Scand J Rehabil Med 1994;26:211–215.

4. Alexandre NM, Nordin M, Hiebert R, Campello M. Predictors of compliance with short-term treatment among patients with back pain. Rev Panam Salud Publica 2002;12:86–94.

5. Beimborn DS, Morrisey MC. A review of the literature related to trunk muscle performance. Spine 1988;13;655–659.

6. Bentsen H, Lindgarde F, Manthorpe R. The effect of dynamic strength back exercise and/or a home training program in 57-year-old women with chronic low back pain. Results of a prospective randomized study with a 3-year follow-up period. Spine 1997;22:1494–500.

7. Biering Soerensen F. Physical measurements as risk indicators for low back trouble over a one year period. Spine 1984;9:106–119.

8. Bolton J, Humphreys BK. Shifts in approaches to continuing professional development: implications for the chiropractic profession. J Manip Physio Ther 1998;21:368–371.

9. Carr-Hyde R, Cook J. The reliability of dynamic endurance testing of the lumbar extensor muscles. Submitted for publication.

10. Croft PR, Macfarlane GJ, Papageorgiou AC, Thomas E, Silman AJ. Outcome of low back pain in general practice. BMJ 1998;316:1356–1359.

11. Danneels LA, Cools AM, Vanderstraeten GG, Cambier DC, Witvrouw EE, Bourgois J, de Cuyper HJ. The effects of three different training modalities on the cross-sectional area of the paravertebral muscles. Scand J Med Sci Sports. 2001;11:335–341.

12. Danneels, LA, Vanderstraeten GG, Cambier DC, Witurouwee EE, Dankaerts W, Decuyper HJ. Effects of three different training modalities on the cross sectional area of the lumbar multifidus in patients with chronic low back pain. Br J Sports Med 2001;35:186–191.

13. Descarreaux M, Normand MC, Laurencelle L, Dugas Evaluation of a specific home exercise program for low back pain. J Manipulative Physiol Ther 2002;25:497–503.

14. Fordyce W, McMahon R, Rainwater G, Jackins S, Quensted K, Murphy T, Delateur B. Pain complaint-exercise performance relationship in chronic pain. Pain 1981;10:311–321.

15. Frost H, Klaber Moffett JA, Moser JS, Fairbank JCT. Randomised controlled trial for evaluation of fitness program for patients with chronic low back pain. BMJ 1995;310:151–154.

16. Graves JE, Pollock M, Foster D, Legget SH, Carpenter DM, Vuoso R, Jones A. The Effect of training frequency and specificity on isometric lumbar extension strength. Spine 1990;15:504–509.

17. Harding VR, Simmonds R, Watson P. Physical therapy for chronic pain. Pain Clin Updates. 1998;1ASP2(3):1–4.

18. Harkapaa K, Jarvikoski A, Mellin G, Hurri H. Controlled study on the outcome of inpatient and out patient treatment of low back pain. Scand J Rehabil Med 1989;21:81–89.

19. Hides JA and Richardson CA. Multifidus muscle recovery is not automatic after resolution of acute, first episode low back pain. Spine 1996;21:2763–2769.

20. Hides JA and Stokes. Evidence of lumbar multifidus wasting ipsilateral to symptoms in patients with acute/sub-acute low back pain. Spine 1994;19:165–172.

21. Hides JA, Richardson CA, Jull GA. Multifidus muscle recovery is not automatic after resolution of acute, first-episode low back pain. Spine. 1996;21:2763–2769.

22. Highland TR, Dreisinger TE, Vie LL, Russell GS. Changes in isometric strength and range of motion of the isolated cervical spine after eight weeks of clinical rehabilitation. Spine. 1992;17(6 Suppl):S77–S82.

23. Hodges P, Richardson CA. Inefficient stabilization of the lumbar spine associated with low back pain. Spine 1996;21:2640–2650.

24. Hodges P. Is there a role for transversus abdominus in lumbo-pelvic stability. Manual Ther 1999;4:74–86.

25. Hodges P. Transverus abdominus: the forgotten muscle. Proceedings of the 3rd interdisciplinary world conference on low back and pelvic pain, Vienna, Austria, 1998.

26. Jordan A, Manniche C. Rehabilitation and spinal pain. J Neuromusculo Sys 1996;4:89–93.

27. Jordan A, Mehlson J, Martin Bulow P, Danneskidd-Samsoe B. A comparison of physical characteristics between patients seeking treatment for neck pain and age-matched healthy people. J Manipu Physio Ther 1997;20:468–475.

28. Jordan A, Mehlson J, Ostergaard K. Strength and endurance measurements of the cervical musculature in 100 healthy subjects. Proceedings of the international conference on spinal manipulation, Toronto, Ontario, 1999.

29. Jordan A, Ostergard K Rehabilitation of neck/shoulder patients in primary health care clinics. J Manipu Physio Ther 1996;19:32–35.

30. Jordan, A, Mehlsen, J, Bulow, P, Ostergaard, K, Danneskiold-Samsoe, B. Maximal isometric strength of the cervical musculature in 100 healthy volunteers. Spine 1999;24:1343–1348.

31. Juker D, McGill SM, Kropf P, Steffen T. Quantitative intramuscular myoelectric activity of lumbar portions of psoas and the abdominal wall during a wide variety of tasks. Med Sci Sports Exercise 1998;30:301–310.

32. Kumar S, Dufrense RM, VanSchor T. Human trunk strength profile in flexion and extension. Spine 1995;20:160–168.

33. Latimer, J, Maher, C, Refschauge, K, Colaco, I. The reliability and validity of the Biering-Soerensen test in asymptomatic subjects and subjects reporting current or non-specific low back pain. Spine 1999;24:2085–2090.

34. Lattika P, Battie MC, Viderman T, Gibbons LE. Correlations of isokinetic and psychophysical back lift and static back extensor endurance tests in men. Clin Biomechanics 1995;10:325–330.

35. Luoto S, Heliovara M, Hurri H, Alaranta H. Static back endurance and the risk of low back pain. Clin Biomechanics 1995;10:323–324.

36. Manniche C, Jordan A. Editorial. Spine 1995;20:1221–1222.

37. Manniche, C Lundberg E, Christensen I, Bentzen L, Hesselsoe G. Intensive dynamic exercises for chronic low back pain: A clinical trial. Pain 1991;47:53–63.

38. Manniche C. Intensive dynamic back exercises with or without hyperextension in chronic back pain after surgery for lumbar disc protrusion: A clinical trial. Spine 1993;18:560–567.

39. Manniche C. Low back pain and exercise. Ugeskr Laeger 1993;155:142–144.

40. McAuley E, Courneya KS, Rudolph DL, Lox CL. Enhancing exercise adherence in middle-aged males and females. J Prev Med 1994;23:498–506.

41. McGill SM. Low back stability: From formal description to issues for performance and rehabilitation. Exercise Sports Sci Rev 2001;29:26–31.

42. McGill S. Low back disorders: evidence-based prevention and rehabilitation. Human Kinetics, 2002.

43. Meyer TG, Gatchel RJ, Mayer H, Kishino ND, Keeley J, Mooney V. A prospective 2 year study of functional restoration in industrial low back injury: an objective assessment procedure. JAMA 1987;258:1763–1767.

44. Ng JK, Richardson CA. Reliability of electromyographic power spectral analysis of back muscle endurance in healthy subjects. Arch Phys Med Rehabil 1996;77:259–264.

45. Pollock ML, Leggett SH, Graves JE, Jones A, Fulton M, Cirulli J. Effect of resistance training on lumbar extensor strength. Am J Sports Med 1989;17:232–238.

46. Reilly K, Lovejoy B, Williams R, Roth H. Differences between a supervised and independent strength and conditioning program with chronic low back syndromes. J Occup Med 1989;31:547–550.

47. Revel M, Minguet M, Gergoy P, Vaillant J, Thomas E, Silman AJ. Changes in cervicocephalic kinaesthesia after a proprioceptive rehabilitation program in patients with neck pain: a randomised controlled trial. Arch Phys Med Rehab 1994;75:895–899.

48. Richardson CA, Snijders CJ, Hides JA, Damen L, Pas MS, Storm J. The relation between the transversus abdominis muscles, sacroiliac joint mechanics, and low back pain. Spine 2002;27:399–405.

49. Rissanen A, Alaranta H, Sainio P, Harkonen. Isokinetic and Non-dynamic tests in low back pain patients related to pain disability index. Spine 1994;19:1963–1967.

50. Rissanen A, Heliovaara M, Alaranta H, Taimela S, Malkia E, Knekt P, Reunanen A, Aromaa A. Does good trunk extensor performance protect against back-related work disability? J Rehabil Med 2002;34:62–66.

51. Saal JA, Saal JS. Non-operative management of herniated cervical intervertebral disc with radiculopathy. Spine 1996;21:1877–1883.

52. Schifferdecker-Hoch F, Denner A. Mobility, strength and endurance parameters of the paraspinal musculature. Age and gender specific reference data. Manuelle Medizin 1999;37:30–33.

53. Vernon H. Muscle strength testing of the neck with a manual modified sphygmomanometer dynamometer. Eur J Chir 1994;44:41–49.

54. Waddell G. Low Back Pain: A twentieth Century Enigma. Spine 1996;21:2820–2825.

28

Weight Training for Back Stability

Chris Norris

Learning Objectives

After reading this chapter, you should be able to understand:

- How to progress patients from floor to isotonic weight machine regimes
- How to incorporate stability principles into health club exercises
- How to vary intensity, sets, and repetitions to achieve strength-training goals
- The basic weight machines that can be used to train endurance and strength in the torso muscles and how to prescribe their use
- The basic free-weight and medicine ball exercises for developing strength and power in the trunk and lower quarter

We have seen in Chapters 2 and 25 that muscles may be categorized into local and global types. Enhancing endurance of the local muscle system and reducing the dominance of the global system has been proposed as a functional method of low back rehabilitation (12,9). However, reducing a patient's reliance on the global system to supply muscle stability to the low back has led to a tendency among some clinicians to forget the global system entirely and seek to enhance the performance of the local muscle system in isolation. However, the use of weight-training to enhance back stability has been shown to be an effective clinical tool (13) and to forbid its use is to withhold a potentially valuable method of treatment in low back pain (see Chapter 27).

Interaction between local and global muscles (2) occurs by the local muscles controlling stability and subtle local movements of the individual lumbar segments, whereas the global muscles balance external forces that would tend to move the spine away from its neutral position. In addition, global muscles act to stabilize in times of extreme need, and both sporting actions and manual handling represent such occurrences.

Weight-training for back stability may be used either as a final progression to a general stability program or for technique instruction of individuals undergoing stability training who currently train in a gym as part of a general fitness regime. One of the essential questions for the clinician is when to move a patient from floor exercise for stability (free exercises and gym balls) to weight-based exercise (machines and free-weights).

When Is Weight-Training Appropriate?

Before beginning a weight-training program, a patient must have good core stability. Techniques to measure this and fundamental exercises to enhance core stability have been described in Chapters 11, 25, 26, and 34. Table 28.1 reiterates the essential requirements before a patient should be allowed to begin a weight-training program.

Back stability training has been described as paralleling the three stages of motor learning (9,10,15). Isolated muscle work (in this case of the deep muscle corset) represents the first stage, and it is essential that this has been completed before weight-training commences. In the second stage the essential feature is that the subjects are now able to recognize and correct their own mistakes in these simple actions. Clinically this means that subjects know when they have moved away from the neutral lumbar position and are able to move back at will. Once this is achieved, complex movements are subdivided into their fundamental components and these are learned while maintaining a neutral spinal position. Limb movements are often used on a stable base during this stage, and basic weight-training movements with machines may also be used. A greater variety of movements are required with free-weight exercises, and so these are used as a progression on the machine exercises. As the subjects move into the third stage of motor learning, the essential feature is that they are now able to control the position of their lumbar region and stabilize with little attention. This represents automatic action and faster explosive exercises may now be used.

Concepts of Resistance Training
Overload

For muscle tissue to strengthen, it must adapt to a resistance that overloads it. Overloading occurs only when muscle contracts at a level greater than that of everyday living. For example, flexing and extending the elbow occurs in everyday activities, so to perform this movement alone will not overload the arm flexors. Overload will only occur when the frequency, intensity, duration, and type of movement is greater

Table 28.1 Before Beginning a Weight-Training Program the Subject Should Be Able to:

- Identify neutral lumbar position
- Identify and maintain neutral position while performing limb movements
- Avoid muscle substitution strategies while maintaining neutral position
- Breath normally (avoid breath holding) while maintaining neutral position
- Maintain neutral lumbar position for 10 repetitions of a 10-second limb movement.
- Perform attention demanding movements while maintaining neutral position
- Perform the hip hinge action (page 695) correctly and for 5 repetitions
- Have a basic knowledge of postural alignment and manual handling techniques associated with gym apparatus.

than that which is familiar to the body. For basic stability work, muscle endurance is required, and exercises must rehearse correct movement patterns. Exercises at this stage have a fairly long duration (10 to 30 seconds) for each repetition, with the aim of recruiting type I fibers. The type of movement chosen must reflect correct lumbo-pelvic alignment. Movements for the main should be performed with the lumbar spine in its neutral position, with the limbs moving on the trunk as a fairly immobile base. The intensity of the actions is low and to familiarize the patient with the movement the frequency is high. For example, actions such as abdominal hollowing and multifidus recruitment (Chapter 25) may be performed throughout the day to build the patients awareness of the action. Through high repetition of movement, the action becomes so familiar that it will eventually become more automatic. When the patient is able to perform these actions automatically (without self-palpation, for example) he/she may use more complex weight-training exercises using free-weights. As the complexity of an exercise increases, the frequency should reduce so the patient does not degrade his/her performance at a particular task.

To increase strength, heavier resistances and fewer repetitions (8 to 10) of an exercise are used. In so doing, larger-diameter muscle fibers are recruited (14) and a greater percentage of type II (fast-twitch) fibers. To maintain muscle balance, it is essential that core stability exercises be maintained. If good core stability is achieved, type I fiber activity should balance type II activity. Should a patient move on to weight-training activities and simply forget core stability work, type II activity is further enhanced but type I activity will degrade through disuse. This will introduce a proportional muscle imbalance that may be detrimental to ultimate performance. Balanced training, at all stages of fitness, is the key.

Fitness Components

There are several components to fitness, and as a training guide the 'S' factor list (Table 28.2) is useful.

All of the fitness components are important to some degree for back stability, and their importance varies depending on the stage of rehabilitation. Stamina, in this case representing local muscle endurance, is important as the holding time of a muscle. Endurance of the back muscles, for example, has been shown to be a predictor for occupational back pain (3,7) and enhancing the holding time of stability muscles has been stressed in Chapters 25 and 26. As the subject progresses to weight-training, there is a tendency to work for strength rather than endurance, whereas both are actually required. In terms of suppleness, both the range of motion and the resistance to motion are important. With functional instability, the stabilizing muscles may lose not only endurance but also their ability to work at full inner range. Performing inner range holding contractions therefore forms an important part of initial stability training and must be extended into the weight-training gym. Similarly, the use of eccentric strength is important. Again, in many popular weight-training programs eccentric actions are rarely used and concentric actions are focused on. From a stability perspective, concentric work must be balanced by an equal emphasis on eccentric (controlled lowering) and isometric (holding) muscle work.

Speed has an important place to play in back stability. Muscle reaction speed in response to a force tending to push a joint away from a stable position is a determining factor in stability of both peripheral joints (6,1) and the spine (5). The ability to detect when such movement is occurring (proprioception) is an aspect of skill. Practicing more complex activities such as free-weight exercises in addition to machine weight-training will enhance movement skill.

The technique used in any exercise will rehearse a specific set of actions that come together to make up a motor program. These actions must accurately reflect the required movement quality that is being sought by the rehabilitation program. Training specificity dictates that the changes occurring in the body as the result of exercise will match the technique

Table 28.2 The Components of Fitness

Component Title	Meaning
Stamina	Cardiovascular and local muscle endurance.
Suppleness	Range of motion and resistance to motion
Strength	Isotonic (concentric and eccentric) and isometric strength
Speed	Rate of movement and muscle reaction time
Specificity	Tailoring an exercise to the patients functional requirements
Spirit	Psychological features of exercise including fear of movement

used. There is said to be a specific adaptation to an imposed demand (the "SAID" pneumonic). Rehearsing incorrect techniques will degrade movement quality. For example, the hip hinge action is used to re-educate a patient's ability to combine stability with pelvic and lumbar movement and to improve general bending and lifting actions. If a squat exercise is practiced as part of a weight-training program, and if a poor technique is used, this will overflow into daily use of bending and lifting and encourage the patient to use poor technique in these actions, increasing the risk of occupational injury. A further aspect of skill that is important is removing fear of movement, so-called fear–avoidance (4,16). With chronic back pain especially, a patient may often consider that an action (for example, lifting or bending) may cause pain and therefore avoid this action. Using movements that involve these actions in a limited and protected way can gradually de-sensitize the patient and improve the functional ability.

Weight-Training Methods

Before an intense exercise program is used, a warm-up is recommended. This should prepare the body for increased levels of activity and rehearse any complex actions before performance with weights. The methods and effects of warm up are not within the remit of this chapter, but further information is available elsewhere (10).

In general terms, larger muscle groups are worked before smaller muscle groups during weight-training. This is because smaller muscles will tend to fatigue more quickly and so will be a limiting factor to training time. Exercises that involve several muscle groups (general exercises) are therefore placed before exercises using single muscles (isolation exercises). One exception to this rule is pre-exhaust training in which isolation movements are performed first.

More complex exercises, and especially free-weight exercises that require high degrees of skill, should be performed early during a routine. They are attention demanding and quality will degrade rapidly as fatigue sets in. Machine exercises are less demanding in terms of complexity and so may be used later in a weight-training program. For basic training with inexperienced users, the body parts that are worked should be alternated, such as arms–legs–trunk and repeat; this is known as circuit format. In this way the muscles worked are allowed an adequate recovery period. As users progress, two further orders may be used. The first is the com-

---

Clinical Pearl

Pre-exhaust training is a technique used purely for strength training to dramatically increase the stress imposed on a muscle and recruit large-diameter muscle fibers. When any muscle contracts to its maximal voluntary contraction (MVC), the point of failure is determined by both central and peripheral mechanisms. Peripheral mechanisms involve a muscle's physiology and include such factors as local phosphocreatine concentration and ATP availability. Central factors are largely the responsibility of mental processes and include motivation and the degree of motor unit recruitment. The point of failure that determines MVC is often the result of central mechanisms especially in the inexperienced user. A patient may therefore feel that they have achieved their maximum when in fact they have not. Using pre-exhaust training is a method of overcoming this limitation. Using the gluteal muscles as an example an isolation movement such as prone lying hip extension is used to the point of MVC. Immediately after this (no rest is allowed) a general exercise such as the squat is used. If the gluteals were truly fatigued the patient would be unable to perform the squat. By changing the muscle emphasis, however, the muscle is "fooled" into working harder.

---

pound set; here, two or more different exercises are used for the same muscle group. The second is the superset, in which two exercises are chosen that work the same body part but for two opposing muscle groups (agonist and antagonist).

In general terms, higher repetitions (12–15) with lighter weights are used for endurance training, and lower repetitions (6–8) with heavier weights are used for strength. A back stability program with weights aims to build strength while maintaining muscle endurance which has already been established by free exercise. Repetition numbers in the region of 10 to 12 are therefore used. Slower movements that take greater time will also improve endurance and allow the user more time to attend to postural alignment. Faster movements that take less time give a more explosive action and less time is available to attend to alignment. For this reason, slower, more precise actions are used in the initial stages of weight-training and faster more explosive exercises are only used when alignment is good and stability has become more automatic and therefore, by definition, less attention-demanding.

To perform intense exercise safely, progressive loading is needed. This enables the user to gradually improve the coordination required by high-intensity muscle work. Several neurogenic changes involving the motor unit are required, including enhanced recruitment, motor unit firing frequency, synchronization, and dis-inhibition (10). These occur in addition to the more complex coordination between muscle groups. To implement this progression in training overload, two to three sets of exercise repetitions are performed. The first set should be of fairly low intensity (40%–50% MVC), the second higher (60%–70% MVC), and the third higher still (80%–90% MVC). In this way the specific coordination involved in a movement is rehearsed at low intensity levels before maximal muscle work is performed. Also, any alignment faults can be identified at low intensity levels in which they are less likely to cause injury. The combination of sets, repetitions, and weight gives a training volume. For example, performing 3 sets of 10 repetitions (30 movements in total) with a weight of 20 kg gives a training volume of 600 kg. Larger training volumes are required for strength and power training and smaller volumes for endurance and speed.

In the initial stages of stability training, exercises are performed regularly throughout the day, on each day, to increase motor learning. This is because repetition is essential to progress motor learning from the cognitive stages (understanding the movement) to the motor stage (movement becoming skillful) and finally to the autonomous stage (action automatic or "grooved"). This frequency of training is only possible because the muscle work involved is not intense and so long recovery periods are not required. With weight-training, however, training intensity (overload) is sufficiently high that microscopic muscle damage (catabolism) is caused. This is intentional and results in tissue regrowth (anabolism) and adaptation. Time is required for these tissue adaptations, however, so weight-training should only be performed on alternate days to allow the worked tissues to recover. In general terms, pain will occur at the time of training through local muscle ischemia and later through delayed onset muscle soreness (DOMS). This pain/stiffness indicates that the muscle is recovering and a second training period should not be begun until muscle pain has reduced considerably. If the training frequency is too great, recovery will not occur and overtraining will result. Selecting training days on Monday, Wednesday, and Friday, for example, with a rest period over the weekend will ensure adequate recovery.

For the experienced user a "split routine" may be used in which separate muscle groups are targeted at each training session to allow a greater training frequency.

Clinical Pearl

A split routine allows muscles to recovery by exercising different muscle groups each day. For example, users can train 4 days each week providing that on Monday and Thursday they exercise the upper body and upper trunk (scapulo-thoracic) stability, and on Tuesday and Friday they work the lower body and lower trunk (lumbar) stability. In this way the same muscle groups are not worked on 2 consecutive days, and adequate recovery is given.

Safety Factors in the Weight Gym

All exercise equipment has risks that must be minimized, and these risks fall broadly into two categories: those associated with moving machinery and those associated with the lifting action itself. A number of simple rules allow the risks to be minimized (Table 28.3).

Control the Weights

Moving weights carry considerable momentum. Unless the weights are kept under control throughout the full range of motion, there is considerable risk to joints and body tissues. When a limb reaches the end of its motion range, the ligaments and muscles surrounding it become tight and limit further movement. Movements that are too rapid lead to loss of control—the joint stops moving at the end of the motion range, but the inertia of the weight forces the joint further against the tightening support tissues.

Table 28.3   Safety Checklist for Weight-Training

- Always warm up before training
- Check machinery before use
- Set up machinery to suit your height and weight
- Tie back long hair and be careful with loose clothing
- Remove jewelry
- Wear serviceable footwear—no flip-flops!
- Use correct exercise techniques and keep the weight under control
- Watch your body alignment—keep a neutral, stable spine
- Keep abdomen hollowed during exercises
- Practice good back care—lift correctly
- Train within your own limitations
- Never train through an injury—see a physical therapist (11)

In turn, this may cause overuse injury, or in some cases severe trauma. When using weight-training equipment, subjects should continually be encouraged to control the movement of the weight rather than allowing it to control them. It is good practice to decelerate the limb towards the end of a movement and avoid hyper extending a joint.

Appropriate Clothing

Even though most machines have guards, fingers and especially hair and clothing can be trapped in the moving weight stack with severe results. Subjects should be instructed to tie back long hair when they use machine weights and keep loose clothing away from the machines. They should remove watches, large rings, and dangling jewelry. Good sports shoes will help protect the feet, and the weight gym is no place for beach shoes or flip-flops! Toes can be stubbed and free-weights dropped onto feet. In addition to protecting against direct injury, good footwear will also keep the feet aligned. Excessive foot pronation encourages the tibia to inwardly rotate and stress the knee especially on exercises such as the squat.

Equipment Adjustment

Most good weight-training machines allow users to adjust the unit for the shape and size of their bodies. Make sure that the machine is set up before it is used, and that the user knows exactly how the machine works before beginning the exercise. Pivot points of machines are normally marked with coloured plastic caps. These should be aligned to the center of rotation of the joint being exercised. Exercising with the joint axis and machine axis out of line will hamper correct movement and stress joints.

Personal Limits

Subjects must be reminded to train well within their limits. An old adage says, "Never sacrifice technique for weight." Lifting a weight that is too heavy can impair both technique and body alignment and increase the risk of injury. In addition, practicing an incorrect technique will rehearse faulty movement patterns, which, when they become habitual, are difficult to modify.

Listen to the Body

Subjects must not train a body part that is injured unless following a structured rehabilitation program. The key is to listen to the body, especially to pain.

Never allow an individual to exercise through increasing pain. If a movement hurts and is continued slowly, the pain may diminish—in which case the person is probably suffering from stiffness that is working loose. If pain increases, however, the movement must stop. Remember that some rapid, repeated actions may "reduce" pain simply because the exercise hurts more than the injury (counter irritant effect) or because the subject simply "gets used to the pain" (habituation or desensitization). Subjects must be warned of this possibility and reminded to stop such movements immediately if they even suspect a masking effect.

Postural Alignment in Weight-Training Practice

A subject's posture may be described in terms of the line of gravity (LOG). In standing, viewed from the side, the LOG passes anterior to the lateral malleolus, anterior to the knee joint axis, and through the greater trochanter, lumbar, and cervical spines, glenohumeral joint, and lobe of the ear. From behind, the body is split into two equal halves with the spine central and the medial borders of the scapula vertical and lying approximately three fingers breadths from the LOG. The center of gravity of the human body lies within the sacrum (S1/2 level). Positioning any weight that is lifted at this level minimizes the forces acting on the body by reducing additional leverage. If the weight is held at a distance from this point, its potentially damaging effects are multiplied. For this reason the pelvis is referred to as the "safe zone" when lifting in an occupational health environment. Subjects should be encouraged to keep the weight they are lifting within or close to the safe zone for as long as possible during a weight-training action. A weight-training movement may take a total of 20 seconds, for example. If during this action the weight can be kept close to the safe zone for 18 of these 20 seconds, the lift is considerably safer than if it can only be kept close to the safe zone for 5 of the 20 seconds. Clearly, however, the time taken to perform the action is exactly the same dispelling the popular notion that "good lifting takes longer." A good lift minimizes muscle work and joint loading and should be performed with a high degree of precision and control.

Movement of body segments away from the LOG introduces a leverage force that must be resisted by passive tissue tension and active muscle contraction. In addition, deviation from the LOG alters joint loading forces. During weight-training the additional forces created by the moving weight make postural alignment doubly important. Any alteration in leverage caused by movement of the LOG will dramatically increase the forces imposed on the body by training weights. In addition, movement of one body part away from the LOG necessitates movement of a neighboring body part in the opposite direction to maintain balance. Constant repetition of incorrect alignment leads to habitual changes in posture that are difficult to modify.

Rehearsing Correct Alignment Patterns

Correct alignment patterns will have been introduced early in the back stability program with free exercise. Each pattern is briefly described in tabulated form, but more detail is located elsewhere (11). In each case subjects must establish the neutral spine position and perform the abdominal hollowing action before the exercise commences. As the subject progresses to the weight gym, the basic exercises must be reinforced using weight-training apparatus for the training to be truly specific. To reinforce correct lumbo-pelvic rhythm during bending the hip hinge action is used (Table 28.4). This may be modified for the weight gym by placing a wooden bar across the shoulders (broom handle), and progressed to a weight-training barbell (Fig. 28.1). This action then becomes the classic "good morning" exercise (Fig. 28.2). The action is useful to develop the hip extensors in the presence of good stability. However, when alignment faults creep in, the leverage and potential intradiscal pressure increase changes a useful movement into a potentially dangerous one.

The sternal lift movement should be used in both sitting and standing (Fig. 28.3). Once the subject is

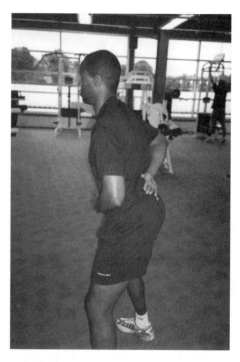

Figure 28.1 Hip hinge.

able to perform the action in isolation to lumbar movement, the action should be incorporated into weight-training exercises. Seated rowing actions are useful either using a rowing machine with a sternal pad (Fig. 28.4) or using a low pulley machine (Fig. 28.5). In each case the subject moves from a posture of thoracic flexion and scapular abduction to one of thoracic extension and scapular depression and adduction to optimal alignment. The optimal position is held for 2 to 3 seconds to emphasize the inner range contraction before lowering the weight.

Table 28.4 Basic Alignment Patterns

Sternal Lift	Hip Hinge	Weight Shift
• Isolate thoracic movement from lumbar movement • Perform thoracic extension to flatten kyphosis • Lift sternal rather than expanding ribcage (discourage subject from taking a deep breath) • Draw scapulae down and in (depression and adduction)	• Unlock knee to reduce stretch on hamstrings • Maintain neutral lumbar position, do not alter depth of lordosis • Anteriorly tilt pelvis on fixed hip, maintaining relative positions of lumbar spine and pelvis • Maintain thoracic alignment, avoiding thoracic flexion and scapular abduction	• Move shoulder girdle and pelvic girdle horizontally • Shift line of gravity from a point between the feet to a point directly over the weight-bearing foot • Do not allow shoulders or hips to "dip" • Maintain alignment as leg is lifted

Chapter Twenty-Eight: Weight Training for Back Stability

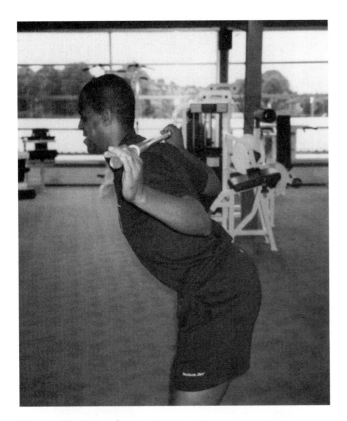

Figure 28.2 Good morning.

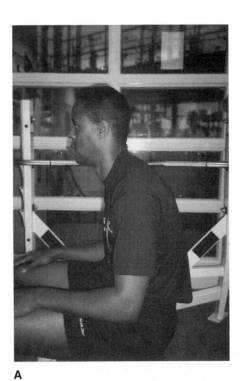

A

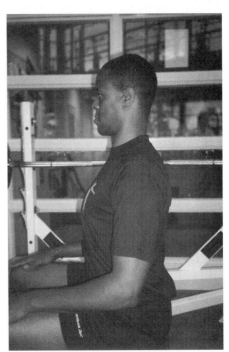

B

Figure 28.3 (A) Sternal lift—start. (B) Sternal lift—finish.

Weight shift movements (Fig. 28.6) are important for exercises using single leg actions such as lunges and hip isolation movements (multi-hip machine). When the subject can accurately control his/her alignment by shifting the pelvis and transferring the LOG over, and away from, the weight-bearing leg the subject should progress to resisted hip movements and lunging. Resisted hip movements may be performed using a low pulley machine fitted with an ankle strap or a purpose built multihip unit (Fig. 28.7). In each case the important factor with respect to back stability is not the leg which is lifting, but the weight-bearing leg. It is essential that the subject maintains their alignment over the weight bearing leg by "standing tall" and not allowing the pelvis to dip toward the moving leg. In the lunging action (Fig. 28.8) (initially performed without weights), the challenge is to control the weight transference throughout the movement without "falling onto" the leading foot or "jumping off" the trailing leg. The pelvis should move close to a horizontal line in the sagittal plane showing that vertical movement of the body's centre of gravity is minimized. Feedback on alignment can be gained by performing the exercise in front of a mirror and comparing the line of the shoulders to the horizontal line. Holding a wooden pole across the shoulders also gives the subject useful feedback

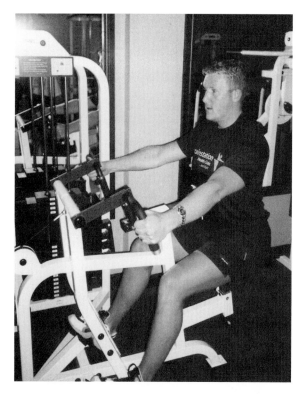

Figure 28.4 Rowing machine with sternal pad.

and makes movement control easier. As weight progression is used, a barbell may be placed across the shoulders or dumbbells held in the hands.

Machine Exercises

A major feature of machine exercises is that they usually allow only single-plane motions and are

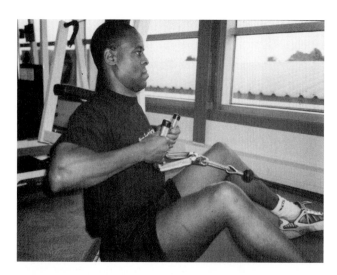

Figure 28.5 Rowing action using low pulley.

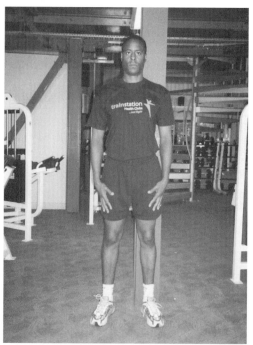

A

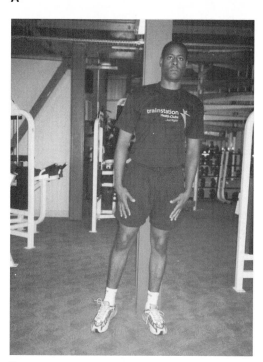

B

Figure 28.6 (A) Weight shift start. (B) Weight shift finish.

therefore easy to coordinate. Pulleys are an exception here. Because they allow tri-plane motion, more complex coordination is possible. For each exercise, the first set of movements is used as part of the warm up to familiarize the subject with the action.

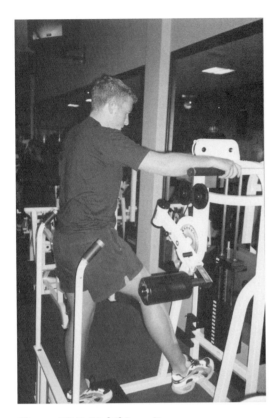

Figure 28.7 Multihip unit.

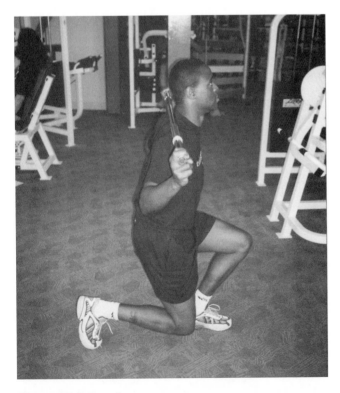

Figure 28.8 Lunging.

For this initial set, 12 to 15 repetitions of a light weight (30% MVC) are used. Two further sets are performed using 10 to 12 and then 8 to 10 repetitions with progressively increasing weight. For endurance and speed work maximum weights of 50% MVC are chosen, but for strength and power higher weights are used up to 80% MVC. During the first set, movements should be slow and controlled. If speed training is to be used, the rate of movement rather than the weight is then progressively increased. Single-sided weight-training exercises are described for the right side of the body. Subjects should perform exercises with both sides of the body, with instructions for the left side being a mirror of those on the right.

Lateral Pull-Down

The latissimus dorsi is one of the muscles (together with the transversus abdominis and gluteals) that tensions the thoracolumbar fascia, an essential component of stabilization. In addition, it is an important lifting muscle and can be strengthened by resisted adduction, pulling the arm into the side of the body from an overhead position, or from a forward reaching position.

For the lateral ("lat") pull-down, the subject lowers the bar either behind the shoulders or to sternal level on the chest (Fig. 28.9A). Either position can be used. Both have advantages and disadvantages. Pulling the bar behind the neck will increase the subject's shoulder mobility, because that position requires a higher degree of external rotation at the shoulder than pulling the bar to the chest. Because external rotation is often limited, this is a desirable form of mobility training. However, the seventh cervical vertebra has a very prominent spinous process and subjects must take care not to strike this point with the bar. To lessen the likelihood of this happening, they should pass the bar behind the head by 2 to 3 inches (5–8 cm) rather than letting it brush the hair. In this way, the bar will miss the cervical spine and come to rest across the shoulders. Individuals unable to adopt this position should pull the bar to the upper chest. The action is a smooth pull downward, placing the bar (in the first case) behind the neck and across the shoulders. The head should be tilted forward slightly, and the bar must not strike the cervical vertebrae but rest across the middle fibers of the trapezius. The lowering action of the weight pulls the bar up again. Instruct your subjects not to permit the weights to rest together at the end of the movement, so that useful traction will be maintained in the latissimus dorsi and the thoracolumbar fascia.

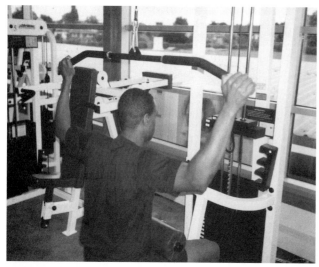

A

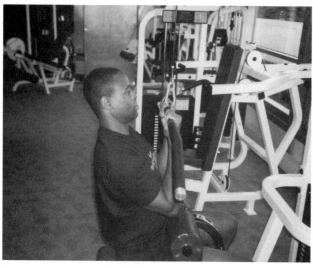

B

Figure 28.9 (A) Lat pull-down to back of neck. **(B)** Lat pull-down to front. Narrow grip.

Bringing the bar in front of the body to the top of the sternum reduces the range of external rotation and extension at the shoulder and is especially useful for less flexible individuals and those with a history of shoulder subluxation or dislocation. Subjects may use whichever grip that seems most comfortable—wide, narrow, pronated, supinated, or midposition, and alteration in the hand position will change the emphasis of the movement. Using a narrow grip (Fig. 28.9B) either on a standard wide bar or a box frame (with elbows in pronated or midposition) will allow the elbows to pass close to the sides of the body as the bar is pulled down. In bodybuilding this is said to thicken the latissimus dorsi rather than broaden it (17). Using a supinated grip

reduces the emphasis on the latissimus dorsi and emphasizes the biceps brachii.

Cable Crossover

The cable crossover again works the latissimus dorsi, but this time in conjunction with the pectoralis major. The starting position is with both arms abducted (Fig. 28.10) and the feet slightly wider than shoulder width apart. The action is to exhale and pull both arms into the sides of the body. An alternate approach is to pull the arms forward across the chest, a technique that increases the adduction range and emphasizes the pectoralis major. The elbows should be slightly bent throughout the movement, to reduce stress on the elbow joint. As the weight is lowered back to its starting position, the abduction must be controlled to reduce the stress on the shoulder joint. Allowing the weight to drop will place a combined abduction and traction force on the joint that could potentially damage the rotator cuff muscles and/or the joint capsule and ligaments.

Back Extension (Machine)

The back extensors are essential to lifting and bending activities, and their importance and retraining has been covered in Chapter 26. The muscles act both to extend the spine and to balance the flexion moment produced by the trunk and weight being lifted. In this action the endurance of the back extensors is a deciding factor for potential injury (3,7). In addition the sequencing of the back extensors with the hip extensors is vital. This sequencing was re-educated by using

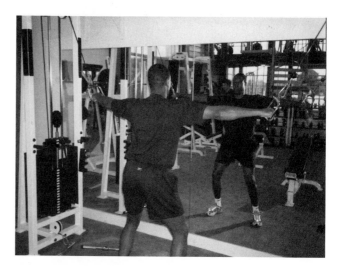

Figure 28.10 Cable crossover.

hip hinge activities. Both the hip extensors and back extensors can be trained using the dead lift action, which is a variation on the hip hinge (see later).

The specialized back extension unit (Fig. 28.11) enables the subject to isolate the back extensors from the hip extensors and to introduce limited range motion, or to re-strengthen only part of the movement range. The machine should only be used once subjects have mastered pelvic tilting and the hip hinge action itself.

Subjects should adjust the machine so that the knees and hips are bent to 70° to 80° and the pivot point of the machine is aligned with the hip joint axis. The movement begins with a posterior tilt of the pelvis, moving the seat contact point from the ischial tuberosities back onto the sacrum. The action is movement of the pelvis on the stationary femur, with the back stabilized and immobile throughout the early part of the movement. Only when the second half of the movement range begins should the spine move into extension.

Inexperienced subjects often lose stability during this exercise and relax the abdominal muscles enabling the lumbar spine to hyperextend. It is vital that the neutral position of the lumbar spine be maintained throughout the first part of the action.

Back Extension (Frame)

Use of the back extension frame (Roman chair or back strong) has been covered in Chapter 27. The

concern here is its use in the weight-training gym (Fig. 28.12A). To ensure correct alignment make sure that the subject maintains the neutral position and performs abdominal hollowing throughout the action. To aid performance with the inexperienced user, place a bench or stool in front of the machine, level with your subject's shoulders. The subject places his/her hands on the stool in a push-up position, with the legs locked onto the machine pads. Instruct the subject to lift first one hand and then both hands from the stool, placing the arms by his sides. Once the subject can perform this action in a controlled manner, spinal movement into extension may be added. Begin in the neutral position (with or without stool support), and move into extension, lifting the shoulders approximately 2 to 3 inches (5–8 cm) above the hip height, and then move back to neutral. Finally move down into flexion.

This action if uncontrolled can place considerable stress on the spinal tissues. At the beginning of the movement, if the abdominal muscles are allowed to relax, the pelvis will anteriorly tilt and the lumbar spine hyperextend, compressing the lumbar facet joints without sufficient intra-abdominal pressure to reduce the load. Back stability and good alignment control are therefore essential pre-requisites for performing this exercise.

When a back extension frame is not available the leg curl bench may be used (Fig. 28.12B and 28.12C). The weight should be set to maximum to provide an immobile fixation point. The subject hooks their feet beneath the machine pads and locks the knees. Abdominal hollowing should be performed and the body straightened while supporting it on the forearms. Finally, the forearms should be lifted from the bench and the body held straight (Fig. 28.12D).

Seated Rowing

The seated row is used to strengthen the scapular stabilizers and thoracic extensors as a progression to the sternal lift action. In addition, the seated row will work the glenohumeral extensors. The starting position (Fig. 28.5) is with the knees bent, to relax the hamstrings and allow the pelvis to anteriorly tilt sufficiently for the lumbar spine to remain in its neutral position. The action is to perform a sternal lift, extending the thoracic spine and on this stable base to introduce upper arm extension, keeping the elbows in to the sides of the body. When the weight is lowered, the stable base must be maintained, making sure that the thoracic spine is not forced into flexion. To effectively extend the thoracic spine, abdominal hollowing must be performed and maintained throughout the exercise to eliminate

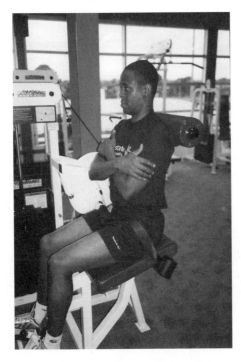

Figure 28.11 Back extension machine.

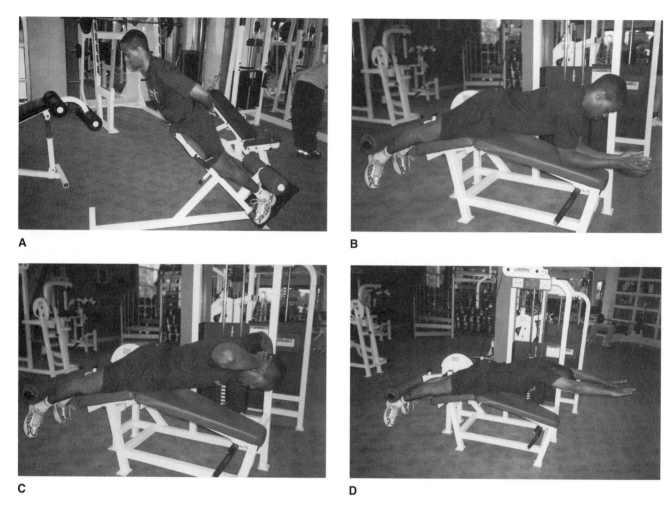

Figure 28.12 (A) Back extension frame. **(B)** Back extension on a leg curl bench, start. **(C)** Short lever. **(D)** Long lever.

unwanted lumbar extension. The exercise should not be used where a subject is unable to stabilize the lumbar spine, because lumbar hyperextension will be used as a "trick movement" to avoid thoracic extension while pressing the chest forwards and upwards.

Single Arm Pulley Row

The single arm pulley row has a similar effect to seated rowing (Fig. 28.13), with the addition that it can be used to gain symmetry between the arms by correcting any unilateral imbalance. In addition, it introduces some rotary stabilization or rotation movement as the trunk is allowed to twist. The combined movements involved present a significant challenge to the stabilizing system of the back.

The starting position is a lunge position to the left of the pulley, with the left foot forward and the D

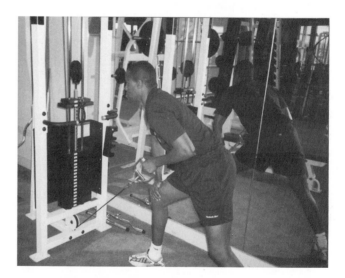

Figure 28.13 Single-arm pulley row.

handle of the low pulley gripped in the right hand. The subject should place his/her left hand on the left knee for support and angle the body forward (trunk on hip) at 45°. The right arm is then pulled into extension at the shoulder and as the pulley hand approaches his chest, the trunk should be rotated slightly to the right, and the thoracic spine extended, as in the sternal lift action. Using a low pulley position (pulley at mid-shin level) requires the subject to lean over slightly, increasing the workload on the spinal extensors. This is suitable only when alignment is good and the subject can keep the spine straight throughout the action. Placing the pulley at waist height negates the requirement to lean forward, taking the workload off the spinal extensors and reducing leverage on the spine. The waist-high position is used if the subject's alignment is poor.

Low Pulley Spinal Rotation

The oblique abdominal muscles are important in controlling rotary forces acting on the spine during manual handling especially. Flexion rotation forces tend to be the most damaging to the spine, and separating these two actions provides a safe and effective method of restrengthening. The low pulley machine is an adaptable unit, which is readily available. However, common resistance tubing may be substituted when weight-training apparatus is not available.

Lying, sitting, or standing starting positions may be chosen. For the lying (Fig. 28.14A) exercise, the subject begins in a half-crook lying position perpen-

dicular to the direction of pull, with the leg closer to the pulley flexed at the knee. The cable of the pulley is attached to the flexed knee with a leather or webbing strap. The action is to rotate the spine so that the bent knee passes over the straight leg and onto the floor.

In the sitting position the subject sits on a stool (Fig. 28.14B), facing perpendicular to the pulley, with the left side approximately 18 inches (0.5 m) from the pulley. The subject should flex their right arm to 90° at the elbow, and hold it across the body. The low pulley is adjusted so that it is level with the subjects elbow and the D handle of the pulley is gripped with the right hand. The action is to rotate the trunk to the right, keeping the hips, legs, and arm immobile so that the weight of the pulley unit if lifted by the trunk action alone. The standing exercise is similar to the sitting. Again, the subject adjusts the pulley to elbow level and folds the outer arm across the body. The feet are placed apart to maintain a wide base of support.

Rotary Torso Machine

The rotary torso machine again strengthens the oblique abdominals but with the added advantage that end-range movements may be avoided, or parts of the range strengthened in isolation. To begin the movement (Fig. 28.15), the rotation lock is positioned to allow full rotation range but not to overstretch the spine. If rotation is painful or the range is limited, the machine lock should be positioned to avoid the painful end-range position. The action is a smooth rotation into full muscular inner range.

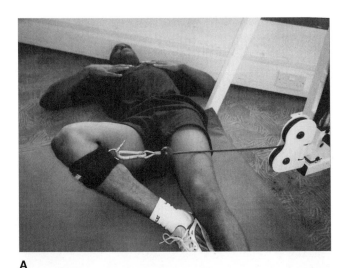

A

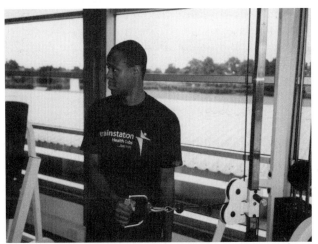

B

Figure 28.14 (A) Low pulley spinal rotation—lying. **(B)** Low pulley spinal rotation—standing.

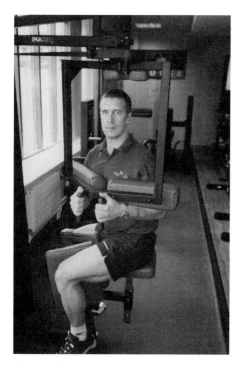

Figure 28.15 Rotary torso machine.

The subject should hold the position and then slowly release it, avoiding the temptation to drop the weights rapidly and spin the machine. Reset the machine for the opposite rotation, remembering that range and strength are not necessarily symmetrical.

Additionally, the full inner-range position into which an individual's muscles can pull the spine (physiological inner range) is generally less than the full inner range into which it can be taken passively (anatomical inner range). As long as the motion is smooth and not too fast, the subject is in no danger of overly stressing the facet joints of the spine during this exercise. If the motion is too rapid, however, the momentum of the machine can take the spine past physiological inner range and into anatomical inner range, loading the facet joints unnecessarily.

Abdominal Machine

Several abdominal machines are available on the market, but most provide resistance to trunk flexion, emphasizing the supraumbilical portion of the rectus abdominis. Some provide additional resistance for the hip flexors working the infraumbilical portion of the rectus abdominis as well (Fig. 28.16). If possible, align the pivot of the machine with the center or lower portion of the lumbar spine rather than the hips. It is important that the rectus abdo-

minis does not bulge outward or "bowstring" during the action, so abdominal hollowing is a vital precursor to this exercise. To begin, the subject grips the machine arms, holding the elbows in throughout the action. The instruction should be to "roll into flexion," keeping the back on the backrest and avoiding the tendency to lean forward. The movement begins by pulling the sternum down rather than forward. The eccentric component of the movement is important, so lowering the weight has to be slow and controlled.

When the lower rollers provide lower abdominal work, the pelvis is posteriorly tilted to cause the hips to lift slightly before the trunk is flexed. In this way the whole of the rectus is worked.

Trunk Flexion with High Pulley (Pulley Crunch)

Trunk flexion may also be performed on a high pulley machine (Fig. 28.17). The subject should either kneel (2-point kneeling) or sit, with their back to the machine, holding the D handle of the machine in both hands behind or in front of the neck (either is correct—the subject should choose the most comfortable position). Encourage the subject to shuffle forward until the slack in the machine cable has been taken up. The action is to flex the trunk alone rather than the trunk on the hip (hip hinging). The correct movement is encouraged by taking the head downward toward the knees rather than forward in front of the knees. The action must be slow and controlled. Because very little movement is available, it is essential that the machine cable is tight before the action begins.

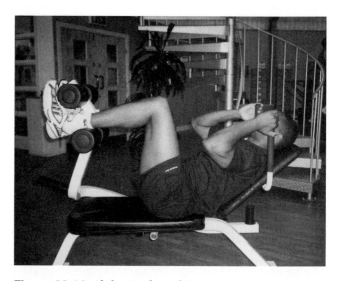

Figure 28.16 Abdominal machine.

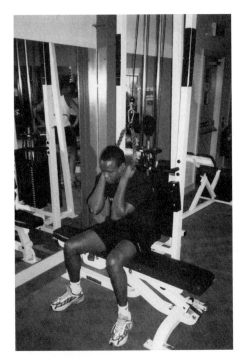

Figure 28.17 Trunk flexion with high pulley.

Free-Weight Exercises

In the context of a back stability program, free-weights are used only for subjects who have heavy demands for strength and speed. Generally this implies individuals who perform either medium or heavy manual handling as part of their job, or who are involved in strenuous sports. Free-weights are particularly useful in these groups as part of late-stage rehabilitation because of the complexity of skills that free-weights require in comparison with machine weights.

In general, free-weight exercises may be seen as a progression on machine weight exercises as those help build the strength needed in these more complex free-weight movements. Subjects must perform the exercises in this section under strict supervision until they have perfected the actions. Special consideration should be give to subjects younger than 18 or older than 60 years of age because bone formation and joint structures is generally more prone to injury. These individuals should exercise only under the supervision of a physical therapist or trainer who is specially trained to teach these groups.

Special Concerns Regarding Free-Weights

Because free-weight exercises combine both speed and weight, they expose the body to high levels of momentum, which are potentially injurious. To minimize the risk of injury the following prerequisites must be met:

- Show good stability and alignment.
- Have good endurance of stability muscles (see chapter 27).
- Have mastered the machine weight exercises described.
- Have performed a warm-up and stretched before each weight session.
- Initially be supervised until their exercise technique is good.
- Within the context of a back stability program, your subjects should perform all the free-weight exercises progressively and non-competitively.

Basic Free-Weight Exercises

For the initial free-weight exercises, the movements should be slow and well controlled. Exercises to develop "explosive power" are described later, and form a progression on the free-weight movements. Because free-weight exercises require more balance and coordination than machine exercises, less weight should be used. Prescribe approximately 10 to 12 repetitions for each exercise, using a final weight that is comfortable for that number of repetitions (i.e., if the individual can perform 20 repetitions, the weight is too light; if he/she can perform only 5 repetitions, it is too heavy). For each exercise, the subject should perform 2 or 3 sets of 10 to 12 repetitions. Use a moderate weight (perhaps half the final weight) for the first set, three-quarters of the final weight for the second, and the full weight only during the third set. In this way, the muscles gradually become accustomed to handling the weight, as the subject increases his/her skill of movement. Subjects should rest after each set until their breathing rates and heart rates return to normal—never let them start a fresh set while their hearts are pounding or they are out of breath. Injury is far more likely if a subject is fatigued.

As a guide, 2 or 3 sets for each exercise should be performed, three sessions per week, resting at least one day between sessions. After 2 weeks, subjects may increase the target weight, again according to how much they can lift comfortably. Let them follow this program—2 or 3 sets of 10 to 12 repetitions, three sessions per week—for a period of at least 16 weeks, never increasing the weights to the points where they feel exhausted.

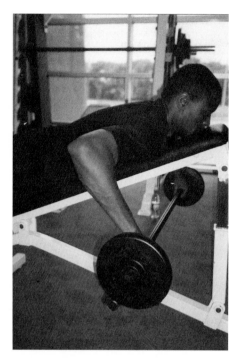

Figure 28.18 Lying barbell row.

Lying Barbell Row

This exercise strengthens the shoulder retractors and helps to increase thoracic spine extension and in so doing may be used in kyphotic posture correction. Because the subject lies on a gym bench, the lumbar spine is prevented from hyperextending, a fault often seen in other rowing exercises.

The subject lies prone on top of a gym bench (Fig. 28.18), which is narrow enough to allow free arm movement. A bench which is too wide will dig into the upper arm and chest of the subject as the arms are lowered. A light barbell (approximately 22.5–32.5 1b, or 10–15 kg) in held in the hands (over grasp) beneath the bench. The subject may hold her elbows either close to the sides of her chest or with arms abducted to 90°—the narrow position places greater work on the latissimus dorsi, whereas the wider grip emphasizes the posterior deltoids and scapular stabilizers.

The action is to pull the bar upwards towards the underside of the bench in a single slow, smooth movement, and at the same time to extend the thoracic spine by performing the sternal lift action. The movement is paused in the upper position for 2 seconds and then the bar is lowered.

Dumbbell Row

The dumbbell row is a single-handed movement, and as such may be used to help correct asymmetry between the should retractors on either side of the body (Fig. 28.19). Typically, asymmetry may be identified by a subject's inability to lift the same amount of weight, or to perform the same number of repetitions, with each arm. The subject begins in a half-kneeling position on a gym bench, with the right arm and right knee on the bench and the left leg straight with the left foot on the ground. The subject grips a dumbbell (whatever weight feels comfortable) with his left hand, then pulls (lifts) it toward him/herself, brushing the side of his body with the elbow. The movement should be stopped when the dumbbell approaches the chest. As the subject pulls the upper arm into extension, the scapula is adducted and the thoracic spine flattened (extended). The inner-range

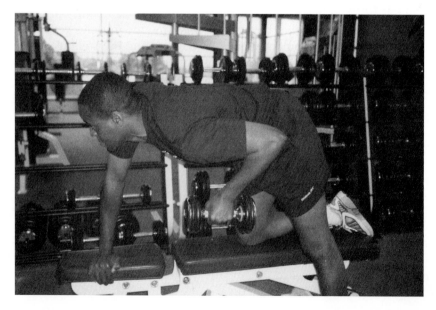

Figure 28.19 Dumbell row.

position should be held for 2 to 3 seconds before lowering the weight under control.

Good Morning

The good morning exercise is basically a hip hinge movement performed with a weight (Fig. 28.2). It works the spinal extensors statically and the hip extensors dynamically, and as such is an excellent movement to develop lifting capacity. It is essential for the subject to have mastered the hip hinge action before performing this exercise.

The subject begins by standing with the feet just wider than shoulder-width apart. The knees should be unlocked slightly (patella over the center of the foot) to relax the hamstrings and allow free pelvic tilt. With a light barbell (approximately 22.5 lb, or 10 kg) across the shoulders, the subject tilts her pelvis interiorly (maintaining the neutral position of the spine) so that her trunk angles forward to 45°. The subjects should be supervised closely to ensure that they do not allow the spine to flex, moving the axis of rotation from the hip joint to the middle of the spine—this stresses the spine considerably, both increasing intradiscal pressure and overstretching the posteriorly placed soft tissues.

Squat

The squat is a fundamental movement in weight-training, and one that can usefully teach correct spinal alignment and strengthen the quadriceps, hamstrings, and gluteals (Fig. 28.20). However, it is also a movement that is often performed incorrectly placing stress on the lumbar spine. Correct technique and close supervision is therefore essential.

To ensure good technique, the subject should practice the action using a light wooden pole (e.g., broom handle) until the technique is perfected. The beginning weight should be 10% to 30% of body weight, depending on body build—stronger subjects can use the larger value. Ideally, subjects should always use a squat rack, so that the bar can be taken in the standing position. Feet should be shoulder-width apart, with the toes turned out slightly. The subject steps under the bar, with the hips directly under his/her shoulders. Gripping the bar with hands slightly wider than shoulder width apart, the subject places it across the back of the shoulders (over the posterior deltoids and trapezius). The sternal left action should be performed to counteract the tendency for the bar to push the subject's thoracic spine into flexion. Both legs are straightened to left the bar off the rack—then a small step is taken backward to clear the bar from the rack.

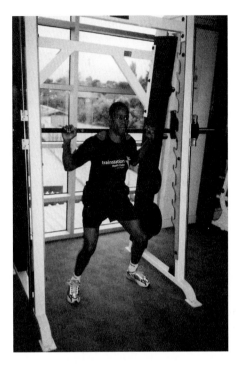

Figure 28.20 Squat.

Throughout the movement, the subject should look up and keep the spine nearly vertical. The action is to flex the hips and knees simultaneously, keeping the weight of the body and bar over the center of the foot rather than the toes. Instruct the subject to lower the bar under control until the thighs are parallel to the ground. After a momentary pause in this lower position to assist balance, the action is reversed to lift the bar. Close supervision should be maintained to ensure that the upward movement is controlled (no increase in speed toward the end of the action) and that her knees stay over the foot rather than moving apart or together.

Barbell Lunge

The squat was said to be one of the basic movements in weight-training. However, it has the disadvantage that it subjects the spine to compression forces that may not be suitable for subjects with discal lesions within the lumbar spine. In these cases especially, the barbell lunge is important (Fig. 28.8). It offers a similar leg motion to the squat, but as a single leg movement is used, less weight is required. The weight reduction results in correspondingly less spinal compression.

The start position is with the bar across the shoulders as for the squat. Because only one leg leads the movement, less than half the weight of a squat is used. The subject stands with the feet shoulder-width apart, with the feet marking the end of an imaginary rectangle on the floor (shoulder-width wide and twice shoulder-width long). As in the squat, the subject performs a sternal left action while maintaining spinal alignment. Instruct him to step directly forward with the right leg (as though placing the foot along the long edge of the rectangle). The knee of the leading leg is bent so that it just obscures the foot, and that of the trailing leg moves toward the ground, stopping when it is 2 to 4 inches (5–10 cm) above the floor. The side of the trailing knee should be 6–14 inches (15–35 cm) from the inner edge of the heel of the leading foot. To stand up again, the subject pushes off the leading leg, bringing the leading foot back to its shoulder-width start position.

The movement must not involve "falling" into the lower position of "jumping" into the upright position. Throughout the movement, the subject should look up and forward, and the bar should remain horizontal. In addition, as the body is lowered into the deep position, the knee should stop short of the floor. It the movement is too rapid, there is a danger that the subject will strike the knee against the floor injuring the patella or pre-patella bursa.

Free-Weight Exercises for Explosive Power

One of the goals of a stabilizing program is to re-instate the control of neutral spinal position during daily tasks, sport, and attention-demanding actions. The requires that the subject re-learns the ability to stabilize the spine with little attention to movement, with the stabilization becoming automatic once more. This stage of training represents the tertiary phase of motor learning, called the "autonomous stage" or stage of automatic action (9,10).

The free-weight exercises in this section are attention-demanding and consist of several combined movements in functional patterns involving lifting. To perform these exercises, your subjects must have progressed through the full back stability program and have good segmental control and spinal alignment. They should have mastered the machine exercises and basic free-weight exercises in the previous section of this chapter. Have them rehearse all of the power movements using a wooden pole first, to ensure that their lumbar stabilization is good.

Although you should still prescribe 2 or 3 sets of 10 to 12 repetitions, the first set should be with an empty bar to be doubly sure that the technique is correct and to train the muscles in the correct move-

ments. Your primary guide for subsequent sets must be spinal alignment rather than the amount of weight the subject can comfortably lift. If alignment is degraded, stop the exercise and reduce the weight, even if the subject feels the resulting weight is "too light." Emphasize to the subject that the aim here is rehabilitation, not competitive weight lifting or body sculpting.

Hang Clean

The clean action is one of the fundamental power movements used in weight-training (Fig. 28.21). Here, it is described in stages to introduce the subject to the movement progressively. The Hang clean forms stage (i) of this sequence.

The subject begins with the barbell (held with hands pronated) resting on the middle of the thighs. For this exercise the instructor should hand the bar to the subject, who is already in the basic position illustrated by (Fig. 28.21A). The subjects body should be angled forward (30°–45°) at the hips, and the spine must be straight, with the lumbar spine in its neutral position. Knees and hips should be flexed, ankles dorsiflexed. The action is divided into two phases: the upward movement and the catch. During the upward movement, the subject holds his/her trunk erect and lifts the bar explosively in a single "jump" action, extending the hips and knees and plantar-flexing the ankles, without allowing her feet to come off the ground. The shoulders should stay directly over the bar, and the path of the bar should be as close to the body as possible. At the point of maximum plantar-flexion of the ankle, the shoulders will begin to shrug to continue in the upward path of the bar (Fig. 28.21B).

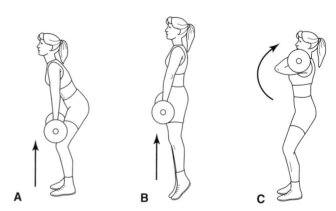

Figure 28.21 Hang clean. Reprinted with permission from Norris CM. Back Stability. Human Kinetics. Champaign, IL, 2000.

During the catch phase, which follows the shoulder shrug as a continuous motion, the subject maintains the upward movement by flexing the arms. The elbows drop under the bar, forcing the wrists into extension to allow the bar to rest on the now horizontal palms (Fig.e 28.21C). The elbows point directly forward, and the bar rests over the anterior aspect of the shoulders. As the bar touches the shoulders, the subject should slightly flex the knees and hips to absorb shock and prevent a sudden jolt of the bar on the shoulders.

The bar is lowered to the ground, by reversing the sequence of actions—the subject dips beneath the bar by bending the knees slightly, and then allows the elbows to drop, with the bar staying close to the body as it is lowered. The knees should bend so that the body is not pulled into spinal flexion as the bar approaches the ground.

Power Clean

The power clean represents stage (ii) of the power movement and is only used when the power clean has been mastered (Fig. 28.22). The movement now is to lift the weight from the floor rather than from the thighs. The barbell rests either on the floor or on two racks approximately 10 to 20 inches (25–50 cm) high. The subject begins standing with the feet shoulder-width apart and knees inside the arms. The feet are flat and turned out slightly. It is important with this exercise that the subject wears supportive training shoes—preferably a weight-lifting boot or high-cut cross training shoes with broad, stable heels. The subject grasps the bar with hands slightly wider than shoulder-width apart, arms straight. He/she should squat down so that the shins are almost in contact with the bar, knees over the center of the feet, and shoulders over or slightly in front of the bar (Fig. 28.22A). A common error with this movement is to get closer to the bar by flexing the spine, using only limited knee and hip flexion. However, this markedly increases the stress on the spine and must be avoided. The lift consists of three uninterrupted phases. First phase—the subject extends the knees and move the hips forward as the shoulders are raised. The shins should stay back (a common error with novices is to hit the knees with the bar), always maintaining the alignment of the back. The line of the bar's movement should be vertical, with the heels staying on the ground and the bar passing close to her body (Fig. 28.22B). The shoulders should stay back, either over or slightly in front of the bar, and the head should be positioned to look straight ahead or slightly up. Second phase—for the "scoop," the subject drives the hips forward, keeping the shoulders over the bar and allowing the elbows to extend fully. The trunk is nearly vertical at this stage (Fig. 28.22C). This movement brings the bar to the midpoint of the thighs. Third phase—the exercise continues as if it were the hang clean, through the upward movement and catch phases of that exercise (see illustrations for hang clean).

The action is one of continuous movement, with no significant pauses between sections. Although the bar maintains its momentum, the subject should never lose control of the movement. The bar should be lowered in a vertical path, bending the knees to prevent the spine from being pulled into flexion.

Dead Lift

The dead lift is a progression on the hip hinge movement, which now adds weight and a pulling action to the basic movement learnt previously. The dead lift is an excellent exercise to develop back and hip strength, and to add the power needed for general lifting actions (Fig. 28.23).

The exercise begins with the bar on the floor (novices may use low racks at first, until they gain control through the full range of the exercise). Your subject should stand with their feet flat on the floor (heels must not lift) and shoulder-width apart. The knees are positioned inside the arms, gripping the bar with hands pronated and slightly wider than shoulder-width apart. The elbows point out to the sides, to allow unimpeded movement as they bend during the lift. Some athletes prefer to use an alternate grip, with one forearm pronated and the other supinated (knuckles down). If the subject finds this grip more comfortable, by all means let him/her use it, but suggest that they alternate which hand is pronated and which supinated to maintain a balanced arm muscle development. The subject should position the bar over the balls of the feet, almost touching the shins. The shoulders should be over or

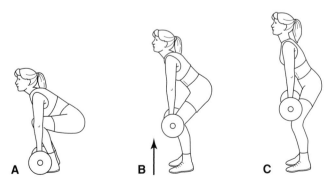

Figure 28.22 Power clean. Reprinted with permission from Norris CM. Back Stability. Human Kinetics. Champaign, IL, 2000.

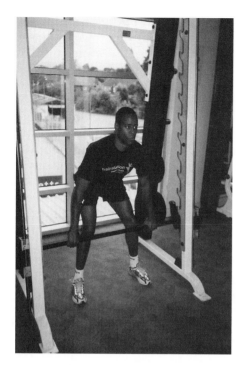

Figure 28.23 Dead lift.

slightly ahead of the bar and they spine aligned in its neutral position.

The movement begins by extending the knees and driving the hips forward. At the same time, your subject raises his shoulders so that the alignment of his back remains unchanged. The path of the bar is initially vertical, and it is held close to the body at all times. The elbows must not bend, because that will cause a loss of power, and the shoulders should stay over or slightly in front of the bar. The head should be placed so that your subject looks forward. Feet should remain flat. As the knees approach full extension, the back begins to move on the hip (hip hinge action), maintaining spinal alignment. Have your subject lower the bar with a squat motion, still maintaining the spine erect, keeping the bar close to the shins.

Power Training Using Plyometrics

Initially, back stability exercises focus on muscle isolation and slow controlled actions to develop the holding (endurance) ability of the core muscles. Weight-training maintains this core work, but adds work for the global muscles which resist the tendency of forces to displace the spine from its neutral position. Initially, these movements themselves are slow, and basic in their complexity, but gradually the complexity of movements is enlarged and the speed of movement increased. The initial muscle adaptation in stability training is one of strength (maximum

force generation) and endurance (maintenance of contraction), and as faster movements are used the adaptation involves changes in power (rate of work performance) and muscle reaction speed. For general usage, and recreational sport the weight-training actions used above are sufficient to build power. For clients who participate in higher levels of sports competition, however, or who simply want greater fitness gains, plyometric exercises specific power exercises called plyometrics are necessary.

Plyometric exercises enhance power development by capitalizing on the stretch–shorten cycle. Rapid actions are used that involve an eccentric action followed by a concentric contraction. Elastic energy results from passive stretching of the elastic components of the muscle during the eccentric phase. In addition the speed of stretch invokes a stretch (myotactic) reflex, which itself generates additional force. The combination of passive and active force generation summates to give a greater power output.

To create maximum power with concentric–eccentric coupling, the subject must be warmed up; and a rapid eccentric movement must be followed immediately by a rapid concentric movement with no rest between the two phases. Any standard exercise can be performed in this way, but not all exercises should be included in a plyometric workout because leverage forces and momentum acting on the spine can be dangerous. Subjects should beware especially of rapid end range motion on the spine and long lever movements.

An additional feature of the use of rapid movements in a stability program is muscle reaction time. Once a certain strength has been gained in a muscle, further strength gains do not necessarily lead to enhanced function. The ability of a muscle to react quickly and stabilize a joint before it is pushed out of alignment is also vital. Such rehabilitation has been used effectively with the ankle (6) and knee (1) and it seems likely that similar activities would be beneficial to the spine.

Before You Start

Before progressing to the following plyometric exercises, your clients must

- Demonstrate good basic stability—be able to perform the basic stability exercises covered in Chapter 26.
- Demonstrate good power and control in the trunk—be able to perform gym ball exercises covered in Chapter 26.
- Have good overall general fitness—demonstrated by regular, moderate to-intense exercise over the previous 6 to 8 weeks.

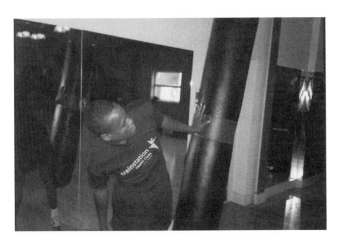

Figure 28.24 Plyometric side bend.

Plyometric Exercises

For each of the exercises make sure that the subject is closely supervised until the correct technique is seen consistently. The movement should be stopped if the exercise technique or back stability is seen to degrade. Subjects should perform each exercise (for both right and left sides of the body if a movement is asymmetrical) a maximum of 20 times per session. They should try from one to three sessions per week for at least 8 weeks, gradually increasing the speed of their movements as they are able. After the 8-week period, subjects may stop using plyometrics unless they are competitive athletes who require explosive strength to aid performance—in which case their strength coach should prescribe the advanced plyometric exercises, tailoring them to the athletes' particular sports or events.

Plyometric Side-Bend Using a Punching Bag

This movement develops power and speed of the trunk side flexors while maintaining back stability (Fig. 28.24). Instruct the subject to stand with his/her left side toward a punching bag, feet shoulder-width apart, with his left arm abducted to 90°. The subject should flex his/her trunk to the left and push (not hit) the bag with the straight arm, then side flexes to the right to decelerate the swing of the bag (stopping short of full range). The left side flexion begins the motion again. The action is reversed with the subject standing with his right side toward the bag.

Plyometric Flexion and Extension Using a Punching Bag

This punch bag exercise develops power and speed in the trunk flexors and extensors while maintaining

back stability (Fig. 28.25). The subject stands facing the punch bag, then pushes the bag with one or both hands. He/she should follow the movement through, using trunk flexion only, to 45°. The subject remains in this flexed position, and, as the bag swings back, takes the bag with his arms straight (but unlocked) and flexes the arms, extending his trunk minimally and transferring his body weight to his back foot to cushion the momentum of the moving bag.

Twist and Throw with Medicine Ball

The twist and throw develops power and speed of the trunk rotators (Fig. 28.26). The subject should stand in an aligned posture, with the trunk stabilized using minimal abdominal hollowing. A training partner, facing in the same direction as the subject, stands approximately 3 feet to the right, holding a medicine ball. While the subject rotates her trunk to the right,

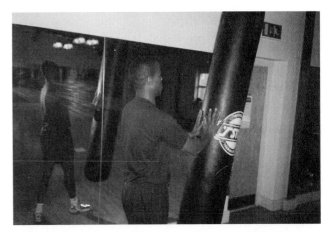

A

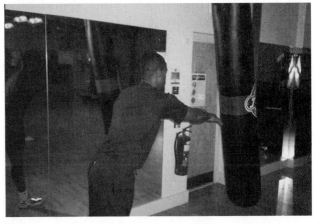

B

Figure 28.25 (A) Plyometric flexion/extension, start. **(B)** Flexion/extension, finish.

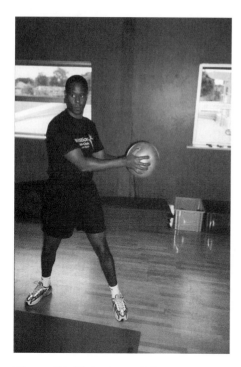

Figure 28.26 Twist and throw.

her partner throws the medicine ball to her. As she catches the ball, she should rotate to the left, pre-stretching the oblique abdominals. She stops the movement short of full range, rotates back to the right, and throws the ball back to her partner.

Medicine Ball Trunk Curl

The trunk curl is a modification of a standard sit-up action (Fig. 28.27). It is designed to reduce the action of the hip flexors and to work the rectus abdominis muscles upon a stable abdominal base by minimally contracting the deep abdominal muscles throughout the movement. The exercise itself is

described elsewhere (11). Here, it is being used as a plyometric action only. Instruct both the subject and his training partner to lie on a mat with their knees bent (crook, or hook lying), such that their ankles are almost touching. They should then raise their trunks (without significantly moving their legs) to a stable upright position. The training partner throws a medicine ball to the subject, who catches it while in the upright position, holding it close to his chest. The subject then moves back into the lower trunk curl position. He should stop the movement short of full range (his back should not touch the ground), then "bounce" back with a concentric trunk curl and throw the ball back to his partner. Increase the range of the curling action by having the subject lie over a cushion—this allows the trunk to move into extension before moving into flexion. Be sure that movement stops short of full range in each direction to reduce joint loading.

Leg Raise Throw

The leg raise action has been heavily criticized as an exercise for the inexperienced user (11). However, for the elite athlete, is has a use to develop power and speed in the lower abdominals (Fig. 28.28). The action described performs a leg raise from a hanging position. This exercise must not be used from a lying position. For a kinesiological comparison between these two movements see (8). The movement must be strictly supervised, and the potential shearing forces

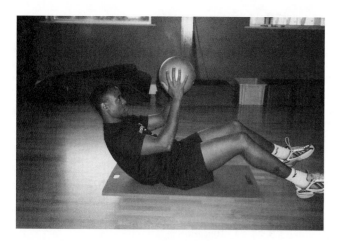

Figure 28.27 Medicine ball truck curl.

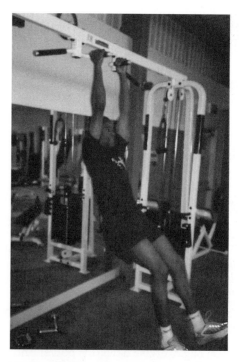

Figure 28.28 Leg raise throw.

on the lumbar spine recognized. Before performing the action using a medicine ball, supervise the action as the subject moves the legs unloaded. Only if alignment is excellent should loading be added.

The subject should hang from a gymnasium beam with a ball beneath him. Instruct him to grip the ball between both feet, then flex his hips and spine to throw the ball forward to a waiting partner. The partner places the ball back between your client's feel while the hips are still flexed to 90°. Your client then lowers his legs to pre-stretch the lower abdominals before repeating the movement.

■ CONCLUSION

Both local and global muscles should be trained to enhance stability of the spine. The use of weight-training is thus clinically useful as well as practical. Weight-training for back stability is an excellent final progression of a stability program, or an adjunct for those individually currently training in a gym as part of a general fitness regime. One of the essential questions that this chapter has addressed is "when to move a patient from floor exercise for stability (free exercises and gym balls) to weight based exercise (machines and free-weights)." The answer is, it depends on when the patient demonstrates appropriate motor control to stabilize the neutral spine position required for safe training. Much of the material for this chapter is based on Norris (2000), to which the reader is referred for further information.

Audit Process
Self-Check of the Chapter's Learning Objectives

• Describe how to determine a patient's readiness to progress to health club exercises.

• How would you incorporate stability principles into health club exercises?

• How can intensity, sets, and repetitions be varied to achieve strength training goals?

• Give advice about how to exercise safely using the popular weight-training machines found in most health clubs.

• What are safe and unsafe techniques for training squats?

■ REFERENCES

1. Beard, DJ, Kyberd PJ, O'Connor JJ, Fergusson CM, Dodd CAF. Reflex hamstring contraction latency in anterior cruciate ligament deficiency. J Orthop Res 1994;12:219–228.

2. Bergmark A. Stability of the lumbar spine. A study in mechanical engineering. Acta Orthop Scand 1989; 230(suppl):20–24.

3. Biering-Sorensen F. Physical measurements as risk indicators of low back trouble over a one year period. Spine 1984;9:106–119.

4. Crombez G, Vlaeyen, JWS, Heuts PHTG, Lyens R. Fear of pain is more disabling than the pain itself. Evidence on the role of pain-related fear in chronic back pain disability. Pain 1999;80:329–340.

5. Hodges PW, Richardson CA. Contraction of transversus abdominis invariably precedes movement of the upper and lower limb. In Proceedings of the 6th international conference of the International Federation of Orthopaedic Manipulative Therapists. Lillehammer, Norway. 1996.

6. Konradsen L, Ravn JB. Ankle instability caused by prolonged peroneal reaction time. Acta Orthop Scand 1990;61(5):388–390.

7. Luoto S, Heliovaara M, Hurri H, Alaranta H. Static back endurance and the risk of low back pain. Clin Biomechanics 1995;10:323–324.

8. Norris CM. Abdominal muscle training in sport. Br J Sports Med 1993;27:19–27.

9. Norris CM. Spinal stabilization. Physiotherapy J. 1995;81(2):1–39

10. Norris CM. Sports injuries. Diagnosis and Management. 2nd ed. Oxford: Butterworth Heinemann, 1998.

11. Norris CM. Back Stability. Human Kinetics. Champaign, IL, 2000.

12. Richardson C, Jull G, Hodges P, Hides J. Therapeutic exercise for spinal segmental stabilization in low back pain. Edinburgh: Churchill Livingstone, 1999.

13. Saal JA, Saal JS. Nonoperative treatment of herniated lumbar intervertebral disc with radiculopathy. Spine 1989;14:431–437.

14. Sale DG. Neural adaptation to strength training. Strength and power in sport. In: Komi PV, ed. IOC medical publication, Blackwell Scientific; Oxford, 1992.

15. Taylor JR, O'Sullivan P. Lumbar segmental instability: pathology, diagnosis, and conservative management. In Twomey LT, Taylor JR, eds. Physical Therapy of the low back, 3rd ed. New York: Churchill Livingstone, 2000.

16. Vlaeyen, JWS, Linton SJ. Fear-avoidance and its consequences in chronic musculoskeletal pain. Pain 2000;85:317–332.

17. Weider J. Ultimate bodybuilding. Chicago: Contemporary books, 1989.

29

Advanced Stabilization Training for Performance Enhancement

Micheal Clark

Learning Objectives
After reading this chapter you should be able to understand:

- The stabilization–strength–power continuum
- The difference between isolated uniplanar strengthening and functional multiplanar strengthening
- How to progress elite athletic patients to core strength and power exercises

Introduction

To bridge the gap between science, and practical application the clinician needs to follow a comprehensive, systematic, and integrated functional approach when training, reconditioning, and/or rehabilitating a client (see Chapters 5, 26, and 32). To develop a comprehensive functional program, the clinician must fully understand the functional kinetic chain. To understand the functional kinetic chain, the clinician must first understand the definition of function. Function is integrated, multidimensional movement (6). Functional kinetic chain training is a comprehensive approach that strives to improve all components necessary to allow a client to return to a high level of function. The clinician must understand that the kinetic chain operates as an integrated, interdependent, functional unit. Functional kinetic chain training and rehabilitation must therefore address each link in the kinetic chain and strive to develop functional strength and neuromuscular efficiency. Functional strength is the ability of the neuromuscular system to reduce force, produce force, and dynamically stabilize the kinetic chain during functional movements upon demand in a smooth coordinated fashion (6). Neuromuscular efficiency is the ability of the CNS to allow agonists, antagonists, synergists, stabilizers, and neutralizers to work efficiently and interdependently during dynamic kinetic chain activities (11).

Traditionally, training and rehabilitation have focused on isolated absolute strength gains, in isolated muscles, utilizing single planes of motion. However, all functional activities are multi-planar (MP) and require acceleration, deceleration, and dynamic stabilization (3,4,17,18,20,26,34). Movement may appear to be one-plane–dominant, but the other planes need dynamic stabilization to allow for optimal neuromuscular efficiency (12,29,35,41). Understanding that functional movements require a highly complex, integrated system allows the clinician to make a paradigm shift. The paradigm shift focuses on training the entire kinetic chain utilizing all planes of movement, and establishing high levels of functional strength and neuromuscular efficiency (3,4,17,18,20,26,34).

A dynamic core stabilization training program is an important component of all comprehensive functional training and rehabilitation programs. A core stabilization program will improve dynamic postural control, ensure appropriate muscular balance and joint arthrokinematics around the lumbo-pelvic-hip complex, allow for the expression of dynamic functional strength and improve neuromuscular efficiency throughout the entire kinetic chain (3,4,14,15,17,18, 26,28,31,34,36,45).

> **Benefits of Core Stabilization Training**
>
> - Improve dynamic postural control
>
> - Ensure appropriate muscular balance and joint arthrokinematics
>
> - Allow for the expression of functional strength
>
> - Provide intrinsic stability to the lumbo-pelvic-hip complex, which allows for optimum neuromuscular efficiency of the rest of the kinetic chain

---

What Is the Core?

The core is defined as the lumbo-pelvic-hip complex (25,40,44,46,49). The core is where our center of gravity is located and where all movement begins. There are 29 muscles that take their attachment to the lumbo-pelvic-hip complex (40,46). An efficient core allows for maintenance of the normal length–tension relationship of functional agonists and antagonists, which allows for the maintenance of the normal force couple relationships in the lumbo-pelvic-hip complex. Maintaining the normal length–tension relationships and force–couple relationships allows for the maintenance of optimal arthrokinematics in the lumbo-pelvic-hip complex during functional kinetic chain movements. This provides optimal neuromuscular efficiency in the entire kinetic chain, allowing for optimal acceleration, deceleration, and dynamic stabilization of the entire kinetic chain during functional movements. This provides proximal stability for efficient lower extremity movements (2,7,9, 19,20,21,22,23).

The core operates as an integrated functional unit, whereby the entire kinetic chain works synergistically to produce force, reduce force, and dynamically stabilize against abnormal force. In an efficient state each structural component distributes weight, absorbs force, and transfers ground reaction forces (44). This integrated interdependent system needs to be trained appropriately to allow it to function efficiently during dynamic kinetic chain activities (Fig. 29.1).

Core Stabilization Training Concepts

Many individuals have developed the functional strength, power, neuromuscular control, and muscular endurance in specific muscles that enable them to perform functional activities (3). However, few people have developed the muscles required for spinal stabilization (19,20,23). The body's stabilization system

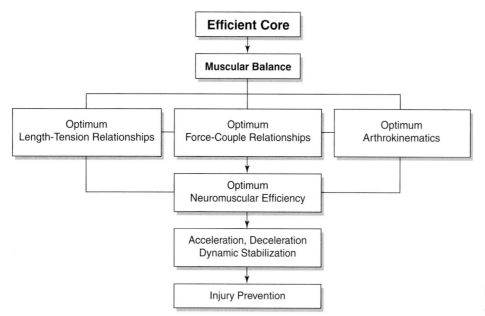

Figure 29.1 Core stabilization concepts.

has to be functioning optimally to effectively utilize the strength, power, neuromuscular control, and muscular endurance that they have developed in their prime movers. If the extremity muscles are strong and the core is weak, then there will not be enough force created to produce efficient movements. A weak core is a fundamental problem of inefficient movements that leads to injury (1,2,3,13,19,20,23,33,37,38,43).

The core musculature is an integral component of the protective mechanism that relieves the spine of deleterious forces that are inherent during functional activities (9,48). A core stabilization training program is designed to help an individual gain strength, neuromuscular control, power, and muscle endurance of the lumbo-pelvic-hip complex. This approach facilitates a balanced muscular functioning of the entire kinetic chain. Greater neuromuscular control and stabilization strength will offer a more biomechanically efficient position for the entire kinetic chain, therefore allowing optimal neuromuscular efficiency throughout the kinetic chain. (3,17,18,26,28,32,34,45).

Neuromuscular efficiency is established by the appropriate combination of postural alignment (static/dynamic) and stability strength, which allows the body to decelerate gravity, ground reaction forces, and momentum at the right joint, in the right plane, and at the right time (6). If the neuromuscular system is not efficient, it will be unable to respond to the demands placed on it during functional activities (11,13,20,23,24). As the efficiency of the neuromuscular system decreases, the ability of the kinetic chain to maintain appropriate forces and dynamic stabilization decreases significantly. This decreased neuromuscular efficiency leads to compensation and substitution patterns, as well as poor posture during

functional activities (11,28). This leads to increased mechanical stress on the contractile and non-contractile tissue, leading to repetitive microtrauma, abnormal biomechanics, and injury (1,2,5,10,12,41, 47). To fully understand functional core stabilization training and rehabilitation, the clinician must fully understand functional anatomy, lumbo-pelvic-hip complex stabilization mechanisms, and normal force couple relationships. (6) (see Chapter 5).

Postural Considerations

The core functions to maintain postural alignment and dynamic postural equilibrium during functional activities. Optimal alignment of each body part is a cornerstone to a functional training and rehabilitation program. Optimal posture and alignment will allow for maximal neuromuscular efficiency because the normal length–tension relationship, force–couple relationship, and arthrokinematics will be maintained during functional movement patterns (Fig. 29.2) (11, 40,44,46). If one segment in the kinetic chain is out of alignment, it will create predictable patterns of dysfunction throughout the entire kinetic chain. These predictable patterns of dysfunction represent the state in which the body's structural integrity is compromised because segments in the kinetic chain are out of alignment. This leads to abnormal distorting forces being placed on the segments in the kinetic chain that are above and below the dysfunctional segment (1,2,11,39,41,44,47,49). To avoid these patterns and the chain reaction that one misaligned segment creates, we must emphasize stable positions to maintain the structural integrity of the entire kinetic

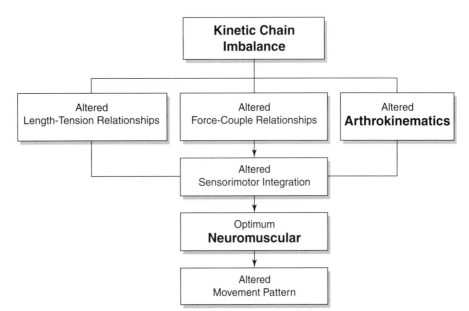

Figure 29.2 Kinetic chain imbalance.

chain (28). A comprehensive core stabilization program will prevent the development of serial distortion patterns and provide optimal dynamic postural control during functional movements.

Before a comprehensive core stabilization program is implemented, an individual must undergo a comprehensive assessment to determine: muscle imbalances, arthrokinematic deficits, core strength, core neuromuscular control, core muscle endurance, core power, and overall function of the lower extremity kinetic chain. It is beyond the scope of this chapter to present a comprehensive kinetic chain assessment (see chapters 10, 11, and 34). The interested reader can also review the National Academy of Sports Medicines Kinetic Chain Assessment home study course for a thorough explanation (www.nasm.org).

Guidelines for Core Stabilization Training

Before performing a comprehensive core stabilization program, each individual must undergo a comprehensive evaluation to determine the following: muscle imbalances, myokinematic deficits, arthrokinematic deficits, core strength/neuromuscular control/power, and overall kinetic chain function. All muscle imbalances and arthrokinematic deficits need to be corrected before initiating an aggressive core-training program. (5,38,39).

When designing a functional core stabilization training program, the clinician should create a proprioceptively enriched environment and select the appropriate exercises to elicit a maximal training response (6). The exercises must be; safe, challenging, stress multiple planes, incorporate a multi-sensory environment, be derived from fundamental movement skills, and be activity-specific (Table 29.1) (see also NASM-OPT Guidelines—www.nasm.org).

The clinician should follow a progressive functional continuum to allow optimal adaptations. The following are key concepts for proper exercise progression: slow to fast, simple to complex, known to unknown, low force to high force, eyes open to eyes closed, static to dynamic, and correct execution to increased reps/sets/intensity (NASM Training Guidelines—www.nasm.org).

The goal of core stabilization should be to develop optimal levels of functional strength and dynamic stabilization. Neural adaptations become the focus of the program instead of striving for absolute strength gains (17,43,45,48). Increasing proprioceptive demand by utilizing a multi-sensory, multimodal (Tubing, Bodyblade, physioball, medicine ball, power sports trainer, weight vest, cobra belt, dumbbell, etc.) environment becomes more important then increasing the external resistance (14,15,30,31). The concept of quality before quantity is stressed. Core stabilization training is specifically designed to improve core stabilization and neuromuscular efficiency. You must be concerned with the sensory information that is stimulating your CNS. If you train with poor technique and poor neuromuscular control, then you develop poor motor patterns and poor stabilization (11,19,20,23). The focus of your program must be on function. To determine if your program is functional, answer to following questions; Is it dynamic? Is it MP? Is it multidimensional? Is it proprioceptively challenging? Is it systematic? Is it progressive? Is it based on functional anatomy and science? Is it activity specific (NASM Guidelines—www.nasm.org)?

Table 29.1   Exercise Training Variables

Plane of Motion	Body Position	Base of Support	Lower Extremity Symmetry	Upper Extremity Symmetry	External Resistance	Balance Modality
• Sagittal • Frontal • Transverse • Combination	• Supine • Prone • Side-lying • Sitting • Kneeling • ½ Kneeling • Double leg Standing • Alternate leg standing • Single leg standing	• Exercise Bench • Stability Ball • Balance Modality • Other	• 2-Leg • Staggered Stance • 1-Leg • 2-Leg Unstable • Staggered Stance Unstable • 1-Leg Unstable	• 2-Arm • Alternate Arms • 1-Arm • 1-Arm w/ Rotation	• Barbell • Dumbbell • Cable Machines • Tubing • Medicine Balls • Power Balls • Bodyblade • Other	• Floor • Sport Beam • ½ Foam Roll • Reebok Core Board • Airex Pad • Dyna Disc • BOSU • Proprio Shoes • Sand

Core Stabilization Training Guidelines

- Progressive
- Systematic
- Activity-Specific
- Integrated
- Proprioceptively Challenging
- Based on Current Science

Core Stabilization Training Functional Continuum

- Multiplanar (3 planes of motion)
- Multidimensional
- Utilize the entire muscle contraction spectrum
- Utilize the entire contraction velocity spectrum
- Manipulate all acute training variables (sets, reps, intensity, rest intervals, frequency, duration)

Program Variables

- Plane of Motion
- Speed of Execution
- Range of Motion
- Loading Parameters (physioball, power ball, Bodyblade, sports trainer, weight vest, dumbbell, tubing, etc.)
- Acute Variables (sets, reps, tempo, time under tension, duration)
- Body Position
- Frequency
- Amount of Control
- Amount of Feedback

Exercise Selection Criteria

- Safe
- Challenging
- Progressive
- Systematic (Integrated Functional Continuum)
- Proprioceptively Enriched
- Activity-Specific

Exercise Progression Continuum

- Slow → Fast

- Known → Unknown

- Stable → Controlled → Dynamic Functional

- Low Force → High Force

- Correct Execution → Increased Intensity

There are 3 levels of training within the National Academy of Sports Medicine's Optimum Performance Training™ model including Stabilization, Strength and Power. A proper integrated core stabilization-training program follows the same systematic progression (Fig. 29.3 and Tables 29.2 and 29.3). (NASM Guidelines).

Stabilization

In the stabilization level of core training, exercises involve little joint motion through the lumbo-pelvic-hip complex. These exercises are designed to improve the functional capacity of the deep stabilization mechanism (9,36,42,43,48) (see Chapters 5, 25, and 26).

Strength

In the strength level of core training, the exercises involve more dynamic eccentric and concentric movements through a full range of motion. The specificity, speed, and neural demand are also progressed in this level. These exercises are designed to improve the neuromuscular efficiency of the entire kinetic chain (14,15,28,31) (see Chapters 27 and 28). See Figures 29.4 to 29.17.

Power

In the power level of core training, the exercises involve the entire muscle action spectrum and contraction velocity spectrum during integrated functional movements. These exercises are designed to improve the rate of force production (3,4,18,26, 32,34,45) (Figs. 29.18 to 29.24).

■ CONCLUSION

A core stabilization program should be an integral component for all individuals participating in a functional training and/or rehabilitation program. A core stabilization training program will allow an individual to gain optimal neuromuscular control of the lumbo-pelvic-hip complex and allow the individual with a kinetic chain dysfunction to return to activity much faster and safer.

Audit Process
Self-Check of the Chapter's Learning Objectives

- How does power training differ from strength training?

- How does strength training differ from stabilization training?

- Give examples of how functional training involves the entire kinetic chain?

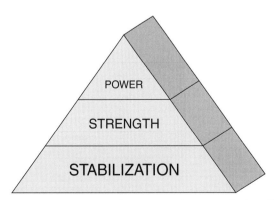

Three Levels of Progression in the Optimum Performance Training™ Model

Figure 29.3 Three levels of progression in the optimum performance training™ model.

Table 29.2   Example: Integrated Core Stabilization Program

	1—Beginner/Slow/Stabilization	2—Intermediate/Moderate/Strength	3—Advanced/Fast/Power
CST	*Core Stabilization*	*Core Strength*	*Core Power*
	Supine Progression	Cable/Tubing Progression	Medicine Ball Progression
	- Single-Leg Slide	Stability Ball Progression	- Pullovers
	- Single-Leg Lift	- Crunch	- Soccer Throws
	- Double-Leg Slide	- Bridge	- Chest Pass
	- Double-Leg Lift	- Curl	- Rotation Pass
	Prone Progression	- Hip Extension	- Oblique Throw
	- Gluteal Squeeze	- Pullovers	- Back Throw
	- Cobra	- Reverse Crunch	- Overhead Throw
	- Leg Raise	- Knee Ups	
	- Arm Raise	- Russian Twists	
	- Opposite Arm/Leg	- Push-Up with Roll	
	Bridging Progression		
	- 2 legs	Bench Progression	
	- Marching	- Reverse Hyper	
	4-Point Progression	- Reverse Crunch	
	- Drawing-In	- Knee-Ups	
	- Arm Raise	- Side Sit-ups	
	- Leg Raise	- Back Extension	
	- Arm Leg Raise	- Back Extension with movement	
	Iso-Ab Progression		
	- Prone	Cable Progression	
	- Prone with Ext	- Chops	
	- Prone with Abd	- Lifts	
	- Side-lying	- Rotations	
	Cable Progression	- Combinations	
	- Supine		
	- Bridging	Dumbbell Progression	
	- Kneeling	- MP Lunge/Curl/Press	
	- Standing	- Squat Press	
		- MP Step Press	

Table 29.3   Acute Variables

1—Beginner/Slow/Stabilization

	Reps	Sets	Tempo	Rest Int.	Frequency	Duration
CST	12–20	1–3	4–2–1 Iso=5–10 seconds	0–90 seconds	2–4 times per week	4–6 weeks

2—Intermediate/Moderate/Strength

	Reps	Sets	Tempo	Rest Int.	Frequency	Duration
CST	8–12	2–4	3–2–1	0–60	2–4 times per week	4–6 weeks

3—Advanced/Fast/Power

	Reps	Sets	Tempo	Rest Int.	Frequency	Duration
CST	8–12	2–4	1–1–1	0–60 seconds	2–4 times per week	4 weeks

For more information on how to use this information in a complete system for all clients, please inquire about our courses (*www.nasm.org*).

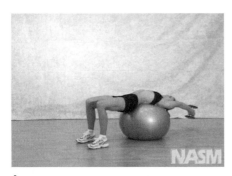

A

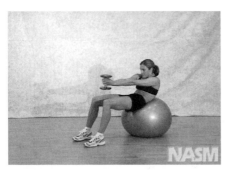

B

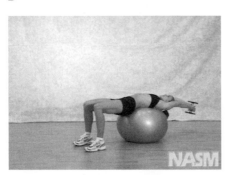

C

Figure 29.4 Ball pullover **(A–C)**.

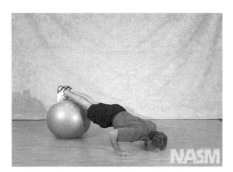

A

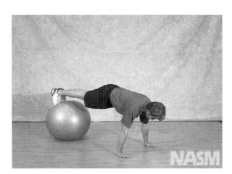

B

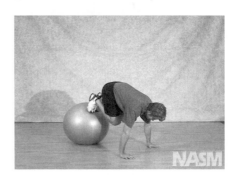

C

Figure 29.5 Ball pushup hands on floor with roll **(A–C)**.

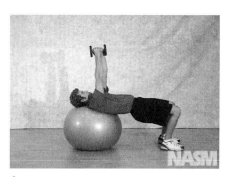

A

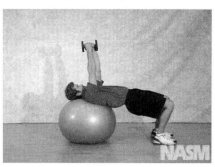

B

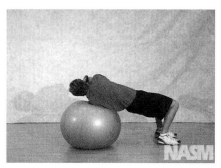

C

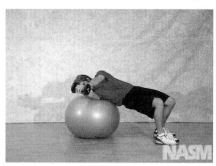

D

Figure 29.6 Ball Russian twist **(A–D)**.

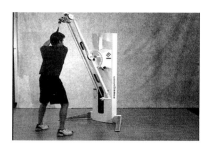

A

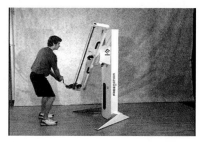

B

Figure 29.7 Cable chop.
(A) Start. **(B)** Finish.

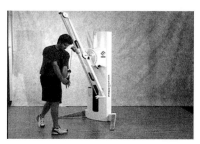

A

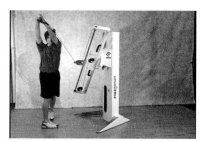

B

Figure 29.8 Cable lift.
(A) Start. **(B)** Finish.

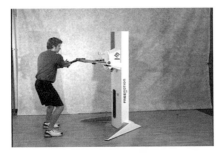

A

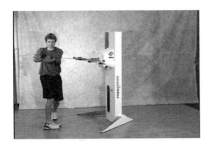

B

Figure 29.9 Cable rotation.
(A) Start. **(B)** Finish.

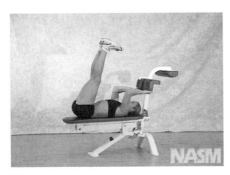

A

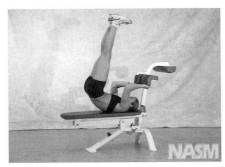

B

Figure 29.10 Knee ups **(A,B)**.

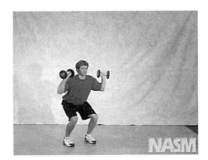

A

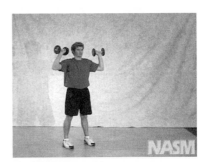

B

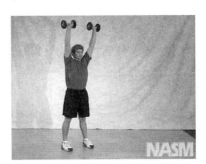

C

Figure 29.11 Lunge to balance
overhead press **(A–C)**.

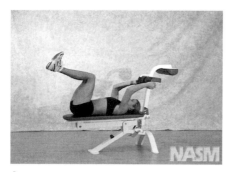

A

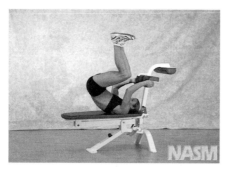

B

Figure 29.12 Reverse crunch with rotation **(A,B)**.

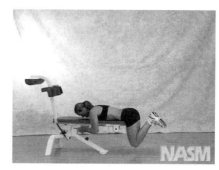

A

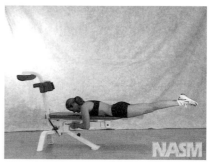

B

Figure 29.14 Reverse hypers **(A,B)**.

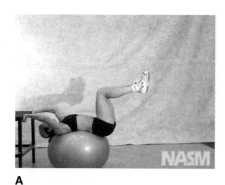

A

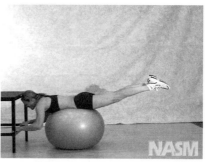

B

Figure 29.13 Reverse crunch with ball **(A,B)**.

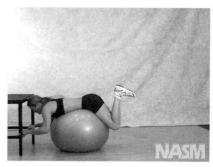

A

B

Figure 29.15 Reverse hypers on ball **(A,B)**.

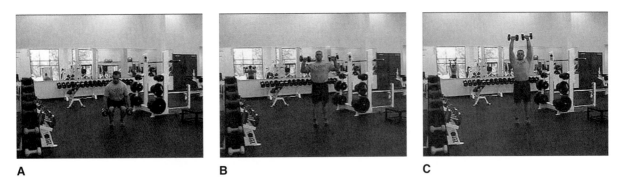

A   B   C

Figure 29.16 Squat to overhead press **(A–C)**.

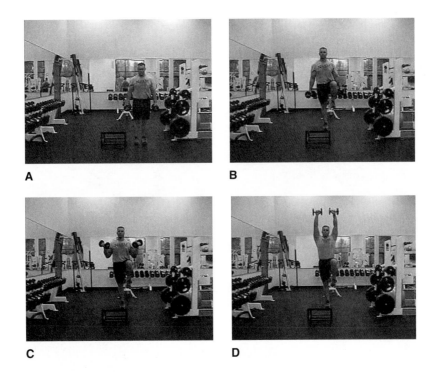

A   B

C   D

Figure 29.17 Step up frontal curl press **(A–D)**.

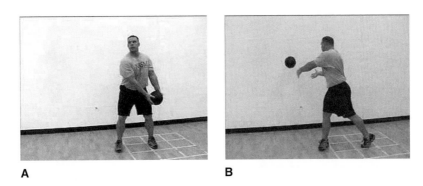

A   B

Figure 29.18 Back extension throw. **(A)** Start. **(B)** Finish.

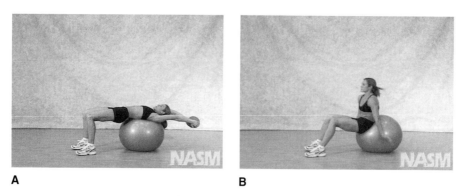

Figure 29.19 Medicine ball pullover on gym ball **(A,B)**.

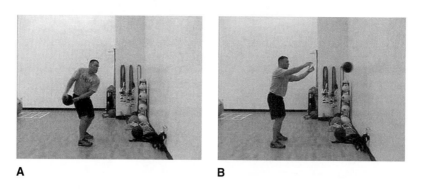

Figure 29.20 Medicine ball front oblique throw. **(A)** Start. **(B)** Finish.

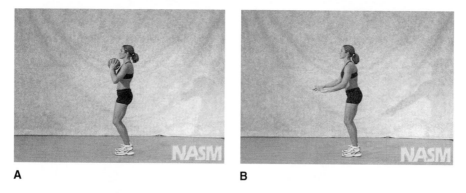

Figure 29.21 Medicine ball chest pass. **(A)** Start. **(B)** Finish.

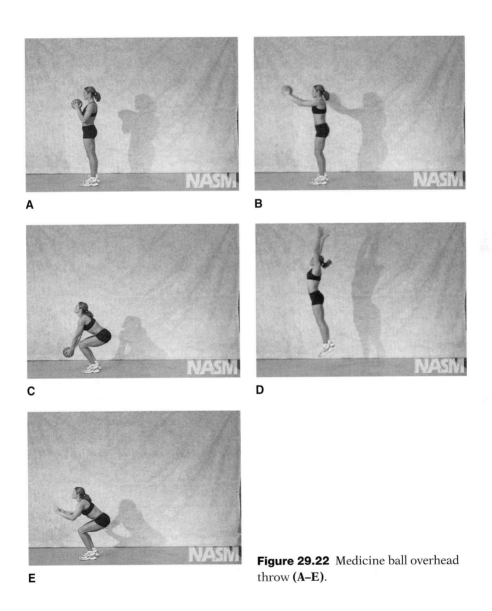

A

B

C

D

E

Figure 29.22 Medicine ball overhead throw **(A–E)**.

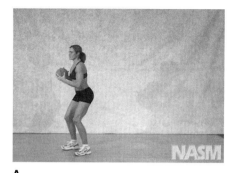

A

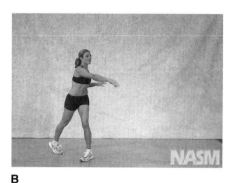

B

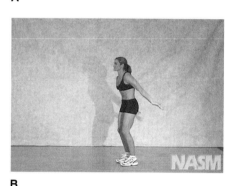

C

Figure 29.23 Medicine ball rotational chest press **(A–C)**.

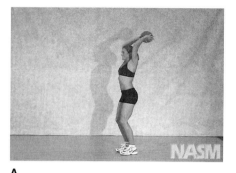

A

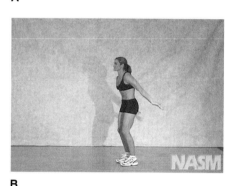

B

Figure 29.24 Medicine ball soccer throw **(A,B)**.

■ REFERENCES

1. Beckman SM, Buchanan TS: Ankle inversion and hypermobility. Effect on hip and ankle muscle electromyography onset latency. Arch Phys Med Rehabil. 76(12):1138-1143, 1995

2. Bullock-Saxton JE. Local Sensation Changes and Altered Hip Muscle Function Following Severe Ankle Sprain. Physical Therapy. 1994; 74(1):17-23

3. Caraffa A, Cerulli G, Projetti M, et al. Prevention of anterior cruciate ligament injuries in soccer. A prospective controlled study of propriocpetive training. Knee Surg Sports Traumatol Artrhrosc. 1996; 4(1): 19-21

4. Chimera NJ, Swanik KA, et al. Effects of plyometric training on muscle-activation strategies and performance in female athletes. J Athl Train. 2004; 39(1):24-31

5. Cibulka MT, Sinacore DR, Cromer GS, et al. Unilateral hip rotation range of motion asymmetry in patients with sacroiliac joint pain. Spine. 1998; 23(9):1009-1015

6. Clark MA. Integrated Training for the new millennium. National Academy of Sports Medicine. Calabasas; 2000

7. Cresswell AG, Grundstrom H, Thorstensson A: Observations on intra-abdominal pressure and patterns of abdominal intra-muscular activity in man. Acta Physiol Scand 144:409-418, 1992

8. Cresswell AG, Oddson L, Thorstensson A: The influence of sudden perturbations on trunk muscle activity and intra-abdominal pressure while standing. Exp Brain Res 98:336-341, 1994

9. Crisco J, Panjabi MM. The intersegmental and multisegmental muscles of the lumbar spine. Spine. 1991; 16:793-799

10. Denegar CR, Hertel J, Fonseca J. The effect of lateral ankle sprains on dorsiflexion range of motion, posterior talar glide, and joint laxity. J Orthop Sports Phys Ther. 2002; 32:166-173

11. Edgerton VR, Wolf S, Roy RR. Theoretical basis for patterning EMG amplitudes to assess muscle dysfunction. Med Sci Sports Exerc. 1996; 28(6):744-751

12. Ford KR, Myer GD, Hewett TE. Valgus knee motion during landing in high school female and male basketball players. Med Sci Sports Exerc. 2003; 35(10):1745-1750

13. Fredericson M, Cookingham CL, Chaudhari M, et al. Hip abductor weakness in distance runners with iliotibial band syndrome. Clinical Journal of Sport Med. 2000; 10(3):169-175

14. Garcia FJ, Grenier SG, McGill SM. Abdominal muscle response during curl-ups on both stable and labile surfaces. Phys Ther. 2000; 80(6):564-569

15. Hahn S, Stanforth D, Stanforth PR, Philips A. A 10 week training study comparing resistaball and tradi-

tional trunk training. Med Sci Sports Exerc. 1998; 30(5):199

16. Hanten WP, Olson SL, Butts NL, Nowicki AL. Effectiveness of a home program of ischemic pressure followed by static stretching for treatment of myofascial trigger points. Phys Ther. 2000; 80(10):997-1003

17. Hewett TE, Lindenfeld TN, Riccobene JV, et al. The effect of neuromuscular training on the incidence of knee injury in female athletes: A prospective study. Am J Sports Med 1999; 27(6):699-706

18. Hewett TE, Stroupe Al, Nance TA, et al. Plyometric training in female athletes. Decreased impact forces and increased hamstring torques. Am J Sports Med 1996; 24:765-773

19. Hides JA, Stokes MJ, Saide M, Jull GA, Cooper DH. Evidence of lumbar multifidus wasting ipsilateral to symptoms in subjects with acute/subacute low back pain. Spine. 1994; 19:165-177

20. Hodges PW, Richardson CA. Inefficient Muscular Stabilization of the Lumbar Spine Associated with Low Back Pain. Spine. 1996; 21(22):2640-2650

21. Hodges PW, Richardson CA, Jull G. Evaluation of the relationship between laboratory and clinical tests of transverse abdominus function. Physiotherapy Research International. 1996; 1:30-40

22. Hodges PW, Richardson CA. Contraction of the abdominal muscles associated with movement of the lower limb. Phys Ther. 1997; 77:132-143

23. Hungerford B, Gilleard W, Hodges P. Evidence of altered lumbopelvic muscle recruitment in the presence of sacroiliac joint pain. Spine. 2003; 28(14): 1593-1600

24. Ireland ML, Wilson JD, Ballantyne BT, McClay I. Hip strength in females with and without patellfemoral pain. J Orthop Sports Phys Ther. 2003; 33(11):671-676

25. Janda V: Muscles, central nervous system regulation and back problems. In Korr IM (ed): Neurobiologic Mechanisms in manipulative therapy. New York, Plennum Press 1978

26. Junge A, Perterson RD, et al. Prevention of soccer injuries: A prospective intervention study in youth amateur players. Am J Sports Med. 2002; 30(5): 652-659

27. Knapik JJ, Bauman CL, Jones BH, et al. Preseason strength and flexibility imbalances associated with athletic injuries in female collegiate athletes. Am J Sports Med. 1991; 19:76-81

28. Kovacs EJ, Birmingham TB, Forwell L, Litchfield RB. Effect of training on postural control in figure skaters: A randomized controlled trial of neuromuscular vs basic off-ice training programs. Clin J Sport Med. 2004; 14(4):215-224

29. Lee TQ, Yang BY, Sandusky MD, McMahon PJ. The effects of tibial rotation on the patellofemoral joint: Assessment of the changes in in situ strain in the peripatellar retinaculum and the patellofemoral contact pressures and areas. J Rehabil Res Dev. 2001; 38:463-469

30. Lephart SM, Pincivero DM, et al. The role of proprioception in the management and rehabilitation of athletic injuries. Am J Sports Med. 1997; 25:130-137

31. Lima LM, Reynolds KL, Winter C, et al. Effects of physioball and conventional floor exercises on early phase adaptations in back and abdominal core stability and balance in women. J Strength Cond Res. 2003; 17(4):721-725

32. Luebbers PE, Potteiger JA, et al. Effects of plyometric training and recovery on vertical jump performance and anaerobic power. J Strength Cond Res. 2003; 17(4):704-709

33. Luoto S, Heliovaara M, Hurri H, et al. Static back endurance and the risk of low back pain. Cinical Biomechanics. 1995; 10:323-324

34. Mandelbaum BR, Silvers HJ, Watanabe D, et al. Effectiveness of a neuromuscular and propriocpetive training program in preventing the incidence of ACL injuries in Female Athletes. American Orthopedic Society of Sports Medicine. 2002

35. McClay I, Manal K. Three-dimensional kinetic analysis of running: Significance of secondary planes of motion. Med Sci Sports Exerc. 1999; 31:1629-1637

36. Mills JD, Taunton JE. The effect of spinal stabilization training on spinal mobility, vertical jump, agility and balance. Med Sci Sports Exerc. 2003; 35(5):S323

37. Nadler SF, Malanga GA, Bartoli LA, et al. Hip muscle imbalance and low back pain in athletes: influence of core strengthening. Med Sci Sports Exerc. 2002; 34(1):9-16

38. Nadler SF, Malanga GA, Feinberg JH, et al. Functional performance deficits in athletes with previous lower extremity injury. Clin J Sport Med. 2002; 12(2):73-78

39. Nicholas JA, Marino M. The relationship of injuries of the leg, foot, and ankle to proximal thigh strength in athletes. Foot and Ankle. 1987; 7(4):218-228

40. Neumann DA. Kinesiology of the Musculoskeletal System; Foundations for Physical Rehabilitation. St. Louis: Mosby; 2002

41. Nyland J, Smith S, Beickman K, et al. Frontal plane knee angles affects dynamic postural control strategy during unilateral stance. Medicine Science Sports and Exercise. 2002; 34(7):1150-1157

42. O'Sullivan PB, Twomey L, Allison GT. Evaluation of specific stabilizing exercises in the treatment of chronic low back pain with radiological diagnosis of spondylosis and spondylolysthesis. Spine. 1997; 22(24):2959-2967

43. O'Sullivan PB, Twomey L, Allison GT. Altered abdominal muscle recruitment in patients with chronic back pain following a specific exercise intervention. J Orthop Sports Phys Ther. 1998; 27(2):114-124

44. Panjabi MM. The stabilizing system of the spine. Part I: Function, dysfunction, adaptation, and enhancement. J Spinal Disord. 1992; 5:383-389

45. Paterno MV, Myer GD, Ford KR, Hewett TE. Neuromuscular training improves single-leg stability in young female athletes. J Orthop Sports Phys Ther. 2004; 34:305-316

46. Porterfield JA, DeRosa C: Mechanical Low Back Pain; Perspectives in functional anatomy. Philadelphia, WB Saunders 1991

47. Powers CM. The influence of altered lower extremity kinematics on patellofemoral joint dysfunction: A theoretical perspective. JOSPT. 2003; 33(11):639-646

48. Richardson CA, Snijders CJ, Hides JA, Damen L, Pas MS, Storm J. The relation between the transversus abdominus muscles, sacroiliac joint mechanics and low back pain; Spine 27(4):399-405, 2002

49. Sahrmann S. Posture and muscle imbalance. Faulty lumbo-pelvic alignment and associated musculolskeletal pain syndromes: Orthop Div Rev- Can Phys Ther. 1992; 12:13-20

30

Nutritional Considerations for Inflammation and Pain

David Seaman

Introduction

Neurophysiology and Biochemistry of Nociception

Hyperalgesia and Allodynia

Pain Is Never "Mechanical"

Diet as a Driver of Inflammation and Pain

Insulin Resistance and Inflammation

Free Radicals and Inflammation

Omega-6 Fatty Acids and Inflammation

Potassium, Magnesium, Dietary pH Regulation, and Inflammation

Learning Objectives

After reading this chapter, you should be able to understand:

- How inflammation affects nociception
- How diet predisposes a person to inflammation
- How pH and inflammation are related
- The value of supplementation as an alternative anti-inflammatory
- How fatty acids affect inflammation

Introduction

Biomechanics and biochemistry are very different and, therefore, practice methods related to biochemistry, such as nutrition, are often difficult to apply for one whose orientation is biomechanics. This chapter is written to help the mechanically oriented practitioner to use nutrition more effectively, and it begins with a general discussion about pain mechanisms related to biomechanics and biochemistry. The production of inflammatory mediators represents the biochemical changes that ignite pain mechanisms, and research has demonstrated that many dietary factors augment the expression of inflammation.

In this chapter, two pro-inflammatory metabolic imbalances are described, including insulin resistance and free radical activity. The specific pro-inflammatory dietary imbalances discussed herein include the following: increased omega-6 fatty acid intake, inadequate potassium intake, inadequate magnesium intake, and inadequate phytonutrient intake. Basic dietary and supplement recommendations are also discussed.

Neurophysiology and Biochemistry of Nociception

Group IV afferents and our other sensory fibers (group I, II, III afferents) are referred to as first-order neurons. Group IV afferents are the most abundant of our sensory fibers and represent the majority of our nociceptive fibers (41,70). They begin in the periphery within musculoskeletal and visceral tissues and they travel to the spinal cord where they synapse with and stimulate second-order neurons in the spinal cord dorsal horn, which become part of the spinothalamic tract that ends in the thalamus. From there, thalamocortical fibers, our third-order neurons, transmit nociceptive information to the limbic system where peripheral noxious stimuli may be realized as pain. In other words, the experience of "pain" is approximately three neurons removed from the original reception of the noxious stimuli. Thus, nociception is the reception of noxious stimuli by group IV afferents, and pain is the cortical realization of such stimuli. It is a great error to equate nociception with pain.

Group IV afferents are nerve cells or neurons, and like all other cells, they have biochemical receptors on their cell membranes. All of our inflammatory mediators, such as prostaglandins, leukotrienes, bradykinin, serotonin, and cytokines, have their own individual receptor on the cell membrane of the group IV afferent. When spinal tissues are injured, inflammatory mediators are liberated from tissues and cells and bind to their respective receptor sites on local group IV afferents. The receptors for inflammatory mediators are coupled to sodium channels, such that when mediators bind to their receptors on group IV afferents, sodium channels open, and sodium rushes into the neuron, resulting in an action potential that is ultimately realized as pain (11,91).

Hyperalgesia and Allodynia

When inflammation persists, group IV afferents are brought closer to threshold, such that innocuous mechanical stimuli associated with activities of daily living become painful. It is important to understand that inflammatory mediators "preload" or "sensitize" group IV afferents, bringing them very close to threshold, which then allows for innocuous stimuli to be realized as pain. In clinical practice, we encounter a sensitized nociceptive system whenever gentle/normal palpation and normal movements are experienced as tender and painful.

Hyperalgesia and allodynia are terms that refer to pain induced by a sensitized group IV afferents. Hyperalgesia refers to abnormally intense pain that is induced by a painful stimulus that would, under normal circumstances, be merely painful. Allodynia is pain that occurs in response to an innocuous stimulus, such that normal movements or normal palpation is experienced as pain, which is a common clinical encounter (90).

Pain Is Never "Mechanical"

The presence of allodynia can lead practitioners to assume that pain is mechanical in nature. When red flags are not present, and when movements associated with normal activities cause back pain, we commonly refer to it as "mechanical" low back pain. While movements and palpation represent mechanical stimuli, the generation of pain with normal mechanical stimuli is typically caused by the sensitization of group IV afferents by biochemical mediators of inflammation.

Clearly, pain is never purely mechanical. Pain is always mechanical, biochemical, and psychological (91), and we should not arbitrarily view one as more important than the other. Complicating the matter a little further is the fact that mechanical, biochemical, and psychological factors are likely to be different from patient to patient, and even different within the same patient depending on the balance of stressors present at a given time (90).

Diet as a Driver of Inflammation and Pain

The inflammatory process occurs after tissue injury and needs to occur after injury if healing is to take place. Clearly, inflammation is part of the healing process; however, chronic inflammation represents a lack of tissue healing and actually, promotes ongoing tissue damage. Cancer, heart disease, hypertension, Alzheimer disease, endometriosis, osteoarthritis, rheumatoid arthritis, diabetes, aging, osteoporosis, chronic obstructive pulmonary disease, and menopause are examples of conditions that develop and exist as a consequence of chronic inflammation (7,8,13,26,38,58,60,61,63,67,68,77,80,84,94,95,97, 104), and this is likely the case for chronic musculoskeletal pain (23,42,57,62,92,98).

Standard physiology and pathology books are responsible for providing us with a segmented view of inflammation. In response to tissue injury, local cells release pro-inflammatory and anti-inflammatory mediators, the balance of which should lead to the resolution of inflammation and facilitate tissue repair. Physiology and pathology texts do not alert us to this fact or that an excess of pro-inflammatory mediators will lead to chronic inflammation and chronic disease (92). Standard texts also do not alert us to the fact that dietary imbalances are responsible for creating a diet-induced, pro-inflammatory state that leads to chronic inflammation (92).

Humans are genetically adapted to eat a diet that consists largely of vegetation (fruits, vegetables, and nuts) and animals that ate vegetation, which represents what is commonly referred to as a Paleolithic or hunter–gatherer diet (16–18,74). In contrast, our modern diet is based largely on grains, animals that ate grains, refined starches, soda, and engineered

foods. Table 30.1 lists anti-inflammatory and pro-inflammatory foods.

Several dietary imbalances result from the consumption of our modern diet that promotes a pro-inflammatory state, such as excessive omega-6 fatty acid intake, inadequate potassium intake, inadequate magnesium intake, and inadequate phytonutrient intake. Related diet-driven metabolic imbalances including insulin resistance, a prediabetic state, and free radical mechanisms are also known to drive inflammation. A concise discussion of each follows.

Before continuing, readers should be aware that the aforementioned dietary imbalances occur simultaneously, are interrelated, and appear to have a cumulative effect, especially in those who are particularly genetically susceptible to a chronic inflammatory disease such as cancer, heart disease, and diabetes (19). Thus, taking magnesium or vitamin E supplements, for example, as a single intervention, will not thoroughly address the diet-induced pro-inflammatory state and is not likely to impart a significant protective or anti-inflammatory effect. In other words, we cannot live on pro-inflammatory foods and expect a single pill, drug, or supplement to have an appreciable anti-inflammatory effect.

Insulin Resistance and Inflammation

Insulin resistance represents a prediabetic state referred to as syndrome X or the metabolic syn-

Table 30.1 Anti-inflammatory and Pro-inflammatory Foods

Anti-inflammatory Foods	Pro-inflammatory Foods
Fruits	Refined grains
Vegetables	Whole grains
Nuts	Grain/flour products
Potatoes	Grain-fed meats/eggs
Fresh fish	Most packaged foods
Wild game	Most processed foods
Grass/pasture-fed meat	Deep fried food
Omega-3 eggs	Trans fats (margarine, and in most packaged/processed foods)
Organic extra virgin olive oil	Corn, safflower, sunflower, soybean oil
Organic coconut oil	Most commercial salad dressings
Organic butter	
Dark chocolate	
Stout beer	
Red wine	
Balsamic vinegar	
Spices: ginger, turmeric, garlic, oregano, marjoram, cumin, etc.	

drome. If patients have three or more of the following risk factors, they are said to have syndrome X: fasting glucose of ≥110 mg/dL; triglycerides of ≥150 mg/dL; HDL cholesterol <40 mg/dL for men and <50 mg/dL for women; blood pressure of ≥130/85 mm Hg; and a waist circumference of >40 inches for men and >35 inches for women (24,105).

Syndrome X is thought to be promoted by a chronic systemic low-grade inflammation (14). Type 2 diabetes is referred to as "pro-inflammatory cytokine-associated disease" (78). Tumor necrosis factor-α (TNF), one of many pro-inflammatory cytokines, is released by both white cells and adipocytes, and as individuals gain additional fat weight, there is an increased release of adipocyte-derived TNF, which serves to inhibit insulin receptor activity that leads to insulin resistance (32,38). As insulin resistance develops, it promotes glycosylation of proteins and DNA, enhances free radical formation (79), and leads to an upregulation of inflammatory protein production (29), and through these mechanisms, insulin resistance will lead to a worsening of inflammation, which leads to a vicious cycle of chronic inflammation (32).

Not surprisingly, insulin resistance is involved in the pathogenesis of many pro-inflammatory diseases such as diabetes, atherosclerosis, stroke, myocardial infarction, and cancer (30,38). In one study (30), 208 apparently healthy, nonobese subjects were evaluated 4 to 11 years after baseline measurements of insulin resistance were made to determine the incidence of various clinical events including hypertension, coronary heart disease, stroke, cancer, and type 2 diabetes. The subjects were divided into tertiles of insulin resistance at baseline, and the development of clinical events was compared among these three groups. A total of 40 clinical events occurred among 37 subjects, including 12 with hypertension, three with hypertension and type 2 diabetes, nine with cancer, seven with coronary heart disease, four with stroke, and two with type 2 diabetes. In contrast, no events occurred in the insulin sensitive tertile.

The pervasiveness of insulin resistance should not be underestimated, because more than 40 million American adults seem to be affected by the syndrome (49), with some estimates reaching as high 75 million Americans (32). The incidence of syndrome X-driven or related diseases is quite high and far and away represent the major health problem in the United States and other Westernized nations (19). This suggests that a significant percentage of patients needing spinal rehabilitation will have syndrome X. Whether syndrome X promotes back pain has yet to be studied; however, it is interesting to note that the same mediators that promote syndrome X are also released from damaged spinal tissues.

Consider, for example, that syndrome X is promoted by TNF and is associated with increased levels of other pro-inflammatory cytokines such as interleukin-6 (IL-6) (78). Intriguingly, increased levels of TNF, IL-6, and interleukin-1 (IL-1) have been found in facet joints of patients with degenerative conditions of the lumbar spine (48). In fact, TNF appears to be a pivotal mediator in disc herniation-induced radicular pain (55).

In general, the best way to treat syndrome X is to eat less and exercise more (24,105), which is a very fundamental and historically recommended practice to help promote long-term health. In recent years, the "Mediterranean diet" has become popular, which focuses on the consumption of fish, lean meats, fruits, vegetables, nuts, whole grains, and olive oil. A 2-year trial was completed in which a Mediterranean-style diet intervention was compared to a control group on prudent diet (50% to 60% carbohydrates, 15% to 20% protein, <30% fat) in patients with syndrome X (28). Subjects on the Mediterranean-style diet lost more weight and had significantly reduced serum concentrations of high-sensitivity C-reactive protein, IL-6, IL-7, and IL-18, as well as decreased insulin resistance. There were 90 subjects in each group, and after 2 years 40 subjects in the intervention group had features of the metabolic syndrome, compared with 78 in the control group.

Clearly, the recommendation to eat high-carbohydrate low-fat diets need to be reconsidered. For many years, we have known that high-carbohydrate diets (60% versus 40%) lead to hypertriglyceridemia, reduction in HDL levels, and hyperinsulinemia, particularly when the carbohydrates are refined sugars and starches (20). At present, it is estimated that refined carbohydrates comprise 36% or more of the daily energy in the typical American diet, which is thought to represent a significant promoter of syndrome X and represents a drastic departure from our Paleolithic dietary heritage, during which syndrome X was unknown (19).

Monounsaturated fatty acids (MUFAs) found in nuts, olive oil, and animal products are increased in a Mediterranean-style diet, and it is known that MUFAs promote insulin sensitivity and have anti-inflammatory properties, which lower insulin resistance (83). Several other specific nutritional factors improve insulin sensitivity including omega-3 fatty acids (95), potassium (22,31), and magnesium (64), which are naturally present in hunter–gatherer and Mediterranean-style diets.

In summary, Paleolithic, hunter–gatherer, and Mediterranean-style diets should be viewed as anti-inflammatory, compared with our modern diet, and represent our best chance at combating syndrome X. Patients should be told that eating vegetation and animals that ate vegetation represents an anti-inflammatory diet. A recent study estimated that consuming a "polymeal" will reduce cardiovascular disease by more than 75% (36). Foods permitted in the anti-inflammatory polymeal include fish, fruits, vegetables, wine, dark chocolate, almonds, and garlic. Foods that should be added to this list include grass-fed animal products, wild game, omega-3 eggs, and spices such as ginger and turmeric.

Grains, cereals, and related flour products, meaning that nearly all packaged foods should be avoided, and this refers to both whole grains and refined grains. The pro-inflammatory nature of grains is discussed in the fatty acid section of this chapter. For snacks, many tend to grab for grain products; a better choice would be fruits, nuts, dark chocolate, or even dark chocolate-covered nuts. Eating an anti-inflammatory diet does not mean that one cannot have tasty snacks.

For cooking, coconut oil is recommended, because it has anti-inflammatory properties (88). Butter is permissible when used in moderation because it has an anti-inflammatory balance of polyunsaturated fatty acids with a 1.5:1 ratio of n-6 to n-3 fatty acids (27) and, as mentioned, olive oil has anti-inflammatory properties (62,83) and should be used in salad dressings and can be used for cooking as well.

Free Radicals and Inflammation

Free radical mechanisms have been implicated in the pathogenesis of more than 100 conditions involving inflammation, such as arthritis, hemorrhagic shock, AIDS, heart disease, aging, Parkinson disease, amyotrophic lateral sclerosis, altered immunity, cataracts, and cancer (92). Even disc degeneration involves free radical pathology. Discal areas showing signs of strong histologic degeneration, such as the nucleus pulposus and the inner/middle layers of the anulus, contain lipofuscin, the aging pigment that is produced by oxidation of lipids or lipoprotein (106).

Free radicals are molecules that have an unpaired electron in their outer orbital, which renders them highly reactive and unstable. Free radicals attempt to restore their stability by interacting with bodily substances that can donate an electron such as lipids, proteins, cell membrane phospholipids, and DNA. This exchange of electrons is very damaging to cellular structures and leads to the development of the pathologies mentioned via the induction of inflammatory processes involving the production of pro-

inflammatory cytokines and pro-inflammatory eicosanoids such as prostaglandin E_2 (92).

In the human body, we possess antioxidant mechanisms that prevent oxidation/free radical activity; we only need to fuel them with proper nutrition. Substances commonly thought of as antioxidants include beta-carotene, vitamin E, vitamin C, and selenium, such that many individuals supplement with these nutrients in the hope that they will be protected against free radical damage. While these substances do function in an antioxidant capacity, it should be understood that our antioxidant defense system is quite complex and involves significantly more nutrients than selenium and the vitamins E and C. In fact, for these antioxidants to function properly, important nutrient-dependent metabolic pathways need to be intact for the purpose of regenerating vitamins E and C so they can actually function as antioxidants. Without intact metabolic pathways, including appropriate glycemic regulation and ATP synthesis, vitamins E and C will oxidize and function as pro-oxidants or free radicals.

Appropriate insulin sensitivity allows for normal glucose entry into cells of the liver, adipocytes, and muscle cells, which is used for the synthesis of ATP, coenzyme Q10, NADPH, and other important substances. In particular, ATP, coenzyme Q10, and NADPH are involved in the recycling of antioxidants such as vitamin E, vitamin C, glutathione, and lipoic acid, a process that is reduced in type 2 diabetes, which significantly increases susceptibility oxidative stress, free radical promotion, and inflammation (29).

In addition to maintaining proper blood sugar balance, patients should also be urged to consume liberal amounts of fruits and vegetables, because they contain numerous phytochemicals that have significant anti-inflammatory and antioxidant properties (92). Overeating must be avoided because it is known to cause oxidative stress and burden our mitochondria. Calorie restriction in all animals studied thus far has shown to reduce oxidative stress and the expression of inflammation (13,68,75, 103). Supplementation with a multivitamin, lipoic acid, acetyl-L-carnitine, and CoQ10 are reasonable options to help improve antioxidant activity (3,4,21, 57,69).

Omega-6 Fatty Acids and Inflammation

Fatty acids are made of carbon, oxygen, and hydrogen. When three fatty acids attach to a three-carbon molecule called glycerol, a triglyceride is formed. When saturated fatty acids are attached to glycerol, the lipid will be solid at room temperature and referred to as a fat. In contrast, when the triglyceride consists of unsaturated fatty acids, the lipid will be liquid at room temperature and referred to as an oil.

Three types of fatty acids are available for us to consume, including saturated, monounsaturated, and polyunsaturated fatty acids. Saturated fatty acids contain only single bonds between carbon atoms, and the carbon atoms are saturated with hydrogen ions. Saturated fatty acids have been unduly blamed for causing heart disease and other diseases. Most saturated fats are actually health-promoting, having anti-bacterial, anti-viral, anti-tumor, and anti-inflammatory qualities (37). Several detailed reviews are available on this subject (37,45,46,54).

Monounsaturated fatty acids contain a single double bond between two carbon atoms, which means that two carbon atoms will not be saturated with hydrogen. Oleic acid and palmitoleic acids are the most common monounsaturated fatty acids, and are referred to as omega-9 fatty acids (n-9). Oleic acid is thought to inhibit the synthesis of pro-inflammatory leukotrienes (57,62). Olive oil is the most well-known source of oleic acid. However, it is important to understand that approximately 40% to 50% of animal fats are made up of oleic acid, the same monounsaturated fatty acid found in olive oil. Approximately 45% of animal fat is saturated, and the remaining 10% is polyunsaturated. Monounsaturated fatty acids constitute the largest percentage of fat in most nuts (27). Nuts are also a rich source of vitamins, minerals, and phytonutrients, which is the likely reason why nuts are known to provide substantial anti-inflammatory benefits (1,65,86,87). The same holds true for olive oil, which is rich in anti-inflammatory oleic acid and phytonutrients (102).

Polyunsaturated fatty acids contain two or more double bonds. The pro-inflammatory potential of our fats is largely dependent on the character of polyunsaturated fatty acids found in the individual foods. The polyunsaturated fatty acids are classified as omega-6 (n-6) or omega-3 (n-3). Linoleic acid, an n6 fatty acid, and α-linolenic acid, an n-3 fatty acid, are referred to as the essential fatty acids, because they must be supplied by the diet.

Ideally, we should consume an n-6:n-3 ratio of 1:1; however, modern humans maintain a 20–30:1 ratio or perhaps greater, which is considered to be significantly pro-inflammatory (95,96). Both linoleic acid (n-6) and α-linolenic acid (n-3) are acted on by desaturation and elongation enzymes that lead to their conversion into arachidonic acid (AA; n-6) and eicosapentaenoic acid (EPA; n-3), respectively, each of which is a precursor to substances known as eicosanoids.

Prostaglandin E2 (PGE2), thromboxane A2 (TXA2), and leukotriene B4 (LTB4) are pro-inflammatory eicosanoids derived from arachidonic acid (n-6), whereas prostaglandin E3 (PGE3), thromboxane A3 (TXA3), and leukotriene B5 (LTB5) are anti-inflammatory eicosanoids derived from EPA (n-3). An n-6–to–n-3 ratio of 4:1 or greater leads to the production of an unbalanced excess of pro-inflammatory eicosanoids and cytokines (IL-1, IL-6, and TNF), and this is thought to drive chronic inflammation (95,96).

As mentioned, Americans consume an average of approximately a 20–30:1 ratio. A favorable dietary ratio is considered to be less than 4:1, with 1:1 being the goal, which means that fruits, vegetables, potatoes, grass-fed animals, n-3–enriched eggs, and wild game have favorable ratios and should represent the majority of foods we consume. Interestingly, these are the foods that represent hunter–gatherer-like and Mediterranean-like diets. See Table 30.2 for a list of n-6:n-3 ratios for common foods.

Grains, grain products (cereal, pasta, bread, desserts, etc.), and processed food have ratios that

Table 30.2 n-6:n-3 Ratios in Common Foods

Food	n-6:n-3 Ratio
Grains	20:1
Seed and seed oils (corn, sunflower, safflower)	70:1 or worse
Soybean oil	7:1
Grain-fed meat	5:1 or worse
Chicken (white meat)	15:1
Chicken (dark meat)	17:1
Farmed-raised salmon	1:1 or worse
Nuts	5:1 or worse
Potato chips (and similar foods with added n-6)	60:1 or higher
Fruit	3:1 or better
Green vegetables	1:1 or better
White potato	3:1
Sweet potato	4:1
Grass-fed meat	2.5:1
Wild game	2.5:1
Fresh fish	1:1 or better

Adapted from Cordain (16), Enig (27), and Hands (40).

reach 20:1 and greater, and are considered pro-inflammatory. A wise choice would be to eat grains sparingly or not at all. Athletes wishing to carbohydrate-load should use potatoes and bananas, both of which have favorable n-6:n-3 ratios and promote an alkaline pH. Grains also contain lectins, gliadin, and an acidic pH, all of which are pro-inflammatory [see Cordain for a review (18)]. Whereas whole grains do offer a positive effect on blood sugar regulation (59,76), this seems to be outweighed by their pro-inflammatory effects (18).

Commonly used cooking oils, including corn, safflower, sunflower, and peanut oils, contain virtually no linolenic acid (n-3), and mostly linoleic acid (n-6), such that n-6:n-3 ratios reach 70:1 or greater (53). Soybean oil has a 7:1 ratio and represents approximately 70% of the oil consumption in the United States (27). Clearly, these cooking oils should be eliminated if one wishes to achieve an n-6:n-3 ratio of less than 4:1. Margarine should also be eliminated because most brands are either made from corn oil or soybean oil. Margarine brings with it a host of additional problems, caused by the partial hydrogenation process that dramatically alters the biochemical character of the corn or soybean oil.

Partially hydrogenated oils, referred to as trans-fats, are found in margarine and nearly all packaged goods found in the grocery store. Trans-fats are structurally similar to saturated fats and have the identical properties of saturated fats when used for cooking and baking. However, from a metabolic perspective, trans-fats have completely dissimilar functions. While natural saturated fats are generally anti-inflammatory (37), trans-fats are pro-inflammatory and, without exception, have no place in the human diet (6,15, 39,71,72). When oils are to be cooked with, or added to the diet, it seems that our best choices are the organic varieties of extra virgin olive oil, coconut oil, and butter, because each has anti-inflammatory properties (27,50,62,88).

Supplementation with EPA/DHA has become popular in recent years for the purpose of attempting to achieve a balance with n-6 fatty acids. It is now possible to buy EPA/DHA in stores such as Walmart and Sam's Club. In fact, a great deal of research has been directed toward EPA/DHA, and so we have insights regarding their impact on musculoskeletal tissues. In the case of articular tissues, inflammatory cytokines such as IL-1 and PGE2 work together and are known to inhibit chondrocyte proliferation and induce cartilage degradation, with the result being a net loss of proteoglycans from articular cartilage. In vitro studies have demonstrated that the incorporation of n-3 fatty acids into articular chondrocyte membranes resulted in a dose-dependent reduction in the expression and activity of proteoglycan-degrading enzymes, the expression of inflammatory cytokines IL-1 and TNF, and expression of the COX2 enzyme. In studies with rheumatoid arthritis patients, EPA/DHA supplementation resulted in a 20% reduction of neutrophil LTB4 production from baseline and a 40% decrease in macrophage IL-1 production (104). This effect can be so profound that certain patients with rheumatoid arthritis are able to discontinue use of medications [see review by Kremer (57)]. Side effects are almost nonexistent in the dosage range of 1 to 3 grams of EPA/DHA per day (57). Only those using powerful anti-coagulants such as Coumadin should be wary of EPA/DHA, as well as other supplements such as ginger, garlic, turmeric, antioxidants, and phytonutrients that have an anti-thrombotic effect.

Concerning ginger and turmeric, they can be used as spices and supplements. They function as natural inhibitors of pro-inflammatory eicosanoids and cytokines, and although more studies are needed, they have demonstrated an ability to reduce pain associated with osteoarthritis, rheumatoid arthritis, and general musculoskeletal pain (2,10,99). Two to four grams of powdered ginger or tumeric, or ginger/turmeric combinations, is the common recommendation.

After reducing inflammation, articular tissues may be helped with supplemental glucosamine sulfate, which helps to build proteoglycans that imbibe water and allow joints to withstand compressive forces. In a 3-year study involving either placebo or 1500 mg of glucosamine sulfate, the 106 patients on placebo had a progressive joint-space narrowing, with a mean joint-space loss after 3 years of −0.31 mm. There was no significant joint-space loss in the 106 patients on glucosamine sulfate (−0.06 mm). Additionally, symptoms worsened slightly in patients on placebo compared with the improvement observed after treatment with glucosamine sulfate (82).

Potassium, Magnesium, Dietary pH Regulation, and Inflammation

Potassium and magnesium are not typically emphasized as dietary constituents with important health benefits. Patients and doctors generally read or hear that we should not fail to get enough calcium and be careful not to take in too much sodium. However, we need to appreciate the health benefits of potassium and magnesium are substantial, with each providing significant anti-inflammatory benefits, and potassium plays a critical role in maintaining acid–base balance.

Most people currently have a low-potassium diet. For example, in the United States, it is estimated that urban whites average approximately 2500 mg per day, whereas southeastern blacks take in approximately 1000 mg per day (73,101). We should urge patients to increase these very low levels to normal, which is 7500 mg per day or more, and it is agreed that this should come from fruits and vegetables, not from supplements (22,44,100).

A low-potassium diet does not result in a classic deficiency syndrome such as with vitamin C or B vitamins; rather, inadequate potassium has a similar outcome as inadequate n-3 fatty acids. A pro-inflammatory state develops that can manifest as diabetes, hypertension, stroke, kidney stones, osteoporosis, cancer, and heart disease (44,100). Recommending that our patients increase their potassium intake by consuming large amount of fruits and vegetables can obviously have long-term beneficial effects; however, most people are motivated to make lifestyle changes when they direct impact immediate problems. In this regard, we can make the argument that inadequate potassium intake is likely promote a metabolic environment that is not friendly toward rehabilitation exercises.

Consider that a deficiency in potassium impairs glucose utilization and reduces glycogen stores in skeletal muscle (52). Reduced potassium promotes free radical release from endothelial cells and macrophages (107). Potassium is also the key element for controlling blood flow during exercise. Without adequate potassium, muscle vessels will not appropriately vasoregulate and the outcome will be hypoxia. These metabolic changes are likely to lead to symptoms of potassium deficiency such as muscle weakness, pain, and cramps. When this scenario is taken to the pro-inflammatory extreme, rhabdomyolysis can occur, which refers to severe ischemic muscle damage (53).

Potassium is also the key element for maintain body pH. The human body is essentially an acid-producing machine, for which we have endogenous buffer systems; however, our body absolutely depends on a continuous flow of exogenous buffer that we derive from food (12,22). This aspect of pH balance is virtually ignored by our current physiology texts; nonetheless, its importance should not be underestimated. Fruits and particularly vegetables contain organic potassium salts, such as potassium malate and potassium citrate. These salts exert an alkalinizing effect by generating potassium bicarbonate (22). Conversely, grains and meat promote an acidic environment, even though meat contains appreciable amounts of potassium. Though meats promote an acidic pH as ingested protein increases the formation of organic acids, and because of the metabolism of sulfer-containing amino acids, the high potassium in meat still offers the other non-pH–related benefits discussed.

There are two significant issues related to diet-induced body acidity that impacts on musculoskeletal practitioners. Researchers maintain that a chronic subclinical acidic pH is a significant promoter of the progressive bone loss and sarcopenia that occurs with aging, and also suggests that a lack of fruit and vegetable consumption during a lifetime is responsible for this degenerative scenario (22,93). Historically, humans consumed meat as the primary source of dietary acid; the remainder of the diet consisted of fruits, vegetables, roots, and tubers, all of which promote an alkaline pH (93). Modern humans now consume additional acid-forming foods including grains, eggs, and yogurt and significantly less fruits and vegetables (93). For perspective, it should be understood that our national consumption of fruits and vegetable is remote from recommended levels. At present, only approximately 20% of children and adolescents and 30% of adults eat 5 serving of fruits and/or vegetables per day (5). To achieve potassium adequacy, we need to consume closer to 10 servings per day (22).

Table 30.3 contains a list of categories of foods with the most favorable potassium levels. Clearly, we need to focus our consumption of fruits, vegetables, and animal products, and the best snack for us all would be an ounce of nuts and ½ cup of dried fruit. Not surprisingly, most of the potassium-rich foods are also excellent sources of anti-inflammatory fatty acids, anti-oxidants, phytonutrients, and magnesium.

In addition to eating more potassium-rich foods, we need to insure magnesium adequacy, because magnesium depletion can profoundly influence potassium homeostasis. During magnesium depletion, the kidney does not conserve potassium adequately and hypokalemia develops. Attempts to replete the potassium a deficit with potassium therapy alone is not successful without simultaneous magnesium therapy (85). A similar pattern exists for hypocalcemia (9), which permits us to see the interrelated nature of our some of our key minerals.

Like potassium, magnesium is a mineral that receives little attention in the media or the doctor's office. This is problematic because inadequacies of magnesium intake are pandemic. A recent study demonstrated that the average American's intake of magnesium is 70 to 140 mg below the recommended dietary allowances (320 mg for women; 420 mg for men) (34), which are likely to represent values that merely maintain magnesium status and cannot replete deficiencies (43). Good food sources of magnesium include vegetables and nuts; however, they are not at levels that would allow for repletion of deficiencies, which is why supplementation of magnesium is recommended.

Magnesium deficiency may influence inflammation from several perspectives. Magnesium is required

Table 30.3 Potassium Levels in Common Foods

Food	mg K+
Fruit	
1 medium banana	500
1 apple	150
1 orange	150
Potatoes	
1 medium potato	500
1 sweet medium potato	350
Vegetables	
1 medium tomato	350
1 cup broccoli	400
5-oz green salad	500
Meat	
3-oz hamburger	300
3-oz steak	300
1 chicken breast	500
1 cod fillet	450
1 flounder fillet	450
1 grouper fillet	900
1 salmon	1000
Dried fruit	
½ cup raisins	600
½ cup dried figs	700
½ cup pitted dates	600
½ cup dried apricots	900
Nuts	
1 oz of almonds	200
1 oz of cashews	150
1 oz of walnuts	150

Adapted from Hands (59).

for ATP synthesis, so deficiencies may lead to compromised mitochondrial function and lead to tissue hypoxia and free radical generation. Magnesium also helps to stabilize cell membrane activity and appears to modulate the phospholipase A2 enzyme that is involved in the generation of pro-inflammatory eicosanoids (89). In most animal models studied, magnesium deficiency leads to an increase in serum substance P levels (25). Nociceptive afferents are a source of substance P, which stimulates immune cells and platelets to release pro-inflammatory mediators (81). It is possible that magnesium deficiency en-

hances nociception and inflammation via this mechanism referred to as neurogenic inflammation. It is also thought that magnesium deficiency will lead to a generalized state of nervous system hyperexcitability, which involves an increase in systemic production of inflammatory mediators and heightened peripheral and central nociceptive activity (25).

Research suggests that magnesium repletion cannot occur by dietary changes alone (43,51). It seems that magnesium balance can be maintained by 375 mg per day in men and women, which can be achieved through diet; however, approximately 1000 mg per day is required to achieve a positive balance (43), suggesting that supplementation of magnesium may be a requirement for many people. Researchers have recently suggested that it is not possible to replete magnesium in patients with syndrome X (51).

■ CONCLUSION

Through the use of medications, we are somewhat conditioned to think that a single pill would be able to solve a painful condition and other health problems. Most individuals quickly learn that this is not the case, although some relief may be afforded by a given pharmacologic intervention. Readers should be aware that there are no natural substitutes for powerful anti-inflammatory drugs or opiates. There is no escaping the fact that diet is perhaps the most important factor in determining our inflammatory status.

A diet that is pro-inflammatory will increase the inflammatory potential of cells and tissues (22,25, 93,95), and the outcome is likely to be the phenotypic expression of a disease or syndrome related to inflammation such as pain, arthritis, cancer, heart disease, diabetes, Alzheimer disease, and most other chronic degenerative diseases (14,33,35,47,56,66,75).

With this information in mind, we can craft a diet that is rich in foods that are known to be anti-inflammatory. As discussed in the body of this chapter, such a diet would be free of simple carbohydrates because they drive hyperinsulinemia and the expression of syndrome X, an inflammatory syndrome. Calories would be restricted to inhibit an increase in fat stores, which serve as a depot of inflammation and a promoter of syndrome X. We would be left with a diet that is similar to the hunter–gatherer diet (74), Mediterranean-like diet (28), and the polymeal (36).

The dietary focus is fruits, vegetables, fresh fish, grass-fed animal meat, wild game, omega-3 eggs, nuts, and minimal grains. This type of diet will increase n-3 fatty acids, potassium, magnesium, antioxidants, and phytonutrients, and create an alkaline pH, all of which are anti-inflammatory.

Table 30.4 Supplemental Options

Supplement	Suggested Amount
Multivitamin/mineral	Depends on product (2–3 pills per day is common)
Magnesium	400–1000 mg per day (mg/d)
EPA/DHA	1–3 gram/d
Coenzyme 10	≥100 mg/d
Lipoic acid	400 mg/d (200 mg twice daily)
Acetyl-L-carnitine	1000 mg/d (500 mg twice daily)
Ginger	1–2 gram/d
Turmeric	1–2 gram/d
Glucosamine sulfate	1500 mg/d

Oils and fats to be included are extra virgin olive oil, butter, and coconut oil. While flaxseed oil is rich in n-3 fatty acids, it may be that grinding flaxseeds immediately before use in foods is the most prudent way to use flax. Oils to be excluded are soybean, safflower, sunflower, corn, and all partially hydrogenated oils/trans-fats.

The appropriate seasoning of meals is a determining factor in palatability. We should choose seasonings that are tasty and known to be anti-inflammatory, such as ginger, garlic, and turmeric. Most spices studied thus far have been shown to have anti-inflammatory activity, unlike table salt, which only adds to our already excessive sodium load.

It is likely that nutritional supplements are best applied to a body that is no longer burdened with a constant inflammatory load from inappropriate foods. In large measure, there are no specific supplements for individual diseases. As with diet, our goal with supplementation should be to improve metabolic function and reduce inflammation. Table 30.4 contains a summary of the supplements discussed in this chapter.

Nutritional applications to reduce inflammation need not be complicated. As described in this chapter, dietary practices are straightforward, as are methods of supplementation. And dietary approaches similar to what is described in this chapter have been used successfully to reduce pain and disability in patients with rheumatoid arthritis and fibromyalgia (23,42,

57,98). This knowledge should be applied to other pain syndromes that affect the musculoskeletal system, and future research will help to guide our applications more specifically.

Audit Process
Self-Check of the Chapter's Learning Objectives

- What foods are pro-inflammatory or anti-inflammatory?
- How can food and/or supplements alter a person's pH?
- How can a normal omega 6:omega 3 fatty acid ratio be achieved?
- How does the Mediterranean-style diet affect insulin resistance?

■ REFERENCES

1. Almario RU, Vonghavaravat V, Wong R, Kasim-Karakas SE. Effects of walnut consumption on plasma fatty acids and lipoproteins in combined hyperlipidemia. Am J Clin Nutr 2001;74(1): 72–79.
2. Altman RD, Marcussen KC. Effects of a ginger extract on knee pain in patients with osteoarthritis. Arthritis Rheum 2001; 44:2531–2538.
3. Ames BN. The metabolic tune-up: metabolic harmony and disease prevention. J Nutr 2003;133: 1544S–15448S.
4. Ames BN. Supplements and tuning up metabolism. J Nutr 2004;134:3164S–68S.
5. Ames BN. DNA damage from micronutrient deficiencies is likely to be a major cause of cancer. Mutat Res 2001;475(1–2):7–20.
6. Baer DJ, Judd JT, Clevidence BA, Tracy RP. Dietary fatty acids affect plasma markers of inflammation in healthy men fed controlled diets: a randomized crossover study. Am J Clin Nutr 2004; 79:969–973.
7. Balkwill F, Mantovani A. Inflammation and cancer: back to Virchow? Lancet. 2001;357:539–545.
8. Ban WQ, Man SF, Senthilselvan A, Sin DD. Association between chronic obstructive pulmonary disease and systemic inflammation: a systematic review and meta-analysis. Thorax 2004;59:574–580.
9. Besser GM, et al. Clinical Endocrinology, 2nd ed. London: Times Mirror, 1994:18.10.
10. Bucci LR. Nutrition applied to injury rehabilitation and sports medicine. Boca Raton: CRC Press, 1995.
11. Byers MR, Bonica JJ. Peripheral pain mechanisms and nociceptor plasticity. In: Loeser JD. Ed. Bonica's management of pain, 3rd ed. Philadelphia: Lippincott Williams & Wilkins, 2001:26–72.
12. Charney AN, Feldman GM. Internal exchanges of hydrogen ions: gastrointestinal tract. In: Seldin DW, Giebisch G, eds. The regulation of acid-base balance. New York: Raven Press, 1989:89–105.

13. Chung HY, Kim HJ, Kim JW, Yu BP. The inflammation hypothesis of aging: molecular modulation by calorie restriction. Ann NY Acad Sci 2001;928: 327–335.

14. Cipollone F, Toniato E, Martinotti S et al. A polymorphism in the cyclooxygenase 2 gene as an inherited protective factor against myocardial infarction and stroke. JAMA. 2004;291:2221–2228.

15. Clifton PM, Keogh JB, Noakes M. Trans fatty acids in adipose tissue and the food supply are associated with myocardial infarction. J Nutr. 2004;134: 874–879.

16. Cordain L, Watkins BA, Florant GL, Kehler M, Rogers L, Li Y. Fatty acid analysis of wild ruminant tissues: Evolutionary implications for reducing diet-related chronic disease. Eur J Clin Nutr 2002;56: 181–191.

17. Cordain L, Eaton SB, Brand Miller J, Mann N, Hill K. The paradoxical nature of hunter-gatherer diets: Meat based, yet non-atherogenic. Eur J Clin Nutr 2002;56(suppl 1):S42–S52.

18. Cordain L. Cereal grains: humanity's double edged sword. World Rev Nutr Diet 1999;84:19–73.

19. Cordain L, Eades MR, Eades MD. Hyperinsulinemic diseases of civilization: more than just syndrome X. Comp Biochem Physiol Part A 2003;136: 95–112.

20. Coulston AM, Liu GC, Reaven GM. Plasma glucose, insulin, and lipid responses to high-carbohydrate low-fat diets in normal humans. Metabolism 1983;32:52–56.

21. Crane FL. Biochemical functions of coenzyme Q10. J Am Coll Nutr 2001;20:591–598.

22. Demigne C, Sabboh H, Remesy C, Meneton P. Protective effects of high dietary potassium: nutritional and metabolic aspects. J Nutr 2004; 134: 2903–2906.

23. Donaldson MS, Speight N, Loomis S. Fibromyalgia syndrome improved using a mostly raw vegetarian diet: an observational study. BMC Comp Alt Med 2001;1:7 (http://www.biomedcentral.com/1472–6882/1/7).

24. Dunbar RL, Rader DJ. Slaying the metabolic syndrome. Are we battling the Hydra or the Chimera? Minerva Endocrinol. 2004; 29:89–111.

25. Durlach J, Bac P, Bara M, Guiet-Bara A. Physiopathology of symptomatic and latent forms of central nervous hyperexcitability due to magnesium deficiency: a current general scheme. Magnes Res 2000;13:293–302.

26. Dvorak HF. Tumors: wounds that do not heal. Similarities between tumor stroma generation and wound healing. N Engl J Med 1986; 315:1650–1659.

27. Enig MG. Know your fats. Silver Spring: Bethesda Press, 2000:280–292, 142, 123.

28. Esposito K, Marfella R, Ciotola M, et al. Effect of a Mediterranean-style diet on endothelial dysfunction and markers of vascular inflammation in the metabolic syndrome. J Am Med Assoc 2004; 292: 1440–1446.

29. Evans JL, Goldfine ID, Maddux BA, Grodsky GM. Oxidative stress and stress-activated signaling pathways: a unifying hypothesis of type 2 diabetes. Endocrinol Rev 2002; 23:599–622.

30. Facchini FS, Hua N, Abbasi F, Reaven GM. Insulin resistance as a predictor of age-related disease. J Clin Endocrinol Metab 2001; 86:3574–3578.

31. Feng JH, Graham AM. The benefits of potassium. Br Med J 2001;323:497–501.

32. Fernandez-Real JM, Ricraft W. Insulin resistance and chronic cardiovascular inflammatory syndrome. Endo Rev 2003;24:278–301.

33. Fernandez-Real JM, Ricart W. Insulin resistance and inflammation in a evolutionary perspective: the contribution of cytokine genotype/phenotype to thriftiness. Diabetologia 1999; 42:1367–1374.

34. Ford ES, Mokdad AH. Dietary magnesium intake in a national sample of US adults. J Nutr 2003;133: 2879–2882.

35. Francheschi C, Bonafe M, Valensin et al. Inflamm-aging: an evolutionary perspective on immunosenescence. NY Acad Sci 2000;908:244–254.

36. Franco OH, Bonneux L, de Laet C, Peters A, Steyerberg EW, Machenbach JP. The polymeal: a more natural, safer, and probably tastier (than the polyp-ill) strategy to reduce cardiovascular disease by more than 75%. Br Med J 2004;329:1447–1450.

37. German JB, Dillard CJ. Saturated fats: what dietary intake? Am J Clin Nutr 2004;80(3):550–559.

38. Grimble RF. Inflammatory status and insulin resistance. Curr Opin Clin Nutr Metab Care 2002;5: 551–559.

39. Han SN, Leka LS, Lichtenstein AH, Ausman LM, Schaefer EJ, Meydani SN. Effect of hydrogenated and saturated, relative to polyunsaturated, fat on immune and inflammatory responses of adults with moderate hypercholesterolemia. J Lipid Res. 2002; 43:445–452.

40. Hands ES. Nutrients in food. Philadelphia: Lippincott Williams & Wilkins, 2000.

41. Hanesch U, Heppleman B, Messlinger K, Schmidt RF. Nociception in normal and arthritic joints: structural and functional aspects. In Willis WD, ed. Hyperalgesia and allodynia. New York: Raven Press, 1992:81–106.

42. Hanninen O, Kaartinen K, Rauma AL, et al. Antioxidants in vegan diet and rheumatic disorders. Toxicology 2000;155:45–53.

43. Hartwig A. Role of magnesium in genomic stability. Mut Res 2001;475:113–121.

44. He FJ, MacGregor GA. Beneficial effects of potassium. BMJ 2001; 323:497–501.

45. Herron KL, Fernandez ML. Are the current dietary guidelines regarding egg consumption appropriate? J Nutr 2004;134:187–190.

46. Herron KL, Lofgren IE, Sharman M, Volek JS, Fernandez ML. High intake of cholesterol results in less atherogenic low-density lipoprotein particles in men and women independent of response classification. Metabolism 2004; 53:823–830.

47. Howel WM, Calder PC, Grimble RF. Gene polymorphisms, inflammatory diseases and cancer. Proc Nutr Soc 2002;61:447–456.

48. Igarashi AI, Kikuchi S, Konno S, Olmarker K. Inflammatory cytokines released from the facet joint tissue in degenerative lumbar spinal disorders. Spine 2004;29:2091–2095.

49. Isomaa B. A major health hazard: the metabolic syndrome. Life Sci 2003;73:2395–2411.

50. James MJ, Gibson RA, Cleland LG. Dietary polyunsaturated fatty acids and inflammatory mediator production. Am J Clin Nutr. 2000; 71(1 Suppl): 343S–348S.

51. Kao WH, Folsom AR, Nieto FJ, Mo JP, Watson RL, Brancatti FL. Serum and dietary magnesium and risk for type 2 diabetes mellitus: The Atherosclerosis Risk in Communities Study. Arch Intern Med 1999;159:2151–2159.

52. Knochel JP. Correlates of potassium exchange. In Seldin DW, Giebisch G. Eds. The regulation of potassium balance. New York: Raven Press, 1989: 31–55.

53. Knochel JP. Clinical expression of potassium disturbances. In Seldin DW, Giebisch G, eds. The regulation of potassium balance. New York: Raven Press, 1989:207–240.

54. Knopp RH, Retzlaff BM. Saturated fat prevents coronary artery disease? An American paradox. Am J Clin Nutr 2004;80:1102–1103.

55. Korhonen T, Karppinen J, Malmivaara A, et al. Efficacy of infliximab for disc herniation-induced sciatica: one-year follow-up. Spine 2004;29:2115–2119.

56. Krauss RM. Atherogenic lipoprotein phenotype and diet-gene interactions. J Nutr 2001;131:340S–343S.

57. Kremer JM. n-3 fatty acid supplements in rheumatoid arthritis. Am J Clin Nutr 2000;71(1 Suppl): 349S–351S.

58. Kushner I. C-reactive protein elevation can be caused by conditions other than inflammation and may reflect biologic aging. Cleve Clin J Med 2001;68:535–537.

59. Liese AD, Roach AK, Sparks KC, Marquart L, D'Agostino RB, Mayer-Davis EJ. Whole-grain intake and insulin sensitivity: the Insulin Resistance Atherosclerosis Study. Am J Clin Nutr 2003;78:965–971.

60. Lim GP, Chu T, Yang F, et al. The curry spice curcumin reduces oxidative damage and amyloid pathology in an Alzheimer transgenic mouse. J Neurosci 2001;21:8370–8377.

61. Linnane AW, Zhang C, Yarovaya N, et al. Human aging and global function of coenzyme Q10. Ann NY Acad Sci 2002;959:396–411.

62. Linos A, Kaklamani VG, Kaklamani E, et al. Dietary factors in relation to rheumatoid arthritis: a role for olive oil and cooked vegetables? Am J Clin Nutr 1999;70:1077–1082.

63. Liu J, Atamna H, Kuratsune H, Ames BN. Delaying Brain Mitochondrial Decay and Aging with Mitochondrial Antioxidants and Metabolites. Ann NY Acad Sci 2002;959:133–166.

64. Lopez-Ridaura R, Willett WC, Rimm EB, Liu S, Stampfer MJ, Manson JE, Hu FB. Magnesium intake and risk of type 2 diabetes in men and women. Diabetes Care 2004;27:134–140.

65. Maguire LS, O'Sullivan SM, Galvin K, O'Connor TP, O'Brien NM. Fatty acid profile, tocopherol, squalene and phytosterol content of walnuts, almonds, peanuts, hazelnuts and the macadamia nut. Int J Food Sci Nutr 2004;55:171–178.

66. Makowski L, Hotamisligil GS. Fatty acid binding proteins—the evolutionary crossroads of inflammatory and metabolic responses. J Nutr 2004;134:24s64S–24s68S.

67. Mathias JR, Franklin R, Quast DC, et al. Relation of endometriosis and neuromuscular disease of the gastrointestinal tract: new insights. Fertil Steril 1998;70:81–88.

68. Mattson MP. Modification of brain aging neurodegenerative disorders by genes, diet, and behavior. Physiol Rev 2002;82:637–672.

69. McKay DL, Perrone G, Rasmussen H, et al. The effects of a multivitamin/mineral supplement on micronutrient status, antioxidant capacity and cytokine production in healthy older adults consuming a fortified diet. J Am Coll Nutr 2000;19:613–621.

70. Mense S, Simmons DG. Muscle pain: understanding its nature, diagnosis and treatment. Philadelphia: Lippincott Williams & Wilkins, 2001:26–30.

71. Mozaffarian D, Pischon T, Hankinson SE, et al. Dietary intake of trans fatty acids and systemic inflammation in women. Am J Clin Nutr 2004; 79:606–612.

72. Mozaffarian D, Rimm EB, King IB, Lawler RL, McDonald GB, Levy WC. Trans fatty acids and systemic inflammation in heart failure. Am J Clin Nutr 2004;80:1521–1525.

73. National Research Council. Recommended dietary allowances, 10th ed. Washington: National Academy Press, 1989:255.

74. O'Keefe JH Jr, Cordain L. Cardiovascular disease resulting from a diet and lifestyle at odds with our Paleolithic genome: how to become a 21st-century hunter-gatherer. Mayo Clin Proc 2004;79:101–108.

75. Otsuka M, Yamaguchi K, Ueki A. Similarities and differences between Alzheimer's disease and vascular dementia from the viewpoint of nutrition. NY Acad Sci. 2002;977:155–161.

76. Pereira MA, Jacobs DR, Pins JJ, et al. Effect of whole grains on insulin sensitivity in overweight hyperinsulinemic adults. Am J Clin Nutr 2002; 75:848–855.

77. Pfeilschifter J, Köditz R, Pfohl M, Schatz H. Changes in proinflammatory cytokine activity after menopause. Endocrine Rev 2002;23:90–119.

78. Pickup JC. Inflammation and activated innate immunity in the pathogenesis of type 2 diabetes. Diabetes Care 2004;27:813–823.

79. Preuss HG, Bagchi D, Bagchi M. Protective effects of a novel niacin-bound chromium complex and a grape seed proanthocyanidin extract on advancing age and various aspects of syndrome X. Ann N Y Acad Sci 2002; 957:250–259.

80. Raisz LG. Physiology and pathophysiology of bone remodeling. Clin Chem 1999;45(8 Pt 2):1353–1358.

81. Rang HP, Bevan S, Dray A. Nociceptive peripheral neurons: cellular properties. In: Wall PD, Melzack R, eds. New York: Churchill Livingstone, 1994:57–78.

82. Reginster JY, Deroisy R, Rovati LC, et al. Long-term effects of glucosamine sulphate on osteoarthritis progression: a randomized, placebo-controlled clinical trial. Lancet 2001;357:251–256.

83. Ros E. Dietary cis-monounsaturated fatty acids and metabolic control in type 2 diabetes. Am J Clin Nutr 2003;78:617S–625S.

84. Ross R. Atherosclerosis—an inflammatory disease. N Engl J Med 1999;340:115–126.

85. Rude RK. Magnesium deficiency: a cause of heterogenous disease in humans. J Bone Min Res 1998;13:749–758.

86. Sabate J. Nut consumption and body weight. Am J Clin Nutr 2003;78(3 Suppl):647S–650S.

87. Sabate J, Haddad E, Tanzman JS, Jambazian P, Rajaram S. Serum lipid response to the graduated enrichment of a Step I diet with almonds: a randomized feeding trial. Am J Clin Nutr 2003; 77: 1379–1384.

88. Sadeghi S, Wallace FA, Calder PC. Dietary lipids modify the cytokine response to bacterial lipopolysaccharide in mice. Immunology 1999;96:404–410.

89. Saris NEL, et al. Magnesium: an update on physiological, clinical and analytical aspects. Clin Chim Acta 2000;294:1–26.

90. Seaman DR, Faye LJ. The subluxation complex. In: Gatterman MI, ed. Foundations of chiropractic: subluxation. 2nd ed. St. Louis: Elsevier 2005: p. 195–226.

91. Seaman DR, Cleveland C. Spinal pain syndromes: nociceptive, neuropathic, and psychologic mechanisms. J Manip Physiol Ther 1999; 22:458–472.

92. Seaman DR. The diet-induced proinflammatory state: a cause of chronic pain and other degenerative diseases? J Manipulative Physiol Ther 2002; 25:168–179.

93. Sebastian A, Frassetto LA, Sellmeyer DE, Merriam RL, Morris RC Jr. Estimation of the net acid load of the diet of ancestral preagricultural Homo sapiens and their hominid ancestors. Am J Clin Nutr 2002; 76:1308–1316.

94. Shacter E, Weitzman SA. Chronic inflammation and cancer. Oncology 2002;16:217–226, 229.

95. Simopoulos AP. Essential fatty acids in health and chronic disease. Am J Clin Nutr 1999;70(3 Suppl):560S–569S.

96. Simopoulos AP. Omega-3 fatty acids in inflammation and autoimmune diseases. J Am Coll Nutr 2002; 21:495–505.

97. Sinaii N, Cleary SD, Ballweg ML, Nieman LK, Stratton P. High rates of autoimmune and endocrine disorders, fibromyalgia, chronic fatigue syndrome and atopic diseases among women with endometriosis: a survey analysis. Hum Reprod 2002;17:2715–2724.

98. Skoldstam L, Hagfors L, Johansson G. An experimental study of a Mediterranean diet intervention for patients with rheumatoid arthritis. Ann Rheum Dis 2003;62:208–214.

99. Srivastava KC, Mustafa T. Ginger (Zingiber officinale) in rheumatism and musculoskeletal disorders. Med Hypotheses 1992;39:342–348.

100. Sueter PM. Potassium and hypertension. Nutr Rev 1998;56:151–153.

101. Tobian L. High potassium diets reduce stokes mortality and arterial and renal tubular lesions and sometimes even the blood pressure in hypertension. In: Seldin DW, Giebisch G, eds. The regulation of potassium balance. New York: Raven Press, 1989:347–368.

102. Visioli F, Galli C. The role of antioxidants in the Mediterranean diet. Lipids 2001;36:S49–S52.

103. Walford RL, Mock D, Verdery R, MacCallum T. Calorie restriction in biosphere 2: alterations in physiologic, hematologic, hormonal, and biochemical parameters in humans restricted for a 2-year period. J Gerontol A Biol Sci Med Sci. 2002;57: B211–B224.

104. Watkins BA, Li Y, Lippman HE, Seifert MF. Omega-3 polyunsaturated fatty acids and skeletal health. Exp Biol Med 2001;226:485–497.

105. Wilson PW, Grundy SM. The metabolic syndrome: practical guide to origins and treatment: Part I. Circulation 2003;108:1422–1424.

106. Yasuma T, Arai K, Suzuki F. Age-related phenomena in the lumbar intervertebral discs: lipofuscin and amyloid deposition. Spine 1992;17:1194–1198.

107. Young DB, Lin H, McCabe RD. Potassium's cardiovascular protective mechanisms. Am J Physiol 1995;268:R825–R837.

31

A Cognitive Behavioral Therapy Program for Spinal Pain

Steven J. Linton

Learning Objectives

After reading this chapter, you should be able to understand:

- How psychological factors can interfere with recovery from acute spinal pain syndromes
- How cognitions, emotions, and behaviors influence self-management
- How a series of cognitive–behavioral classes can be used with patients with chronic pain

Introduction

This chapter deals with early interventions that may prevent the development of long-term work disability caused by back pain problems. Although psychological factors are known to be related to the development of chronic pain, the implementation of an approach that includes such factors has been hampered by a lack of clearly described programs. Among the successful psychological approaches to pain is cognitive–behaviorally oriented interventions (7,14,24). However, the cognitive behavioral approach does not refer to one specific intervention, but rather to a class of intervention strategies. These may vary considerably and include methods to engage clients (e.g., goal setting, motivational interviewing), relaxation (e.g., applied relaxation), cognitive restructuring, fear reduction, coping strategies, activity training (e.g., graded activity), stress management, problem solving, and assertiveness training. Furthermore, because many health care professionals have limited education in psychology, the details of how and why these interventions are used may be unclear. As a result, the purpose of this chapter is to describe a cognitive–behavioral group intervention program designed for early implementation.

There is good reason to consider a cognitive–behavioral approach for patients at risk for long-term disability. Basically, if psychological variables catalyze the development of persistent disability, then using cognitive behavioral interventions is logical and should have great value. In fact, such programs have demonstrated their value in treating chronic back pain problems (24,33). Through the years, it has become apparent that early interventions might be more effective and actually prevent persistent disability from developing. The setting has varied, but these programs are often used in conjunction with other treatments, including manipulation and physical therapy.

Let us briefly examine some programs to underscore their potential as well as the variety of content. In one program, van den Hout and associates (32) studied the effects of teaching problem-solving skills to participants off work less than 6 months for back pain. Subjects were randomized to a group receiving graded activity training and education or to a group receiving graded activity and problem-solving. The long-term results indicated that those receiving problem-solving skills training were significantly more successful at returning to work. This indicates, then, that the specific technique of problem solving was quite helpful in preventing long-term disability. Using a similar design, Marhold and co-workers (23) examined the effects of teaching specific return-to-work skills. They reasoned that one problem for those off work might be a lack of skills concerning how to actually return to work. Participants off work an average of 3 months were randomized to a treatment as usual control group or a cognitive–behavioral group that included specific return-to-work skills training such as making contact with the employer, overcoming barriers, and coping with anticipated increased pain. Results demonstrated that participants in the CBT program had significantly less absenteeism at the 1-year follow-up than did the treatment as usual control group.

Although most programs are limited to one facility, a community-based program designed to prevent pain disability has recently been tested in Canada (29). Here again, the intervention is specific to certain risk factors. In fact, individuals were selected for treatment if they were off work for back pain and had elevated scores on risk factors addressed by the intervention program. The program systematically works with goal-directed activity training and in minimizing psychological barriers to return to work. This program specifically focuses on reducing catastrophizing, fear, and avoidance. Although the study did not have a randomized design, the results were encouraging because 65% returned to work as compared to an 18% base rate of return.

In a primary care setting, von Korff and associates (37) screened back pain patients approximately 2 months after their visit for functional difficulties. Those with significant functional problems were randomized into a control group versus a group receiving early activation and efforts to reduce fear. Although there were no differences between the groups at the follow-up on disability compensation benefits, the intervention group was more active and had less functional disability.

In our own work, we have used a cognitive behavior group therapy as secondary prevention and evaluated it in several studies (18,22,23). In the most recent evaluation, we selected participants with short-term back pain in a primary care setting who had "at risk" profiles on a screening instrument and then provided the cognitive–behavioral group intervention designed to address these risk factors (20). These participants (n=185) were randomly assignment to either a standardized, guideline-based, treatment as usual, or to a cognitive–behavioral group (alone), or to the combination of a cognitive–behavioral group and physical therapy (assessment plus exercise). The results showed that for work absenteeism, the two groups receiving cognitive–behavioral interventions had fewer days off work for back pain during the 12-month follow-up than did the guideline-based treatment as the usual group. The risk for developing long-term sick disability leave was more than five-fold higher in the guideline-based treatment as usual group than the other two groups receiving the cognitive–behavioral intervention. Thus, there is some evidence that using a psychologically oriented intervention may help prevent future disability.

Because few lucid descriptions of cognitive–behavioral interventions for early prevention exist, let us now turn to a more detailed description of the cognitive behavioral group intervention. The description begins with a closer look at the psychological risk factors that such interventions are designed to deal with. This is important, because the intervention is only provided for patients with relatively high levels of psychological risk factors. That is, it is offered to patients "at risk" for disability.

Psychological Risk Factors Deserve Psychological Interventions

Psychological factors are powerful risk factors linked to the development of persistent disability (see Chapter 9). Even though psychological factors are often found to be potent risk factors, most treatments offered to patients early on are nevertheless medical in nature. Consequently, patients displaying such psychological risk factors seem to deserve an intervention that addresses these. Let us examine this idea more closely.

Although many factors may be related to the development of disability, psychological factors appear to be particularly relevant. Other chapters in this book cogently show that a host of factors are related to the development of persistent pain and disability. These involve medical or biological factors, such as ischias pain, and sensitization, in addition to previous history of treatment (25). Furthermore, the work environment is important in terms of physical work (34,35) and in terms of psychosocial factors such as stress, control, and demands (8,15). Social factors akin to educational level, income, race, and family situation are complex, but certainly may also influence the development of a pain problem (25,30). However, psychological factors have been found to have a clear relationship to the development of persistent pain (5,6,13,26,27,28). Moreover, psychological factors are integrally related to the transition from acute to chronic pain (16). Thus, psychological factors seem to be of great importance for the understanding of the development of chronic disability.

There is considerable logic in providing psychologically oriented interventions for a problem characterized by psychological aspects. For example, providing a psychological intervention would help to match the treatment to the patient's unique needs. Further, the identification of psychological factors might provide guides for defining intervention targets and barriers to recovery. Finally, the identification of psychological factors might also enhance the development of interventions by providing insight into the mechanisms that are maintaining the problem. For example, if depressed mood were identified, appropriate measures might be taken.

Although it would seem logical to use psychologically oriented interventions, this seldom happens in the current health care system (see Chapter 4). For a variety of reasons, most health care units fail to identify psychosocial factors let alone implement an early psychologically oriented intervention (1). Consider the fact that although psychological factors are often present, it is still common to only provide medical treatments (36). This appears to be related to an approach of providing "more of the same" if a treatment is not successful. In other words, as the problem progresses toward chronic disability, there is a tendency to prescribe more of the same therapies tried early on. Consequently, the "dose" of the treatment is increased rather than viewing the progression as a risk situation that needs to be tackled in an alternative way. However, if psychological factors are catalyzing the problem toward chronicity, these treatments may be ineffective because they do not address the problem. Unfortunately, before the clinician realizes that this "normal" treatment is not successful, the problem may well be on the way to a persistent disability. To be successful, then, changes in the system of health care may need to be taken to implement an alternative that can address psychological aspects of the problem.

Determining Risk

The CBT program is designed to help patients with back pain who are at risk for persistent disability, but how might this risk be determined in the clinic? Fortunately, a number of screening instruments to assess yellow flags exist (31) (see Chapter 9). We developed the Örebro Musculoskeletal Pain Screening Questionnaire as a tool for clinicians in the early identification of problem cases (2,21,18). It is used as a tool to help determine proper candidates who would be likely to benefit from the CBT program. Thus, it is a clinical instrument designed to complement medical examinations and provide information concerning the likelihood that a patient will have disability develop. It consists of 25 items focusing on psychological factors. It provides information about various aspects of the problem including fear–avoidance beliefs, function, experienced pain, beliefs about the future, stress, mood, work, and coping. The items contain statements or assertions that patients rate on

0- to 10-point Likert scales. This instrument is self-administered and most patients complete it within 7 or 8 minutes. A trained health care provider can score and evaluate it in a few minutes. The questionnaire provides an overall score from which risk may be approximately judged as well as ratings on each item. The latter may be used in discussing and communicating with the patient. Several studies have shown that this questionnaire is reliable and valid (2,4,9,10,19,21). Those at risk may be invited to participate in an intervention that focuses on these risk factors such as the CBT group intervention.

The Cognitive-Behavioral (CBT) Group Intervention

To provide an early, secondary preventive intervention, a program was developed in our clinic that builds on experiences from programs provided for chronic pain patients (3,14,24,33). However, we paid close attention to the risk factors identified in the screening assessment described. As a result, the content focuses on the prevention of persistent pain and disability and not simply pain treatment. The intervention is provided in groups of 6 to 10 people and encompasses six 2-hour sessions.

The CBT intervention is geared to help each participant develop her/his own coping program. We ask participants to learn, and apply, all the skills presented during the course so that a tailored program that bests suits each person's needs is developed. Naturally, from a provider's point of view, we hope to prevent pain related disability, the need for health care services, as well as to improve quality of life. Because back pain is recurrent in nature, we do not attempt to eliminate all back pain but rather to decrease recurrences and reduce their impact.

Sessions are organized to activate participants and promote coping. Each session begins with a short review of homework assignments. Subsequently, the therapist introduces the topic for the session and provides information for a maximum of 15 minutes. Issues concerning how one might control pain intensity, participate in activities, or problems encountered with work or leisure are examples of topics. Participants work with a case description in which they are asked to solve problems concerning the case. This allows participants to analyze the "case" and compare it with their own situation. Solutions are presented in the group and discussed. Subsequently, the therapist introduces new coping skills and participants practice them. These included pain control measures such as relaxation and distraction. However, most skills are oriented toward activity and function. These range from problem solving skills and graded activity to social and stress management skills. Homework assignments are then made and these are tailored to the participant's needs. Every participant is asked to apply all of the skills learned in their everyday life to evaluate their use. Finally, the session is reviewed, underscoring what the participants have learned and strengths and weaknesses of the session are discussed. During the course of the group meeting, participants develop their own personal coping program based on the techniques they believed are most effective for their problem.

Strategies for Behavioral Change

Changing cognitions, emotions, and behaviors are central to self-management, but how might this be achieved? Our CBT course is designed to help participants actively alter current cognitions and behaviors. For example, beliefs about the relationship between pain and activity ("The more I do, the more it will hurt") or beliefs about stress ("I must do everything asked of me and exactly on time") may need to be revised. Likewise, behaviors may need to be changed, e.g., increasing activity levels or being able to say "no" to certain demands. Our program uses several strategies to promote such changes.

First, the program engages the participant. Learning by doing is emphasized. Therefore, much of the session consists of practicing new skills and working with the cognitions and emotions surrounding them. Even for discussions, *every* participant is asked individually to provide input. Above all, each person is given the mission of developing his or her personal coping program. Second, restricted amounts of information are used to prime behavioral changes. Thus, this part of the session is used to model appropriate behaviors as well as to challenge common beliefs. A third strategy is behavioral tests. For patients we conceptualize this as learning through experience. Thus, we ask patients to "test" each skill they learn to assess its possible value for them. This is one basis participants use for the selection of skills to be included in their personal coping program.

Problem solving is a fourth strategy. This skill is honed in a special problem-based learning module, and it is used whenever patients describe a "problem" or hindrance. Fifth, the group leader is taught to shape new thoughts and behaviors by reinforcing successive approximations of good coping behavior. Positive reinforcement such as in the form of encouragement is contingently provided when participants correctly approximate a goal behavior. Thus, gradual change is encouraged.

A sixth method is to enhance each patient's self-efficacy, that is, the patient's belief that he/she can impact on the pain and its course. This is a logical goal because many patients have low self-efficacy levels and do not believe that they can change their health behavior. For example, we might ask a person who has successfully completed a homework assignment (e.g., practiced relaxation and decreased pain) to tell the entire group how he/she has accomplished this, to share the "secret" of their success.

Finally, enjoyment is used to enhance learning, engagement, maintenance, and pleasure. It is an important strategy to ensure that every participant feels good about his/her accomplishments. People should have the opportunity to laugh and to receive social support. Thus, encouragement is contingently delivered in a rich schedule and humor is used to provide a good learning atmosphere.

Organization of the Sessions

The intervention encompasses a six-session structured program in which participants meet in groups of 6 to 10 people, six times, once per week for 2 hours. A manual guides therapy to standardize the intervention (12). Therapists to date have had previous training in behavior therapy and in addition they have received special training in administering this intervention.

In turn, each session has several parts. First, an introduction to the session is provided lasting approximately 15 minutes. During the first session, this deals mainly with helping participants feel comfortable and getting to know one another. Information about the course is provided. For the remaining ses-

sions, this time is used to set the tone for the session as well as to review homework. Next, a short presentation (maximum 15 minutes) is given by the therapist to introduce the topic of the session and to provide modern scientific facts. The third part of the session is problem-solving (30 minutes), in which pairs solve problems from a case study. Fourth, skills training is provided (30 minutes) to give participants the opportunity to learn or improve on their coping skills. Homework assignments are discussed and the session is evaluated during the final 15 minutes of the session.

Each session focuses on a particular area of relevance and participants develop a personal coping program; an overview is provided in Table 31.1. The first session deals with the causes of back pain and how it might be prevented from becoming a chronic, disabling problem. The role of structural and soft tissue injuries in relation to activity is stressed. In particular, the difference between "hurt" and "harm" is brought forth in the lecture. Further, the consequences of pain are described and the fact that some will have persistent problems. A model is presented in which gradual lifestyle changes are underscored and the role of work, family, and psychological factors are mentioned. Thus, it becomes clear that prevention is a very worthwhile endeavor. The problem-solving focuses on why the individual in the case study has chronic pain and what could have been done to prevent it. The skills for the session include problem-solving and pain control, including cognitive and applied relaxation skills.

The subsequent sessions deal with activities, self-care, work, and leisure. The sessions share basic

Table 31.1 An Overview of the Content of the CBT Intervention

Session	Focus	Skills
1.	Causes of pain and the prevention of chronic problems	Problem-solving, applied relaxation, learning, pain
2.	Managing your pain	Activities, maintain daily routines, scheduling activities, relaxation training
3.	Promoting good health, controlling stress at home and at work	Warning signals, cognitive appraisal, beliefs
4.	Adapting for leisure and work	Communication skills, assertiveness, risk situations, applying relaxation
5.	Controlling flare-ups	Plan for coping with flare-up, coping skills review, applied relaxation, developing own coping program
6.	Maintaining and improving results	Risk analysis, plan for adherence, own program finalized

aspects. First, participant's cognitive beliefs are challenged through the problem-solving case study and in discussion. Second, alternate ways of thinking (e.g., self-statements) and behavioral skills are taught as possible ways of coping better. Third, the new cognitive–behavioral skill is tested in real life through homework assignments. In this way, a wide variety of common beliefs and behaviors may be dealt with in a group format.

The task of planning a coping program begins in session five. In addition, the session includes planning for eventual flare-ups. Consequently, a focus is on application of the skills over time. Participants work on developing their coping program with a special section on dealing with a flare-up. The final session is used to fine-tune the coping program and deal with long-term maintenance. We discuss adherence to the program from a self-help point of view where conscious decision is underscored. In essence, we challenge patients to make their own decisions about the content of their coping program, even in the future. To promote this, we encourage participants to make active decisions rather than waking up to the fact that the program has changed. Therefore, reviews are planned and scheduled so individuals will review their own program and decide on possible changes.

In session six, the final coping plan is reviewed and the focus turns to maintaining the plan over time. Rather than prodding participants a self-determination approach is used. As participants have chosen the content of their coping package, they are also given charge of maintenance. Work centers on making planned changes only in the program. Thus, if an element of the program does not seem to be working, then it could be eliminated from the program. Likewise, in some situations, such as flare-ups, more coping strategies may be needed and thus could be added to the program. However, having a part of the program inadvertently disappear is not good because this would not be a conscious choice. As a result, a key is to periodically make a progress check. To enhance this process, participants book progress checks into their calendar. This check only takes a few minutes and basically is a review of how well the program is working. It is concluded with a decision as to whether the program should be changed in any way or be continued as is. Again, the rule is planned changes only. To assist in identifying factors that may be beneficial to or hinders doing the coping program as planned, participants also complete an adherence roadmap (11). Participants liken their future to a car trip, in which one destination is relapse and the other is success. Thus, they try to identify "the road" to each of these. The identified factors may then be used in developing the maintenance plan for the coping program.

A follow-up session may be scheduled. Some groups also may choose to meet on their own periodically.

Potential Problems

Although the system described here offers many advantages, there are also potential problems. The methods reviewed here are very recent and considerable research is needed to develop and assess their effectiveness. Perhaps the most frequent problem is that the program in a sense goes "against the grain" of the medical model and is therefore difficult for staff to administer without training. Training should not be underestimated because it takes time and effort to understand why the methods should work as well as to hone the skills. Consequently, it is advantages to work in teams, e.g., with a doctor, chiropractor, physical therapist, and psychologist. In this way, efforts may be coordinated and training may be incorporated into clinical practice.

Related to training, is the problem of inadvertently reinforcing "sick behavior." By focusing on screening and early intervention, personnel might actually reinforce concern and inappropriate behaviors. If this happens, the overall results would be worse than treatment as usual. Thus, it is important to practice interactions with patients in training settings to ensure that the program is administered properly.

Another potential difficulty is the logistics of delivering the program in health care settings such as a chiropractic practice. Many such units do not have psychologists and the amount of time afforded each patient is limited. The procedure in this chapter is designed to fit into routines for providing these patients medical care. In part, the problem may involve "beliefs" concerning the psychological nature of the program. This may create a bias in which a variety of factors are said to prevent implementation such as costs, and the time involved. Consider, however, that a new chiropractic or medical treatment procedure that relieved back pain might well be incorporated even if some costs and time were involved in administering it. While planning and time are necessary for the proper administration of the cognitive–behavioral program, most patients will not be at risk and contacts may be developed for obtaining qualified group leaders. Thus, only a minority of the patients will have screening profiles that dictate more consideration. And, of those with a "risk" profile, only a limited number will be candidates for an early intervention. Consequently, the time and resources needed for the program are limited.

The potential for incorrectly classifying the risk of patients may generate concern. The screening procedure is relatively crude and both false-negatives and false-positives will undoubtedly be generated. Although the goal of future research is to reduce the number of these, such "errors" are present in virtually all tests including biological ones. Fortunately, the consequences of such a mistake should not be particularly large. First, if a false-negative is identified and the problem does not remit, the patient will seek additional care and this should trigger a warning flag to reassess the situation. Some time is lost, but there should still be ample opportunity to deal with prevention. Certainly, applying the program may be an improvement on the current situation in which patients may not be identified until the problem is chronic. Second, if a false-positive is identified and early intervention is given to someone who would have recovered anyway, the prevention may still be of some value. Because back pain is recurrent, the person may in fact nevertheless have been on his/her way to developing a persistent problem even if the current episode would have resolved. Moreover, the intervention suggested in this chapter focuses on coping skills that presumably are of value even if the problem is not dire. Finally, by adjusting the cut-off level, the number of "misses" may be adjusted. Thus, although we need to improve accuracy, the consequences of mistakes do not seem to be large. One scenario is that extra costs are incurred by providing the intervention to someone not truly in need of it.

A final potential problem is the coordination of the program between different professionals. Chiropractors, doctors, nurses, physical therapists, psychologists, and other health care professionals may be involved. This is, again, why working in a team may have advantages. The team may initiate the program with special training that identifies roles for each member and teaches skills. Periodic meetings allows for monitoring and adjustment of the program. It also provides an opportunity for continuing education in that special cases may be brought up for discussion.

working toward prevention. Good clinical practice skills combined with excellent communication skills will be very helpful in meeting patients with an early back pain problem. Having a clear conception of the problem including the medical and also the psychosocial consequences of the problem will also be valuable for developing clear goals and engaging the patient in treatment. For certain patients, however, chronic disability gradually develops and becomes a problem in itself. To prevent this, there is a need to assess the psychological risk factors early on to get a sense of the level of risk. Fortunately, most patients will have relatively low levels of these factors. However, for those "at risk," adding psychologically oriented interventions early on can be helpful as a preventive tool. A description of a particular cognitive–behavioral program has been provided here. It provides in-depth information that is helpful in developing such a program and also in evaluating potential programs that you may wish to refer patients to or coordinate treatment with. Adding such a psychological perspective to a chiropractic practice may prove to be challenging, exciting, and above all may provide better care for your patients.

Audit Process
Self-Check of the Chapter's Learning Objectives

- What psychological factors are proven to be related to the transition from acute to chronic pain?

- What specific cognitions, emotions, and behaviors should be addressed clinically in a cognitive–behavioral program?

- Can the components of cognitive–behavioral classes be incorporated into single clinician encounters with chronic pain patients?

- How are pain flare-ups addressed from a cognitive–behavioral perspective?

■ CONCLUSION

This chapter has described a cognitive–behavioral group intervention that may be useful in preventing the development of chronic disability for selected back pain patients. This intervention is not magical. However, there is mounting evidence that psychological factors may catalyze the development of chronic disability. Given that back pain patients often seek the care of chiropractors, these professions are in an excellent position to engage the patient into

■ REFERENCES

1. Armstrong MP, McDonough S, Baxter G. Clinical guidelines versus clinical practice in the management of low back pain. Int J Clin Practice 2003; 57(1):9–13.

2. Boersma K, Linton SJ. Early assessment of psychological factors: The Örebro Screening Questionnaire for Pain. In: Linton SJ, ed. New avenues for the prevention of pain, vol. 1. Amsterdam: Elsevier, 2002:205–213.

3. Compas BE, Haaga D, Keefe AF, Leitenberg H, Williams DA. A sampling of empirically supported

psychological treatments from health psychology: Smoking, chronic pain, cancer, and bulimia nervosa. J Consult Clin Psychol 1998;66: 89–112.

4. Ektor-Andersen J, Örbaek P, Ingvarsson E, Kullendorff M. Prediction of vocational dysfunction due to musculoskeletal symptoms by screening for psychosocial factors at the social insurance office. Paper presented at the 10th World Congress on Pain, San Diego, CA, 2002.

5. Gatchel RJ. Psychological disorders and chronic pain: Cause and effect relationships. In: Gatchel RJ, Turk DC, eds. Psychological approaches to pain management: A practitioner's handbook, vol. 1. New York: Guilford Press, 1996:33–54.

6. Gatchel RJ, Polatin PB, Kinney RK. Predicting outcome of chronic back pain using clinical predictors of psychopathology: a prospective analysis. Health Psychol 1995;14(5):415–420.

7. Gatchel RJ, Turk DC. Psychosocial factors in pain: Critical perspectives. New York: Guilford Publications, Inc, 1999.

8. Hoogendoorn WE., van Poppel MNM, Bongers PM, Koes BW, Bouter LM. (2000). Systematic review of psychosocial factors at work and in the personal situation as risk factors for back pain. *Spine, 2000;25(16)*, 2114–2125.

9. Hurley D, Dusoir T, McDonough S, Moore A, Baxter G. How effective is the Acute Low Back Pain Screening Questionnaire for predicting 1-year follow-up in patients with low back pain? Clin J Pain 2001;17: 256–263.

10. Hurley D, Dusoir T, McDonough S, Moore A, Linton SJ, Baxter G. Biopsychosocial screening questionnaire for patients with low back pain: Preliminary report of utility in physiotherapy practice in Northern Ireland. Clin J Pain 2000;16(3), 214–228.

11. Keefe FJ, Beaupré PM, Gil KM. Group therapy for patients with chronic pain. In: Gatchel RJ, Turk DC, eds. Psychological approaches to pain management: A practitioner's handbook, vol. I. New York: Guilford Press, 1996:259–282.

12. Linton S J. Cognitive-behavioral therapy in the early treatment and prevention of chronic pain: A therapist's manual for groups. Örebro Sweden: Department of Occupational and Environmental Medicine, 2000.

13. Linton SJ. Psychologic risk factors for neck and back pain. In: Nachemsom A, Jonsson E, eds. Neck and back pain: The scientific evidence of causes, diagnosis, and treatment. Philadelphia: Lippincott Williams & Wilkins, 2000:57–78.

14. Linton SJ. Utility of cognitive-behavioral psychological treatments. In: Nachemson A, Jonsson E, eds. Neck and back pain: The scientific evidence of causes, diagnosis, and treatment. Philadelphia: Lippincott Williams & Wilkins, 2000:361–381.

15. Linton S J. Occupational psychological factors increase the risk for back pain: A systematic review. J Occup Rehab 2001;11(1), 53–66.

16. Linton SJ. Why does chronic pain develop? A behavioral approach. In: Linton SJ, ed. New avenues for the prevention of chronic musculoskeletal pain and disability. Amsterdam: Elsevier Science, 2002:67–82.

17. Linton SJ. Understanding pain for better clinical practice: A psychological perspective. London: Elsevier, 2005.

18. Linton SJ, Andersson T. Can chronic disability be prevented? A randomized trial of a cognitive-behavior intervention and two forms of information for patients with spinal pain. Spine 2000;25(21): 2825–2831.

19. Linton SJ, Boersma K. Early identification of patients at risk of developing a persistent back problem: The predictive validity of the Örebro Musculoskeletal Pain Questionnaire. Clin J Pain 2003;19:80–86.

20. Linton SJ, Boersma K, Jansson M, Svärd L, Botvalde M. The effects of cognitive-behavioral and physical therapy preventive interventions on pain related sick leave: A randomized controlled trial. Clin J Pain (Accepted for publication).

21. Linton SJ, Halldén K. Can we screen for problematic back pain? A screening questionnaire for predicting outcome in acute and subacute back pain. Clin J Pain 1998;14(3):209–215.

22. Linton SJ, Ryberg M. A cognitive-behavioral group intervention as prevention for persistent neck and back pain in a non-patient population: A randomized controlled trial. Pain 2001;90:83–90.

23. Marhold C, Linton SJ, Melin L. Cognitive behavioral return-to-work program: effects on pain patients with a history of long-term versus short-term sick leave. Pain 2001;91:155–163.

24. Morley S, Eccleston C, Williams A. Systematic review and meta-analysis of randomized controlled trials of cognitive behavior therapy and behavior therapy for chronic pain in adults, excluding headache. Pain 1999;80(1–2):1–13.

25. Nachemson A, Jonsson E. Neck and back pain: The scientific evidence of causes, diagnosis, and treatment. Philadelphia: Lippincott Williams & Wilkins, 2000.

26. Pincus T, Burton AK, Vogel S, Field AP. A systematic review of psychological factors as predictors of chronicity/disability in prospective cohorts of low back pain. Spine 2002;27(5):E109.120.

27. Pulliam CB, Gatchel RJ. Employing risk factors for screening of chronic pain disability. In: Linton SJ, ed. New avenues for the prevention of chronic musculoskeletal pain and disability. Amsterdam: Elsevier Science, 2002:183–204.

28. Schultz IZ, Crook JM, Berkowitz J, Meloche GR, Milner R, Zuberbier OA, et al. Biopsychosocial multivariate predictive model of occupational low back disability. Spine 2002;27(23):2720–2725.

29. Sullivan MJL, Stanish WD. Psychologically based occupational rehabilitation: The Pain-Disability Prevention program. Clin J Pain 2003;19:97–104.

30. Waddell G, Aylward M, Sawney P. *Back pain, incapacity for work and social security benefits: An international literature review and analysis.* London: The Royal Society of Medicine Press, 2002.

31. Waddell G, Burton AK, Main CJ. Screening to identify people at risk of long-term incapacity for work: A conceptual and scientific review. London: Royal Society of Medicine Press, 2003.

32. van den Hout JHC, Vlaeyen JWS, Heuts PH, Zijlema JHL, Wijnen JA. Secondary prevention of work-related disability in nonspecific low back pain: Does problem-solving therapy help? A randomized clinical trial. Clin J Pain 2003;19(2):87–96.

33. van Tulder MW, Ostelo R, Vlaeyen JWS, Linton SJ, Morely SJ, Assendelft WJJ. Behavioral treatment for chronic low back pain: A systematic review within the framework of the Cochrane Back Review Group. Spine 2000;25(20):2688–2699.

34. Westgaard RH, Winkel J. On occupational ergonomic risk factors for musculoskeletal disorders and related intervention practice. In: Linton SJ, ed. New avenues for the prevention of chronic musculoskeletal pain and disability, vol. 1. Amsterdam: Elsevier Science, 2002:143–164.

35. Wickström GJ, Pentti J. Occupational factors affecting sick leave attributed to low-back pain. Scand J Work Environment Health 1998;24(2):145–152.

36. Vingård E, Mortimer M, Wiktorin C, Pernold G, Fredriksson K, Németh G, et al. Seeking care for low back pain in the general population. Spine,2002;27(19):2159–2165.

37. von Korff M, Balderson BHK, Miglioretti DL, Lin EHB, Berry S, et al. A trial of an activating intervention for chronic back pain in primary care and physical therapy settings. Pain 2005;113:323–330.

Practical Application by Region

Editor's Note

This section integrates the specific assessment and treatment methods presented in the book thus far in a region-by-region look at the emergent functional reactivation model. Diagnostic triage, functional assessment, reactivation methods, and outcomes tools are relevant throughout the locomotor system. In showing how the same step-by-step process can be applied throughout the body it should bring into sharper focus the ease by which practitioners of all stripes (physical therapy, chiropractic, orthopedics, physiatry, etc.) can utilize the universal principles and methods of the functional self-management approach.

32

An Integrated Approach to Regional Disorders

Craig Liebenson

Introduction
Clinical Framework (CF)
Clinical Challenges
On Finding the "Key Link"
  The Art
Atlas of Key Tests and Exercises
"Best Practice" Keys to Recovery—The 7 Rs
Principles of Evidence-Based Neuro-Musculoskeletal Care

Learning Objectives
After reading this chapter you should be able to understand:

- The individual steps required to implement a self-management approach for spinal symptoms
- How to record relevant patient data on a patient profile
- The process of linking clinical symptoms, the diagnosed pain generator, and the actual source of biomechanical overload
- The systematic continuum of care involving palliative, sparing, stabilizing, and functional strategies

Introduction

The management of back and neck disorders has been revolutionized by recent scientific evidence. International guidelines recommend a shift from the medicalization of spine problems (medication, imaging, and surgery) to a self-management strategy. The clinical framework for how to promote this includes an emphasis on functional goals, self-care, a biopsychosocial approach, and outcome-based care.

This chapter presents a step-by-step model of care that can be applied to the majority of patients seeking care for activity limiting spinal problems. Practice tools for easing the integration of this new paradigm into daily practice are recommended. The steps outlined in this chapter are reinforced in the regional chapters that follow in this section (Chapters 34 and 35). This will guide clinicians from the initial assessment and diagnostic triage through release from care.

Clinical Framework (CF)

The Victorian WorkCover Authority in Australia has developed a training system to facilitate evidence-based practice for the management of work-related musculoskeletal disorders (42). The pillars of this Clinical Framework (CF) approach are summarized in Table 32.1.

Evidence-based practice means that practice is current with latest literature. Chapter 3 reviews many current international guidelines for management of back and neck disorders. Often, the scientific literature is very weak, so Sackett the Godfather of the evidence-based movement says, "clinical expertise should be informed but not replaced by evidence" (34). Excellent resources for the latest evidence can be found from the Cochrane Library and the National Guideline Clearinghouse (11,31).

It is important to measure the effectiveness of treatment and a patient's progress under care. An outcome-based practice must decide what to measure (Chapter 8). Treatment effectiveness can be measured with tools that are reliable, valid, and sensitive to change. The measurements chosen should be related to the patient's own functional goals. Impairments (e.g., range of motion), activities (e.g., Oswestry,

Table 32.1 The Clinical Framework

- Evidence-based
- Outcome-based
- Biopsychosocial
- Promoting self-care
- Focused on the patient's functional goals

Table 32.2 SMART Outcomes

- **S**pecific—variable
- **M**easurable—reliable
- **A**chievable—realistic
- **R**elevant—related to work/sport/home
- **T**imed—responsive, sensitive to change

NDI), and participation (return to work) can all be measured.

According to the Victorian WorkCover group outcomes should meet a certain minimum standard (Table 32.2).

Chronic illnesses like back pain require a shift from a biomedical to a biopsychosocial paradigm (see chapter 4). Back problems are multi-factorial, having to do as much with attitude and beliefs as pathology. The physician's role as teacher may be at least as important as his/her role as treater. For back problems, just as for diabetes or asthma, the patient's active involvement in his/her own care is a great determinant of quality of life, participation, and activity restrictions (43).

The goal in acute care is to decrease pain, enhance tissue healing, and promote early resumption of near normal activities. In contrast, the goals in chronic care are to focus on activity limitations, impairments, and self-care strategies. For chronic patients it is important to help shape appropriate expectations. For instance, informing them that flare-ups are normal and inevitable. Many "weekend warriors" require advice about appropriate pacing. A key is to mutually agree on the goals of care and to arrive at an exercise prescription that is customized for each individual patient.

Because back problems tend to recur, a self-care prescription should be a primary component of care (see Chapter 14). Patient empowerment to self-manage encompasses education about what is causing the pain, the prognosis for recovery, functional goal setting, activity modification advice or precautions to spare the spine, the risks with inappropriate treatment (e.g., bed rest, narcotics), and the benefits with appropriate treatment.

Patients who embrace active coping strategies have a speedier recovery than those adopting passive coping strategies (9,10). Active copers take responsibility, whereas passive copers expect their health care provider (HCP) to fix or cure them. Active coping is a behavior not a personality trait, and is thus amenable to change. It is important that patients attribute to self-care instead of "hands-on" treatment of the HCP. This will build self-efficacy or confidence and reduce dependency.

Patients typically would rather have someone "fix" their problem than have to learn to cope with it or to control it. How can patient compliance with self-care be enhanced?

- Mutually establish functional goals (eliminating activity intolerances) as the aim of care

- Identify the patient's "weak link"—functional diagnosis—as a key predisposing or perpetuating factor in their painful activity intolerance

- Perform a post-training audit as in the McKenzie system to adjudicate for the patient a reduction in pain and improvement in function after performance of exercise

- If the patient is fearful of exercise administer "graded exposures" to feared stimuli in a comfortable range to disprove their belief

Modern care focuses on the patient's functional goals not just the symptoms. These should be mutually agreed upon and matter to the patient. According to the World Health Organization's International Classification of Function (ICF) document functional status should be defined in terms of (1,41,48):

- **Impairments**
  - Physical Limitations
    - Loss or abnormality in structure or function of a body part
      - Range of motion, strength
- **Activity limitations**
  - Limitations at the Personal level
    - Difficulties in performing activities, e.g., walking, climbing, etc.
      - Mobility, self-care, domestic life
- **Participation restrictions**
  - Limitations at the Societal level
    - Work absence, leisure activities
      - Interpersonal, major life, community, social, civic life

Functional goals should relate more to activities and participation than to impairments (17). However, intermediate goals might include the impairments. It is important that regular goal revision is undertaken.

Because many functional disability questionnaires fall short of measuring participation a new question-

naire has been developed (38). Five questions relating to participation were taken from the Chronic Pain Grading Scale and validated for this purpose (44) (Fig. 32.1).

Clinical Challenges

The modern CF described is designed to minimize chronicity and disability. This section describes a set of action steps for HCPs wishing to put the CF into practice. These action steps are termed clinical challenges (Table 32.3).

An important Practice Tool for recording the Clinical Challenges is the Patient Profile. This is designed to be used on both initial evaluations as well as during re-evaluations. It has a place for each action step—goals, AIs, MI, MS, AMC, as well as the self-care prescription (Fig. 32.2). It provides the HCP with all the relevant information for managing the case on a single page. It is invaluable in multi-practitioner settings to facilitate communication. For instance, at a quick glance the HCP can see what the CC, AI, and MS are.

Clinical Challenge #1a

Can you uncover from the patient's history what their fears, worries, concerns, and goals are?

Most people cope with pain without seeking health care (8). Patients usually seek care if they are getting worse, not getting better, or have severe pain. Many patients are concerned their pain is caused by something serious (e.g., cancer) (24). Others, that their pain will become chronic or require surgery. Patients are often fearful that the wrong movement will make it much worse (27,43). Patients not only want to know what is causing their pain, but what can be done for it and how long it may take (40).

Practice Tool

Are you using the yellow flags form? (see chapter 9)

Clinical Challenge #1b

Can you provide reassurance and gradual reactivation advice to a distressed patient so they won't catastrophize their illness?

After the initial history mutually establish the goals of care with the patient, for instance, to reduce pain and activity intolerances. Reassure and reactivate the patient by explaining that their care will include palliative measure to make them more comfortable, tissue-sparing strategies to help them avoid

Participation Questionnaire

1. To what extent did you perform any activities in or around your home during this episode of low back pain (not being work or household activities)?

| 0 | 1 | 2 | 3 | 4 | 5 | 6 | 7 | 8 | 9 | 10 |

No
participation

full
normal
participation

2. To what extent did you participate in any work and/or household activities during this episode of low back pain?

| 0 | 1 | 2 | 3 | 4 | 5 | 6 | 7 | 8 | 9 | 10 |

No
participation

full
normal
participation

3. To what extent did you participate in sport activities during this episode of low back pain?

| 0 | 1 | 2 | 3 | 4 | 5 | 6 | 7 | 8 | 9 | 10 |

No
participation

full
normal
participation

4. To what extent did you participate in any leisure time activities, besides sports, during this episode of low back pain?

| 0 | 1 | 2 | 3 | 4 | 5 | 6 | 7 | 8 | 9 | 10 |

No
participation

full
normal
participation

5. To what extent did you participate in any social and/or family activities during this episode of low back pain?

| 0 | 1 | 2 | 3 | 4 | 5 | 6 | 7 | 8 | 9 | 10 |

No
participation

full
normal
participation

Scoring:

■ *Calculate the mean of the 5 scores*

■ *If the patient does not engage in sports (question #3) then the mean of the other scores is used.*

Figure 32.1 Participation Questionnaire. Reproduced from Swinkels-Meewisse IEJ, Roelofs J, Verbeek ALM, Oostendorp RAB, Vlaeyen JWS. Fear of movement/(re)injury, disability and participation in acute low back pain. Pain. 2003;105:371–379.

Table 32.3   Clinical Challenges

Are you . . .

History
1. Identifying patient fears, worries and goals?
   - Offering reassurance
2. Identifying activity intolerances (AI)?
   - Establishing mutual functional goals
3. Identifying mechanism of injury (MI)
   - Rx spine sparing advice

Examination
4. Identifying mechanical sensitivity (MS)
   - Rx palliative exercises
5. Identifying relevant abnormal motor control (AMC)
   - Rx spine stabilizing exercises
   - Rx functional training specific to the patients home, sport and work activities?

---

adding to the problem, thorough evaluation to rule out "red flags" of serious disease, and if necessary tissue stabilizing strategies to increase their fitness level so that it exceeds the physical demands of their lifestyle/occupation (Tables 32.4 and 32.5).

An excellent application of this new paradigm is through Working Backs Scotland (35). They have emphasized that recovery depends on reactivation. They have utilized a large public education marketing campaign focused on three messages:

- stay active
- try simple pain relief
- if you need it, get advice

This approach has been successful in achieving a reversal in health care beliefs. The majority favored rest at first, but afterwards the majority favored staying active. This change took 1 to 2 months to accomplish, and improvement continued for more than 2 years afterwards.

It is important to engage in "shared decision-making" with patients (2,3). According to social-cognitive theory of change the following steps in patient communication are essential (see Chapter 14) (2,3).

- Health promotion should begin with goals, not means
  - Biomedical interventions are not the only means
- Social cognitive theory specifies a set of core determinants
  - Knowledge of health risks and benefits of health practices/behaviors

- Perceived self-efficacy that one can exercise control over health habits
- Outcome expectations about costs/benefits of different health habits
- Health goals and concrete plans/strategies for achieving them
- Perceived facilitators and impediments to the changes being sought

Practice Tool

The Back Book, Explain Pain, The Neck Book, and The Whiplash Book (5,7,46,47) (Chapters 14, 15, and 31).

Clinical Challenge #2

Can you uncover from the patient's history what specific activity intolerances are present?

The history should identify the patient's functional limitations, specifically what activities aggravate the patient's symptoms. The most fundamental limitations are those that interfere with basic activities like sitting, standing, and walking. Eliminating these intolerances can usually be established as a mutually agreed on goal of care. This helps focus the patient on clinically relevant dysfunction instead of pain. These can be measured in reliable and responsive ways and become markers of the patient's progress over time.

Practice Tool

Outcome forms (e.g., Oswestry, Patient Specific Functional Scale, etc.) (see Outcome chapter 8).

Clinical Challenge #3

Can you identify the patient's mechanism of injury and provide appropriate tissue sparing advice?

Patients generally want to know what caused their pain. Frequently, there is no specific trauma which leaves the patient perplexed as to the cause of their pain. Before the HCP can confidently recommend therapeutic interventions a clear understanding of how the pain arose is needed.

Usually pain is caused by some form of repetitive strain. An end-range postural load such as from sitting in kyphosis will over time irritate the back. Such postural pain is usually relieved by avoiding the static positions of cumulative overload. Lewit says, "the first treatment is to teach the patient to avoid what harms him." McKenzie has theorized that when such postural strain is encountered frequently enough

Patient Profile

Name _____ Date _____

CC _____ Initial Onset _____ Episode Duration _____

Acute_____ Recurrent _____ Chronic _____ VAS _____ OM _____ Yellow Flags _____

Goals/ Fears/ Worries/ Concerns *Activity intolerances (AI)*	*Mechanism of injury (MI) & Past history* *Neuro signs & Red flags*
Mechanical sensitivities (MS) (ROM, ortho, TrP)	*Abnormal motor control (AMC)* (incoordination, balance)
Posture	*Joint palpation/Muscle length*
1-leg balance (10 – 30 secs) *Side bridge* (41 secs) *Sorenson* (62 secs) *C0 – C1 flexion* (26 mmHg, 10 reps, 10 secs)	*Home exercise list*

Figure 32.2 The patient profile.

Table 32.4 Acute Patients Require a Simple Information (43)

- Reassurance that they do not have a serious disease
- Encouragement that gradual resumption of normal activities is safe and effective
- Basic biomechanical advice

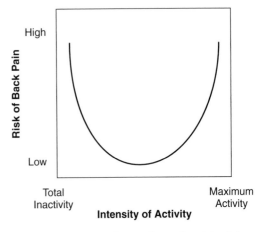

Figure 32.3 The relationship of activity history and injury. From Abenheim L, Rossignol M, Valat JP, Nordin M, Avouac B, Blotman F, Charlot J, et al. The role of activity in the therapeutic management of back pain: Report of the International Paris Task Force on Back Pain. Spine 2000;25:1S–33S.

that tissues will "adaptively shorten" to protect themselves (Chapter 15). The resultant dysfunctional pain can be re-created whenever the shortened structures are stretched, even if briefly. According to McKenzie a third classification of mechanism of injury is when tissues become so dysfunctional that discal derangement occurs. This pain is not only caused by sustained or brief static overload, but can be triggered by mid-range movements or even movements in various directions.

According to McGill injury can occur from either too much or too little of anything (Fig. 32.3) (see Chapters 2 and 5). Too little activity results in deconditioning, which predisposes to overload from even trivial trauma. Too much activity results in incomplete healing and a cycle of repetitive strain. Repetitive strain injury depends on three main factors (Table 32.6).

One particularly pernicious mechanism of injury for the low back is prolonged or early morning flexion (36). In fact, avoidance of early morning flexion has been shown to accelerate recovery from acute low back pain (36)

An understanding of the patient's mechanism of injury should lead to a prescription of tissue sparing strategies. These might include:

- Micro-breaks from prolonged sitting
- Hip hinging when bending or lifting
- Ergonomic advice about the computer workstation

Practice Tool

Utilize patient hand-outs of self-care advice for specific tissue sparing strategies relevant to the patient (www.lasportsandspine.com).

Clinical Challenge #4a

Can you uncover from the patient's examination what specific movements and positions provoke or peripheralize symptoms—mechanical sensitivity (MS)?

Once red flags of serious disease are ruled out the primary role of the physical examination is to find the movements or positions that reproduce the patient's characteristic symptoms. This generally includes range of motion, orthopedic and even myofascial tests. The McKenzie system of evaluation involving repetitive and/or sustained end-range tests of cardinal ranges of motion is a well-validated method for identifying the patients MS (see Chapter 15)(26).

Practice Tool

Record the findings on the patient profile.

Table 32.5 Subacute Patients Require Stepped-up Information (43)

- Discussion of "red flags" vs. more common and less worrisome sources of back pain
- Identification of factors that increase or decrease pain
- Posture and body mechanics advice
- Identify activity limitations related to back pain
- Set personal goals to overcome those limitations

Table 32.6 Three Aspects of Repetitive Strain Disorders (37)

1. Magnitude of load
2. Duration of load
3. Frequency of such loads

Clinical Challenge #4b

Can you prescribe introductory exercises which are safe and effective movements for the acute phase?

McKenzie's chief contribution to clinical decision making for acute patients is that self-treatments can be prescribed on the basis of a valid and easily testable classification system (23,26,33). A recent study by Long et al reported that individualized care was superior to evidence based care (26). The individualized care sought the patient's directional preference. This is defined as the posture or repeated end-range movement(s) in a single direction (flexion, extension, or side-glide/rotation), which decrease or abolish lumbar pain, or cause referred pain to retreat in a proximal direction. The McKenzie style approach led to matched treatments with the following results

- 95% of matched patients improved
- 56% of evidence-based care group improved
- 75% of opposite direction group were not improved or were worse

In another related study within-session reassessment of mechanical sensitivity was shown to predict between-session improvement (18). If post-treatment audit within-session of MS showed improvement those patients were at least 3.5 times more likely to have between-session improvement. Linear regression analysis shows that within-session changes predicted 12% to 64% of between-session improvement in ROM.

Practice Tool

Utilize patient hand-outs of self-care advice for specific palliative exercise strategies relevant to the patient (www.lasportsandspine.com).

Clinical Challenge #5a

Can you identify relevant abnormal motor control findings in your patients?

When the acute phase has passed functional tests of relevant impairments are of value. Enthoven et al. found that strength, endurance, and coordination tests are all influenced by pain and are thus not predictive of recovery in acute patients; however, they are in subacutes (12). Both single leg standing balance ability and trunk extensor endurance have been shown to predict future back pain (4,28,39).

Practice Tool

Record the findings on the patient profile.

Clinical Challenge #5b

Can you prescribe safe, effective exercises to isolate and "groove" relevant stability patterns?

Appropriate stability exercises involve fine motor control training that reduces the patient's MS (Chapter 26). Such exercises are described as in the patient's "functional range." This is defined by Dennis Morgan as "the range which is painless and appropriate for the task at hand" (30). These exercises should address specific impairments the patient has.

Hides reported that isolated stability exercise training prevents recurrences in acute low back pain patients (19–21). O'Sullivan found that these exercises were valuable for treating chronic back pain as well (32) (Chapter 25). McGill has shown which exercises have the widest margins of safety and how to progress patients by gradually increasing load (29) (see Chapter 5). Patient's are progressed through the stages of motor learning from the cognitive–kinesthetic to associative, and finally to autonomous learning (see Chapter 26).

The prescription of stability exercises should always be audited in a similar fashion to the McKenzie program. This means that the exercises should not peripheralize symptoms and post-exercise audits of the patient's MS should empirically validate within-session improvement for each individual patient.

Practice Tool

Utilize patient hand-outs of self-care advice for specific spine stabilizing exercise strategies relevant to the patient (www.lasportsandspine.com).

Clinical Challenge #5c

How can we progress training to a functional stage so it will stabilize the patient in their home, sport and occupational activities?

Functional integrated training (FIT) is specific to the patient's activity and participation goals, and usually triplanar (Chapter 26). The best exercises are those that require the least amount of conscious control or hypervigilance. If an exercise can be found which the patient performs well automatically or with a minimum of cueing this is ideal.

Practice Tool

Utilize patient hand-outs of self-care advice for functional training exercise strategies relevant to the patient (www.lasportsandspine.com).

Table 32.7 Goals of Functional Examination (22)

History
Identify the clinical symptom complex

Examination
Identify the tissue injury complex (or pain generator(s))
Identify the source of biomechanical overload
Identify the dysfunctional kinetic chain
Identify the functional adaptations

Summary

Find the patient's AI, MS, and AMC. Expand the patient's "functional range" through advice, manipulation, and exercise. Perform post-treatment audits by:

- Recheck AI
- Recheck MS (painful ROM's, orthopedic, and myofascial findings)
- Recheck AMC (key functional pathology)

On Finding the "Key Link"

All clinicians are faced with the problem of identifying what area to treat first. The locomotor system is made up of mechanical links that function to performed an infinite variety of tasks. Central nervous system control, somato-sensory input, and muscular output frame the potential for this powerful machinery of life. When we treat pain in the locomotor system the threat of persistence or recurrence of activity limitations associated with the pain hangs over our craft. The challenge is to rule out "red flags" of serious disease (tumor, infection, fracture), "yellow flags" of psychosocial predisposition to chronic pain or disability, and then to move full throttle towards reactivation of the patients activity tolerance and functional capacity.

Treatment of the site of pain may provide relief of pain, but it is often temporary. The art of treatment of locomotor system disorders consists of seeing the mechanical linkage system and it's underlying neurologic control and finding patterns of dysfunction responsible for the eventual (or inevitable!) onset of pain. This is a functional approach rather than a symptomatic one. We attempt to determine where mechanical load is most pernicious to the body. A history of constrained postures or repetitive activities should be uncovered. Additionally, examination of how the body moves should seek to identify where the linkage system is not handling even simple movements efficiently.

According to Lewit (25), "Many doctors whose methods include treating only function and concomitant reflex changes are thinking only in terms of the method, not in terms of the clinical object to which the method is applied, i.e. to disturbed function, which seems very elusive. Yet to treat mainly at the site of symptoms, or pain, is to fail, if the trouble is disturbed function . . . The practitioner may well feel the ground slipping from under him that is why the patterns of chains based on empirical observation help by providing a rational approach to systematic clinical examination directed at disturbed function."

Treatment should not be aimed at the site of symptoms, but to the source of biomechanical overload. The body should be viewed as a linkage system whereby one link in the chain can have an effect on even distant links. Kibler describes a functional approach to distinguishing the source of pain from the pain generator and functional adaptations (Tables 32.7 and 32.8) (22). In this way, for example, subtalar hyperpronation can be understood to affect not only the foot and ankle but also the knee, lumbar spine, or even shoulder stability.

The regional chapters that follow (Chapters 34 and 35) utilize this approach to frame care in a consistent manner. Functional rehabilitation should focus on the source of biomechanical overload rather than the site of symptoms. Too often patients receive an endless array of treatments to "fix" the problem or cure their symptoms. For instance, a knee problem will be treating with the very best and latest manipulation, massage, medication, injection, acupuncture, modality, or surgery but not respond because the problem was coming from another link in the kinetic chain! If subtalar hyperpronation is the cause of medial collapse of the knee and valgus overload then no treatment of the knee itself is going to help. Therefore, a functional evaluation should identify the source of biomechanical overload in the kinetic chain before a treatment plan commences so that the "key link" can be unmasked.

The Art

That local lesions have widespread effects throughout the locomotor system cannot be overestimated. Foot dysfunction (subtalar hyperpronation) affects the lower extremity kinetic chain (valgus overload of

Table 32.8 An Example of the Kinetic Chain

- Chief symptom—shoulder pain
- Pain generator—rotator cuff tendon
- Source of biomechanical overload—kyphosis→ stiff posterior capsule→impingement
- Dysfunctional kinetic chain—poor balance and mobility of lower extremity kinetic chain
- Functional adaptation—tightness in upper trapezius and levator scapulae

the knee) and pelvis (lower crossed syndrome). Mid-thoracic dysfunction (fixed kyphosis) effects the upper quarter (altered scapulo-humeral rhythm) and cervical spine (head forward posture). Treating muscles affects joints and vice versa.

Clinical Pearl

According to Lewit, "I don't touch a patient until I have examined everything. I want to know what is the relevant chain. I begin with a general picture, not a single lesion."

In other words, think globally, but act locally.

The clinician should look diligently for a pattern of dysfunction. Look to see if the primary problem is due to the foot (hyperpronation), hip (gluteus medius insufficiency), or trunk (poor control of twisting torques). Try to find out where to enter the dysfunctional program. The criteria are from the history, the clinical findings or a diagnostic "hunch". The history may reveal an important onset (i.e., trauma), progression (i.e., repetitive strain), or provocative behavior of the symptoms (i.e., worse with forward bending). The clinical findings may reveal that a key region is dysfunctional such as the feet or mid-thoracic region. Also, a particular tissue may be markedly dysfunctional such as a blocked joint or very weak muscle. Finally, an area may be treated as a "key link" merely to pursue a hunch. For instance, an old scar may be treated to empirically see what happens to related structures in the kinetic chain.

Performing a screening examination of AMC is the quickest way to identify areas of increased strain (Table 32.9). This will also enable the clinician to see patterns of compensation and thus determine the "key link" through empirical trial.

Once we have identified a faulty movement pattern, we can see the holistic picture of dysfunction for our patient. For instance, if the lower back is sensitive and during the Janda hip extension test hip extension is limited, but hypermobility is occurring in the lumbar spine in hyperextension and rotation

---

Table 32.9 Examples of Screening Tests for Abnormal Motor Control

- Single-leg standing balance
- Squat test
- Vleeming hip flexion test
- Janda's hip extension test
- Side bridge endurance
- Sorenson's trunk extensor endurance test
- C0-C1 flexion coordination/endurance
- Scapulo-humeral rhythm

---

then clear treatment targets emerge. Rather than manipulating the lumbar spine or offering soft tissue manipulation to tender areas, treatment will be focused at the key dysfunctional links in the kinetic chain. The hip stiffness would be addressed with hip joint mobilization and/or psoas lengthening. The spine instability would be addressed with bracing training and "neutral" spine control exercises during twisting or extension challenges such as pushing, pulling, squat, and balance reach training.

Practice-Based Problem

Because impairments (dysfunction) are so common how can the clinician avoid over-treating coincidental functional pathology?

According to Lewit, "the objective of remedial exercise is a faulty motor pattern or stereotype which has been diagnosed and is considered relevant to the patient's problem." However, "remedial exercise is always time consuming, and time should not be wasted . . . We should not attempt to teach patients ideal locomotor patterns, but only correct the fault that is causing the trouble."

A select group of patients who you feel are most likely to relapse should be singled out for more intensive rehabilitation.

Many dysfunctions (impairments) are secondary and should be audited for improvement, but they should not be targeted with specific interventions. For instance, tight upper trapezius are typically secondary to faulty workstation ergonomics and a stiff upper thoracic kyphosis. The trapezius tightness is a functional adaption and not a cause of biomechanical overload. Treatment should be aimed at the workstation and kyphosis. There is a systematic approach—a continuum of care for addressing this functional pathology of the locomotor system (Table 32.10).

Clinical Pearl

According to Lewit, "For remedial gymnastics: do not indicate them before you have analyzed the chain or chains, and then treat according to the essential link which will also be decisive for the method of rehabilitation, whether sensory-motor, just self-mobilization, exteroceptive stimulation, or even McKenzie! There is no single approach!"

There are many approaches in rehabilitation—McKenize, stabilization, cognitive–behavioral, etc. It is important to keep the purpose of rehabilitation in mind when determining the self-care strategy. The main goals of care are to reduce activity intolerances and increase participation associated with pain. By

Table 32.10   The Continuum of Care

1. **Advice**—Teach the patient spine sparing strategies reduce repetitive strain
2. **Manipulation**—Mobilize or release adverse tension in joint, muscle, fascia, nerve, or skin
3. **Exercise**
   a) Reassure the patient that reactivation is the road to recovery
   b) Train stability patterns to isolate the "weak link"
   c) Train functional patterns relevant to the individual's work, home, and sport activities

auditing care the HCP will find which exercise(s) are required to achieve the goals.

Atlas of Key Tests and Exercises

With 90% of patients being labeled as having "non-specific" back pain, there is a great need to perform a functional assessment leading to a functional diagnosis. The Fourth International Forum on Low Back Pain Research in Primary Care in Israel in March 2000 concluded that patients are dissatisfied with the "non-specific" label (6). Achieving a validated classification system for "non-specific" LBP was their top research priority. Since that time, matching treatment to the specific subgroup has been found to outperform unmatched or generic guideline based treatments (14–16,26).

When a report of findings is being given to the patient it is important to offer a concrete plan of action. The major types of care offered should be described and the goals specified. Because patients are seeking relief of pain and the modern approach is to focus on activity intolerances associated with pain a simple framework is to explain care as being related to one of the following goals: palliative, sparing, stabilizing, or functional (Table 32.11).

Most patients—approximately 80%—recover quickly and require a minimalist approach. If a person is seeking care, a simple palliative approach is often all that is required (13,45). However, in more complex cases the effectiveness of such measures is unfortunately short-term. Rather than continue to offer medication, manipulation, or modalities (e.g., hot packs, massage, ultrasound, etc.), it is wise to identify the perpetuating factor in a person's lifestyle (i.e., mechanism of injury) and teach the patient spine-sparing strategies. This gets to the actual source of the patient's biomechanical overload and trains the patient in more efficient ergonomic approaches. Examples of spine sparing strategies include taking micro-breaks when working at a desk for prolonged periods, or learning to hip hinge when bending or lifting.

Table 32.11   Goals of Care

- Palliative
  • Pain relief measures (McKenzie, NSAIDs, Tylenol, Manipulation, etc.)
- Spine-Sparing Strategies
  • micro-breaks, lifting advice, etc.
- Spine-Stabilizing Strategies
  • Exercises to improve spinal fitness
- Functional Integrated Training (FIT)
  • Exercises to enhance performance and function

In the more chronic or recurrent cases deconditioning may also need to be addressed. Sparing the spine may not be sufficient because the individual's spinal fitness or functional capacity is not adequate for the demands of their occupational, recreational, or home activities (see figure 2.5). In such cases stability training is needed to give the patient a stability margin for error. For athletes or others involved in more strenuous or repetitive tasks, stability training should be progressed to functional integrated training (FIT) exercises so they are specific to the task. This will give a higher likelihood of success and can be viewed as a form of "work hardening."

What follows is an atlas of the most promising functional tests along with major sparing, palliative, stabilizing, and functional self-care techniques (Tables 32.12 and 32.13). These are shown in more detail in Chapters 26, 34, and 35 (Fig. 32.4 to 32.45).

Table 32.12   Functional Screening Tests

1. One-leg standing balance
2. Vele's reflex stability test
3. Two-leg squat
4. One-leg squat
5. Lunge
6. Modified Thomas test
7. Hip internal rotation mobility
8. Vleeming's active and resisted SLR
9. Janda's hip abduction test
10. Janda's hip extension test
11. Side bridge endurance
12. Trunk extensor endurance
13. Janda's trunk flexor test
14. Trunk flexor endurance
15. T4 screen (wall angel)
16. Arm abduction
17. Push up
18. C0-C1 flexion
19. Mouth opening test

Table 32.13 The Exercises

 Palliative
1. McKenzie

Spine-Sparing Strategies
2. Brügger
3. McGill's standing overhead arm reach
4. Cat camel
5. Bracing
6. T4-8 extension mobilizations
7. Piriformis stretch
8. Psoas stretch

Spine-Stabilizing Strategies
9. Respiration
10. Quadruped leg/arm reach
11. Side bridge
12. Curl-up

13. Dead bug
14. Bridge
15. Hamstring curls
16. Back extensions
17. Sphinx/chin tuck
18. Push-up
19. Twister

FIT
20. Sensory–motor training
21. Squat
22. Lunge
23. Balance reach
24. Bosu
25. Pulley

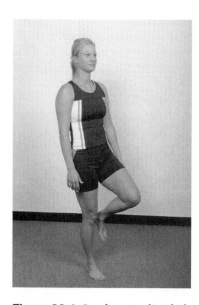

Figure 32.4 One leg standing balance test.

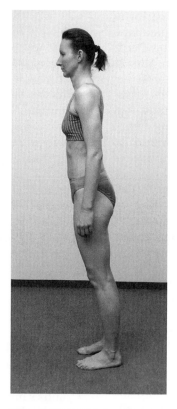

Figure 32.5 Vele's reflex stability test.

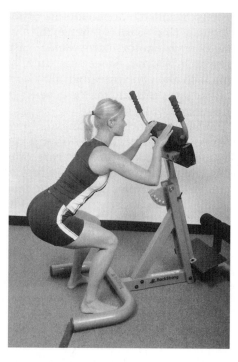

Figure 32.6 Two-leg squat.

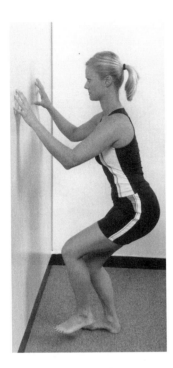

Figure 32.7 One-leg squat.

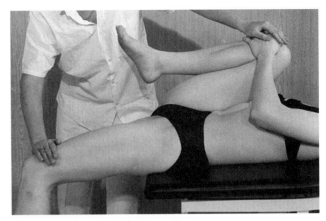

Figure 32.9 Modified Thomas test.

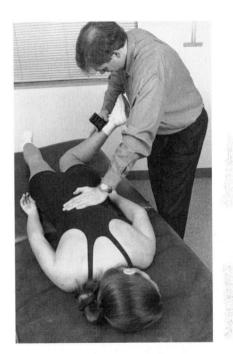

Figure 32.10 Hip internal rotation mobility.

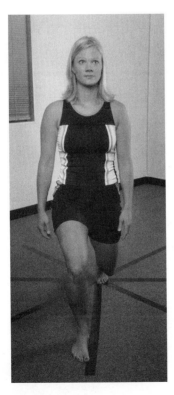

Figure 32.8 Lunge.

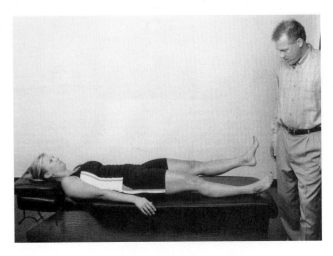

Figure 32.11 Vleeming's active straight leg raise.

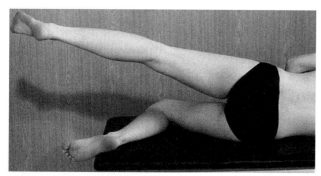

Figure 32.12 Janda's hip abduction test.

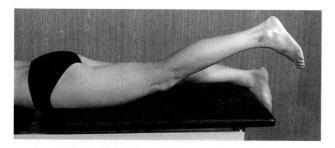

Figure 32.13 Janda's hip extension test.

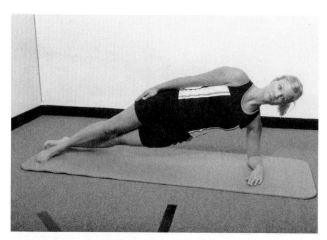

Figure 32.14 Side bridge endurance.

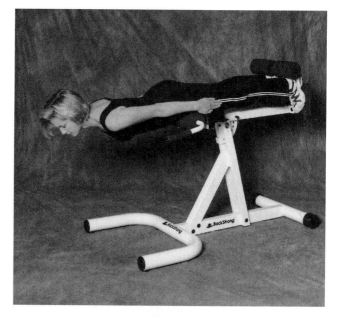

Figure 32.15 Trunk extensor endurance.

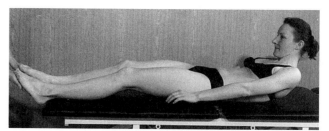

Figure 32.16 Janda's trunk flexor test.

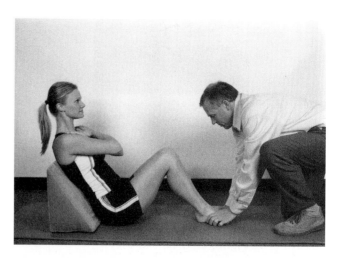

Figure 32.17 Trunk flexor endurance.

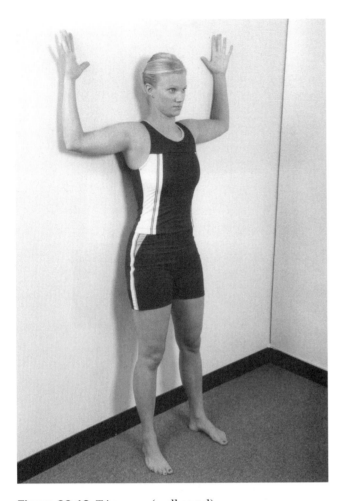

Figure 32.18 T4 screen (wall angel).

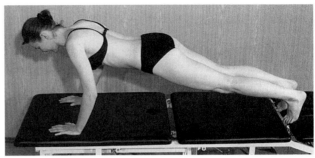

Figure 32.20 Push up.

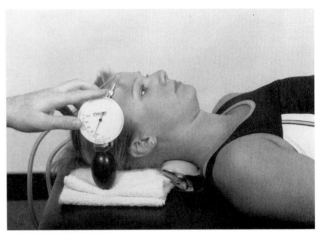

Figure 32.21 C0-C1 flexion.

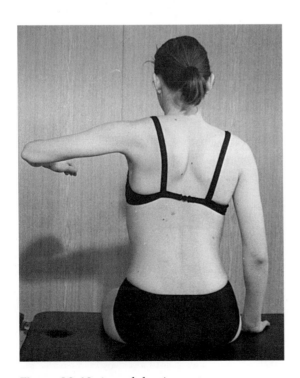

Figure 32.19 Arm abduction test.

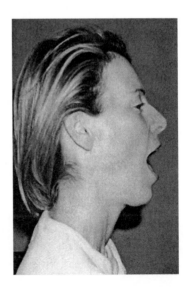

Figure 32.22 Mouth opening test.

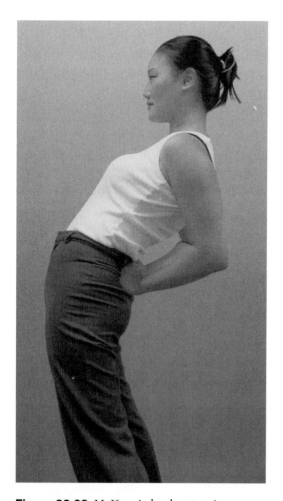

Figure 32.23 McKenzie back extension.

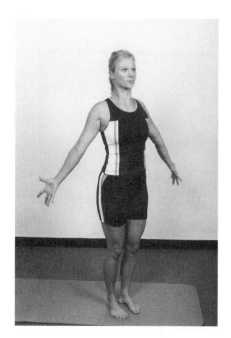

Figure 32.24 Brügger.

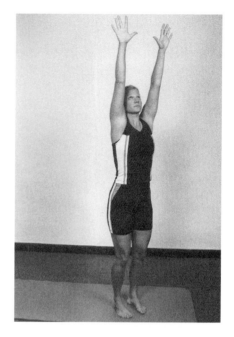

Figure 32.25 McGill's standing overhead arm reach.

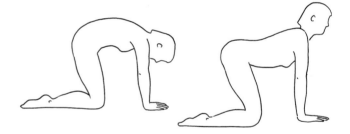

Figure 32.26 Cat camel.

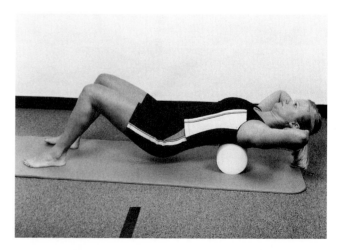

Figure 32.27 Foam roll for T4.

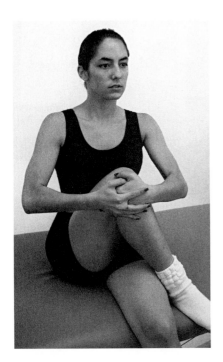

Figure 32.28 Piriformis stretch.

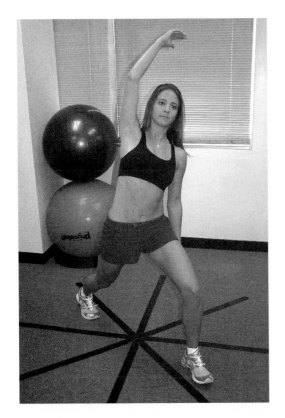

Figure 32.29 Psoas stretch.

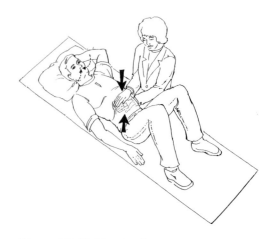

Figure 32.30 Respiration.

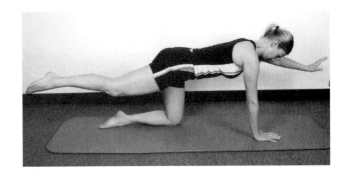

Figure 32.31 Quadruped leg reach.

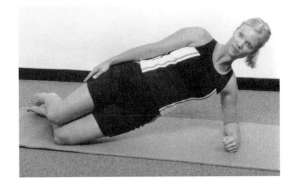

Figure 32.32 Side bridge.

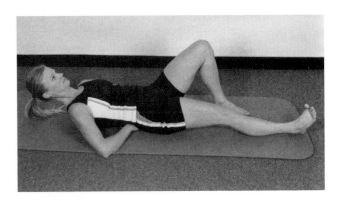

Figure 32.33 Curl-up.

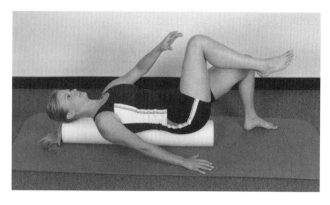

Figure 32.34 Dead bug.

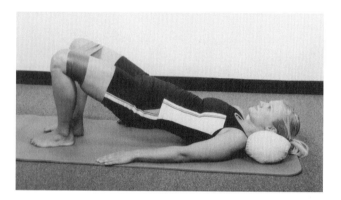

Figure 32.35 Bridge.

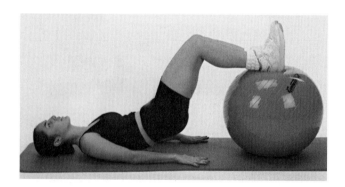

Figure 32.36 Hamstring curls.

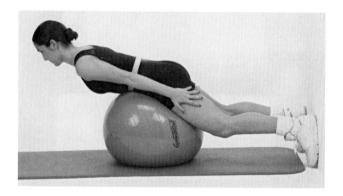

Figure 32.37 Back extensions.

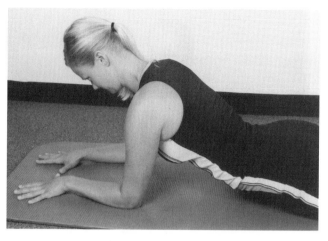

Figure 32.38 Sphinx/chin tuck.

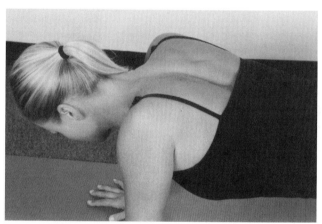

Figure 32.39 Push-up.

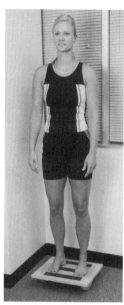

Figure 32.40 Sensory–motor training.

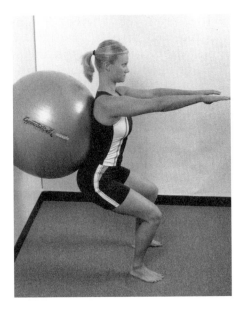

Figure 32.41 Squat.

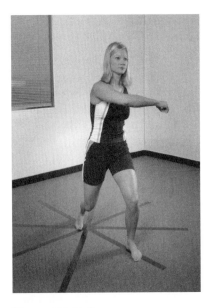

Figure 32.42 Lunge.

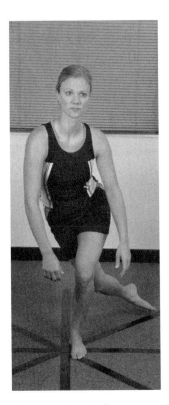

Figure 32.43 Balance reach.

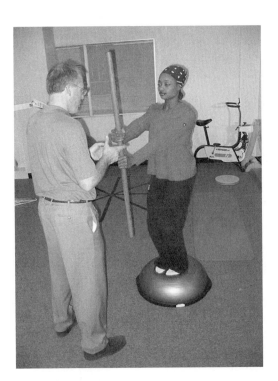

Figure 32.44 Bosu.

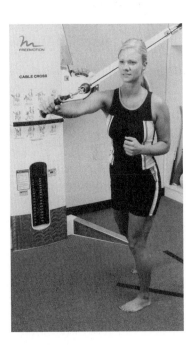

Figure 32.45 Pulley.

"Best Practice" Keys to Recovery—The 7 Rs

There are a discreet set of decision points in patient care (Chapter 4) that are recommended for the bio-psychosocial management of neuromusculoskeletal symptoms.

The first step is ruling out "red flags" of serious disease. Patient reassurance naturally follows in this revolutionary management paradigm. For instance, that recovery is likely and that hurt does not necessarily equal harm. Fortunately, diagnostic triage is very sensitive for ruling out "red flags" of serious disease. Those patients requiring additional testing to rule out sinister causes of spine pain such as tumor, infection or fracture are easily identified by a focused history and examination.

Most acute pain patients begin recovering quickly. Imaging should generally be avoided because most pathology that is identified is misleading and focusing on it only promotes patient anxiety, excessive diagnostic testing, and inappropriate treatment. In fact, the main reason acute pain becomes chronic is caused by the patient taking on the "sick role" instead of viewing their pain as a temporary illness like a common cold.

Functional reactivation of the patient is the next step in the patient centered approach. Focusing on functional issues rather than structural problems is a key to reactivating the patient. Patients are normally apprehensive about the safety of normal activities for their painful back. Reactivation advice about the safety of resuming normal activities is the single most important key both emotionally and physically to a successful recovery. In contrast, the presription of bed rest except in the most severe cases carries with it the risk of reinforcing illness behaviors and promoting deconditioning.

Patients want to know what can be done for their pain and what they should and should not do on their own. If significant pain is present the physician has reached a key decision point at which simple pain relief approaches including manipulation and non-narcotic medication should generally be recommended. Patients with lower back problems can learn to modify risky behavior such as early morning flexion, but generally should be advised not to overly protect their back or they risk weakening and stiffening their spine.

Reevaluation is needed if patients are not adequately recovering within 1 month of care. The natural history is excellent for most people, but if an individual is not responding they likely require a change in management to prevent the onset of chronic, disabling pain. Thus, a key decision point is reached when after 3 to 4 weeks the patient has not begun to improve yet. Whereas, minimal management is required early on the ideal time for more aggressive intervention is in the subacute phase. Screening for "yellow flags" early on can help to identify patients at risk of a poor recovery. This can help clinicians to direct patients requiring more aggressive treatment to the appropriate management. This typically includes treatment by a rehabilitation specialist—an individual or team—trained in reconditioning and cognitive–behavioral approaches.

A very important decision point arises in patients with nerve root compression syndromes who are not recovering within 1 month of onset. If the symptoms are not improving satisfactorily this is a clear indication for advanced imaging and a referral for surgical consultation. However, the question about of a patient's surgical candidacy is not solved by taking an MRI. Clear surgical indications include disabing symptoms or neurological progression of the case. But most patients present with a more vague clinical picture where the progress is merely stalled. In such instances, the question about surgery may be more of a social one, with highly active individuals opting for a "sooner rather than later" operation whereas others may choose to wait since the long-term outcome of conservative care is on par with that of surgery.

Table 32.14 summarizes the 7 Rs decision points in patient care.

The regional Chapters 34 and 35 in this section follow a common format incorporating the key components of care into a repeatable practice model.

1. Initial assessment and diagnosis
   - diagnostic triage
   - yellow flags
   - activity intolerances
   - goals/concerns/worries
2. Kinetic chain functional assessment
   - Clinical symptom complex
   - Pain generator (Tissue injury complex)
   - Source of biomechanical overload
   - Kinetic chain dysfunction
   - Functional adaptation
3. Treatment/Rehabilitation
   - Palliative
   - Sparing
   - Stabilizing
   - Functional

Principles of Evidence-Based Neuro-Musculoskeletal Care

Modern care for spinal symptoms requires a new perspective. The following principles have emerged as keystones of this new paradigm.

Table 32.14 The 7 Rs Decision Points

1. Rule out "red flags" of serious disease
2. Reassurance that no serious disease is present and that improvement is likely to begin rapidly (within a few weeks)
3. Reactivation advice that normal activities can be resumed (walk, swim, bike, etc.) and education about simple activity modifications to reduce bio-mechanical strain (i.e., hip hinge, cats, abdominal bracing)
4. Relieve pain with manipulation, modalities, or medication
5. Re-evaluation of those entering the subacute phase for structural, functional, or psycho–social pathology
6. Rehabilitate/recondition/re-educate muscles with McKenzie, stabilization, progressive strengthening, or cognitive-behavioral (indicated if high "yellow flags" score) approaches
7. Refer for specialist tests (i.e., diagnostic imaging) or treatments (multidisciplinary rehabilitation) when indicated (i.e., "red flags" or "yellow flags")

1. Evidence-based guidelines are used as a framework for making clinical decisions.

2. Cases are managed in a biopsychosocial context by providing "patient-centered" care cognizant of the patient's support structure, job dissatisfaction, economic situation, distress level, coping mechanisms, and other appropriate personal social factors.

3. A diagnostic triage is performed on all patients to rule out "red flags" of serious disease and identify the need for specialist referral or additional diagnostic testing.

4. For patients without "red flags" of serious disease, reassurance is provided regarding the positive prognosis for most neuromusculoskeletal (NMS) conditions.

5. Patient's goals, fears, worries, and concerns are identified and respected regarding their NMS condition.

6. Information about the cause of the pain is provided as far as is possible, even when the exact pain generator cannot be pinpointed.

7. A prognosis for the patient's condition is provided.

8. The patient is informed of general precautions—sparing strategies—with regard to their condition.

9. Patients receive information about specific pain relief measures that are available on their own or from the health care provider.

10. "Yellow flags" risk factors predictive of a prolonged recovery are identified and discussed with the patient.

11. Gradual reactivation advice is provided. For example, that hurt does not necessarily equal harm and the merits of pacing activity.

12. Patients receive advice that recovery is stepwise and that "flare-ups" are normal.

13. Self-care exercises are prescribed which have been demonstrated to be both safe and effective. New exercises are tested post-treatment to confirm that they successfully reduce the patient's mechanical sensitivity.

14. Reliable, valid, and responsive outcomes will be regularly utilized to determine the patient's progress over time.

■ CONCLUSION

The atlases of selected functional screening tests and functional–stability exercises are anchors to the rehabilitation of the spine pain patient. The modern approach does not focus on pain. Rather, it focuses on functional restoration and a self-management strategy.

The essential components of this model are the identification of the patients AIs, MS, AMC, and self-care prescription. None are more significant to facilitate the administration of this functional approach than is the McKenzie method of auditing the patients "within-session" improvement (MS) to motivate the patient to perform the adjudicated self-care prescription. This coupled with identifying the patient's AIs—functional goals; and AMC—functional deficits; are the key steps in establishing the patients intermediate and final goals (end points of care).

Audit Process
Self-Check of the Chapter's Learning Objectives

- What are the key components of the modern clinical framework?

- Why are the patient's fears, worries, or concerns so important to identify?

- How is the patient's mechanical sensitivity identified and utilized in patient care?

- How are tests of the patient's abnormal motor control used differently than those of mechanical sensitivity?

- What is the limitation of stabilizing and functional training versus sparing strategies?

- Why is identification of the pain generator not sufficient for case management?

■ REFERENCES

1. Australian Institute of Health and Welfare. Disability Data Briefing. The International Classification of Functioning, Disability and Health, ICF, ICIDH, Canberra 2002; (http://www.aihw.gov.au/publications/dis/ddb20/ddb20.pdf) accessed 20 February 2004]

2. Bandura A. Health promotion by social cognitive means. Health Education & Behavior 2004;31:143–164.

3. Bandura A. The anatomy of stages of change. Am J Health Prom 1997;12:8–10.

4. Biering-Sorensen F. Physical measurements as risk indicators for low-back trouble over a one-year period. Spine 1984;9:106–119.

5. Bigos S, Roland M, Waddell G. The Back Book (American Edition). The Stationary House. London: The Stationary House, 2004.

6. Borkan J, Van Tulder M, Reis S, Schoene ML, Croft P, Hermoni D. Advances in the field of low back pain in primary care: A Report from the Fourth International Forum. Spine 2002;27:E128–E132.

7. Butler D, Moseley L. Explain Pain. Noigroup Publications, Adelaide, Australia, 2003.

8. Carey TS, Mills Garret J, Jackman AM. Beyond the good prognosis. Spine 2000:25:115–120.

9. Carroll L, Mercado AC, Cassidy JD, Cote P. A population-based study of factors associated with combinations of active and passive coping with neck and low back pain. J Rehabil Med 2002;34:67–72.

10. Carroll LJ, Cassidy JD, Cote P. Depression as a risk factor for onset of an episode of troublesome neck and low back pain. Pain 2004;107:134–139.

11. Cochrane Collaboration. http://www.cochrane.org/index0.htm accessed June 8, 2005.

12. Enthoven P, Skargren E, Kjellman G, Oberg B. Course of back pain in primary care: a prospective study of physical measures. J Rehabil Med 2003;35:168–173.

13. European Commission Research Directorate General: Low back pain guidelines for its management. http://www.backpaineurope.org/. Accessed June 8, 2005.

14. Erhard RE, Delitto A. Relative effectiveness of an extension program and a combined program of manipulation and flexion and extension exercises in patients with acute low back syndrome. Phys Ther 1994;74:1093–1100.

15. Fritz JM. George S. The use of a classification approach to identify subgroups of patients with acute low back pain. Spine 2000;1:106–114.

16. Fritz JM, Delitto A, Vignovic M, et al. Interrater reliability of judgments of the centralization phenomenon and status change during movement testing in patients with low back pain. Arch Phys Med Rehabil 2000;81:57–60.

17. Grotle M, Borx JI, Vollestad NK. Functional status and disability questionnaires: what do they assess? A systematic review of back-specific outcome questionnaires. Spine 2004;30:130–140.

18. Hahne A, Keating JL, Wilson S. Do within-session changes in pain intensity and range of motion predict between-session changes in patients with low back pain. Australian Journal of Physiotherapy 2004;50:17–23.

19. Hides JA, Jull GA, Richardson CA. Long-term effects of specific stabilizing exercises for first-episode low back pain. Spine 2001;26:e243–e248

20. Hides JA, Richardson CA, Jull GA 1996. Multifidus muscle recovery is not automatic after resolution of acute, first-episode of low back pain. Spine 1996;21:2763–2769.

21. Hides JA, Stokes MJ, Saide M, Jull Ga, Cooper DH 1994. Evidence of lumbar multifidus muscle wasting ipsilateral to symptoms in patients with acute/subacute low back pain. Spine 1994;19:165–172

22. Kibler WB, Herring SA, Press JM. Functional Rehabilitation of Sports and Musculoskeletal Injuries. Aspen, 1998.

23. Kilpikoski S, Airaksinen O, Kankaanpaa M, Leminen P, Videman T, Alen M. Interexaminer reliability of low back pain assessment using the McKenzie method. Spine 2002;27:E207–E214.

24. Klassen AC, Berman ME. Medical care for headaches. A consumer survey. Cephalgia 1991;11(supp 11):85–86.

25. Lewit K. Manipulative therapy in rehabilitation of the motor system. 2nd edition. London: Butterworths, 1991:129.

26. Long A, Donelson R, Fung T. Does it matter which exercise? Spine 2004;29:2593–2602.

27. Moore JE, Von Korff M, Cherkin D, et al. A randomized trial of a cognitive-behavioral program for enhancing back pain self-care in a primary care setting. Pain 2000;88:145–153.

28. Luoto S, Heliovaara M, Hurri H, Alaranta H. Static back endurance and the risk of low-back pain. Clin Biomech 1995;10:323–324.

29. McGill, S. M., Low Back Exercises: Evidence for improving exercise regimens, Physical Therapy 1998;78:754–765.

30. Morgan D. Concepts in functional training and postural stabilization for the low-back-injured. Top Acute Care Trauma Rehabil 1988;2:8–17.

31. National Guideline Clearinghouse. http://www.guideline.gov/. http://www.cochrane.org/index0.htm Accessed June 8, 2005.

32. O'Sullivan P, Twomey L, Allison G. Evaluation of specific stabilizing exercise in the treatment of chronic low back pain with radiologic diagnosis of spondylolysis or spondylolysthesis. Spine 1997;24:2959–2967.

33. Razmjou H, Kramer JF, Yamada R. Intertester reliability of the McKenzie evaluation in assessing patients with mechanical low back pain. J Orthop Sports Phys Ther 2000;30:368–383.

34. Sackett DL, Rosenberg WMC, Muir Gray JA, Haynes BA, Richardson W. Evidence based medicine: What it is and what it isn't. British Medical Journal 1996;312:71–72.

35. Scotland's Working Backs Partnership 2000. Working-Backs Scotland. www.workingbacksscotland.com. Accessed June 8, 2005.

36. Snook SH, Webster BS, McGorry RW, Fogleman MT, McCann KB. The reduction of chronic nonspecific low back pain through the control of early morning lumbar flexion, Spine 1998;23: 2601–2607.

37. Solomonow M, Hatipkarasulu S, Zhou B, Baratta RV, Aghazadeh F. Biomechanics and EMG of a common idiopathic low back disorder. Spine 2003;28:1235–1248.

38. Swinkels-Meewisse IEJ, Roelofs J, Verbeek ALM, Oostendorp RAB, Vlaeyen JWS. Fear of movement/(re)injury, disability and participation in acute low back pain. Pain. 2003;105:371–379.

39. Takala EP, Vikari-Juntura E. Do functional tests predict low back pain? Spine 2000;25:2126–2132.

40. Turner JA. Educational and behavioral interventions for back pain in primary care. Spine 1996;21: 2851–2859.

41. United Nations. World program of action concerning disabled persons. Division for Social and Policy Development, United Nations; 2003 [http://www.un.org/esa/socdev/enable/diswpa01.htm. Accessed 16 February 2004].

42. Victorian WorkCover Authority. http://www.workcover.vic.gov.au/dir090/vwa/home.nsf/pages/chiropractors. Accessed June 8, 2005.

43. Von Korff M, Moore JE, Lorig K, et al. A randomized trial of a lay-led self-management group intervention for back pain patients in primary care. Spine 1998;23:2608–2615.

44. Von Korff M, Ormel J, Keefe FJ, Dworkin SF, Grading the severity of chronic pain. Pain 1992;50:133–149.

45. Waddell G. The Back Pain Revolution, 2nd edition. 2004. Edinburgh: Churchill Livingstone.

46. Waddell G, Burton K, McCline T, Derebery J. The Whiplash Book. London: The Stationary House, 2004.

47. Waddell G, Burton K, McCline T, Derebery J. The Neck Book (American Edition). London: The Stationary House, 2004.

48. World Health Organization. International Classification of Functioning, Disability and Health: ICF, World Health Organization, Geneva (2001).

33

Managing Common Syndromes and Finding the Key Link

Karel Lewit

Introduction

The Functional Approach

The "Holistic" Principle

Chain Reactions: Up to Date

Brügger's Approach

The Forward Drawn Posture

The "Nociceptive" Chain

The Chain of the Deep Trunk Stabilizers

The Stereotype of Lifting the Thorax When Breathing

The Chain of Food Intake—Mastication

The Chain of Grasping (Epicondylar Pain)

The Chain of Restricted Trunk Rotation

Visceral Chains or Patterns

Finding the Key Link

Body Statics and Pelvic Obliquity

Learning Objectives

After reading this chapter you should be able to understand:

- How to differentiate functional from structural pathology
- The key role of antagonist co-activation patterns of trigger points
- How motor programs relate to specific patterns of muscle imbalance and joint dysfunction

Introduction

By far the most common painful conditions of the motor system are those usually called "nonspecific" or "idiopathic," because no pathology can be found (9). The vast and ever-increasing number of patients labeled in this way are in no way malingerers, and adequate clinical examination furnishes a wealth of signs and symptoms to prove the somatic origin of their complaints. Because some motor function can be shown to be impaired, this being "mechanical," disturbed biomechanics are thought to be the cause, hence the term "mechanical disorder" is frequently used. This term, however, is inadequate, because the organism invariably reacts through its nervous system: in fact, any mechanical change is a source of information processed by the nervous system, which makes the motor system react in a coordinated fashion. Therefore, however, a mechanical disorder may be prominent or even measurable, and we have to deal with disturbed function or dysfunction (1,18).

If we apply the methods of rehabilitation, including manipulation, relaxation etc., our objective is dysfunction, even in cases in which we find pathology, i.e., in disc lesions, treated by conservative methods. In rehabilitation, therefore, our task is to improve or if possible normalize function. Hence a good understanding of the functioning of the motor system, and of "functional pathology," is essential. Motor activity in everyday life consists not of simple movements like flexion or extension of a limb, but of learned activities like driving a car, writing, craftsmanship, playing an instrument, or sport. To perform such activities, motor programs have to be established (19,21). It is essential to understand this if we are to understand motor dysfunction. However, it can be explained only by an analysis of motor learning. The example of the tennis player may serve for illustration. If we try to explain it by conventional neurology, we will certainly fail; the tennis player sees the approaching ball, the visual stimulus travels from his retina via the midbrain to the occipital lobe, from there to the sensomotor area in the parietal lobe, then to the prerolandic motor area, then by the cerebro-spinal pathway to the ventral horn, and by the peripheral nerves to the muscles; the muscular activity must be fine tuned by the afferents going to the cerebellum and from there back to the parietal area (feed-back loop). In addition, the player must also run and perhaps leap in the right direction. If we take into account that the fastest nerve fibers work at a speed hardly ever exceeding 100 m/sec, the ball would never be caught or hit by our tennis player.

Only motor learning, more precisely, forming a program, can explain what happens. First, we place a ball into the cupped hands of the small child. Later on, we carefully throw the ball so that it falls into his hands. It will take weeks or months before the child learns to reach with both hands for the ball and/or to run for it. Much later he learns how to reach and catch it with one hand. Finally, he is provided with a tennis racket and has to learn how to hold the racket and how to assess its length so that the ball hits its center, etc. But by that time a program has been formed and well-established: the moment the eye perceives the ball, the whole program is ready and represents a coordinated response of eyes, head, posture, and upper and lower extremities, within a fraction of a second. Something similar will happen when a piano player reads music or a driver sees a curve in the road. In each case, the program concerns the motor system as a whole.

The Functional Approach (14)

What then are the most frequent changes in function, i.e., reversible lesions without structural changes? There is the (not too chronic) myofascial trigger-point (TrP), reversible joint movement restriction, hyperalgesic skin zones, and dysfunctional changes in the deep connective tissues such as fascias, the scalp, and the tissues covering painful periosteal points (7); this also applies to "active scars" (see Chapter 18). In all these lesions we find pathological restrictive barriers and obtain immediate relief on normalization of these barriers. In addition to these local changes there are disturbances of body statics and motor stereotypes (31) or motor patterns. These can be the result of structural changes or changes in function and affect the motor system as a whole.

Our first task when dealing with a patient is therefore to decide whether he suffers (mainly) from a disturbance of function or one of structure.

- We have to insist that function (physiology) is as real as anatomy (pathology).
- Pathology has to be determined both as to localization and nature. Function, however, is the outcome of the correlation and interplay of a whole chain of different structures of various localization.
- Even if there is structural pathology there are also changes in function which cause clinical symptoms.
- The clinical picture correlates mainly with changes in function, much less with structural pathology. Very frequently pathological changes do not manifest themselves so long as function is not impaired. However, changes in

function by themselves may cause clinical changes in the absence of any (structural) pathology.

- For the same reasons, even clearly diagnosed pathology can be clinically irrelevant (disc herniations at CT, spondylolisthesis), whereas dysfunction that can usually be diagnosed only by clinical means can be of decisive importance.

- If we directed our therapeutic efforts at the pathological changes, our therapy would fail in such cases; however, even if the pathological changes are important, we may still improve the patient's condition if we improve function, because this is exactly what can be achieved by rehabilitation. It is, however, necessary to be aware of the limits of what can be achieved.

- The diagnostic task in pathological diagnosis is to localize the lesion exactly and to determine its nature (principle of localization).

- The diagnostic task in dysfunction is to determine the pathogenetic chain and to assess the correlation and relevance of the individual links (holistic principle).

- The mechanism producing pain caused by pathological changes corresponds to the nature of the pathology in the case; however, if function is changed, the mechanism is mainly caused by increased tension, the regular result of dysfunction. We find clinically increased tension in tissues (TrPs, hyperalgesic zones) wherever the patient feels pain, and relief, whenever we succeed in releasing tension.

- If therapy is successful in conditions caused by pathological changes, it is continued until the lesion has healed, or the decision to operate is taken.

- If therapy is successful in changes caused by dysfunction, we shall probably decide to treat another link of the pathogenetic chain. If we have to treat the same lesion again, we should first consider whether there is not a more important lesion that we have missed or underestimated at first examination. Because the lesion is reversible by definition, changing treatment after each control examination is the routine approach.

- In pathological conditions, success is achieved by effective drugs, or possibly by surgery. In dysfunction, success depends on the correct choice of the relevant link, or links, of a chain at the right moment.

- From what has been said, it follows that the functional approach is much more difficult. We may compare pathology to the "hardware" and dysfunction to the "software" of the motor system.

- Therefore, he who only treats dysfunction at the point where pain is felt is lost, and certainly his patient is.

- Because changes in function are reversible in nature. it can be expected that, if adequately treated (and the case is not complicated), the effect of treatment is immediate, giving the impression of a "miracle cure," which, however, is predictable.

- The relationship between cause and effect usually presents no major problem in conditions caused by structural pathology. However, it can be very subtle in changes caused by dysfunction; what was originally the cause may become secondary and vice versa. Chronic pain of any origin will produce changes in motor patterns or stereotypes, which, in turn, will cause dysfunction perpetuating pain. Chronic joint movement restriction and trigger points cause impaired mobility of fasciae, which, in turn, produce joint movement restriction and muscular trigger points.

- Statistical methods are very useful in well-defined pathology and should be mandatory in this field. It is, however, much more difficult to apply them in changes of function. Even for diagnosis, the same clinical condition (e.g., headache) can be the result of a long chain of various disturbances, the relevance of each link constantly changing. In therapy, if we have treated one link successfully, it would be nonsensical to repeat the same treatment. If, therefore, there are still symptoms left, we have to treat another link in the chain. If the patient is then without symptoms, this by no means implies that the first treatment was of no avail. However, this is very difficult to assess by statistics.

- Psychology is very important in every type of patient for its influence on the autonomous nervous system, e.g., stress. In dysfunction, however, psychology is part of the pathogenetic chain because the locomotor system is the effector of our mental activity, the organ of voluntary movement. This is further borne out by the fact that pain is the most constant symptom, and that tension and relaxation play a very important role. It is, however, necessary to decide how relevant the psychological factor is in each case and how amenable to treatment.

- Modern technology enables us to diagnose pathological lesions much more effectively, even if irrelevant, and also to objectify them. In dysfunction, technology is usually of little use and very cumbersome. Clinical skill remains decisive. This, however, is considered "subjective" (Fig. 33.1).

The "Holistic" Principle

This approach was characteristic for all ancient medical systems based on "humours," and for herbal medicine. It is most prominent in traditional Chinese medicine, with its system of "meridians" stressing connections and interplay between, e.g., internal organs and points at the extremities and the importance of physical exercise and diet. The shortcomings of this approach were its pure empiricism, sometimes bordering on superstition, and the complete lack of scientific proof. This was also true for diagnosis, considered in modern times to be the basis for rational therapy. It was the success of pathological anatomy that has seemed to prove the true cause of disease in structural, well-defined, and localized changes, which could be demonstrated and verified. This became the hallmark of scientific medicine. Therapy, mainly by drugs or surgery, was judged by its effectiveness in normalizing these well-defined and verifiable changes. Modern technology not only greatly

enhanced our ability to diagnose structural changes but also provided drugs that were much more powerful in specific situations, and made surgery much more effective and safe at the same time. These incontestable successes brought about the current belief of the medical establishment, that all medical problems will be solved when we find the pathological (structural) cause of every disease and the specific drug to cure it and, hence, their complacence. Anyone who does not accept this model is branded as denying "modern science," trying to revive the old obsolete empiricism and promote some sort of "alternative" or "complementary" medicine, held to be "unscientific," even if treatment by their methods proves to be successful.

This is the reason why many of those who practice methods considered "alternative" are not prepared to adopt whole-heartedly the "Functional Approach" or "Functional Pathology," although they are aware that (at least) 90% of their cases with motor symptoms have to be classified as "non specific" (9). They still hope that the "true pathology" will be revealed at any moment. For the same reason, most adherents of the numerous sects of alternative medicine who proclaim a holistic approach do not really know how to implement it. This is no mere coincidence. We have pointed out that the "functional approach" is more complicated, i.e., more demanding than structural pathology, comparing it to software in contrast to hardware. This also explains why most schools or sects of alternative medicine are system-forming and dogmatic, i.e., they simplify the more demanding functional, truly holistic approach. This can only be an open system, based on physiology, which after all is even more complicated than anatomy.

D. D. Palmer's "hole in one" theory offers a good example from chiropractic history. He thought that all the problems of the spinal column (if not of the whole organism) can be solved by adjusting atlas/ axis, or of Illi (the Swiss chiropractor) who believed in the supreme importance of the pelvis. Earlier chiropractors and osteopaths believed that all health problems were the result of spinal "subluxation" or "osteopathic lesion," interfering with the flow of "energy" from the brain to internal organs: simple and satisfying. Once we practice manipulative techniques, however, we sooner or later find that the changes we diagnose (mainly by manual methods) are not just haphazard, but follow certain rules. Very frequently when we treat the craniocervical junction, we observe responses throughout the motor system, which seem to follow a certain pattern. More importantly, the responses are by no ways limited to a particular segment of the spinal column, an accepted tenet of neurology. No less frequently, and quite regularly, we see responses at all levels of the motor sys-

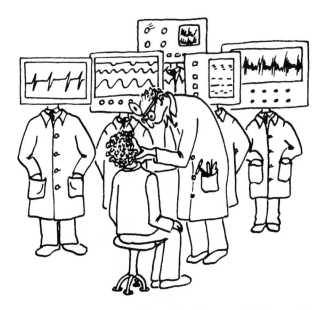

Figure 33.1 Cartoon. Clinical medicine and advanced technology.

tem. We thus learned to distinguish "key regions" (7) of the spinal column where treatment was particularly effective in producing such reactions. For a long time these observations were limited to the spinal column, ignoring feet, hands, and the orofacial system, putting the emphasis on joints and under-rating muscles and soft tissues.

It therefore seemed important to find out whether there is a rule governing these "repercussions" involving the motor system as a whole. We first speculated that what we called chain reactions corresponded to some "basic" functions of the motor system. These appeared to be gait, body statics, respiration, and prehension and food intake. This was certainly an important step explaining a good many clinical phenomena, but the predictive value was still limited. Gait seemed too centered on the lower extremities, prehension on the upper and food intake on the orofacial and neck region. From what we have learned now, this was not a sufficiently holistic approach. Thanks to developmental kinesiology we now have a better understanding of the correlation and interplay of all sections of the motor system.

Chain Reactions: Up to Date

Developmental kinesiology has been the subject of Chapter 23 (11,31). I can therefore point out briefly only those conclusions that seem essential to understand the chains that will be given in some detail.

The most important is the co-activation pattern, which is essential for human bipedal posture. Under normal conditions there is a well-balanced activity of the older, mainly tonic trunk (flexors) and the younger phasic (extensors), and the mainly tonic extremity flexors, adductors, and inward rotators, and the mainly phasic extremity extensors, abductors, and outward rotators. Disturbance of this equilibrium regularly results in a preponderance of the older tonic system, i.e., of trunk flexion and flexion with adduction and inward rotation of the extremities. Another very recent development is the postural function of the diaphragm (28) and the pelvic floor, which appear particularly prone to dysfunction. Another function found only in humans is active trunk rotation.

It may appear from these lines that chain reactions concern only muscles. This would of course be a gross error. The muscles are, however, under direct control of the nervous system and therefore responsible for the co-activation pattern. In dysfunction at any level, joints, too, become involved and so become the soft tissues (22). They then enhance and perpetuate the dysfunction. Disturbance of the co-activation patterns shows itself in painful lesions mainly in the form of trigger points (TrPs). This is a highly specific phe-

nomenon. Only a few muscle fibers harbor TrPs, and if a TrP is in a large muscle like the pectoralis it is regularly linked or chained-up with a TrP in its "antagonist" or more precisely in its "co-activation partner," in this case in the erector spinae. But here, too, it will be only in some muscle fibers—a specific localization in the pectoralis corresponding to a specific localization in the erector spinae. The same is true, e.g., for TrPs in the adductors and abductors at the hip.

This "patterning" of TrPs in antagonists has recently found confirmation in a paper by Radebold and Cholewicki et al. entitled "Muscle response pattern to sudden trunk loading in healthy individuals and in patients with chronic low back pain." The authors registered the reaction time of abdominal and back muscles to sudden loading and release and found an increase both on the ventral and on the dorsal aspect in the patients with low back pain (28).

There are also chain reactions in which the co-activation partners are in equilibrium and in which they are out of balance. If out of balance, we invariably find that the tonic muscles prevail over the mainly phasic muscles, and that posture is changed. Dysfunctional chains are an expression of an altered motor program; this takes time. Hence, we find them mainly in complicated patients with a lengthy history.

Imbalance of these muscle groups can result from stimulation (by Vojta's technique) in an unfavorable position, e.g., in reclination of the head; however, we find it also in many conditions that are stressful: depression and mere tiredness, as well as painful conditions, and also upper motor neuron lesions. In all these conditions we see the preponderance of the tonic over the phasic system. For rehabilitation, the first step was obviously inhibition of the tonic and stimulation of the phasic system. Dealing with (painful) chain reactions, we can distinguish those in which muscles with their TrPs are in balance, i.e., without alteration of posture, and those chains in which this equilibrium is disturbed in favor of the mainly tonic muscles.

Brügger's Approach (1,17)

In many ways, Brügger's approach is similar to ours: he, too, stresses the primary and fundamental importance of function. He also emphasizes the role of the periphery, particularly of the hands, the feet, and the eye (muscles), in which the most differentiated movements take place, and also that every function or dysfunction wherever it originates will affect the motor system as a whole. In full agreement with developmental kinesiology, he divides the spinal column into two sections: the upper to Th5 and the lower, lordotic from Th5 to the sacrum. The cervical section should be mainly straight. In Brügger's view, these are the best conditions for load-bearing. His clinical approach is determined by what he mostly finds in modern society, i.e., that the work force is sitting at the writing desk, in front of a computer or a panel, driving cars or tractors—in each case in a crooked position. For this state he uses the term "homo curvatus" and describes the entire clinical syndrome under the term "sterno-symphyseal syndrome." He speaks of "painfully tense and painfully week" muscles. Brügger, however, does not explain his findings by muscular imbalance, but by the position of joints and of the spinal column.

If the fingers and hands are in flexion and internal rotation, it is not possible to lift your arms to a full 180 degrees, and your shoulders tend to be drawn forward; if the arms are crossed in front of the chest, you cannot fully extend the spinal column in the thoracolumbar region and therefore tend to overextend the lumbar spine when attempting to straighten up. If your feet are in pronation and internal rotation, full extension is inhibited at the knees, and there is a tendency to adduction at the hip joint. In this position of the hip, extension of the lumbar spine is restricted; on trying to straighten up while sitting, there is overextension in the thoracolumbar region.

For therapy, the following principles should be followed: the trunk is in an erect posture with thoracolumbar lordosis up to Th5, and the neck is held erect with no reclination of the head. If the subject is seated, the upper extremity should be held in external rotation—(abduction), the shoulder girdle in retroposition, the lower extremities also in external rotation and abduction. This position corresponds exactly to that of a normal 3-month-old infant (prone or supine).

For specific treatment, stimulation of the most distal sections of the extremities is recommended, i.e., of the sections of the most differentiated phasic movements, which is also the region with the greatest number of afferents. Consequently active movement is recommended with the extremities extended and fingers (toes) stretched out and separated. Using passive movement, the hands (feet) are extended and in this position the patient extends the fingers (toes) against resistance, or resists the therapist's attempt to force them into flexion (Fig. 33.2). Resisted extension of the distal parts of both hands and feet inhibits not only the flexors at the hand or feet but also all flexor activity throughout the motor system, including, e.g., the hamstrings, thus improving the straight leg raising test! Mainly for self-treatment, Brügger makes use of an elastic band, with the patient exercising into extension against the resistance of the band (Fig. 33.3).

For postural training, the cog wheel principle (Fig. 33.4) is applied: the patient sits with knees apart and legs in external rotation. This places the pelvis in a slightly forward tilted position, allowing for a lordotic curve that culminates in the thoraco-lumbar area and ends in the mid-thoracic region. The cervical region (above Th4) should be mainly straight. Trunk stabilization results from the activity of the deep abdominal muscles from below and the descending fibers of the pectoralis from above (cog wheel mechanism).

To facilitate mobility in the cervical region, Brügger recommends following the moving hands with the eyes. Stiffness in the thoracic region is overcome by a rocking movement in the mid thoracic region (Fig. 33.5) with the patient seated and his/her legs apart in external rotation.

It is obvious that what Brügger expresses in terms of posture and joint function (dysfunction) corresponds exactly to what we and Janda, in particular, express in terms of muscle imbalance as summarized in Table 33.1.

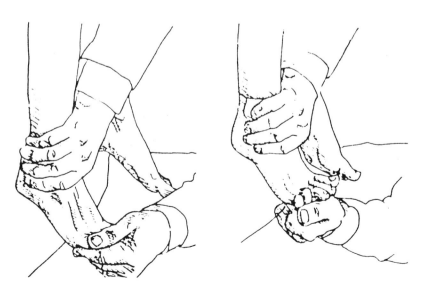

Figure 33.2 Plantar-resisted toe flexion-producing inhibition of flexor activity locally and generally.

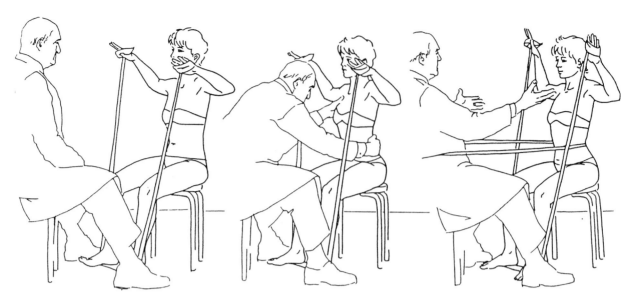

Figure 33.3 Exercise with the aid of the "Thera-band" inhibiting flexor activity (tonic muscles).

The Forward Drawn Posture (2) (Fig. 33.6).

Here, too, we are dealing with a chain in which the co-activation pattern is out of balance. Observing the patient from the side, we see the pelvic girdle in front of the cuboid and the shoulder girdle in front of the pelvic girdle while the head and neck, too, are in a forward drawn position. This full pattern, however, need not be present in all cases. We therefore have to rely clinically on muscle tension: if the point of gravity is shifted forward, balance has to be maintained by contraction of the back and neck muscles to prevent the patient from falling. The following clinical test, therefore, is diagnostic: if we find tension in the back and neck muscles with the patient standing and

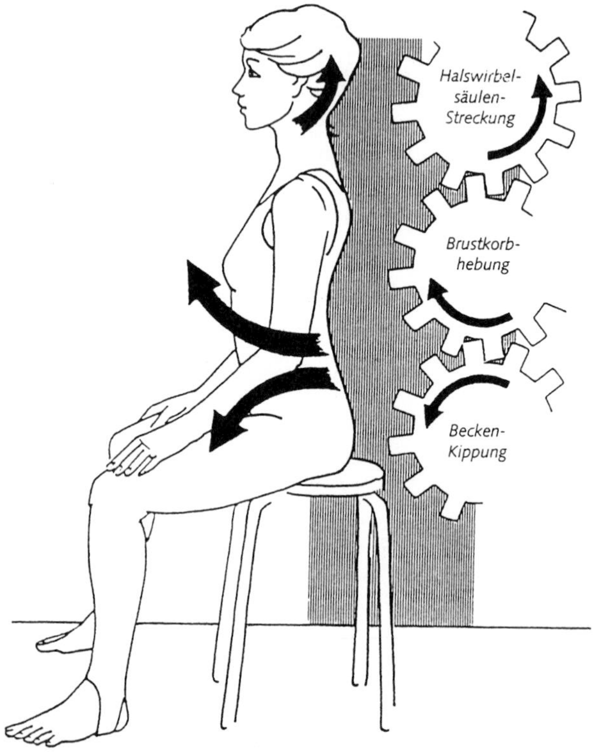

Figure 33.4 Diagram. Brügger's cog wheel principle.

Halswirbel-säulen-Streckung

Brustkorb-hebung

Becken-Kippung

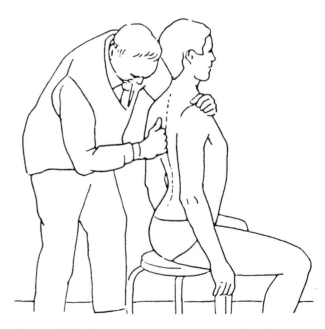

Figure 33.5 Brügger's rocking technique (for diagnosis and mobilization).

Table 33.1 (Mainly) Tonic Aphasic Muscles (3,8)

Hypertonus	Hypotonus
Short neck extensors, sterno-M. longus colli, capitis cleidomastoideus, scaleni rectus capitis anterior	
M. trapezius (upper part)	M. trapezius (lower part)
Levator scapulae	
M. pectoralis maior	m. infraspinatus, teres min.
M. subscapularis	deltoideus, rhomboidei
M. pectoralis minor	thoracic erector spinae
M. biceps brachii	triceps brachii
Forearm pronators and flexors forearm supinators and extensors	
Lumbar erectores spinae	recti abdominis
Hip flexors	gluteus maximus
Hip adductors	gluteus medius + minimus
Tensor fasciae latae	external thigh rotators
Hamstrings	m. vastus lat. & med.
Foot flexors	foot extensors

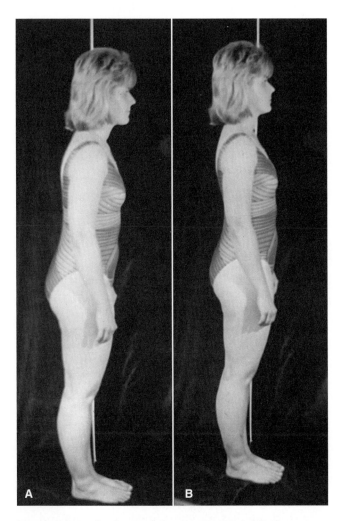

Figure 33.6 The forward drawn posture **(A)** before **(B)** after treatment.

looking at a point at eye level, and if tension is relieved when the patient is seated, looking at a point at eye level, the forward drawn posture is clinically relevant. Not only is it relevant but also can we conclude that the cause is not in the upper cervical region, but much lower down. The most constant finding in this syndrome is TrPs in the straight abdominal muscles. We are likely to find the following TrPs and joint dysfunctions (Table 33.2).

Because of tension at the attachment points at the symphysis and the tuber ossis ischii, the tuber ossis ischii appears lower and the pubic bone close to the symphysis higher on palpation where tension is increased (palpatory illusion!). In the literature this is frequently described as "upslip," "downslip," or "shear dysfunction" (after treatment, e.g., at the fibular head there is "reposition" and X-rays of the tubera ischiadica never change, although the difference on palpation can be up to 2 cm). Because forward drawn posture affects the motor system as a whole, symptoms can be present in all its sections: head and neck pain, less frequently chest pain, frequently low back pain, and even pain in the legs.

The proof that this is a chain lies in treatment of the most relevant link. This is usually the most caudal dysfunction found in this syndrome: at the feet, the fibula, the gluteal muscles, and even at the straight abdominals.

The "Nociceptive" Chain

Chains take some time to develop, particularly in patients with very painful chronic lesions like root

Table 33.2 TrPs and Joint Dysfunction in the Forward Drawn Posture

- In the cervical area at the SCM and the short extensors of the craniocervical junction, with reclination of the head and movement restriction at the craniocervical junction. On the dorsal aspect mainly TrPs in the upper trapezius with movement restriction at the cervico-thoracic junction

- In the thoracic area TrPs in the pectoralis and possibly at the diaphragm and in the dorsal erector spinae

- In the lumbar region most prominently TrPs in the rectus abdominis with painful attachment points at the lower arch of the ribs and the xiphoid, and at the symphysis, in the erector spinae, the gluteus maximus, sometimes at the pelvic floor and the psoas with the quadratus

- In the lower extremity in the biceps femoris with movement restriction at the fibular head and the short plantar flexors with movement restriction at the tarso-metatarsal joints

syndromes. In such patients we frequently observe that they have symptoms mainly on one side. That TrPs (muscular dysfunction) spread throughout one side is related to postural balance. If we stand and lean on or push with the right arm contracting the pectoralis, we also have to contract the right adductors, with the right shoulder-girdle being stabilized by the right pelvic girdle and lower extremity. The shoulder girdle is also stabilized by the head, i.e., the neck muscles, mainly on the right. This chain is therefore mainly one-sided, more frequently on the right side, and characteristic for chronic painful conditions. On careful examination we also find a much less marked reaction on the other side. In this chain the co-activation pattern is in balance and posture need not be altered. With the patient supine, we see, however, his shoulder, more frequently his right, jutting forward because of TrPs in the pectoralis. In typical cases we find TrPs mainly on one side in the following muscles (Table 33.3).

This chain need not be always complete; abortive cases (as in other clinical fields) are not uncommon. More importantly, we regularly find joint movement restrictions corresponding to the muscular TrPs: at the cranio-cervical junction related to the sternomastoid and the short extensors of the cranio-cervical junction; most of the cervical spine related to the diaphragm; the cervico-thoracic junction is

closely related to the muscles of the shoulder girdle; the mid thoracic spine to the pectorales and rhomboids; the upper ribs to the subscapularis; the psoas, quadratus, and the thoracolumbar erector spinae (with the latissimus dorsi?) to trunk rotation (the thoracolumbar junction), the rectus femoris to the segment L3-4, the piriformis to the segment L4-5, the iliacus to L5-S1; the tibio-fibular joint to the biceps femoris, the plantar muscles to the tarsometatarsal joints; and the biceps, triceps, supinator, and finger extensor to the elbow joint and to the mid cervical spine.

In addition, we find in the affected segments hyperalgesic skin zones. The most important soft tissue lesions, particularly in chronic cases, are dysfunctional fascias that do not easily move against bone. If this is the case, the "stuck" fascias inhibit the joints to move freely and thus perpetuate both joint and muscle dysfunction, i.e., the entire chain reaction (13).

Table 33.3 The "Nociceptive" Chain

TrPs in the cervical region

Sternocleidomastoids, scaleni, the short extensors of the craniocervical junction, the splenius, the upper trapezius, levator scapulae (on the same side)

TrPs in the thoracic region

Pectoralis major (with attachment point at Th4,5, pectoralis minor, diaphragm, subscapularis, serratus anterior, iliocostalis

TrPs in the lumbar (abdominal) region

Oblique abdominals, (rectus abdominis), longissimus, quadratus lumborum, psoas major

TrPs in the pelvic girdle

Pelvic diaphragm, short adductors, hamstrings, glutaei (maximus, medius), piriformis, rectus femoris, iliacus, tensor fasciae latae

TrPs in the leg and foot

Long toe extensors, tibialis ant., soleus, short flexors and extensors of the toes

TrPs in the shoulder girdle

Subscapularis (diaphragm) infraspinatus, supraspinatus, deltoideus, teres major, triceps (long head)

TrPs at the forearm and hand

Pronators, supinators (biceps brachii) long finger extensors and flexors, short finger extensors and flexors

The Chain of the Deep Trunk Stabilizers (24,32)

Stabilization training is the subject of some of the previous chapters. In this connection, it is very important that the muscles with a stabilizing function are linked, forming a chain that enables the therapist to choose the link most relevant and amenable to treatment. In our experience, the role of these muscles is such that this constitutes the most important and frequently treated chain, and because it is frequently found in combination with other chains it then represents the most important links (Table 33.4).

This conclusion is the result of a different approach to a problem that is quite rightly considered with the greatest interest in spinal rehabilitation. In 1989 Silverstolpe (18,25,26) published a paper in which he described the following reflex: by snapping palpation of a trigger point in the thoracic erector spinae, he induced a twitch reaction in the lumbar region, producing dorsiflexion of the pelvis. At the same time he usually found a pain point in the buttock laterally, at the level of the upper end of the tip of the coccyx. When this was so, pressure by his forefinger in the direction of the sacrotuberous ligament produced a sharp pain. If, however, he massaged this pain point, he obtained release and both the pain point at the buttock and the TrP in the thoracic erector spinae vanished. At the same time, many other symptoms the patient reported were improved (Fig. 33.7).

Pain in the low back, visceral pain, and even pain in the cervical region improved. Most curiously, as we then thought in many singers whose voice was dis-

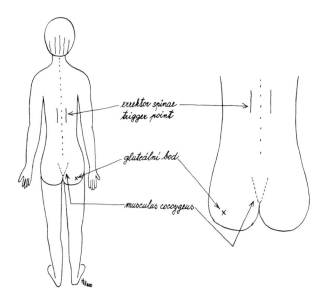

Figure 33.7 Diagram. The Silverstolpe reflex.

turbed he obtained immediate, spectacular results. He ascribed this to the sacro-tuberous ligaments.

When we had gained some experience with his method, we noticed that when we palpated what was supposed to be a painful sacro-tuberous ligament, we were met with resistance. Because massage produced much pain, we tried gentle pressure only, and obtained release, as is typical for myofascial TrPs! This made us suspect that the painful structure Silverstolpe (and we) was treating was not the sacro-tuberous ligament, but the underlying m. coccygeus on the pelvic floor. This seemed more probable, because the pelvic floor provided a much better explanation for the spectacular effects of the treatment.

The pelvic floor is one of the walls of the abdominal cavity and is essential for the respiratory function of the diaphragm. This readily explains the effect of the voice of his singers. While the Australian physiotherapists rightly stress the role of the transverse abdominis in trunk stabilization, it was obvious that this is also true for the pelvic floor and the diaphragm, because it is not a single muscle that stabilizes the lumbar spine, but the abdominal cavity with all its walls (Fig. 33.8). This then also explains why the TrPs in the (superficial) thoracic erector spinae immediately disappear with Silverstolpe's method: they are a compensatory mechanism in dysfunction of the deep stabilization system.

We were soon able to obtain clinical proof of our hypothesis. However effective the pressure in the direction of the sacro-tuberous ligament (M. coccygeus), the patient's symptoms recurred. In fact, some patients I saw in Silverstolpe's office had been there repeatedly. Therefore, we developed a method to

---

Table 33.4   The Chain of the Deep Stabilization System

- The core is formed by the pelvic floor, the deep abdominal muscles, the diaphragm, the deep layers of the erector trunci and the deep neck flexors;
- In close connection are the iliopsoas, the quadratus lumborum and the superficial layers of the thoracolumbar erector trunci.
- In a caudal direction we find TrPs in the adductors, the hamstrings (fibula) and in the muscles of the feet;
- In a cranial direction in the pectoralis, subscapularis, the scaleni, trapezii, the sternomastoids and in the masticatory muscles.
- Movement restriction is regularly found at the feet, the fibula, in the lumbo-sacral and thoracolumbar region, at the cervico-thoracic junction, in the cervical region, in particular at the cranio-cervical junction.

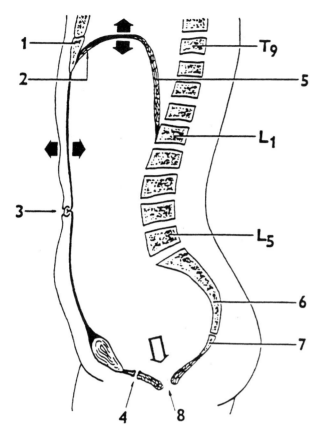

Figure 33.8 Diagram. The abdominal cavity and its walls.

on his/her side and is told to do the same at his anal region, warning him/her not to pull the buttocks together, but on the contrary to keep them relaxed and try to make a "sucking" movement, similar to that at the navel, which should be performed at the same time (Fig. 33.10). The patients have to concentrate on this and when they think that they can sense it, they are told to hold their nose and try to inhale against resistance, thus producing negative pressure in the abdominal cavity. This maneuver facilitates their attempt and they should sense it more distinctly. When this is so, we know that they have succeeded. Then, of course, we check up on the whole chain, which should be greatly improved, and of course the pelvic floor should be no longer be painful or at least be less painful at palpation. If this is so, we tell the patient to exercise the transverse abdominis and the pelvic floor several times daily, slowly and seated.

The next logical step was to bring the diaphragm into play. We knew, of course, that a painful gall bladder produces pain referred to the shoulder blade, and if palpation in the corresponding area was painful, we had the patient's gall bladder examined. The results were, however, frequently negative. This gave us the idea that not the gall bladder but rather the diaphragm was the source of referred pain. A simple experiment proved that this hypothesis was correct. Postisometric relaxation (PIR) of the diaphragm immediately stopped the pain. This is performed very easily: the patient sits and holds his/her nose, trying to inhale with his/her mouth shut. In this way an isometric contraction of the diaphragm is produced and held for approximately 10 seconds. After this he breathes out slowly, and the diaphragm relaxes. This is repeated. The patient should be taught to make the isometric contraction simply by shutting his/her glottis. At the end he/she makes a maximum exhalation (reciprocal inhibition). This technique is so effective that if pain

make our patients contract and relax their pelvic floor actively: once the patient had learned to do it himself, the effect was as prompt and intense as after the inevitably painful pressure. It is obvious that patients did not contract their sacro-tuberous ligaments.

The patient is first told to pull in his navel (Fig. 33.9), and we insist that this is not related to respiration. Once this can be done smoothly, the patient lies

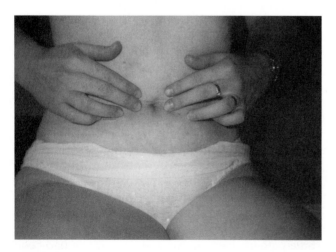

Figure 33.9 Pulling in the navel.

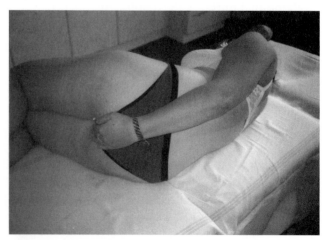

Figure 33.10 Pulling ("sucking") in the pelvic floor.

does not disappear we can exclude the diaphragm as a cause of pain.

The best way to diagnose TrPs of the diaphragm is with the patient seated in a slightly kyphotic position. The examiner stands behind the patient and palpates with his fingers under the arch of the ribs in a cranial direction. He then performs a snapping palpation by moving his fingers in a latero-lateral direction (Fig. 33.11). After PIR, no resistance should be felt at palpation.

To return to the chain reaction: we have mentioned the effect of the pelvic floor on the erector spinae and via the diaphragm on respiration (singing). We also find a similar correlation between the diaphragm and the pelvic floor, which of course is mutual.

The Australian physiotherapists approached the problem of the deep stabilizing system by training the transverse abdominis (24). The patient is supine and a cushion with a manometer is placed under the lumbar spine. He/she lifts the right and left leg in turn and has to maintain pressure on the cushion (Fig. 33.12A). This exercise has proved very effective, even statistically. It took the patients a few weeks to learn it. Training the pelvic floor and the diaphragm is usually achieved after one thorough instruction session, after which it is only necessary to check for

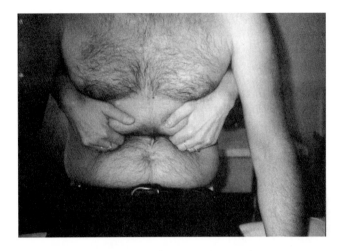

Figure 33.11 Palpation of TrPs at the diaphragm.

mistakes. Some patients are fit enough to use the Australian method of exerting pressure against a cushion. We now advise such patients to place their pronated cupped hand below their lumbar spine with the palm on the table. A soft layer of cloth on the hand makes it more comfortable (Fig. 33.12B). The patient should try to increase pressure with the hand and counter-pressure with the lumbar spine.

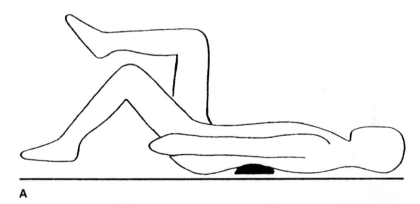

A

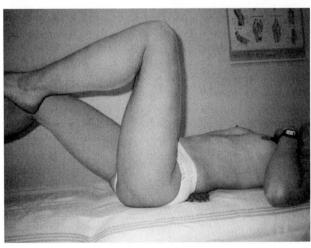

B

Figure 33.12 (A) Exerting pressure on a cushion placed underneath the lumbar spine, while lifting the legs. **(B)** Self-treatment using the cupped hand.

The deep stabilizing system would not be complete without mention of the deep neck flexors. Here the technique described by Jull (10) seems optimal. She again used a cushion placed under the cervical spine and measured the pressure the patient was able to exert on it without contraction of the sternocleido-mastoid (SCM), registered by EMG. This method can be very easily used for rehabilitation: with the fingers of the therapist placed under the patient's neck, he/she is told to press down on them; at the same time, the therapist palpates the SCM, which the patient is told not to contract. Once the patient has understood this, he/she can do it alone, placing the fingers under his/her neck and palpating the SCM with the other hand (Fig. 33.13).

The chain is usually more marked on one side than the other and it is not always complete. TrPs cannot be detected in the transverse abdominis and in the multi-fidi. We know by now that there is frequently no S-reflex and yet we find TrPs in the m. coccygeus and the diaphragm, which have to be treated. If there are adductor TrPs on both sides and TrPs in the quadrati lumborum and iliopsoas, we should suspect the pelvic floor and, in most of the cervical syndromes, the diaphragm. Obviously, TrPs in the diaphragm are more frequent in patients with symptoms in the cervical and the cervico-thoracic region and TrPs in the pelvic floor with symptoms in the lumbo-sacral region. The most important chains described so far frequently overlap, and we cannot exclude some arbi-trariness in deciding which chain was the most rele-vant in a given case. It seems, however, that what has recently been called the stabilization system is partic-ularly frequent; therefore, examination of TrPs of the diaphragm and the pelvic floor should become part of

routine examination. From July 1999 to July 2000, 390 new patients were examined in our office, of whom 112 presented typical chain reactions. In 73 cases, the decisive role was played by dysfunction of the pelvic floor and the diaphragm.

Not only do chains overlap but also are they fre-quently not complete; they may involve only the upper or lower part of the body or may even cross over to the opposite side. In the framework of the "big chains" described earlier, there are what we may call smaller chains of great constancy. One of the most important is the chain related to faulty breathing.

The Stereotype of Lifting the Thorax When Breathing

This is a very frequent and harmful stereotype linked to a large extent to the crooked sitting position. In fact, when sitting in such a position with the head in ante-flexion, it is difficult not to breathe in this way. In this type of respiration, the thorax is lifted instead of broadened. According to Kapandji, broadening of the thorax is mainly caused by contraction of the descending parts of the diaphragm, lifting the lower ribs, thus broadening the thorax from below (from the waist). This type of respiration is further enhanced by the activity of the obliqui externi lifting the middle ribs. In the crooked sitting position, the thorax cannot be broadened; instead of this, the scaleni lift the tho-rax as a whole, reversing the normal mechanism of respiration. In extreme cases there is even "paradoxi-cal respiration": the patient draws in the abdominal wall during inhalation and relaxes it on exhalation (Fig. 33.14).

The thorax can be compared to an upturned cylin-der with the diaphragm acting like a piston and the scaleni fixing the bottom. When, however, the thorax cannot broaden and is lifted, it is the scaleni that work like a piston. In this case, the punctum fixus is the cervical spine and the first ribs, which must be stabilized. The scaleni with the SCM pull the cervical spine forward, causing reclination of the head at the cranio-cervical junction. We therefore obtain the fol-lowing chain reaction:

TrPs in the SCM, the short extensors of the cranio-cervical junction, the scaleni, the upper trapezii, and levatores scapulae, the pectorales, the subscapularis, the diaphragm, and the upper section of the abdomi-nal muscles.

Therefore there is movement restriction in the upper cervical spine, in the cervico-thoracic junc-tion, and the upper ribs. In the chronic stage, the cervico-thoracic fasciae become adherent.

This chain is frequently connected through the diaphragm to the pelvic floor etc., or by the action of the upper part of the abdominal muscles to a forward

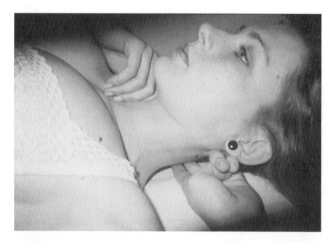

Figure 33.13 The patient exerts pressure on his own fin-gers placed underneath the cervical spine and with the other hand palpates his own SCM, which must stay relaxed, supine or standing against the wall.

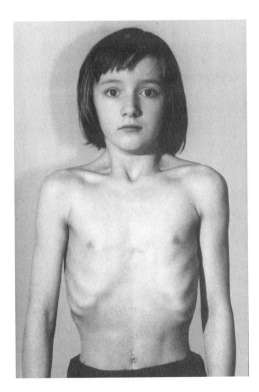

Figure 33.14 Paradoxical respiration.

drawn posture. It causes overstrain of all structures of the cervical region. It is best treated with the patient sitting erect with legs apart and in external rotation, the arms relaxed in supination, while he/she checks the position of the collarbones in a mirror: they must not lift!

The Chain of Food Intake—Mastication (16,17)

There is a very constant chain connecting the temporomandibular joint, the masticatory muscles, the digastricus, and the hyoid to the craniocervical junction with the short extensors and the SCM; this is further linked to the cervico-thoracic junction, the diaphragm, etc. This is the reason why the mandibulo-cranial syndrome is not easily distinguished from the cervico-cranial.

The Chain of Grasping (Epicondylar Pain)

Another short and constant chain is found in lateral epicondylar pain. It affects the following muscles attached there: the supinator, the biceps, and the long finger and wrist extensors; in addition, we regularly find a TrP in the triceps (the antagonist of the biceps). There is also restricted joint play at the elbow and dysfunction of the mid cervical spine. The muscles attached to the lateral epicondyle are essential for gripping, the basic function of the upper extremity (hence "tennis elbow").

The Chain of Restricted Trunk Rotation (15,27)

Another chain is related to trunk rotation. If we find TrPs in the psoas, the quadratus lumborum, and the thoraco-lumbar section of the erector trunci of one side, trunk rotation with the patient seated astride the table is restricted to the opposite side. Relaxation of any of these muscles will produce relaxation of the other two and restore trunk rotation. This short chain is frequently part of other chains, particularly of the deep stabilizers. Because active trunk rotation is only found in humans, it is very easily disturbed and frequently chained up with cervical rotation; in such cases, it is often the cause of cervical dysfunction and has to be treated first.

The feet and the fibular head can be key links in the nociceptive chain, in the chain of trunk stabilizers, and also in forward drawn posture! TrPs in the foot accompany movement restriction of the tarso-metatarsal joints. Restriction at the fibular head goes with TrPs in the biceps femoris, the main stabilizer of the pelvis.

Most of the chains discussed can be triggered by soft tissue lesions, particularly of fascias or by active scars (see Chapter 18). This is particularly true of the scalp and the fascias around the thorax, which can be even more important than the diaphragm and the subscapularis. Active scars are frequently more important than any other link in the chain.

Visceral Chains or Patterns

Visceral disease is another factor that may modify and even produce chain reactions in the motor system. Every nociceptive stimulus from the periphery (including the viscera) produces both a somatic and an autonomous response. In this respect, the motor system mirrors the entire organism. The clinical expression of this fact is what we call visceral patterns, i.e., typical patterns of motor system dysfunction characteristic of a specific visceral organ, and are therefore of considerable diagnostic value.

The Heart. If muscles work under ischemic conditions, pain is the result. The heart muscle, which must never stop working, is therefore frequently the source of nociceptive input, typically localized in the motor system, i.e., in the chest, left shoulder, and arm. This involves the following structures: the pectoralis, the serratus anterior, the subscapularis, the upper trapezius, frequently also the scaleni, and the SCM and the erector spinae, particularly in the segments Th3-5. There is movement restriction at the cervico-thoracic junction, the movement segments Th3-5 with the 3rd to 5th ribs. Side-bending to the left is restricted in the mid thoracic region. This pattern or chain is frequently part of larger chains, e.g., via the diaphragm to the pelvic floor, or via the SCM to the craniocervical junction (the nociceptive chain).

The Kidneys. Diseased kidneys become painful only if there is also reflex muscular involvement. The muscles harboring TrPs are most constantly the quadratus lumborum, the psoas, and the thoraco-lumbar part of the erector spinae, producing restriction of trunk rotation to the opposite side of the affected kidney (and TrPs). Here, too, we may have involvement of the pelvic floor producing TrPs also in the adductors, iliacus, etc. This is regularly the case in what is called nephroptosis. This condition results from generalized ligament laxity in particular in the pelvic region, i.e., instability causing the stabilization system to react. Hence, it should be mainly treated by methods of motor rehabilitation including the deep stabilization system.

Pain in Gynecological Conditions. Gynecological affections were formerly considered the main cause of low back pain in women. They should not be underrated even at present. They involve, most regularly, the following structures: the iliacus, the pelvic floor, the adductors and the lumbosacral, the sacroiliac joint, and the coccyx. Obviously, involvement of the pelvic floor will trigger off widespread chain reactions, as we have seen.

These very well known reflex conditions in visceral disease may serve as an example.

Finding the Key Link

The importance of chain reactions lies in the effectiveness of treatment if the (or a) key link can be found, because treatment of the key link brings about the normalization of the entire chain, or at least of most of it. This enables us not only to work more effectively but also to apply further treatment and rehabilitation to the region of that key link, which may be far from the site of the patient's symptoms.

This has far-reaching consequences for daily practice:

- Always examine the whole patient.
- Do not treat anything before completing the examination.
- Make a thorough analysis of your findings and choose which link to treat first.
- After this, re-examine the patient, in the first place the chain.

- If the result of your treatment is satisfactory, the patient should be taught self-treatment (if possible) or be sent for rehabilitation; if this is not the case, treat another link in the chain. Hence, choosing what seems to be the key link is also a diagnostic measure!
- If there are some additional findings outside the chain, or one minor remaining link in the chain that remains dysfunctional, treat them.

Criteria for the Key Link

- The importance of the dysfunctional structure. In the field of manipulation we use the term "key segment" (7). It covers the cranio-cervical, the cervico-thoracic, the thoraco-lumbar, and the lumbo-sacro-iliac regions. We now also include the feet and the mid thoracic spine, where the two lordotic curves meet and the spinal erector is weakest.
- But we also have to stress key muscles or key muscle groups: the masticatory muscles, the scaleni, the subscapularis, the diaphragm, the transversus abdominis and the pelvic floor, the adductors and the hamstrings, and the small muscles of the feet and the hands.
- No less important are soft tissue lesions, particularly adherent fascias on the back, around the thorax and neck, and the scalp. Perhaps most important of all are "active scars" (see Chapter 18).
- Disturbance of afferent impulses has been neglected so far. The striking effectiveness of exteroceptive stimulation in cases of disturbed sensitivity of the sole of the foot may reveal another most important key link (see Chapter 18 Appendix).
- The intensity of the lesion.
- Anamnestic data, where and how symptoms began, what made them recur, and what is the overall trend of the disease.

When choosing the first therapeutic step, it is good to bear in mind that if this choice proves wrong, it is of minor importance, for nothing or only very little has been changed, and we can immediately try another link. In fact, because the first step is as much of diagnostic as of therapeutic importance, we frequently make the first choice to disprove or to confirm our hypothesis. This chapter deals with chain reactions formed in the first place by TrPs. To put it into the right perspective, some explanation of the pathophysiology is appropriate. Because TrPs are the most relevant expression of pain, the reader may get the impression that their main role is to make patients suffer. The real cause of pain is, of course, dysfunction, and the typical response to pain in the motor system is immobilization. TrPs, as we know, go hand-in-hand with movement restriction. This explains why TrPs are usually found in the antagonists, restricting joint movement.

The same principle, although in a much more complicated way, applies to chains of TrPs that immobilize or stabilize erect posture, mainly in the sagittal plane. Stable equilibrium above the ball-shaped femoral heads at the hip joints, of the thorax above the pelvis, and of the head on the atlas is the result of muscular co-activation in the sagittal plane. One muscle provides the punctum fixus of its cranial partner in that plane, down to the feet. Chain reactions, as we have seen, can be traced throughout the whole length of the motor system. They give stability to erect posture. This is why dysfunction with TrPs of the deep stabilization system is particularly liable to provoke widespread reactions. For the same reason, it cannot be sufficient only to suppress these reactions but also to normalize function by active rehabilitation in the end.

Body Statics and Pelvic Obliquity

As we have seen, chain reactions are closely related to the co-activation pattern of flexor and extensor muscles in bi-pedal human posture, as developmental kinesiology shows. Similarly, pelvic obliquity can play a role only in bi-pedal posture, i.e., only in humans. In the frontal plane, however, balance (body statics) is not a problem only of muscular activity above the spherical femoral condyli; there are two supporting legs and the center of gravity of the human body should be between them.

Just as the ever-changing pelvic tilt in the sagittal plane has to be compensated by muscular activity, pelvic obliquity in the coronal plane may be held in balance by muscles. In fact, we do not usually stand with both legs stretched (at attention), but we stand at ease on the supporting leg, which is stretched at the knee, while the other leg is slightly bent. Pelvic obliquity is therefore a perfectly normal condition when standing at ease (the normal position). The same is, of course, true during walking, when bi-pedal support takes place only for a fraction of a second.

What actually happens in cases with a difference in leg length is that on walking, the person lifts his/her body (more) when stepping on the longer leg, which thus may be overstrained. From this introduction, it can be seen that pelvic obliquity has to be seen in its functional aspects. This implies that obliquity (while walking or standing at ease) has to be constantly compensated by lumber scoliosis

towards the lower side and (usually) above the thoracolumbar junction to the opposite side. Under normal conditions, the ensuing curvatures are in a state of static equilibrium. When the patient marks time in front of an X-ray screen, the scoliotic curves of the spine can be seen to oscillate from side to side around a fixed point at approximately Th12 (15).

The most frequent fallacy is to identify disturbed body statics with pelvic obliquity and with leg length difference (LLD), making LLD the main problem.

The first problem is that LLD cannot be measured by clinical means: measuring from the trochanters, we omit the femoral necks; measuring from the spina iliaca anterior superior, we include the hip bone; measuring from the navel, we include even part of the abdominal wall. But even X-ray measurement, "scanography," is not as reliable as may be thought because of (ante)torsion, which distorts the femoral neck. Only a difference between leg length below the knees can be measured reliably, but this may be compensated by a longer thigh, as happens during growth. Therefore, pelvic obliquity is usually examined by palpation of the iliac crests.

At first sight palpation of the iliac crests seems very simple. There are, however, two major pitfalls:

1. The iliac crests can be much higher than the upper end of the buttocks, and the most frequent mistake is to look for them by palpating just above the contour of the buttocks. Correct palpation calls for sliding from the ribs downwards, "landing" on top of the iliac crests! There may be very little space between the lowest ribs and the iliac crests. This is particularly so in hefty men with hardly any waistline and buttocks lower by several centimeters.

2. The second pitfall threatens when the pelvis is even slightly shifted to one side. In this case, the entire crest is deviated, too. Therefore, we must follow the deviating crest with the palpating hands, i.e., on the side from which the pelvis deviates; we must dig much deeper above the thigh. Without this, the side to which the pelvis deviates will always appear to be higher. Because a slight prominence of the hip on one side is very frequent, we find publications quoting a majority of patients as having "LLDs" (5).

Last but not least, it is frequently questionable whether there is any relevance in a LLD or, for that matter, in pelvic obliquity. The relevant problem is body statics and only if this is disturbed by pelvic obliquity, it may become clinically relevant. This, however, need not be the case for at least two reasons.

The relevant structure on which body statics depend is the promontorium, even L5, L4, and not the iliac crests. The promontorium can be oblique while the pelvis is straight and vice versa. Therefore, if pelvic obliquity or LLD is corrected when the promontorium is level, this can only disturb body (spinal) statics (Fig. 33.15). The position and the tilt of the promontorium in both planes can only be assessed by X-rays. This is very important for yet another reason: the iliac crests can be level and the length of both legs equal, but there is obliquity at the promontorium or even at L5. There will then be the same static reaction as if there was pelvic obliquity including the promontorium (4,6,12,20).

> **Clinical Pearl**
>
> Some patients present with leg length inequality or pelvic obliquity (e.g., unleveling). Some of these patients may be decompensated by a lift. The reason is because the promontorium is level and there is no scoliosis; therefore, the lift could only destabilize the patient.

Even if there is obliquity of the promontorium, body statics need not be disturbed. The criterion of normal body statics in bi-pedal humans is that a minimum of muscle activity should be sufficient for its maintenance. Obliquity goes hand in hand with scoliosis and if this is in balance, body statics are nor-

mal (Fig. 33.16A). In fact, in cases of scoliosis, pelvic obliquity is frequently a compensation resulting in normal body statics. Scoliosis unless very marked is usually symptom-free. If this is corrected with a lift, the appropriate compensation is disturbed (Fig. 33.16B).

> **Clinical Pearl**
>
> In cases in which pelvic and promontorium obliquity are in balance with scoliosis, a lift can only decompensate the patient.

What then are the clinical criteria of disturbed body statics related to LLD and to pelvic-promontorium obliquity? If the patient's symptoms arise mainly in a situation of static load, e.g., standing. If disturbance of statics is caused by obliquity at the promontorium (L5, L4), correction may be indicated even with the patient seated (Fig. 33.17).

> **Clinical Pearl**
>
> Clinically significant pelvic or promontorium unleveling presents with symptoms that arise in static postures such as standing or sitting.

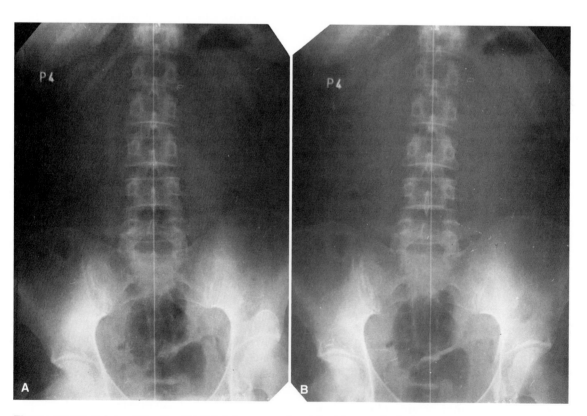

Figure 33.15 Pelvic obliquity. **(A)** Pelvis lower on the right (short right leg) with a horizontal promontorium and a straight lumbar spine. **(B)** With a right heel pad, obliquity appears at the promontorium and deviation of the lumbar spine to the left.

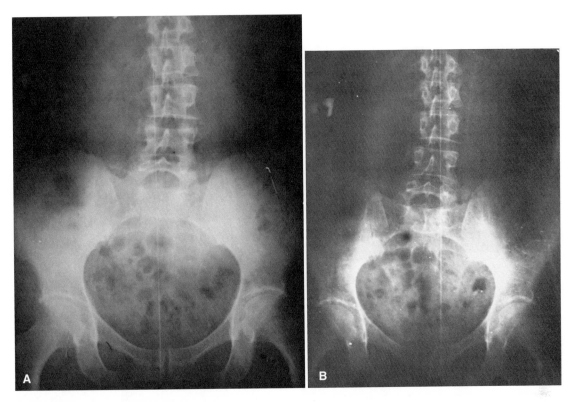

Figure 33.16 Pelvic and sacral obliquity caused by a short left leg. **(A)** Left scoliosis with deviation of the thoracolumbar junction to the left. **(B)** Less pelvic obliquity after application of a left heel pad, but no improvement in lumbar statics.

For correction of obliquity, we first have to decide its clinical relevance. We should then see whether there is also obliquity at the promontorium (L5, L4). This is only possible by using X-rays with the patient standing. If there is LLD, we should diagnose its cause. If it is the consequence of a fracture, we know that the organism may not yet be adapted and that correction is very probably needed. If it is because of leg deformity, this can be another problem requiring special measures.

There is, however, one frequent lesion, which should never be missed: a one-sided (relatively) flat foot. With the patient standing, we insert a finger under the foot from the medial aspect of either side. On the side of the flat foot, the finger penetrates less far. If the patient is then told to stand on the outer margin of his feet, the pelvis levels up! If this is the case, we know that pelvic obliquity is because of the flat foot, which requires our attention (rehabilitation, support).

If, after all, we still believe that LLD is the relevant cause of the patient's symptoms, we decide to correct it. This is an important decision, because it is only effective if the patient permanently wears the correction when standing or walking. In functional pathology, even differences of 1 cm may play a role,

as can be easily seen on X-rays (standing). The following criteria are important.

- The physiological reaction to LLD is deviation of the pelvis to the higher side. Therefore, putting a sole of approximately 1 cm under the short leg should correct that deviation (Fig. 33.18).

- The patient's reaction to the correction: a normal subject resents even 0.5 cm under one leg if told to put the same weight on both stretched legs. Hence, if the patient feels better with the heel pad or does not resent it, it confirms our assumption that correction is indicated. If, however, he feels worse, adaptation may be attempted, but not forced.

- It is advisable to check the correction on two scales: the patient stands on two scales, again being told to put the same weight on each foot. The normal error in our experience is up to 4 kg. If the difference improves with the heel pad, this is considered favorable; if it increases, it is not.

- As pointed out earlier, body statics are determined by the position of the promon-

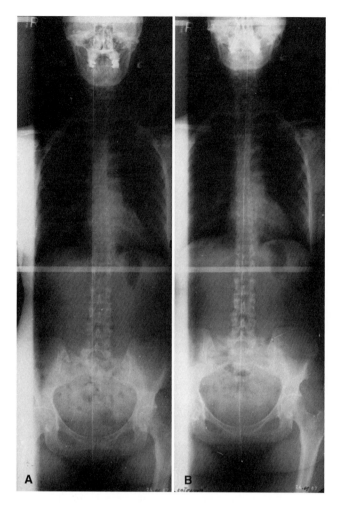

Figure 33.17 Sacral obliquity without pelvic obliquity. **(A)** Before correction. **(B)** After correction.

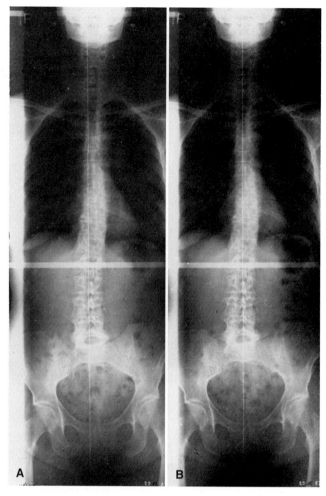

Figure 33.18 Pelvic and sacral obliquity caused by a short leg. **(A)** Before correction. **(B)** After correction.

torium, which can be assessed only by X-rays. Because correction has to be worn permanently, this is a far-reaching decision. Therefore, X-ray examination, preferably of the entire spinal column, with the patient standing is strongly recommended. His/her feet must be placed so that both heels are symmetrically below the center of the X-ray screen and he/she has to stretch the legs, putting the weight equally on both feet (Fig. 33.19).

Under normal static conditions, obliquity is followed by scoliosis to the lower side and deviation of the pelvis to the higher side; the thoracolumbar junction should be straight above the lumbosacral junction (on the same plumb-line), and the same applies to the odontoid and the occipital spur. It is particularly important to repeat the X-ray with the heel-pad to obtain objective confirmation of the patient's response to correction, because the patient's

spinal column may or may not "accept" the correction offered.

If correction is finally indicated, a simple heel-pad has the disadvantage of interfering with the fit of the shoes. It is therefore better to shorten the heel of the shoe on the longer leg or make the heel on the other side longer. This is for differences up to 1 cm. If differences of approximately 2 cm and more are to be corrected, there should be a higher sole on the shoe of the short leg, because lifting the heel only changes the function to the foot.

If obliquity is only at the promontorium (L5, L4), correction is advisable even with the patient seated, by placing a pad under the buttock (ischial tuberosity) on the lower side (Fig. 33.20).

As we have seen, the problem of LLD is closely related to the problem of spinal curvature. When dealing with chain reactions, the problem of muscular and joint dysfunction was our main interest. But here, too, spinal curvature, especially in the sagittal plane, plays a role.

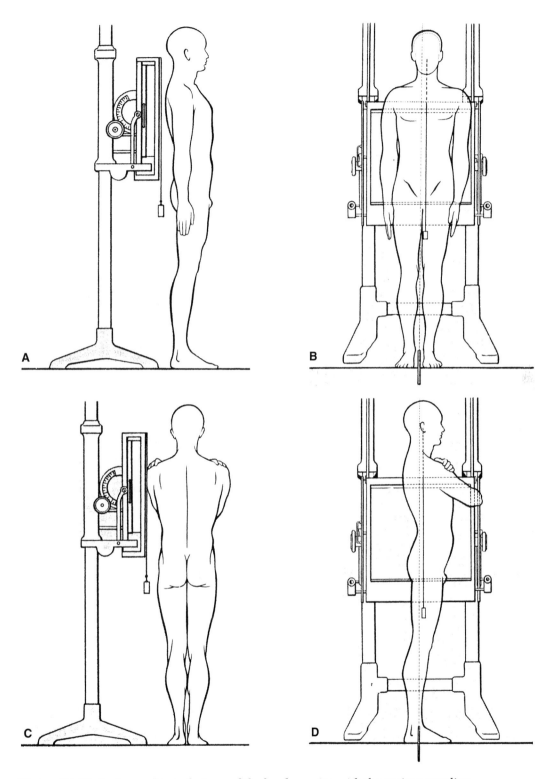

Figure 33.19 Radiographic technique of the lumbar spine with the patient standing. **(A)** Positioning of the movable plumb line. **(B)** Device prepared for radiographic examination, anteroposterior view. **(C)** Positioning of the plumb line. **(D)** Device prepared for radiographic examination, lateral view. (From Gutmann G. Klinisch-roentgenologishe Untersuchungen zur Wribelsule. In: Wolff HD, ed. Manuelle Medizin und ihr wissenschaftlihen Grundlagen. Heidelberg: Physikalishe Medezin, 1970:109–127.)

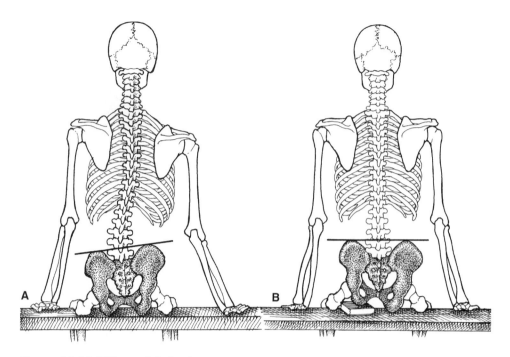

Figure 33.20 Effects of skeletal asymmetry due to a smaller left hemipelvis. **(A)** The tilted pelvis causes compensatory scoliosis, which tilts the shoulder - girdle axis. **(B)** A small ischial lift levels the pelvis on a hard surface. (From Figure 48.10 B & C, p. 932 from Travell & Simons' Myofascial Pain and Dysfunction: The Trigger Point Manual, Volume 1, second edition. Baltimore: Lippincott Williams & Wilkins, 1999 with permission.)

From textbook diagrams we are very prejudiced and believe in something like an "ideally normal" spinal column with a lordotic curve down to Th4-5 and another one down to the sacrum in the sagittal plane, and with an "ideal" straight spinal column in the coronal plane. Sollmann and Breitenbach (29) have shown on 1000 X-rays of the entire spinal column that such a view is untenable and that there is only what we should call an "individual" norm.

Also, that a spinal column without any minor scoliosis (and some rotation) is exceptional, as anyone familiar with X-ray pictures will readily agree.

What then are the relevant criteria? They are to be found in the physiological function of the spinal column and body statics. Rash and Burke (23) and Vele and Gutmann (30) have shown that body statics are normal if equilibrium is maintained with a minimum of muscle activity. This is precisely the case if the co-activation pattern, the physiological basis of chain reactions, functions normally.

For much the same reasons, we may conclude that spinal curvature can be considered normal if it subserves static function to the effect that equilibrium is maintained with a minimum of muscle activity. This is true for both the sagittal as well as the coronal plane, unless curvature is excessive, which then is not simply a problem of function. There is, however, one important point to be made from the view point of function: a flat spine (little curvature) tends to be more mobile or hypermobile, whereas increased curvature increases stability.

■ CONCLUSION

Correct pelvic obliquity only if there is clinical evidence of disturbed body statics after treating clinically diagnosed chain reactions including the deep stabilization system and respiration. Pelvic obliquity must then also correspond to obliquity of the promontorium (L5, L4), bearing in mind all the possible errors and pitfalls.

Audit Process
Self-Check of the Chapter's Learning Objectives

- Does treatment of relevant dysfunction depend on treatment of pathology or pain?

- How are Brügger's and Janda's patterns of muscle imbalance similar?

- What is the typical key link in the forward drawn posture?

- What is the relationship between abdominals, diaphragm, pelvic floor, and deep spinal intrinsics?

■ REFERENCES

1. Brügger A. Lehrbuch der funktionellen Störungen des Bewegungssystems. Zollingen und Benglen, Brügger Verl. GmbH, 2000.
2. Brügger A. Das Sternale Syndrom. Bern: Huber, 1971.
3. Chaitow L, Walker DeLany J. Clinical Application of Neuromuscular Techniques, vol 1. The upper body. Edinburgh: Churchill Livingstone, 2000:98–99.
4. Cyriax J. Textbook of Orthopaedic Medicine, 8th ed, vol 1. Diagnosis of Soft Tissue Lesions. London: Bailliere Tindall, 1988:262.
5. Edinger A, Biedermann F. Kurzes Bein, schiefes Becken. Fortschr. R"ntgenstr. 1957;86:754.
6. Greenman PE. Verkrzungsausgleich. Nutz und Unnutz. In: Neumann HD, Wolff HD, eds. Theoretische Fortschritte und Praktische Erfahrungen der Manuellen Medizin. Konkordia: Bohl, 1979:333–341.
7. Gutmann G. Die obere Halswirbelsle im Krankheitsgeschehen. Neuralmedizin. 1953:1.
8. Janda V. Introduction to functional pathology of the motor system. Physiother Sport 1982;3:39.
9. Jayson MIV. The problem of backache. Practitioner. Symposium on the rheumatic diseases. 1970;205:615.
10. Jull G. Deep flexor muscle dysfunction in whiplash. J Musculoskeletal Pain 2000;8:143.
11. Kolar P. The sensomotor nature of postural functions. Its fundamental role in rehabilitation of the motor system. J Orthop Med 1999;21:40–45.
12. Lewit K. Röntgenologische Kriterien statischer Störungen der Wirbelsäule. Manuelle Med. 1982;28:26.
13. Lewit K. Verspannungen von Bauch und Gesässmuskulatur mit Auswirkung auf die Körperhaltung. Manuelle Med. 1992;38:75.
14. Lewit K. The Functional Approach. J Orthop Med 1994;16:73.
15. Lewit K. X-ray of trunk rotation. J Manipul Physiol Ther 1997;20:454–458.
16. Lewit K. Manipulative Therapy in Rehabilitation of the Locomotor System, 3rd ed. Oxford: Butterworth-Heinemann, 1999.
17. Lewit K. Chain reactions in the locomotor system in the light of the co-activation patterns based on developmental neurology. J Orthop Med 1999;21:52–57.
18. Lewit K. Stabilisierung der Wirbelsule. Manuelle Therapie 1999;3:117.
19. Lewit K. Vztah struktury s funkce v pohybove, soustave (Relationship between structure and function in the locomotor system). Rehabilitace a fyzikalni lekarstvi 2000;7:99.
20. Logan HB, Hulti LJ. Textbook of Logan Basic Methods: Clinical Application of Basic Technique, 2nd ed. Chesterfield, MO: L.B.M., Inc., 1998.
21. Pribram KH. Language of the Brain. Englewood Cliffs: Prentice-Hall Inc, 1971.
22. Radebold A, Cholewicki J, Panjabi MM, Patel TCH. Muscle response patter to sudden trunk loading in healthy individuals and in patients with chronic low back pain. Spine 2000;25:947–954.
23. Rash PJ, Burke RK. Kinesiology and Applied Anatomy. Philadelphia: Lea & Febiger, 1971.
24. Richardson L, Jull G, Hodges P, Hides J. Therapeutic Exercise for Spinal Stabilization in Low Back Pain. Edinburgh: Churchill Livingstone, 1999.
25. Silverstolpe L. A Pathological erector spinae reflex— a new sign of mechanical pelvis dysfunction. J Manual Med 1989;4:28.
26. Silverstolpe L, Hellsing G. Cranial and visceral symptoms in mechanical pelvic dysfunction. In: Paterson JK, Burn L, eds. Back Pain, an International Review. Dordrecht: Kluwer, 1990:255.
27. Singer KP, Giles LGF. Manual therapy consideration at the thoracolumbar junction. J Manipul Physiol Ther 1990;13:83.
28. Skladal J, Skavran K, Ruth C. Posturalni funkce branice (the postural function of the diaphragm). Ceskoslovenska Fyziologie 1970;19:279.
29. Sollmann, AH, Breitenbach H. Röntgenanalyse und Klinik von 1000 seitlichen Röntgenganzaufnahmen. Fortschr. Röntgenstr 1961;94:704.
30. Vele F, Gutmann G. Die Beeinflussung der Posturalreflexe ober die Gelenke. Z Physiother 1971;23:383.
31. Vojta V, Peters A. Das Vojtaprinzip. Heidelberg: Springer, 1992.
32. Ward RC. Myofascial release concepts. In: Basmajian JV, Nyberg R, eds. Rational Manual Therapies. Baltimore: Williams & Wilkins, 1993:223–242.

34

Integrated Approach to the Lumbar Spine

Craig Liebenson, Scott Fonda, and Sylvia Deily

Learning Objectives

After reading this chapter you should be able to understand:

- How to evaluate functional stability
- The functional classification systems available for patients with "nonspecific" lower back pain
- The different rehabilitation methods to consider when a specific functional test is positive
- The continuum of care for the most common clinical symptom or tissue injury complexes

Introduction

Low back pain (LBP) and sciatica are common problems. They are usually self-limiting, but recurrent. Patients who seek professional health care usually have severe pain, are getting worse, or are simply not getting better in a reasonable time. These patients require a diagnostic triage to rule out "red flags" of serious disease. While necessary, this is not sufficient to properly manage the case. Other steps that are essential for the promotion of a self-management approach are identification of the patient's activity intolerances, functional deficits, work status, and "yellow flags" indicative of a poor prognosis.

Evidence is accumulating that specific impairment (functional deficits) clusters can be used to classify patients into meaningful treatment subgroups. This chapter integrates the functional assessment and treatment methods necessary for promoting self-management of activity limiting LBP and sciatica.

Diagnosis and Classification

The World Health Organization's classification of health and disease suggests a comprehensive strategy for patient assessment (4,63,67,74). An assessment of impairment (structural and functional), disability (activity intolerance), and participation (social/work) should be performed (Chapters 1 and 32) (27,67). Structural impairment is identified by a diagnostic triage (Chapter 7). Functional impairments screened for by a functional assessment will be reviewed in this chapter (Chapters 10 and 11). Disability is screened for by a history of activity intolerances. This can be quantified with outcome tools such as the Oswestry questionnaire (Chapter 8). Participation can be assessed with a subset of questions from the Chronic Pain Grading Scale (Chapter 32) (27,61,70).

Each patient's goals, concerns and worries should be identified (Chapters 14 and 32) (67). Finally, an assessment of yellow flags should be performed to determine the patient's future risk of chronicity (Chapter 9).

Diagnostic Triage

Current "state of the art" guidelines suggest performing a diagnostic triage to classify patients with low back problems into three distinct groups (see Chapter 3). The first group is patients with LBP caused by "red flags" of serious disease—e.g., tumor, infection, fracture, serious medical disease (<2%); second, caused by nerve root compression (<10%); or third, caused by "nonspecific" mechanical factors (85%–90%) (1,16,59) (Tables 34.1 and 34.2).

Table 34.1 Red Flags of Serious Disease (tumor, infection, fracture, serious medical disease)

- Age <20 or >50 years
- Trauma related to pain
- History of cancer
- Night pain
- Fevers
- Weight loss
- Pain at rest
- Immune suppression (i.e., significant corticosteroid use)
- Recent infection
- Generalized systemic disease (diabetes)
- Failure of 4 weeks of conservative care
- Cauda equina
- Saddle anesthesia
- Sphincter disturbance
- Motor weakness lower limbs

Subclassification of Nonspecific Back Pain

A limitation of this diagnostic triage approach is that, the overwhelming majority of patients are labeled with nonspecific or idiopathic LBP. Hopefully this will evolve because the most crucial of all "stake holders"—the patient—is dissatisfied with the diagnosis nonspecific back pain (6, 9). A report from the 2nd International Forum of Primary Care Researchers on LBP concluded that achieving a validated classification system for nonspecific LBP was their top research priority (7).

University of Pittsburgh Subclassification Approach

Over the past decade, evidence has gradually grown showing that back pain patients can be subclassified into meaningful treatment groups. Work at the University of Pittsburgh has shown that subclassification of the "nonspecific" group is possible with an evaluation consisting of a thorough history, disability questionnaires, and examination utilizing a battery of low-tech yet reliable tests (i.e., sacroiliac [SI], lumbar, pain centralization) (17–19,22,24–26,52,62). Initial research showed that treatment matched to the appropriate subclassification is superior to unmatched treatments (22). A randomized clinical trial (RCT) has confirmed that treatment driven by this subclassification is superior to the "generic" treatment recommended by the Agency for Health Care Policy and Research (1) for the broad "nonspecific" category (26).

The classification system is based on placing the patient in one of four mutually exclusive treatment categories (Table 34.3).

Table 34.2 Differential Diagnosis for LBP and Sciatica

Differential Diagnosis List for LBP of Musculoskeletal Origin

Discogenic Pain
   Herniated Nucleus Pulposus with or without
      radicular involvement
   Internal Derangement (annular tearing, etc.)
Facet-Mediated Pain
   Capsulitis/synovitis
   Osteoarthritis
Sacroiliac Joint-Mediated Pain
Myofascial Pain
   Muscular Strain (acute)
   Muscular Overload
Compression Fracture
Posterior Element Fracture
Acute Spondylolysis (adolescent—stress fracture;
   adult—traumatic)
Instability (spondylolisthesis)

Degenerative Disorders
   Osteoarthritis
   Degenerative Disc Disease
   Central or Lateral Canal Stenosis
Radiculopathy
   Compressive
   Inflammatory
Sciatic Nerve Entrapment/Irritation
   Piriformis Syndrome
Infection
   Discitis
   Osteomyelitis
Malignancy
   Metastasis, Multiple Myeloma . . .
Ankylosing Spondylitis

Fritz et al. reported moderate inter-rater reliability for the tests used in the subclassification (65% agreement) (19). The individual tests have been looked at by others. The presence of a lateral shift can be reliably identified (k = 1.0) (62). When three out of four reliable SI tests are positive a high level of intertester agreement has been reported (k = 0.88) (13) (Table 34.4). Whereas this study used two observers, another study using 34 observers could not confirm the reliability—only 39% agreement (k = 0.26) (58). Figures 34.1 to 34.6 show these SI tests as well as common alternatives. The centralization phenomenon has been identified as an important clinical finding that can be reliably identified (24,25,35,57).

1. **Manual Therapy:** Patients with signs and symptoms that suggest movement restrictions of the lumbar or sacroiliac region are treated with joint mobilization–manipulation techniques and range of motion exercises.

2. **Self-Treatment:** Patients exhibiting the centralization phenomenon during lumbar range of motion testing are treated with the specific exercises (flexion or extension) that promote central-

ization of symptoms. Lateral shift is based on visible frontal plane deformity and asymmetric standing side bending.

3. **Stabilization:** Numerous findings from the patient's history or physical examination (e.g. frequent previous episodes with minimal perturbations, "instability catch") reportedly are associated with clinical instability, and patients with these findings are treated with a trunk strengthening and stabilization exercise program.

- A unique test for stability of the lumbar spine is a shear test where the patient is prone with the upper body supported on the table and feet on the ground. Posterior to anterior pressure is applied over the spinous processes. Then the patient lifts their legs in the air and pressure is re-applied. If the patient feels pain when the feet are on the ground and no or less pain with the feet in the air then it is concluded that they have instability which may respond to trunk extensor training (Fig. 34.7).

4. **Traction:** Patients with signs of nerve root compression who do not demonstrate centralization during the examination are treated with spinal traction.

Table 34.3 Treatment-Based Classification System (19,24,26)

- Manual Therapy (Lumbar or SI Mobilization)
- Self-Treatment (extension, flexion, lateral shift centralizers)
- Stabilization
- Traction

Table 34.4 Reliable Sacro-Iliac Tests

1. Standing Flexion Test
2. Sitting PSIS Palpation (asymmetry)
3. Supine Long-Sitting Test
4. Prone Knee Flexion Test

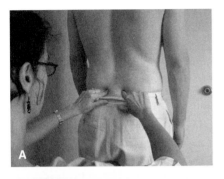
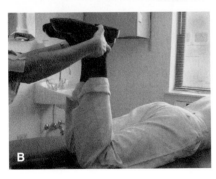

Figure 34.1A, B Standing flexion test.

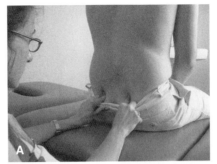
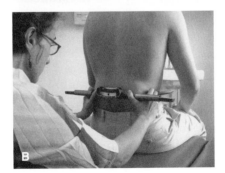

Figure 34.2A, B Sitting PSIS palpation.

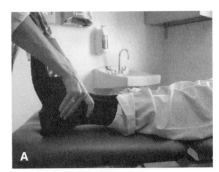
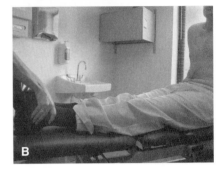

Figure 34.3A, B Supine long-sitting test.

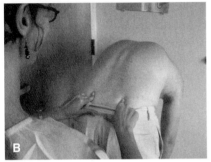
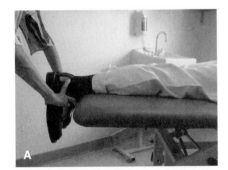

Figure 34.4A, B Prone knee flexion test.

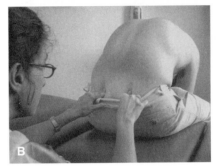
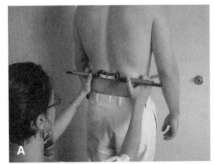

Figure 34.5A, B Iliac crest height standing and sitting.

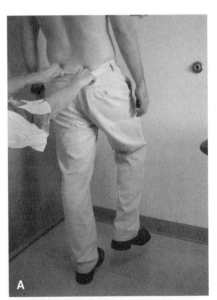

Figure 34.6A, B Gillet's test.

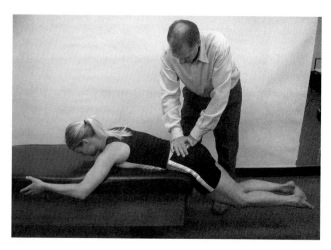

Figure 34.7 Shear stability test.

The manipulation category has been subjected to further analysis by investigating if a clinical prediction rule which can predict success with treatment by manipulation exists. It has been shown that there are five factors, which if any four of five is present in an acute LBP patient, the probability of success with manipulation rises from 45% to 95% (Table 34.5) (23). These five factors predicted who would improve at least 50% in 1 week with a maximum of two manipulations.

A more recent outcome based study found that 36% of LBP patients were positive on the rule (10). A patient who was positive on the rule and received manipulation has a 92% chance of a successful outcome, with an associated number needed to treat for benefit at 4 weeks of 1.9 (CI, 1.4 to 3.5). Patients who were positive on the rule and received manipulation outperformed those positive on the rule who received exercise or those negative on the rule who received manipulation. This was true initially as well as at 6-month follow-up.

McKenzie Classification

The McKenzie method by itself has been shown to be a promising classification system (reviewed in Chapters 1 and 15). Based on three types of studies, those reporting high reliability in classifying patients into subgroups (14,15,24,25,35,57); those showing out-

Table 34.5 The Clinical Prediction Rule for Low Back Pain

1. Pain less than 16 days
2. Not having symptoms distal to the knee
3. Fear–Avoidance Beliefs Questionnaire (FABQ) <16 points on the work scale
4. ≥1 hypomobile segment in the lumbar spine
5. ≥1 hip with >35° hip internal rotation

come predictability for centralization and non-centralization subgroups (20,33,39,60,71,72); and in a recent RCT (40) reporting that the large subgroup found at baseline to have a directional preference had superior outcomes using their concordant direction of exercise compared with evidence-based care or patients treated with the opposite direction of exercise.

Patients are classified into postural, dysfunction, or derangement syndromes based on distinctly different responses to a standardized clinical assessment. The derangement syndrome with directional preference is by far the most common category of LBP patients.

Postural Syndrome

Assessment—Typical pain provoked by sustained end-range, static loading (the history is typically decisive, as sustained loading is required for a variable period of time to reproduce the patient's characteristic symptoms). The portion of the physical examination that confirms postural pain includes the absence of symptoms:

- in neutral positions
- with full range of movement
- with repeated test movements in any direction

The only positive examination finding would be reproduction of concordant (e.g. consistent with pain of chief symptom) pain with prolonged (sustained) end-range positioning, usually slouched sitting.

Treatment—Self-care utilizing postural advice to avoid prolonged end-range loading in the direction which reproduced the symptoms

Outcome—Immediate reduction in pain

Dysfunction Syndrome

Assessment—Concordant pain provoked only at end-range, usually in a single direction of limited or restricted mobility in any direction.

Treatment—Frequent end-range stretching of painful, hypothesized adaptively shortened structures performed repeatedly over weeks in order to remodel and lengthen painful shortened structures.

Outcome—Short-term discomfort with stretching followed by improvement in end-range symptoms and mobility

Derangement Syndrome

Assessment—Concordant pain produced, worsened, or peripheralized in some end-range direction(s), but reduced, centralized, and/or abolished in another single direction of end-range motion (referred to as the patient's "directional preference"). This is the only syndrome with mid-range pain.

Treatment—Repeated end-range exercises (loading) in direction which reduces, centralizes, and/or abolishes pain. Avoidance of repeated or static end-range loading in the direction found to produce, worsen, or peripheralize symptoms.

Outcome—Centralization of referred symptoms and elimination of local symptoms. Restoration of normal mobility.

Active Limb Movement Testing Classification

Shirley Sahrmann has proposed a testing system based on specific movement impairments related to provocation of the patients' typical pain (Figs. 34.8 to 34.13). Positive test findings have been shown to be related to pain intensity and functional disability in a group of patients with LBP or sciatica more than 7 weeks (n = 188) (66). The tests used have been shown to be reliable (64). Preliminary evidence suggests that classification based on this assessment can be valuable for guiding treatment decisions in LBP patients (41,66).

Canadian Back Institute Classification Approach

The Canadian Back Institute demonstrated the reliability of a pain pattern system utilizing key elements from the history and examination (73). They demonstrated 78.9% agreement amongst examiners utilizing their approach. Furthermore, unlike the successful McKenzie study mentioned, only minimal training was required. This approach is only in the preliminary stages of validation.

A Functional Screen

It is frequently difficult to pinpoint the specific pain-generating tissue responsible for LBP syndromes. Even in cases where a tissue-specific diagnosis is attained, the reasons behind its generation are often elusive. For these reasons, and to guide the rehabilitation effort, a thorough functional evaluation is needed. In fact, various functional deficits (impairments) have been shown to correlate with LBP (see Chapters 1 and 5). An adequate diagnosis for LBP patients must include both tissue-specific and functional elements.

Functional deficits may be categorized as quantitative or qualitative. Quantifiable functional tests have been covered in detail in Chapter 11. This section will provide an atlas of both quantitative and qualitative test of motor control. Deficits in strength, balance, coordination, and endurance represent the spectrum of motor control, which when lacking can place undue mechanical stress on pain-sensitive tissues, or lead to biomechanically unfavorable compensatory motor strategies.

The Lower Crossed Syndrome and the Spine

Janda emphasized the importance of muscle balance in function. The relationships between agonists, antagonists and synergists can be looked at in terms of coordination or timing. Deficits in mobility of joints near or remote from the lumbar spine can impact function. Pelvic, hip, knee, and foot/ankle joints should be evaluated for these deficiencies. For instance, poor hip mobility will cause a compensatory reaction in the spine. Subtalar hyperpronation is another example of a lower quarter functional deficit which can lead to compensatory movements throughout the kinetic chain. Observation of functional activities, either in isolated motions, or more complex weight-bearing functions can show these different motor control strategies at work, leading to a better understanding of individual patient function and a customized rehabilitation prescription.

A classic example of muscle imbalance is the lower crossed syndrome (Fig. 34.14). This is a typical postural overstress resulting from muscle imbalance (Table 34.6). The overactive/shortened muscles include the gastro-soleus, hip flexors, hamstrings, adductors, TFL, and piriformis. The underactive/inhibited muscles include the gluteus maximus, gluteus medius, quadratus plantae, peronei, and abdominal wall muscles. The erector spinae is often tight, but also loses endurance. Agonist-antagonist-synergist muscle imbalances are predictable. For instance, an ankle sprain will lead to inhibition of the gluteus maximus that will persist even after the ankle has healed (8).

A key concept for spine stability is load sharing. The hip joints are designed to handle high loads. The deep acetabulum and large surrounding musculature are capable of supporting these forces. However, if hip joint mobility is compromised, loads may transfer to the next available motion segment, typically the lumbar spine. It has been shown that decreased passive hip extension mobility is related to LBP (36,44,65), as is decreased hip internal rotation (12,21). Preliminary data from McGill suggest that decreased hip extension mobility may be predictive of disabling LBP (44). Van Dillon reported that chronic LBP subjects had less passive hip extension mobility than asymptomatic subjects (65). Studies in adolescents have documented that future episodes of LBP are correlated with decreased hip extension ROM (36).

Nadler et al. demonstrated that hip muscle imbalance is associated both retrospectively and prospectively with LBP in female athletes (48, 49). In particular, asymmetric hip extensor strength was significantly correlated with LBP incidence. Those with

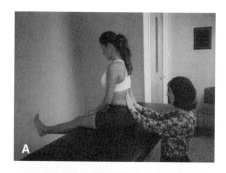

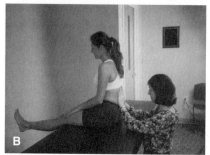

Figure 34.8A, B Knee extension in sitting.

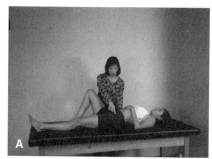

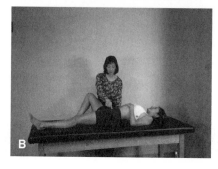

Figure 34.9A, B Hip abduction and lateral rotation in partial hook-lying.

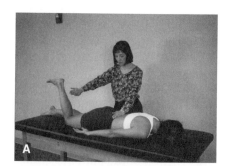

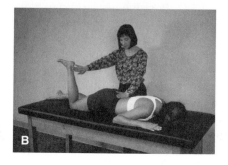

Figure 34.10A, B Knee flexion in prone.

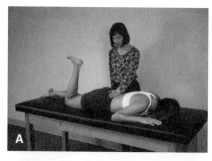

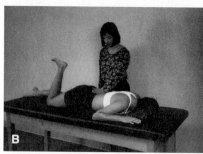

Figure 34.11A, B Hip rotation prone.

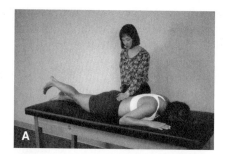

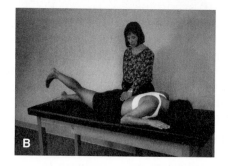

Figure 34.12A, B Hip extension prone.

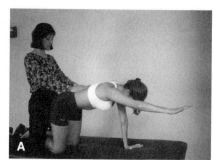

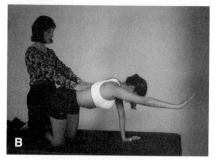

Figure 34.13A, B Quadruped arm reach.

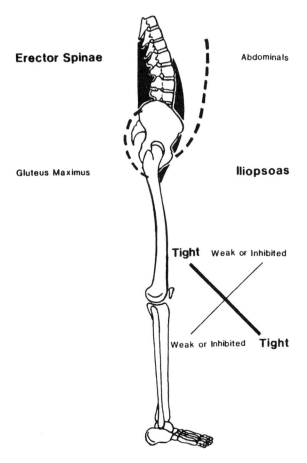

Erector Spinae

Abdominals

Gluteus Maximus

Iliopsoas

Tight Weak or Inhibited

Weak or Inhibited **Tight**

Figure 34.14 Lower crossed syndrome.

LBP had a 15% strength imbalance compared with only a 5.3% imbalance in those without LBP. This same asymmetry was not found in male athletes, but it is interesting to note that National Collegiate Athletic Association Injury Surveillance Data from 1997 to 1998 showed that female athletes were almost twice as likely as males to develop LBP (National Collegiate 1997–1998). Other consistent findings include increased fatigability of the gluteus maximus in individuals with chronic LBP (32,38). Vogt et al. found that reduced active hip extension (Janda's test) range of motion (ROM) and delayed relaxation of the gluteus maximus and lumbar erector spinae muscles can distinguish back pain subjects from asymptomatic individuals (68,69). Similarly, delayed relaxation of trunk agonist and antagonist muscles during func-tional tasks has been shown to distinguish LBP indi-viduals from asymptomatic people (11,55,56).

A positive active straight leg raise (hip flexion) has been shown to be associated with postpartum sacro-iliac (SI) pain (46). Sensitivity was 0.87 and specificity was 0.94 (45). It has been shown that altered kine-matics of the diaphragm and pelvic floor are present in those with a positive test (51).

A key factor in the lower quarter kinetic chain is gluteus medius weakness (54). Mascal et al. have demonstrated that a pelvic drop and excessive knee valgus during a step down task is indicative of con-tralateral gluteus medius weakness (42). Ireland et al. has showed this weakness is common in patients with knee pain (31). Specifically, deficits of 26% in hip abduction strength and 36% hip external rota-tion strength were found. Hewett et al. have shown in female collegiate athletes that supinatory training during plyometric squats prospectively reduced the incidence of injury in the coming season (28).

Gait abnormalities have been found to be associ-ated with LBP. Arendt-Nielson found both over- and under-activity in muscles during different phases of gait in chronic LBP subjects, but not in asymptomatic subjects (3). Overactivity of back muscles was found during the swing phase of gait and decreased agonist peak muscle activity during the double stance phase was found in LBP patients (3). Hussein has reported that stride length is decreased in the gait of LBP indi-viduals compared to normals (29,30). Lamoth and col-leagues recently found that pelvis-thorax coordination in the LBP group differed significantly from that in the control group (37). Specifically, they reported that a more rigid, less flexible pelvis–thorax coordination, and slower gait velocity characterized the gait of LBP patients versus asymptomatics. In asymptomatic indi-viduals as gait accelerates transverse plane rotation of the pelvis and thoracic regions becomes uncoupled because of counter-rotation. However, in LBP subjects this uncoupling did not occur.

Hyperpronation of the subtalar joint has been asso-ciated with the development of many musculoskeletal conditions. The mere presence of hyperpronation does not predict LBP; however, it may add to or perpetuate existing biomechanical stresses on the system, leading to overload elsewhere. Hyperpronation will create lower extremity internal rotation. If uncontrolled by

Table 34.6 Muscle Imbalance and Altered Movement Patterns

Weak Agonist	Overactive Antagonist	Overactive Synergist	Movement Pattern
Gluteus maximus	Psoas, RF	Erector spinae, hamstrings	Hip extension
Gluteus medius	Adductors	QL, TFL, piriformis	Hip abduction

Table Key: RF, rectus femoris; QL, quadratus lumborum; TFL, tensor fascia latae.

eccentric motor control, this can lead to mechanical stresses at the knee, hip, and lumbar spine (47). Ankle dorsiflexion of at least 10 degrees is also required for normal gait. The typical compensation for inadequate ankle dorsiflexion is increased pronation.

At least 60 degrees of dorsiflexion at the first metatarsal phalangeal (MTP) joint is required for normal gait. Less than this amount will change gait mechanics; typically a reduction in stride length and altered lower extremity rotation at toe off. Hip rotation demands then change and hip/spine mechanics are altered. First MTP dorsiflexion is inhibited in the hyperpronated foot.

Adequate dorsiflexion of the first MTP joint is also necessary to create sufficient tension in the plantar fascia, which in turn creates greater medial longitudinal arch stability. This process is known as the windlass mechanism and is essential for efficient toe off. Failure to attain adequate supination during terminal stance may lead to compensatory kinetic chain reactions contributing to not only foot/ankle problems, but potentially knee, hip or low back pain syndromes as well.

When combined in closed-chain functional activity, such as lunges, squats, or lifting tasks, these mechanical aberrancies can be observed throughout the lower extremity and spine. As hyperpronation or genu valgus are observed during single-leg squatting, the evaluation must attempt to measure how much and judge how well controlled? This is the essence of the quantitative and qualitative evaluation of movement.

Atlas of Functional Screens

The purpose of functional assessment is to identify a patient's functional or performance deficits and capabilities. The modern management of neuromusculoskeletal problems focuses on functional reactivation, restoration and rehabilitation. Structural problems such as herniated discs or arthritis are relevant in just a small percentage of cases, typically they are coincidental findings. Therefore, the functional assessment has become a pivotal and often misunderstood component in patient care.

For each test the patient's mechanical sensitivity (MS) and abnormal motor control (AMC) is noted. This atlas follows a consistent format for describing each test:

- Indications
- Procedure
- Score
- If positive, possible treatments to consider

  - Tissue to relax/stretch
  - Tissue to adjust/mobilize
  - Tissue to facilitate/strengthen

This functional assessment does not replace the initial diagnostic triage of patients, but rather complements it. Evidence-based consensus panel guidelines conclude that for over 80% of back pain the exact pain generator cannot be identified and the label nonspecific or mechanical back pain is applied. It is precisely because of this situation that the functional assessment is so important. Patients want to know what is causing their pain, and while a functional diagnosis does not pinpoint causality it does give the clinician essential targets for functional reactivation as well providing simple, inexpensive tests that can be used to audit the patient's progress towards functional goals and recovery.

Choosing the correct functional tests is an art not a science. Acute patients will receive a functional assessment limited mostly to range of motion (ROM) and orthopedic tests. Identifying the movements or positions that reproduce the patient's characteristic pain—their MS—is essential on an initial visit. This becomes an essential audit tool (e.g., post-treatment check) for adjudicating and legitimizing the treatment or exercise prescription, and thus motivating the patient. Once acute pain settles a more comprehensive functional assessment evaluating AMC can also be performed (Table 34.7). The tests chosen will be based on the functional goals or activity intolerances (AI) of the patient. In other words, identify what activities they want or need to do that they are having difficulty with. For instance if walking is an AI then assessment of balance, psoas length, Vleeming's SLR, hip abduction and hip extension coordination would be appropriate tests.

Table 34.7 Functional Screening Tests for the Lumbo-Pelvic and Lower Quarter Regions

1. Single-leg standing balance
2. Vele's reflex stability test
3. Squat
4. Single-leg squat
5. Lunge
6. Modified Thomas test
7. Vleeming's active & resisted SLR
8. Janda's hip abduction test
9. Janda's hip extension test
10. Side bridge endurance
11. Trunk extensor endurance
12. Janda's trunk flexion test
13. Trunk flexor endurance
14. T4 mobility—arms overhead test

1. Single Leg Standing Balance Test

Indications

- Elderly/fall prevention
- Poor balance
- History of ankle sprains
- Subacute musculoskeletal pain (MSP)
- In particular:
  - Lower extremity pain
  - Low back pain (LBP)

Procedure

- Instruction: Stand on one leg and look straight ahead (Fig. 34.15A)
- Patient chooses preferred one-leg stance position
- If they can do 10 seconds eyes open (EO), then use this instruction:
  - Stand on one leg and look straight ahead, focusing on spot on the wall in front of you.
  - Now, keep balancing and close your eyes (EC)
- Janda's variation
  - Eyes open
  - Foot of raised leg is at knee height and not allowed to touch stance leg

Score

- Patient gets up to five tries on each leg
- Pass if they can last 10 seconds with EC on both legs (optional, test up to 30 seconds)
- Fail if:
  - Stance foot hops or twists on floor
  - Either hand reaches for support
  - Foot is put down
- Normative data (5)—20 to 49 years 24 to 28 seconds; 50 to 59 years 21 seconds; 60 to 69 years 10 seconds; 70 to 79 years 4 seconds
- Janda's variation: Fail if there is a pelvic side shift of greater than 1 inch during the single leg standing balance test with eyes open (Fig. 34.15B)

If Positive, Possible Treatments to Consider

- Model "small foot" (passive, active-assistance, active) (Fig. 34.15C)
- Sensory–motor training
  - Single-leg balance (Figs. 34.15D, E)
  - Rocker board in all three planes
    - Static (holding still and level) (Fig. 34.15F)
    - Dynamic (moving)
  - Balance sandals (Fig. 34.15G)
    - Tiny steps without sandals
    - Supported tiny steps with sandals
    - Unsupported tiny steps with sandals
  - Balancing on Bosu
  - Balance reaches (arm or leg) (Fig. 34.15H)
- Functional training
  - Lunges (Figs. 34.15I, J)
  - Pulleys (Fig. 34.15K)

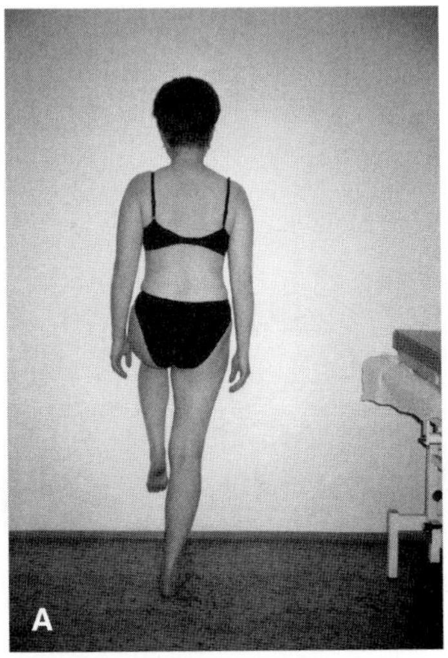

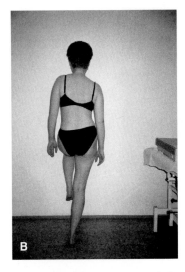

Figure 34.15A Janda's variation, single leg balance test.

Figure 34.15B Pelvic side shift.

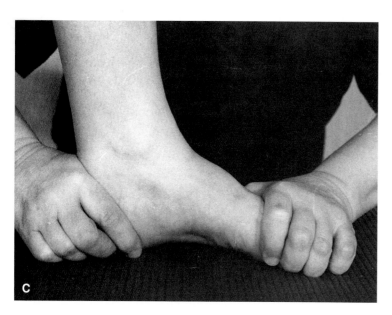

Figure 34.15C Passive modeling of the small foot.

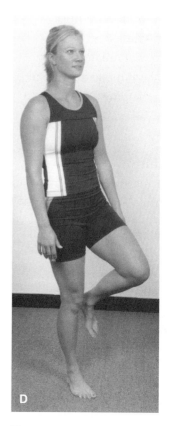

Figure 34.15D Single-leg balance on floor.

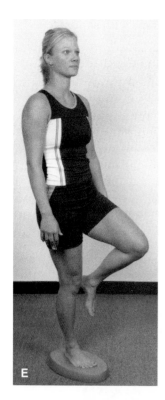

Figure 34.15E Single-leg balance on foam pad.

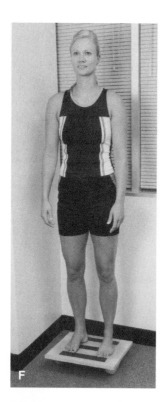

Figure 34.15F Rocker board.

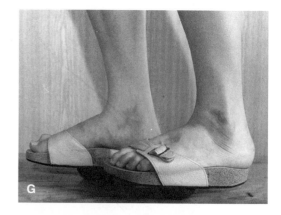

Figure 34.15G Walking with balance sandals.

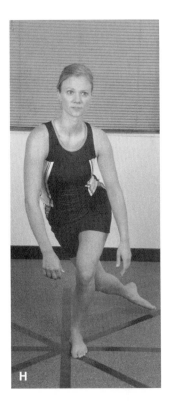

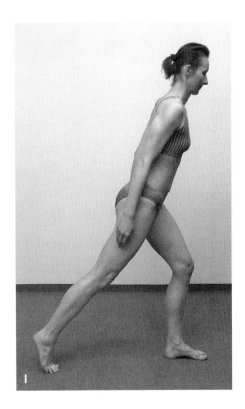

Figure 34.15H Balance reach (arm or leg).

Figure 34.15I Forward lean and step (Janda lunge).

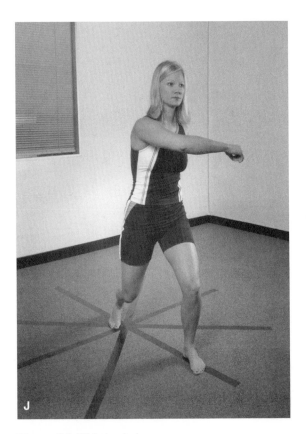

Figure 34.15J Angle lunge.

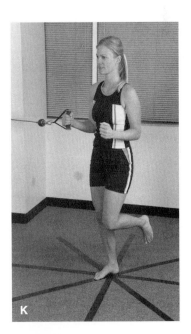

Figure 34.15K Single leg punch.

2. Vele's Reflex Stability Test of the Transverse Arch
(Fig. 34.16A)

Indications
- Stratification (Layer) syndrome
- Acute or subacute MSP
- In particular
  - Lower extremity pain
  - LBP

Procedure
- Lean forward from the ankles without bending at the waist

Score
- Fail if delayed or absent gripping of toes

If Positive, Possible Treatments to Consider
- Relax/stretch
  - Calf (Fig. 34.16B)
- Adjust/mobilize
  - Foot (Fig. 34.16C)
- Facilitate/strengthen
  - Intrinsic muscles of the foot (Fig. 34.16D)
    - Inchworm
    - Rolling towel
    - Picking up pencil
- Sensory motor training
  - Forward lean with toe gripping and side-to-side swaying (same as Fig. 34.16A)

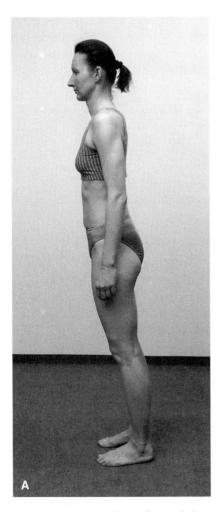

Figure 34.16A Vele's reflex stability test.

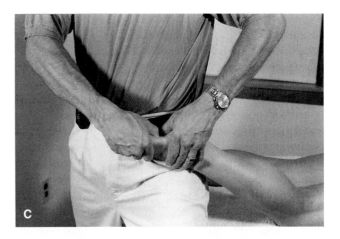

Figure 34.16C Foot adjustment.

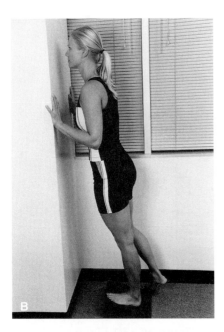

Figure 34.16B Calf stretch.

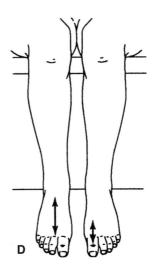

Figure 34.16D Inchworm. Reproduced with permission from Liebenson CS. Sensory-motor training. Journal of Bodywork and Movement Therapies. 2001;5;1:21–25.

3. Squat

(Fig. 34.17A)

Indications

- Lower quarter pain, in particular knee pain
- Back and neck pain
- Elderly
- Lifting occupation

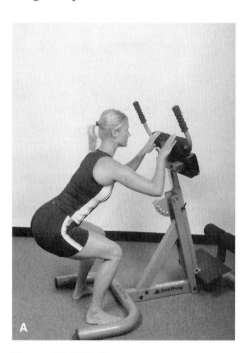

Figure 34.17A Squat test.

Procedure

- Stand with feet hip width apart
- Arms straight ahead, or supported
- Squat down until thighs are nearly parallel to the floor (less if acute or elderly)

Score

- Fail if:
  - Decrease depth of squat
  - Subtalar hyper pronation (Fig. 34.17B)
  - Knee valgus (Fig. 34.17B)
  - Knee flexion beyond line of toes (Fig. 34.17C)
    - Possibly due to restricted posterior hip capsule tightness
  - Lumbar hyperextension
  - Lumbar flexion (Fig. 34.17D)

If Positive, Possible Treatments to Consider

- Facilitate/strengthen
  - Bridges (Fig. 34.17E)
- Functional training
  - Squats (Figs. 34.17F, G, H)
  - Lunges (Figs. 34.17I, J)

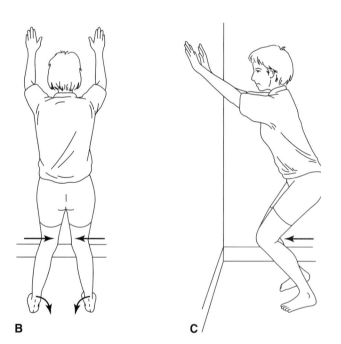

Figure 34.17B, C (B) Squat with hyperpronation and knee valgus. **(C)** Squat with knee beyond line of toes.

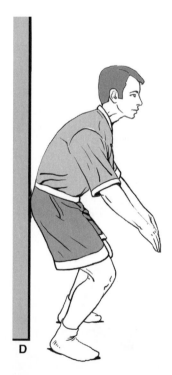

Figure 34.17D Lumbar flexion.

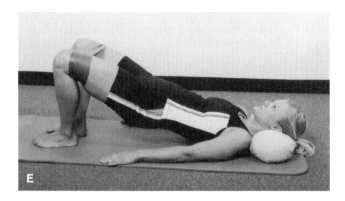

Figure 34.17E Bridge with band.

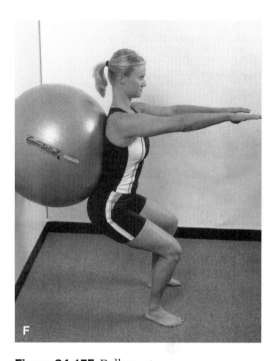

Figure 34.17F Ball squat.

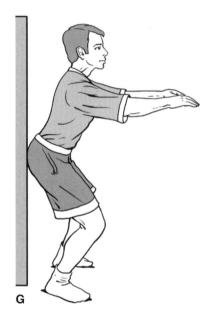

Figure 34.17G Squat with back to wall.

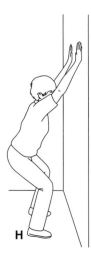

Figure 34.17H Squat facing wall.

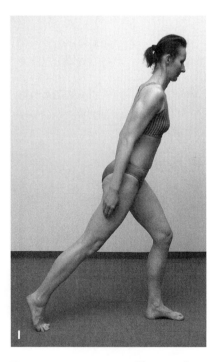

Figure 34.17I Forward lean and step.

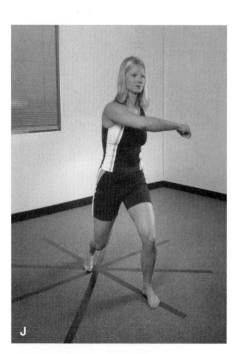

Figure 34.17J Angle lunge.

4. Single-Leg Squat Test

(Fig. 34.18A)

Indications
- Lower quarter pain
- LBP

Procedure
- Stand on one leg
- Perform a mini-squat

Score
- Fail if:
  - Inability to perform
  - Subtalar hyperpronation (Fig. 34.18B)
  - Knee valgus (Fig. 34.18B)
  - Knee flexion beyond line of toes
  - Trendelenberg sign (Fig. 34.18C)

If Positive, Possible Treatments to Consider
- Relax/stretch
  - Piriformis (Fig. 34.18D)
  - TFL and IT Band (Fig. 34.18E)
  - Posterior hip capsule release (Fig. 34.18F)
- Facilitate/strengthen
  - Gluteus medius (Fig. 34.18G)
  - Single-leg bridge (Fig. 34.18H)
- Sensory–motor balance training (Fig. 34.18I)
- Functional training
  - Single-leg squats (Fig. 34.18J, K)

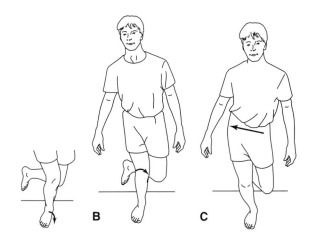

Figure 34.18B, C Single-leg squat with knee valgus, single-leg squat with Trendelenburg sign.

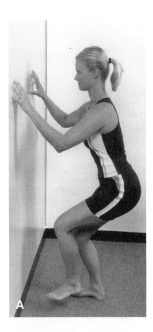

Figure 34.18A Single-leg squat test.

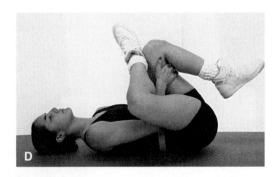

Figure 34.18D Piriformis stretch.

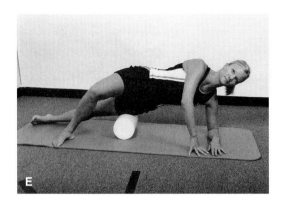

Figure 34.18E IT band release with foam.

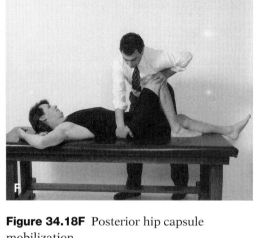

Figure 34.18F Posterior hip capsule mobilization.

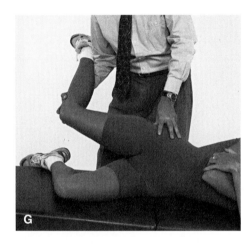

Figure 34.18G Sister Kenny gluteus medius facilitation.

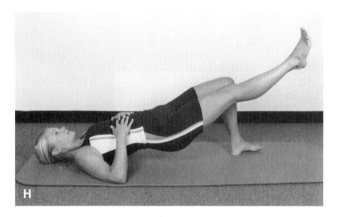

Figure 34.18H Single-leg bridge.

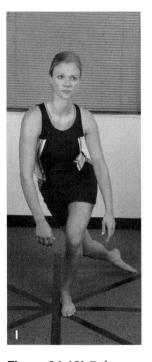

Figure 34.18I Balance reach.

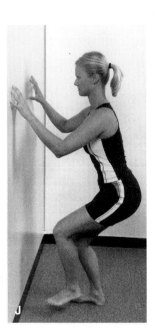

Figure 34.18J Single-leg squat.

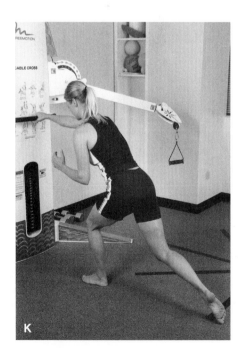

Figure 34.18K Supported running man.

5. Forward Lunge

(Fig. 34.19A)

Indications

- Lower extremity pain
- LBP

Procedure

- Step forward and kneel on the floor with one knee down
- Then, rise back up to a standing position

Score

- Fail if:
  - Inability to reach the floor with the back knee
  - Poor balance
  - Subtalar hyperpronation
  - Knee valgus
  - Knee flexion beyond line of toes
  - Trunk flexion (Fig. 34.19B)

If Positive, Possible Treatments to Consider

- Relax/stretch
  - Hip flexors (Fig. 34.19C)
  - Anterior hip capsule (Fig. 34.19D)
- Sensory–motor balance training (Fig. 34.19E)
- Functional training
  - Lunges (Figs. 34.19F, G, H)

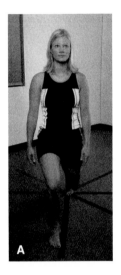

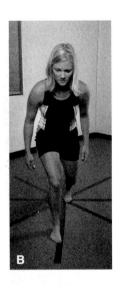

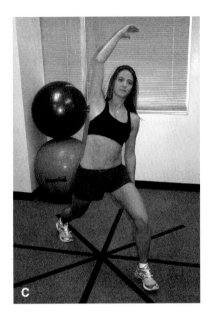

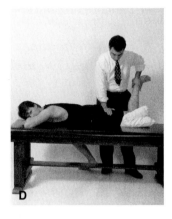

Figure 34.19A Forward lunge test.

Figure 34.19B Forward lunge with trunk flexion.

Figure 34.19C Psoas stretch.

Figure 34.19D Anterior hip capsule mobilization.

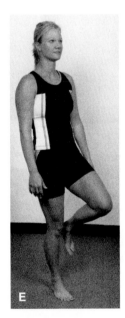

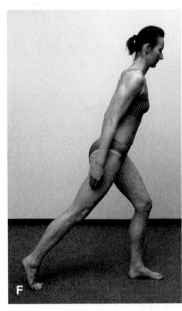

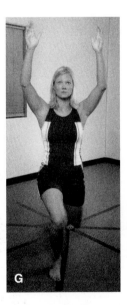

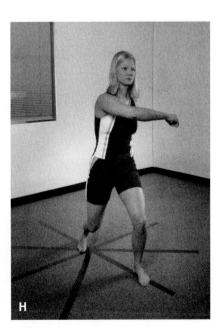

Figure 34.19E Single-leg balance on floor.

Figure 34.19F Forward lean and step.

Figure 34.19G Forward lunge with arms overhead.

Figure 34.19H Angle lunge.

6. Modified Thomas Muscle Length Test (see also Chapter 11)

(Fig. 34.20A)

Indications

- Subacute MSP

Procedure

- Patient perching at edge of table, bring one knee to chest
- Slowly lower him or her to the table
- Keep knee close to the chest so that the back remains flat
- Allow the opposite (tested) leg to dangle freely from the table

Score

- If the thigh is horizontal or above horizontal the hip flexors are shortened or hypertonic
- If the knee extends beyond 90°, the rectus femoris is shortened
- If the thigh does not extend below horizontal, but the knee falls at 90°, then the iliopsoas is shortened
- If the thigh abducts beyond neutral then the TFL is shortened
- If the thigh adducts beyond neutral then single joint adductors are shortened

If Positive, Possible Treatments to Consider

- Relax/stretch
  - Hip flexors (Fig. 34.20B)
  - Anterior hip capsule (Fig. 34.20C)
- Adjust/mobilize
  - Femoral nerve (Fig. 34.20D)
- Facilitate/strengthen
  - Bridge (Fig. 34.20E)
- Functional training
  - Squats (Fig. 34.20F)
  - Lunges (Fig. 34.20G)

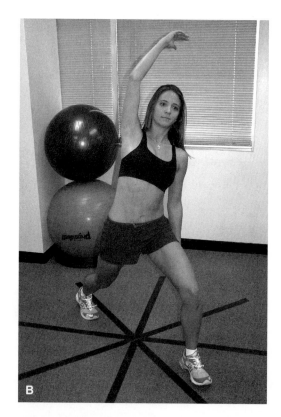

Figure 34.20B Psoas stretch.

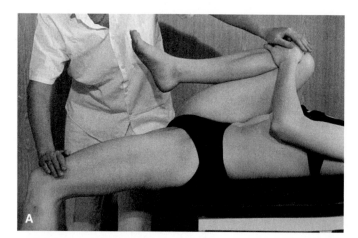

Figure 34.20A Modified Thomas test.

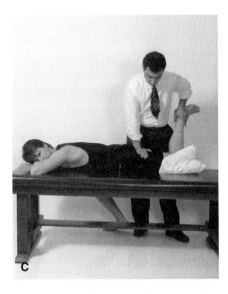

Figure 34.20C Anterior hip capsule mobilization.

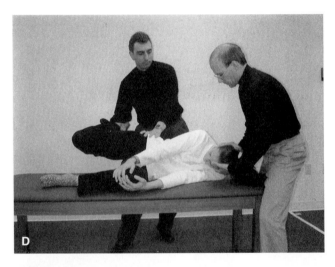

Figure 34.20D Femoral nerve mobilization.

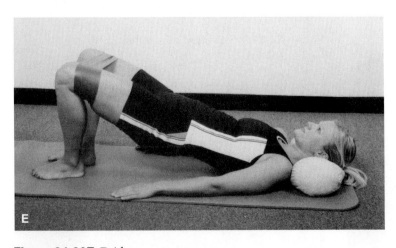

Figure 34.20E Bridge.

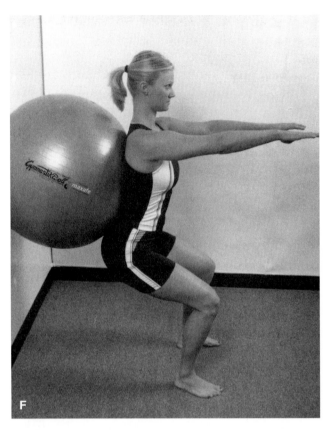

Figure 34.20F Ball squat.

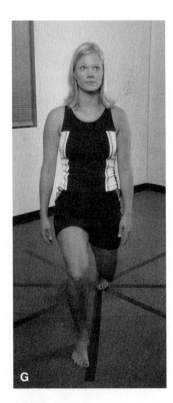

Figure 34.20G Forward lunge.

7. Vleeming's Active Straight Leg Raise

(Fig. 34.21A)

Indications
- Subacute LBP or posterior pelvic pain (45,53)

Procedure
- Supine, have patient perform a straight leg raise 20 cm up from table

Score
- Fail if:
  - Sacroiliac joint pain
  - Significant trunk rotation toward raised leg usually indicating inhibited/weak oblique abdominals
- Assess if active bracing improves response
- Grade muscle strength
  - Perform resisted strength test (with leg raised 20 cm from the table)

Note: Patient may place hands under small of back in order to palpate loss of pressure and trunk rotation with their hands.

If Positive, Possible Treatments to Consider
- Relax/stretch
  - Piriformis and hip flexors (Fig. 34.21B)
- Adjust/mobilize
  - Sacroiliac joint (Fig. 34.21C)
- Facilitate/strengthen
  - Bridge (Fig. 34.21D)
- Stabilization training
  - Core/trunk (Figs. 34.21E, F, G, H)
- Functional training
  - Squats (Fig. 34.21I)
  - Lunges (Fig. 34.21J)
  - Two-handed twist with cable (Fig. 34.21K)

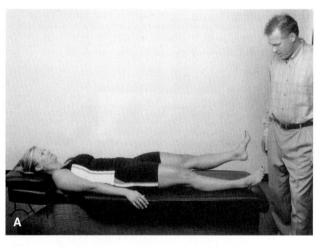

Figure 34.21A Vleeming's active straight leg raise.

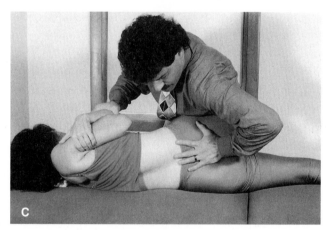

Figure 34.21C Sacroiliac adjustment.

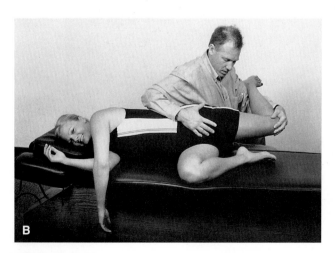

Figure 34.21B Psoas PIR.

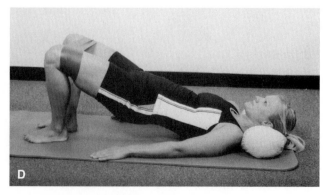

Figure 34.21D Bridge.

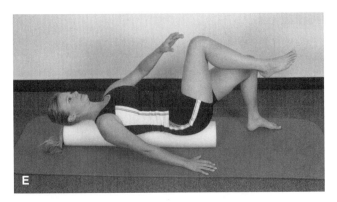

Figure 34.21E Beginner dead bug on foam.

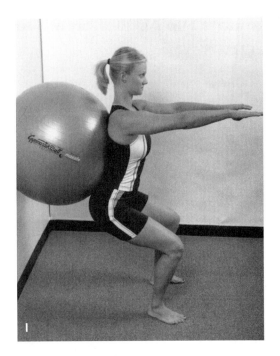

Figure 34.21I Ball squat.

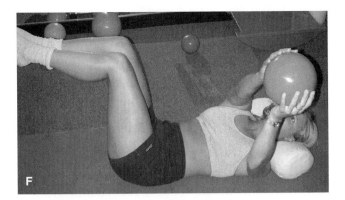

Figure 34.21F Dead bug with twist.

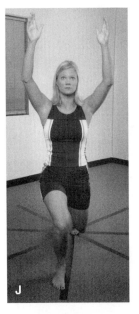

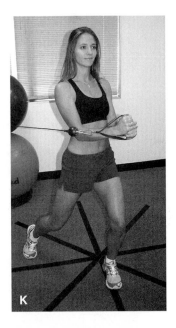

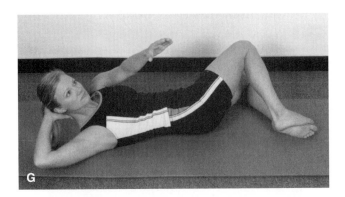

Figure 34.21G Oblique curl-up.

Figure 34.21J Forward lunge.

Figure 34.21K Two-handed twist with cable.

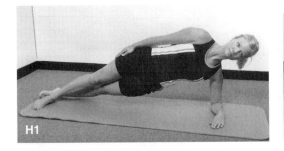
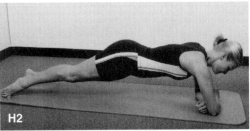

Figure 34.21H Side bridge from ankles with roll.

8. Janda's Hip Abduction Movement Pattern
(Fig. 34.22A)

Indications
- Lower extremity pain
- Ankle sprain
- IT Band syndrome
- Patello-femoral pain syndrome
- LBP
- Gait dysfunction such as hip hiking
- Quadratus lumborum trigger points

Procedure
- Side lying with lower leg flexed at hip and knee
- Pelvis perpendicular to the table
- Slowly raise leg straight up to the ceiling

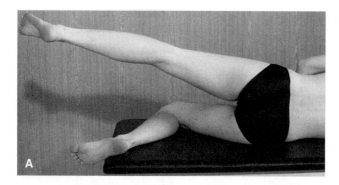

Figure 34.22A Janda's hip abduction test.

Score
- Fail if:
  - At initiation of movement, cephalad shift of pelvis indicates QL substitution (Fig. 34.22B)
- Fail if the first 40° occurs with:
  - Hip flexion—TFL substitution (Fig. 34.22C)
  - Hip external rotation—piriformis substitution
  - Pelvic rotation—substitution pattern indicating gluteus medius weakness
  - Reduced range of motion in abduction—adductor tightness
- Grade muscle strength
  - Perform resisted strength test with leg pre-positioned in 20° to 30° of pure hip abduction

If Positive, Possible Treatments to Consider
- Relax/stretch
  - TFL, piriformis (Fig. 34.22D), adductors (Fig. 34.22E), quadratus lumborum, IT band (Fig. 34.22F)
- Facilitate/strengthen
  - Gluteus medius (Figs. 34.22G, H, I)
- Sensory–motor balance training (Figs. 34.22J, K)
- Functional training
  - Gluteus medius (Figs. 34.22L, M)

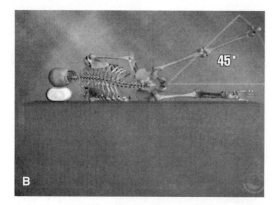

Figure 34.22B Cephalad shift of pelvis, quadratus lumborum substitution Liebenson CS, Chapman S. Lumbar Spine: Making a Rehabilitation Prescription. Lippincott Williams and Wilkins, 1998.

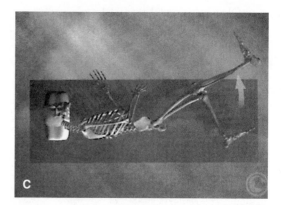

Figure 34.22C Hip flexion, TFL substitution Liebenson CS, Chapman S. Lumbar Spine: Making a Rehabilitation Prescription. Lippincott Williams and Wilkins, 1998.

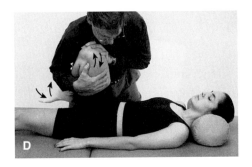

Figure 34.22D Piriformis PIR.

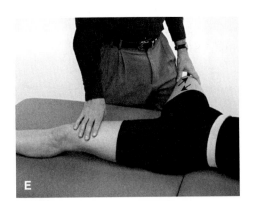

Figure 34.22E Adductor PIR.

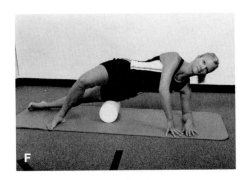

Figure 34.22F IT band release with foam.

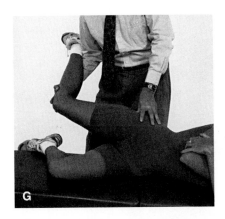

Figure 34.22G Sister Kenny gluteus medius facilitation.

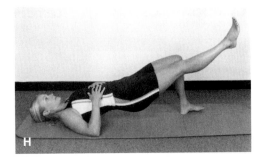

Figure 34.22H
Single-leg bridge.

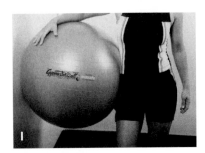

Figure 34.22I Wall ball.

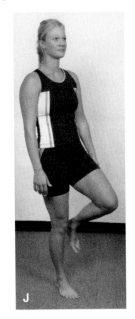

Figure 34.22J
Single-leg stance.

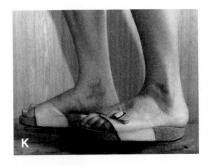

Figure 34.22K Walking with balance sandals.

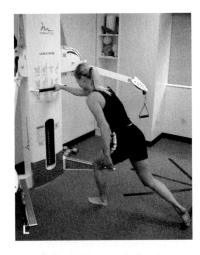

Figure 34.22L Single-leg squat.

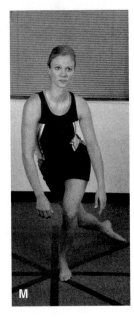

Figure 34.22M
Balance reach.

9. Janda's Hip Extension Movement Pattern

(Fig. 34.23A)

Indications

- Gait dysfunction such as lumbar hyperextension or decreased stride length.
- Subacute MSP
  - LBP
  - Ankle sprain
  - Neck pain

Procedure

- Prone
- Raise leg towards ceiling

Score

- Fail if:
  - At initiation of movement, anterior pelvic tilt occurs
- Fail if within the first 10° of leg raising:
  - Lumbar hyperextension or trunk rotation occurs (Fig. 34.23B)
  - Delayed activation of the gluteus maximus
  - Knee flexes indicates hamstring substitution (Fig. 34.23C)

Note: Patient may place hands under pelvis (ASIS) and palpate loss of pressure and trunk rotation with their hands.

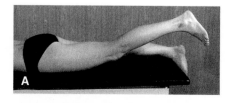

Figure 34.23A Janda's hip extension test.

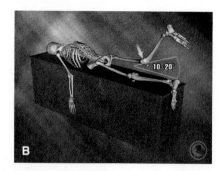

Figure 34.23B Anterior pelvic tilt. Liebenson CS, Chapman S. Lumbar Spine: Making a Rehabilitation Prescription. Lippincott Williams and Wilkins, 1998.

- Grade muscle strength
  - Perform resisted strength test (with leg in approximately 10° of hip extension)

If Positive, Possible Treatments to Consider

- Relax/stretch
  - Hip flexors (Fig. 34.23D), hamstrings
- Adjust/mobilize
  - Hip joint (Fig. 34.23E)
  - Femoral nerve (Fig. 34.23F)
  - Thoracic spine (T4–8) (Fig. 34.23G)
- Sensory–motor training (Fig. 34.23H)
- Facilitate/strengthen
  - Bridges (Fig. 34.23I)
- Stabilization training
  - Core/trunk (Figs. 34.23J, K, L, M)
- Functional training
  - Squats (Fig. 34.23N)
  - Lunges (Fig. 34.23O)

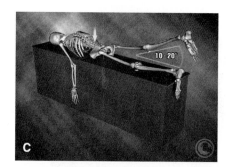

Figure 34.23C Hamstring substitution. Liebenson CS, Chapman S. Lumbar Spine: Making a Rehabilitation Prescription. Lippincott Williams and Wilkins, 1998.

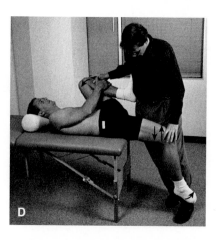

Figure 34.23D
Psoas PIR.

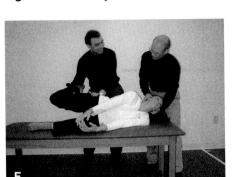

Figure 34.23E Hip traction.

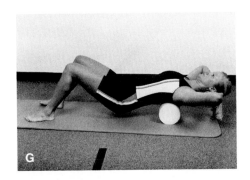

Figure 34.23F Femoral nerve mobilization.

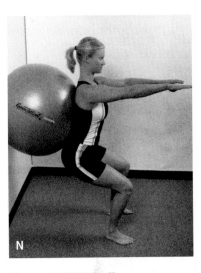

Figure 34.23G Thoracic spine mobilization.

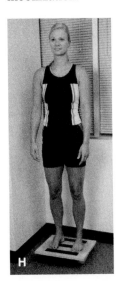

Figure 34.23H Rocker board.

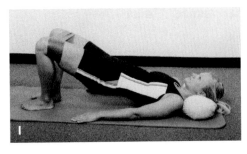

Figure 34.23I Bridge.

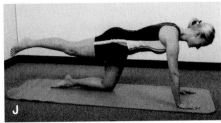

Figure 34.23J Quad leg reach.

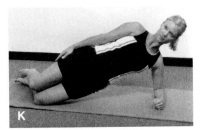

Figure 34.23K Side bridge from knees.

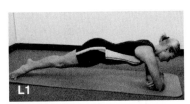

Figure 34.23L Side bridge from ankles, with roll.

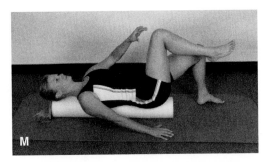

Figure 34.23M Beginner dead bug on foam.

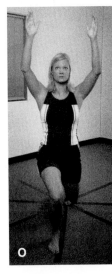

Figure 34.23N Ball squat.

Figure 34.23O Forward lunge with arms overhead.

10. Side Bridge Endurance Test

(Fig. 34.24A)

Indications
- LBP

Procedure
- Perform test on each side
- Raise pelvis from floor until spine is aligned
- Only feet and forearm/hand are on floor
- Ability to maintain position is timed

Score
- Record time to failure
  - When pelvis begins to lower, cue them to raise up again. The second time pelvis drops from it's peak height the time is recorded as the failure time.

- Quantitative data (see Chapter 11) (43)
  - Less than 45 seconds is dysfunctional
  - A side-to-side difference in time of greater than 5% is dysfunctional

If Positive, Possible Treatments to Consider
- Relax/stretch
  - Hip flexors (Fig. 34.24B)
  - Anterior hip (Fig. 34.24C)
- Stabilization training
  - Side bridges (Fig. 34.24D)

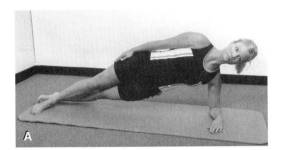

Figure 34.24A Side bridge endurance test.

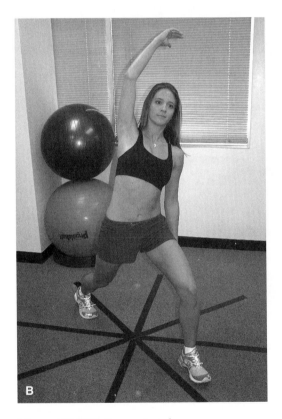

Figure 34.24B Psoas stretch.

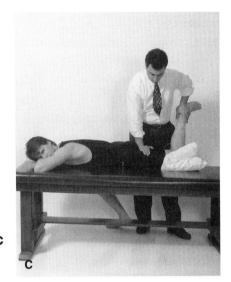

Figure 34.24C Anterior hip mobilization.

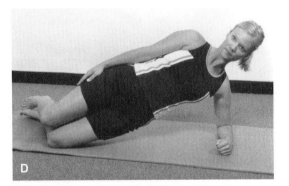

Figure 34.24D Side bridge from knees.

11. Trunk Extensor Endurance Test—Sorensen's Test

(Fig. 34.25A)

Indications

- Subacute or chronic LBP
- Prevention of LBP

Procedure

- ASIS supported at edge of treatment table or BackStrong machine
- Arms at sides or across chest
- Raise up until trunk is horizontal
- Ability to maintain position is timed

Score

- Record time to failure
  - When trunk begins to lower, cue them to raise up again. The second time back drops from its peak height the time is recorded as the failure time.
- Quantitative Data (see Chapter 11)
  - Less than 60 seconds is dysfunctional (2,43)
  - A back extensor endurance time that is less than a trunk flexor endurance time or side bridge endurance times is dysfunctional (43)

If Positive, Possible Treatments to Consider

- Relax/stretch
  - Hip flexors (Fig. 34.25B)
- Facilitate/strengthen
  - Trunk extensors (Figs. 34.25C, D, E)
  - Gluteus maximus (Fig. 34.25F)
  - Hamstrings (Fig. 34.25G)

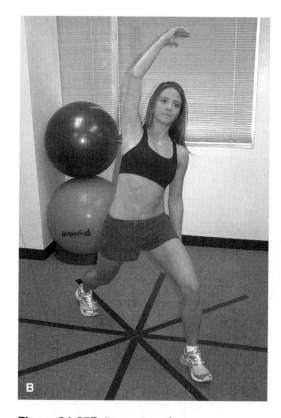

Figure 34.25B Psoas stretch.

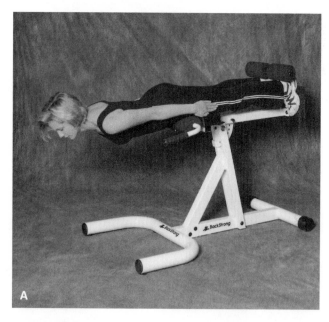

Figure 34.25A Trunk extensor endurance test.

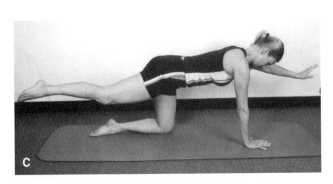

Figure 34.25C Quadruped opposite arm and leg reach.

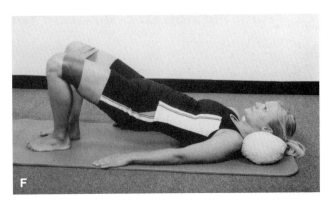

Figure 34.25F Bridge.

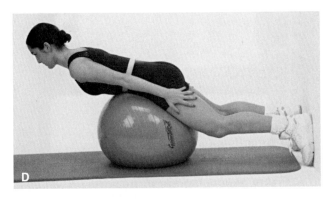

Figure 34.25D Superman on ball.

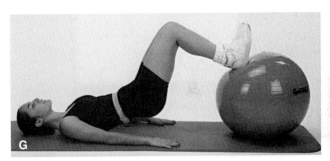

Figure 34.25G Hamstring curl.

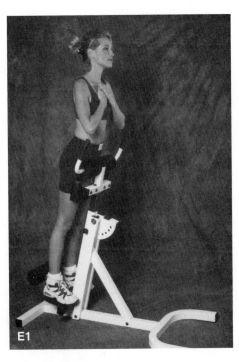

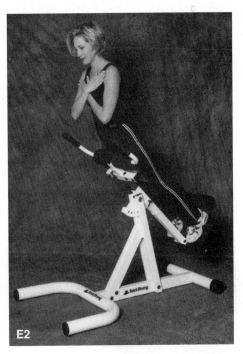

Figure 34.25E Back strong, beginner.

12. Trunk Flexion Coordination Test

(Fig. 34.26A)

Indications
- Subacute or chronic LBP

Procedure
- Supine with knees slightly flexed
- Perform curl-up until scapulae are off the table/floor
- Alternative test:
  - Cup heels and ask subject to exert downward pressure with heels and then perform curl-up

Score
- Fail if:
  - Feet rise up from table before scapulae come off the table (major dysfunction) (Fig. 34.26B)
  - Downward pressure lost prior to scapulae lifting completely up (minor dysfunction)

Note: Hyperlordotic patients may have a false positive since it takes much more effort to curl-up

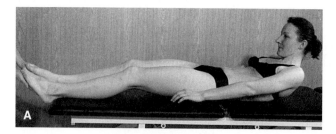

Figure 34.26A Trunk flexion test.

If Positive, Possible Treatments to Consider
- Relax/stretch
  - Hip flexors (Fig. 34.26C)
- Stabilization training
  - Core/trunk (Figs. 34.26D–H)
- Functional training
  - Core/trunk (Figs. 34.26I–K)

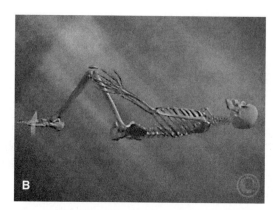

Figure 34.26B Feet rise up from table before scapulae come completely off, Liebenson CS, Chapman S. Lumbar Spine: Making a Rehabilitation Prescription. Lippincott Williams and Wilkins, 1998.

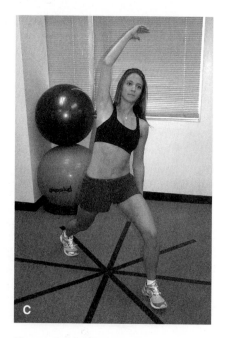

Figure 34.26C Psoas stretch.

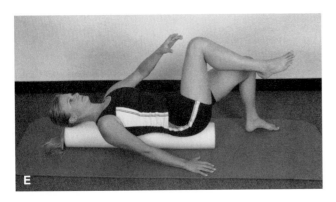

Figure 34.26D Basic curl-up.

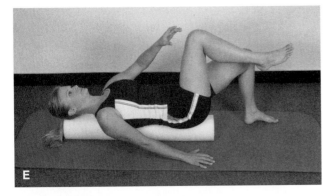

Figure 34.26E Beginner dead bug on foam.

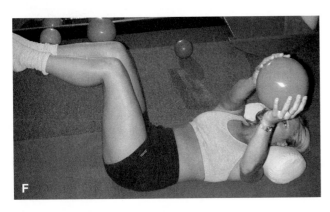

Figure 34.26F Dead bug with twist.

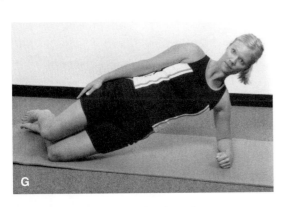

Figure 34.26G Side bridge from knees.

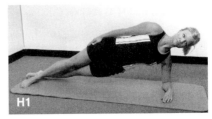

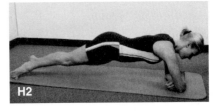

Figure 34.26H
Side bridge from
ankles, with roll.

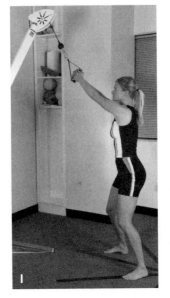

Figure 34.26I, J Wood chops.

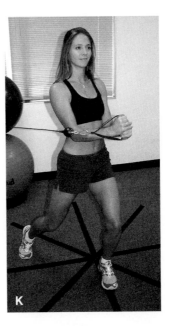

Figure 34.26K Two-
handed twist with cable.

13. Trunk Flexor Endurance

(Fig. 34.26L)

Indications

• Subacute or chronic LBP

Procedure

• Leaning supported on 50° wedge
• Feet anchored by tester
• Wedge is pushed back 4 inches, patient must maintain spinal alignment
• Ability to maintain position is timed

Score

• Record time to failure (when trunk leans back into wedge)
  ◦ Patient is given cues if position is lost, multiple cues can be given until failure occurs
  ◦ Less than 50 seconds is dysfunctional (43)
• Quantitative Data (see Chapter 11)
  ◦ Less than 50 seconds is dysfunctional (43)
• Trunk flexor endurance time should be longer than the side bridge endurance time, but weaker than the trunk extensor endurance time

If Positive, Possible Treatments to Consider

• (similar treatments as previous test)

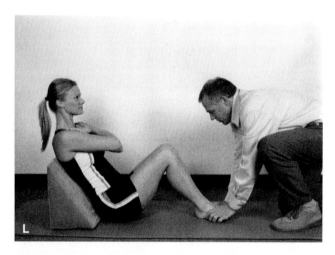

Figure 34.26L Trunk flexor endurance test.

14. T4 Mobility Screen—Arm Overhead Test (50)

(Fig. 34.27A)

Indications

- Subacute or chronic MSP
- Poor posture
- Osteoporosis

Procedure

- Stand with back against a wall and feet slightly forward
- Instruct patient to raise their arms overhead

Score

- Fail if:
  - Lumbopelvic junction hyperextends (Fig. 34.27B)
  - Arms don't reach vertical plane (Fig. 34.27B)
  - Thoracic kyphosis remains

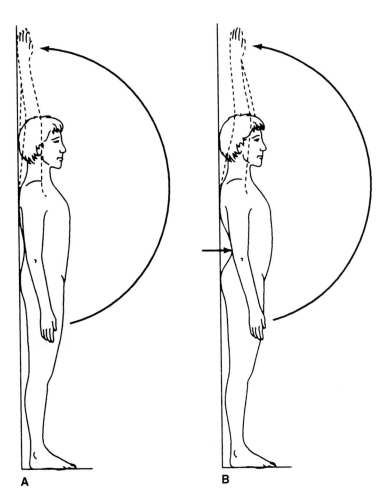

A   **B**

Figure 34.27A, B Arm overhead test. Lumbar hyperextension and reduced glenohumeral range of motion.

If Positive, Possible Treatments to Consider

- Relax/stretch
  - Latissimus dorsi, pectoralis major/minor
  - Breathing exercises
- Adjust/mobilize
  - Thoracic spine (T4–8) (Figs. 34.27C, D)

- Stabilization training
  - Core/trunk (Figs. 34.27E, F, G)
- Functional training
  - Backhand (Figs. 34.27H, I)
  - Overhead cable pull down (Fig. 34.27J)

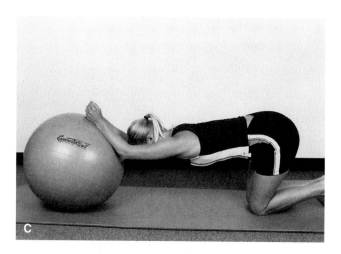

Figure 34.27C Upper back cat on ball.

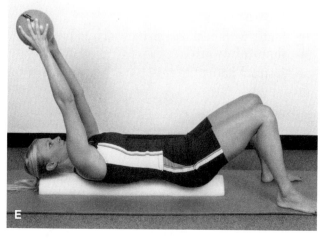

Figure 34.27E Dead bug on foam with medicine ball overhead.

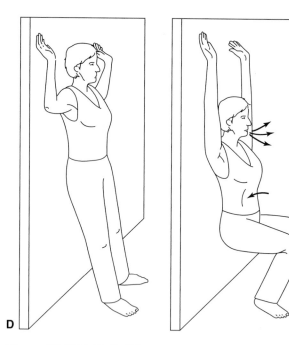

Figure 34.27D Wall slide.

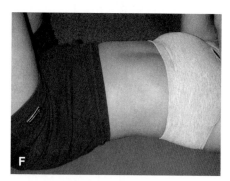

Figure 34.27F Crunch start position with ribs elevated, inhalation position.

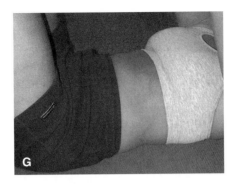

Figure 34.27G Crunch start position with ribs depressed, exhalation position.

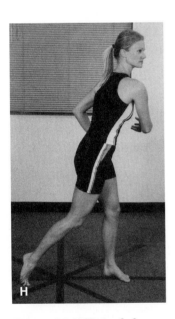

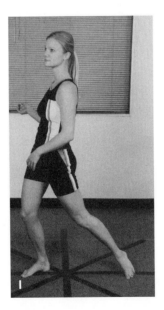

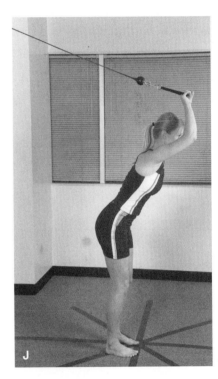

Figure 34.27H Angle lunge backhand, start position.

Figure 34.27I Angle lunge backhand.

Figure 34.27J Overhead cable pull down.

Cases

This section details a few examples of common clinical presentations. A common format incorporating the different key elements of care in a repeatable practice model will be shown (34). Kibler's functional kinetic chain model is presented for each case to show how management should not be limited to merely an orthopedic assessment of the pain generator, but should be predicated on a functional assessment (Tables 32.7 and 32.8). Additionally, the goals of care will be presented for each case (palliative, tissue-sparing, tissue-stabilizing, and functional training) (Table 32.11). Within the goals of care are subsumed the continuum or steps of care (advice, manipulation, and exercise) (Table 32.9). For example, sparing strategies include *advice* on ergonomic modifications or *manipulations* of joints or soft tissues; and *exercise* is included in both stabilizing and functional training.

Clinical Pearl

The Prague school of manual medicine (Lewit & Janda) espoused the general rule that tight muscles should be relaxed PRIOR to a strengthening program being initiated. The purpose being to avoid unwanted substitution patterns occurring during strength training with synergists compensating for agonists. This is consistent with stabilization training approaches of Waterloo, Canada (McGill) and Queensland, Australia (Richardon, Jull, Hodges). The Waterloo approach recommends that lower quarter mobility deficits are addressed to ensure load-sharing of the spine during stability training. The Queensland approach emphasizes the importance of addressing "global" muscle overactivity during "local" stabilization training to avoid synergist substitution.

Case 1: Herniated Disc

Kinetic Chain Approach

Clinical symptom complex: Nerve root symptoms below the knee worse with sitting, flexion and in the morning (Fig. 34.28A)

Tissue injury complex: Nerve root compression or tension due to disc herniation (Fig. 34.28B)

Source of biomechanical overload: End range loading of disc during ADLs (i.e., sitting, lifting, and forward bending) (Fig. 34.28C).

Pertinent factors include:

- Temporal—pain in morning or after prolonged flexion (i.e., sitting and stooping)
- Poor physical fitness and respiratory challenge leading to loss of abdominal stabilization of low back
- Coupled flexion and rotation; reduced mobility of peripheral joints of the lower extremity and compensatory hypermobility of lumbar spine in flexion
- Reduced coordination or endurance of spinal stabilizers (deep spinal extensor muscles, QL, deep abdominal stabilizer muscles)

Dysfunctional kinetic chain:

- Inadequate lumbar segmental stability in the sagittal plane with flexion overload during bending and lifting activities due to back extensor fatigue (e.g., multifidus).
- Poor lateral stability caused by QL fatigue
- Forward lunge with trunk flexion
- Squat with trunk flexion (Fig. 34.28D)

Goals of and Continuum of Care

Palliative care: reduce irritability of nerve root (McKenzie, traction, modalities) (Figs. 34.28E, F, G)

Sparing Strategies:

- Activity modification advice (postural awareness training) (Fig. 34.28H)
- Mobilize lower extremity peripheral joints and T4–8
- Release gastro-soleus, hamstring, hip flexors
- Consider neuromobilization of the sciatic nerve (Fig. 34.28I)
  - This should be performed as a slider not a tensor.

Stabilizing Strategies:

- Facilitate back extensors and side support muscles (Fig. 34.28J, K)

Functional Training:

- Reeducate postural awareness of neutral spine during lifting, bending, and sitting. (Fig. 34.28L)

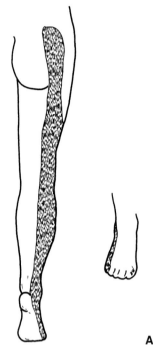

A

Figure 34.28A Referred pain from an irritated or compressed S-1 nerve root.

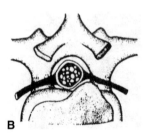

B

Figure 34.28B Nerve root compression caused by disc herniation.

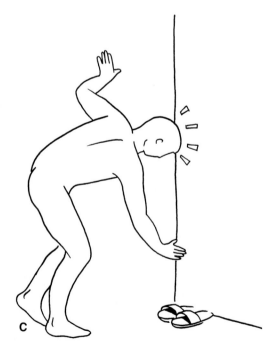

C

Figure 34.28C End range loading of disc during ADLs.

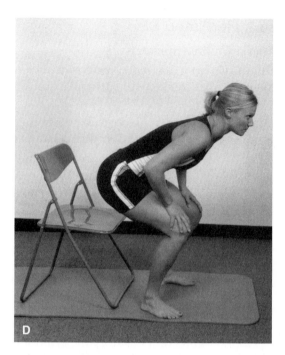

D

Figure 34.28D Squat with trunk flexion.

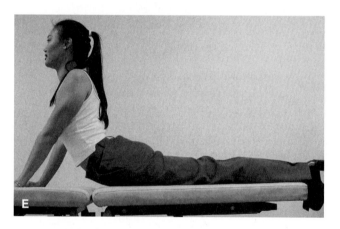

E

Figure 34.28E McKenzie prone extension exercise.

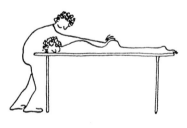

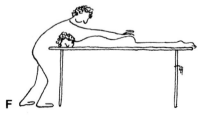

F

Figure 34.28F Manual traction of the pelvis.

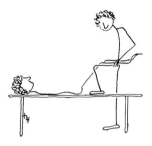

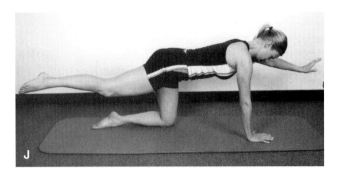

Figure 34.28J Quadruped arm and leg reach.

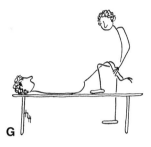

Figure 34.28G
Supine rhythmic
traction of the lum-
bar spine.

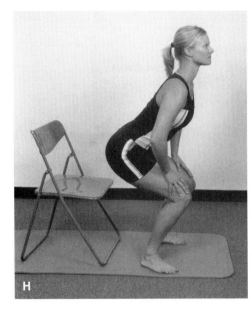

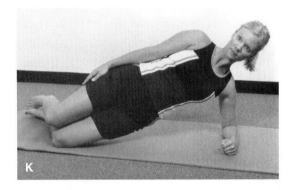

Figure 34.28K Side bridge.

Figure 34.28H Hip hinge.

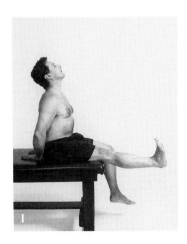

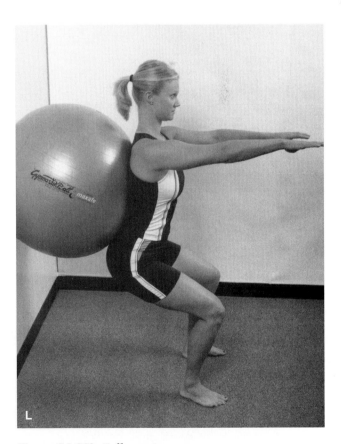

Figure 34.28I Sciatic nerve
slider neuromobilization.

Figure 34.28L Ball squat.

Case 2: Facet Syndrome

Kinetic Chain Approach

Clinical symptom complex: Low back pain (Fig. 34.29A)

Tissue injury complex: Facet syndrome (Fig. 34.29B)

Source of biomechanical overload: End range loading of facets during ADL's (i.e., gait, reaching overhead, etc.) due to altered axis of hip extension or thoracic extension with primary fulcrum in low back. Facet overstrain is also common if the deep abdominals don't stabilize the spine in a "neutral range" during ADLs such as lifting or exercises such as sit-ups (Fig. 34.29C).

Dysfunctional kinetic chain:

a. Reduced hip extension mobility (Differential diagnosis (DDx)—anterior hip joint capsule, hip flexor muscle tightness, femoral nerve tension) with compensatory lumbo-sacral hypermobility in extension (Fig. 34.29D)

b. Reduced thoracic (T4–8) extension mobility during trunk straightening or arm flexion (Fig. 34.29E) (DDx—muscle tightness: pectoral, lat, subscapularis; brachial plexus tension; and joint mobility restrictions: upper thoracic extension or anterior rib depression)

c. Inadaquate lumbar segmental stability in the sagittal plane with extension overload during lifting activities.

Goals of and Continuum of Care

Palliative:

- Reduce irritability of facet joints (adjustments, modalities, soft tissue manipulation) (Figs. 34.29F, G, H, I)

Sparing:

- Activity modification advice (postural awareness training) (Fig. 34.29J)

Stabilizing

- Bridge (Fig. 34.29K)
- Basic curl–up (Fig. 34.29L)
- Crunch with ball overhead (Fig. 34.29M)

Functional

- Wall slide (Fig. 34.29N)
- Overhead pull down with cable (Fig. 34.29O)

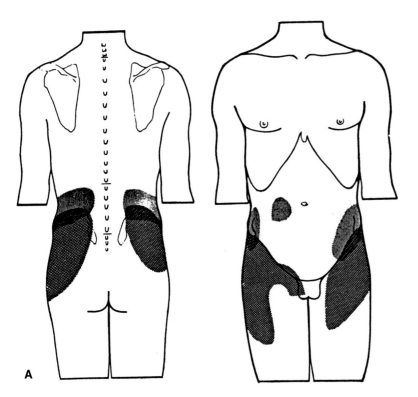

Figure 34.29A Referred pain from lumbar spine joints.

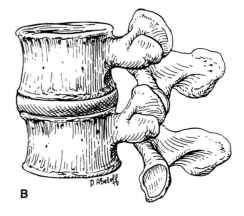

Figure 34.29B Lumbar vertebral and facet joints.

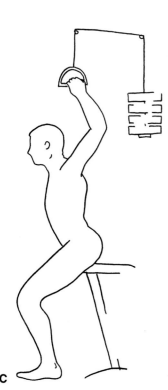

Figure 34.29C Facet over-strain with exercise.

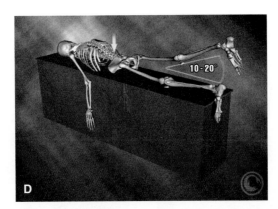

Figure 34.29D Faulty hip extension.

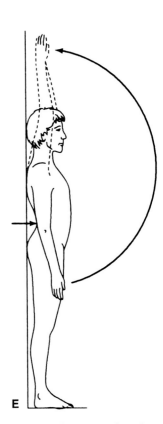

Figure 34.29E Reduced thoracic (T4) extension mobility during arm flexion.

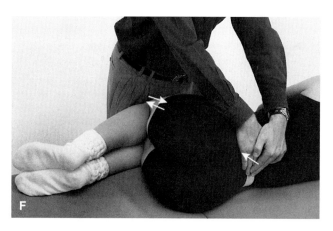

Figure 34.29F Lumbar spine extension PIR mobilization.

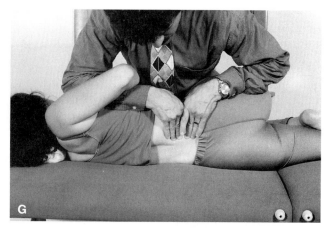

Figure 34.29G Lumbar lateral flexion manipulation.

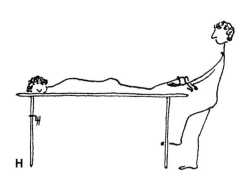

Figure 34.29H Prone rhythmic traction of the lumbar spine.

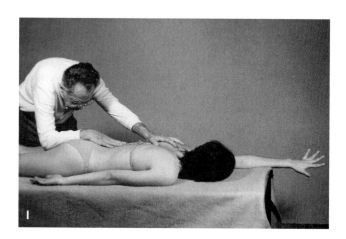

Figure 34.29I Lewit fascial release.

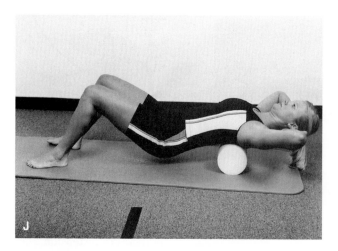

Figure 34.29J T4 mobilization with foam roll.

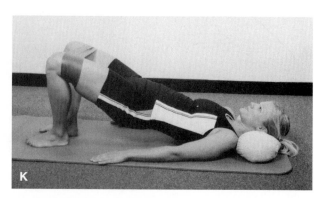

Figure 34.29K Bridge.

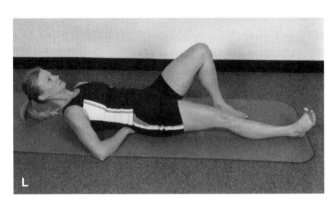

Figure 34.29L Basic curl-up.

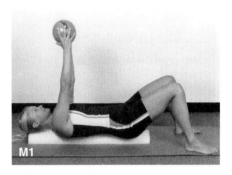

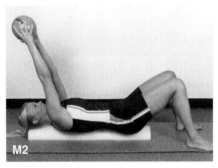

Figure 34.29M Crunch with ball overhead.

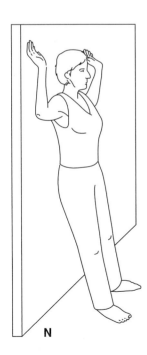

Figure 34.29N Wall slide.

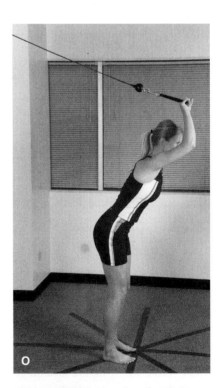

Figure 34.29O Overhead pull down with cable.

Case 3: Spinal Stenosis

Kinetic Chain Approach

Clinical symptom complex: Nerve root symptoms below the knee worse with standing, and walking and in the elderly (Figs. 34.30A and B)

Tissue injury complex: Nerve root compression or tension due to spinal stenosis (narrowing of the spinal canal caused by degenerative joint disease) (Fig. 34.30C)

Source of biomechanical overload: Similar to facet syndrome

Dysfunctional kinetic chain: Similar to facet syndrome

Goals of and Continuum of Care

Palliative care: Reduce irritability of nerve root (Fig. 34.30D)

Sparing Strategies:

- Activity modification advice (postural awareness training) (Fig. 34.30E)
- Mobilize lower extremity peripheral joints, T4–8, and lumbar spine in flexion
- Release gastro-soleus, hamstring, hip flexors (Fig. 34.30F)
  - If necessary release the relevant nerve, sciatic or femoral (Fig. 34.30G)

Stabilizing Strategies:

- Similar to facet syndrome

Functional Training:

- Similar to facet syndrome

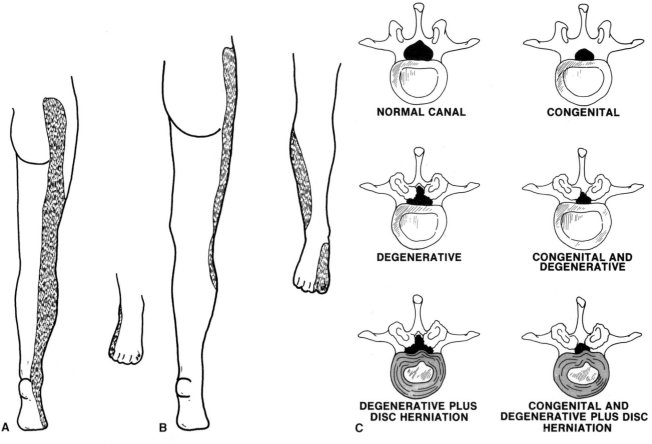

Figure 34.30A Referred pain from an irritated or compressed SI nerve root.

Figure 34.30B Referred pain from an irritated or compressed L5 nerve pain. Reproduced with permission from Cox JM, Low Back Pain: Mechanism, Diagnosis and Treatment, 6th edition, Baltimore: Lippincott Williams & Wilkins, 1999; obtained from fig 10.74, p 419.

Figure 34.30C Normal spinal canal and various combinations of conditions that may cause spinal stenosis (narrowing of the spinal canal due to DJD). Reprinted with permission from White AA, Panjabi MM. Clinical Biomechanics of the Spine, 2nd ed. Philadelphia: JB Lippincott, 1990:403. Obtained from fig 6.17, p 403.

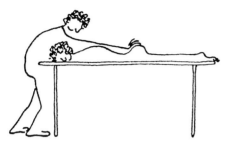

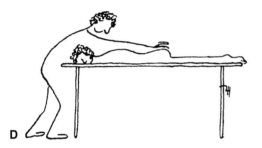

Figure 34.30D Isometric manual traction of the pelvis.

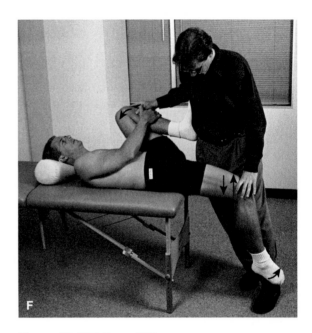

Figure 34.30F Psoas PIR.

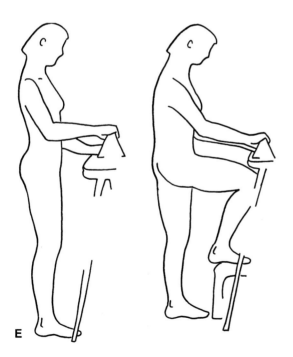

Figure 34.30E Use of footstool to reduce low back strain.

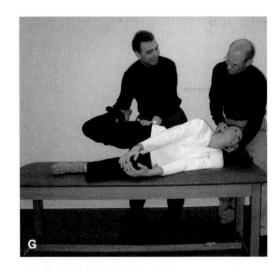

Figure 34.30G Femoral nerve slider neuro-mobilization.

Case 4: Sacroiliac Syndrome

Kinetic Chain Approach

Clinical symptom complex: Sacro-iliac (SI) pain (Fig. 34.31A)

Tissue injury complex: Sacro-iliac joint

Source of biomechanical overload: Sacro-iliac instability during ADLs (i.e., gait, climbing stairs, forward bending, etc.)

Dysfunctional kinetic chain: Poor pelvic stability in stance phase of gait (Fig. 34.31B) (weak gluteus medius & overactive TFL, QL, adductors, piriformis) with resultant lumbo-sacral and SI hypermobility

Goals of and Continuum of Care

Palliative care: Reduce irritability of SI joint—SI mobilizations (Figs. 34.31C, D, E)

Tissue sparing: Activity modification advice, adductor, piriformis (Fig. 34.31F), IT band releases

Stabilizing:

- Facilitate gluteus medius
  - Sister Kenny gluteus medius facilitation (Fig. 34.31G)
  - Single-leg bridge (Fig. 34.31H)
  - Wall ball (Fig. 34.31I)
  - Balance reach (Fig. 34.31J)

Functional:

- Running man (Fig. 34.31K)
- Single-leg pull down with cable (Fig. 34.31L)

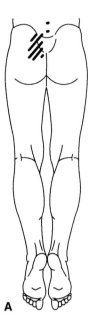

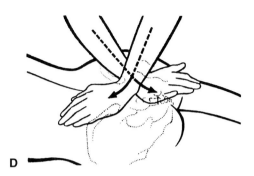

Figure 34.31A Sacro-iliac joint pain referral pattern. Obtained from SIJ referral pattern fig 1, p 1484 Fortin JD, Aprill CN, Ponthieux B, Pier J. Sacroiliac Joint: Pain Referral Maps Upon Applying a New Injection/Arthrography Technique, Part II: Clinical Evaluation, Spine 1994;19:1483–1489.

Figure 34.31D Mobilization of the sacro-iliac joint.

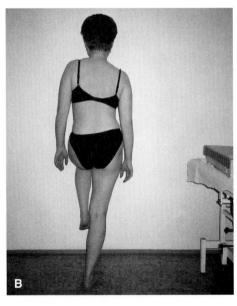

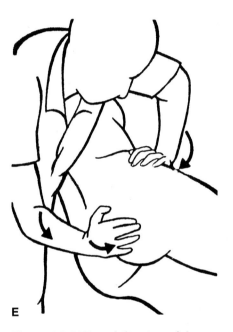

Figure 34.31B Trendelenberg sign.

Figure 34.31E Mobilization of the lower part of the sacroiliac joint.

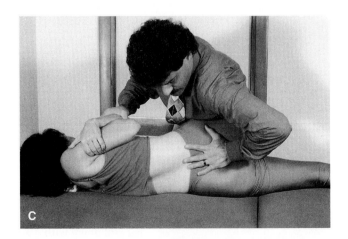

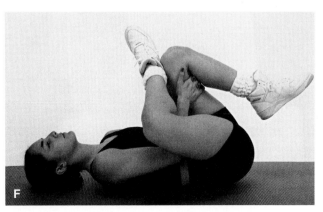

Figure 34.31C Sacroiliac joint manipulation.

Figure 34.31F Piriformis stretch.

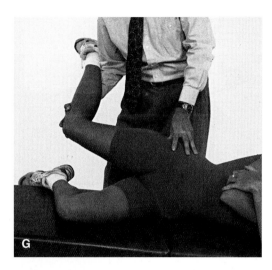

Figure 34.31G Sister Kenny gluteus medius facilitation.

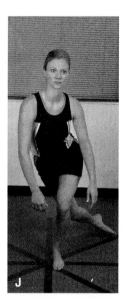

Figure 34.31J Balance reach.

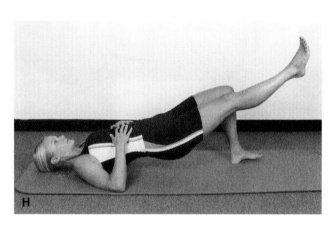

Figure 34.31H Single-leg bridge.

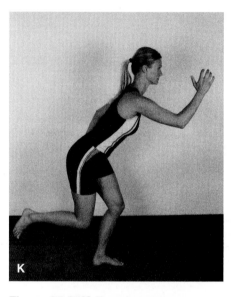

Figure 34.31K Running man.

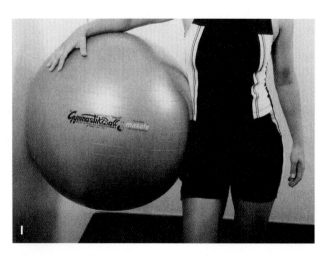

Figure 34.31I Wall ball.

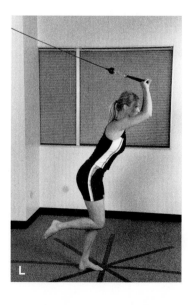

Figure 34.31L Single-leg pull down with cable.

Audit Process
Self-Check of the Chapter's Learning Objectives

• How are the different University of Pittsburgh low back pain subclassifications determined?

• What rehabilitation methods should be considered for dysfunctional hip extension or abduction?

• What rehabilitation methods should be considered for a dysfunctional Vleeming's test?

• What is the continuum of care for nerve root syndromes

• What is the continuum of care for facet and sacroiliac problems?

■ REFERENCES

1. Agency for Health Care Policy and Research (AHCPR). Acute low-back problems in adults. Clinical Practice Guideline Number 14. Washington DC, US Government Printing, 1994.

2. Alaranta H, Hurri H, Heliovaara M, et al. Non-dynamometric trunk performance tests: Reliability and normative data. Scand J Rehab Med 1994;26: 211–215.

3. Arendt-Nielson L, Graven-Nielson T, Svarrer H, Svensson P. The influence of low back pain on muscle activity and coordination during gait. Pain 1995;64: 231–240.

4. Australian Institute of Health and Welfare. Disability Data Briefing. The International Classification of Functioning, Disability and Health, ICF, ICIDH, Canberra 2002. (http://www.aihw.gov.au/publications/dis/ddb20/ddb20.pdf). Accessed February 200, 2004.

5. Bohannon RW, Larkin PA, Cook AC, Gear J, Singer J, Decrease in timed balance test scores with aging. Physical Therapy 1984;64;7:1067–1070.

6. Borkan J, Reis S, Hermoni D, et al. Talking about the pain: a patient-centered study of low back pain in primary care. Soc Sci Med 1995;40:977–988.

7. Borkan JM, Koes BW, Reis R, Cherkin DC. A report from the second international forum for primary care research on low back pain: Reexamining priorities. Spine 1998;23:1992–1996.

8. Bullock -Saxton JE, Janda V, Bullock MI. Reflex activation of gluteal muscles in walking. Spine 1993;18: 704–708.

9. Burton K, Waddell G. Information and advice to patients w/ back pain can have a positive effect. Spine 1999;24:2484–2491.

10. Childs JD, Fritz JM, Flynn TW, Irrgang JJ, Johnson KK, Majkowski GR, Delitto A. A clinical prediction rule to identify patients with low back pain most likely to benefit from spinal manipulation: a validation study. Ann Intern Med. 2004;141:920–928.

11. Cholewicki J, Simons APD, Radebold A. Effects of external loads on lumbar spine stability. Journal of Biomechanics 2000;33:1377–1385.

12. Cibulka MT, Sinacore DR, Cromer GS, Delitto A. Unilateral hip rotation range of motion asymmetry in patients with sacroiliac joint regional pain. Spine 1998;23:1009–1015.

13. Cibulka MT, Koldehoff R. Clinical usefulness of a cluster of sacroiliac joint tests in patients with and without low back pain. 1999;29(2):83–92.

14. Clare H, Adams R, Maher C. Reliability of the McKenzie spinal pain classification using patient assessment forms. Physiotherapy 2004;90:114–119.

15. Clare H, Adams R, Maher C. Reliability of McKenzie classification of patients with cervical and lumbar pain. JMPT 2005;28:122–127.

16. Danish Health Technology Assessment (DIHTA). Manniche C et al. Low back pain: Frequency Management and Prevention from an HAD Perspective, 1999.

17. Delitto A, Shulman AD, Rose SJ, et al. Reliability of a Classical Examination to Classify Patients with Low Back Syndrome. Physical Therapy Practice 1992; 1(3):1–9.

18. Delitto A, Cibulka MT, Erhard RE, et al. Evidence for use of an Extension-Mobilization Category in Acute Low Back Syndrome: A Prescriptive Validation Pilot Study. Phys Ther 1993;73:216–228.

19. Delitto A, Erhard RE, Bowling RW. A Treatment-Based Classification Approach to Low Back Syndrome: Identifying and Staging Patients for Conservative Treatment. Phys Ther 1995;75:470–89.

20. Donelson R, Silva G, Murphy K. The centralization phenomenon: its usefulness in evaluating and treating referred pain. Spine 1990;15:211–213.

21. Ellison JB, Rose SJ, Sahrmann SA: Patterns of rotation range of motion: a comparison between healthy subjects and patients with low back pain. Phys Ther 1990;70:537–541.

22. Erhard RE, Delitto A. Relative effectiveness of an extension program and a combined program of manipulation and flexion and extension exercises in patients with acute low back syndrome. Phys Ther 1994;74:1093–1100.

23. Flynn T, Fritz, J, Whitman J, Wainner R, Magel J, et al. A Clinical Prediction Rule for Classifying Patients with Low Back Pain Who Demonstrate Short-Term Improvement With Spinal Manipulation [Exercise Physiology and Physical Exam]. Spine 2002;27:2835–2843.

24. Fritz JM. George S. The use of a classification approach to identify subgroups of patients with acute low back pain. Spine 2000;1:106–114.

25. Fritz JM, Delitto A, Vignovic M, et al. Interrater reliability of judgments of the centralization phenomenon and status change during movement testing in patients with low back pain. Arch Phys Med Rehabil 2000;81:57–60.

26. Fritz JM, Delitto A Erhard RE. Comparison of classification-based physical therapy with therapy based on clinical practice guidelines for patients with acute low back pain: a randomized clinical trial. Spine, 2003;28:1363–1371.

27. Grotle M, Borx JI, Vollestad NK. Functional status and disability questionnaires: what do they assess? A systematic review of back-specific outcome questionnaires. Spine 2004;30:130–140.

28. Hewett T, Lindenfeld TN, Roccobene JV, Noyes FR. The effect of neuromuscular training on the incidence of knee injury in female athletes: a prospective study. Am J Sp Med 1999;27:699–706.

29. Hussein TM, Simmonds MJ, Olson SL, et al. Kinematics of gait in normal and low back pain subjects. American Congress of Sports Medicine 45th Annual Meeting. Boston, MA, 1998.

30. Hussein TM, Simmonds MJ, Etnyre B, et al. Kinematics of gait in subjects with low back pain with and without leg pain. Scientific Meeting & Exposition of the American Physical Therapy Association. Washington, DC, 1999.

31. Ireland ML, Wilson JD, Ballantyne BT, McClay Davis I. Hip strength in females with and without patellofemoral pain. J Ortho Sp Phys Ther 2003;33:671–676.

32. Kankaapaa M, Taimela S, Laaksonen D, et al. Back and hip extensor fatigability in chronic low back pain patients and controls. Arch Phys Med Rehabil 1998;79:412–417.

33. Karas R, McIntosh G, Hall H, et al. The relationship between nonorganic signs and centralization of symptoms in the prediction of return to work for patients with low back pain. Physical Therapy 1997;77:354–360.

34. Kibler WB, Herring SA, Press JM. Functional Rehabilitation of Sports and Musculoskeletal Injuries. Aspen, 1998.

35. Kilpikoski S, Airaksinen O, Kankaanpaa M, Leminen P, Videman T, Alen M. Interexaminer reliability of low back pain assessment using the McKenzie method. Spine 2002;27:E207–E214.

36. Kujala UM, Taimela S, Salminen JJ, Oksanen A. Baseline anthropometry, flexibility and strength characteristics and future low-back-pain in adolescent athletes and nonathletes. A prospective, one-year, follow-up study. Scand J Med Sci Sports 1994;4:200–205.

37. Lamoth CJC, Meijer OG, Wuisman PIJM, van Dieën J H, Levin MF, Beek PJ. Pelvis-thorax coordination in the transverse plane during walking in persons with nonspecific low back pain. Spine 2002;27:E92–E99.

38. Leinonen V, Kankaanpaa M, Airaksinen O, et al. Back and hip flexion/extension: effects of low back pain and rehabilitation. Arch Phys Med Rehabil 2000;81:32–37.

39. Long A. The centralization phenomenon: its usefulness as a predictor of outcome in conservative treatment of chronic low back pain. Spine 1995;20:2513–2521.

40. Long A, Donelson R, Fung T. Does it matter which exercise? A randomized controlled trial of exercise for low back pain. Spine 2004;29:2593–2602.

41. Maluf KS, Sahrmann SA, Van Dillen LR: Use of a classification system to guide non-surgical treatment of a patient with chronic low back pain. Physical Therapy 2000;80:1097–1111.

42. Mascal CL, Landel R, Powers C. Management of patellofemoral pain targeting hip, pelvis, and trunk muscle function: 2 case reports. J Ortho Sp Phys Ther 2003;33:647–660.

43. McGill S, Childs A, Liebenson C. Endurance times for low back stabilization exercises: Clinical targets for testing and training from a normative database. Arch Phys Med Rehabil, 1999;80:941–944.

44. McGill S, Grenier S, Bluhm M, Preuss R, Brown S, Russell C. Previous history of LBP with work loss is related to lingering deficits in biomechanical, physiological, personal, psychosocial and motor control characteristics. Ergonomics 2003;46:731–746.

45. Mens JM, Vleeming A, Snijders CJ, et al. Reliability and validity of the active straight leg raise test in posterior pelvic pain since pregnancy. Spine 2001;26:1167–1171.

46. Mens JM, Vleeming A, Snijders CJ, et al. Validity of the active straight leg raise test to measure disease severity in posterior pelvic pain since pregnancy. Spine 2002;27:196–200.

47. Michaud T. Foot Orthoses. Baltimore: Williams & Wilkins, 1993.

48. Nadler SF, Malanga GA, DePrince ML, Stitik TP, Feinberg JH. The relationship between lower extremity injury, low back pain, and hip muscle strength in male and female collegiate athletes. Clin J Sports Med 2000;10:89–97.

49. Nadler SF, Malanga GA, Feinberg JH, Prybicien M, Stitik TP, DeFrince M. Relationship between hip muscle imbalance and occurrence of low back pain in collegiate athletes: a prospective study. Am J Phys Med Rehabil 2001;80:572–577.

50. Norris, CM: Back Stability. London: Human Kinetics, 2000.

51. O'Sullivan PB, Beales DJ, Beetham JA, Cripps J, Graf F, Lin IB, Tucker B, Avery A. Altered motor control strategies in subjects with sacroiliac joint pain during the active straight-leg-raise test. Spine 2002;27:E1–E8.

52. Piva SR, Erhard RE, Childs JD, Hicks G, Al-Abdulmohsin H. Reliability of measuring iliac crest level in the standing and sitting position using a new measurement device. J Manipulative Physiol Ther. 2003;26:437–441.

53. Pool-Goudzwaard A, Vleeming A, Stoeckart C, Snijders CJ, Mens MA. Insufficient lumbopelvic stability: a clinical, anatomical and biomechanical approach to "a-specific" low back pain. Man Ther 1998:3;12–20.

54. Powers CM. The influence of altered lower-extremity kinematics on patellofemoral joint dysfunction: a theoretical perspective. J Ortho Sp Phys Ther 2003;33:639–646.

55. Radebold A, Cholewicki J, Panjabi MM, Patel TC. Muscle response pattern to sudden trunk loading in healthy individuals and in patients with chronic low back pain. Spine 2000;25:947–954.

56. Radebold A, Cholewicki J, Polzhofer BA, Greene HS. Impaired postural control of the lumbar spine is associated with delayed muscle response times in patients with chronic idiopathic low back pain. Spine 2001;26:724–730.

57. Razmjou H, Kramer JF, Yamada R. Intertester reliability of the McKenzie evaluation in assessing patients with mechanical low back pain. J Orthop Sports Phys Ther 2000;30:368–383.

58. Riddle DL, Freburger JK. Evaluation of the presence of sacroiliac joint region dysfunction using a combination of tests: a multicenter intertester reliability study. Phys Ther. 2002;82:772–781.

59. Royal College of General Practitioners (RCGP). Clinical Guidelines for the Management of Acute Low Back Pain. London, Royal College of General Practitioners (www.rcgp.org.uk). 1999.

60. Sufka A, Hauger B, Trenary M, et al. Centralization of low back pain and perceived functional outcome. J Orthop Sports Phys Ther 1998;27:205–212.

61. Swinkels-Meewisse IEJ, Roelofs J, Verbeek ALM, Oostendorp RAB, Vlaeyen JWS. Fear of movement/(re)injury, disability and participation in acute low back pain. Pain. 2003;105:371–379.

62. Tenhula JA, Rose SJ, Delitto A. Association between direction of lateral lumbar shift, movement tests, and side of symptoms in patients with low back pain syndrome. Phys Ther. 1990;70:480–486.

63. United Nations. World program of action concerning disabled persons. Division for Social and Policy Development, United Nations; 2003 [http://www.un.org/esa/socdev/enable/diswpa01.htm. Accessed February 16, 2004.

64. Van Dillen LR, Sahrmann SA, Norton BJ, Caldwell CA, Fleming DA, McDonnell MK, Woolsey NB: Reliability of physical examination items used for classification of patients with low back pain. Physical Therapy 1998;78:979–988.

65. Van Dillen LR, McDonnell MK, Fleming DA, Sahrmann SA: The effect of hip and knee position on hip extension range of motion measures in individuals with and without low back pain. Journal of Orthopedic and Sports Physical Therapy 2000;30(6):307–316.

66. Van Dillen LR, Sahrmann SA, Norton BJ, McDonnell MK, Fleming DA, Caldwell CA, Woolsey NB: The effect of active limb movements on symptoms in patients with low back pain. Journal of Orthopedic and Sports Physical Therapy 2001; 31:402–413.

67. Victorian WorkCover Authority. http://www.workcover.vic.gov.au/dir090/vwa/home.nsf/pages/chiropractors. Accessed June 8, 2005.

68. Vogt L, Banzer W. Dynamic testing of the motorial stereotype in prone hip extension from the neutral position. Clinical Biomechanics 1997;12:122–127.

69. Vogt L, Pfeifer K, Banzer W. Neuromuscular control of walking with chronic low-back pain. Manual Therapy 2003;8:21–28.

70. Von Korff M, Ormel J, Keefe FJ, Dworkin SF, Grading the severity of chronic pain. Pain 1992;50:133–149.

71. Werneke M, Hart DL, Cook D. A descriptive study of the centralization phenomenon. A prospective analysis. Spine 1999;24:676–683.

72. Werneke M, Hart DL. Centralization phenomenon as a prognostic factor for chronic low back pain and disability. Spine 2001;26:758–765.

73. Wilson L, Hall H, McIntosh G, Melles T. Intertester reliability of a low back pain classification system. Spine 1999;24:248–254.

74. World Health Organization. International Classification of Human Functioning, Disability and Health: ICF. Geneva: WHO, 2001.

35

Integrated Approach to the Cervical Spine

Craig Liebenson, Clayton Skaggs, Scott Fonda, and Sylvia Deily

Learning Objectives
After reading this chapter you should be able to understand:

- How to evaluate functional stability
- The different rehabilitation methods to consider when a specific functional test is positive
- The continuum of care for the most common clinical symptom or tissue injury complexes

Introduction

Head, neck, upper back and referred arm pain are common problems. They are usually self-limiting, but recurrent. Patients who seek professional health care usually have severe pain, are getting worse, or are simply not getting better in a reasonable time.

These patients require a diagnostic triage to rule out "red flags" of serious disease. While necessary, this is not sufficient to properly manage the case. Other steps that are essential for the promotion of a self-management approach are identification of the patient's activity intolerances, functional deficits, work status, and "yellow flags" indicative of a poor prognosis.

This chapter will integrate together the functional assessment and treatment methods necessary for promoting self-management of activity limiting cervico-thoracic complaints.

Diagnostic Triage

Red Flags

The term 'Red Flags' was coined and popularized by the AHCPR Guidelines in 1994 (5). Diagnostic triage refers to the process of evaluating and determining initial management strategies for presenting complaints. In first contact provider situations, emphasis is placed on securing a diagnosis and implementing the most conservative and reasonable treatment options. The likelihood of encountering sinister causes for cervical spine pain complaints is low, but always present. Most epidemiological studies noting the likelihood of encountering a sinister or non-benign cause have focused on low back pain instead of cervical spine complaints, primarily due to the higher incidence of low back pain in the general population. In this section, general red flags will be outlined, followed by brief sections on special considerations for the cervico-thoracic region and some specific conditions (see also Chapter 7).

It is the intention of red flags to act as screening procedures which would prompt the clinician toward further investigation. The majority of red flags are points noted during the history taking process, thus making thorough history taking of great importance in raising the clinician's index of suspicion to any potential sinister causes for the presenting complaints (see Table 35.1).

Differential Diagnosis

The conditions which red flags and diagnostic triage are most focused upon can be divided into etiological categories. These include fracture/dislocation,

Table 35.1 General Red Flags from the History

- Age <18 without precipitating event or onset age >45
- Prior history of cancer
- Significant trauma onset
- Constitutional symptoms: fever, chills, night sweats, nausea, vomiting, fatigue, diarrhea
- Night pain
- Pain unrelieved by rest or position
- Pain or pattern of symptoms disproportionate to typical musculoskeletal disorders
- Unexplained weight loss
- Bowel or bladder habit change
- Systemic illness (e.g. diabetes)
- Immunosuppressed states (corticosteroid use, HIV, etc . . .)
- Failure of conservative management

neoplasm (malignancy), infection, visceral referral, myelopathy, and radiculopathy (30). Once the general index of suspicion is raised, additional lines of questioning, physical examination procedures, and diagnostic testing can be administered with greater specificity toward a single category.

Fracture/Dislocation

The presentation of fracture or dislocation is rather straight forward, but a caveat to keep in mind is that in order to cause fracture, one must sustain major trauma if healthy, however, even minor trauma in an at risk individual may be sufficient for fracture. At risk individuals may include the elderly or others with osteoporosis. Major risk factors for osteoporosis include (13,18,75,81).

- Female with:
  - Age over 55 years
  - Low weight (<127 lbs.)
  - Post-menopausal NOT taking ERT (estrogen replacement therapy)
  - Asian or Caucasian
  - Smokers
- Males with hypogonadism

Intraspinal/Intracranial Considerations

Stroke and vertebro-basilar syndromes often present as headache and dizziness, similar to upper cervical spine mediated complaints. A history of hypertension or current elevated blood pressure is a red flag for ischemic stroke. Although often clinically silent, vertigo, visual disturbances and headache are clinical manifestations of vertebro-basilar insufficiency. A presentation of headache with fever and cervico-thoracic complaints must be considered for meningitis.

Neoplasm (Malignancy)

The most typical red flags alerting the clinician to the possibility of malignancy include age >50, prior history of cancer, unexplained weight loss, no relief with rest, and failure of conservative therapy. Metastatic disease can present in any number of ways and is the most common neoplastic consideration. Other considerations include primary benign bone tumors (osteochondroma, osteoblastoma, aneurismal bone cyst, hemangioma, and osteoid osteoma). Other neoplastic considerations include extra- and intra-medullary spinal cord tumors.

Infection

Infectious processes which can affect the cervical region include osteomyelitis, discitis, meningitis and perivertebral abscess formations. The index of suspicion should be particularly high in the immunosuppressed (HIV +, chronic corticosteroid use, or other immunosuppressive therapy). Other higher risk factors include: co-existing urinary tract infection (UTI), IV drug use, recent surgical or invasive procedures (including dental procedures), or a known penetrating wound (abscess). Diabetics are also known to have a higher incidence of infection.

Myelopathy

The presence of signs of myelopathy demands delineation of the cause and extent of the neurologic deficit. Historical detail regarding impotence and bowel or bladder continence is extremely important. Examination should include a thorough upper and lower extremity neurological examination, to include notation of motor coordination and signs of spasticity. Causes can include instability, vertebral degenerative changes, disc herniation, or other space occupying lesions of the spinal canal (benign or malignant). Trauma may play a role in the development of myelopathy, particularly if congenital stenosis exists, or there are other risks of instability (i.e. rheumatoid arthritis).

Radiculopathy

The presence of radiculopathy is not an immediate cause for surgical referral, but persistence or progression of neurologic deficit despite conservative management warrants additional consideration. Initial examination must include upper and lower extremity muscle stretch reflexes, dermatomal light touch and sharp sensibility, and motor strength. Atrophy should be measured if possible and fasciculation should be noted if present. This will not only define the extent of the radiculopathy, but also serve as a baseline for interval comparison. Advanced imaging and/or electro-diagnostic studies are the most useful diagnostic modalities for further evaluation.

Visceral Referral

One of the signs not previously listed is the failure of neuromusculoskeletal examination procedures to reproduce the presenting complaints. Various visceral conditions can create referred pain to the neck and cervical region, upper thoracic region, scapular area, and perhaps the upper extremity (27). Some of the more common origins and their referral patterns are listed below (see Table 35.2).

Summary

There are numerous conditions which can cause neck or mid back pain. Tables 35.3 and 35.4 review the most common of these.

The Functional Model

The Biopsychosocial (BPS) Approach

The natural history of neck pain is poorly understood, and amazingly very little research about its causes or treatments has been performed (9,73). The severity of symptoms and the severity of trauma are not always directly related. Very few objective findings are correlated with the symptoms reported in the head, neck, or upper quarter. In a survey of over 10,000 cases of Whiplash Associated Disorders (WAD) pain it persisted in 25% of the cases for 5 years after the accident (20).

The BPS approach recognizes the importance of reassurance and reactivation for promoting a quick recovery and minimizing the risk of chronicity (65, 73,95).

A helpful tool for classifying neck related disorders emerged from the Quebec WAD Guidelines (see Table 35.5) (87). It does not hypothesize about the specific cause of pain, but enables different researchers to compare similar groups of patients. It has been pointed out that a common category like WAD II should be considered to include a heterogeneous group of patients (88).

Table 35.2   Sources and Features of Visceral Referred Pain

Origin	Conditions	Historical Features	Referred Pain Region
Cardiac	Angina, myocardial infarction, pericarditis	Chest pain, and risk factors (hyperpension (HTN), Coronary artery disease (CAD), hyperlipidemia, smoking)	Chest, left shoulder/medial arm, anterior neck
Pulmonary	Pleurisy, pulmonary embolus, pneumothorax	SOB/dyspnea, and history of respiratory disease	Tracheobronchial—anterior neck/chest Pleural—neck, ipsilateral trap/shoulder
Hepatic	Hepatitis, cirrhosis, abscess, hepatic metastasis	Positive risk factors (alcohol abuse, IV drug use, multiple sexual partners)	Right shoulder, interscapular/subscapular
Biliary	Cholecystitis, cholelithiasis	Prior history of cholelithiasis, epigastric/RUQ pain, fever, nausea	Epigastric/RUQ, right scapula
Gastric	Peptic ulcer disease (Gastric or duodenal)	Epigastric pain, temporal assoc. with meals	Epigastric/LUQ, with referral to back/scapula
Pancreatic	Pancreatitis, pancreatic carcinoma	Positive history alcohol abuse, history of cholelithiasis	Epigastric/RUQ, with referral to back/scapula

Table 35.3   Differential Diagnosis List for Neck Pain of Musculoskeletal Origin

Discogenic
    Herniated nucleus pulposus with or without radiculopathy or myelopathy
    Internal disc derangement (annular tear)
Facet-mediated pain
    Capsulitis/synovitis
    Osteoarthritis
Myofascial pain
    Muscular strain (acute)
    Muscular overload
Trauma
    Ligamentous sprain
    Vertebral fractures
    Instability
Degenerative disorders
    Osteoarthritis
    Degenerative disc disease
    Central or lateral canal stenosis
Cervical radiculopathy
    Compressive
    Inflammatory
Thoracic outlet syndrome
    Supraclavicular (scalene syndrome)
    Costoclavicular
    Infraclavicular
Other peripheral entrapment neuropathy
Brachial plexus injuries ("stingers & burners")

The BPS reactivation model espouses that pain and disability are not synonymous. The patient should receive reassurance that they are not in danger of making their neck worse with gradual reactivation, but actually will speed recovery and lessen the likelihood of developing a chronic pain syndrome (see Chapter 14) (65,73,95).

Course and Prognosis

What Predisposes a Person to Acute Neck Pain? (See Chapter 3)

The incidence of neck pain is quite high. Hill (35) estimates that as many as 31% of individuals have had neck pain in the past month. A number of factors have been shown to predispose a person to having an

Table 35.4   Differential Diagnosis List for Thoracic Regional Pain of Musculoskeletal Origin

Thoracic disc herniation
Facet mediated pain
Costovertebral joint mediated pain
Compression fracture
Rib fracture
Myofascial pain
    Muscular strain (acute)
    Muscular overload

Table 35.5 Quebec Whiplash Associated Disorders (WAD) Guidelines Classification System Based on Signs and Symptoms (87)

Grade	Clinical Presentation
0	No complaint or physical sign*
I	Neck complaint of pain, stiffness or tenderness. No physical signs
II	Neck complaint and musculoskeletal signs*
III	Neck complaint and neurological signs
IV	Neck complaint and fracture or dislocation

*physical or musculoskeletal signs—range of motion loss or tenderness.

episode of neck pain. Siivola (82) reported that adolescent neck pain predicts adult neck pain. Also, that psychological stress is a risk factor for neck pain incidence. While a reduced risk of neck pain was found amongst those engaged in sports activities involving the upper extremities. Carroll (15) et al. also found that depression is an independent risk factor for an episode of neck or back pain.

What Predisposes a Person to Chronic Neck Pain? (See Chapters 3 and 9)

Hill et al. (35) found that 48% of neck pain patients report persistent pain even 1 year after onset. Many risk factors of chronicity are shared by the neck and low back (62). Feuerstein et al. (26) reported that acute neck/shoulder patients who use catastrophizing as a pain coping mechanism were 1.5 to 2 times more likely to have pain at 1, 3 and 12 months. According to Carroll et al. (14) high levels of passive coping strategies are associated with disabling neck or back pain. In particular:

• Inability to function with pain
• Not taking responsibility for care
• Low self-rated health

Kjellman et al. (50) distinguished between predictors of one year persistence of neck pain or disability and found the following:

Predictors of Future Disability
• High pain intensity
• Low self-rated health

• Low expectations of treatment
• Lengthy duration of current episode

Predictors of Future Pain
• High disability score
• Lengthy duration of current episode
• Similar problem during the previous five years

Both Hoving and Hill reported that individuals above 40 years of age are more likely to develop persistent neck pain (35,36). Although compensation has been shown to be predictive of prolonged recovery from whiplash, however Scholten-Peters (80) in a systematic review of prospective studies concluded that there is "strong evidence that compensation has no prognostic value for delayed functional recovery".

Limitations of Structural Pathology

When considering imaging for the cervical spine it is important to know what findings may be relevant or may be misleading. In the neck, the false positive rate for imaging has been reported to be as high as 75% with an asymptomatic population (7,91). When comparing patients with radiographic evidence of cervical spine degeneration to those without (mean age 49 years old), there is no difference in reported pain and disability levels (74).

Imaging is also used to study spinal alignment and vertebral relationships. However, the degree of cervical lordosis, or lack thereof, has no predictive value for future neck pain or future degenerative changes (28).

Imaging tests have high sensitivity (few false negatives) but low specificity (high false positive rate) for identifying disc problems. Such poor specificity marks imaging as an inappropriate screening method. Bush found that most cervical disc herniations regress with time without resorting to surgery (12). Additionally, he found that the larger the disc herniation the more likely it is to reduce in size over time. Therefore, it is important to avoid "labeling" patients as being damaged since this may have disabling effects by promoting the "sick role" and interfering with functional reactivation (65).

Panjabi theorized that most WAD patients experience mild soft-tissue injury which does not cause tissue failure and thus is undetected by static imaging procedures (72). In these sub-failure injuries the soft tissues are not torn, but are stretched beyond their elastic limit resulting in functional instability and poor healing.

Impairments Associated with Pain and Disability

A number of different functional impairments have been shown to be associated with neck related problems. For instance, decreased cervical range of motion (ROM) is present to a greater extent in neck pain than asymptomatic individuals (52,53,89). However, most relevant impairments are related to abnormal motor control; for instance, increased activity in the upper trapezius, repositioning error, and poor control of cervico-cranial flexion motion.

Edgerton et al. studied altered muscle activation ratios of synergist spinal muscles during a variety of motor tasks in whiplash patients (21). They discovered that underactivity of agonists and overactivity of synergists was able to discriminate chronic neck pain patients from those who had recovered with 88% accuracy. They concluded that, "The nervous system apparently can detect a reduced capacity to generate force from a specific muscle or group of muscles and compensate by recruiting more motoneurons. This compensation can be made by recruiting motor units from an uninjured area of the muscle or from other muscles capable of performing the same task."

Lauren et al. discuss the associations between motor skills and coordination as it relates to neck pain (51). This study described appropriate timing and amplitude of muscle reactions and how poor motor control of arm motion was correlated with neck pain. Bansevicious and Sjaastad (3) reported increased EMG activity of the upper trapezius in patients with cervicogenic headache while performing computer tasks requiring concentration. Babyar (2) reported that faulty arm abduction related to a disturbed scapulo-humeral rhythm was present in neck/shoulder pain patients. Nederhand et al. demonstrated that a decreased ability to relax the upper trapezius muscles during static tasks and following exercise distinguished chronic WAD II patients with marked disability (Neck Disability Index (NDI) = 26, SD 8.5) from healthy control subjects (69).

Nederhand showed in less disabled patients that upper trapezius underactivity is the norm (NDI = 19, SD 8.1) (70). Increased activity of the sternocleidomastoid (SCM) and anterior scalene muscles during low load repetitive upper limb tasks was found in both whiplash or idiopathic neck pain patients compared to asymptomatic subjects. (6)

Bilenkij et al. reported poor motor control (i.e., impairment) was associated with greater disability (i.e., functional loss) (6).

Kinesthetic awareness of position sense has been shown to be compromised in neck pain individuals (16,32,33,63,76–78,89,93). The ability to find or return to a specific position of the head in space and is called repositioning ability or error. Neck pain patients typically error in repositioning by at least 5° (3 cm), whereas normal control subjects error by less than 2° (63). Cervical mechanoreceptor dysfunction is a likely cause of dizziness in WAD. Increased neck repositioning error has also been found in WAD patients that present with associated dizziness (93). Severity of injury seems significant to joint position error, with deficits noted only in moderate to severely disabled individuals, as measured with the NDI (89).

Jull and others have shown that a cranio-cervical flexion test can differentiate asymptomatic individuals from patients with various neck related presentations: acute and chronic post-whiplash neck pain patients, chronic headache patients, and non-traumatic neck pain patients (42,43,25,45). Jull has concluded that the test correlates with pain (45). During the test both types of patients showed overactivation of the superficial neck muscles (SCM) (25,45,89). They also displayed an inability to hold the head at a constant pressure against a pressure sensor at all test levels, as well as an inability to target higher pressure levels (26–30 mmHg) (42,43,45,89). Falla et al. confirmed that reduced performance of the craniocervical flexion test is associated with dysfunction of the deep cervical flexor muscles (25). Falla et al. has also demonstrated that neck pain subjects had significant difference in reaction time for the deep neck flexors in experimental arm elevation. Interestingly, they reported possible bleed over from the suprahyoid muscles during the collection on subjects. Manual therapy and exercise to improve the strength and coordination of this movement has been shown to achieve lasting results both in improved function and reduced symptoms.

Numerous studies have shown that decreased endurance of neck flexors (cranio-cervical flexion test) (42,43,92, 97) or extensors (modified Biering-Sorensen Test) (52,53) can distinguish neck pain or headache patients from asymptomatic individuals. Watson and Trott found that forward head posture is correlated with decreased isometric strength and endurance of neck flexors (97). Silverman found that individuals with neck pain had reduced neck flexor strength than asymptomatics (83). Yllinin et al. (99) reported decreased isometric strength in neck flexion, extension, and rotation distinguished female chronic neck pain subjects from those without pain. The authors concluded in a related study that the decreased strength may reflect reduced pain tolerance not an actual strength deficit (100).

Neural provocation tests have been studied for their reliability and diagnostic accuracy for patients with cervical radiculopathy or carpal tunnel syndrome. The upper limb tension test, which is designed to tension and provoke symptoms in the median nerve and/or the brachial plexus, can be considered the "straight leg raise" of the upper extremity. It has been found to have greater diagnostic accuracy than a neurological evaluation including sensory, motor and reflex testing (96).

Effectiveness of Reactivation

The Quebec WAD guideline recommended early, active intervention (including manipulation) as a basic approach to managing symptoms (73,87). Treatment following these guidelines has been shown to be much more effective than traditional passive based care (79). Clinically important symptoms at 6 months post-accident were present in only 10% of properly managed patients (early active intervention with submaximal movements identified by McKenzie evaluation) as compared with >50% of those given standard care (e.g., soft collar, initial rest, gradual mobilization).

Similar positive results for early activation were found in other studies. Encouragement to continue with activities of daily living (ADL's) had a superior outcome than prescription of sick leave and immobilization (8). Physical therapy or exact instruction in self-mobilization were both better than 2 weeks rest with a soft collar at 1 month, 2 month and 2 year follow-ups (66). A recent randomized control trial (RCT) showed that general exercise treatments or McKenzie treatments were slightly more effective than low-intensity ultrasound (49). McKenzie treatment led to significantly greater improvement than ultrasound at 3 week and 6 month follow-up period. Chronic pain patients also receive benefit from exercise or exercise plus manual therapy programs.

A recent study found that chronic neck pain patients receive more benefit from a combination of low-technology exercise and manipulation than with either high-technology exercise or manipulation alone (10,24). Most outcomes were similar for the two exercise groups, except that patient satisfaction was higher for the combined exercise and manipulation group. Jull demonstrated that manual therapy combined with exercise training aimed at improving deep neck flexor function improved recovery in chronic neck pain patients following a whiplash injury (44). Mobilization, manipulation, and exercise were found to be equally effective by Jordan, et al. (41).

Ahlgren et al. demonstrated that any of 3 types of active care (strength, endurance or coordination training) was superior to a group that received only ergonomic and relaxation advice for improving chronic work-related neck shoulder pain (1). Yllinin '03 studied the effectiveness of exercise for women with chronic neck pain (98). Endurance training was most effective, followed by strength training, and lastly flexibility with aerobic conditioning was the least effective.

Outcomes

The NDI is a very simple, reliable and responsive tool for measuring functional status in individual neck pain patients (90). Other scoring tools can be utilized and are reviewed in Chapter 8. Tuttle showed that "within-session" auditing of patient care with tests of the patients mechanical sensitivity is a valid way to empirically identify manual interventions that will have lasting "between-session" effectiveness (94).

A Functional Screen

It is frequently difficult to pinpoint the specific pain-generating tissue responsible for head/neck and upper back syndromes. Even in cases where a tissue-specific diagnosis is attained, the reasons behind its generation are often elusive. For these reasons, and to guide the rehabilitation effort, a thorough functional evaluation is needed. In fact, various functional deficits (impairments) have been shown to correlate with neck pain (see Chapters 1 and 25). An adequate diagnosis for neck patients must include both tissue-specific elements and functional elements.

Functional deficits may be categorized as quantitative or qualitative. Quantifiable functional tests have been covered in detail in Chapter 11. This section will provide an atlas of both quantitative and qualitative test of motor control. Deficits in strength, balance, coordination, and endurance represent the spectrum of motor control, which when lacking can place undue mechanical stress on pain-sensitive tissues, or lead to biomechanically unfavorable compensatory motor strategies.

The Upper Crossed Syndrome and the Spine

Janda emphasized the importance of muscle balance in function (37–40). Agonist-antagonist-synergist relationships should occur with proper coordination and synergy (54,55,56,68,84). Alterations of this muscle balance occur in characteristic, predicatable patterns (see Table 35.6). Additionally, deficits in mobility of joints near or remote from the cervical spine can impact function. Cervical, thoracic, glenohumeral, and tempero-mandibular joints should be evaluated for these deficiencies. For instance, poor thoracic mobility will cause a compensatory reaction in the cervico-cranial region or gleno-humeral joints

Table 35.6 Key Myofascial or Osteoligamentous Pain Syndromes and Muscle Imbalances Associated with Head and Neck Dysfunction

Painful Joints	Trigger Points	Shortened Muscle	Inhibited Muscle
Cervico-cranial	SCM	Suboccipitals	Deep neck flexors
Gleno-humeral	Upper trapezius	Levator scapulae	Lower trapezius or subscapularis
Upper ribs	Scalenes	Pectorals	Diaphragm
TMJ	Lateral pterygoids	Masseter	Suprahyoids

(4,11,47,57–60,64). Observation of functional activities, either in isolated motions, or more complex weight-bearing functions can show these different motor control strategies at work, leading to a better understanding of individual patient function and a customized rehabilitation prescription.

A classic example of muscle imbalance is the upper crossed syndrome (see Fig. 35.1). This is a typical postural overstress resulting from muscle imbalance (see Table 35.7). The overactive/shortened muscles include the pectorals, upper trapezius, levator scapulae, sternocleidomastoid (SCM), masseters, and lateral pterygoids. The underactive/inhibited muscles include the serratus anterior, lower trapezius, deep neck flexor, and suprahyoids muscles. The suboccipitals are often tight, but also lose endurance. (52,53) For instance, whiplash will lead to inhibition of the deep neck flexors that will persist for some time after the injury (43,45,92). The result of this muscle imbalance is increased kyphosis, rounded shoulders, flexion of the lower cervical spine, exten-

sion of the upper cervical spine and anterior head carriage.

The maintenance of spinal stability and integrity requires efficient load sharing along the kinetic chain. The glenohumeral joint is designed to have great mobility but is inherently unstable, and can be easily upset into functional instability. This leads to the alteration of mechanics and the development of impingement or repetitive strain disorders. If thoracic mobility is compromised, loads may increase in adjacent segments, typically the cervical spine and shoulder complex. Associations have been shown between decreased thoracic extension mobility and both neck pain (4) and shoulder pain (64). Cleland et al. reported that thoracic spine manipulation results in immediate analgesic effects in patients with mechanical neck pain. (17)

Muscle imbalances are not limited to the axial region. The pattern of over- and under-active muscles extends throughout the extremity (54). Overactive/shortened muscles include the scapular elevators, shoulder internal rotators, shoulder/elbow/wrist flexors, and forearm pronators. The underactive/inhibited muscles include the scapular adductors, scapular depressors, shoulder external rotators, shoulder/elbow/wrist extensors, and forearm supinators. The result of this muscle imbalance on the upper extremity is altered scapulo-humeral rhythm, anterior/superior migration of the glenohumeral joint, internal rotation and flexion of the upper extremity, and pronation of the forearm.

The scapulothoracic mechanism is the crossroads of the axial and appendicular components of the upper quarter. Impaired functional mechanics and scapular stability are frequently the result of various muscle imbalances and changes in mobility. Key elements in a treatment approach include the restoration joint mobility, normalization of muscle activity and endurance, and functional stabilization of cranio-cervical, scapulo-thoracic and glenohumeral mechanics.

Manipulation and mobilization techniques are of great benefit in the restoration of upper thoracic extension and improving other articular restrictions.

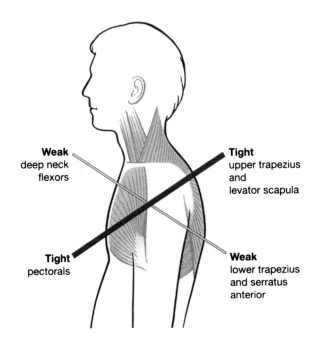

Figure 35.1 Upper cross syndrome.

Table 35.7 Relationship Between Key Sources of Biomechanical Overload and Painful Joints

Painful Joints	Faulty posture	Faulty Movement Pattern
Cervico-cranial	Head forward	Neck flexion
Gleno-humeral	Rounded shoulder	Arm Abduction
Upper ribs	Slumped posture	Respiration
TMJ	Chin protrusion	Mouth opening

Overactive or hypertonic muscles respond well to muscle relaxation techniques. In cases of adaptive shortening or fibrous adhesion, more aggressive connective tissue or myofascial release-type treatments may be necessary.

Stabilization exercises are designed to improve motor control and endurance. Common elements include lower trapezius/serratus anterior synergy, deep neck flexor activity, and thoracic extensor endurance. Closed kinetic chain strategies are often helpful in establishing muscle activation and coordination. Progression can then be made to more dynamic, functional activities. The ultimate goal of patient-specific functional restoration must be kept in mind when designing and progressing exercise.

The Upper Crossed Syndrome and the Orofacial Region

The orofacial region has a number of functional responsibilities. Mastication, swallowing, and speech are three of the most important functions (19). The primary joint complex in this region is the temperomandibular joint (TMJ), however the hyoid bone and the cervico-cranial junction are also crucial to function of this region (19,46,67). There are many important muscles, but perhaps most important are the suprahyoids, masseters and lateral pterygoids.

The main actions of the jaw are to open and close. Mouth opening couples mandible depression with chin retrusion, while mouth closing is coupled with chin protrusion. The suprahyoids produce the action of mouth opening, while the lateral pterygoids bilaterally stabilize the TMJ. The masseter is the chief muscle responsible for closing the mouth while it is assisted by the synergistic medial pterygoids and temporalis (71).

An individual with a forward head posture typically also has their chin protruded and cervicocranial junction hyperextended (61,84,85). In this posture the deep neck flexors are lengthened while the suboccipitals are shortened (19,46). The masseter becomes shortened due to increased gravitational challenge while the antagonistic suprahyoids become further inhibited. Centration of the TMJ and cervico-

cranial junction is compromised, thus making the region less stable (19).

Recent studies have identified significant relationships, biomechanical and neurophysiologic, that demonstrate functional interplay between the head, neck and jaw (23,31,34). The first movement during chewing and speaking seems to be extension of the upper neck (22,101). Importantly, in WAD patients this movement is absent.

The suprahyoids have received little attention in cervical and TMJ research and/or clinical instruction. Several new studies have shown that they act synergistically with the deep neck flexors in providing stability to the cervical spine (29,86)

Atlas of Functional Screens

The purpose of functional assessment is to identify a patient's functional or performance deficits and capabilities. The modern management of neuromusculoskeletal problems focuses on functional reactivation, restoration and rehabilitation. Structural problems such as herniated discs or arthritis are relevant in a small percentage of cases and are often coincidental findings. Therefore, the functional assessment has become a pivotal and often misunderstood component in patient care.

For each test the patient's mechanical sensitivity (MS) and abnormal motor control (AMC) is noted. This atlas follows a consistent format for describing each test:

- Indications
- Procedure
- Score
- If positive possible treatments to consider
  - Tissue to relax/stretch
  - Tissue to adjust/mobilize
  - Tissue to facilitate/strengthen

This functional assessment does not replace the initial diagnostic triage of patients, but rather complements it. Evidence-based consensus panel guidelines conclude that for over 80% of back pain the exact pain generator cannot be identified and the label non-specific or mechanical back pain is applied. It is precisely because of this situation that the functional assessment is so important. Patients want to know what is causing their pain, and while a functional diagnosis does not pinpoint causality it does give the clinician essential targets for functional reactivation as well providing simple, inexpensive tests that can be used to audit the patient's progress towards functional goals and recovery.

Choosing the correct functional tests is an art not a science. Acute patients will receive a functional assessment limited mostly to range of motion (ROM) and orthopedic tests. Identifying the movements or positions that reproduce the patient's characteristic pain—their MS—is essential on an initial visit. This becomes an essential audit tool (e.g., post-treatment check) for adjudicating and legitimizing the treatment or exercise prescription, and thus motivating the patient. Once acute pain settles a more comprehensive functional assessment evaluating AMC can

also be performed (see Table 35.8). The tests chosen will be based on the functional goals or activity intolerances (AI) of the patient. In other words, what activities they want or need to do that they are having difficulty with. For instance, if sitting is an AI then assessment of mid-thoracic mobility, scapulo-humeral rhythm, and C0-C1 coordination would be appropriate tests.

Table 35.8 Functional Screening Tests for the Cervico-Thoracic and Orofacial Regions

1. Respiration
2. T4–8 screen (wall angel)
3. Push-up
4. Arm abduction
5. Janda's neck flexion test
6. C0–C1 flexion
7. Mouth opening

1. Respiration Assessment

Test A—Seated

Indications

- Subacute or chronic musculoskeletal pain (MSP)
- Poor posture

Procedure

- Visually observe the patients normal, relaxed breathing pattern
- Manually palpate the lateral rib cage from T6-T10

Score

- Failure if during normal inhalation:
  - Clavicles or shoulders elevate
  - Lower rib cage does not widen in the horizontal plane (can be monitored with palpation)

Test B—Supine

Procedure

- Visually observe the patients normal, relaxed breathing pattern

Score

- Failure if during normal inhalation:
  - Chest breathing predominates over abdominal breathing (minor dysfunction) (Fig. 35.2A)
  - Abdomen moves in, rather than out (paradoxical respiration–major dysfunction)

If Positive Possible Treatments to Consider

- Relax/stretch
  - Scalene PIR (Fig. 35.2B)
  - Breathing re-education (Fig. 35.2C, D)
- Adjust/mobilize
  - Thoracic spine T4–8 (Fig. 35.2e)
  - Upper costo-vertebral joints (Fig. 35.2F)
- Facilitate/strengthen
  - Brügger (Fig. 35.2G)
  - Scapular depressors (Fig. 35.2H)
- Functional training
  - Breathing during exertional exercise

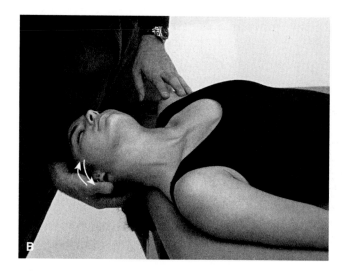

Figure 35.2B Scalene PIR.

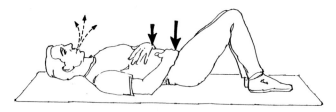

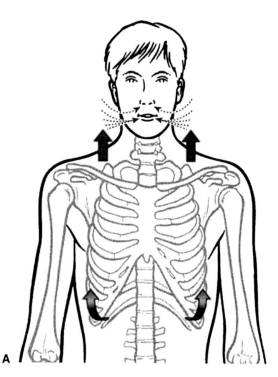

Figure 35.2A Faulty pattern of chest breathing.

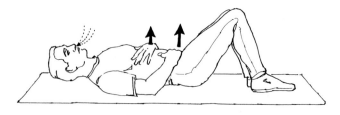

Figure 35.2C Abdominal breathing.

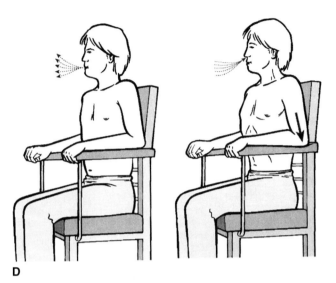

D

Figure 35.2D Self exercise to inhibit chest breathing.

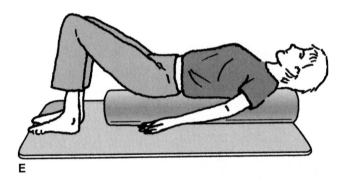

E

Figure 35.2E Thoracic spine mobilization/relaxation, foam roll—vertical.

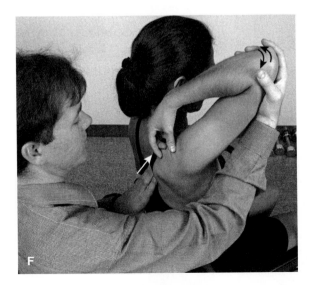

F

Figure 35.2F Upper rib PIR mobilization.

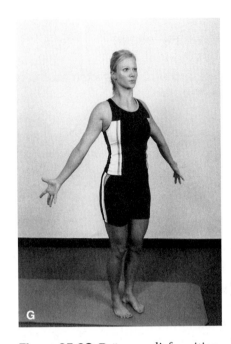

G

Figure 35.2G Brügger relief position.

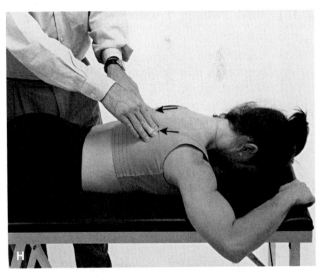

H

Figure 35.2H Scapular depressors.

2. T4—8 Mobility Screen—Wall Angel

Indications

- Subacute or chronic musculoskeletal pain (MSP)
- Poor posture
- Osteoporosis

Procedure (Fig. 35.3A)

- Stand against wall with arms abducted 90°, elbows bent 90°, palms supinated & feet slightly forward
- Try to flatten back
- Ask patient to nod so as to tuck their chin
  - Give passive overpressure to aid cervico-cranial flexion testing

Score

- Fail if
  - Thoraco-lumbar junction does not flatten
- Record where patient feels tension or pain (mid-back, left or right side, neck).
- Note if any symptoms occur when
  - Flattening back
  - Tucking chin
  - With passive overpressure into cervico-cranial flexion

If Positive Possible Treatments to Consider

- Relax/stretch
  - Pectoralis major (Fig. 35.3B)/minor, sub-scapularis (Fig. 35.3C), upper trapezius, levator scapula (Fig. 35.3D)
  - Breathing re-education
- Adjust/mobilize
  - Thoracic spine (T4–8) (Fig. 35.3E)

- Facilitate/strengthen
  - Thoracic spine extensors (Fig. 35.3F)
  - Scapular depressors (Fig. 35.3G)
- Stabilization training
  - Core/trunk (Fig. 35.3H, I)
- Functional training
  - Backhand (Fig. 35.3J)
  - Sword (Fig. 35.3K)

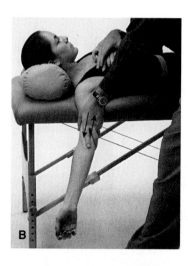

Figure 35.3B Pectoralis major.

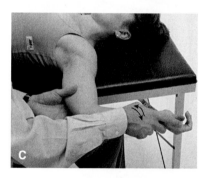

Figure 35.3C Subscapularis.

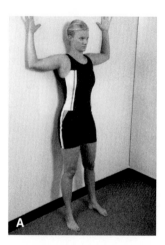

Figure 35.3A T4–8 mobility screen (wall angel).

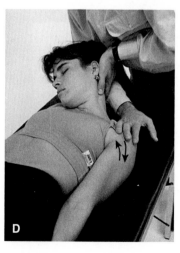

Figure 35.3D Levator scapula.

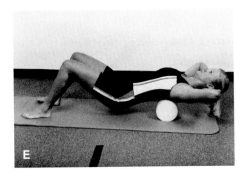

Figure 35.3E Thoracic spine mobilization, foam roll—horizontal.

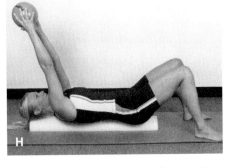

Figure 35.3H Dead Bug on foam with medicine ball overhead.

Figure 35.3F
Prayer position. Reproduced with permission from Liebenson CS. *Mid-thoracic dysfunction (Part Three): Patient self-help.* Journal of Bodywork and Movement Therapies, 2001;5;269.

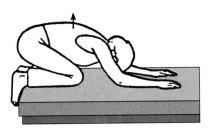
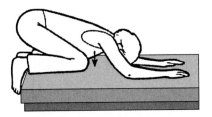

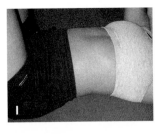

Figure 35.3I Crunch start position—ribs elevated/inspiration position, Crunch final position—ribs depressed/exhalation position.

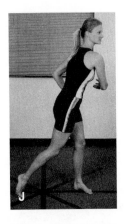
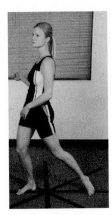

Figure 35.3J Backhand.

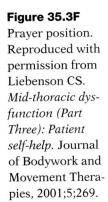
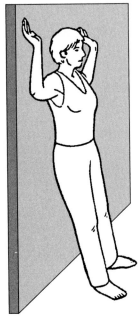
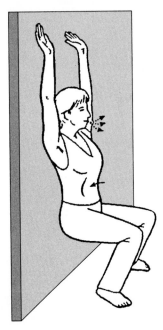

Figure 35.3G Wall slide. Reproduced with permission from Liebenson CS. *Mid-thoracic dysfunction (Part Three): Clinical Issues.* Journal of Bodywork and Movement Therapies, 5;269: 2001.

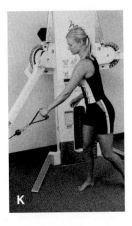
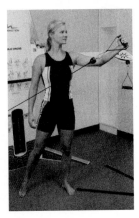

Figure 35.3K Sword.

3. Push-Up Test

Indications

- Shoulder pain
- Scapular or mid-thoracic pain

Procedure (Fig. 35.4A)

- In a push-up position from toes or knees
- Slowly lower and then raise the trunk up

Score

- Fail if:
  - Scapulae retracts
  - Scapulae wings
  - Shoulders shrug

If Positive Possible Treatments to Consider

- Relax/stretch
  - Pectoralis major (Fig. 35.4B)/minor, upper trapezius, levator scapulae
- Adjust/mobilize
  - Thoracic spine (T4–8) (Fig. 35.4C)
  - Scapulo-thoracic articulation (Fig. 35.4D)
  - Glenohumeral joint (Fig. 35.4E)
- Facilitate/strengthen
  - Scapular protraction (Fig. 35.4F, G)
- Functional training
  - Backhand (Fig. 35.4H)
  - Punch with cables (Fig. 35.4I)

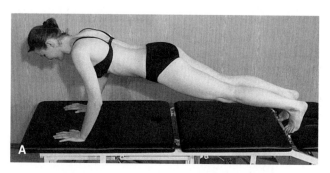

Figure 35.4A Push-up test.

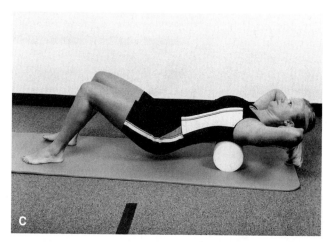

Figure 35.4C Thoracic spine mobilization, foam roll—horizontal.

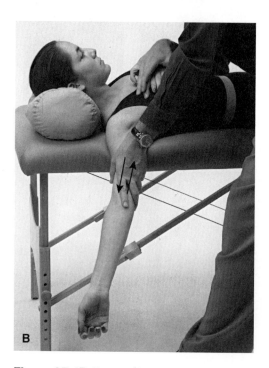

Figure 35.4B Pectoralis major PIR.

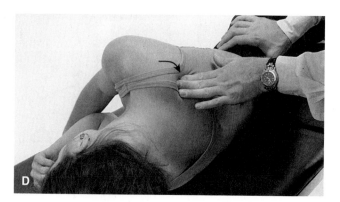

Figure 35.4D Scapulo-thoracic facilitation.

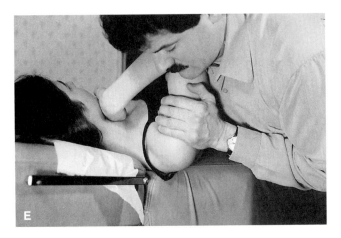

Figure 35.4E Glenohumeral manipulation, caudal glide.

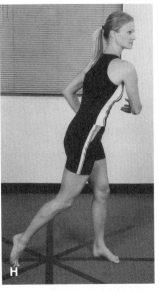

Figure 35.4H Backhand.

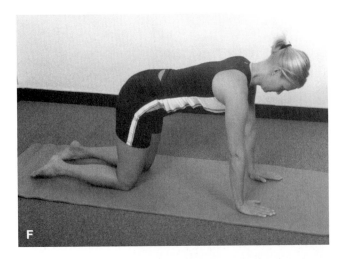

Figure 35.4F Push-up with plus, all fours rock.

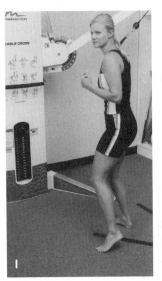

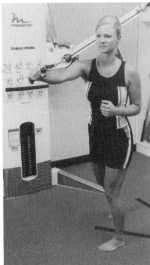

Figure 35.4I Punch.

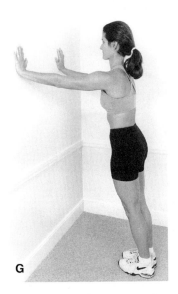

Figure 35.4G Push-up with a plus on wall.

4. Arm Abduction—Scapulo Humeral Rhythm

Indications
- Shoulder or upper quarter pain
- Neck pain, whiplash, or headaches

Procedure (Fig. 35.5A)
- Arm at side, elbow bent 90°, and wrists in neutral position
- Slowly raise arm (abduction)

Score
- During the "setting phase", first 60°, the shoulder should not elevate

If Positive Possible Treatments to Consider
- Relax/stretch
  - Upper trapezius (Fig. 35.5B) and levator scapula (Fig. 35.5C)
- Adjust/mobilize
  - Thoracic spine (T4–8) (Fig. 35.5D)
  - SC joint (Fig. 35.5E) and AC joint (Fig. 35.5F)
  - GH joint
- Facilitate/strengthen
  - Scapulo-thoracic (Fig. 35.5G)
  - Scapular depressors (Fig. 35.5H)
- Functional training
  - Ergonomic advice (Fig. 35.5I)
  - Sword pull (35.5J)

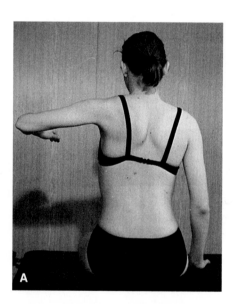

Figure 35.5A Arm abduction test.

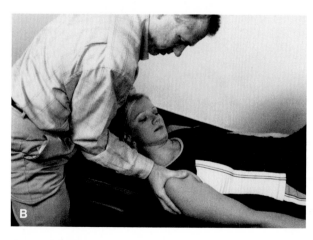

Figure 35.5B Upper trapezius PIR.

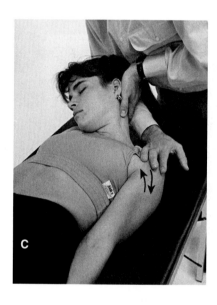

Figure 35.5C Levator scapula PIR.

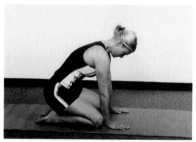

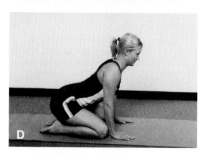

Figure 35.5D Yoga sphinx on hands.

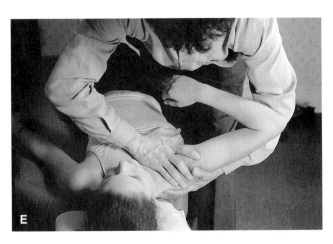

Figure 35.5E SC joint, long axis distraction.

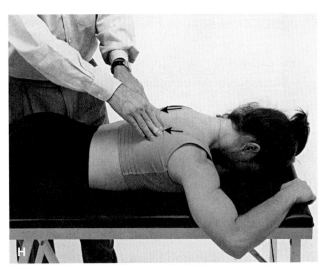

Figure 35.5H Scapular depression facilitation.

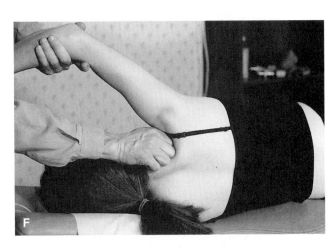

Figure 35.5F AC joint manipulation.

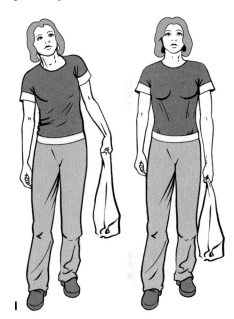

Figure 35.5I Carrying a bag, incorrect, correct.

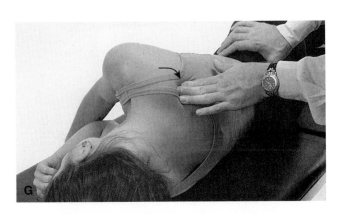

Figure 35.5G Scapulo-thoracic facilitation.

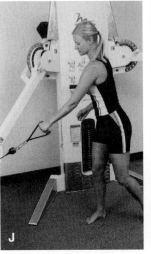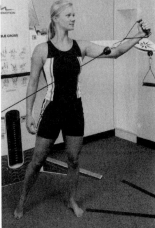

Figure 35.5J Sword.

5. Janda's Neck Flexion Coordination Test

Indications
- Neck, whiplash or headache pain

Procedure (Fig. 35.6A)
- Slowly raise head up from table toward chest

Score
- Fail If
  - Chin protrusion
  - SCM overactivity
  - Shaking

If Positive Possible Treatments to Consider
- Relax/stretch
  - SCM (Fig. 35.6B), suboccipitals, upper trapezius (Fig. 35.6C)
  - Breathing reeducation

- Adjust/mobilize
  - Occiput, upper cervical spine (Fig. 35.6D)
  - Cervico-thoracic junction (Fig. 35.6E)
  - Thoracic spine (T4–8) (Fig. 35.6F, G)
- Sensory-motor training (Fig. 35.6H, I)
- Facilitate/strengthen
  - Brügger (Fig. 35.6J)
  - Cervico-cranial flexion motor control and endurance training (nodding in supine, prone, sitting & standing positions) (Fig. 35.6K, L, M)
- Functional training
  - Postural exercises (Fig. 35,6N, O)
  - Ergonomic advice (Fig. 35.6P)

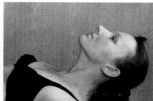

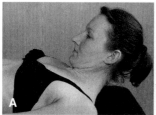

Figure 35.6A Janda's neck flexion test.

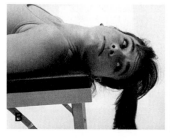
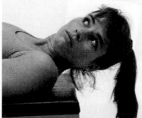

Figure 35.6B SCM PIR.

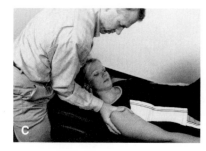

Figure 35.6C Upper trapezius PIR.

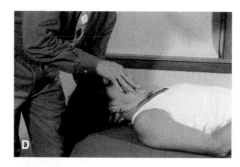

Figure 35.6D Occiput, upper cervical spine.

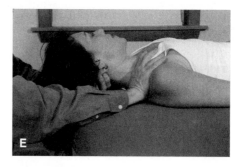

Figure 35.6E Cervico-thoracic junction.

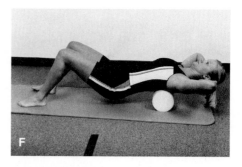

Figure 35.6F Thoracic spine mobilization, foam roll—horizontal.

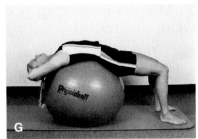

Figure 35.6G Back stretch over ball.

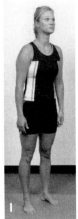

Figure 35.6H Rocker board.

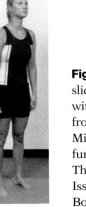

Figure 35.6I Forward lean.

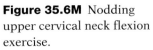
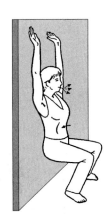

Figure 35.6M Nodding upper cervical neck flexion exercise.

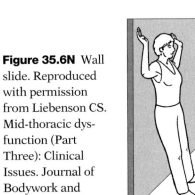

Figure 35.6N Wall slide. Reproduced with permission from Liebenson CS. Mid-thoracic dysfunction (Part Three): Clinical Issues. Journal of Bodywork and Movement Therapies, 5;269: 2001.

Figure 35.6J Brügger relief position.

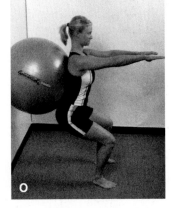

Figure 35.6O Ball squat.

Figure 35.6K Cervico-cranial flexion with stabilizer cuff.

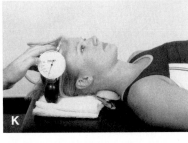

Figure 35.6L Prone sphinx with chin tuck.

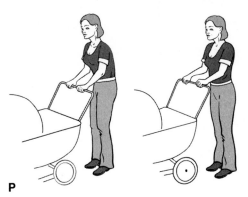

Figure 35.6P Pushing a stroller, correct, incorrect.

6. Cervico-Cranial Flexion

Indications

• Neck pain, whiplash, or headaches

Procedure (Fig. 35.7)

• Patient demonstrates nodding motion
  ○ If patient is unable then clinician models motion on patient until they are able
• Inflate cuff to 20 mmHG
• With the chin nod motion, patient increases pressure to 22 mmHG & holds for 10 seconds
• Patient tries to increase pressure to 24, 26, 28 and 30 mmHg holding for 10 seconds with a rest period after each new level

Score

• Fail if:
  ○ Overactivation of the superficial neck muscles (SCM)
  ○ Iinability to hold a constant pressure at specific test level
  ○ Inability to achieve higher pressure levels (26–30mmHg).

If Positive Possible Treatments to Consider

• (similar treatments as Janda's neck flexion coordination test)

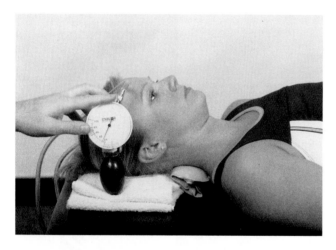

Figure 35.7 C0-C1 flexion test.

7. Mouth Opening (Orofacial Coordination)

Indications

• TMJ/orofacial pain, headache, neck pain

Procedure: (Fig. 35.8A)

• Patient is instructed to open their mouth fully

Score

• Fail if:
  ○ Chin protrusion (Fig. 35.8B)
  ○ Decreased ROM (less than 3 knuckles vertical clearance)
  ○ Head extension

If Positive Possible Treatments to Consider

• Relax/stretch
  ○ Sub occipitals, lateral pterygoids, masseters (Fig. 35.8C)
• Adjust/mobilize
  ○ TMJ (Fig. 35.8D)
  ○ Hyoid mobilization (Fig. 35.8E)
  ○ Occiput, upper cervical spine (Fig. 35.8F)
  ○ Thoracic spine (T4–8) (Fig. 35.8G)
• Facilitate/strengthen
  ○ Retrusion re-training (Fig. 35.8H)
  ○ Suprahyoids

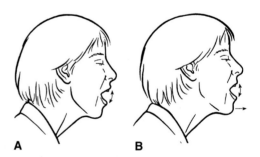

Figure 35.8A,B (A) Mouth opening test **(B)** mandibular protrusion. Liebenson CS. Advice for the clinician and patient: Mid-thoracic dysfunction (Part One): Overview and Assessment. Journal of Bodywork and Movement Therapies, 2001:5;96.

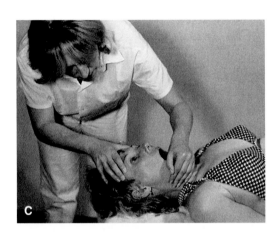

Figure 35.8C Masseter PIR.

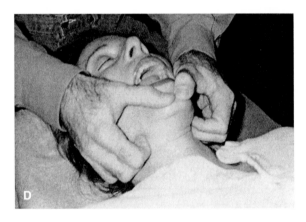

Figure 35.8D TMJ mobilization.

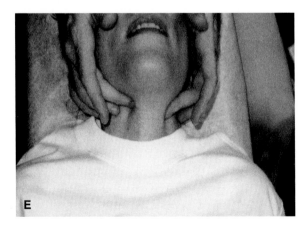

Figure 35.8E Hyoid mobilization.

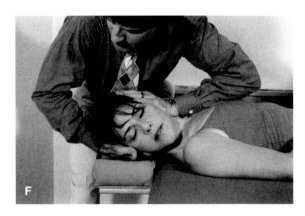

Figure 35.8F Occipital lift.

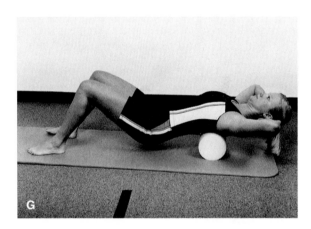

Figure 35.8G Thoracic spine mobilization, foam roll—horizontal.

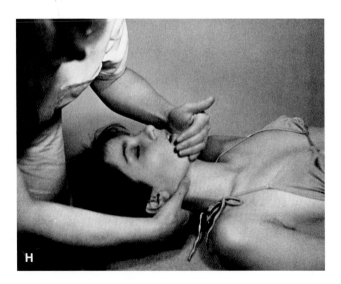

Figure 35.8H Mandibular retrusion re-training.

Cases

This section will detail a few examples of common clinical presentations. A common format incorporating the different key elements of care into a repeatable practice model will be shown (see Tables 32.7, 32.9 and 32.10) (48). Kibler's functional kinetic chain model will be presented for each case to show how management should not be guided only by an orthopedic assessment of the pain generator, but be predicated on a functional assessment (see Table 32.7) (48). Additionally, the goals of care will be presented for each case (palliative, tissue sparing, tissue stabilizing, and functional training) (see Table 32.10). Within these goals of care are subsumed the continuum or steps of care (advice, manipulation, and exercise) identified/discussed in Chapter 32 (see Table 32.9). For example, sparing strategies include advice on ergonomic modifications or manipulations of joints or soft tissues; and exercise is included in both stabilizing and functional training.

Case 1: Neck Pain and Non-Migrainous Headache

Kinetic Chain Approach

Clinical symptom complex: Head pain bilaterally, typically localizes in the supraorbital or suboccipital region, often presents with restricted cervical ranges of motion and associated neck pain (Fig. 35.9A, B, C)

Tissue injury complex: Differential diagnosis (DDx)—myofascial, zygapophyseal

Source of biomechanical overload: Forward head with cervico-cranial hyperextension and cervico-thoracic kyphosis (Fig. 35.9D), and/or shrugged shoulders due to faulty scapulo-humeral rhythm (SHR) during:

- Prolonged sitting (Fig. 35.9E), and computer activity (Fig. 35.9F)
- Sleep ergonomics (Fig. 35.9G)
- Carrying (Fig. 35.9H)
- Push-up, curl up, bench press, latissimus pull-down (Fig. 35.9I)

Dysfunctional kinetic chain:
- Inhibited deep neck flexors, faulty SHR, faulty push-up
- Hypomobility of mid/upper thoracic spine
- Hypertonic SCM, cervical extensors (suboccipitals), upper trapezius and levator scapula

Goal and Continuum of Care

Palliative care: Reduce irritability of cervicocranial and related myofascial tissues

Sparing strategies:
- Activity modification advice (avoid prolonged reading, writing, computer activities and postural awareness training) (Fig. 35.9J)
- Sleep ergonomics (Fig. 35.9K)
- Adjust/mobilize thoracic spine (T4–8) (Fig. 35.9L)
- Relax/lengthen upper trapezius (Fig. 35.9M), levator scapula, cervical extensors & SCM

Stabilizing strategies:
- Facilitate deep neck flexors (Fig. 35.9 N, O, P)
- Scapular depressors (Fig. 35.9 Q, R, S)

Functional training:
- Reeducate postural awareness during reaching overhead, pulling, pushing, lifting, bending (Fig. 35.9 T, U, V)

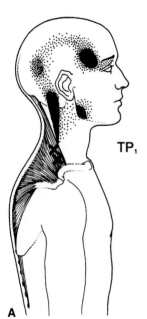

Figure 35.9A Referred pain from upper trapezius.

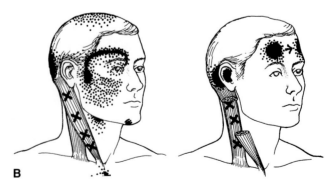

Figure 35.9B Referred pain from SCM.

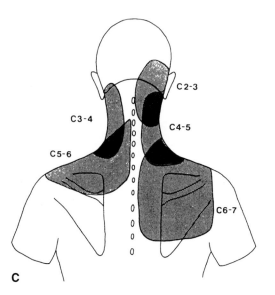

C

Figure 35.9C Referred pain from cervical spine joints.

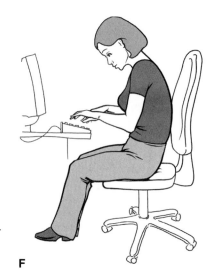

Figure 35.9F Typical slouched desk posture. **F**

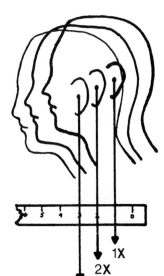

Figure 35.9D Effects of posture on neck muscle activity. **D**

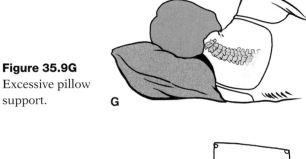

Figure 35.9G Excessive pillow support. **G**

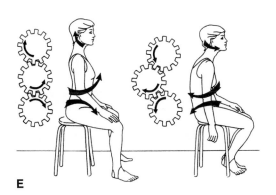

E

Figure 35.9E Slouched posture.

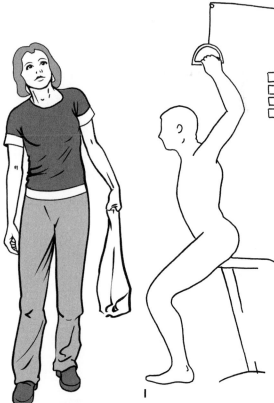

H
Figure 35.9H Carrying a bag incorrectly.

I
Figure 35.9I Improper form during "lat pull down" exercise.

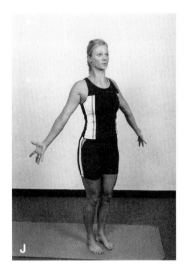

Figure 35.9J Brügger relief position.

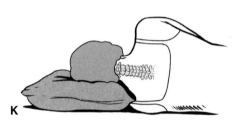

Figure 35.9K Ideal pillow support.

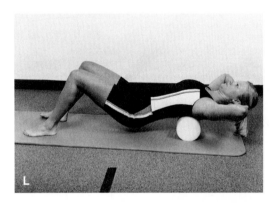

Figure 35.9L Thoracic spine mobilization, foam roll—horizontal.

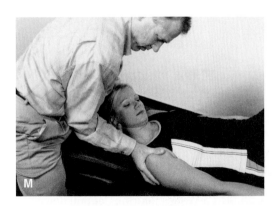

Figure 35.9M Upper trapezius PIR.

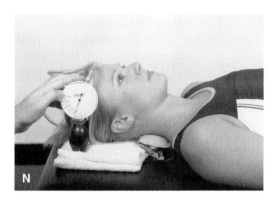

Figure 35.9N Cervico-cranial flexion with stabilizer cuff.

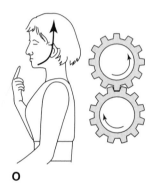

Figure 35.9O Nodding upper cervical neck flexion exercise.

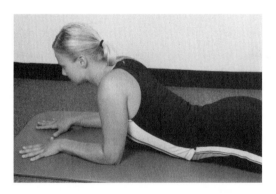

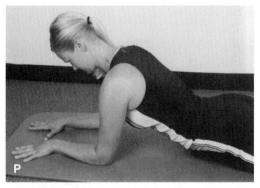

Figure 35.9P Prone sphinx with chin tuck.

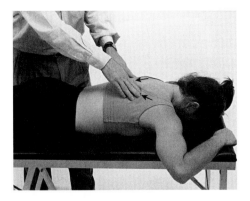

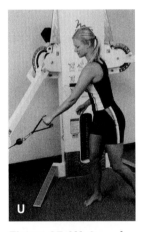

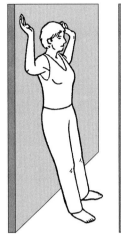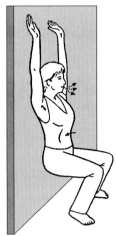

Figure 35.9T Wall slide. Reproduced with permission from Liebenson CS. Mid-thoracic dysfunction (Part Three): Clinical Issues. Journal of Bodywork and Movement Therapies, 5;269: 2001.

Figure 35.9Q Scapular depression facilitation.

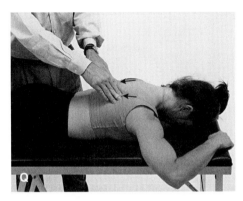

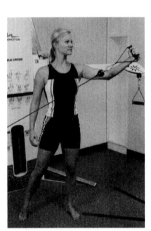

Figure 35.9U Sword.

Figure 35.9R Scapulo-thoracic facilitation.

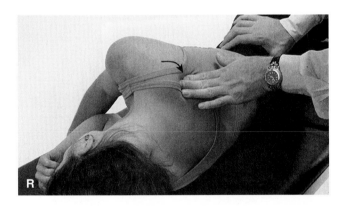

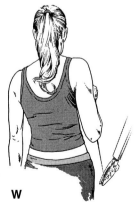

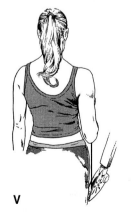

Figure 35.9V Single arm row, **(V)** correct **(W)** incorrect. Reproduced with permission from Liebenson CS. Self-management of shoulder disorders. Journal of Bodywork and Movement Therapies, 2005; 9:201.

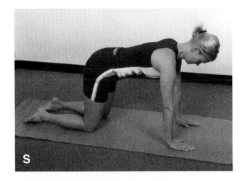

Figure 35.9S Push-up, all fours rock.

Case 2: Temporomandibular Joint Syndrome

Kinetic Chain Approach

Clinical symptom complex: Pain and clicking during mouth opening and closing (Fig. 35.10A)

Tissue injury complex: DDx—condyle/disc complex, myofascial

Source of biomechanical overload: Mandibular protrusion (Fig. 35.10B), overactive mandibular elevators and upper cervical extensors.

Dysfunctional Kinetic Chain:
- Weak activation of suprahyoid muscles
- Poor cranio-cervical stability and endurance for head/neck tasks (e.g., sitting, curl up, speaking)
- Poor swallowing
- Poor respiration (Fig. 35.10C)

Goals and Continuum of Care

Palliative Care:
- Reduce irritability condyle-disc complex (e.g., moist heat, ice)
- Activity modifications (i.e., teach mandibular rest position)
- Behavior modifications (e.g., clenching, bruxism, tongue habits)

Sparing Strategies:
- Release masseter (Fig. 35.10D), lateral pterygoid, sub-occipitals
- Mobilize condyle-disc complex (Fig. 35.10E)
- Mobilize C0-C1 junction

Stabilization Strategies:
- Facilitate suprahyoid muscles

Functional Training:
- Reeducate mandibular opening and resting positions (Fig. 35.10F)

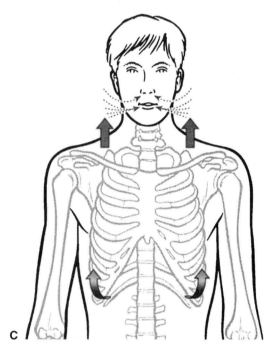

Figure 35.10C Faulty pattern of chest breathing.

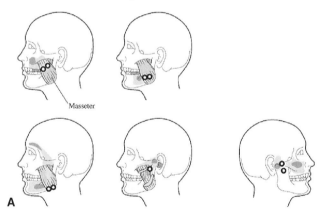

Figure 35.10A Masseter trigger point referral pattern. Masseter trigger point reprinted with permission from Chaitow L. Clinical Application of Neuromuscular Techniques, Vol 1, Churchill Livingstone, Edinbrgh 2000.

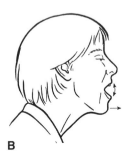

Figure 35.10B Mandibular protrusion. Liebenson CS. Advice for the clinician and patient: Mid-thoracic dysfunction (Part One): Overviw and Assessment. Journal of Bodywork and Movement Therapies, 2001:5;96.

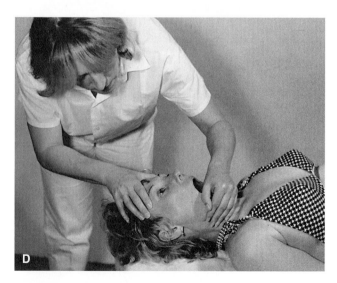

Figure 35.10D Masseter PIR.

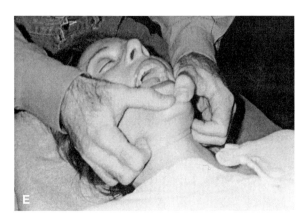

Figure 35.10E TMJ mobilization.

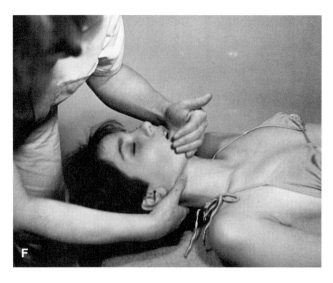

Figure 35.10F Mandibular retrusion re-training.

Case 3: Cervical Discogenic Radiculopathy

Clinical symptom complex: Nerve root symptoms down the arm and/or medial scapular pain aggravated by various neck postures and movements

Tissue injury complex: Nerve root compression or tension due to disc herniation

Source of biomechanical overload:

- End range loading of disc during ADL's - poor sitting or sleeping ergonomics (Fig. 35.11A, B)
- Pertinent factors include:
  - Temporal - morning or after prolonged flexion (sitting, stooping)
  - Poor postural and breathing habits leading increased thoracic kyphosis and head forward posture

Dysfunctional kinetic chain:

- Identify centralizing and peripheralizing maneuvers (Fig. 35.11C, D)
- Perform upper limb tension tests (Fig. 35.11 E, F, G)

McKenzie practitioners will likely attest to the frequent difficulty in initially attaining a centralizing position or movement in the acute case (see Chapter 15). Perhaps this can be attributed to a more active inflammatory component (chemical radiculitis). This will certainly limit, but does not exclude functional examination. Mechanical directional sensitivity should be noted, if present. Sensitivity to neural tension tests may be helpful in establishing what movements are safe to pursue, and what should be initially avoided (see Chapter 20). As time and early pain-based interventions take effect, a clearer picture of functional deficits will emerge, and a more specific reactivation and functional restoration program can be administered.

Goal and Continuum of Care

Palliative care:

- Ice, anti-inflammatories, cervical collar, traction (Fig. 35.11H)

Sparing Strategies:

- Ergonomic workstation (Fig. 35.11I), sitting (Fig. 35.11J), and sleep (pillow) (Fig. 35.11K) advice
- Avoid peripheralizing positions/movements (e.g., cervical extension) and perform centralizing positions/movements (e.g., cervical retraction) (Fig. 35.11L)
- Perform centralizing activities (e.g., sleep with arm overhead (Bakody's position)

Stabilizing Strategies:

- Increase mid-thoracic extension mobility
- Train scapular setting
- Train deep neck flexors

Functional Training:

- Squats/lunges
- Push/pull

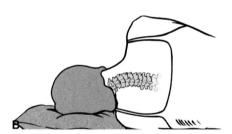

Figure 35.11B Lack of pillow support.

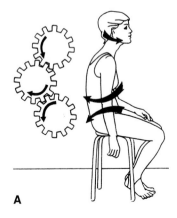

Figure 35.11A Slouched posture.

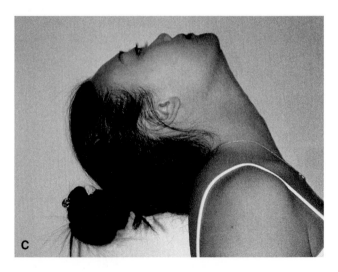

Figure 35.11C Sitting retraction-extension.

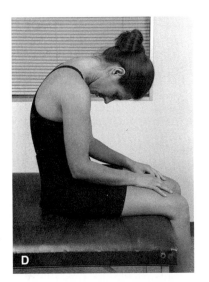

Figure 35.11D Promotion of cervical flexion.

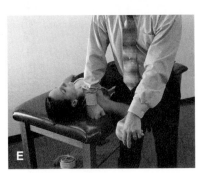

Figure 35.11E Upper Limb Neural Tension Test (ULNT), median nerve.

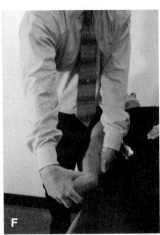

Figure 35.11F ULNT test, radial nerve.

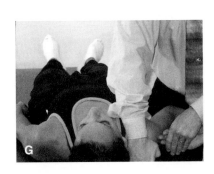

Figure 35.11G ULNT test, ulnar nerve.

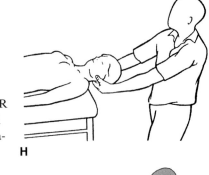

Figure 35.11H PIR traction of cervical spine using respiration only.

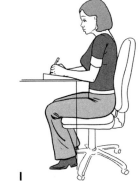

Figure 35.11I Proper desk posture.

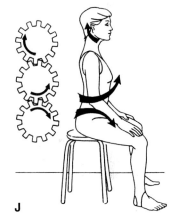

Figure 35.11J Upright posture.

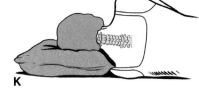

Figure 35.11K Ideal pillow support.

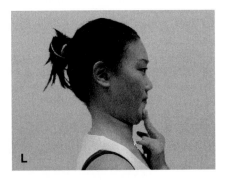

Figure 35.11L Cervical retraction.

Audit Process
Self-Check of the Chapter's Learning Objectives

• What rehabilitation methods should be considered for dysfunctional neck flexion?

• What rehabilitation methods should be considered for a dysfunctional scapulo-humeral rhythm?

• What is the continuum of care for cervical nerve root syndromes

• What is the continuum of care for orofacial problems?

■ REFERENCES

1. Ahlgren C, Waling K, Kadi F, Djupsjobacka M, Thornell LE, Sundelin G. Effects of physical performance and pain from three dynamic training programs for women with work-related trapezius myalgia. J Rehabil Med 2001;33:162–169.
2. Babyar SR. Excessive scapular motion in individuals recovering from painful and stiff shoulders: causes and treatment strategies. Phys Ther 1996; 76:226–238.
3. Bansevicius D, Sjaastad O: Cervicogenic headache: The influence of mental load on pain level and EMG of shoulder-neck and facial muscles. Headache 1996;36:372–378.
4. Barton PM, Hayes KC. Neck flexor muscle strength, and relaxation times in normal subjects and subjects with unilateral neck pain and headache. Arch Phys Med Rehabil 1996; 77:680–687.
5. Bigos SJ, Bowyer O, Braen G, et al.: Acute low back problems in adults. Clinical Practice Guideline No. 14. Washington, DC, US Department of Health and Human Services, Agency for Health Care Policy and Research, December 1994.
6. Bilenkij G, Falla D, Jull G. Patients with chronic neck pain demonstrate altered patterns of muscle activation during performance of a functional upper limb task. Spine. 2004 Jul 1;29:1436–40.
7. Boden SD. McCowin PR, Davis Do, Dina TS, Mark AS, Wiesel S. Abnormal magnetic-resonance scans of the cervical spine in asymptomatic subjects. J Bone Joint Surg 1990;72A:1178–1184.
8. Borchgrevink GE, Kaasa A, McDonoagh D, et al. Acute treatment of whiplash neck sprain injuries. Spine 1998;23:25–31.
9. Borghouts JAJ, Koes BW, Bouter LM. The clinical course and prognostic factors of nonspecific neck pain: A systematic review. Pain 1998;77:1–13.
10. Bronfort G, Evans R, Nelson B, Aker P, Goldsmith CH, Vernon H. A randomized clinical trial of exercise and spinal manipulation for patients with chronic neck pain. Spine 2001;26:788–799.
11. Bullock MP, Foster NE, Wright CC. Shoulder impingement: the effect of sitting posture on shoulder pain and range of motion. Man Ther 2005;10:28–37.
12. Bush K, Chaudhuri R, Hillier S, Penny J. The pathomorphologic changes that accompany the resolution of cervical radiculopathy. Spine 1997;22:183–187.
13. Cadarette S, Jagdal S, Kreiger N, McIsaac W, Darlington G, Tu J. Development and validation of the Osteoporosis Risk Assessment Instrument to facilitate selection of women for bone densitometry. Canadian Medical Association Journal 2000;162: 1289–1294.
14. Carroll L, Mercado AC, Cassidy JD, Cote P. A population-based study of factors associated with combinations of active and passive coping with neck and low back pain. J Rehabil Med 2002;34:67–72.
15. Carroll LJ, Cassidy JD, Cote P. Depression as a risk factor for onset of an episode of troublesome neck and low back pain. Pain 2004;107:134–139.
16. Christensen HW, Nilsson N. The ability to reproduce the neutral zero position of the head. J Manipulative Physiol Ther 1999;22:26–28.
17. Cleland JA, Childs JD, McRae M, Palmer JA, Stowell T. Immediate effects of thoracic manipulation in patients with neck pain: a randomized clinical trial. Man Ther. 2005;10:127–35.
18. Davidson M, DeSimone E. Osteoporosis Update. Clinician Reviews 2002;12:75–82.
19. Dawson, PE. A classification system for occlusions that relates maximal intercuspation to the position and condition of the temporomandibular joints. J Prosthetic Dent 1996;75:60–66.
20. Dvorak J, Valach L, Schmidt S. Cervical spine injuries in Switzerland. J Manual Med 1989;4:7–16.
21. Edgerton VR. Wolf SL, Levendowski DJ, Roy RR. Theoretical basis for patterning EMG amplitudes to assess muscle dysfunction. Med Sci Sp Exer 1996;28:744–751.
22. Eriksson PO, Haggman-Henrikson B, Nordh E, Zafar H. Co-ordinated mandibular and head-neck movements during rhythmic jaw activities in man. J Dent Res. 2000;79:1378–84.
23. Eriksson PO, Zafar H, Haggman-Henrikson B. Deranged jaw-neck motor control in whiplash-associated disorders. Eur J Oral Sci. 2004;112:25–32.
24. Evans R, Bronfort G, Nelson B, Goldsmith CH. Two-year follow-up of a randomized clinical trial of spinal manipulation and two types of exercise for patients with chronic neck pain. Spine. 2002;27:2383–2389.
25. Falla DL, Jull GA, Hodges PW. Patients with neck pain demonstrate reduced electromyographic activity of the deep cervical flexor muscles during performance of the craniocervical flexion test. Spine. 2004;29:2108–14.
26. Feuerstein, M., Huang, G. D., Miller, J. & Haufler, A. J. Development of a screen for predicting clinical outcomes in patients with work-related upper extremity disorders. Journal of Occupational and Environmental Medicine, 2000;42:749–761.
27. Gray J, Skaggs CD, McGill SM. Assessment of Orofacial Activation and Head Position on Neck and Trunk Muscle Activity During Abdominal Exercise. J Orthop Sports Phys Ther 2005. In review.
28. Goodman CC, Snyder TEK: Differential Diagnosis in Physical Therapy: 2nd edition. Philadelphia, W. B. Saunders, 1995.

29. Gore DR. Roentgenographic findings in the cervical spine in asymptomatic persons. A ten-year follow-up. Spine 2001;26:2463–2466.

30. Haldeman S: Diagnostic Tests for the Evaluation of Back and Neck Pain. Neurol Clin 1996;14:103–117.

31. Haggman-Henrikson B, Zafar H, Eriksson PO. Disturbed jaw behavior in whiplash-associated disorders during rhythmic jaw movements. J Dent Res. 2002;81:747–51.

32. Heikkila H, Astrom PG. Cervicocephalic kinesthetic sensibility in patients with whiplash injury. Scand J Rehab Med 1996;28:133–138.

33. Heikkila HV, Wenngren BI. Cervicocephalic kinesthetic sensibility, active range of cervical motion, oculomotor function in patients with whiplash injury. Arch Phys Med Rehabil 1998;79:1089–1094.

34. Henrikson T, Ekberg EC, Nilner M. Masticatory efficiency and ability in relation to occlusion and mandibular dysfunction in girls. Int J Prosthodont. 1998 M;11:125–32.

35. Hill J, Lewis M, Papageorgiou AC, Dziedzic K, Croft P. Predicting persistent neck pain. Spine 2004;29:1648–1654.

36. Hoving JL, de Vet HCW, Twisk JWR, Deville WLFJ, van der Windt D, et al. Prognostic factors for neck pain in general practice. Pain 2004;110:639–645.

37. Janda V. Some aspects of extracranial causes of facial pain. J Prosthet Dent. 1986;56:484–7.

38. Janda, V. : Muscles and Cervicogenic pain syndromes. In Twomey, LT, Taylor, JR, (eds) : Physical Therapy of the Cervical and Thoracic Spine, Clinics in Physical Therapy. Churchill Livingston, New York 1987.

39. Janda V. Muscle strength in relation to muscle length, pain and muscle imbalance. In Harms-Rindahl K (ed): Muscle Strength. New York, Churchill Livingstone, 1993.

40. Janda V. Chapter 6, Evaluation of muscle imbalance in Liebenson C. Rehabilitation of the Spine: A Practitioner's Manual, Liebenson C (ed). Williams and Wilkins, Baltimore, 1996.

41. Jordan A, Bendix T, Nielsen H, et al. Intensive training, physiotherapy, or manipulation for patients with chronic neck pain: A prospective single-blinded randomized clinical trial. Spine 1998;23:311–19.

42. Jull G, Barret C, Magee R, Ho P : Further clinical clarification of the muscle dysfunction in cervical headache. Cephalgia 1999;19:179–185.

43. Jull GA. Deep cervical flexor muscle dysfunction in whiplash. Journal of Musculoskeletal Pain 2000;8:143–154.

44. Jull G, Trott P, Potter H, Zito G, Niere K, Emberson J, Marschner I, Richardson C. A randomised control trial of physiotherapy management of cervicogenic headache. Spine 2002;27:1835–1843.

45. Jull G, Kristjansson E, Dalll'Alba P. Impairment in the cervical flexors: a comparison of whiplash and insidious onset neck pain patients. Man Ther 2004;9:89–94.

46. Just J, Ayer W, Greene C et al. Treating TM disorders: A survey on diagnosis, etiology and management. J Am Dent Assoc. 1991;122:56–60

47. Kebaetse M, McClure P, Pratt NA. Thoracic position effect on shoulder range of motion, strength, and three-dimensional scapular kinematics. Arch Phys Med Rehabil 1998;80:945–950.

48. Kibler WB, Herring SA, Press JM. Functional Rehabilitation of Sports and Musculoskeletal Injuries. Aspen, 1998.

49. Kjellman G, Oberg B. A randomized clinical trial comparing general exercise, McKenzie treatment and a control group in patients with neck pain. J Rehabil Med 2002;34:183–190.

50. Kjellman G, Skargren E, Oberg B. Prognostic factors for perceived pain and function at one-year follow-up in primary care patients with neck pain. Disabil Rehabil. 2002;24:364–70.

51. Lauren H. Luoto S, Alaranta H, Taimela S, Hurri H, Heliovaara M: Arm motion speed and risk of neck pain. Spine 1997;22:2094–2099.

52. Lee H, Nicholson LL, Adams RD. Cervical range of motion associations with subclinical neck pain. Spine 2003;29:33–40.

53. Lee H, Nicholson LL, Adams RD. J Manipulative Physiol Ther. 2005;28:25–32.

54. Lewit K. Manipulative therapy in rehabilitation of the motor system. 3rd edition. London: Butterworths, 1999.

55. Liebenson C. Rehabilitation of the Spine: A Practitioner's Manual. Lippincott/Williams & Wilkins, Baltimore, 1996.

56. Liebenson C, DeFranca C, Lefebvre R. Rehabilitation of the Spine: Functional Evaluation of the Cervical Spine—videotape, Lippincott/Williams & Wilkins, Baltimore, 1998.

57. Liebenson CS. Advice for the clinician and patient: Mid-thoracic dysfunction (Part One): Overview and Assessment. Journal of Bodywork and Movement Therapies 2001;5;2.

58. Liebenson CS. Advice for the clinician and patient: Mid-thoracic dysfunction (Part Two): Treatment. Journal of Bodywork and Movement Therapies 2001;5;3.

59. Liebenson CS. Advice for the clinician and patient: Mid-thoracic dysfunction (Part Three):Clinical Issues. Journal of Bodywork and Movement Therapies 2001; 5;4.

60. Liebenson CS. Advice for the clinician and patient: Functional reactivation for neck pain patients. Journal of Bodywork and Movement Therapies 2002; 6;1:59–68.

61. Liebenson CS, Skaggs C. The role of chiropractic treatment in whiplash injury. In Whiplash. Eds. Malanga G, Nadler S. Hanley and Belfus, Philadelphia 2002.

62. Linton SJ. A review of psychological risk factors in back and neck pain. Spine 2000;9:1148–1156.

63. Loudon JK, Ruhl M, Field E. Ability to reproduce head position after whiplash injury. Spine 1997;22:865–868.

64. Lukasiewicz AC, McClure P, Michener L, et al. Comparison of 3-dimensional scapular position and

orientation between subjects with and without shoulder impingement. J Orthop Sports Phys Ther 1999;29:574–586.

65. Main CJ, Watson PJ. Psychological aspects of pain. Manual Therapy 1999;4:203–215.

66. McKinney LA. Early mobilisation and outcome in acute sprains of the neck. BMJ 1989;299:1006–8.

67. McNamara JA, Seligman DA, Okeson JP. Occlusion, orthondontic treatment, and temporomandibular disorders: A review. J Orofacial Pain 1995;9:73–90.

68. Murphy D. Conservative Care of Cervical Spine Disorders. McGraw Hill, New York, 1999.

69. Nederhand MJ, Ijzerman MJ, Hermens HK, Baten CTM, Zilvold G. Cervical muscle dysfunction in the chronic whiplash associated disorder Grade II(WAD-II). Spine 2000;15;1938–1943.

70. Nederhand MJ, Hermens HK, Ijzerman MJ, Truk DC, Zilvold G. Chronic neck pain disability due to an acute whiplash injury. Pain 2003;102:63–71.

71. Okeson, JP.: Management of Temporomandibular Disorders and Occlusion. 3rd edition, Mosby Year Book; 1993.

72. Panjabi MM, Nibu K, Cholewicki J. Whiplash injuries and the potential for mechanical instability. Eur Spine J 1998;7:484–492.

73. Peeters GGM, Verhsgen AP, de Bie RA, OOstendorp RAB. The efficacy of conservative treatment in patients with whiplash injury. Spine 2001;26: E64–E73.

74. Peterson C, Bolton J, Wood AR, Humphreys BK. A cross-sectional study correlating degeneration of the cervical spine with disability and pain in United Kingdom patients. Spine 2003;28:129–133.

75. Physician's guide to prevention and treatment of osteoporosis. National Osteoporosis Foundation, Washington DC, 1998.

76. Revel M, Minguet M, Gergoy P, Vaillant J, Manuel JL. Changes in cervicocephalic kinesthesia after a proprioceptive rehabilitation program in neck pain: A randomized controlled study. Arch Phys Med Rehabil 1994;75:895–899.

77. Rix GD, Bagust J. Cervicocephalic kinesthetic sensibility in patients with chronic, nontraumatic cervical spine pain. Arch Phys Med Rehabil. 2001;62: 911–919.

78. Rogers RG. The effects of spinal manipulation on cervical kinesthesia in patients with chronic neck pain: a pilot study. J Manipulative Physiol Ther 1997;20:80–85.

79. Rosenfeld M, Gunnarsson R, Borenstein P. Early intervention in whiplash-associated disorders: A comparison of two treatment protocols. Spine 2000;25:1782–1787.

80. Scholten-Peeters, G., Verhagen, A., Bekkering, G., van der Windt, D., Barnsley, L., Osstendorp, R. and Hendriks, E. Prognostic factors of whiplash associated disorders: a systematic review of prospective cohort studies. Pain 2003;104:303–322.

81. Scientific Advisory Board. Clinical practice guidelines for the diagnosis and management of osteoporosis. Canadian Medical Association Journal-supplement 1996;155:1113–1133.

82. Siivola SM, Levoska S, Latvala K, Hoskio E, Vanharanta H, Keinanen-Kiukaanniemi S. Predictive factors for neck and shoulder pain: a longitudinal study in young adults. Spine 2004;29: 1662–1669.

83. Silverman JL, Rodriguez AA, Agre JC. Quantitative cervical flexor strength in healthy subjects and in subjects with mechanical neck pain. Arch Phys Med Rehabil 1991;72:679–81.

84. Skaggs C, Diagnosis and Treatment of Temporomandibular Disorders In Murphy D. Conservative Care of Cervical Spine Disorders. McGraw Hill, New York, 1999.

85. Skaggs C, Liebenson CS. Orofacial Pain. Top Clin Chiropr 7: 43–50, 2000.

86. Skaggs CD, Gray JR, McGill SM. Orofacial Contraction Does Not Affect Neck Muscle Activity in a Clinical Test. International Society of Electrophysiology and Kinesiology. Boston, MA. 2004.

87. Spitzer WO, Skovron ML, Salmi LIR, et al. Scientific monograph of the Quebec Task Force on Whiplash-Associated Disorders: Redefining "Whiplash" and its management. Spine;20(Supp):S1–73, 1995.

88. Sterling M. A proposed new classification system for whiplash associated disorders–implications for assessment and management. Man Ther 2004;9: 60–70.

89. Sterling M, Jull G, Vicenzino B, Kenardy J Characterization of acute whiplash-associated disorders. Spine 2004;29:182–188.

90. Stratford PW, Riddle DL, Binkely JM, Spadoni G, Westaway MD, Padfield B. Using the Neck Disability Index to make decisions concerning individual patients. Physiother Canada 1999; Spring: 107–119.

91. Teresi LM, Lufkin RB, Reicher MA, et al. Asymptomatic degenerative disk disease and spondylosis of the cervical spine: MR Imaging. Radiology.;164: 83–88, 1987.

92. Treleavan J, Jull G, Atkinson L. Cervical musculoskeletal dysfunction in post-concussion headache. Cephalalgia 1999; 14: 273–279.

93. Trelealvan J, Jull G. Sterling M. Dizziness and unsteadiness following whiplash injury: characteristic features and relationship with cervical joint position error. J Rehabil Med 2003;35:36–43.

94. Tuttle N. Do changes within a manual therapy treatment session predict between-session changes for patients with cervical spine pain? Aust J Physiother. 2005;51:43–8.

95. Waddell G, Burton K, McClune T. The Whiplash Book: How you can deal with a whiplash injury–based on the latest medical research. The Stationary Office, Norwich, England, 2001.

96. Wainner RS, Fritz JM, Irrgang JJ, et al. Reliability and diagnostic accuracy of the clinical examination and patient self-report measures for cervical radiculopathy. Spine 2003;28:52–62.

97. Watson, DH, Trott PH. Cervical Headache: an investigation of natural head posture and cervical flexor muscle performance. Cephalgia 1993;13; 272–284.

98. Ylinen J, Takala EP, Nykanen M, Hakkinen A, Malkia E, Pohjolainen T, Karppi SL, Kautiainen H, Airaksinen O. Active neck muscle training in the treatment of chronic neck pain in women: A randomized controlled trial," JAMA 2003;289: 2509–2516.

99. Ylinen J, Salo P, Nykanen M, Kautiainen H, Hakkinen A. Decreased isometric neck strength in women with chronic neck pain and the repeatability of neck strength measurements. Arch Phys Med Rehabil. 2004;85:1303–8.

100. Ylinen J, Takala EP, Kautiainen H, Nykanen M, Hakkinen A, Pohjolainen T, Karppi SL, Airaksinen O. Association of neck pain, disability and neck pain during maximal effort with neck muscle strength and range of movement in women with chronic non-specific neck pain. Eur J Pain. 2004;8:473–8.

101. Zafar H, Nordh E, Eriksson PO. Spatiotemporal consistency of human mandibular and head-neck movement trajectories during jaw opening-closing tasks. Exp Brain Res. 2002;146:70–6.

PART VII

Implementing the Functional Paradigm

Editor's Note

This section offers a multidisciplinary vision of how the self-management model presented in this book is applicable to all specialists in the neuro-musculoskeletal field. In fact, the core competencies required of conservative care specialists can now be outlined so that both small private practices and larger multidisciplinary clinics can benchmark themselves according to the modern clinical framework. "Best practice" approaches require best evidence synthesis, practice integration, outcome assessment, and finally re-evaluation. Through this process, leaders in the musculoskeletal field can offer practitioners in the trenches a vision of excellence. Each individual practitioner can utilize the simple audit process presented in the book's final chapter to evaluate how close they come and what changes are required to achieve a "best practice" approach.

36

The Patient and the Doctor

William H. Kirkaldy-Willis

Learning Objectives

After reading this chapter you should be able to:

- Understand the importance of the doctor–patient relationship to positive outcomes
- Understand how to respond to patients presenting with different emotional make-ups or attitudes
- Gain insight into the value of enhanced listening skill
- Appreciate the role of prayer and coping

From Chaos to Order. We remind ourselves that heavy doors move on small well-oiled hinges. Study of chaos theory teaches us that small changes at the beginning of a sequence often lead to large changes at the end, as a state of chaos leads to one of new order. This is particularly true in the case of rehabilitation of spinal disorders and allied lesions. In this we have to deal with a number of nudges, listening, compassion, caring, understanding, and togetherness that have such a big effect in healing and, on the other hand, ripples such as stress, anger, anxiety, and uncertainty that hinder the patient's recovery. The attitude of the patient and of the physician is as important as the modality of treatment that may be chosen.

Our Relationships

The interaction between medical doctor and patient, chiropractor and patient, and medical doctor and chiropractor embraces these three and their environment. These relationships to one another matter more than any individual factors.

John Macmurray (1,2), professor of philosophy at London University in the 1930s, defines the scope of human relationships.

> "In the realm of science, the unbiased observer records facts from the world around us . . . In the field of art, the observer is involved in a personal assessment of the objects studied . . . In the sphere of religion, two or more people are involved in personal interaction."

In other words, it is better to rely on simple kinds of therapy than on major interventions such as another operation. Recovery from major surgery is largely dependent on simple methods of rehabilitation. Treatment of a patient by one therapist in a simple friendly setting is more likely to enhance recovery than treatment by many different therapists in a large impersonal setting. We see this in the world around us equally well. The transistor, initially small and crude, has replaced the thermionic valve. Small steel mills, initially looked on with disdain, now produce as mush steel as the remaining large mills. The personal computer has, to a large extent, replaced the large departmental computer. In rehabilitation, for the most part, small is beautiful. The use of the so-called disruptive techniques initially are for convenience, ease of use, and cost-effectiveness and only later for improved performance.

The Individual

It is convenient to regard each person as made of four different, yet interconnected, parts: the physical, the cognitive (logical), the emotional (intuitive), and the mental (spiritual). This can be illustrated simply by drawing a circle that represents the individual, dividing it into four quadrants, and imagining a door between each division to illustrate the connection between the parts (Fig. 36.1). A practical application follows. Each one of the four parts influences the others. There is a big difference between the treatment of a disk herniation in a person who is in good mental, emotional, and spiritual health and one in an individual who has mental or emotional problems. A complete diagnosis includes the other three components as well as the physical findings.

It is often easy to treat a patient with a sacroiliac syndrome who is otherwise in good health, but the same treatment is difficult in an individual who is resentful toward her employer.

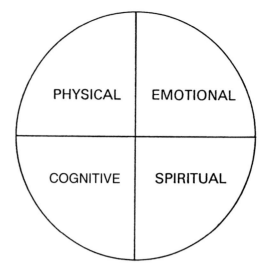

Figure 36.1 Four aspects of personality.

The Environment

The environment also can, for convenience, be considered in four parts (Fig. 36.2): the workplace; the home; the social gathering, consisting of activities in the club or the church; and the patient's hobbies and interests. There is further interaction between the individual and the different parts of the environment. A simple practical application follows. The diagnosis must include not only the physical or mental problems within the individual but also how the patient feels about life at work, at home, and in the external environment. A facet syndrome may be a minor problem in a person who is happy at work and at home. A sacroiliac syndrome may present a difficult problem for a person whose spouse is unsympathetic.

In prescribing treatment, the answer may be found by introducing a change in the workplace or adjustment to life in the home rather than in chiropractic manipulation or drug, injection, or other therapy. The writer recalls the case of a young man with symptoms suggestive of a cauda equina syndrome who recovered rapidly when plans were made for his mother-in-law to take a long vacation in a distant part of the country.

The wise physician, chiropractor, or physical therapist sees the patient as someone with these four parts to their make-up living in a four-part environment. Practitioners cannot help every patient with all possible aspects of their problem, but they may need to approach the problem in greater detail sometimes. Often it is helpful to allow the patient time to tell all he or she wants to say about himself or herself. We should be as prepared to refer a patient to a social worker, industrial adviser, or psychologist as we would to a neurosurgeon or orthopedic surgeon.

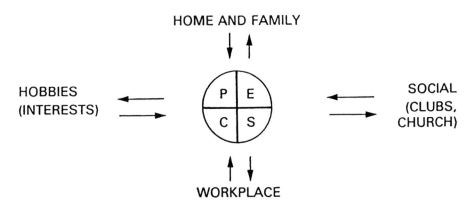

Figure 36.2 The individual and the environment.

Listening: An Essential Skill

In this it is helpful to accept the framework of the whole creation, the actual nature of our world, and of all of us in it and to appreciate our place in it. This is difficult to do. For our good fortune, "epistemology models ontology." What we can know is a good guide to the way things really are.

A study at the University of Minnesota suggests that 60% of misunderstandings in business result from poor listening. Eight percent of all business communications must be repeated. Rarely is more than 20% of what top management says understood five levels below. Sixty percent of customers who stopped buying from a company did so because of poor listening, an attitude of indifference to the client. Eighty percent of the day in business is spent in communication, but time spent in listening is often at only a 25% efficiency level (3). Poor listening skills are responsible for many of our failures and for much dissatisfaction felt by our patients.

Dr. Bernard Lown of Harvard, cardiologist and Nobel Prize winner, has stressed the importance of taking time to listen to the patient. In his opinion it is essential to spend an hour with the patient on his or her first attendance.

Frank discussion of religion has often been difficult, awkward, and sometimes taboo. It has taken three or four hundred years to recover from the dictum propounded by Descartes, who taught that the mind and the body are two separate entities in any individual. For many years, both doctor and patient have felt uncomfortable discussing religious matters.

This attitude is changing, however. Many of us now feel at ease when talking about our world, our universe, and our Creator. The approach of many, particularly younger people, to this subject is often one that differs from beliefs once considered orthodox. As physicians, we need to keep open minds with respect to different ideas and beliefs. The good physician sits beside the patient prepared to listen, rather than standing over the patient or sitting behind the desk, prepared to make pronouncements about the individual's health.

Managing Several Problems at the Same Time

Although a great deal of our work helping people back to health is quite straightforward, it often can be difficult and tax our capacities to the limit. Ackhoff, an expert adviser and writer on the subject of business and industrial management, commented, as quoted by Dixon, (4) that problems in these areas rarely occur in isolation. In a plant or factory, several problems typically exist at the same time: they are constantly changing and interacting with another. Ackhoff calls this continuing process a "mess." In his opinion, a good chief executive officer is not merely someone who can manage a problem, but one who maintains control when coping with a "mess."

From this discussion of the individual and the environment, it is easy to see the common ground between the business executive and the health care professional. In helping his or her patients, the physician or chiropractor must be prepared to deal with this "mess" frequently. To realize that health care provider- patient situations often are fraught with this kind of difficulty is to minimize the stress experienced by the therapist. In addition, it enables him or her to understand more easily the thoughts, feelings, and attitudes of the patient.

It is curious that we human beings have two opposing facets within us. On the one hand, we want to be different, stand out among our fellows as brilliant football player, top of the class, or receiving early promotion; on the other hand, we want to merge with the crowd, have the same ideas and habits, and wear the same sort of clothes. These warring factors make the "mess" more complex.

Of the many ways to deal with this "mess," the most valuable is laughter, with and not against someone else, often about something ridiculous. We can sit beside our patients, chatting naturally, getting them to laugh, laughing with them, sometimes when necessary being ourselves the butt of the joke to enhance the interaction.

The Hawthorne Effect (5,6)

The management at the Western Electric Plant at Hawthorne in the western United States was anxious to improve the output of the workers. They employed a team of sociologists who visited the plant, talked to the workers, and inspected the workshops. Among other things, they decided to increase the lighting in several areas. At once, the output from the workers increased dramatically. Everyone was delighted. At this point, one of the visitors suggested a further change. They told the workers that they planned to help them further but were careful not to say what they intended to do. They then decreased the strength of the lighting to a point below the original level. To the surprise of the management, the output of the workers increased still further. In fact, the workers had been influenced not by the strength of the light but by the feeling that both management and the team of sociologists were interested in their welfare.

In commenting on the Hawthorne effect, Dixon notes that the scientist, in designing experiments, does his or her best to minimize or eliminate this phenomenon, which is one kind of placebo effect. Dixon thinks that using this effect forms the basis of a good deal of his practice and is a central feature of family medicine. The author concurs in regard to his practice as well.

Obtaining the Patient's Confidence

The effect of putting the preceding principles into practice in our office and clinics is to build up a patient's confidence in him or herself as well as in the provider of health care.

Our interaction with each patient should begin with a friendly greeting, a handshake, walking with him or her from the waiting room to the office, and sitting beside him or her and not behind our desk. These things are little but very important, and represent the invaluable combination formed when patient and therapist work together.

Legend has it that in teaching his apprentices, Hippocrates stressed the value of obtaining the patient's confidence. It is reported that he went so far as to say that even in cases of the direst of diseases, the contentment engendered by the patient's conviction of the real concern of the physician could be the main factor responsible for a cure. To this, Sir William Osler, Professor of Medicine first at McGill, then at Hopkins, and finally at Oxford University, added that in his opinion the character of the patient with a particular disease was more important than the nature of that disease.

Chiropractors have an advantage in that their particular skill requires them to lay hands on their patients. This action itself induces confidence. The rest of us should share this advantage, by touching the patient with our hands during the examination and placing a reassuring hand on his or her shoulder when saying goodbye. In referring to a specialist, one patient said, "He never laid a hand on me to examine me. He came into the room, greeted me briefly and then asked his resident to tell him what he had found. Then he told me I would need a CT scan, a myelogram, and an operation. I was not satisfied. I said I would think it over. I didn't go back to see him again."

Interaction

Discussion of the ways in which one may increase the patient's confidence leads us to consider the interaction that takes place between the doctor and the patient. We would like to be able to make a concise and complete objective diagnosis in every case but this is often not possible. One of my patients was an elderly widow who lived by herself in a small prairie town in Saskatchewan. She first presented with a sacroiliac syndrome that did not respond to manipulation but became symptom free after an injection to the sacroiliac joint. She returned with the same symptoms a few months later, which again responded to injection. This happened several times over the months, always with the same satisfactory result. Eventually I realized that the real problem was loneliness and boredom. This was in fact relieved temporarily by a trip on the local bus, a visit to the hospital, and some talk and encouragement from me, incidentally accompanied by an injection to the sacroiliac joint, the whole giving her an enjoyable outing. This kind of problem is not uncommon. The counterpart to this phenomenon is found in quantum physics. At the beginning of this past century, Max Plank and Albert Einstein made the discovery that light, energy, and mass all could be described as waves or as small particles (quanta), depending on how the experiment was set up. The Danish physicist, Nils Bohr, solved the problem when he postulated that the right approach was a subjective one in which the interaction of the observer, looking for waves or for particles, was the determining factor. Einstein found this difficult to accept!

The Whole Person

Obtaining the patient's confidence stems from our regarding him or her as an entire, integrated being, a unity, someone of value, with the physical, mental, emotional, and spiritual working in combination. This draws attention to an important observation, already considered to some extent: as we look on our patients, set out to diagnose their ills, and attempt to treat them, we must think of them, all the time, as a whole man or woman, an individual person in their own particular environment. In so doing, we try to exert empathy to get alongside the patient, almost as a part of him or her, to help solve the problem.

How Symbols and Metaphors Work

The use of symbols and metaphors has a powerful effect on the patient. They help the patient overcome the feelings of loss of wholeness and oneness, loss of control, vulnerability, and isolation from friends, relatives, and colleagues. Jung found that the subconscious of his patients was teeming with symbols!

Symbols and metaphors are very personal. Each individual has the ability to make his or her own symbols. Sometimes, external events over which we seem to have no control make symbols for us. Groups of people and nations also have their symbols. A symbol often, perhaps always, carries more weight than logic.

The situation in which we find ourselves is not always friendly. Friends, acquaintances, doctors, nurses, and even chiropractors can disturb the working of our symbols and metaphors by their attitude, their thoughts, their words, and their actions. All of us to our shame can recall examples of being abrupt, unkind, or unfeeling in treating a patient. Reminding ourselves of such occurrences encourages us to do better in the future.

The following scenario occurred in a major teaching hospital. A patient was taken to the operating room for a cystoscopy, from the ward, without any preoperative medication. He had to get himself across from the stretcher to the operating table. His legs were placed in stirrups, with all of him in full view of all persons in the brightly lightly room. The surgeon then injected a local anesthetic per urethram. A few minutes later, the cystoscope was passed, a painful procedure. This experience of both pain and embarrassment affected the patient adversely, leaving a permanent scar, with fear of and dislike for the urologist. A few changes in procedure, a few minutes of explanation by the surgeon the previous evening, and some arrangements for more privacy could have made the whole procedure less traumatic, both physically and symbolically.

Restoring the Patient's Self-Respect

Fortunately, it is usually not difficult for the caring physician or chiropractor to help the patient regain his or her feeling of wholeness, belonging, and worth. The physician or other health care provider can listen carefully and with concern to the patient's account of the assault on his or her dignity. Some sample exchanges follow:

- He or she can then say "I agree, this is thoroughly bad, let's see what we can do about it together."
- The patient can be seen as often as is necessary to help him or her feel happy, free from embarrassment and at ease again.
- The practitioner can put himself or herself in the patient's shoes, saying, "Yes, if that happened to me I would be really mad."
- The practitioner can say, "After what you have told me, I would be reluctant to undergo that procedure. I can imagine how you felt."
- Another patient said, "Once I had a catheter passed by a rough, inexperienced assistant. It was very painful. In my case, I was told not to be a sissy. I decided not to go to that surgeon ever again unless driven to it." The physician replied, "I'd make the same decision myself."
- A physician said to a patient, "Yes, some years ago, like you, I had on one occasion to take all my clothes off and wait for the doctor while standing in front of five or six men and women. They seemed to be enjoying my predicament."

All of these situations sound ridiculously simple. The reader may think that they are not helpful. I believe they are extremely important for ensuring a fruitful interaction between patient and physician, chiropractor, or other provider of health care. Certainly, the patient can do some things for the doctor or chiropractor: having a bath before their appointment; washing the feet thoroughly; and wearing clean underwear.

It is good to follow Dr. Craig Liebenson's advice. He often asks the chronic pain patient if he or she is frustrated or angry about their pain or disability. They usually say yes. It is a relief to have their emotions validated.

Prevention: Promoting Health

The most important measures for the future are in the realm of prevention. Fortunately, individuals now involved in health care are concerned with the promotion of active health and not just with the correction of a disease process. This cogent lesson has been learned mostly in the field of sports medicine. The rest of us owe a debt of gratitude to the pioneers in this field. Our motto should be "health through activity." The writer made this simple but vital discovery while treating African patients with tuberculosis of the spine. While lying in a plaster of Paris shell during recovery after a spinal fusion, the patient was instructed to move arms and legs to music several times per day. Rest was essential for the healing of the spinal lesion. Activity of arms and legs was very important for promotion of the circulation and thus for a sense of well-being and of the general health of the whole patient.

The tools and resources needed for disease prevention are well known. We need to now refine and develop them. That chiropractors and medical practitioners have learned to work together in harmony is probably the most significant advance in the field of musculoskeletal illness and its treatment. These professionals have different yet complementary skills and attitudes. For the past 25 years of practice, my work, in increasing cooperation with chiropractors, has turned out to be of great benefit to chiropractor, physician, and patient, and was of great assistance in teaching and in research. When chiropractor and physician work together, almost in symbiosis, the result is something of far greater power than the sum of the two working alone. An analogy can be helpful. The power resulting from fusion of interests on the mental and spiritual plane is akin to that released by the fusion of hydrogen atoms on the physical.

Sometimes the chiropractor takes the lead and sometimes it is the physician. Each should learn from the other. The chiropractor can help the physician by making treatment simpler and more cost-effective. Quick, almost immediate, intervention by the physician makes things better for both patient and chiropractor if something suddenly goes wrong in the management of a disk herniation or spinal stenosis, or sudden development of cauda equina syndrome.

Education

The back school or self-care program is an essential part of this. The reader is referred to Chapters 14 and 31. The physician or chiropractor should be able to send a patient at any time with delay of no more than 2 or 3 days. A back school may be staffed by physical and/or occupational therapists, sometimes with volunteer help, or by two or three chiropractors. It may be in the office of a chiropractor, physical therapist, or physician, or in a gymnasium or hospital outpatient department. In many instances the knowledge that the patient acquires in the back school is in due course of benefit to the community as well.

The Fitness Center

Even small North American cities have one or two fitness centers, and large cities have many. This type of venture is usually run by a trained therapist or exercise physiologist. These centers were started for the benefit of those engaged in athletic activities of all kinds, to both promote fitness and help the resolution of minor musculoskeletal injuries. The client attends at his or her own volition, does his or her own workout, and asks for help and advice as necessary. Many providers of health care use the fitness center to supplement what they can do for the patient in their office and what the patient can do at home. They refer the patient to the therapist in charge, being careful to let the latter know by phone or written note the nature of the problem, with perhaps some suggestions as to the type of exercise likely to be useful. The therapist has free rein to direct and advise the patient and to control his or her activity.

While the patient is attending a fitness center, the health care practitioner and therapist can have frequent discussions about the progress made. The chiropractor or physician sees the patient at regular intervals. Sometimes, the professional personally attends the same fitness center, which provides additional valuable contact with both patient and demonstrates that the doctor does the things that he or she advises patients to do. Every chiropractic or medical office should have access to such a supportive program.

Coulehan outlined the dimensions of treatment outcome (7). The doctor–patient interaction is expressed in three ways: (1) focal, the treatment method; (2) symbolic, resulting from both cognitive and affective influences; and (3) behavioral, again from these two influences. The routine of the fitness center affords all three. It provides the incentive to develop both the physical and the spiritual well-being of the client.

The Spandex Bodysuit

The rationale for wearing an elastic bodysuit for the prevention and treatment of low back pain is similar to that put forward by athletes engaged in many different kinds of sporting activities: downhill and cross-country skiing: bobsledding; rowing; water skiing; and scuba diving, among other things. Elastic trunks or suits are often worn by football, tennis, and basketball players and by cyclists. Weight lifters wear a similar garment. This type of garment supports trunks and pelvis (focal), gives confidence and endurance (behavioral), and expresses the idea that the athlete is a combination of body, mind, and spirit, all working in harmony (8).

Physicians, chiropractors, and others have been slow to grasp the fact that an elastic bodysuit is not a rigid corset but something that enhances activity exactly as this type of garment does for the athlete. We need to rethink this means of making extra provision for prevention and treatment. In the context of doctor–patient interaction, it is the symbolic aspect that is the most important.

Spiritual Factors in Healing

A series of steps lead upward from what might be considered the purely physical (if such a state existed) to the completely spiritual (something not seen in this world). In our work as health care practitioners, we are concerned with the spectrum that lies between these two extremes.

Help From New Scientific Advances

Recent information on the Internet lends support to the thought that the membrane between this universe and the cosmos beyond is a thin and tenuous one. Scientific investigators of repute believe that there is much sound evidence to support the existence of an "Intelligent Designer" behind the origin and development of the universe. Darwin does not any longer have it all his own way. Natural selection through the inheritance of acquired characteristics alone does not give an adequate explanation of the origin of species or the arrival of homo sapiens on the scene. These writers say that it is far more difficult to postulate that the evolution of the universe and of life on our planet had natural causes, taking place "out of the blue," than to believe in the existence of an Intelligent Designer who planned and initiated the whole process. They have described in some detail the ways in which the known forces (such as gravity and electromagnetism) and constants (such as the speed of light) operate in our universe, interact, and are dependent on one another.

Those who look for further details are referred to two articles on the Internet:

1. The Intelligent Design Movement by William A. Dembski http://www.origins.org/offices/dembski/docs/bd-idesign.html
2. The Designed Just So Universe by Walter L. Bradley, PhD http://www.origins.org/offices/bradley/docs/universe.html

They lend credence to any discussion of spiritual factors in healing.

Religion and Healing

Abdul Baha writes, "Religion and Science are the two wings on which man's intelligence can soar to the heights. It is not possible to fly with one wing alone. With the wing of religion alone an individual would fall into the quagmire of superstition. With the wing of science alone he or she would fall into the despairing slough of materialism" (9).

Edison patented 1,093 inventions and turned the inventions of others into a success. For example, in 1879, after many unsuccessful attempts, he made the first electric light bulb. Later on his team produced latex from goldenrod after examining hundreds of plants. When asked where his ideas came from, he used to smile and point to the sky.

Quite ordinary men and women like us believe in the existence of a God who is all-powerful and prepared under certain conditions to intervene in our affairs, provided this intervention does not compromise our free will. We seek this help through what we call "prayer." It is wise to do this more often than we do.

Either/Or: Both/And

Something is lacking in the way we think. Perhaps it has always been that way. In most situations, we think in terms of either/or. The chiropractor or osteopath thinks in terms of manual therapy; the physician thinks in terms of medication or surgery. In Saskatoon, the process of chiropractors and orthopedic surgeons learning to work together was at first painful for both sides. Out of this effort came a "both/and" approach, resulting in a synthesis of both disciplines, something new for us, to the benefit of both ourselves and our patients.

Turning to consideration of the physical and the spiritual, we encounter the same difficulty. Many spiritually minded health care professionals see no need for anything other than physical and material methods of treatment. Priests and ministers who have a concern for healing often tend to think in spiritual terms only. The best approach is a synthesis of the two. Intermediate steps on the journey from the physical to the spiritual contain elements of both and are mentioned only briefly.

Chaos Theory, Nudges, and Ripples

Chaos theory teaches us that in many situations with minor changes at the beginning of a particular situation we encounter major changes as we reach the end. Here for convenience we refer to the factors that promote health as "nudges" and those that prevent health as "ripples." These factors are pertinent in nearly every human situation. The contrasting two types of factor, ripples and nudges are listed in the box below.

Nudges and Ripples

Ripples	Nudges
Fear	Listening
Anxiety	Laughter
Anger	Explaining
Uncertainty	Encouraging
Boredom	Attention
Hurry	Prayer

Other Resources

The back school or self-management program, already mentioned, deals not only with material facts but also with the interaction of instructors and clients and with the whole group in the class. Discussion of their problems during breaks is as important as any instruction given.

Meditation, relaxation, and imagery can be a part of self-management or they can be taught individually, both with great benefit. An integral part of this process is how to manage stress. This subject is discussed at length by Zahourek (10).

To use the imagination is most helpful. Sanford (11) tells how she was able to help a small boy with a serious heart condition. She discovered that he was fascinated by football. She said, "Let's play a game." He nodded and agreed. "Billy, imagine that you are playing football and that you are getting better and better at it. One day your team is playing against the best team in the league. You play so well that you score more goals than anyone else and win the game for your side. You hear some of the onlookers say 'Just look at Billy, how fast he can run, how well he tackles, how strongly he kicks the ball. We'd like to be like him. He must be so fit and well.' Billy was thrilled." Sanford continues, "Can you make a picture of that in your mind three or four times every day." Once again, Billy nodded vigorously. He did this every day. After a few months, he became perfectly fit and well again, with no problem with his heart. He later became a great football player.

The Institute for the Advancement of Human Behavior, another resource, is situated in Stamford, Connecticut. This organization of psychologists, psychiatrists, and other practitioners plans seminars and meetings dealing with the psychologic and immunologic aspects of both wellness and disease.

Publications

Siegel wrote of lessons learned about self-healing from a surgeons experience with exceptional patients (12). His approach combines orthodox medicine with the spiritual. The American Cancer Society has produced a pamphlet entitled "Say It With the Heart" to help those with cancer. It is full of helpful suggestions and emphasizes the importance of the patient's attitude and feelings. Another book by Simonton, Matthews-Simonton, and Creighton appeals equally to health care professionals and patients with cancer (13). The underlying philosophy is that we are all responsible for our own health and illnesses, and that we participate, consciously or unconsciously, in creating our own physical, emotional, and spiritual health. The knowledge gained from reading this book can also be applied to the management of many other conditions, be they physical, emotional, and/or spiritual ("Getting Well Again" is also available on video cassette).

The Power of Prayer

Many of us believe that the natural indwelling defenses against foreign invaders and disease, including the immune system, were given to us by God as part of our make-up; that our environment contains many resources for healing, substances like penicillin and digitalis; and that health care professionals and others have their source of training directly from Him—it is no accident that hospitals and clinics had their origin in the monasteries of the Middle Ages.

It is not too great a stretch of the imagination to believe in the existence of an all-powerful being, prepared under certain circumstances to intervene in our affairs. Again, we seek this help through prayer. It is easy to ignore the existence of a power greater than ourselves when the sun is shining. Then our god may well be golf, our savior the computer, our inspiration gained from thoughts of sex. When ill health and disaster loom ahead, we are more inclined to look above and beyond ourselves for help. Fortunate is the man or woman, health care professional, or patient who seeks to take advantage both of the natural provisions for health and wellness and of those from the supernatural realm.

The same sort of interaction can take place when someone has severe low back pain at a time when both patient and doctor are at their wit's end. A priest in the Episcopal Church developed severe back and leg pain of sudden onset. He contacted a friend who in turn called his friend, an orthopedic surgeon. The surgeon examined the man and thought he had an acute L4–5 disk herniation. This suspicion was confirmed by a CT scan. Members of the priest's church prayed for him that night. On his next visit, the surgeon prayed for him as well, with some reluctance (surgeons do not usually pray for priests!). In the middle of that night, the patient woke up and realized all his pain had gone. From that point, he had a rapid and uneventful recovery. The priest later said that he had experienced two miracles: the first was that a surgeon had visited him in his own home, and the second was the healing of his back.

■ CONCLUSION

Interaction between physician, chiropractor, and patient is both fundamental and complex. The resulting relationships are the phenomena of most importance. They depend on something more than science alone. The raw materials of which they are built come from a variety of sources:

- A careful study of science and its branches
- The humanities
- Philosophy
- Myth, the story with a meaning
- Behavior, symbol, and metaphor

The combinations of these sources with the greatest significance are those with a strong symbolic content. Good relations stem from our seeking the best for one another. The search may involve us in efforts to understand aspects of a persons psyche that range from slight differences in dress to grasping the nature of an individual's reaction to a situation of life and death. At times, it is not difficult for the discerning physician to empathize with the distress felt by a patient, sharing the symbolic content and the behavioral aspects of the situation. The practitioner must shift from time to time from close identity on the stage to standing back in the wings.

In the process of traveling with a client from a state of distress to one of complete well-being, we should be prepared to seek help from other sources. Complete rapport between the physician and the chiropractor is of greatest significance and also is rewarding. The convergence of ideas and beliefs held by students and teachers from two different backgrounds produces within them the stimulation required to conquer new areas in the spectrum of musculoskeletal illness.

Given the large a number of different approaches to spiritual healing, it is essential to respect beliefs that are different from our own. It is good to be aware of the presence and involvement of the Creator in any and every scenario in which client and helper seek health and wholeness. This statement does not imply that we are always talking about such awareness. When we ourselves do not have access to this kind of help, we should feel free to refer the client to someone else who has. The One who sits on the throne is able to come "alongside" us just as we are taught to come alongside our clients in their need.

Audit Process
Self-Check of the Chapter's Learning Objectives

- What are patient's expecting on the first visit?
- How does good or bad listening skill impact patient satisfaction?
- What are some good ways to gain a patient's trust or confidence?
- What are some resources that can help the patient maintain spiritual balance?

■ REFERENCES

1. Macmurry J. Reason and Emotion. London: Faber and Faber, 1935.
2. Macmurry J. Creative Society. London: Faber and Faber, 1935.
3. Blanchard K. Listening: a Basic Business Skill. Inside Guide, Newsletter for Canadian Plus. Toronto: Grant N. R. Geall; June, July, and August, 1992.
4. Dixon T. The philosophies of family medicine (editorial) Can Fam Physician 1989;35:743.
5. Chapman-Smith D. Reflections on the Hawthorne effect. Chiropractic Report (editorial). 1989;4:1.
6. Dixon T. In praise of the Hawthorne Effect (editorial). Can Fam Physician 1989;35:703.
7. Coulehan L. The treatment act: An analysis of the clinical art in chiropractic. J Manipulative Physiol Ther 1990;14:1.
8. Kirkaldy-Willis WH. Energy stored for action: The elastic bodysuit. In: Kirkaldy-Willis WH, Burton CV, eds. Managing Low Back Pain. New York: Churchill Livingstone, 1992.
9. Abdul B. Paris talks. London: Bahai Public Trust, 1973:143.
10. Zahourek R. Relaxation and Imagery. Philadelphia: WB Saunders, 1988.
11. Sanford A. The Healing Light. New York: Ballantine Books, 1983.
12. Siegel BS. Love, Medicine and Miracles. New York: Harper & Row, 1986.
13. Simonton OC, Matthews S, Creighton JL. Getting Well Again. New York: Bantam Books, 1980.

37

The Role and Safety of Activity in the Elderly

Craig Liebenson

Learning Objectives
After reading this chapter you should be able to:

- Understand how activity in the elderly is associated with all causes mortality
- Understand how activity in the elderly can be better promoted by health care providers

- Screen for risk factors with exertion in the elderly
- Organize rehabilitation services for patients with osteoarthritis, osteoporosis, joint arthroplasty, and spinal stenosis
- Offer osteoporosis, balance and frailty prevention services

Introduction

Healthy lifestyles incorporating physical activity and exercise have been shown to be highly beneficial for persons aged 75 and older. Reductions in functional decline (frailty), coronary heart disease (CHD), and disability before death along with increased life expectancy have all been demonstrated (31,48,72,113). Specific exercise programs have also been shown to prevent falls in the elderly (42,134,135) and improve function and quality of life in individuals with osteoarthritis (44,97,121,128).

A recent Surgeon General's report indicates that only 22% of adults in the United States are active enough to derive benefits from activity (100). Meanwhile, The American College of Sports Medicine and the Centers for Disease Control and Prevention (CDC) recommend that all Americans should engage in a minimum of 30 minutes of moderate physical activity daily (95). The National Institute of Health (NIH) also issued similar recommendations (101).

In a landmark report, the Surgeon General of the United States stated that older people regardless of gender or socioeconomic class are not exercising as much as they should, with women generally less active than men; 30% of women ages 60 to 69 engage in no leisure time activity compared with 17% of men (100). In 80-year-olds, 62% of women and 40% of men engage in no leisure time activity. The Surgeon General calls for at least 30 minutes of physical activity per day.

Exercise has even been shown to be related to increased life expectancy. Inactive men 60 years of age who become active have a mortality rate 50% lower than their peers who remain inactive (11). A study of Harvard University alumni confirmed this result. Men who were initially sedentary but later began engaging in vigorous sports had a 23% lower rate of mortality than their inactive counterparts (92). A Honolulu Heart program found that retired men who walked more than 2 miles per day had half the mortality rate (22%) than those who walked less than 1 mile per day (43%) (47). A follow-up study by Hakim reported that men who walked less than 0.25 miles per day had a 2-fold increased risk of coronary heart disease than those who walked 1.5 miles per day. Also, men who walked more than 1.5 miles per day experienced even

greater preventive benefit. Women nurses have also been shown to reduce their risk of cardiovascular disease from walking (48).

Many physicians counsel patients about smoking and body weight, but not about inactivity (18). In the past it was believed that unless exercise intensity was fairly high (60%–80% maximal heart rate) that health benefits would not accrue. A 3- to 4-mph walk is now acknowledged as beneficial (4). Additionally, exercise does not have to be at one time; therefore, for instance three 10-minute walks will be of benefit (33).

The factors that limit physical performance in the elderly are either immutable or modifiable. Immutable characteristics include such things as gender, race, age, or chronic health problems. Modifiable include behavioral (i.e., moderate exercise), social network characteristics, and psychological characteristics (i.e., self-efficacy beliefs) (see chapter 14) (113). Both physical exercise and emotional support from one's social network predict physical performance over a 2.5-year follow-up period (113). In fact, moderate activities (leisure walking) are as effective as strenuous activities (brisk walking).

Cardiovascular Risks and Benefits

Cardiovascular Benefits Associated With Activity and Exercise in the Elderly

The Cochrane Collabertation reviewed randomized, controlled trials and found there was a 27% reduction in all-causes mortality in the exercise-only intervention groups (odds ratio, 0.73; 95% confidence interval [CI], 0.54–0.98). Total cardiac mortality was reduced by 31% (odds ratio, 0.69; 95% CI, 0.51–0.94)(55). The European Society of Cardiology has provided age-specific recommendations for exercise (35).

Regular activity decreases the risk of MI and death, and low cardiovascular (CV) fitness if measured as endurance is well-correlated with CHD and mortality (69,132). This may be the most important single independent risk factor. Aging and decreased CV fitness as measured by maximal oxygen consumption (VO_2max) are directly associated.

In a long-term (16-year) follow-up study, The Multiple Risk Factor Intervention Trial study found that a moderate exercise program reduced mortality from heart disease (71). The study population included men at relatively high risk for CHD caused by being sedentary. Data showed that a relatively small amount (10–36 minutes per day) of moderate intensity leisure time exercise reduced premature mortality from CHD. The intensity of physical activity relative to effort and cardiovascular fitness may also be relevant (70).

Cardiovascular Risks Associated With Activity and Exercise in the Elderly

With such clear benefits of physical activity and exercise among older persons, issues of the safety and risks of re-activation in the elderly or health compromised need to be detailed. Only when the risks and benefits are explained clearly can a change in behavior be expected (see Chapter 14).

The Myocardial Infarction Onset Study was performed to identify activities that trigger an acute myocardial infarction (MI) in elderly individuals. The relative risk of MI in the hour after vigorous physical exertion was 12.7 (relative risk is the ratio of incidence rates for a condition in two distinct populations—in this case for MI after vigorous exertion versus normal activity). Vigorous physical exertion is equivalent to six metabolic equivalents (METS), which include slow jogging, speed walking, tennis, heavy gardening, and shoveling snow. The relative risk of MI within 2 hours of sexual intercourse (3–4 METS) was 2.5 (81,84).

The Cardiovascular Health Study—the only population-based, longitudinal study of cardiovascular diseases in older individuals—reported that regular vigorous exercise 3 days per week increased the risk of MI from 1.3% to 1.6% in a 79-year-old woman, and from 3.9% to 4.8% in a 90-year-old man. However, over time the risk would fall because those who exercise regularly have a lower relative risk that an MI will be triggered by heavy physical exertion (43,81). In fact, regular activity or exercise has been shown to reduce the risk of MI and death in older adults (47,48).

Osteoporosis

Risk Factors

Loss of bone mass occurs with aging. This leads to bone fragility and an increased incidence of fracture, especially to the hip, spine, and wrist. The incidence varies with sex, geography, and ethnicity. The postmenopausal white female is at particular risk. Regional variations exist, with American women in the southeast being at highest risk (99). The lifetime incidence of a hip fracture in a 50-year-old white American female is 17%, whereas for a similar white male it is just 6% (24).

Strong evidence has accumulated that physical activity (aerobic and progressive strengthening) helps maintain bone mass in premenopausal and significantly slows bone loss in postmenopausal women (130). The effect was approximately 1% per year favoring exercisers as seen by decreased rates of bone loss in the lumbar spine and femoral neck (130).

Role of Exercise

Ideal exercises are weight-bearing. Examples include walking, hiking, jogging, stair climbing, tennis, and dancing. Although more recent studies suggest high-intensity exercise can increase or maintain bone density in premenopausal women (8) as well as elderly men (73).

It has been shown that certain exercises are more risky than others. Postmenopausal women with low spine bone mineral density have a greater incidence of further wedge or compression fractures if they perform trunk flexion rather than trunk extension exercises (110,116).

The Young Female Athlete and Osteoporosis

Young women participating in high-intensity exercise (i.e., runners, triathletes, ballet dancers) are vulnerable to numerous adverse effects similar to elderly women

1. Reduction in estrogen levels similar to postmenopausal state
2. Menstrual abnormalities
   - Present in 50% of competitive female athletes versus 5% of normal population (16)
   - Oligomenorrhea (irregular menstrual cycles)
   - Amenorrhea (cessation of menstrual function)
3. Osteoporosis
   - Despite high levels of physical activity bone loss is common particularly in the lumbar spine (27,109)
   - Increased risk of stress fractures (86)
   - Increased risk of osteoporosis later in life

Knee Osteoarthritis

Function

Patients with knee osteoarthritis have a lower walking speed, shorter stride, reduced ankle power at terminal stance, and dysfunctional knee kinematics when walking at a paced speed (78). They have increased muscle activity and muscle co-activation during gait and stair descent on a 20-cm step (21). It has been suggested that this step height may be too high for the elderly (21). Poor balance has been found in individuals with bilateral knee osteoarthritis more so than in an age-matched control group (131). Pandya et al. reported that knee OA reduces obstacle avoidance strategies and increased the propensity to trip on an obstacle (the greater the pain the greater the risk) (93)

Activity levels and functional performance (self-paced walk test, timed up-and-go test, and timed stair performance) measures in individuals awaiting total knee arthroplasty (TKA) are much lower than in fit elderly (124). OA patients had the following disabilities compared to age-matched non-sufferers (124).

- Household score only 16% compromised
- OA patients climbed fewer stairs, shopped less often
- OA patients sports participation was 10% of asymptomatics

OA patients walked at a 62% slower pace. Female patients had 46% the muscle endurance. Of note is the fact that the performance tests were not more painful in the symptomatic group.

Rehabilitation

OA often leads to sedentarism and thus can increase the risk of CVD, yet historically patients with OA were advised to avoid activity (12,100). It is now recognized that exercise programs for patients with knee or hip OA are beneficial (7,22,28,100). In a large study of 439 individuals older than the age of 60 with radiologic knee OA, either aerobic or resistance exercise improved function and reduced pain without increasing any signs of radiographic arthritis (28). Petrella reported that increases in physical capacity and physical activity are achieved with exercise (97). Such rehabilitation may be preventive of end-stage OA requiring total knee arthroplasty (TKA). Specific approaches found to be effective include:

- Isometric quadriceps training (44,97,89)
- Supervised walking (127)
- General aerobic conditioning (96,128)

Patients whose self-efficacy improves with treatment experienced the greatest improvement (59,60,128). The combination of psycho-social approaches with exercise was superior to either alone. Keefe recently reported that spouse assisted coping skills training enhances the effectiveness of the treatment program for knee OA (61).

Total Knee Arthroplasty

Demographics

Joint replacements of the hip and knee are typically performed on individuals between 65 and 80 years old (94). Joint replacement surgery is now being performed on individuals as young as 40 or as old as 90. Individuals in their 40s and 50s have more rapid aseptic loosening from polyethylene wear. Survivorship of the implants is better in women than men.

Recovery Expectations

Pain relief usually begins 1 week postoperatively (54). Rissanen reported a 55% reduction in pain intensity at 2 and 5 years (104). Noble recently reported TKA patients continue to experience significant disability compared to their age and gender matched peers. Table 37.1 summarizes the major areas where difficulty can be expected

Shai reported that after TKA all patients could kneel under supervision, but, their perceived ability to kneel was less than their observed ability (111). Those who had difficulty kneeling had scar pain or back related problems as major factors limiting kneeling ability. Noble also reported that TKA patients had similar function as their asymptomatic peers with swimming, stationary biking, and golfing (88).

Kinematic and electromyographic assessment of function during the timed up and go test, 6-meter walk, and stair ascent revealed a number of pre-TKA deficits, which all persisted postsurgically (90). Specific impairments that were identified include increased hip mobility and decreased knee and ankle mobility. More intensive postsurgical rehabilitation was recommended to address these functional deficits.

Rehabilitation

Munin found that early rehabilitation (day 3) was superior to a usual care group (85). The rehabilitation group had a shorter duration hospital stay, lower total cost of care, and more rapid attainment of functional goals.

Hip Osteoarthritis

Function

Patients with hip OA typically have a number of functional deficits. Reduced hip strength compared to

Table 37.1 Expected Residual Functional Deficits After TKA

- Kneeling
- Squatting
- Moving laterally
- Turning and cutting
- Carrying loads
- Stretching
- Leg strengthening
- Tennis
- Dancing
- Gardening
- Sexual activity

Table 37.2 Residual Functional Deficits After THR

- Doublestance time during gait is significantly longer compared to normal
- Gait velocity is slower
- There is a slight lean toward the operated limb throughout the doublestance phase

age-matched controls and marked muscle atrophy compared to the contralateral hip (5). Those with end-stage OA have severe CV deconditioning (98), and altered gait pattern in individuals (65). Poorer physical and social functioning has been documented in those awaiting total hip replacement (THR) compared to population norms (62). Patients with end stage hip OA were found to have decreased hip muscle strength compared to age and gender matched peers: 51% for thigh extensors and 68% for thigh flexors (37).

Exercise

An 8-week exercise program with strength training and lifestyle advice for older adults (older than 55 years) with hip OA was studied (121). The program had a positive effect on pain, hip function, self-reported disability, and performance (timed up-and-go test). General aerobic training has also been found to be beneficial (128).

Total Hip Replacement

Recovery Expectations

Pain relief usually begins 1 week postoperatively (54). Improvement is well-established by 3 months (68). Rissanen reported a 55% reduction in pain intensity at 2 and 5 years (104).

Patients and surgeons have different expectations and define success and failure based on different criteria (14,15,94). Surgeons define failure as need for revision while patients define failure as persistant pain that limits function. Preoperative expectation of pain reduction exceeds what is achieved (26). Patient's satisfaction with surgery depends more on preoperative expectations regarding symptom relief and return of function (74). If the patient's criteria for surgical failure (satisfaction) is used as a criteria for success, then 20% of THRs fail, whereas if surgeon's criteria of revision is used then only 7% fail (94). Success with THR is usually based on revision rates or a scoring system including assessments of pain, walking ability, joint mobility, and radiologic findings (30,32). Residual functional deficits are summarized in Table 37.2 (117).

Medicare data suggest that 52% of hip replacement and 77% of revisions are performed by surgeons who do fewer than 10 procedures per year (56–58). Similar data exist for hospitals. Morbidity and mortality data show an inverse relationship to hospital procedure volume.

Patients felt they were ready for discharge following THR if they felt safe (50). This was related to their confidence and the support of family and friends.

Rehabilitation

Berge found that that non-rehabilitation patients had a 43% reduction in pain intensity, whereas rehabilitation patients experienced a 55% decrease (10). Function was not benefited, but quality of life was. Table 37.3 summarizes a pre-habilitation program that demonstrated promising effectiveness (37).

Maire has shown that an upper extremity exercise program is effective in postsurgical rehabilitation for THR (75). Passive physical therapy after THR has been shown to lead to deterioration of both exercise capacity and physical condition. The upper extremity exercise program starts 1 week postoperatively. It involves 30 minutes per session at a frequency of three times per week for a duration of 6 weeks. Each session consists of:

- 6 consecutive periods of 5 minutes
- 4 minutes of low-intensity "base" work
  - Ventilatory threshold
- 1 minute of intense "peak" work
  - Maximum tolerated power

Table 37.3 The Best Outcomes With Surgery Occur in Patient Who Participate in Preoperative Rehabilitation

- Fit, strong patients rehabilitate more quickly after surgery than those less fit
- 4.2 days in hospital vs 7.2 days for prerehabilitation vs non-prerehabilitation patients
- Preoperative hip strength was an independent predictor of length of hospital stay
- 30-minute aerobic and strength program followed by 30-minute mobility and gait in hydrotherapy pool program
- Start with 5-minute warm-up on cycle
- Control subjects at 24 weeks postoperatively had more disability than prerehabilitation patients at 12 weeks.

- Avoid flexion past 90°
- Avoid adduction past neutral
- Avoid hip internal rotation

Fall Prevention

The Problem

Few areas of medicine are more important than reducing the burden of health care problems in the elderly. In Canada, nearly one-third of all seniors will fall this year (123). Falls are responsible for nearly 40% of the Canada's senior health care costs! The California Department of Aging in the Department of Health Services has created a No More Falls! Program. The self-care advice is responsible for a 20% reduction in falls 1 year after completion of program (105,106). Public health organizations such as the Rand Corporation and Cochrane Collaboration have mobilized recently to address this preventable health care dilemma (2,20,42,108,112).

A study of Australians found that one-third of fallers are multiple fallers (83). Most of these are elderly women with co-morbidities, perceived difficulty walking, poor self-rated eyesight, and back pain.

Associated Functional Deficits

A number of functional deficits (impairments) have been shown to increase the incidence of falls. Decreased single leg standing balance time (less than 30 seconds) has been shown to correlate with a history of falling, whereas a longer balance time suggests a much lower risk (53). Pandya et al. reported that knee OA reduces obstacle avoidance strategies and increased the propensity to trip on an obstacle (the greater the pain the greater the risk) (93). Reduced peak hip extension mobility and increased anterior pelvic tilt distinguishes elderly fallers from young adults (63). Kneeling hip extension stretching was later shown to improve hip extension mobility and ankle plantarflexion mobility and power generation (64).

Falls on stair descent outnumber ascent 3:1 (67). Eccentric contraction is utilized. Nadeau has studied the task of stair climbing (87). It requires concentric action of hip abductor muscles. Elevation of the contralateral hip is necessary for the swing phase leg to avoid the step. It is important to assess this. Decreased knee flexion is also a problem with stair climbing. Strength of the knee extensors is needed also to raise the body weight up. The extension moment in knee is doubled in stair climbing versus level walking; 11 weeks of eccentric leg muscle training in elderly individuals at high risk improved stair descent performance by 21%, balance by 7%, strength by 60%, and significantly decreased the risk of falling (67).

Interventions

An intervention including exercise was superior to one without exercise in reducing the incidence of falls. When balance training was added the effectiveness was even greater (103).

Brandt et al. have found that elderly with ataxia can be treated successfully with balance training (13). Two weeks of training was shown to lead to significant improvement 9 months later without any home maintenance program. Thick foam is used on the floor to deprive the feet of sensory feedback and the eyes are closed, thus facilitating the vestibular and somatosensory systems. Similarly, you can facilitate optokinetic and mechano receptor (feet) function by leaving the eyes open, but tipping the head back (taking the otoliths out of their functioning range).

- Eliminate loose rugs and wire
- Ensure handrails on all stairs
- Recommend use of handrail especially when going down stairs
- Practice balance training
- Increase CV fitness with aerobic training
- Increase dynamic strength especially of legs

In another 5-week balance program, only shorter-term results were achieved, thus suggesting for maintenance of results that training may need to continue (114). Two different trials of Tai Chi showed that a longer term program improves balance abilities of older adults and that improvement persisted after training stopped (134,135).

Frailty

The Problem

Decreases in muscle strength and mass are an inevitable consequence of aging. A consistent feature of age and inactivity is limb muscle atrophy and the loss of peak force and power (125,126). However, recent studies show that the rate of age-related muscle loss—sarcopenia—can be slowed down with increased activity (aerobic and resistance) and nutrition (androgens and growth hormone) (107,129). Insulin resistance has been shown to have a possible link to the development of sarcopenia (129). Sacropenia is especially risky for older individuals facing acute or chronic illnesses. It is important to maximize muscle mass and protein stores to maintain quality of life with advancing age. Health care professionals and the public have focused much attention on age-related changes in bone density, but have ignored these muscle changes. Yet, muscle changes are extremely important when one considers risk of falls, fractures, and general well-being.

Consistent with the benefits of physical activity and exercise are the debilitating effects of prolonged bed rest. McGuire et al. showed in 1966 that in healthy 20-year-old men, 20 days of complete inactivity led to serious deconditioning (79). An 8-week dynamic training program largely reversed the negative effects of bed rest. A recent follow-up study on this cohort demonstrated that nearly equivalent amounts of deconditioning as occurred with 20 days of bed rest occurred from 30 years of aging in largely sedentary individuals (79)! Significant increases in body weight (25%), body fat (100%), and decreases in maximum oxygen consumption (VO_2max), maximal heart rate, and maximal stroke volume occurred. Again, a conditioning program—this time for 6 months—focusing on endurance reversed the deconditioning of 30 years (80).

A few points emerge from this work. First, that 20 days of bed rest is as deleterious as 30 years of sedentary lifestyle. Second, deconditioning is reversible! McGuire reported that "100% of the age-related decline in aerobic power . . . was reversed . . ." (80).

Physical frailty (as determined by gait speed) was the only factor that was associated significantly with the development of insidious disability (odds ratio: 2.4, 95% confidence interval: 1.4 to 4.1) (41). A recent report found that habitual physical activity is an independent predictor of successful recovery of independent activities of daily living (ADL) function (bathing, dressing, walking inside the house, and transferring from a chair) among newly disabled community-dwelling older persons (49).

Interventions

Gill et al. tested a 6-month home care exercise program for a physically frail group of community-living older persons (39). Physical frailty was determined by

two tests shown to be most predictive of functional decline (102,132):

- Rapid gait (back and forth as fast as possible over a 3-meter course)
- Single chair stand (standing up from a hard back chair/arms folded)
- Score: frail if more than 10 seconds on rapid gait and unable to do single chair stand with arms folded
  ○ Severe—if failed both tests
  ○ Moderate—if failed one test

The program was home-based and targeted specific impairments in physical capacity. There was an emphasis on adherence by describing the impairment and how this could affect the person's abilities. The patient was asked if they agreed and if they would like to work to overcome this impairment. Interventions were explained and the patient asked to rate their belief in the chances of success with the intervention. The patients preferences were explicitly incorporated into the program

The control group received only education vs the intervention group's exercise. The exercise group realized significantly greater improvement in disability, mobility, and physical performance at 7- and 12-month follow-ups. ADL improvement was 45% greater at 7 months and 37% greater at 12 months in the exercise versus education group. In a follow-up to this study, Gill found there was no increase in adverse events in the exercise group versus the education group (40).

Chandler et al. found that a lower extremity strengthening program improved mobility, chair rise performance, gait speed, and falls efficacy in a group of frail community-dwelling elders (19). The more impaired the individual the greater the improvement in strength.

Spinal Stenosis

Diagnosis

Spinal stenosis is a clinical term not a radiologic finding (120). A narrow canal does not necessarily cause symptoms. Spine problems often restrict activities, for instance, individuals with spinal stenosis have reduced walking tolerances. Inactivity is itself a cardiac risk factor. Neurogenic claudication associated with spinal stenosis is the number one symptomatic spine problem in the elderly and reason for spine surgery. In fact, low back surgery for individuals older than age 65 is increasing dramatically. Such surgeries are not without risk and cardiac complications are recognized as the leading cause of death in such operations (29).

Leg pain with walking is the hallmark of spinal stenosis and must be differentiated from vascular claudication. Pain with walking that is relieved with stooping while walking is diagnostic. A patient with stenosis will be worse on a treadmill than a bicycle whereas vascular claudication will not. A 20-minute treadmill test on a level surface correlated strongly with spinal stenosis symptoms with 88% of pre-operative patients having a significant increase of their symptoms (122). In contrast only 41% of patients had significant symptoms with a 10-minute bicycle test when holding handle bars. On repeat testing 2 years postoperatively there was significant improvement in the treadmill test, but not in the bicycle test.

Potential Complications

The overall complication rate was 40%; however, serious complications were less common, occurring in 12% of patients (9). Deyo found that if the surgical procedure included arthrodesis patients had an increased risk of morbidity as well as an increased length of hospital stay (25).

Results

Atlas et al. has compared conservative to surgical care for spinal stenosis and found at 8- to 10-year follow-up that low back pain relief, predominant symptom improvement, and satisfaction with the current state were similar in patients initially treated surgically or non-surgically (6). However, relief of leg symptoms and improved back-related functional status were present in those initially receiving surgical treatment.

Simotas et al. utilized a flexion-based stabilization exercise program with analgesics and epidural steroid injections in a group of patients all considered to be surgical candidates (115). At 3 years follow-up, 80% of patients were at least somewhat satisfied with the results. Degree of spinal cord narrowing was not significantly correlated with outcome. Age and degree of scoliotic deformity were both positively correlated with poorer outcomes.

Katz studied patients who elected to have surgery and reported on long-term follow-up data at 10 years that 60% to 80% of patients are satisfied enough that they would have the surgery again (56,57). According to Padua et al., 4 years after spinal stenosis surgery, although referred pain was improved, physical aspects of health-related quality of life continued to show severe impairment (91). Additionally, there

were no significant EMG differences before and after surgery (91).

A number of factors have been found to be associated with surgical outcome—co-morbidities, degree of spinal cord narrowing, female sex, and Waddell's non-organic signs (52,57,77,120) (see Table 37.4).

According to Katz et al. the most important predictor of greater walking capacity, milder symptoms, and greater satisfaction with surgery was pre-operative self-rated health as good or excellent (57). It was concluded that co-morbidities are an important risk factor of a poor recovery (57).

Hurri et al. found that the degree of spinal canal narrowing correlates more with disability (as measured with the Oswestry index) than does the choice of treatment (conservative or surgical), age, sex, or body mass index (52). Mariconda et al. reported that canal diameter influences the response to conservative care, but not surgical care (77). Surgical patients who had a poorer outcome were more likely to be female, whereas having a narrower canal was not relevant.

Sprat et al.'s follow-up study focused on the following outcomes: leg pain, pain with walking, and Waddell's non-organic signs (see Chapter 9) (120); 58.3% patients who underwent operation were deemed a success. Using exact logistic regression analysis, Waddell's non-organic signs (NOS) were the only significant risk factor (odds ratio: 0.648, 95% CI: 0.362–0.9901). The authors concluded, "This suggests that illness behavior can play an important role in determining results of treatment, even in such a highly organic disorder as spinal stenosis."

More detailed analysis revealed that for females without aorta calcification outcome is predicted based on canal diameter (less than 0.305 predicted failure) (120). For males without aorta calcification, outcome is predicted based on Waddell's NOS (higher score more failure). For females with calcification, no predictors were found. For males with calcification pretreatment VAS predicted outcome (higher score 66/100 predicted failure). Thus, subclinical vascular factors are inferred to be important such as arterial insufficiency at the spinal level. The study recommended that stenosis patients undergo color echo Doppler (duplex scan) examination.

Table 37.4 Factors Related to a Poorer Outcome With Spinal Stenosis Surgery

---

- Co-morbidities
- Degree of spinal cord narrowing
- Female sex
- High Waddell non-organic signs score

Practice-Based Problem

Because long-term data suggest that surgical outcomes are somewhat better than those for conservative care, is it unwise to recommend a trial of conservative care before surgery?

Amundsen et al. showed that whereas surgical outcome is slightly better than for conservative care, there is no difference in surgical outcome in individuals who have it sooner versus after an unsatisfactory outcome with conservative care for 3 to 27 months (3). Thus, conservative care is still advisable since there is no deterioration in surgical outcome as a result of waiting and surgery always carries an iatrogenic risk, especially in the elderly.

Exertional Risk Assessment

ACSM and AHA Risk Assessment Recommendations

With the benefits of exercise and physical activity so clear, it is important that the risks associated with activity be identified. Silent myocardial ischemia is believed to affect between 2 and 5 million individuals (76). Thus, screening asymptomatic individuals for risk of cardiac complications with activity is important. Two major national organizations have issued guidelines for screening for risk factors associated with exertional activities, the American College of Sports Medicine (ACSM) (1) and the American Heart Association (AHA) (33) (see Tables 37.5 to 37.8).

Limitations of ACSM and AHA Risk Assessment Recommendations

The ACSM and AHA both recommend exercise stress testing for older individuals before starting a vigorous exercise program. They also recommend such testing

Table 37.5 Health Screening for Physical Activity (1)

- Physical Activities Readiness Questionnaire (PAR-Q) (17) (see appendix)
- Identify patients for whom physical activity might be inappropriate or should have medical advice
- Evaluate for signs and symptoms suggestive of cardiopulmonary disease or coronary artery disease

Table 37.6 Symptoms or Signs Suggestive of Cardiopulmonary Disease

- Ischemic pain, discomfort in the chest, neck, jaw, arms
- Shortness of breath at rest or with mild exertion
- Dizziness or syncope
- Orthopnea or paroxysmal nocturnal dyspnea
- Ankle edema
- Palpitations or tachycardia
- Intermittent claudication
- Known heart murmur
- Unusual fatigue or shortness of breath with usual activities

for most older persons before starting a moderate exercise program. However, most forms of exercise stress testing were not designed for individuals older than 75 (38). Therefore, screening tests to identify those people at risk with physical exertion need to be reviewed for their applicability across the age spectrum.

The ACSM distinguishes moderate from vigorous activity based on maximal rate of oxygen consumption (VO_2max), but this is difficult to measure in older individuals (38,102). Furthermore, the mathematical calculations required are not sufficiently accurate in this population (38,66). The AHA guidelines use maximum capacity to define exercise intensity but do not describe the method of its assessment. Gill concludes that these guidelines are designed for identifying risk factors associated with exertion in young and middle-aged adults NOT in older persons (38)!

A major problem with exercise stress testing in those older than 75 is that many individuals with asymptomatic coronary artery disease (CAD) would be identified leading to an escalation of invasive cardiac procedures (133). In fact, there is a lack of evidence of health benefit supporting such aggressive evaluation and intervention, whereas there is evidence of iatrogenic risk (23,82).

Table 37.7 Coronary Artery Risk Factors

- Age: men older than 45; women older than 55
- Family history: MI or sudden death younger than 55 years in father/brother or younger than 65 in mother/sister
- Current cigarette smoking
- Hypertension: more than 140/90 mm Hg
- Hypercholesterolemia: Total serum cholesterol more than 200 mg/dL or HDL less than 35 mg/dL
- Diabetes mellitus
- Sedentary lifestyle

Table 37.8   Initial Risk Stratification

- Apparently healthy: asymptomatic and no more than one major coronary risk factor
- Increased risk: signs & symptoms of cardio-pulmonary disease or two or more coronary risk factors
- Known disease

Exercise stress testing in the elderly is limited by another factor. Most older persons cannot satisfactorily complete a treadmill exercise test. Only 26.4% of a group of individuals 75 years or older without known cardiovascular disease, medical contraindications, or physical impairments achieved a maximal exercise effort (51). This was defined at a minimum of 2 minutes of exercise involving a respiratory exchange rate of 1.10 or more (51).

Thus, the high prevalence of asymptomatic CAD and the low ability to complete an exercise stress test make requiring such testing as a prerequisite to recommending physical activity in the elderly a major impediment to health care providers wishing to promote physical activity and exercise in the elderly.

Two-dimensional echocardiography (e.g., sestamibi or dobutatimine echocardiography) has been recommended to screen for silent heart disease in prospective older spine surgery patients. A significant number of patients—18%—scheduled for spinal stenosis surgery were found to have evidence of coronary artery disease (29). Such testing for surgical patients may be a wise use of resources but it is of questionable usefulness because of its high cost as a screen for individuals embarking on an exercise program.

Gill's Recommendations for Screening Elderly Individuals for Cardiac Risk With Exertional Activities

Because exercise has proven benefits in the elderly but exertional risk factors for cardiac events are also present, some form of evaluation is necessary. VO_2max a standard for measuring exercise capacity is unfortunately not an appropriate measure for the elderly. Maximal heart rate, heart rate reserve, and subjective ratings of perceived exertion may have a role to play, but they have not been adequately studied (38). Pharmacological stress testing combined with radionuclide imaging can detect asymptomatic, myocardial ischemia, but its high cost and uncertain benefits limit its usefulness. Despite these problems and in the absence of any standard of care, Gill makes the following recommendations for evaluating sedentary older persons

without a history of symptomatic cardiovascular disease:

1. Complete history and examination to identify cardiac contraindications to exercise
   - MI in past 6 months
   - Angina
   - Physical signs and symptoms of congestive heart failure
     1. Bilateral rales
     2. Shortness of breath
     3. Resting systolic blood pressure of at least 110 mm Hg
   - Cardiovascular reserve
     a. Chest pain or shortness of breath triggered by any of the following
     b. Walking 15 m
     c. Climbing one flight of stairs
     d. Cycling in the air for 1 minute (supine)
     e. Getting up and down from examination table (1 minute)
   - Resting ECG
     - New Q waves
     - ST-segment depressions
     - T-wave inversions
2. Individuals with cardiovascular disease should be risk stratified (36)
   - Risks versus benefits of exercise should be considered

If any risk factors are identified then exercise outside of a monitored environment is not recommended without approval of the patients cardiac specialist. According to Gill, in the absence of any of these risk factors the benefits of a low-intensity unsupervised exercise outweigh the risks.

Recommendations for Initiating and Progressing Mild to Moderate Exercise Programs in the Elderly

According to Gill, all sedentary older persons without cardiovascular disease as screened should start with a low-intensity exercise program (38). Examples include:

- Gait training
- Balance exercises
- Tai Chi
- Self-paced walking
- Lower extremity resistance training with elastic tubing or ankle weights

Instruction in proper technique is recommended in all cases. Supervision is recommended on at least one occasion. Intensity and dosage of exercise should be gradually increased as tolerated by the individual. Warm-up and cool-down periods should be included. Balance, hearing, and vision dysfunctions are typical in the elderly. These should be taken into account when recommending exercise in order to ensure safety (119). Also, the effects of warmer weather on fatigue and weakness should be considered (119).

Individuals should be given the following warning signs to look out for (38):

- Chest pain
- Shortness of breath
- Dizziness

If any of these occur, the patient should be instructed to rest. If they persist or recur, then a physician visit is warranted (38).

If low-intensity exercises are well-tolerated, then progression toward moderate intensity exercises is acceptable (38). Examples include:

- Strength training with weight machines
- Fast walking
- Swimming
- Bicycling

Again monitoring or supervision is recommended initially. Blood pressure and heart rate should be checked. Abnormal cardiac responses include (38):

- Decrease in systolic blood pressure at least 20 mm Hg
- Increase in systolic blood pressure of at least 250 mm Hg
- Increase of diastolic blood pressure of at least 120 mm Hg
- Repeated increase in heart rate of at least 90% of age-specific maximum

Any of these findings should necessitate specialist re-evaluation and limitation to low-intensity exercise.

Despite the limitations of using VO_2max measurements as an index of CV fitness in the elderly a number of studies have shown that aerobic training is superior to strength training for increasing the VO_2max in the elderly. Hagberg reported a 22% increase in VO_2max in healthy 70- to 79-year-old men and women after 6 months of aerobic training at 70% to 75% of VO_2max (45). Strength training has not shown similar gains in VO_2max (34,46). When aerobic and strength training have been compared head-to-head, VO_2max has consistently been shown to be increased greater by aerobic training (45,118).

Only a minority of persons aged 75 years or older are capable of high-intensity or vigorous exercise (51). Such high-functioning individuals should be taught to

- Rate their perceived exertion
- Monitor their heart rate

Although, as Gill points out, the usefulness of this approach is not demonstrated (38).

■ CONCLUSION

Many physicians counsel patients about smoking and body weight, but not about inactivity (4). In the past it was believed that unless exercise intensity was fairly high (60%–80% maximal heart rate) that health benefits would not accrue. A 3- to 4-mph walk is now acknowledged as beneficial (4). Additionally, exercise does not have to be performed all at one time; for instance, three 10-minute walks will be of benefit.

Exercise is extremely valuable for individuals of all ages. Yet there is increased risk associated with exertional activities with increasing age. Thus, an age-appropriate evaluation of risk factors with exertion is necessary to sort out the risks and benefits of increasing an individuals activity level.

Activity and exercise are beneficial for a wide variety of conditions in the elderly such as cardiovascular, arthritis, osteoporosis, fall prevention, frailty prevention, and spinal stenosis. Promotion of appropriate self-management methods in the elderly can reduce the consequences of chronic illness and slow the debilitation of age.

Audit Process
Self-Check of the Chapter's Learning Objectives

- What is the relationship between inactivity and cardiovascular disease?
- What type or intensity of activity is required to prevent heart cardiovascular disease?
- What factors can help promote compliance with a self-management program?
- What are the risk factors for the elderly with exertion?
- What are the key functional deficits requiring improvement in hip and knee arthritis and arthroplasty?
- What type of exercise can be utilized for prevention of falls or frailty?
- What type of exercises are best to slow down the onset of osteoporosis?

■ REFERENCES

1. ACSM's Guidelines for Exercise Testing and Prescription, 5th ed. Williams and Wilkins, 1995.
2. American Geriatrics Society, British Geriatrics Society, Academy of Orthopaedic Surgeons Panel on Falls Prevention. Guideline for the prevention of falls in older persons. J Am Geriatr Soc 2001;49:664–772.
3. Amundsen T, Weber H, Nordal HJ, et al. Lumbar spinal stenosis: conservative or surgical management? A prospective 10-year study. Spine 2000;25: 1424–1436.
4. Andersen RE, Blair SN Cheskin LJ, Bartlett SJ. Encouraging patients to become more physically active : the physician's role. Ann Intern Med 1997; 127:395–400.
5. Arokoski MH, Arokoski JPA, Haara M, Kankaanpaa M, Vesterinen M, et al. Hip muscle strength and muscle cross sectional area in men with and without hip osteoarthritis. Journal of Rheumatology 2002;29:2185–2195.
6. Atlas SJ, Keller RB, We UA, Deyo RA, Singer DE. Long-Term Outcomes of Surgical and Nonsurgical Management of Lumbar Spinal Stenosis: 8 to 10 Year Results from the Maine Lumbar Spine Study. Spine 2005;30:936–943.
7. Bashaw RT, Tingstad EM. Rehabilitation of the osteoarthritic patient: Focus on the knee. Clin Sports Med 2005;24:101–131.
8. Bassey EJ, Rothwell MC, Littlewood JJ, Pye DW. Pre- and postmenopausal women have different bone mineral density responses to the same high-impact exercise. J Bone Miner Res. 1998;13: 1805–13.
9. Benz RJ, Ibrahim ZG, Afshar P, Garfin SR. Predicting complications in elderly patients undergoing lumbar decompression. Clin Orthop Relat Res. 2001;384:116–121.
10. Berge DJ, Dolin SJ, Williams A CdeC, Harman R. Pre-operative and post-operative effect of a pain management programme prior to total hip replacement: a randomized controlled trial. Pain 2004;110: 33–39.
11. Blair SN. Kohl HW, Barlow CE, et al. Changes in physical fitness and all-cause mortality: A prospective study of healthy and unhealthy men. JAMA 195;273:1093–1098.
12. Brady TJ, Kruger J, Helmick CG, Callahan LF, Boutaugh ML. Intervention programs for arthritis and other rheumatic diseases. Health Education and Behavior 2003;30:44–63.
13. Brandt T, Krafczyk S, Malsbendend I. Postural imbalance with head extension: improvement by training as a model for ataxia therapy. Ann NY Acad Sci 1981;374:636–649.
14. Brokelman RB, van Loon CJ, Rijnberg WJ, Patient versus surgeon satisfaction after total hip arthroplasty. The Journal of Bone Joint Surgery British Volume 2003;85:495–498.
15. Bullens PH, van Loon CJ, de Waal Malefijt MC, Laan RF, Veth RP, Patient satisfaction after total knee arthroplasty: a comparison between subjective and objective outcome assessments. J Arthroplast 2001;16:740–747.

16. Carbon RJ. Exercise, amenorrhea and the skeleton. Br Med Bull 1992;48:546–560.
17. Cardinal BJ, Esters J, Cardinal MK. Evaluation of the revised Physical Activities Readiness Questionnaire in older adults. Med Sci Sports Exer 1996; 28:468.
18. Caspersen CJ, Powell KE, Christenson GM. Physical activity, exercise and physical fitness: Definitions and distinctions for health-related research. Public Health Rep 1985;100:126–131.
19. Chandler JM, Duncan PW, Kochersberger G, Studenski S. Is lower extremity strength gain associated with improvement in physical performance and disability in frail, community-dwelling elders? Arch Phys Med Rehabil 1998;79:24–30.
20. Chang JT, Morton SC, Rubenstein LZ, Mojica WA, Maglione M, Suttorp MJ, Roth EA, Shekelle PG. Interventions for the prevention of falls in older adults: systematic review and meta-analysis of randomized clinical trials. BMJ 2004;328:680.
21. Childs JD, Sparto PJ, Kelley Fitzgerald G, Bizzini M, Irrgang JJ. Alterations in lower extremity movement and muscle activation patterns in individuals with knee osteoarthritis. Clin Biomechanics 2004; 19:44–49.
22. Christmas C, Andersen RA. Exercise and older patients: guidelines for the clinician. J Am Geriatr Soc 2000;48:318–324.
23. Creditor MC. Hazards of hospitalization of the elderly. Ann Intern Med 1993;118:219–223.
24. Cummings SR, Melton LJ. Epidemiology and outcomes of osteoporotic fractures. Lancet 2002; 359:1761–7.
25. Deyo RA, Ciol MA, Cherkin DC, Loeser JD, Bigos SJ. Lumbar spinal fusion. A cohort study of complications, reoperations, and resource use in the Medicare population. Spine 1993;18:1463–70.
26. Dolin SJ, Williams ACC, Ashford N, George J, Pereira L, Perello A. Factors affecting medical decision-making in patients with osteoarthritis of the hip: allocation of surgical priority. Disabil Rehabil 2003;25:771–777.
27. Drinkwater BL, Nilson K, Chenut CH, Bremner WJ, Shainholtz S, Southworth MB. Bone mineral content of amenorrheic and eumenorrheic athletes. N Engl J Med 1984;311:277–281.
28. Ettinger Jr WH, Burns R, Messier SP, et al. A randomized trial comparingaerobic exercise and resistance exercise with a health education program in older adults with knee osteoarthritis. The Fitness Arthritis and Seniors Trial (FAST). JAMA 1997;277: 25–31.
29. Faciszewki T, Jensen R, Rokey R, Berg R. Cardiac risk stratification of patients with symptomatic spinal stenosis. Clin Orth Rel Res 2001;384: 110–115.
30. Faulkner A, Kennedy L, Baxter K, Donovan J, Wilkinson M, Bevan G. Effectiveness of hip prostheses in primary total hip replacement: a critical review of evidence and an economic model. Health Technol Assess 1998;2:1–133.
31. Ferucci L, Izmirlina G, Leveille S, et al. Smoking, physical activity, and life expectancy. Am J Epidemiol 1999;149:645–653.

32. Fitzpatrick R, Shortall E, Sculpher M, Murray D, Morris R, et al. Primary total hip replacement surgery: a systematic review of outcomes and modelling of cost-effectiveness associated with different prostheses. Health Technol Assess 1998;20:1–64.

33. Fletcher GF, Balady G, Froelicher VR, et al. Exercise standards: A statement for healthcare professionals from the American Heart Association. Circulation 1995;91:580–615.

34. Frontera W, Meredith CN, O'Reilly K, et al. Strength training and determinants of VO_2max in older men. J Appl Physiol 1990;68:329–333.

35. Giannuzzi P, Mezzani A, Saner H, et al. Physical activity for primary and secondary prevention. Position paper of the Working Group on Cardiac Rehabilitation and Exercise Physiology of the European Society of Cardiology. Eur J Cardiovasc Prev Rehabil 2003;10:319–327.

36. Gibbons RJ, Chatterjee K, Daley J, et al. Guidelines for the management of patients with chronic stable angina: a report of the American College of Cardiology/American Heart Association Task Force on Practice Guidelines. J Am Coll Cardiol 1999;33: 2092–2197.

37. Gilbey HJ, Ackland TR, Wang AW, Morton AR, Trouchet T, Tapper J. Exercise improves early functional recovery after total hip arthroplasty. Clin Orthop Rel Res 2003;408;193–200.

38. Gill TM, Dipietro L, Krumholz HM. Role of exercise stress testing and safety monitoring for older persons starting an exercise program. JAMA 2000;284: 342–349.

39. Gill TM, Baker DI, Gottschalk M, et al. A program to prevent functional decline in physically frail elderly persons living at home. N Engl J Med 2002;347:1068–1074.

40. Gill TM, Baker DI, Gottschalk M, Gahbauer EA, Charpentier PA, et al. A prehabilitation program for physically frail community-living older persons. Arch Phys Med Rehabil 2003;84:394–404.

41. Gill TM, Allore H, Holford TR, Guo Z. The development of insidious disability in activities of daily living among community-living older persons. Am J Med. 2004;117:484–491.

42. Gillespie LD, Gillespie WJ, Robertson MC, Lamb SE, Cumming RG, Rowe BH 2001. Interventions for preventing falls in elderly people. Cochrane Database Syst Rev. 2001;3:CD000340.

43. Giri S, Thompson PD, Liernan FJ, et al. Clinical and angiographic characteristics of exertion-related acute myocardial infarction. JAMA 1999;282: 1731–1736.

44. Gur H, Cakin N, Akova B, Okay E, Kucukoglu S. Concentric versus combined concentric-eccentric isokinetic training: Effects on functional capacity and symptoms in patients with osteoarthrois of the knee. Arch Phys Med Rehabil 2002;83: 308–316.

45. Hagberg J, Graves J, Limacher M. Cardiovascular responses of 70- to 79-year old men and women to exercise training. J Appl Physiol 1989;66:2589–2594.

46. Hagerman FC, Walsh SJ, Staron RS, et al. Effects of high-intensity resistance training on untrained older men. J Gerontol 2000;55:B336–B346.

47. Hakim AA, Petrovitch H, Burchfiel CM, et al. Effects of walking on mortality among nonsmoking retired men. N Engl J Med 1998;30:922–1008.

48. Hakim AA, Curb D, Petrovitch H, Rodrigues BL, Yano K, Ross W, et al. Effects of walking on coronary heart disease in elderly men: The Honolulu Heart Program. Circulation 1999;100:9–1013.

49. Hardy SE, Gill EM. Factors associated with recovery of independence among newly disabled older persons. Arch Intern Med. 2005;165:106–112.

50. Heine J, Koch S, Goldie P. Patients' experiences of readiness for discharge following a total hip replacement. Aust J Physiother 2004;50:227–33.

51. Hollenberg M, Ngo LH, Turner D, Tager IB. Treadmill exercise testing in an epidemiologic stud of elderly subjects. J Gerontol A Biol Sci Med Sci 1998;53A:B259–B267.

52. Hurri H, Slatis P, Soini J, et al. Lumbar spinal stenosis: assessment of long-term outcome 12 years after operative and conservative treatment. J Spinal Disorders 1998;11:110–115.

53. Hurvitz EA, Richardson JK, Werner RA, Ruhl A, Dixon MR. Unipedal stance testing as an indicator of fall risk among older outpatients. Arch Phys Med Rehabil 2000;81:587–591.

54. Irens H, Hall G, Hughes S, Salmon B. Short term recovery from hip and knee arthroplasty. J Bone Joint Surg Br 1996;78:555–558.

55. Jolliffe JA, Rees K, Taylor RS, et al. Exercise-based rehabilitation for coronary heart disease. (Cochrane Review) In: Cochrane Library. London, England: John Wiley & Sons, Ltd, 2003:4.

56. Katz JN, Lipson SJ, Chang LC, Levine SA, Fossel AH, Liang MH. Seven- to 10-year outcome of decompressive surgery for degenerative lumbar spinal stenosis. Spine 1996;21:92–8.

57. Katz JN, Stucki G, Lipson SJ, Fossel AH, Grobler LJ, Weinstein JN. Predictors of surgical outcome in degenerative lumbar spinal stenosis. Spine 1999;24: 2229–33.

58. Katz JN, Losina E, Barrett J, et al. Association between hospital and surgeon procedure volume and outcomes of total hip replacement in the United States medicare population. J Bone Joint Surg Am 2001;83:1622–1629.

59. Keefe FJ, Caldwel DS, Baucom D, et al. Spouse-assisted coping skills training in the management of osteoarthritis knee pain. Arthritis Care Res 1996a;9: 279–291.

60. Keefe FJ, Kashikar-Suck S, Opiteck J, et al. Pain in arthritis and musculoskeletal disorders: The role of coping skills training and exercise interventions. J Orthop Sports Phys Ther 1996b;24:279–290.

61. Keefe FJ, Blumenthal J, Baucom D, Affleck G, Waugh R, et al. Effects of spourse-assisted coping skills training in patients with osteoarthritis knee pain: a randomized controlled study. Pain 2004;110: 539–549.

62. Kelly KD, Voaklander DC, Johnston DW, Newman SC, Suarez-Almazor ME. Change in pain and function while waiting for major joint arthroplasty. Journal of Arthroplasty 2001;16:351–359.

63. Kerrigan DC, Lee L, Collins J, Riley P, Lipsitz L, Reduced hip extension mobility during walking:

healthy elderly and fallers versus young adults. Arch Phys Med Rehabil 2001;82:26–30.

64. Kerrigan DC, Xenopoulos-Oddsson A, Sullivan MJ, Lelas JJ. Riley PO. Effect of hip flexor-stretching program on gait in the elderly Arch Phys Med Rehabil 2003;84:1–6.

65. Lafuente R, Belda JM, Sanchz-Lacuesta J, Soler C, Poveda R, Prat J. Quantitative assessment of gait deviation: contribution to the objective measurement of disability. Gait Posture 2001;11:191–198.

66. Lakatta EG. Cardiorespiratory regulatory mechanisms in advanced age. Physiol Rev 1993;73:413–467.

67. LaStayo PC, Ewy GA, Pierotti DD, Johns RK, Lindstedt S. The positive effects of negative work: increased muscle strength and decreased fall risk in a frail elderly population. J Gerontol A Biol Sci Med Sci 2003;58:M419–M424.

68. Laupacis A, Bourne R, Rorabeck C, Feeny D, Wong C, et al. The effect of elective total hip replacement on health-related quality of life. J Bone Joint Surg Am 1993;75:1619–1626.

69. Lee CD, Blair SN, Jackson AS. Cardiorespiratory fitness, body composition, and all cause mortality in men. Am J Clin Nutr 1999;69:373–380.

70. Lee IM, Sesso HD, Oguma Y, et al. Relative intensity of physical activity and risk of coronary heart disease. Circulation. 2003;107:1110–1116.

71. Leon AS, Myers MJ, Connell J. Leisure time physical activity and the 16–year risks of mortality from coronary heart disease and all-causes in the Multiple Risk Factor Intervention Trial (MRFIT). Int J Sports Med.1997;18(suppl 3):S208–S215.

72. Leveille SG, Guralnik JM, Ferrucci L, Langlois JA. Aging successfully until death in old age: opportunities for increasing active life expectancy. Am J Epidemiol 1999;149:654–664.

73. Maddalozzo GF, Snow CM. High intensity resistance training: effects on bone in older men and women. Calcif Tissue Int 2000;66:399–404.

74. Mahomed NN, Liang MH, Cook EF, et al. The importance of patient expectations in predicting functional outcomes after total joint arthroplasty. The Journal of Rheumatology 2002;29:1273–1279.

75. Maire J, Faillenet-Maire AF, Grange C, Dugue B, Tordi N, et al. A specific arm-interval exercise program could improve the health status and walking ability of elderly patients after total hip arthroplasty: a pilot study. J Rehabil Med 2004;36:92–94.

76. Mangano DT. Perioperative cardiac morbidity. Anesthesiology 1990;72;153–184.

77. Mariconda M, Zanforlino G, Celestinon GA, et al. Factors influencing the outcome of degenerative lumbar spinal stenosis. J of Spinal Disorders 2000;13:131–137.

78. McGibbon CA, Krebs DA. Compensatory gait mechanics in patients with unilateral knee arthritis. J Rheumatol 2002;29:2410–2419.

79. McGuire DK, Levine BD, Williamson JW, Snell PG, Blomqvist CG, Saltin B, Mitchell JH. 30-year follow-up of the Dallas Bedrest and Training Study: I. Effect of age on the cardiovascular response to exercise. Circulation. 2001;104:1350–1357.

80. McGuire DK, Levine BD, Williamson JW, Snell PG, Blomqvist CG, Saltin B, Mitchell JH. A 30-year follow-up of the Dallas Bedrest and Training Study: II. Effect of age on cardiovascular adaptation to exercise training. Circulation. 2001a;104:1358–1366.

81. Mittleman MA, Maclure M, Tofler GH, Sherwood JB, Goldberg RJ, Muller JE. Triggering of acute myocardial infarction by heavy physical exertion: protection against triggering by regular exertion. N Engl J Med 1993;329:1677–1683.

82. Mold JW, Sten HF. The cascade effect in clinical care of patients. N Engl J Med 1986;314:512–514.

83. Morris M, Osborne D, Hill K, Kendig H, et al. Predisposinug factors for occasional and multiple falls in older Australians who live at home. Aust J Physiother 2004;50:153–159.

84. Muller JE, Mittleman MA, Maclure M, Sherwood JB, Tofler GH. Triggering myocardial infarction by sexual activity: low absolute risk and prevention by regular physical exertion. JAMA 1996;275:1405–1409.

85. Munin MC, Rudy TE, Glynn NW, et al. Early inpatient rehabilitation after elective hip and knee arthroplasty. JAMA 1998;279:847–852.

86. Myburgh KH, Hutchins J, Fataar AB, Hough SF, Noakes TD. Low bone density is an etiologic factor for stress fractures in athletes. Ann of Internal Med 1990;113:754–759.

87. Nadeau S, McFadyen BJ, Malouin F. Frontal and sagittal plane analyses of the stair climbing task in healthy adults aged over 40 years: what are the challenges compared to level walking? Clin Biomech 2003;10:950–959.

88. Noble PC, Gordon MJ, Weiss JM, Reddix RN, Conditt MA, Mathis KB. Does total knee replacement restore normal knee function? Clin Orthop Relat Res. 2005;431:157–65.

89. O'Reilly SC, Muir KR, Doherty M. Effectiveness of home exercise on pain and disability from osteoarthritis of the knee: a randomized controlled trial. Ann Rheum Dis 1999;58:15–19.

90. Ouellet D, Moffett H. Locomotor deficits before and two months after knee arthroplasty. Arthritis Rheum 2002;47:484–493.

91. Padua L, Padua R, Mastantuoni G, Pitta L, Caliandro P, Aulisa L. Health-related quality of life after surgical treatment for lumbar stenosis. Spine 2004;29:1670–1675.

92. Paffenberger RS Jr, Hyde RT, Wing AL, et al. The association of change sand physical-activity level and other lifestyle characteristics with mortality among men. N Engl J Med 1993;328:538–545.

93. Pandya NK, Draganich LF, Mauer A, Piotrowski GA, Pottenger L. Osteoarthritis of the knees increases the propensity to trip on an obstacle. Clin Orthop Relat Res. 2005;431:150–156.

94. Parsons IM, Sonnabend DH. What is the role of joint replacement surgery? Best Practice & Research Clinical Rheumatology 2004;18:557–572.

95. Pate R, Pratt M, Blair Sn, Haskell WL, Macera CA, Bouchard C, et al. Physical activity and public health. A recommendation from the Centers for Disease Control and Prevention and the American College of Sports Medicine. JAMA 1995;273:402–407.

96. Penninx BW, Messier SP, Rejeski WJ, Williamson JD, DiBari M, et al. Physical exercise and the prevention of disability in activities of daily living in older persons with osteoarthritis. Arch Int Med 2001;161:2309–2316.

97. Petrella R, Bartha C. Home based exercise therapy for older patients with knee osteoarthritis: a randomized clinical trial. J Rheumatol 2000;27: 2215–2221.

98. Philbin EF, Groff GD, Ries MD, Miller TE. Cardiovascular fitness and health in patients with end-stage osteoartritis. Arthritis Rheum 1995;38: 799–805.

99. Phillips EM, Bodenheimer CF, Roig RL, Cifu DX. Geriatric rehabilitation. 4. Physical medicine and rehabilitation interventions for common age-related disorders and geriatric syndromes. Arch Phys Med Rehabil 2004;85(Suppl 3):S18–S22.

100. Physical Activity and Health: A Report of the Surgeon General. Atlanta, GA: U.S. Department of Health and Human Services, Centers for Disease Control and Prevention, National Center for Chronic Disease Prevention and Health Promotion; 1996.

101. Physical activity and cardiovascular health. NIH Consensus Development Panel on Physical Activity and Cardiovascular Health. JAMA 1996;276:241–246.

102. Posner JD, Gorman KM, Klein HS, Woldow A. Exercise capacity in the elderly. Am J Cardiol 1986;57:52C–58C.

103. Province MA, Hadley EC, Hornbrook MC, et al. The effects of exercise on falls in elderly patients. A pre-planned metaanalysis of the FICSIT Trials. Frailty and Injuries: Cooperative Studies of Intervention Techniques. JAMA 1995;273:1341–1347.

104. Rissanen P, Aro S, Slatis P, Sintonen H, Paavolainen P. Health and quality of life before and after hip or knee arthroplasty. J Arthroplasty 1995;10:169–175.

105. Rose DJ. FallProof balance and mobility program developed by Center for Successful Aging at Cal State Univ, Fullerton, 2003a.

106. Rose DJ. Fallproof. A Comprehensive Balance and Mobility Training Program. Champaign, IL: Human Kinetics, 2003b.

107. Roubenoff R. Sacropenia: effects on body composition and function. J Gerontol A Biol Sci Med Sci 2003;58:1012–1017.

108. Rubenstein L, Powers CM, MacLean CH. Quality indicators for management and prevention of falls and mobility problems in vulnerable elders. Ann Intern Med 2001;135:686–693.

109. Rutherford OM. Spine and total body mineral density in amenorrheic athletes. J of Applied Physiol 1993;74:2904–2908.

110. Rutherford OM. Bone density and physical activity. Proceedings of the Nutrition Society 1997;56:1–8.

111. Schai PA, Gibbon AJ, Scott RD. Kneeling ability after total knee arthroplasty. Clin Orthop Rel Res 1999;367:195–200.

112. Scott VJ, Dukeshire S, Gallagher E, Scanlan A. A best practices guide for the prevention of falls among seniors living in the community. Report prepared on behalf of the Federal/Provincial/Territorial Committee of Officials Seniors) for the Ministers Responsible for Seniors, Ottawa. Available at: www.hc-sc.gc.ca/seniorsaines/pubs/best_practices/ intro_e.htm. Accessed May 11, 2004.

113. Seeman TE, Berkman LF, Charpentier PA, Blazer DC, Albert MS, Tinetti ME. Behavioral and psychosocial predictors of physical performance: MacArthur studies of successful aging. J Gerontol A Biol Sci Med Sci 1995;50:M177–M183.

114. Seidler R, Martin PE. The effects of short term balance training on the postural control of older adults. Gait Posture 1997;6:224–236.

115. Simotas AC, Dorey FJ, Hansraj KK, Cammisa F. Nonoperative treatment for lumbar spinal stenosis: Clinical and outcome results and a 3-year survivorship analysis. Spine 2000;25:197–204.

116. Sinaki M, Mikkelsen BA. Postmenopausal spinal osteoporosis: flexion vs extension exercises. Archives of Phys Med and Rehab 1984;65: 593–596.

117. Sliwinski MM, Sisto SA, Batavia M, Chen B, Forrest GF. Dynamic stability during walking following unilateral total hip arthroplasty. Gait Posture 2004;19: 141–147.

118. Smutok M, Reece C, Kokkinos P, et al. Aerobic vs strength training for risk factor intervention in middle-aged men at high risk for coronary heart disease. Metabolism 1993;42:177–184.

119. Snow L. Aging with a physical disability: Is it safe to exercise? Orth Phys Ther Clin North Am 2001;10:251–263.

120. Sprat KF, Keller TS, Szpalski M, Vandeputte K, Bunzburg R. A predictive model for outcome after conservative decompression surgery for lumbar spinal stenosis. Eur Spine J 2004;13:14–21.

121. Tak E, Staats P, van Hespen A, Hopman-Rock M. The Effects of an Exercise Program for Older Adults with Osteoarthritis of the Hip. J Rheumatol 2005;32:1106–1113.

122. Tenhula J, Lenke LG, Bridwell KH, Gupta P, Riew D. Prospective functional evaluation of the surgical treatment of neurogenic claudication in patients with lumbar spinal stenosis. J of Spinal Disorders 2000;13:276–282.

123. The Falls Prevention Initiative. Division of Aging and Seniors Public Health Agency of Canada. http://www.phac-aspc.gc.ca/seniors-aines/pubs/injury_prevention/falls_factsheets/ fallsprevtn8_e.htm. Accessed in 2004.

124. Thomas SG, Pagura SMC, Kennedy D. Physical Activity and its Relationship to Physical Performance in Patients With End Stage Knee Osteoarthritis. J Orthop Sports Phys Ther 2003;33:745–754.

125. Thompson LV. Aging muscle: Characteristics and strength training. Issues Aging 1995;331;821–827.

126. Thompson LV. Physical activity and exercise: Identification of benefits. Orth Phys Ther Clin North Am 2001;10:193–211.

127. Toda, Y. The effect of energy restriction, walking, and exercise on lower extremity lean body mass in obese women with osteoarthritis of the knee. J Orthop Sci 2001;6:148–154.

128. van Baar ME, Dekker J, Oostendorp RA, Voorn TB, Bijlsma JW. Effectiveness of exercise in patients with osteoarthritis of the hip or knee: nine months follow-up. Ann Rheum Dis 2001;60:1123–1130.

129. Volpi E, Nazemi R, Fufita S. Muscle tissue changes with aging. Curr Opin Clin Nutr Metab Care 2004;7:405–410.

130. Vuori IM. Dose-response of physical activity and low back pain, osteoarthritis, and osteoporosis. Med Sci Sports Exerc. 2001;33(Suppl):S551–S586.

131. Wegener L, Kisner C, Nichols D. Static and dynamic balance responses in persons with bilateral knee osteoarthritis. J Orthop Sports Phys Ther 1997;25:13–18.

132. Wei M, Kampert JB, Barolow CE, et al. Relationship between low cardiorespiratory fitness and mortality in normal-weight, overweight, and obese men. JAMA 1999;282:1547–1553.

133. Wennberg DE, Kellett MA, Dickens JD, Malenka DJ, Keilson LM, Keller RB. The association between local diagnostic testing intensity and invasive cardiac procedures. JAMA 1996;275:1161–1164.

134. Wolf SL, Barnhart HX, Kutner NG, et al. Reducing frailty and falls in older persons: An investigation of Tai Chi and computerized balance training. JAGS 1996;44:489–497.

135. Wolfson L, Whipple R, Derbe C, et al. Balance and strength training in older adults: Intervention gains and Tai Chi maintenance. JAGS 1996;44:498–506.

Physical Activity Readiness Questionnaire

PAR-Q reproduced with permission from Gordon NF. Pre-participation health appraisal in the non-medical setting in ACSM's Resource Manual for Guidelines for Exercise Testing and Prescription (3rd edition). American College of Sports Medicine. Baltimore: Lippincott Williams & Wilkins, 1998:343.

Table 40.2 Physical Activity Readiness Questionnaire (PAR-Q)

For most people, physical activity should not pose any problem or hazard. PAR-Q has been designed to identify the small number of adults for whom physical activity might be inappropriate or those who should have medical advice concerning the type of activity most suitable.

Yes No

☐ ☐ 1. Has a doctor ever said that you have a heart condition *and* that you should only do physical activity recommended by a doctor?
   (**Significance/Clarification:** Persons with known heart disease are at increased risk for cardiac complications during exercise. They should consult a physician and undergo exercise testing before starting an exercise program. The exercise prescription should be formulated in accordance with standard guidelines for cardiac patients. Medical supervision may be required during exercise training.)

☐ ☐ 2. Do you feel pain in your chest when you do physical activity?

☐ ☐ 3. In the past month, have you had chest pain when you were not doing physical activity?
   (**Significance/Clarification:** A physician should be consulted to identify the cause of the chest pain, whether it occurs at rest or with exertion. If ischemic in origin, the condition should be stabilized before starting an exercise program. Exercise testing should be performed with the patient on his or her usual medication and the exercise prescription formulated in accordance with standard guidelines for cardiac patients. Medical supervision may be required during exercise training.)

☐ ☐ 4. Do you lose your balance because of dizziness or do you ever lose consciousness?
   (**Significance/Clarification:** A physician should be consulted to establish the cause of these symptoms which may be related to potentially life-threatening medical conditions. Exercise training should not be undertaken until serious cardiac disorders have been excluded.)

☐ ☐ 5. Do you have a bone or joint problem that could be made worse by a change in your physical activity?
   (**Significance/Clarification:** Existing musculoskeletal disorders may be exacerbated by inappropriate exercise training. Persons with forms of arthritis known to be associated with a systemic component (for example, rheumatoid arthritis) may be at an increased risk for exercise-related medical complications. A physician should be consulted to determine whether any special precautions are required during exercise training.)

☐ ☐ 6. Is your doctor currently prescribing drugs (for example, water pills) for your blood pressure or heart condition?
   (**Significance/Clarification:** See question 1. Medication effects should be considered when formulating the exercise prescription. The exercise prescription should be formulated in accordance with guidelines for the specific cardiovascular disease for which medications are being used. A physician should be consulted to determine whether the condition/factor requires special precautions during exercise training or contraindicates exercise training.)

☐ ☐ 7. Do you know of any other reason why you should not do physical activity?
   (**Significance/Clarification:** The exercise prescription may need to be modified in accordance with the specific reason provided. Depending on the specific reason, a physician may need to be consulted.)

If a person answers yes to any question, vigorous exercise or exercise testing may need to be postponed. Medical clearance may be necessary.

38

Role of Non-Operative Spinal Specialist in Managing the Spine Patient

Joel Press, John J. Triano,
Craig Liebenson, and Robert Watkins

Learning Objectives
After reading this chapter you should be able to:

- Understand the role of interventional diagnostic and therapeutic techniques
- Understand the role of different medications and injections for back and neck problems
- Understand the expected recovery for different spinal surgeries
- Gradually reactivate post-surgical patients
- Recommend invasive pain management options for chronic pain patients

Introduction

The purpose of this chapter is to discuss the non-operative treatment options for patients with musculoskeletal spinal disorders who are not responding to reactivation advice, manipulation, or rehabilitative exercises. What, if any, contribution interventional techniques such as spinal injections, medications, and invasive pain management procedures may make and their appropriate use will be presented. More important than the single benefit of any, or all, of the above treatments, is how they can be integrated into a treatment approach in a cost-effective, patient-oriented approach.

Patients who have severe symptoms or complex pathology often require care coordination and/or co-management. Complementary to conservative procedures are a number of interventional techniques obtained through this multidisciplinary management. The key to improving quality of care and outcomes is the appropriate and timely recognition of the patient's need for these services for the purpose of controlling extreme symptoms and/or diagnosing and improving the response for patients who have prolonged symptoms.

Interventional techniques in general offer two advantages for those patients who need them. First, is the improvement of diagnostic specificity as well as the promotion of symptom relief that may empower active coping, return to activity, and social participation (66). As is well known, diagnostic certainty is a rarity in spine pain. The exact source of the patient's pain and symptoms is often ambiguous. A number of different tissues are known to create overlapping pain patterns. For example, lumbosacral facet disease, sacroiliac disease and discopathy may have sclerotomal pain distribution patterns that overlap and can be confusing. Additionally, central sensitization (see Chapter 2) can even cause non-noxious stimuli to healthy tissue to be perceived as painful. In patients whose symptoms are severe or prolonged introduction of appropriate interventional procedures can improve the patient's compliance with functional restoration. They can promote greater confidence in the approach by successful identification/confirmation of the source of pain and providing short-term, immediate relief that can facilitate progress in rehabilitation and therapy.

This chapter will give the authors' perspective on how some of these treatment options can be used to assist difficult cases with the care of their disabling spine problems. Some of the information is based on the limited scientific literature available for non-surgical treatment for spine pain. Certain procedures have stronger evidence than others. For instance, microdiscectomy for lumbar nerve root compression has far greater evidence of efficacy than does lumbar fusion for either nerve root compression or chronic back pain (24,26). Clinicians must make informed choices about how to facilitate coping and/or recovery in stubborn, disabling, chronic spine patients. Such choices should be informed by the evidence, but often evidence is minimal. In such instances, helpful guides such as provided by the Cochrane Collaboration should be used, but also taken with a grain of salt when a limited number of randomized, controlled trials are used from which to draw conclusions (24,31,43,45,46,51,63,64).

When it is all said and done, we have to treat the patient and do the best we can with the information available. Sometimes that will mean trying things that are unconventional. Other times it means not doing anything to them at all, but giving them some direction and hope for managing their problems. This chapter may be as much editorial as literature review. Regardless, hopefully it will be useful to clinicians treating back pain.

A health care provider (HCP) specializing in conservative care of neuromusculoskeletal (NMS) disorders must have broad based knowledge of the decision points for various diagnostic and treatment steps for uncomplicated and complicated cases. Spine care requires most of the same core competencies as for NMS care in general.

Basic Principles

First, and foremost, when treating patients with musculoskeletal disorders, especially back pain, ultimately it is the patient's responsibility to get better. Our job is to provide the therapeutic milieu, appropriate counseling and home program for the patient. We may provide treatment to decrease nociceptive pain (i.e., manual treatments, medications, modalities, etc.) with the goal of promoting increased patient participation and activity in the healing process. With chronic back pain the chances of passive treatment alone providing lasting pain relief is very slim. An important key to providing the right type of activity and/or home program is to understand the musculoskeletal system as a whole and the ability for compensatory interaction within its many parts. Treatment needs to address stability and self-efficacy. Exercise should be as functional as possible, meaning it should resemble, at least in some way, the activity or sport that the patient engages in. Straight leg raises may strengthen the quadriceps muscles, but very few of us lie on our back and lift our legs up as part of our daily activities. Loading all components of the kinetic chain such as in a squat most closely simulates real life and therefore function.

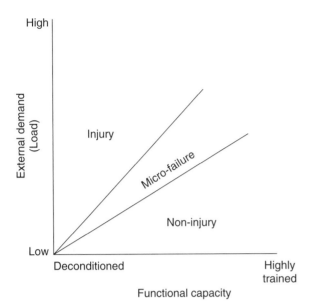

Figure 38.1 Relationship of functional capacity and external demand.

Secondly, treatment should be active, meaning that the patient participates and ultimately is independent within the program (see Chapter 14). Our job is to teach spine sparing activity modifications and spine stabilizing exercises to help them handle their normal activities of daily living with a wide margin of error. The more effective way to know if a patient is compliant with the prescribed exercise is to ask them to demonstrate the program when you see them on follow up. Only then can adequate assessment of their report of usefulness be made. Patients will often say they are compliant, "doing those back exercises . . . you know. . . ." However, if they are unable to demonstrate proper form and function then either they are not doing them or are doing them incorrectly, potentially aggravating their problems. The only people that will continue to perform an exercise or treatment program are those that perceive they are getting some benefit from it.

In becoming active, patients should be encouraged to pace themselves. An athlete will need a more aggressive rehabilitation program while a sedentary person a less aggressive one, but all patients require sufficient functional capacity to meet or exceed their functional demands (Figs. 38.1 and 38.2).

A corollary to this is that back booklets with pages and pages of exercises and back tips, rarely are read, often are inappropriate for a given patient and disorder. Many patients, without adequate supervision and coaching, lack sufficient motivation to follow-through with generic exercise sheet use, even if the exercises are appropriate. To improve patient compliance, keep exercises simple, customized, and focused to the immediate needs, progressing from one set to the next as the patient progresses. Further, with a larger series, should one exercise aggravate symptoms, the patient will have a difficult time differentiating which exercise is responsible and may abandon all of them.

Third, the more effective approach to musculoskeletal problems is eclectic. As complex as these disorders may be, no one clinical specialty can provide all the answers; although many individuals may think that they do. Different clinicians and HCPs offer separate skill sets that may be more or less appropriate for different types of problems—i.e., nerve irritation vs. joint dysfunction versus muscle restriction or imbalance vs. psychosocial issues. Complex or chronic cases may have more than one of these contributing elements to their clinical presentation. The value of understanding and coordinating integrated care across multiple disciplines for patients of this type is the improvement of quality of life (61,62). For uncomplicated cases the knowledge and skills set is presented in Table 38.1 (see also Chapter 4). For complicated cases the knowledge and skill set is presented in Table 38.2.

Advanced Diagnostic Steps

Most patients presenting with acute neck or back related disorders do not require any advanced diagnostics (imaging, serological testing, EMG, diagnostic needling, etc.) (see Chapters 3, 4, and 7) and (Fig. 4.8a). However, if the history or examination produces suspicion of serious injury or disease (e.g., "red flag" findings) additional testing is necessary. For persistent, undiagnosed symptoms advanced studies may prove useful to confirm the absence of serious disease and empower the patient's confidence and acceptance of their treatment plan. Should underlying treatable pathology by found, more invasive procedures (e.g., injections, surgery) may be appropriate. Imag-

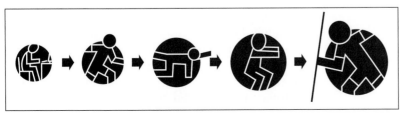

Figure 38.2 The reactivation/rehabilitation/ functional performance continuum.

Table 38.1 Uncomplicated Spine Care
Core Competencies

1. Diagnostic triage
2. Reassurance
3. Reactivation advice
4. Medication
5. Manipulation/manual therapy

ing, serology, and EMG have been covered elsewhere in this text (see Chapter 7) (see Tables 7.7, 7.8, 7.9, 7.10, and 7.11). This section will emphasize the indications and utility of interventional diagnostic injection (needling) methods.

Diagnostic Needling Procedures

There are five primary diagnostic techniques utilized within interventional procedures (see also Chapters 6 and 7). They include:

1. Facet and costovertebral joint blocks
2. Discography
3. Nerve blocks
4. Epidural injections
5. Sacroiliac joint blocks

Most of these methods provide both diagnostic and therapeutic benefit by identifying the pain generator relieved or provoked by the injected material

and by providing a vehicle to transport medication directly to the specific tissue. Except for discography, the diagnostic application is discussed along with the therapeutic procedure in the section on the role of therapeutic injections.

Under no circumstances should diagnostic or therapeutic injection procedures be performed without the use of videofluoroscopy for direct visualization of the placement of the needle, visualization of contrast at the targeted site, and successful injection of the diagnostic/therapeutic agent into the tissue in order to insure proper interpretation of the results.

Discography

Indication: Central axis pain which has failed non-operative management, including medication, physical therapy and chiropractic procedures. In general use, discography is not used, because of its extreme invasive nature, until and/or unless the patient has had six months of therapy without adequate recovery and all other probable pain generators have been ruled out. Discography is often used in patients who have MRIs showing multiple areas of pathology including the possibility of multiple level disc bulge/protrusion and/or degenerative disease and in which surgery (e.g., arthroplasty disc replacement and/or fusion procedures) is being contemplated.

Discography is a controversial procedure. Carragee et al. showed that discography or MRI (i.e., annular disruption) are not good predictors of future back

Table 38.2 Complicated Spine Care Core Competencies

1. Advanced Diagnostic steps
   a. Imaging
      i. Radiology
      ii. Advanced imaging
   b. Serology
   c. EMG
   d. Diagnostic needling
2. Basic role and limitations of medication
   a. Analgesics
      i. Non-narcotic
      ii. Narcotic
      iii. Topical agents
   b. Anti-inflammatories
      i. NSAIDs
      ii. Steroids
   c. Muscle relaxants
   d. Anti-depressants
   e. Anti-convulsants/Neuropathic agents

3. Role of interventional injection techniques
   a. Muscle injections
   b. Joint blocks
      i. Facet
      ii. Sacroiliac
      iii. Costovertebral
   c. Rhizotomy
   d. Epidural steroids
      i. Caudal
      ii. Translaminar
      iii. Transforaminal (nerve root block)
4. Post-surgical management
   a. Course
   b. Rehabilitation
5. Chronic pain management interventions
   a. Cognitive–behavioral approach
   b. Multidisciplinary pain management
   c. Interventionist methods

pain, disability, or medical care, whereas psychosocial risk factors were very robust (12,13). Carragee et al. have also shown that discography is positive on a similar percentage (40%) of asymptomatic as symptomatic individuals who had previously had disc surgery (11). Patients with abnormal psychological profiles have significantly higher positive findings with discography than either asymptomatic volunteers or symptomatic subjects with normal psychological screening.

Discography should not be used in patients who have significant psycho-social overlay, multiple pain sites within the body, or previous musculoskeletal surgery. The procedure should be performed using fluoroscopic guidance, and the patient's pain response should be carefully noted. A positive test is one that shows reproduction of the patient's symptoms (concordance) with morphologic change within the injected disc, although the high false-positive rate with this test should always be borne in mind.

The Role of Medication

There is not a single medication nor one class of medication that works best for all spine pain patients. To understand when a medicine or nutraceutical may contribute to case management, some knowledge of the indications, contraindications, mechanism of action, side effect profile, and interactions with other medications is essential. Although rare, severe reactions can occur with combined use of herbal and prescription medications.

A rational pharmacologic approach for severe acute or chronic spine pain and may include the use of nonsteroidal anti-inflammatory medications, oral steroids, and opioids. Over time, should simple

pharmacologic management fail, or levels of analgesia and function reach a plateau, a more comprehensive medication pain management along with other interventional strategies may be necessary. A mechanistic approach to rational pharmacology is an important component of the spine practitioner's armamentarium for managing acute and chronic pain. This approach incorporates the use of various medications including newer generation and traditional antidepressants, neuropathic and sleep agents, and, in carefully selected cases, chronic opioid therapy. The mechanistic approach requires an understanding of basic physiologic and neurotransmitter function that helps to target the use of single or a combination of agents to reduce inflammation, alter excitability and block pain peripherally or centrally.

Goals for pharmacotherapy should focus on decreasing pain, maximizing independent physical function (activity level), and improving psychosocial or emotional state (social participation). This section reviews current updates in pharmacotherapy as it applies to a broad range of spine related conditions including neuropathic pain (a model for treatment of radiculopathy) and manifestations of chronic pain conditions (pain, affective distress, and sleep disturbance). The sections will include an overview related to controversies in the use of cyclooxygenase (COX)-2 inhibitors, pharmacological use of opioids, traditional and novel antidepressants, anticonvulsant medications, and topical analgesics.

A few simple, common questions should be included in the patient history to protect against iatrogenic medical complications (Table 38.3). Inclusion of this information when obtaining an interdisciplinary consultation will facilitate successful co-management of the patient.

Table 38.3 Most Common Questions for Directing Interdisciplinary Consultation for Medication to Manage Back Pain

Clinical History	Application
Known drug allergies or adverse reactions?	Avoid allergy inducing medications
Stomach sensitivity/ulcer symptoms/	Avoid NSAIDs, aspirin
Diabetic history?	Avoid steroids
Hypertension history?	Avoid certain NSAIDs and others with hypertensive complications
Glaucoma history?	Avoid agents that can increase ocular pressure
Seizure history?	Avoid medications that create central excitability

Analgesics

Non-Narcotic (Acetaminophen)

A generally accepted first-line medication for patients with low back or neck pain is acetaminophen (Tylenol) (18,39,42). Acetaminophen is inexpensive, is available over the counter, and has a good safety profile. Serious side effects including liver toxicity can occur with prolonged use of high doses, particularly in association with substantial alcohol intake (42). Toxicity at doses less than 4 g daily is rare. Acetaminophen prescribed at regular intervals is effective in mild to moderate low back pain. Comparisons of effectiveness in contrast to non-steroidal anti-inflammatory medications (NSAIDs) are inconsistent.

Indication: Front line non-prescription medicine for pain relief.

Risk: Minimal with short-term use. Liver toxicity with long-term use.

Narcotic (Opioid Analgesics)

Opioid analgesics act primarily by binding with opiate receptors in the central nervous system and are indicated for the treatment of acute, moderate to severe pain. Long-term use may be associated with tolerance, toxicity, addiction and illicit use. Treatment of patients with low back pain with narcotic analgesics should be limited to pain that is unresponsive to alternative medication, such as appropriately prescribed NSAIDs, or when other analgesics are contraindicated. To be effective, they should be used on a defined dosing schedule and not as needed. This dose should be individualized and not arbitrarily established because the latter approach can result in inadequate pain control and the possibility of pseudo-addictive behavior by the patient. Prolonged or repeated use of opioids is not necessary in most patients with acute low back pain.

Indication: Short-term specific dosage for severe pain unresponsive to other medications.

Risk: Tolerance, toxicity, addiction, and illicit use. Risk is increased if used "as needed."

Topical Analgesics

The use of over-the-counter and prescription topical analgesics continues to grow. Increased understanding of nociceptor physiology has demonstrated greater involvement of thermosensation than previously known. Recently, a new thermosensitive transreceptor protein channel family has been identified. Included in this, the vanilloid receptor (VR), a nonselective cation channel that is activated by capsaicin, the pungent agent found in chili peppers, now marketed in a number of analgesic creams. The cold and menthol sensitive receptor (CMRI), also has been identified and may result in the development of targeted cold producing analgesics. Over-the-counter topical analgesics include capsaicin-based products (heat-activated) and menthol (cooling effects by inhibiting calcium currents and decreasing temperature thresholds). Pharmacologic studies of menthol have suggested a possible kappa opioid receptor effect, contributing additional analgesic properties to this substance.

Prescription medications include lidocaine 5% patches (Lidoderm Patch, Endo Pharmaceuticals) indicated for postherpetic neuralgia (PHN). Randomized placebo controlled studies have demonstrated efficacy in PHN dosed 12 hours per day. Recent studies demonstrated safety and decreased risk for systemic effects with multiple patches worn 24 hours at a time with no significant systemic toxic effects. Although lidocaine's mechanism of action (peripheral sodium channel blockade) has long been understood, recent studies have demonstrated physiologic changes at the dorsal horn and changes in fMRI after patch use suggesting additional effects on central sensitization. Open-label studies in osteoarthritis demonstrated reduced stiffness and pain with local application in osteoarthritis and chronic low back pain.

Topical tricyclic antidepressants, including doxepin (FDA approval for dermatologic condition eczema) has been used more widely in Europe in the management of neuropathic pain. Compounding pharmacies may serve a unique service in providing a number of compounds for topical use including ketamine (NMDA receptor antagonist), gabapentin, and cyclobenzaprine. Tropical medications can serve as an adjunct to other pharmacologic treatments especially for well localized areas of pain.

Indication: Short-term use for chronic, intractable pain.

Risk: Minimal for short-term use.

Anti-Inflammatories

NSAIDs and Cox-2 Inhibitors

Conventional (i.e., non-specific) NSAIDs have been first-line treatment for analgesia and the treatment of inflammatory conditions including osteoarthritis and rheumatoid arthritis (Naproxen, Naprosyn) (39,42). Acute spine pain may benefit from anti-inflammatory effects of these agents as related to lumbar radiculopathy, facet joint irritation, and related soft tissue injury (18). A Cochrane Collaboration review involving 51 clinical trials concluded that

NSAIDs are effective for short-term symptomatic relief in patients with acute LBP (63). An NSAID in common use is Aleve, which is the over-the-counter version of naproxen.

All NSAIDs are analgesic, antipyretic, and anti-inflammatory. No significant differences have been demonstrated among currently available NSAIDs in numerous clinical trials (9,30). Considerable variability in efficacy and toxicity is observed from patient to patient, and even within the same chemical class of NSAIDs. Similar patients express marked variation in preference for various NSAIDs (29,57). Therefore, there is no perfect NSAID or the definite "one" to try first. Because of the similar efficacy and significant variability in response to a particular agent, choice of NSAID is empiric. Choices should be made on physician preference (what have you used and are comfortable with), cost, that patient's prior experience with various NSAIDs, and possible side effects given a specific patients medical history. An adequate trial of any NSAID is 2 to 3 weeks. If one class showed no response of an ill effect, changing to a different class of NSAID would be appropriate.

The biggest concern with NSAIDs in clinical practice are toxic side effects (22,40). Although several rare, but serious, side effects including clinical hepatitis, aplastic anemia, and agranulocytosis can occur, gastrointestinal side effects are by far the most common and occur in approximately 25% of NSAID uses, though silent endoscopically demonstrated lesions occur in as many as 60% (40,25). The relative risk of serious GI disease or complications (ulcer, bleeding, death) has been reported to range from 1.4 to 10.5 in NSAIDs users (58). A meta-analysis concluded that the overall risk of serious gastrointestinal bleeding in patients who took NSAIDs is approximately 1 per 1,000 patients, with the risk being significantly greater in patients older that 65 years of age. (63). Risk for GI problems are greater in patients older than 60, patients with prior ulcer disease, concomitant corticosteroid therapy, and higher-dose NSAID use (58). Unfortunately, not all patients with GI problems with NSAIDs will present initially with mild or even moderate GI symptoms.

Conventional NSAIDs were found to offer effective analgesic responses but are limited by potential upper gastrointestinal (GI) bleeding and ulceration, renal toxicities, and platelet dysfunction. A recent effort to resolve the common gastric side-effects of NSAIDs has been the development of the COX-1 and COX-2 inhibitors. These isoforms catalyze the conversion of arachidonic acid to prostaglandins. More recent classification of NSAIDS include: (1) conventional or non-selective (NS-NSAID), those that inhibit both the cyclooxygenase-1 (COX-1) isoenzyme and the COX-2 isoenzyme; and (2) those that are more selective for COX-2 isoenzyme (COX-2 inhibitors). Recent evidence suggests that these preparations may have higher incidence of cardiovascular adverse reactions.

Indication: NSAIDs are a front line non-prescription medicine for pain relief.

Risk: With NSAIDs GI side effects are common, especially in patients older than 60.

Corticosteroids

Theoretically, oral corticosteroids may be useful as a strong anti-inflammatory agent for patients with radicular symptoms due to a disk herniation. The inhibition of the inflammatory process by corticosteroid is more complete than that by NSAIDs because the leukotriene-mediated response is also diminished. The risk of serious complication of steroid therapy is related to the dose and duration of treatment. Short-term use (7–10 days) of even high-dose (30–40 mg prednisone or equivalent) corticosteroid has not been associated with major adverse side effects (44). Oral steroids maybe helpful in patients with an acute inflammatory musculoskeletal problem i.e. radiculopathy who can not tolerate NSAIDs or who have had NSAIDs and not gotten significant relief.

Indication: If front line non-prescription medicines are ineffective for radiculopathy.

Risk: Minimal with short-term use (7–10 days).

Muscle Relaxants

All of the muscle relaxants are centrally acting drugs that alter polysynaptic supraspinal and spinal pathways, which modulate stretch reflexes (54). These preparations basically produce non-specific sedation which accounts for their muscle relaxation. According to a Cochrane Collaboration review, muscle relaxants are effective in the management of non-specific low back pain, but the adverse effects require that they be used carefully (64). Muscle relaxants are more effective than placebo in relief of symptoms in the treatment of acute musculoskeletal disorders. However, in studies comparing muscle relaxant therapy with pure analgesics, no significant differences in outcomes has been demonstrated. Muscle relaxants have been commonly used in combination with analgesics or NSAIDs. Studies support a modest short-term advantage of use of combinations of medications over single agents. The most significant side effects of muscle relaxants are drowsiness and dizziness. Use of muscle relaxants should be incorporated before bedtime, when possible, to take advantage of their sedating effects and reduce daytime sedation. Muscle relaxants are often not tolerated when used during the day time hours when the patient needs to be alert. It is not known if muscle relaxants are more effective than analgesics or non-steroidal anti-inflammatory drugs (64).

Indication: If front line non-prescription medicines are ineffective for acute LBP.

Risk: Drowsiness and dizziness require their careful use during the daytime.

Anti-Depressants

Although tricyclic antidepressants have demonstrated a role in the treatment of chronic low back pain, they are not indicated for acute episodes (21,23,32,56,62). Benefits of this class of medication may be due to analgesic effects, anti-depressant effects, or even improvement of sleep (44). Tricyclic antidepressants should definitely be considered when pain, depression, or sleep disturbances coexist. Initial doses should be low, and subsequent doses can be slowly increased, as necessary to minimize adverse effects of dry mouth, daytime sedation, constipation, urinary retention, and orthostatic hypotension. Endpoints of treatment include improvement of restorative sleep, reduction in pain, improvement of mood, and improvement in ability to participate in reconditioning and rehabilitative activities (44).

The tricyclic antidepressants (TCAs) are effective agents in selected neuropathic pain states. Their use as both potent antidepressants and sedating medications may fit into a number of therapeutic targets related to symptom management of chronic pain syndrome (pain, depression, disturbed sleep). Dosing these medications initially at night may be of benefit for the relatively potent serotonin (5-HT) and norepinephrine (NE) effects. Slow titration to higher antidepressant doses may lead to additional antidepressant effects and analgesia. Although selective serotonin reuptake inhibitors (SSRIs) have proven effects as potent antidepressants and anxiolytics in general anxiety states, with less side effects than traditional TCAs, limited analgesic effects have been reported.

The newest class of antidepressants, dual monoamine reuptake inhibitors (serotonin/norepinephrine reuptake inhibitors), were developed for the treatment of depression with a goal of providing shorter onset of antidepressant effects and less side effects due to their relatively selectivity. Mirtazapine (Remeron®) is a potent antagonist of central α_2 adrenergic receptors, an antagonist of 5-HT_2 and 5-HT_3 receptors and enhances NE and 5-HT neurotransmission. Mirtaza-

pine is indicated for the treatment of depression and may be used to enhance the efficacy of SSRIs. Its relatively sedating effects may have additional benefits for improving sleep in chronic pain patients. Venlafaxine (Effexor, Wyeth) is a potent reuptake inhibitor of 5-HT, with less potent effects on NE and dopamine. Higher doses (> 150mg) have been found to have additional analgesic effects and may be efficacious in a number of neuropathic pain states. Duloxetine (Cymbalta, Eli Lily) is a potent balanced reuptake inhibitor of both 5-HT and NE. It is indicated for depression, diabetic peripheral neuropathy, and post-herpetic neuralgia (PHN).

Tricyclics and other anti-depressants are very helpful in chronic pain conditions, in lower doses and taken at bedtime, in patients with disturbed sleep patterns related to their pain.

Indication: If pain, depression, and sleep disturbances co-exist in chronic pain patients.

Risk: Minimal in small doses for short-term use.

Anticonvulsants/Neuropathic Agents

The important pathophysiological mechanism underlying chronic neuropathic pain, including radiculopathy, is central sensitization (see Chapter 2). The use of newer generation anticonvulsants has made their incorporation into outpatient management more practical given their more favorable metabolic and interaction profiles as compared to traditional anticonvulsants. New generation agents demonstrate limited enzyme induction, relatively longer half-lives, and strong protein binding, limiting the necessity of ongoing serum monitoring.

Gabapentin (Neurontin, Pfizer) approved for post-herpetic neuralgia and diabetic peripheral neuropathy has found wide off-label use for spine related pain conditions including radiculopathy, as well as migraine headache, spasticity, and a number of psychiatric conditions. Many of the anticonvulsant/neuropathic agents can be used in pain symptoms when postoperative neuropathic symptoms persist or in some cases of chronic radiculopathy or other nerve related pain.

Indication: Chronic pain apparently involving central sensitization if other medications have not been effective.

Risk: Minimal in short-term use.

Summary

Pain relief is generally better in patients treated with analgesics compared to placebo in RCT's (18). Acetaminophen or NSAIDs can be used acutely for episodes of low back pain. If these agents do not produce adequate pain relief, muscle relaxants may be added. At times, a short course (5 to 7 days) of relatively low doses of oral corticosteroids, or narcotic analgesics may be beneficial in order to get the patient over a pain barrier and facilitate reactivation and engagement in a rehabilitation program. Antidepressant medications (which are generally very well tolerated at low doses) can be an excellent adjunct to other components of a treatment program for the patients with more subacute and chronic pain, especially when sleep disturbances are associated. With all medication use, knowledge of medication profiles, drug interactions, and toxic side effects is essential.

The Role of Injections

Spinal injections can be a helpful tool in the evaluation and treatment of spine disorders. Injections can be placed in a number of potential pain generating structures to relieve pain and facilitate a rehabilitation program. Injections should not be used in isolation. The rationale for using epidural corticosteroid injections is supported by the evidence of an inflammatory basis for radicular pain due to disk herniation. Although epidural injections have been effective in reducing pain in patients with radicular pain, the results in some controlled, prospective studies are variable (45). The benefit of facet joint injections and sacroiliac injections are also controversial (45). However for chronic pain, when the pain generating tissue is clearly diagnosed—such as by double anesthetic block technique—there is a definite role (see chapter 6). Injections may provide an adjunct to other treatments (i.e., manipulation, mobilization, exercise) by reducing inflammation and facilitating joint movement in otherwise hypomobile joints or segments.

Proper patient selection is the key to gaining benefit form these procedures. Patients with radicular symptoms and clear cut radiculopathy with consistent imaging studies, who have failed to respond to appropriate measures usually will benefit from epidural injections. Similarly, other pain sources, i.e., facet mediated pain and sacroiliac pain, when clinical history, physical exam, and provocative tests are suggestive (because no specific historical feature or exam finding are definitive) can be addressed with fluoroscopically guided injections to insure proper needle placement.

To think that any type of spinal injections, used a sole treatment for a chronic spinal disorder, will be of significant benefit is unrealistic. Concurrent cognitive–behavioral management is advised to avoid the patient placing too much emphasis on fixing or curing the problem, without sufficient orientation on learning improved coping and rehabilitation strategies (see Chapter 31). Contraindications for these procedures include infection, diabetes, pregnancy, bleeding disorders and anticoagulation therapy.

Muscle/Trigger Point Injections

Indication: Patients with recalcitrant local pain which can be reproduced by soft tissue palpation:

Trigger point injections utilize saline, local anesthetic, or corticosteroid (42). More than three injections are usually not required.

Joint Blocks

There are some risks associated with these procedures, thus the requirement that fluoroscopy be used as a directive tool. In the cervical spine the most risky is that of possible vertebral artery damage from an errant approach. If the nerve itself should be violated, then a traumatic neuropathy may develop that may be transient or may become chronic with possible development of complex regional pain syndrome. Occasional steroidal side effects are noted which can include several days of a flu-like syndrome with low grade fever, generalized aches and pains. This may also range to full anaphylactic reaction in patients who are sensitive to the carrier medication. Improper needle insertion may result in dural puncture, spinal cord trauma, infection, intervascular injection, spinal anesthesia, chemical meningitis, neural trauma and hematoma formation.

In final comment, indications for these joint block procedures would include high suspicion of a joint source non-responsive to care and/or extreme joint irritation preventing adequate care over time, and non-responsive to medication management.

Facet (see Chapter 6)

Indication: A patient suspected of having facet capsulitis or symptomatic facet degenerative joint disease that is severe, non-responsive or recurrent may benefit from a joint block.

The procedure tests the hypothesis that the target joint is the source of the patient's pain. The joint blocks can be accomplished by either injecting local anesthetic into the articulation itself or adjacent to the medial branch of the dorsal rami that innervate the target joint. Successful response is rather quick and significant relief of the patient's pain. If the patient does not achieve significant reduction in symptoms, then an alternate hypothesis for the pain generation should be considered.

Assessing the joint in locating the site for these procedures to be applied should include physical stressing of the articulation itself using provocative maneuvers in an effort to identify the most painful site. It is not uncommon for the physician to identify the joint through facet loading with posterior/anterior pressure using a single digit to apply the load to the most painful site. This can be marked with an radiopaque marker and appropriately directed radiographs utilized to get an accurate count of the site for requesting the procedure (Fig. 38.3).

On occasion it may be found that an articular capsule is torn and radiopaque materials and medication will leak from the capsule itself. Under these circumstances the prospect for resolution of the patient's problem is dim, because the articulation has become a dry joint.

Facet/costovertebral joint blocks may be administered at three possible sites: interarticular, medial branch block and medial branch neurotomy (rhizotomy). A Cochrane Collaboration metaanalysis found that few studies were methodologically strong and concluded that "convincing evidence is lacking on the effects of injection therapies for low back pain. There is a need for more, well designed explanatory trials in this field" (45). Short-term response from injection procedures is the resolution or significantly improved symptoms in less than a three-month interval. Patients that tend to receive good response but for shorter term relief (days to weeks) may benefit from a series of up to three injections. If the patient's symptomatology returns despite the use of a series with interventional management and the patient is non-responsive to other conservative care, then a neurotomy procedure may be appropriate.

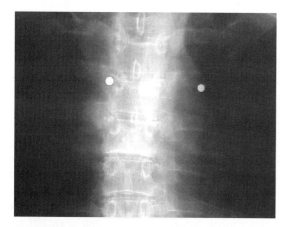

Figure 38.3 Radiopaque marking of painful tissue.

Sacroiliac Joint (see Chapter 6)

Indication: The indications for sacroiliac joint block are essentially the same as that of a facet block but for patients in whom there is high suspicion of the sacroiliac joint being the cause of the patient's symptoms.

The sacroiliac joint is a large, primarily weight-bearing, facet articulation in many respects. There are few good physical findings clearly indicating that it is a source of pain. The intent, like that of facet joint block, of these procedures is to identify the joint as the source of symptoms and to provide symptomatic management.

Costovertebral

See Facet section.

Rhizotomy

Rhizotomy/percutaneous radiofrequency neurotomy generally incorporates multi-level cauterizations due to the fact each facet joint may have multiple innervations. For the sacroiliac joint, neurotomy of the lateral branch for L2–S1 is required as the joint is innervated by branches from all of these levels. A Cochrane review concluded that there is "limited evidence that radiofrequency denervation offers short-term relief for chronic neck pain of zygapophyseal joint origin and for chronic cervicobrachial pain; conflicting evidence on the short-term effect of radiofrequency lesioning on pain and disability in chronic low-back pain of zygapophyseal joint origin; and limited evidence that intradiscal radiofrequency thermocoagulation is not effective for chronic discogenic low-back pain" (46).

Epidural Steroids

Indication: Patients who may benefit from these procedures most are those who have radicular pain and whose initial response to conservative, non-operative or interventional management has been poor. Generally, these are patients whose symptoms are disabling and either not improving or worsening at 4 to 6 weeks.

The specific approach to be utilized will be determined by the physician who will perform the procedure and may be based upon physician preference and/or technical anatomical constraints that limit or make a different approach more preferable. Epidural injections are available through three different portals. They include caudal injections through the sacral hiatus, interlaminar epidural injections and transforaminal injections (selected nerve root block). Fluoroscopically guided interlaminar or caudal lumbar epidural injections have a low complication rate (5,6).

Fluoroscopically guided lumbar transforaminal epidural steroid injections are effective for patients with radicular leg pain due to lumbar spinal stenosis (7); 75% of patients had successful 1-year outcomes, with more than 50% reduction in pain, 64% of patients had improved walking tolerance, and 57% had improved standing tolerance.

Neck Pain With or Without Radicular Symptoms

A recent Cochrane Collaboration meta-analysis concluded injections can play a potent role in cervical spine pain management (51). Local anesthetics were found to be effective for chronic neck pain. Corticosteroid injection effective for acute whiplash. Epidural injection of a corticosteroid helpful for chronic neck patients with associated arm symptoms. Botwin et al. found that fluoroscopically guided interlaminar cervical epidural injections have been found to be 38% to 75% effective (8). There is a low incidence of complications with this procedure (8). However, because of the proximity to the spinal cord, greater skill is required in this area.

Post-Injection Care

Patient behavior in the 48 hours after a procedure can make all the difference between a successful and a failed outcome. For optimal results, the patient should avoid bending, lifting, and twisting, but be encouraged to walk after the procedure. Periodic (Q2 waking hours) ice treatments are also valuable. This provides time for the maximum therapeutic effect and to minimize the dispersion of the medication by activity.

The Postsurgical Management

Skill Set for a Conservative Care Spine Specialist

A HCP wishing to specialize in care of complicated spine patients must be familiar with surgical indications, complications, and postoperative care. Such a specialist need not be expert in all skills, but must be knowledgeable about the methods of other experts from the multidisciplinary fraternity who co-manage such cases (e.g., physiatry, physical therapy, chiropractic) (Table 38.4).

Spine surgery is generally an elective procedure. Patients with primarily leg symptoms who are not responding to a gradual step-ladder approach with

Table 38.4 Conservative Spine Specialist Core Knowledge Set Regarding Surgical Patients (60)

- Indications for microdiscectomy
- General indications for instrumented anterior interbody fusion
- Indications for spinal stenosis decompression
- Indications for cervical spine surgery
- Expected pathoanatomic weakness from various spine surgeries
- Expected postsurgical course
- Postoperative activity modification advice/restrictions
- Ability to diagnose postfusion nonunion/pseudoarthrosis
- Familiarity with early and late phase complications
- Rehabilitation methods, limitations, and contraindications

conservative care (e.g., McKenzie, traction, stabilization exercise, NSAIDs, oral steroids, and epidurals) are candidates for surgery. Table 4-2 and 4-3 review leading expert opinion about the indications for lumbar spine surgery.

Postsurgical Course and Outcomes

Lumbar Spine

According to Atlas et al. 10 year results on 400 patients with sciatica revealed that 69% of patients initially treated surgically reported improvement in their predominant symptom (back or leg pain) versus 61% of those initially treated nonsurgically (P = 0.2) (2). A larger proportion of surgical patients reported that their low back and leg pain were much better or completely gone (56% vs. 40%, P = 0.006) and were more satisfied with their current status (71% vs. 56%, P = 0.002) than non-operated patients. Work and disability status at 10 years were comparable among those treated surgically or nonsurgically. 25% of both groups eventually had either a second or first back operation.

Hakkinen et al. reported that 2 months after lumbar disc surgery average back pain was 67% lower and leg pain 70% lower than preoperatively (26); 5% to 8% did report severe pain at 2- and 14-month follow-ups.

According to Ostelo (2005) the occurrence of residual symptoms after lumbar disc surgery ranges from 22% to 45%, and 30% to 70% of patients report residual sciatica and residual low back pain, respectively, after surgery (49). According to Hakkinen, at 2 months after surgery, significant decreases in trunk muscle strength and decreased mobility remained (27). Thus, active rehabilitation is recommended.

In patients receiving interbody cage lumbar fusion (ICLF) nearly half were dissatisfied with their results (38). Functional status was worse than expected in most and 38% were totally disabled at 18-month follow-up. A 2005 Cochrane Collaboration review of surgery for degenerative lumbar spondylosis (degenerative disc disease) reported that new trials on the effectiveness of fusion showed conflicting results (24). While one study showed that fusion was superior to conventional physiotherapy, the other showed it was not better than a modern exercise/rehabilitation program. There is also evidence that fusion may be associated with higher complication rates than other surgeries.

The outcomes and course for spinal stenosis surgery is addressed in detail in Chapter 37. Spinal stenosis is a clinical term not a radiologic finding (59). A narrow canal does not necessarily cause symptoms. Neurogenic claudication associated with spinal stenosis is the number one symptomatic spine problem in the elderly. Low back surgery for individuals older than age 65 is increasing dramatically. Such surgeries are not without risk and cardiac complications are recognized as the leading cause of death after non-cardiac operations (19).

The overall complication rate was 40%, however serious complications were less common, occurring in 12% of patients (4). Deyo found that if the surgical procedure included arthrodesis patients had an increased risk of morbidity, as well as an increased length of hospital stay (15).

Atlas et al. has compared conservative to surgical care for spinal stenosis and found at 8- to 10-year follow-up that relief of leg symptoms and back-related functional status were better in those initially receiving surgical treatment (3). Amundsen noted that patients who elect to delay surgery do not have a lower chance of surgical success (1).

Katz found that at 10-year follow-up after surgery that 60% to 80% of patients are satisfied enough that they would have the surgery again (35). According to Padua et al., 4 years after spinal stenosis surgery, although referred pain was improved, physical aspects of health-related quality of life continued to show severe impairment (50). Additionally, there were no significant EMG differences before and after surgery (50).

Cervical Spine

Ylinen et al. reported that the outcomes for anterior cervical diskectomy are very good (68). However, 43%

of patients reported experiencing moderate to severe pain (VAS score >30 mm) at follow-up. Pain, disability, and impairment (ROM and strength) were all well-correlated. Both ROM and strength were lower in surgery patients than in healthy controls. The most limited ROM was cervical extension. Grip strength was equal when comparing surgical patients to healthy subjects.

Fouyas et al. performed a systematic review of surgery for cervical spondylotic radiculopathy or myelopathy and stated that "it is not clear whether the short-term risks of surgery are offset by any long-term benefits" (20). A recent Cochrane group review reported that "discectomy alone has a shorter operation time, hospital stay, and postoperative absence from work than discectomy with fusion, while there is no statistical difference for pain relief and rate of fusion. It also appears that fusion techniques that use autograft give a better chance for fusion than interbody fusion techniques that use a cage, but other outcome variables could not be combined" (31).

Risk Factors for a Poor Recovery

According to Ostelo et al. (2005) it was found that high treatment expectancy was associated with a favorable outcome on perceived recovery and functional status at the 3- and the 12-month follow-ups (49). The patient's treatment expectations also have been shown to be important in predicting outcomes in low back pain (34), as well as for surgery for sciatica (41).

Taking pain medication and a poor functional status at baseline were associated with poor perceived recovery and functional status at both follow-up measurements (49). Leg pain and back pain at baseline were associated with residual leg and back pain at the 3- and the 12-month follow-up, respectively.

Depressive symptoms and the presence of pain in multiple regions of the body both predicted a poor outcome with lumbar discectomy at 2-year follow-up (33). It was suggested that such patients be referred for cognitive–behavioral management not surgery.

Early pre-operative outcome—at 2 months—is a reliable indicator of 1-year outcome in lumbar disc surgery patients (26)

According to Rompe et al. (55) those at risk for difficult recovery post-surgery are:

- Individuals older than 50 vs 35 to 45
- More than 20% overweight
- Increased motor dysfunction
- Long delay before surgery
- Multiple surgeries

LaCaille (38) reported that predictors of poorer outcome following ICLF included tobacco use, depression, and litigation.

According to Craton (see Chapter 7), the complications of fusion surgery include hardware malalignment, hardware failure, pseudarthrosis, adjacent segment disk degeneration, and infection. Plain radiographs are typically the first diagnostic technique in this patient population. Lucent areas noted adjacent to pedicle screw hardware suggest hardware loosening.

For spinal stenosis surgery, the most important predictor of greater walking capacity, milder symptoms, and greater satisfaction with surgery was preoperative self-rated health as good or excellent (36). It was concluded that co-morbidities are an important risk factor of a poor recovery (36).

For anterior cervical decompression and fusion male sex, non-smoking, greater segmental kyphosis, and a low pain and disability level are preoperative predictors of a good outcome (52). In particular the magnitude of the cervical kyphosis was the most significant predictor of outcome.

Postoperative Restrictions

Microdiscectomy

Watkins (65) has described the basic activity restrictions postoperatively. From the minute they wake up from the surgery, they should walk as much as possible. There are no restrictions on the limit and type of walking that they do. They are not to perform bending or lifting. Nothing heavier than a coffee cup for 2 weeks, not more than 20 pounds for 6 weeks, and no bending forward without flexing the knees and squatting. They are to limit their seating to 20 minutes and get up, walk around, and sit back down. No sitting on low, soft couches/chairs. No driving for 3 weeks. They can be driven, but the increased intradiscal pressure with driving and the potential of being caught on the freeway and having their back start to hurt could cause flair-up.

The key is to wait until annular disruption has had a chance to begin healing before increasing spinal stress. At 2 weeks postoperatively, an introductory core stabilization program is introduced. The wound is checked at 2 weeks and then activity levels are increased from the onset of physical therapy according to what their capabilities are.

Clinical Pearl

A Cochrane Collaboration systematic review concluded that there is no evidence that patients need to have their activities restricted after a first lumbar micro-discectomy surgery (48).

Carragee et al. reported that by lifting postoperative restrictions return to work was accelerated and there were no increased complications (10). Most even went back to work within 1 to 2 weeks. Eck and Riley suggest return to play can occur within 6 to 8 for non-contact sports and 4 to 6 months for contact sports after microdiscectomy (17).

Lumbar Fusion

Lumbar fusion patients are encouraged to get out of bed the morning after their surgery. They walk as much as possible from that point on. The restrictions postoperatively are to do no bending, lifting, or twisting (BLT). Lifting restrictions are similar to the microscopic discectomy. Rehabilitation is not begun in the first 3 months after spinal fusion. The patient is encouraged to walk as much as possible. The driving restrictions are similar to microscopic discectomy.

Eck and Riley suggest return to play can occur after 1 year for non-contact sports and is not recommended at all for contact sports following spinal fusion (17).

Spinal Stenosis Decompression

Spinal stenosis decompression patients are encouraged to stand and walk immediately after surgery and walk as much as possible from that point on. Rehabilitation is normally begun at 6 weeks with a gentle core stabilization training program and restrictions postoperatively are similar to microscopic lumbar discectomy.

Eck and Riley suggest return to play can occur after 4 to 6 months for a laminectomy and after 1 year for a fusion (17). Contact sports are not recommended.

Cervical Fusion

One level cervical fusion does not require the patient to wear a brace. The patient is encouraged not to do any lifting more than 10 pounds for 6 weeks, avoid overhead work, and to begin rehabilitation at 6 weeks doing a basic stability exercise program. No cervical strengthening or cervical ranges of motion exercises are encouraged in the first 6 months. The exercises should emphasize neutral postural alignment (e.g., Brügger relief position). Cervical retraction and dorsal gliding mobilizations are strictly avoided. They are encouraged to work from the bottom up. Use of the trunk, hips, and chest to produce proper cervical alignment. At two to three months post-op, the patient is assessed with x-ray and/or CT scan for solid fusion. After 3 months, the patient begins rehabilitation and is progressed back to normal activities. No head contact sports are allowed in the first 6 months. Every sports activity proceeds according to their ability to do the core stabilization chest-out exercises.

In terms of return to professional sports, after a cervical fusion microscopic discectomy, we insist that the patient be able to do advanced stabilization and functional training prior to return to competition. Moderate stabilization training allows some sports specific exercises and a return to practice. It is important to emphasize core stabilization with cervical problems, because of the partial alignment capability for head contact sport; leg strengthening and leg flexibility is critical for proper position of the body in order to play head contact sports. Neck strengthening is a component of return to head contact sports, but this is one of the last things to be begun. Normal pain free range of motion is a prerequisite to return.

Rehabilitation

Numerous studies have shown the beneficial effects of rehabilitation for postoperative recovery. A Cochrane Collaboration systematic review concluded that there is strong evidence for intensive exercise programs after 4–6 weeks postoperative (47). There is no evidence such programs increase the re-operation rate.

Ostelo et al. reported that behavioral graded activity after first-time lumbar disc surgery was not superior to traditional physical therapy (48). It was concluded that such patients should not be viewed as similar to chronic pain patients. A functionally based rather than psychologically oriented training program may be all that is required.

It appears that supervised training is superior to a home-based program (14,16,37,67). Dolan et al. studied exercise vs. reactivation advice and found that exercise gave superior results (16). All patients had sciatica with MRI documented herniated disc. All patients had either failed 6 weeks trial of conservative care or had severe motor loss. Treatment postoperatively the first 6 weeks all patient received advice about exercise and return to activity. They received encouragement to return to full activities as soon as possible.

- Specifically informed they could return to full activities as soon as they could tolerate the specific activity
- Patients were told that most people return to work in 1 to 2 weeks
- Aside from wound precautions no other postoperative restrictions were given
- Patients were told to expect some back and leg pain postoperatively, that this was "normal"

At 6 weeks randomization to exercise or a control group occurred. The control group received no more care. The exercise group performed a 4-week exercise program consisting of two 1-hour exercise classes/week which included aerobics, stretching, and trunk conditioning. Pain, disability, and spinal function improved more in the exercise group than the non-exercise group at follow-ups between 6 and 52 weeks postoperatively.

Danielson et al. compared a vigorous stabilization program to a mild home exercise routine for patients receiving microdiscectomy for sciatica (14). The stabilization program was 8 weeks in length. The home program consisted of two to three home exercises. The results were that the stabilization training group reported more improvement at both 6- and 12-month follow-ups.

Yilmaz et al. compared three groups after their first lumbar microdiscectomy (67). One group received supervised stabilization exercises, another home exercise, and a third no exercise advice. All patients were examined once before the exercise program and again 8 weeks later. The supervised exercise group improved the most in terms of pain relief and functional parameters (trunk, abdominal, and low back strength; back mobility).

Kjelby-Wendt and Styf compared early active training (EAT) versus simple activity modification (SAM) advice for patients having a microdiscectomy for sciatica (37). SAM patients received pre-operative advice about how to rise from bed from a side-lying position, to assume side lying, supine lying, and semi-Fowler positions. Postoperatively in the first 6 weeks they were trained in mild exercises focused on the abdominals and thighs. After 6 weeks the exercises progressed to include mobility training in spine flexion and lateral flexion. They were given recumbent exercises, but not upright or functional ones.

EAT patients received pre-operative training in sitting, standing, and lying advice to maintain lordosis. They were taught how to rise from bed from a prone position and encouraged to increase daily activities postoperatively such as daily walks. Postoperatively they received training in pain coping, passive nerve mobilization (first day postoperatively), passive extension exercises (5 days postoperatively (cobra); and passive flexion (8 weeks postoperatively). Functional stabilization training started at 6 weeks.

At 6- and 12 -eek follow-ups the EAT group had significantly less pain and increased mobility. At 2-year follow 88% of EAT group were satisfied with their outcome versus 67% in the control group.

Hakkinen et al. reported disappointing long-term compliance with home exercise prescriptions and suggested, "Progressive loading, supervision of training, and psychosocial support is needed in long-term rehabilitation programs to maintain patient motivation" (28).

Chronic Pain Management Interventions

In severe, chronic neck and back pain patients fusion surgery is often considered. However, alternatives should be explored before recommending fusion for chronic spine pain without leg or arm symptoms. Such alternatives include a CB program, multidisciplinary pain management, or interventionist methods.

Cognitive–Behavioral Approach

A CB approach is necessary for intractable chronic pain patients (see Chapters 14 and 31). This approach typically involves patient education classes along with therapeutic exercise incorporating quota-based, graded exposures to specific feared stimuli. CB classes or sessions address the patient's worries and fears and teaches them simple, safe, and effective methods to reduce these apprehensions.

Clinical Pearl

A recent, randomized controlled trial showed that intensive rehabilitation is more cost-effective than surgical stabilization for chronic back pain patients (53). The rehabilitation was more successful in returning patients to work.

Multidisciplinary Pain Management

A comprehensive, multidisciplinary biopsychosocial approach involves the above CB model along with strategies which address return to work obstacles (employer, compensation system, etc.) as well as co-morbid psychological illness. Multidisciplinary care (psychologist, pain management specialist, physical therapist) and workplace involvement are keys to success in these most complex cases.

Interventionist Methods

There are a number of invasive options other than surgery for chronic back pain. Intradiscal electrothermal therapy and implantable therapies, which include spinal cord stimulation and implantable intrathecal drug administration systems are available for pain management associated with chronic, unrelenting pain.

Intradiscal Electrothermal Therapy (IDET)

Intradiscal electrothermal therapy is strictly for patients with central axial pain and evidence of internal disc derangement determined by flexion/extension studies showing significant vacuum phenomenon and discogram procedure identifying the level of concordant pain. The most recent evidence on intradiscal electrothermal therapy shows that the results are at best a 50–50 proposition and in many locations they are no longer performed.

In brief, intradiscal electrothermal therapy involves the insertion of the catheter into the disc. A probe is advanced which is self-coiling following the laminations of the annulus. The coil is then heated expecting to denature the collagen fibers of the disc shrinking them and enhancing their stiffness.

Complications from this procedure are generally related to the possibility of infection by penetrating the skin, misdirecting of the probe with potential damage to associated nerve and/or spinal cord.

Implantable Therapies

Implantable therapies consist primarily of two modes. They include spinal cord stimulation systems that are placed inside the spinal canal posterior to the dorsal columns. The second is the use medication pumps, which are placed again inside the spinal canal. Both of these approaches are used in patients with intractable pain that has not been able to be managed effectively through medication or conservative manual procedures, and the patient has failed or is no longer a surgical candidate.

Patients who have implanted electrical stimulators can be treated effectively with manual methods for other complaints; however, no use of electrical or ultrasound modalities should be considered because they may interact with the implanted bodily system causing damage to the patient.

■ CONCLUSION

It is important for HCPs who specialize in spine problems to understand the continuum from minimalist care, such as reassurance and reactivation, to interventionist care, such as injections and spinal surgery. HCPs caring for patients with chronic, unremitting pain must be aware of diagnostic and treatment options that are outside of their own specialty. Patient-centered care mandates that the diagnostic or therapeutic methods should serve the patient's goals—such as increasing social participation and physical function. Ideally, the least invasive procedures would be attempted first, but if these are unsuccessful more aggressive strategies should be discussed with the patient in a shared-decision making manner.

<table>
<tr><td>

Audit Process
Self-Check of the Chapter's Learning Objectives

- What are the indications for lumbar epidural injections?

- What is the role of oral steroid medications?

- What is the success rate for different spinal surgeries?

- How would patients who are less likely to have a good outcome with surgery be identified?

- What specific activity restrictions should be given to patients following various spinal surgeries?

</td></tr>
</table>

■ REFERENCES

1. Amundsen T, Weber H, Nordal HJ, et al. Lumbar spinal stenosis: conservative or surgical management? A prospective 10-year study. Spine 2000;25:1424–1436.

2. Atlas SJ, Keller RB, Wu YA, Deyo RA, Singer DE. Long-Term Outcomes of Surgical and Nonsurgical Management of Sciatica Secondary to a Lumbar Disc Herniation: 10 Year Results from the Maine Lumbar Spine Study. Spine. 2005;30:927–935.

3. Atlas SJ, Keller RB, We UA, Deyo RA, Singer DE. Long-Term Outcomes of Surgical and Nonsurgical Management of Lumbar Spinal Stenosis: 8 to 10 Year Results from the Maine Lumbar Spine Study. Spine 2005;30:936–943.

4. Benz RJ, Ibrahim ZG, Afshar P, Garfin SR. Predicting complications in elderly patients undergoing lumbar decompression. Clin Orthop Relat Res. 2001;384:116–121.

5. Botwin KP, Gruber RD, Bouchlas CG, Torres-Ramos FM, Freeman TL, Slaten WK. Complications of fluoroscopically guided transforaminal lumbar epidural injections. Arch Phys Med Rehabil. 2000;81: 1045–1050.

6. Botwin KP, Gruber RD, Bouchlas CG, Torres-Ramos FM, Hanna A, Rittenberg J, Thomas SA. Complications of fluoroscopically guided caudal epidural injections. Am J Phys Med Rehabil. 2001;80:416–424.

7. Botwin KP, Gruber RD, Bouchlas CG, Torres-Ramos FM, Sanelli JT, Freeman ED, Slaten WK, Rao S. Fluoroscopically guided lumbar transformational epidural steroid injections in degenerative lumbar stenosis: an outcome study. Am J Phys Med Rehabil. 2002;81:898–905.

8. Botwin KP, Castellanos R, Rao S, Hanna AF, Torres-Ramos FM, Gruber RD, Bouchlas CG, Fuoco GS. Complications of fluoroscopically guided interlaminar cervical epidural injections. Arch Phys Med Rehabil. 2003;84:627–633.

9. Brooks PM, Day RO. Nonsteroidal antiinflammatory drugs—differences and similarities. N Engl J Med. 1991;324:1716–1725.

10. Carragee EJ, Han MY, Yang B, Kim DH, Kraemer H, Billys J. Activity restrictions after posterior lumbar discectomy. A prospective study of outcomes in 152 cases with no postoperative restrictions. Spine. 1999;24:2346–2351.

11. Carragee EJ, Chen Y, Tanner CM, Truong T, Lau E, Brito JL. Provocative discography in patients after limited lumbar discectomy: A controlled, randomized study of pain response in symptomatic and asymptomatic subjects. Spine. 2000;25:3065–3071.

12. Carragee EJ, Barcohana B, Alamin T, van den Haak E. Prospective controlled study of the development of lower back pain in previously asymptomatic subjects undergoing experimental discography. Spine. 2004;29:1112–1117.

13. Carragee EJ, Alamin TF, Miller JL, Carragee JM. Discographic, MRI and psychosocial determinants of low back pain disability and remission: a prospective study in subjects with benign persistent back pain. Spine J. 2005;5:24–35.

14. Danielson JM, Johnsen R, Kibsgaard SK, Hellevik E. Early aggressive exercise for postoperative rehabilitation after discectomy. Spine. 2000;25:1015–1020.

15. Deyo RA, Ciol MA, Cherkin DC, Loeser JD, Bigos SJ. Lumbar spinal fusion. A cohort study of complications, reoperations, and resource use in the Medicare population. Spine. 1993;18:1463–1470.

16. Dolan, P, Greenfield K, Nelson RJ, Nelson IW. Can exercise therapy improve the outcome of micro-discectomy? Spine. 2000;15:1523–1532.

17. Eck JC, Riley LH 3rd. Return to play after lumbar spine conditions and surgeries. Clin Sports Med. 2004;23:367–379.

18. European Guidelines for the management of acute nonspecific low back pain in primary care–preliminary draft—http://www.backpaineurope.org

19. Faciszewki T, Jensen R, Rokey R, Berg R. Cardiac risk stratification of patients with symptomatic spinal stenosis. Clin Orth Rel Res 2001;384:110–115.

20. Fouyas IP, Statham PFX, Sandercock PAG, Lynch C. Surgery for cervical radiculomyelopathy. The Cochrane Database of Systematic Reviews 2001, Issue 2.

21. France RD, Houpt JL, Ellinwood EH. Therapeutic effects of antidepressants in chronic pain. Gen Hosp Psychiatry. 1984;6:55–63.

22. Gabriel SE, Jaakkimainen L, Bombardier C. Risk for serious gastrointestinal complication related to use of nonsteroidal anti-inflammatory drugs: A meta-analysis. Ann Intern Med 1991;115: 787–796.

23. Getto CJ, Sorkness CA, Howell T. Issues in drug management. Part I. Antidepressants and chronic nonmalignant pain: a review. J Pain Symptom Manage. 1987;2:9–18.

24. Gibson JNA, Waddell G. Surgery for degenerative lumbar spondylosis. The Cochrane Database of Systematic Reviews 2005 Issue 3.

25. Greene JM, Winickoff RN. Cost-conscious prescribing of nonsteroidal anti-inflammatory drugs for adults with arthritis. A review and suggestions. Arch Intern Med. 1992;152:1995–2002.

26. Hakkinen A, Ylinen J, Kautiainen H, Airaksinen O, Herno A, Kiviranta I. Does the outcome 2 months

after lumbar disc surgery predict the outcome 12 months later? Disabil Rehabil. 2003;25:968–972.

27. Hakkinen A, Kuukkanen T, Tarvainen U, Ylinen J. Trunk muscle strength in flexion, extension, and axial rotation in patients managed with lumbar disc herniation surgery and in healthy control subjects. Spine. 2003;28:1068–1073.

28. Hakkinen A, Ylinen J, Kautiainen H, Tarvainen U, Kiviranta I. Effects of home strength training and stretching versus stretching alone after lumbar disk surgery: a randomized study with a 1-year follow-up. Arch Phys Med Rehabil. 2005;86:865–870.

29. Huskisson EC, Woolf DL, Balme HW, Scott J, Franklin S. Four new anti-inflammatory drugs: responses and variations. Br Med J. 1976;1:1048–1049.

30. Huskisson EC. How to choose a non-steroidal anti-inflammatory drug. Clin Rheum Dis. 1984;10:313–323.

31. Jacobs WCH, Anderson PG, Limbeek J, Willems PC, Pavlov P. Single or double-level anterior interbody fusion techniques for cervical degenerative disc disease. The Cochrane Database of Systematic Reviews 2004, Issue 3.

32. Jenkins DG, Ebbutt AF, Evans CD. Tofranil in the treatment of low back pain. J Int Med Res. 1976;4:28–40.

33. Junge A, Dvorak J, Ahrens S. Predictors of bad and good outcomes of lumbar disc surgery. A prospective clinical study with recommendations for screening to avoid bad outcomes. Spine. 1995;20:460–468.

34. Kalauokalani D, Cherkin DC, Sherman KJ, Koepsell TD, Deyo RA. Lessons from a trial of acupuncture and massage for low back pain: patient expectations and treatment effects. Spine. 2001;26:1418–1424.

35. Katz JN, Lipson SJ, Chang LC, Levine SA, Fossel AH, Liang MH. Seven- to 10-year outcome of decompressive surgery for degenerative lumbar spinal stenosis. Spine. 1996;21:92–98.

36. Katz JN, Stucki G, Lipson SJ, Fossel AH, Grobler LJ, Weinstein JN. Predictors of surgical outcome in degenerative lumbar spinal stenosis. Spine. 1999;24:2229–2233.

37. Kjelby-Wendt G, Styf J. Early active training after lumbar discectomy. Spine. 1998;23:2345–2351.

38. LaCaille RA, DeBerard MS, Masters KS, Colledge AL, Bacon W. Presurgical biopsychosocial factors predict multidimensional patient: outcomes of interbody cage lumbar fusion. Spine. 2005;5:71–78.

39. Lipetz JS, Malanga GA. Oral medications in the treatment of acute low back pain. Occup med. 1998;13:151–166.

40. Loeb DS, Ahlquist DA, Talley NJ. Management of gastroduodenopathy associated with use of non-steroidal anti-inflammatory drugs. Mayo Clin Proc. 1992;67:354–364.

41. Lutz GK, Butzlaff ME, Atlas SJ, Keller RB, Singer DE, and Deyo RA, The relation between expectations and outcomes in surgery for sciatica. J Gen Intern Med 1999;14:740–744.

42. Malanga G, Nadler S. Nonoperative Treatment of Low Back Pain. Mayo Clin Proc, November 1999:74;1135–1148.

43. Manchikanti L, Staats P, Singh V, Schultz DM, Vilims BD, Jasper JF et al. Evidence-based practice guidelines for interventional techniques in the management of chronic spinal pain. Pain Physician 2003;6:3–81.

44. Mazanec DJ. Medication use in sports rehabilitation in Functional Rehabilitation of Sports and Musculoskeletal Injuries. Kibler WB, Herring SA Press JM (eds). Aspen, Gaithersburg, Maryland, 1998.

45. Nelemans PJ, de Bie RA, de Vet HCW, Sturmans F. Injection therapy for subacute and chronic benign low-back pain. The Cochrane Database of Systematic Reviews 1999, Issue 4.

46. Niemisto L, Kalso E, Malmivaara A, Seitsalo S, Hurri H,. Radiofrequency denervation for neck and back pain. The Cochrane Database of Systematic Reviews 2002, Issue 3.

47. Ostelo RW, de Vet HC, Waddell G, Kerckhoffs MR, Leffers P, van Tulder M. Rehabilitation following first-time lumbar disc surgery: a systematic review within the framework of the Cochrane collaboration. Spine. 2003;28:209–18.

48. Ostelo RWJG, de Vet HCW, Berfelo MW, Kerchhoffs MR, Vlaeyen JWS, et al. Effectiveness of behavioral graded activity after first-time lumbar disc surgery: short term results of a randomized controlled trial. Eur Spine J. 2003;12:637–644.

49. Ostelo WJGR, Vlaeyen JWS, van den Brandts PA, de Vet CWH. Residual complaints following lumbar disc surgery: prognostic indicators of outcome. Pain. 2005;114:177–185.

50. Padua L, Padua R, Mastantuoni G, Pitta L, Caliandro P, Aulisa L. Health-related quality of life after surgical treatment for lumbar stenosis. Spine 2004;29:1670–1675.

51. Peloso P, Gross A, Haines T, Trinh K, Goldsmith CH, Aker P, Cervical Overview Group. Medicinal and Injection therapies for mechanical neck disorders. The Cochrane Database of Systematic Reviews 2005 Issue 3.

52. Peolsson A, Hedlund R, Vavruch L, Oberg B. Predictive factors for the outcome of anterior cervical decompression and fusion. Eur Spine J. 2003;12:274–280.

53. Rivero-Arias O, Campbell H, Gray A, Fairbank J, Frost H, Wilson-MacDonald J. Surgical stabilization of the spine compared with a program of intensive rehabilitation for the management of patients with chronic low back pain: cost utility analysis based on a randomized controlled trial. BMJ. 2005;330:1239.

54. Robinson JP, Brown PB. Medications in low back pain. Phys Med Rehabil Clin North Am. 1991;2:97–126.

55. Rompe JD, Eysel P, Zollner J, Heine J. Prognostic criteria for work resumption after standard lumbar discectomy. Eur Spine J. 1999;8:132–137.

56. Rosenblatt RM, Reich J, Dehring D. Tricyclic antidepressants in treatment of depression and chronic pain: analysis of the supporting evidence. Anesth Analg 1984;63:1025–1032.

57. Scott DL, Roden S, Marshall T, Kendall MJ. Variations in responses to non-steroidal anti-inflammatory drugs. Br J Clin Pharmacol. 1982;14:691–694.

58. Soll AH, Weinstein WM, Kurata J, McCarthy D. Non-steroidal anti-inflammatory drugs and peptic ulcer disease. Ann Intern Med. 1991;114:307–319.

59. Sprat KF, Keller TS, Szpalski M, Vandeputte K, Bunzburg R. A predictive model for outcome after conservative decompression surgery for lumbar spinal stenosis. Eur Spine J 2004;13:14–21.

60. Triano JJ, Rashbaum RF, Hansen DT. Opening access to spine care in the evolving market: integration and communication. Top Clin Chiro. 1998;5:44–52.

61. Triano JJ. Chiropractic personnel in the 21st century depends on strategy today. Top Clin Chiro. 2000;7:27–32.

62. Turner JA, Denny MC 1993 Do antidepressants medications relieve chronic low back pain? Journal of Family Practice 37:545–553 (systematic review).

63. van Tulder MW, Scholten RJ, Koes BW, Deyo RA. Nonsteroidal anti-inflammatory drugs for low back pain: a systematic review within the framework of the Cochrane Collaboration Back Review Group. Spine. 2000;25:2501–2513.

64. van Tulder MW, Touray T, Furlan AD, Solway S, Bouter LM. Muscle relaxants for non-specific low back pain. Cochrane Database Syst Rev. 2003;2.

65. Watkins R. Lumbar disc injury in the athlete. Clinics in Sports Medicine 2002;21:147–164.

66. World Health Organization. International Classification of Functioning, Disability and Health: ICF, World Health Organization, Geneva, 2001.

67. Yilmaz F, Yilmaz A, Merdol F, Parlar D, Sahin F, Kuran B. Efficacy of dynamic lumbar stabilization exercise in lumbar microdiscectomy. J Rehabil Med. 2003;35:163–167.

68. Ylinen JJ, Savolainen S, Airaksinen O, Kautiainen H, Salo P, Hakkinen A. Decreased strength and mobility in patients after anterior cervical diskectomy compared with healthy subjects. Arch Phys Med Rehabil. 2003;84:1043–1047.

39

From Guidelines to Practice: What is the Practitioner's Role?

Alan Breen

Learning Objectives

After reading this chapter you should be able to:

- Appreciate the cultural values surrounding clinical practice guidelines
- Explain the different ways in which guidelines are produced and used
- Appreciate the issues that lead to controversy in the selection of research evidence
- Evaluate a guideline for practice use
- Identify why a guideline may be difficult to implement
- Devise ways to implement guidelines
- Audit practice against a guideline

Clinical Practice Guidelines

"Systematically developed statements to assist practitioner and patient decisions about appropriate health care for specific clinical circumstances" (19).

Clinical Vignette

An American lady with a high public profile tells the story of her frustrated quest for effective treatment for her painful shoulder. From the start her friends insisted that she must have "the best" and arranged a next-day appointment with an orthopedic surgeon who specialized in the exact placement of steroid injections. This helped, but the pain returned. Unable to sleep, but not wishing to offend her friends, she contacted a sports physiotherapist whose skills were widely sought by world-class athletes. The physiotherapist also saw her quickly in his clinic and diagnosed a muscle imbalance as the underlying impediment to recovery. He then applied muscle energy techniques and electrical stimulation. That night she was in great pain. She returned to the physiotherapist the next day and was given cold treatment and ultrasound, which eased things slightly. Still seeking the right treatment, and on the recommendation of yet another close friend, she saw that friend's chiropractor, who examined her whole spine as well as both shoulders and told her he believed the actual site of the problem to be in her neck. After six treatments consisting of spinal manipulation she was no worse, but no better, and she did not go again.

This lady was not only in constant pain, without sleep and rapidly succumbing to depression, but also anxious at the thought of having to tell her three closest friends, who constantly inquired about her shoulder, that their unshakable faith in their favorite practitioners had done her no good at all. When she could no longer avoid it and to muster the strength to face them, she finally went to her general practitioner (GP) in pursuit of sleeping pills and stronger analgesics. Suspicious of joint pain that wakes in the night, the GP ordered an ESR and a test for rheumatoid factor, which came back positive. The cause of her symptoms was not tendonitis, muscle imbalance, or cervical dysfunction, but acute rheumatoid arthritis.

The rest of her story is about coming to terms with what was to become an aggressive form of rheumatoid disease that completely changed her life and career and made pain, deformity, and the juggling of anti-inflammatory drugs the dominant feature of it. Of course, no other initial care could have prevented the inevitable, but her story is a dramatic illustration of the cost of inappropriate and fragmented care, based on the misguided belief that specialist reputations should displace the basic principles of good practice.

Clinical practice guidelines are about current best practice and generally address basic principles. It is because they are "tools and not rules" that they only replace clinical decision-making when these decisions are extremely bad (19). By contrast, guidelines are there to sit comfortably with decision making for individual patients (52). The practitioner's role in care remains central. This chapter explores that role in the context of spinal rehabilitation when guidelines and clinicians come into contact.

A Brief History of Clinical Practice Guidelines

Health care has traditionally been guided by the collective wisdom of clinicians, often based on whatever research was available but, until relatively recently, without a way of verifying cause and effect. In the 1940s, with the development of statistical methods, this changed. When Sir Austin Bradford-Hill used a randomized controlled trial (RCT) to compare streptomycin and PAS (para-aminosalicylic acid) with usual care in the treatment of tuberculosis in 1948, the dramatic results established the RCT as a new aid to clinical decision-making; especially in the field of pharmacotherapeutics (28).

Tuberculosis has since, however, come to be regarded as the last great epidemic and decisive conclusions from single RCTs have become rarer. Furthermore, the limitations of RCTs are still a source of controversy. Nevertheless, the pressure to make choices between competing treatments in the face of limited budgets made their prominence inevitable (22). During the "clinical outcomes" movement of the 1980s, evidence was sought (usually unsuccessfully) to substantiate many drug claims, leading to an explosion of research. From then until the time of writing, health care policy in all treatment areas, both at practitioner and organizational level, has been increasingly influenced by such research. By the early 1990s, the volume of literature was so great that the need to summarize and interpret for practice was apparent. The age of "evidence-based health care" had arrived.

Another factor that occupied the thoughts of health planners was the explosion of costs. Commissioners of care sought order in the form of written guidelines to contain unrestrained choice. In America especially, many guidelines were based on the consensus of local groups rather than systematically evaluated research, which caused governments to appoint groups of experts to produce guidelines that were "evidence-based" and develop a methodology for using them (19).

Main Methods of Guideline Development

- Informal consensus

- Formal consensus (Delphi, etc.)

- Evidence-based

- Explicit approach (details time, cost, etc.)

The Route From Research to Practice Standards

Guidelines are specific to the encounter between patient and practitioner, but they are not the only route from research to practice standards (see box) (21).

Other Approaches to Practice Standards

- Total Quality Improvement/Management

- Managed Care Systems

- Health Technology Assessment

- Health Care Needs Assessment

Other schools of thought hold that rather than offer evidence-based recommendations for treatment decisions, it may be more appropriate to take a Total Quality Improvement (TQI) approach and establish an actual protocol to be followed, evaluate the outcomes, and then revise the protocol in the light of this (13). This is a more top-down approach that also addresses costs, but allows the practitioner and patient less freedom of choice. It is appealing to health care commissioners because of its accessibility to direct management under a Total Quality Management (TQM) scheme that decides the important outcome measures and manages the process of care by data. The outcomes chosen as being desirable tend to depend on national cultures and funding processes. In the United States' managed care systems, for example, the outcomes are (37):

- Functional health status (including risks and well being)

- Clinical outcomes

- Satisfaction against need

- Costs (direct, indirect, of health and social care)

National policies towards different interventions are sometimes based on a Health Technology Assessment exercise (HTA), which is an internationally recognized term that covers any method used by those working in health services to promote health, prevent and treat disease, and improve rehabilitation and long-term care ("technologies" in this context are not confined to new drugs or pieces of sophisticated equipment). The purpose of HTA is to try to ensure that high-quality research information on the costs, effectiveness, and broader impact of health technologies is produced in the most effective way for those who use, manage, and provide care. It also tends to be performed on a national scale.

A more local (and liberal) approach to care standards is Health Care Needs Assessment (see box) (1). This is a tool for a managed route to care that also incorporates the effects of costs and clinical effectiveness but is based on the existing impact of the condition(s), the local community's view on what is important, and on the nature of existing services. Here, care standards can be audited against the need identified by the Needs Assessment. However, when there are complex service issues (e.g., multifaceted interventions, important social and occupational influences, and multiple provider types) local consensus can be difficult to reach.

Health Care Needs Assessment

- Incidence/Prevalence/Natural History (without intervention)

- Cost without intervention

- Local culture on:
  - Most important impact
  - Most important measures
  - Existing services

Evidence-based guidelines influence practice in a different way by addressing the clinical encounter itself (47). As such, they are much more patient-centered and somewhat less threatening to the clinician. The disadvantage of often not addressing cost is balanced against giving the flexibility to take individual patient circumstances into account. The route from research to the eventual improvement of practice standards through guidelines (Fig. 39.1) has a number of stages, from the evaluation and synthesis of evidence into coherent statements, to linking these statements to recommendations for practice and the formulation of criteria for use in assuring care quality. At each stage when judgments on points of view are needed, there should be a consensus, or appraisal process.

Once a guideline's development is complete, its recommendations can be translated into review criteria

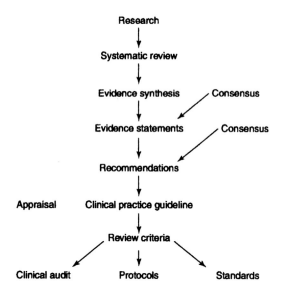

Figure 39.1 The route from research to practice standards.

(4). These are statements on which the implementation of recommendations can be tested. For example:

> Recommendation: "Carry out diagnostic triage."
>
> Review criterion: "The records show that diagnostic triage was done and the patient's back complaint was categorized as either serious pathology, root pain, or unclassified back pain."

It is desirable that review criteria are based on research evidence, prioritized on the strength of this and the influence on patient outcomes, measurable, and appropriate for the setting for which they are recommended. It may be desirable to group criteria into protocols, or attributable actions, that follow in sequence. This is helpful when the guideline user is not likely to be familiar with the basis for a set of recommendations, or what order to approach them in.

The development of review criteria is necessary to be able to audit guideline use. Practitioners can then see, in a group of actual patients, where they are consistent with guidance and where they are not, and be able to critically reflect on this. The proportion of times that events agree is called "standards" (see the box.). Again reflecting the "tools and not rules" ethos of guidelines, it may not be advisable to always expect standards to reach 100%. This applies, for example, when the review criteria do not cover all contingencies (40). Standard setting is a process that must be carefully managed as a partnership between practitioners and the other stakeholders in care. It sometimes follows an initial audit round of practitioner

groups to expose the "baseline" findings before engaging in discussion of what the standards should be. For practitioners, this can be a very valuable educational exercise (25).

From Recommendations to Practice Standards

Review Criteria

Systematically developed statements that can be used to assess the appropriateness of specific health care decisions.

Protocol

Comprehensive set of criteria for a single clinical condition or aspect of organization.

Standard

Percentage of events that should comply with the criterion.

Guidelines and Gurus: The Problem of RCTs

The pursuit of certainty in health care is one problem of naivety (see the box) in that modern empirical science, and particularly statistics, provides only estimates in domains that may themselves be the subject of dispute. This puts pressures on guideline developers born of the biases and political interests that are generated. This combined with the non-uniformity of patient characteristics means that good guidelines should keep to simple concepts with clear limitations. The conventional view of the RCTs as a "gold standard" is less easy to sustain in rehabilitation disciplines.

Problems of Naivety

- Limitations of science
- Bias/politics in the production of guidelines
- Non-uniformity of patients

However, RCTs are still probably the best way to compare the effectiveness of treatments and infer a causal relationship between intervention and outcome. Unfortunately, their profile in health science is such that much more is often expected. They are particularly well-suited to the comparison of interventions with very clear outcomes (such as survival), with test treatments that are simple to apply (such as pharmaceuticals) in patients whose diagnoses are well-defined (such as tuberculosis). When these margins are blurred, there is a tendency to reject randomized trials as being too rigid of a method of assessment. This applies in such heterogeneous conditions and treatments as are presented in rehabilitation. A better approach is to understand these limitations and their solutions, as well as the fact that they are not the only source of research evidence for guidelines (7). Table 39.1 suggests alternative methods and their indications. For example, cohort and case-control studies are preferred options for research to inform recommendations about natural history, diagnosis, and risk of rare events. A key concept is that RCTs do not evaluate treatments but differences between treatments. Because benefits are relative, it is necessary to interpret their results in this light.

The Development of Guidelines

The context for clinical guidelines is determined by their professional use. That requires discussion between professionals and that discussion is most productive if it centers around how clinical judgment operates, and what constitutes good standards of care.

The process begins with the identification of a manageable number of key clinical decisions that the guideline is to inform. This is a balance between the importance of the decisions and the availability and quality of the research evidence. Once the key clinical decisions have been decided on, the steps that follow are:

1. Finding the evidence (using an explicit literature search strategy)
2. Appraising the evidence by:
   • Characterizing the studies
   • Grading the studies
3. Formulating evidence statements
4. Grading the evidence statements
5. Formulating evidence-linked recommendations

Evidence, however, is not just that which comes from research (see the box) (42). Guidelines that deny the value and participation of clinical experts and the preferences of patients start at a disadvantage when it comes to implementation. Furthermore, there is still debate about the relative merits of unidisciplinary versus multidisciplinary guidelines, both in development and use (15,44).

Components of Evidence

• Research (e.g., natural history, treatment effects etc.)

• Clinical expertise

• Patient preferences

(From Sackett, Rosenberg & Grey, 1996)

To complete the guideline development process can take considerable resources and if these are absent the feasibility is weakened (see the box). The time required depends a lot on how many decisions and circumstances the guideline is meant to cover and how complex the evaluation of interventions needs to be. This will determine the skills required of the guideline development group and how the work is to be divided between its members. It is also necessary to look towards the implementation of the final product when considering developing it. A guideline that suggests a change from what has become standard practice needs to be very transparent about the reasons for its recommendations. Similarly, recommendations that could have legal penalties if not followed (such as a recommendation to adhere to new legislation) must be properly authorized (23). The following box shows some of the issues to be considered in deciding of the feasibility of developing any guideline.

Feasibility of Developing a Guideline

• Time

• Complexity

• Skills

• Local standards

• Coverage

• Legal implications

• Implementation

Table 39.1 Methodological Limitations of RCTs and Their Solutions

Limitation	Solution
1. Do not address subgroups	Research subgroups for RCTs separately
2. Do not address complex treatments	Factorial trial designs
3. Seldom address long-term outcomes	Large cohort studies tracking outcomes
4. Seldom address risk	Case-control studies

(from Breen & Feder, 1999)

The development of evidence-linked guidelines does not remove the need for consensus, nor does their validity depend principally on the clinical, or even the research, expertise of the development group but on finding a reproducible and relatively unbiased method of identifying the relevant evidence, and explicitly linking recommendations to it. The following box shows the techniques commonly used.

Techniques for Processing the Evidence for Guideline Production

- Systematic reviews
- Narrative summaries of evidence
- Evidence tables
- Meta-analysis
- Decision analysis
- Balance sheets listing benefits, harms, or costs for each recommendation

---

Tools, Rules, and Relevance: Good and Bad Guidelines

The practitioner in receipt of a guideline has the crucial role in deciding whether it is good or bad for patient care. Often, however, this is limited to considerations other than those of methodological quality, such as whether they sit comfortably with practice procedures (see Implementation below). A summary of what to look for is shown in the following box.

Characteristics of Good Guidelines

- Based on reliable and up-to-date evidence and professional consensus
- Address key clinical decisions
- Deal with heterogeneity

Because it is the practitioner who ultimately determines the appropriateness and use of guidelines, it is best to be clear about what benefits and harms they can promote (53). The main ones are suggested in Table 39.2.

The assessment of the validity of clinical practice guidelines is an important, and legitimate, educational exercise for practitioners. Once guidelines are disseminated for clinical use, however, it is too late to amend them. Furthermore, many practitioners are inundated with guidelines. It is therefore worth investing in an appraisal process to ensure that implementation stands a chance through acceptance by the people they will affect. For example, work has been underway through a collaborative group for the Appraisal of Guidelines, Research, and Evaluation in Europe to establish criteria on which guidelines can be appraised (see the box) (2). This paves the way for the production of international guidelines. In preparation for this in the area of back pain, Koes et al. compared low back pain guidelines from 11 different countries published between 1994 and 2000 and found generally similar diagnostic and therapeutic recommendations (24). This comparison was vital to the development of the European Commission's Acute Low Back Pain Guidelines (18).

Criteria for Appraisal of Clinical Guidelines (Version 1)

- Scope and purpose
- Stakeholder involvement
- Rigor of development process
- Clarity and presentation
- Applicability
- Editorial independence

(AGREE collaborative group, 2000)

Table 39.2 Benefits and Harms of Guidelines

Potential Benefits of Guidelines	Potential Harms of Guidelines
- Continuous professional development - Inform research agenda - Reduce poor quality care - Improve care - Decrease health care costs - Reduce medico-legal liability	- Poor patient care (biggest risk) - Inflexibility - Disruption of practice - Threat to livelihood - Medico-legal liability (if not following)

Semantic Discrepancies

In a field as diverse as musculoskeletal pain, some acknowledgment of hermeneutical problems is needed. What, for example, is meant by the term "specific back exercises," and how does the evidence help us? The UK Acute Back Pain Guideline Development group of the 1990s considered these to be exercises that were specific in the muscle groups that they targeted, or in the sequence or nature of the regime (50). The trial evidence was that they were, as a whole, less effective for acute back pain than the interventions to which they had been compared. The evidence statements agreed on was therefore, "From the evidence available at present, it is doubtful that specific back exercises produce clinically significant improvement in <u>acute low back pain,</u> (author's underlining) or that it is possible to select which patients will respond to which exercises." A second evidence statement continued: ". . . there is some evidence that exercise programs and physical reconditioning can improve pain and functional levels in patients with <u>chronic low back pain</u>" (author's underlining). By "specific," the guideline was attempting to indicate exclusion of regimes aimed at overall strength and endurance and to make clear where such regimes could be helpful. This was broadly accepted in the appraisal process of the Guideline and its subsequent Audit Tool in light of the recommendation: "Consider arranging reactivation/rehabilitation for patients who have not returned to ordinary activities and work by 6 weeks."

By contrast, a subsequent Cochrane review entitled "Exercise Therapy for Low Back Pain" offered the evidence against specific back exercises for acute back pain without such a qualification, provoking critical comment objecting to the unqualified inference (49,30) The lesson from this is that a guideline, or HTA process, requires a consensus, as well as a systematic review process, followed by a recommendation that reflects the evidence in clinical scenarios, whereas an evidence statement in a systematic review lacks the protection of such contextual clarification.

A further example is in the evidence on manipulation. Most of the reviewers of trials of this interven-

tion ignored the study by Meade that showed a decisive, if modest, superiority of chiropractic over fast-track hospital outpatient management for subacute and chronic low back pain (33,34). This has often been objected to on the basis that an important manipulation trial was ignored, whereas in this trial, both treatment arms used manipulation at least sometimes. Reviewers of manipulation as an intervention would have found this to be outside of their criteria for the selection of studies.

In the European Acute Back Pain Guideline, the evidence on manipulation had been summarized in one Cochrane review, which characterized the intervention negatively as being no better than other treatments which were found effective (3). This evidence was strong for the subacute and chronic phases, with less availability of acute studies with acceptably long-term follow-up (50). However, the patient types, interventions, and outcome measures varied greatly and, despite the weight of evidence, a few trials of reasonable quality had a negative result. This rendered the evidence conflicting, making it impossible to produce an unequivocal evidence statement about manipulation. Instead, the recommendation agreed on was:

"Consider (referral for) spinal manipulation for patients who are failing to return to normal activities."

Guideline developers, therefore, have an obligation to contextual logic and its communication and semantics can conspire to defeat this. It is here that the strength of multidisciplinary guidelines over unidisciplinary ones becomes apparent, for these have to find a way of expressing recommendations in terms that are clear and logical to practitioners from a variety of backgrounds, as well as their patients.

Implementing Guidelines

In a survey of local audit groups in England, audit administrators were asked about the attitudes toward the problem of back pain and the use of the UK Acute Back Pain Guideline. The results (Table 39.3) are instructive. To use guidelines one must first

Table 39.3   Attitudes and Use of the UK/RCGP Back Pain Guidelines by NHS Audit Groups

Attitude to Problem		Use of RCGP Guideline*	
See LBP as a significant health problem	51/57	Raising awareness	10/27
Received a copy of RCGP Guideline	47/57	Clinical Audit	8/27
Made use of RCGP Guideline*	27/57	Setting standards	2/27
Intend to use in future	11/57	Local guidelines	11/27
Priority levels of back pain care:		Change services	3/27
Low: 21%; Medium: 51%; High: 44%		Local education	10/27

(n = 57, response rate: 59%)[8]

receive them. Ten out of 57 respondents said they had not. Of those who had, only approximately half had used them for any purpose, even though a substantial majority saw the problem as significant and 79% regarded it as a medium or high health care priority. Of the many choices available to local groups about when to use guidelines, the most popular were: education, raising awareness, or making local guidelines. Very few had actually used them to audit standards, set standards, or change services.

Guidelines, even if they do survive rigorous appraisal processes intact, do not, therefore, automatically change behavior. The UK Acute Back Pain Guidelines and the Clinical Standards Advisory Group report and Epidemiology Review of the subject that preceded it, were thought to have made little difference to general practitioner behavior or to the availability of many of the services it recommended (50,11,12,29,5).

One problem with implementing guidelines on musculoskeletal rehabilitation is the relative newness of the psychosocial elements in care. The debate about whether practitioners should have these responsibilities started in the 1970s and has probably not ended yet (17). Learning about psychosocial assessment and intervention is an educational issue, which fits well with the evidence about successful implementation and suggests that professionals must be personally engaged in the process before practitioner behavior will change. They must have some kind of resonance with usual practice (51,21). However, it may be better to target a number of barriers concurrently, rather than rely on single initiatives (39). Practitioners could, for example, implement guidelines into their practices within a public awareness, educational, or research program in which they have a part (especially if these are highly interactive). The educational power of vignettes illustrating "what works" within the system is becoming increasingly appreciated. Change management techniques can be especially effective where practitioners work in groups (14), especially with their closest colleagues present. This makes learning about new ways of working "collectively reinforced, internalized, and tacit" within the practice itself (20). The theoretical model for this is the "Communities of Practice" model (27), in which novices to the new evidence become owners of it by virtue of their participation. This implies a work-based learning approach that benefits the organization and the learner (10). The Guidelines for the Evidence-Based Management of Acute Musculoskeletal Pain produced by the Australian Acute Musculoskeletal Guidelines Group (35) contain similar themes to the European Back Pain Guidelines (18), but spreads across all musculoskeletal areas. The Australian Guideline also uses concise information sheets for each complaint, summaries of findings, and their limitations and summaries of the key messages for each topic. It is more amenable to

holding the attention of its clients in a work-based learning scenario than most evidence-based guidelines. This kind of approach has been shown to result in improvement in back pain management (13) and may also equip practitioners to help shape local services together to better meet patient needs.

Key Points in the Implementation of Guidelines

- Operate directly on the consultation process through:
  - Restructured records
  - Patient-specific reminders (e.g., note if patient has acute back pain)
  - Audit system for guideline in operation
- Absence of bias
- Resonance with usual practice
- Multi-faceted initiatives to promote implementation
- Use in educational, public awareness, or research programs
- Group practice "change management" process

There remain, however, significant barriers, foremost among which are patient preferences (43). A good example of this is the desire for X-rays when patients do not realize that it adds little but a radiation risk to most cases of acute undifferentiated back pain (48). In practice, this is an opportunity to formulate a response that promotes patient confidence, compliance with care recommendations, and strategy for re-activation by demonstrating knowledge, concern, and commitment when explaining the true nature of the symptom. Readiness to undertake special investigations when necessary combined with emotional support and reassurance is the other side of this coin that assumes that patients are equal partners in their care and must have the opportunity to understand the reasons for the clinical decisions which affect them.

Frequently, guidelines do not address the management decisions that professionals regard as important (43). Here, the practitioner may lose interest. This is, however, less likely if the guideline contains agreed recommendations based on up-to-date evidence about care that will affect clinical outcomes. It is important to understand the reasons for the omissions, which are usually that there is either insufficient evidence to support a recommendation or agreement by peers that it is not fundamental in care. The practitioner is then at liberty to make decisions based on her/his own clinical judgment. A special case of this is when the practitioner does not see the patients to which the guidelines refer, such as physiotherapists working in hospitals with waiting lists which excludes them from seeing patients with acute back pain (38).

Barriers to Implementation of Guidelines

- Patient preferences
- Management decisions not addressed
- Does not apply to patients seen
- Practitioner desire to "tailor" information
- Poor ability to use recommendations
- Poor access to facilities
- Information not standardized
- Comfort with current practice
- Other pressures
- Inconsistent/absent leadership
- Poor interprofessional integration

(from Bird 2000)

Generalists may fail to implement guidance about rehabilitation, simply because they do not have an interest in the area and are comfortable with current practice (6). This can be addressed with consistent leadership that promotes integration with other services and funding and support for evidence-based care and education. It can be part of a practice outreach program which, although it has been shown to improve knowledge and understanding, is less able to change attitudes (31).

Organized quality improvements can, therefore, change practice, improving patient outcomes, linking professionals through common goals, and reducing tribalism and isolation (46). The rewards include getting access to wider services and support while sharing skills and data. Unfortunately, this is all new and there are few examples to follow—only principles and applying steep learning curves over a short time. Additionally, there is an undeniable decrease in clinical autonomy and an increase in accountability that pits the professional's self-esteem against the spirit of clinical quality improvement. This raises thoughts about whether future health care is to be corporate or isolationist. There is, however, emerging evidence that the successful implementation of guidelines does improve both processes and patient outcomes, particularly with regard to limiting the need for (generally more expensive) secondary care services (41,32,26,45).

Guidelines and Musculoskeletal Rehabilitation

In the rehabilitation of the spine, it is essential to evaluate the relationship between neuromuscular performance, distress, and disempowerment in patients to be able to intervene at the appropriate levels. Current research addresses these fairly explicitly and, therefore, there is scope for evidence-based recommendations for practice. However, evidence in this field is also plagued by heterogeneity, notably in the characteristics of the subjects, the way their conditions are differentiated, the instruments used to evaluate treatment outcomes, in the methodologies deployed by researchers and the way results are analyzed This is the current weakness of the evidence. Although unidisciplinary research and guidelines reduce the variations and semantic discrepancies, they do not assist continuity of care when it crosses disciplines. Multidisciplinary guidelines, however, are immediately confronted by all the factors brought about by the sources of heterogeneity. Imprecise descriptors, intangible variables, and the persistent use of metaphors confound this process even further. An advocate from the profession concerned who can promote the messages of a multidisciplinary guideline may be one solution to this (9).

As impenetrable as these obstacles may seem, and recalling the vignette with which this chapter opened, if there is one approach that is optimal for a person at a given point in their condition, it should be available regardless of which practitioner that person sees first. The need for integrated care is well-recognized (16).

A possible solution to the fragmentation of care is to return to the issue of key clinical decisions. For example, for acute undifferentiated back pain, most guidelines advise triage, avoidance of X-rays, psychosocial assessment, pain control with analgesics at regular intervals, avoidance of bed rest, advice to stay active, and the consideration of manipulation and/or strengthening and reconditioning if symptoms are persisting beyond a few weeks. Discipline-specific practice habits might, for example, dictate that all patients receive analgesics and none receive manipulation, or the converse. A more sensible approach would be to arrange analgesia for patients who need pain control to remain active and have no contraindications for their use, and to use manipulation as a pain control and arresting measure for patients who meet the criteria for its use and show signs of not recovering early in the episode. It is sensible for evidence-based interventions to be used according to patient need rather than practitioner preference.

Audit and Guideline Implementation

Audit is the final stage in the route to practice standards based on guidelines, but it is not a way of implementing them. Clinical audit was devised as a continuous process of self-appraisal, recommended especially for continuous professional development programs. The audit cycle (Fig. 39.2) is repeated until the desired standard of each audit (review) criterion is reached.

To get the best out of audit, collaboration is highly desirable. If performing an off-the-shelf audit within a practice or professional group, there should be a meeting to discuss why it is being done and how. There should be a clear data collection strategy that is specific to the clinical setting and it is best, if possible, to involve an audit support or advisory group and to engage all stakeholders. Health care authorities, be they regulatory bodies, commissioners of health care, or practitioner groups can decide the proportion of times a guideline recommendation should be met and audit practice to reveal the match with their ideal standard. The following box describes a typical activity list for facilitating guideline audit by a group.

Auditing Guideline Use by a Group

Stage 1—Preparation for the Audit

- Convert the guideline's recommendations to review criteria (Figure 39.1) (or access an off-the-shelf audit)
- Decide when the audit will occur, who it is aimed at, what the inclusion and exclusion criteria are, number of patient records to be audited, what educational material should accompany it, etc.

- Construct data collection form to record compliance with criteria against patient records
- Initiate discussion about the audit (e.g., practice meeting, study group meeting, large group mailing of materials)

Stage 2—First Audit Round

- Circulate audit forms and instructions for first audit round
- Practitioners sample patient records, complete forms, and return for processing
- Audit data compiled and fed back to practitioners (see example)
- Group discussion of audit findings followed by changes to improve standards before second audit round (e.g., 6 months later)

Stage 3—Second Audit Round

- Circulate audit forms and instructions for second audit round
- Practitioners sample patient records, complete forms, and return for processing
- Audit data compiled and fed back to practitioners (completion of audit loop)
- Group discussion of audit findings followed by changes to improve standards and when to repeat audit cycle in the future

(For further examples of audit systems in musculoskeletal rehabilitation, see www.imrci.ac.uk/Audit/audit.html)

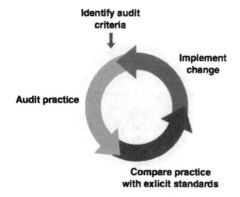

Figure 39.2 The audit cycle.

The first round of such an audit gives a baseline return on which to consider improvements, serving the aims of continuous professional development. Table 39.4 shows a concise example of how the results might be reported to practitioners. This is the time to think about what the standards should be and how to reach the target needed to achieve the necessary change. After a period of time, a second audit round is conducted and the findings reported, which completes the audit loop.

Although audit is the final stage in the route to practice standards based on guidelines, it is a vehicle for guideline implementation, not a strategy in itself. Audit and feedback are useful processes on which to promote compliance with guidelines but feedback alone is generally insufficient to achieve implementation (36).

Table 39.4 Example of Clinician Report Form
Acute Low Back Pain Audit in Primary Care

First Audit Round	January 2003 Audit Population: Practitioners— 86 Patients (1st 6 weeks of episode)—843	
Review Criterion	*Cohort Findings*	*My Findings*
The record shows that:		
1. Diagnostic triage was carried out	98%	99%
2. Psychosocial factors were considered	67%	96%
Patients with nonspecific back pain were:		
3. Not X-rayed	87%	92%
4. Advised to stay active	85%	93%
5. Not prescribed bed rest	97%	95%
. . . and if not resolving at 4–6 weeks from onset:		
6. Rehabilitation was initiated	67%	72%

The Future

The rapid increase in the availability of systematic reviews through organizations such as the Cochrane Collaboration, the growth of guideline networks in many nations, and international collaboration in guideline development and appraisal all mean that the ownership of guidelines may, in the future, become much more global. Patients, health professionals, and care commissioners will be able to benefit from the experiences of implementation in other countries and avoid reinvention of solutions to getting evidence into practice. Recently, audit has ceased to be always a paper exercise, because Internet-based audit has become a reality in the care of coronary heart disease and acute back pain, providing the possibility of crossing borders and more effectively sharing solutions to clinical problems.

The unavoidable fact that health care costs money (and "every cost is somebody's salary") will probably continue to be the main inhibiting factor; yet, since guidelines address interventions and not professions, care overlap and fragmentation could hopefully diminish if good guidelines are implemented successfully. This will require considerable interprofessional collaboration and, to some extent, the subordination of market rivalries to evidence-based practice. In a new model of service provision for spinal pain, the "preferred provider" could eventually be the individual who can demonstrate expertise against agreed criteria rather than simply claim it by virtue of a qualification. Furthermore, the cooperation of practitioners and patients alone is not enough to ensure practice standards. Policy makers including educators, licensing bodies, insurers, employers, state welfare agencies, professional associations, and trade unions also have major parts to play.

■ CONCLUSION

In the rehabilitation of painful musculoskeletal disorders, tolerances and well-being are important concepts. On the part of the patient, tolerance can be to pain, disability, impairment, handicap, distress, or cost. On the part of the practitioner, the patient's perceived tolerances apply, plus the practitioner's own, which may include symmetry and perceived normality of osseous position and movement, clinical course and progress, ranges of motion, strength, and endurance. Closer to home, the pressures of self-image, income, influence, and interest all impact on processes of care. In the real world, these will never be optimal; therefore, it is important to identify clearly the aims of rehabilitation treatment.

Clinical practice guidelines, as suggested at the beginning of this chapter, give mainly basic guidance, intended to help us to avoid catastrophes, fragmented care, and poor outcomes. The key benefits to practitioners lie in their being up-to-date, reflecting the opinions of peers and experts, and addressing key issues while taking into account that no two patients are the same. This protects patient and practitioner against the consequences of basic omissions and errors in rehabilitation. They can unite professionals both within and between disciplines. However, this only works if they are implemented effectively. Effective implementation depends on a conclusive environment that promotes positive attitudes towards improving care and provides both the resources and time to do this (36). Its success depends on the support of a much wider church than practitioners.

Audit Process
Self-Check of the Chapter's Learning Objectives

- What are the steps in the route from research to practice?

- How does a systematic review differ from a meta-analysis?

- What criteria should be used to determine when a guideline be updated?

- Why would a guideline be difficult to implement and what methods increase the likelihood of practitioner implementation?

- How can a practitioner audit that they are practicing in a manner consistent with a guideline?

■ REFERENCES

1. Acton C, Newbronner E. Health Needs Assessment: A Step by Step Guide. York: York Health Economics Consortium, 1997 (http://www.actonshapiro.co.uk).
2. AGREE Collaborative Group. Guideline Development in Europe. Int J Technol Assess Health Care 2000;16(4):1039–1049.
3. Assendelft WJJ, Morton SC, Yu EI, Suttorp MJ, Shekelle PG. Spinal manipulative therapy for low back pain: a meta-analysis of effectiveness relative to other therapies. Ann Intern Med 2003;138:871–881.
4. Baker R, Fraser RC. Development of review criteria: linking guidelines and assessment of quality. BMJ 1995;311:370–373.
5. Barnett AG, Underwood MR, Vickers MR. Effect of UK national guidelines on services to treat patients with acute low back pain: follow-up questionnaire survey. BMJ 1999;318:919–920.
6. Bird C. Commissioned R&D Programmes: Implementation of low back pain guidelines in North Thames. London: NHS Executive London Regional Office, 2000.
7. Breen A, Feder G. Where does the evidence come from? In: Hutchinson A, Baker R, eds. Making use of Guidelines in Clinical Practice. Oxford: Radcliffe Medical Press Ltd, 1999:15–28.
8. Breen AC, Langworthy JM, Sutherland G, et al. Testing an audit process for the Royal College of General Practitioners' Acute Back Pain Guidelines. Presented at the 4th International Forum for Primary Care Research on Low Back Pain. Eilat, March 2000.
9. Breen A, van Tulder M, Koes B, Jensen I, Reardon R, Bronfort G. Mono-disciplinary or multidisciplinary back pain guidelines? How can we achieve a common message in primary care? Eur Spine J 2005; (in press).
10. Breen, R. What kind of work-based learning simultaneously benefits organizations and learners?

A review of the literature. NHSU Internal report, 2004.
11. Clinical Standards Advisory Group (CSAG). Back Pain. London: Department of Health, 1994.
12. Clinical Standards Advisory Group (CSAG). Epidemiology Review: The epidemiology and cost of back pain. London: Department of Health, 1994.
13. Deyo RA, Schall M, Berwick DM, Nolan T, Carver P. Innovations in education and clinical practice: continuous quality improvement for patients with back pain. J Gen Intern Med 2000;15:647–655.
14. Donleavy GD. A basic law of management? In: Sanchez R & Heene A, eds. Theory Development for competence-based management. Stamford, Connecticut: Jai Press Inc, 2000:57–67.
15. Eccles M, Clapp Z, Grimshaw J, Adams PC, Higgins B, Purves I, Russell I. Developing valid guidelines: methodological and procedural issues from the North of England evidence based guideline development project. Quality Health Care 1996;5:44–50.
16. Eisenberg DM, Kessler RC, Foster C, Norlock FE, Calkins DR, Delbanco TL. Unconventional medicine in the United States: prevalence, costs and patterns of use. N Engl J Med 1993;328(4):246–252.
17. Engel GL. The need for a new medical model: a challenge for biomedicine. Science 1977;196(4286):129–136.
18. European Commission COST B13 Management Committee. European guidelines for the management of low back pain. Acta Orthop Scand 2002;73(Suppl. 305):20–25.
19. Field MJ, Lohr KN (eds). Guidelines for Clinical Practice: from development to use. Washington DC: Institute of Medicine/National Academy Press, 1993.
20. Gabbay J, le May A. Evidence based guidelines or collectively constructed "mindlines?" Ethnographic study of knowledge management in primary care. BMJ 2004;329:1013–1017.
21. Grol R, Dalhuijsen J, Thomas S, in't Veld C, Rutten G, Mekkink H. Attributes of clinical guidelines that influence use of guidelines in general practice: observational study. BMJ 1998;317:858–861.
22. Hine D. For the good that it will do: issues confronting healthcare in the UK. J Royal Soc Med 1999;92:332–338.
23. Hurwitz B. Legal and political considerations of clinical practice guidelines. BMJ 1999;318:661–664.
24. Koes BW, Van Tulder MW, Ostelo R, Burton AK, Waddell G. Clinical guidelines for the management of low back pain in primary care. Spine 2001;26(22):2504–2514.
25. Langworthy JM. Development of a clinical audit program in chiropractic. Eur J Chiropractic 1998;46:31–39.
26. Lattimer V, Sassi F, George S, Moore M, Turnbull J, Mullee M, Smith H. Cost analysis of nurse telephone consultation in out of hours primary care; evidence from a randomized controlled trial. BMJ 2000;320:1053–1057.
27. Lave J, Wenger E. Situated Learning: Legitimate Peripheral Participation. New York: Cambridge University Press, 1991.
28. Le Fanu J. 1950: Streptomycin, smoking and Sir Austin Bradford Hill. In: The Rise and Fall of

Modern Medicine. London: Little, Brown and Company, 1999:29–59.

29. Little P, Smith L, Cantrell T, Chapman J, Langridge J, Pickering R. General practitioners' management of acute back pain: a survey of reported practice compared with clinical guidelines. BMJ 1996;312: 485–488.

30. Manniche C. Letter to the Editor. Spine 2001;26: 840–844.

31. Markey P, Schattner P. Promoting evidence-based medicine in general practice–the impact of academic detailing. Family Practice 2001;18(4):364–366.

32. McGuirk B, King W, Govind J, Lowry J, Bogduk N. Safety, efficacy and cost effectiveness of evidence-based guidelines for the management of acute low back pain in primary care. Spine 2001;26(23): 2615–2622.

33. Meade TW, Dyer S, Browne W, Townsend J, Frank AO. Low back pain of mechanical origin: randomized comparison of chiropractic and hospital outpatient treatment. BMJ 1990;300:1431–1437.

34. Meade TW, Dyer S, Browne W, Frank AO. Randomized comparison of chiropractic and hospital outpatient management for low back pain: results from extended follow-up. BMJ 1995;311:349–351.

35. National Health Medical Research Council, Australian Acute Musculoskeletal Pain Guidelines Group. Evidence-based management of acute musculoskeletal pain. Brisbane: Australian Academic Press Pty Ltd, 2003.

36. National Institute for Clinical Excellence. Principles for best practice in clinical audit. Oxford: Radcliffe Medical Press Ltd, 2002. (www.nice.org.uk)

37. Nelson EC, Mohr JJ, Batalden PB, Plume SK. Improving Health Care, Part 1: The Clinical Value Compass. J Quality Improvement 1996;22(4): 243–256.

38. Newton-John T, Ashmore J, McDowell M. Early intervention in acute back pain. Physiotherapy 2001;87(8):397–401.

39. Oxman AD, Thomson MA, Davis DA, et al. No magic bullets: a systematic review of 102 trials of interventions to improve professional practice. CMAJ 1995;153:1423–1431.

40. Royal College of General Practitioners' Clinical Guidelines Working Group. The development and implementation of clinical guidelines. Exeter: Royal College of General Practitioners, 1995.

41. Rossignol M, Abenhaim L, Seguin P, Neveu A, Collet J-P, Ducruet T, Shapiro S. Co-ordination of Primary Health Care for Back Pain: a randomized controlled trial. Spine 2000;25(2):251–259.

42. Sackett DL, Rosenberg WMC, Gray JAM, Haynes RB, Richardson WS. Evidence based medicine: what it is and what it isn't. BMJ 1996;312:71–72.

43. Schers H, Braspenning J, Drijver R, Wensing M, Grol R. Low back pain in general practice: reported management and reasons for not adhering to the guidelines in the Netherlands. Br J Gen Pract 2000;50: 640–644.

44. Shekelle PG, Woolf SH, Eccles M, Grimshaw J. Clinical guidelines: developing guidelines. BMJ 1999;318: 593–596.

45. Smith RB. Gatekeepers and sentinels: their consolidated effects on inpatient medical care. Evaluation Review 2001;25(3):288–330.

46. Sweeney G, Stead J, Sweeney K, Greco M. Exploring the implementation and development of clinical governance in primary care within the South West Region: views from PCG Clinical Governance Leads. Exeter: NHS Executive South West Region-R&D Support Unit, 2000.

47. University of York, NHS Centre for Reviews & Dissemination. Effective Health Care: Getting evidence into practice. London: Royal Society of Medicine 1999;5(1).

48. van Tulder MW, Assendelft WJJ, Koes BW, Boulter LM. Spinal radiographic findings and nonspecific low back pain: a systematic review of observational studies. Spine 1997;22(4):427–434.

49. van Tulder MW, Malmivaara A, Esmail R, Koes BW. Exercise therapy for low back pain (Cochrane Review). In: The Cochrane Library, Issue 1, Oxford: 2001.

50. Waddell G, McIntosh A, Hutchinson A, Feder G, Lewis M. Low back pain evidence review. London: Royal College of General Practitioners, 1999.

51. Watkins C, Harvey I, Langley C, Gray S, Faulkner A. General practitioners' use of guidelines in the consultation and their attitudes to them. Br J Gen Pract 1999;49:11–15.

52. Wilson MC, Hayward RSA, Tunis SR, Bass EB, Guyatt G. Users' guides to the medical literature. VIII: How to use clinical practice guidelines. B: What are the recommendations and will they help you in caring for your patients? JAMA 1995;274(20): 1630–1632.

53. Woolf SH, Grol R, Hutchinson A, Eccles M, Grimshaw J. Potential benefits, limitations and harms of clinical guidelines. BMJ 1999;318:527–530.

Index

Page numbers followed by t indicate table; those in *italics* indicate figure.